Principles and Practice of Veterinary Technology

Fourth Edition

Margi Sirois, EdD, MS, RVT, CVT, LAT
Program Director, Veterinary Technician Program
Ashworth College
Norcross, Georgia

With 702 illustrations

ELSEVIER

ELSEVIER

3251 Riverport Lane
St. Louis, Missouri 63043

PRINCIPLES AND PRACTICE OF VETERINARY TECHNOLOGY,
FOURTH EDITION
ISBN: 978-0-323-35483-7

Library of Congress Cataloging-in-Publication Data

Names: Sirois, Margi, editor.
Title: Principles and practice of veterinary technology / [edited by] Margi Sirois.
Description: Fourth edition. | St. Louis, Missouri : Elsevier, [2017] | Includes bibliographical references and index.
Identifiers: LCCN 2016016043 | ISBN 9780323354837 (pbk. : alk. paper)
Subjects: | MESH: Veterinary Medicine--methods | Animal Welfare | Animal Technicians | Animal Diseases--nursing
Classification: LCC SF774.4 | NLM SF 774.4 | DDC 636.089--dc23 LC record available at https://lccn.loc.gov/2016016043

Content Strategist: Brandi Graham
Content Development Manager: Luke Held
Senior Content Development Specialist: Diane Chatman
Publishing Services Manager: Jeff Patterson
Book Production Specialist: Carol O'Connell
Design Direction: Julia Dummitt

Printed in China

Last digit is the print number: 9 8 7 6 5 4 3 2 1

For my family, especially Dan-the-wonder-husband, and my amazing children, Jen and Daniel. I would be lost without your constant support.

Contributors to the Previous Editions

Carrie Jo Anderson, CVT
Tampa, Florida

Elaine Anthony, MA, CVT
Pinellas Park, Florida

Ron E. Banks, DVM, DACVPM, DACLAM
Denver, Colorado

Jane Baron-Sorensen, BSN, MA
Santa Rosa, California

Susan A. Berryhill, BS, RVT
Topeka, Kansas

Robert L. Bill, DVM, PhD
West Lafayette, Indiana

James T. Blackford, DVM, MS, DACVS
Knoxville, Tennessee

Christine Bretz, RVT
West Lafayette, Indiana

Regina Brotherton, DVM, CCRP, PhD
Slidell, Louisiana

Linda J. Brown, AAS, CVT
Urbana, Illinois

Marg Brown, RVT, BEd AD ED
Scottsdale, Arizona

Maria L. Calabrese, CVT
Philadelphia, Pennsylvania

Mary Tefend Campbell, CVT, VTS (ECC)
Montgomery, Alabama

Lisa A. Centonze, DVM
Tampa, Florida

Vincent Centonze, DVM
Plant City, Florida

Phillip E. Cochran, MS, DVM
Portland, Oregon

Joann Colville, DVM
Fargo, North Dakota

Thomas P. Colville
Fargo, North Dakota

Markiva Contris, LVT, BA
Lakewood, Washington

†Michael D. Cross, DVM
Grand Blanc, Michigan

Autumn P. Davidson, AHT, DVM, DACVIM
Davis, California

Harold Davis Jr., BA, RVT, VTS (ECC)
Davis, California

Barbara J. Deeb, DVM, MS
Shoreline, Washington

Jacqueline Ann De Jong, LVT, BS
Corvallis, Oregon

Gael L. De Longe, DVM
Weyers Cave, Virginia

Donald R. Dooley
Los Gatos, California

John T. Ervin, BS, DVM
St. Petersburg, Florida

Samuel M. Fassig, DVM, MA
Bennett, Colorado

David J. Fisher, DVM, DACVP (Clinical Pathology)
West Sacramento, California

Theresa W. Fossum, DVM, MS, PhD, DACVS
College Station, Texas

Ruth Francis-Floyd, DVM
Gainesville, Florida

Laurie J. Gage, DVM
Vallejo, California

Franklyn B. Garry, DVM, MS, DACVIM
Fort Collins, Colorado

Peter J. Gaveras, DVM, MBA
Milwaukee, Wisconsin

Madonna E. Gemus, DVM
East Lansing, Michigan

Richard A. Goebel, DVM
West Lafayette, Indiana

Elizabeth A. Gorecki, LVT
East Lansing, Michigan

Shashikant Goswami, BVSc, PhD
St. Petersburg, Florida

Sheila Grosdidier, BS, RVT, MCP
Evergreen, Colorado

Connie M. Han, RVT
West Lafayette, Indiana

Guy Hancock, DVM, MEd
St. Petersburg, Florida

Christi Hayes, BS
Yorba Linda, California

Suzanne Hetts, PhD
Littleton, Colorado

Bruce Hopman, MS, DVM
Portland, Oregon

Karen Hrapkiewicz, DVM, MS, Dipl ACLAM
Detroit, Michigan

Cheryl D. Hurd, RVT
West Lafayette, Indiana

Muhammed Ikram, DVM, MSc, PhD
Fairview, Alberta, Canada

Eileen M. Johnson, DVM, MS, PhD
Davis, California

Tina Kemper, DVM, DACVIM
Yorba Linda, California

Linda R. Krcatovich, LVT
East Lansing, Michigan

Michel Levy, DVM, DACVIM
West Lafayette, Indiana

Bertram Lipitz, DVM
Stratford, New Jersey

Heidi B. Lobprise, DVM, DAVDC
Dallas, Texas

Roger L. Lukens, DVM
West Lafayette, Indiana

Danielle Mauragis, AS, CVT
Gainesville, Florida

Michelle Mayers, VMD
Charleston, South Carolina

Shawn Patrick Messonnier, DVM
Plano, Texas

Seyedmehdi Mobini, DVM, MS, DACT
Fort Valley, Georgia

Sharyn Niskala, CVT, RVT, LVT
Palm Bay, Florida

Jody Nugent-Deal, RVT
Davis, California

Donna A. Oakley, CVT, VTS (ECC)
Philadelphia, Pennsylvania

Sarah Okumura, MA, RVT, CVPM
San Leandro, California

Kristina Palmer-Holtry, RVT
Davis, California

Catherine Ann Picut, VMD, JD, DACVP
Nutley, New Jersey

Stuart L. Porter, VMD
Weyers Cave, Virginia

Heather Prendergast, BS, AS, RVT, CVPM
Las Cruces, New Mexico

Rose Quinn, CVT, BA
Glenwood Springs, Colorado

Angel M. Rivera, CVT
Milwaukee, Wisconsin

Bernard E. Rollin, PhD
Fort Collins, Colorado

Rebecca Rose, AAS, CVT
Gunnison, Colorado

Cheri Barton Ross, MA
Santa Rosa, California

Christine Royce-Bretz, RVT
West Lafayette, Indiana

Kathy Ruane, BS, RVT
Scottsdale, Arizona

Scott W. Rundell, DVM
Morehead, Kentucky

Katie Samuelson, DVM
Scottsdale, Arizona

Philip J. Seibert Jr., CVT
Calhoun, Tennessee

Howard B. Seim III, DVM, DACVS
Fort Collins, Colorado

Sally B. Smith, LVT
Blairstown, New Jersey

Teresa Sonsthagen, BS, LVT
Fargo, North Dakota

Kathy A. Sylvester, BA, RVT, VDT
Paramus, New Jersey

Terry N. Teeple, DVM
Fort Steliacoom, Lakewood, Washington

Amy E. Thiessen, DVM
Stillwater, Oklahoma

Vivian Tiffany, CVT
St. Petersburg, Florida

Mary E. Torrence, DVM, PhD, DACVPM
Blacksburg, Virginia

C.L. Tyner, DVM
Mississippi State, Mississippi

Wendy E. Vaala, VMD, DACVIM
Kennett Square, Pennsylvania

Steven D. Van Camp, DVM, DACT
Raleigh, North Carolina

Robert J. Van Saun, DVM, MS, PhD, DACT, DACVN
Corvallis, Oregon

M. Randy White, DVM, PhD, DACVP
West Lafayette, Indiana

Sheila M. Wing-Proctor, LVT
East Lansing, Michigan

Cathy Winters, LVT
East Lansing, Michigan

Preface

The roles and responsibilities of the veterinary technician and nurse have continued to evolve and expand, and veterinary technicians and nurses are increasingly expected to perform as independent yet interconnected members of the veterinary health care team. The knowledge required of veterinary technicians and nurses today has increased exponentially since the first edition of this text. This fourth edition has been designed primarily for the veterinary technician student with a particular focus on providing a ready reference on the diverse information that will be needed once the student graduates and begins working in the field. Discussions present the fundamental information veterinary technicians and nursing students should know and entry-level technicians and nurses will find useful.

This edition is organized into four sections representing the four major areas of responsibility for the practicing veterinary technician and veterinary nurse. Chapters related to veterinary diagnostics and therapeutics represent the latest advancements in veterinary medicine. Comprehensive information on nursing care of a wide variety of species is also presented with a particular focus on providing procedural details for a vast array of techniques. The increased numbers of avian and exotic animal species seen in companion animal practice is addressed, with greatly expanded chapters on nursing and medicine in these species.

The text has been amply illustrated with color photos throughout. Large numbers of tables are used to provide a summary and handy reference for vital information. More than 80 procedures, many of them illustrated, show students exactly how to accomplish complex skills. Each chapter begins with learning objectives, a chapter outline, and key terms. "Technician Notes" throughout each chapter highlight important points and provide helpful tips to improve knowledge and skill. Recommended readings provide additional sources of detailed information on the topics.

It is my hope that this new edition will become an essential reference in the teaching of veterinary technicians and veterinary nurses and will be utilized in their daily practice of veterinary nursing technology.

Margi Sirois

Acknowledgments

Many people are involved in the production of a book. I am grateful for the hard work of the contributors to the previous editions. I have been blessed to benefit from the expertise of many mentors throughout my career and am grateful to all of them. I thank God every day for blessing my life with the world's most amazing husband, Dan, and my children, Jen and Daniel. I am truly blessed to have them by my side. Finally, to all my friends at Elsevier that have helped and encouraged me through the years. Thank you!

Contents

How to Use This Learning Package

Principles and Practice of Veterinary Technology is the ultimate learning package for preparing students to become veterinary technicians. It provides a solid foundation for the basic and advanced clinical skills students must master to achieve competence, and its student-friendly style clarifies even the most complex concepts and procedures to help prepare for the VTNE and certification.

TEXTBOOK FEATURES

A simple chapter outline introduces you to the chapter material as a whole, allowing you to see at a glance how the subject material is organized. It also helps you focus on one topic at a time by showing you the relationship to other topics in the chapter.

Learning Objectives help you focus on key concepts and procedures for mastery on completion of the chapter.

Key Terms listed on the chapter opening page reinforce new terminology and are defined in a glossary at the back of the text.

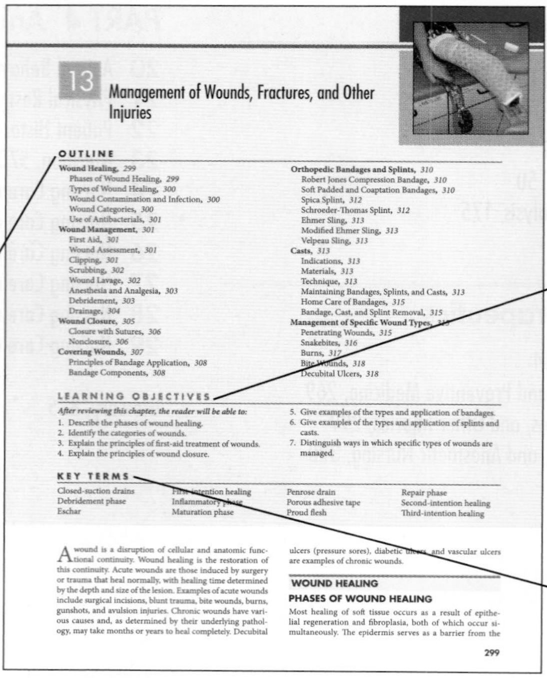

13

Management of Wounds, Fractures, and Other Injuries

OUTLINE

LEARNING OBJECTIVES

After reviewing this chapter, the reader will be able to:
1. Describe the phases of wound healing.
2. Identify the categories of wounds.
3. Explain the principles of first-aid treatment of wounds.
4. Explain the principles of wound closure.
5. Give examples of the types and application of bandages.
6. Give examples of the types and application of splints and casts.
7. Distinguish ways in which specific types of wounds are managed.

KEY TERMS

Closed-suction drains
Debridement phase
Eschar
First-intention healing
Inflammatory phase
Maturation phase
Penrose drain
Porous adhesive tape
Proud flesh
Repair phase
Second-intention healing
Third-intention healing

A wound is a disruption of cellular and anatomic functional continuity. Wound healing is the restoration of this continuity. Acute wounds are those induced by surgery or trauma that heal normally, with healing time determined by the depth and size of the lesion. Examples of acute wounds include surgical incisions, blunt trauma, bite wounds, burns, gunshots, and avulsion injuries. Chronic wounds have various causes and, as determined by their underlying pathology, may take months or years to heal completely. Decubital ulcers (pressure sores), diabetic ulcers, and vascular ulcers are examples of chronic wounds.

WOUND HEALING

PHASES OF WOUND HEALING

Most healing of soft tissue occurs as a result of epithelial regeneration and fibroplasia, both of which occur simultaneously. The epidermis serves as a barrier from the

299

Full-color format helps you easily visualize microscopic images.

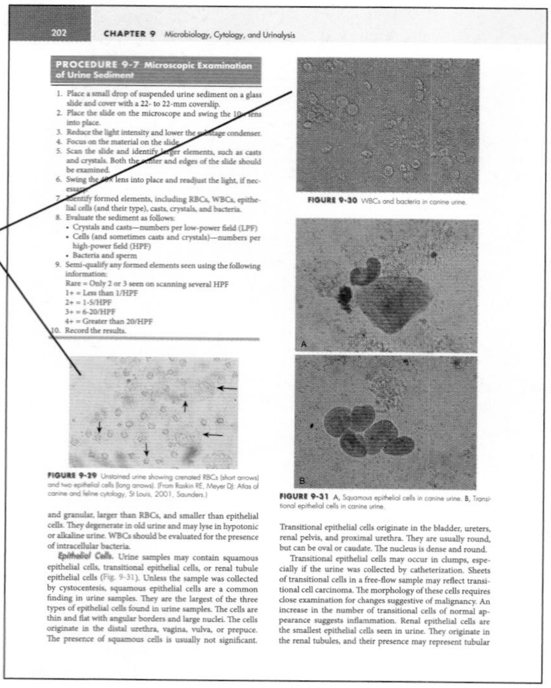

202 CHAPTER 9 Microbiology, Cytology, and Urinalysis

PROCEDURE 9-7 Microscopic Examination of Urine Sediment

1. Place a small drop of suspended urine sediment on a glass slide and cover with a 22- to 22-mm coverslip.
2. Place the slide on the microscope and swing the 10× lens into place.
3. Reduce the light intensity and lower the substage condenser.
4. Focus on the material on the slide.
5. Scan the slide and identify larger elements, such as casts and crystals. Both the center and edges of the slide should be examined.
6. Swing the 40× lens into place and readjust the light, if necessary.
7. Identify formed elements, including RBCs, WBCs, epithelial cells (and their type), casts, crystals, and bacteria.
8. Evaluate the sediment as follows:
   - Crystals and casts—numbers per low-power field (LPF)
   - Cells (and sometimes casts and crystals)—numbers per high-power field (HPF)
   - Bacteria and sperm
9. Semi-qualify any formed elements seen using the following information:
   Rare = Only 2 or 3 seen on scanning several HPF
   1+ = Less than 1/HPF
   2+ = 1-5/HPF
   3+ = 6-20/HPF
   4+ = Greater than 20/HPF
10. Record the results.

FIGURE 9-29 Unstained urine showing crenated RBCs (short arrows) and two epithelial cells (long arrows). (From Raskin RE, Meyer DJ: Atlas of canine and feline cytology, St Louis, 2001, Saunders.)

and granular, larger than RBCs, and smaller than epithelial cells. They degenerate in old urine and may lyse in hypotonic or alkaline urine. WBCs should be evaluated for the presence of intracellular bacteria.

Epithelial Cells. Urine samples may contain squamous epithelial cells, transitional epithelial cells, or renal tubule epithelial cells (Fig. 9-31). Unless the sample was collected by cystocentesis, squamous epithelial cells are a common finding in urine samples. They are the largest of the three types of epithelial cells found in urine samples. The cells are thin and flat with angular borders and large nuclei. The cells originate in the distal urethra, vagina, vulva, or prepuce. The presence of squamous cells is usually not significant.

FIGURE 9-30 WBCs and bacteria in canine urine.

FIGURE 9-31 A, Squamous epithelial cells in canine urine. B, Transitional epithelial cells in canine urine.

Transitional epithelial cells originate in the bladder, ureters, renal pelvis, and proximal urethra. They are usually round, but can be oval or caudate. The nucleus is dense and round.

Transitional epithelial cells may occur in clumps, especially if the urine was collected by catheterization. Sheets of transitional cells in a free-flow sample may reflect transitional cell carcinoma. The morphology of these cells requires close examination for changes suggestive of malignancy. An increase in the number of transitional cells of normal appearance suggests inflammation. Renal epithelial cells are the smallest epithelial cells seen in urine. They originate in the renal tubules, and their presence may represent tubular

Dozens of illustrated, step-by-step procedures help you learn processes from start to finish.

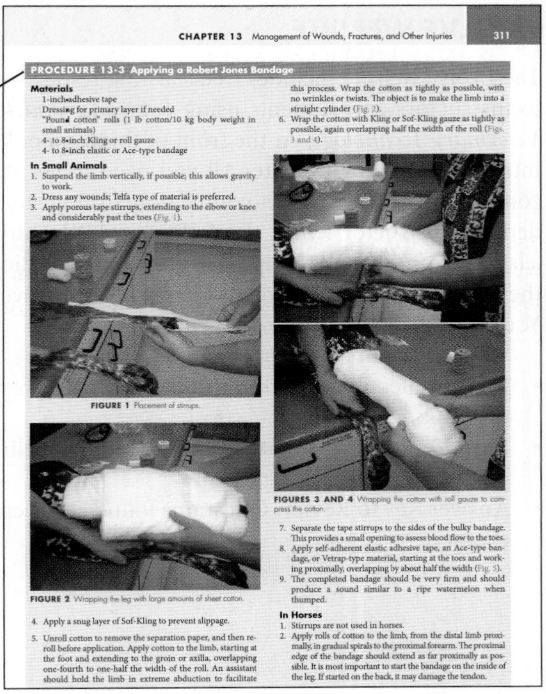

CHAPTER 13 Management of Wounds, Fractures, and Other Injuries 311

PROCEDURE 13-3 Applying a Robert Jones Bandage

Materials
1-inch adhesive tape
Dressing for primary layer if needed
"Pound cotton" rolls (1 lb cotton/10 kg body weight in small animals)
4- to 8-inch Kling or roll gauze
4- to 8-inch elastic or Ace-type bandage

In Small Animals
1. Suspend the limb vertically, if possible; this allows gravity to work.
2. Dress any wounds; Telfa type of material is preferred.
3. Apply porous tape stirrups, extending to the elbow or knee and considerably past the toes (Fig. 1).

FIGURE 1 Placement of stirrups.

FIGURE 2 Wrapping the leg with large amounts of sheet cotton.

4. Apply a snug layer of Sof-Kling to prevent slippage.
5. Unroll cotton to remove the separation paper, and then reroll before application. Apply cotton to the limb, starting at the foot and extending to the groin or axilla, overlapping one-fourth to one-half the width of the roll. An assistant should hold the limb in extreme abduction to facilitate this process. Wrap the cotton as tightly as possible, with no wrinkles or twists. The object is to make the limb into a straight cylinder (Fig. 2).
6. Wrap the cotton with Kling or Sof-Kling gauze as tightly as possible, again overlapping half the width of the roll (Figs. 3 and 4).

FIGURES 3 AND 4 Wrapping the cotton with roll gauze to compress the cotton.

7. Separate the tape stirrups to the sides of the bulky bandage. This provides a small opening to assess blood flow to the toes.
8. Apply self-adherent elastic adhesive tape, an Ace-type bandage, or Vetrap-type material, starting at the toes and working proximally, overlapping by about half the width (Fig. 5).
9. The completed bandage should be very firm and should produce a sound similar to a ripe watermelon when thumped.

In Horses
1. Stirrups are not used in horses.
2. Apply rolls of cotton to the limb, from the distal limb proximally, in gradual spirals to the proximal forearm. The proximal edge of the bandage should extend as far proximally as possible. It is most important to start the bandage on the inside of the leg. If started on the back, it may damage the tendon.

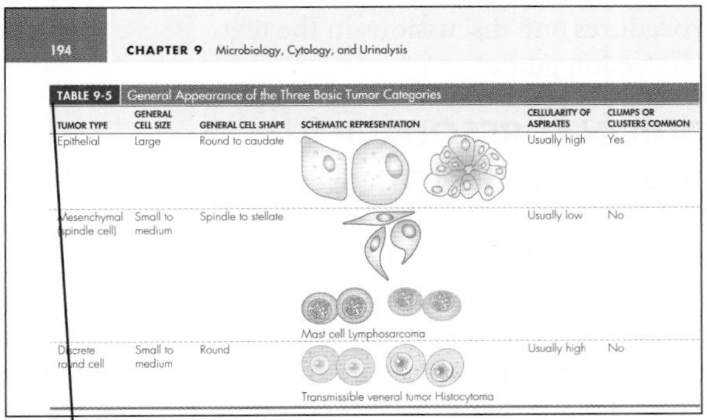

194 CHAPTER 9 Microbiology, Cytology, and Urinalysis

TABLE 9-5 General Appearance of the Three Basic Tumor Categories

TUMOR TYPE	GENERAL CELL SIZE	GENERAL CELL SHAPE	SCHEMATIC REPRESENTATION	CELLULARITY OF ASPIRATES	CLUMPS OR CLUSTERS COMMON
Epithelial	Large	Round to caudate		Usually high	Yes
Mesenchymal (spindle cell)	Small to medium	Spindle to stellate	Mast cell Lymphosarcoma	Usually low	No
Discrete round cell	Small to medium	Round	Transmissible veneral tumor Histocytoma	Usually high	No

Many tables and boxes are illustrated to help you visualize information.

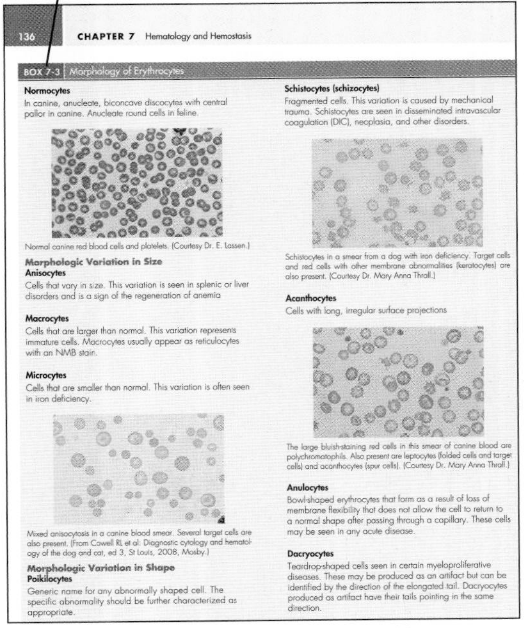

136 CHAPTER 7 Hematology and Hemostasis

BOX 7-3 Morphology of Erythrocytes

Normocytes
In canine, anucleate, biconcave discocytes with central pallor in canine. Anucleate round cells in feline.

Normal canine red blood cells and platelets. (Courtesy Dr. E. Lassen.)

Morphologic Variation in Size
Anisocytes
Cells that vary in size. This variation is seen in splenic or liver disorders and is a sign of the regeneration of anemia

Macrocytes
Cells that are larger than normal. This variation represents immature cells. Macrocytes usually appear as reticulocytes with an NMB stain.

Microcytes
Cells that are smaller than normal. This variation is often seen in iron deficiency.

Mixed anisocytosis in a canine blood smear. Several target cells are also present. (From Cowell RL et al: Diagnostic cytology and hematology of the dog and cat, ed 3, St Louis, 2008, Mosby.)

Morphologic Variation in Shape
Poikilocytes
Generic name for any abnormally shaped cell. The specific abnormality should be further characterized as appropriate.

Schistocytes (schizocytes)
Fragmented cells. This variation is caused by mechanical trauma. Schistocytes are seen in disseminated intravascular coagulation (DIC), neoplasia, and other disorders.

Schistocytes in a smear from a dog with iron deficiency. Target cells and red cells with other membrane abnormalities (keratocytes) are also present. (Courtesy Dr. Mary Anna Thrall.)

Acanthocytes
Cells with long, irregular surface projections

The large bluish-staining red cells in this smear of canine blood are polychromatophils. Also present are leptocytes (folded cells and target cells) and acanthocytes (spur cells). (Courtesy Dr. Mary Anna Thrall.)

Anulocytes
Bowl-shaped erythrocytes that form as a result of loss of membrane flexibility that does not allow the cell to return to a normal shape after passing through a capillary. These cells may be seen in any acute disease.

Dacryocytes
Teardrop-shaped cells seen in certain myeloproliferative diseases. These may be produced as an artifact but can be identified by the direction of the elongated tail. Dacryocytes produced as artifact have their tails pointing in the same direction.

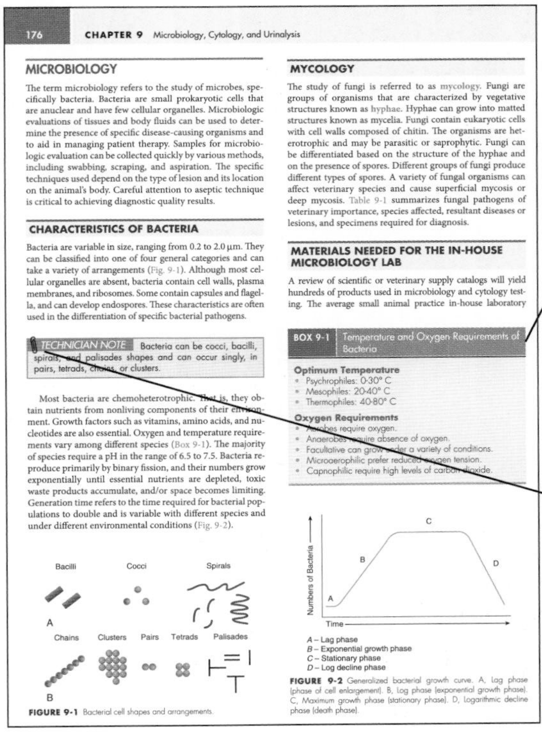

176 CHAPTER 9 Microbiology, Cytology, and Urinalysis

MICROBIOLOGY

The term microbiology refers to the study of microbes, specifically bacteria. Bacteria are small prokaryotic cells that are anuclear and have few cellular organelles. Microbiologic evaluations of tissues and body fluids can be used to determine the presence of specific disease-causing organisms and to aid in managing patient therapy. Samples for microbiologic evaluation can be collected quickly by various methods, including swabbing, scraping, and aspiration. The specific techniques used depend on the type of lesion and its location on the animal's body. Careful attention to aseptic technique is critical to achieving diagnostic quality results.

CHARACTERISTICS OF BACTERIA

Bacteria are variable in size, ranging from 0.2 to 2.0 μm. They can be classified into one of four general categories and can take a variety of arrangements (Fig. 9-1). Although most cellular organelles are absent, bacteria contain cell walls, plasma membranes, and ribosomes. Some contain capsules and flagella, and can develop endospores. These characteristics are often used in the differentiation of specific bacterial pathogens.

TECHNICIAN NOTE Bacteria can be cocci, bacilli, spirals, and palisades shapes and can occur singly, in pairs, tetrads, chains, or clusters.

Most bacteria are chemoheterotrophic. That is, they obtain nutrients from nonliving components of their environment. Growth factors such as vitamins, amino acids, and nucleotides are also essential. Oxygen and temperature requirements vary among different species (Box 9-1). The majority of species require a pH in the range of 6.5 to 7.5. Bacteria reproduce primarily by binary fission, and their numbers grow exponentially until essential nutrients are depleted, toxic waste products accumulate, and/or space becomes limiting. Generation time refers to the time required for bacterial populations to double and is variable with different species and under different environmental conditions (Fig. 9-2).

FIGURE 9-1 Bacterial cell shapes and arrangements.

MYCOLOGY

The study of fungi is referred to as mycology. Fungi are groups of organisms that are characterized by vegetative structures known as hyphae. Hyphae can grow into matted structures known as mycelia. Fungi contain eukaryotic cells with cell walls composed of chitin. The organisms are heterotrophic and may be parasitic or saprophytic. Fungi can be differentiated based on the structure of the hyphae and on the presence of spores. Different groups of fungi produce different types of spores. A variety of fungal organisms can affect veterinary species and cause superficial mycosis or deep mycosis. Table 9-1 summarizes fungal pathogens of veterinary importance, species affected, resultant diseases or lesions, and specimens required for diagnosis.

MATERIALS NEEDED FOR THE IN-HOUSE MICROBIOLOGY LAB

A review of scientific or veterinary supply catalogs will yield hundreds of products used in microbiology and cytology testing. The average small animal practice in-house laboratory

BOX 9-1 Temperature and Oxygen Requirements of Bacteria

Optimum Temperature
- Psychrophiles: 0-30° C
- Mesophiles: 20-40° C
- Thermophiles: 40-80° C

Oxygen Requirements
- Aerobes require oxygen.
- Anaerobes require absence of oxygen.
- Facultative can grow under a variety of conditions.
- Microaerophilic prefer reduced oxygen tension.
- Capnophilic require high levels of carbon dioxide.

A – Lag phase
B – Exponential growth phase
C – Stationary phase
D – Log decline phase

FIGURE 9-2 Generalized bacterial growth curve. A, Log phase (phase of cell enlargement). B, Log phase (exponential growth phase). C, Maximum growth phase (stationary phase). D, Logarithmic decline phase (death phase).

Boxes make studying easier.

Technician Notes are interspersed throughout each chapter to help you retain key information related to the technician's role.

EVOLVE WEBSITE

The Evolve website includes free learning resources available to instructors and students using *Principles and Practice of Veterinary Technology.* At the front of this textbook is a page introducing the Evolve site. All you need to get started is a computer with an internet connection. To register as a Student or Instructor, enter the following URL: http://evolve.elsevier.com/Sirois/principles/. Follow the directions for either "Instructors" or "Students" to create an Evolve account. You will have to do this only one time.

Student resources include:

- Image collection containing all of the images from within the book
- Exercises including matching, illustration labeling, multiple-choice questions, and more
- Answer Key to Review Questions found at the end of each chapter

Instructor resources include:

- TEACH Lesson Plans
- PowerPoint Lecture Presentations
- Test Bank in Examview including more than 1400 questions
- Image collection containing all of the images from within the book
- Access to all the student resources
- AVMA-required tasks and competencies are mapped to procedures and discussions in the text
- Conversion guide

ADDITIONAL RESOURCE

Mosby's Veterinary PDQ, Second Edition (ISBN: 978-0-323-24066-6)

Margi Sirois, EdD, MS, RVT

You will be able to enter the clinical setting confidently with this full-color, pocket-sized reference that offers instant access to hundreds of veterinary medicine facts, formulas, drug calculations, lab values, procedures, and photographs of parasites, laboratory diagnostic samples, and instruments for easy identification.

Principles and Practice of Veterinary Technology

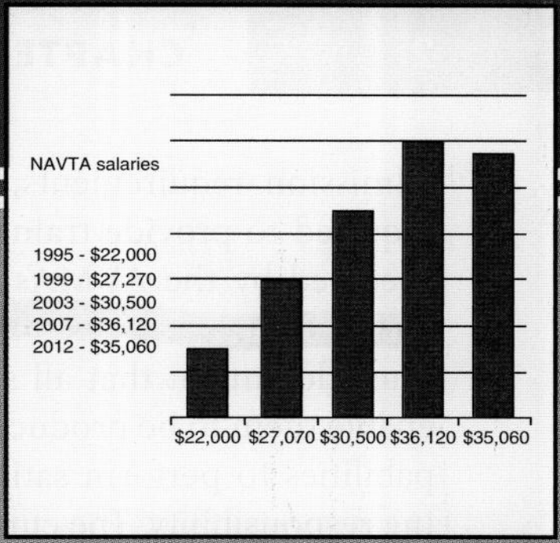

1 Overview of Veterinary Technology

OUTLINE

LEARNING OBJECTIVES

After reviewing this chapter, the reader will be able to:

1. Describe educational requirements of veterinary technicians.
2. Define appropriate nomenclature describing veterinary personnel.
3. Identify veterinary technician duties.
4. Differentiate between certification, registration, and licensing.
5. Compare career opportunities and salary ranges.
6. Recognize professional organizations supporting veterinary technicians.
7. Define Veterinary Technician Specialist (VTS) and identify paths to specialty certification.
8. Define trends in veterinary technology.

KEY TERMS

Academy
Accreditation Policies and Procedures of the AVMA CVTEA Manual
Certification
Committee on Veterinary Technician Education and Activities
Credentialed veterinary technician
Licensure
Registration
Society
Veterinarian
Veterinary Assistant
Veterinary Practice Acts
Veterinary team
Veterinary Technician
Veterinary Technician Specialist
Veterinary Technologist
Veterinary technology

Veterinary technology is a relatively new group of paraprofessionals in veterinary medicine, similar in many respects to nurses in human medicine. The first class of Animal Health Technician students in the United States graduated in 1972. The National Association of Veterinary Technicians in America (NAVTA) began representing veterinary technicians in 1981.

By the American Veterinary Medical Association's (AVMA) definition, a veterinary technician must be a graduate of an AVMA-accredited college program in veterinary technology and work under a licensed veterinary practitioner (DVM or VMD).

The emergence of educated veterinary technicians as members of the veterinary team has been an important development for the veterinary profession. This change was in its infancy in the 1960s, in the developmental stage in the 1970s, dynamically improving in the 1980s, and matured in the 1990s. Now, heading toward 2016, veterinary technology is projected to grow 30% and is considered one of the fastest growing careers. Veterinary technicians will continue to play an increasingly important role in the veterinary profession, such as nurses do in human medicine.

EDUCATION OF VETERINARY TECHNICIANS

At the present time there are over 200 AVMA-accredited veterinary technology programs, including 9 accredited distance education programs. To attain AVMA accreditation, veterinary technology education programs must meet 11 minimum standards pertaining to facilities, faculty, admission requirements, and curricula. All programs are required to provide training in a variety of clinical tasks as specified by the AVMA's Committee on Veterinary Technician Education and Activities (CVTEA). Each program must document that all students acquire technical skills to enable them to be productive employees and develop the capabilities to perform satisfactorily in a position of increasing responsibility. The curricula must be designed to provide hands-on experience to ensure that each student performs all essential tasks listed in the Accreditation Policies and Procedures of the AVMA CVTEA Manual. Proficiency outcomes for each procedure depend on the program emphasis and the number of times students have practiced these tasks. Students are required to complete an internship at a veterinary hospital (or similar setting), honing their technical skills and learning the fundamental structure of working in a hospital. For the 2014-2015 academic year more than 27,000 students were enrolled in AVMA CVTEA-accredited programs, representing campus and distance education programs. More than 5000 veterinary technicians graduated in 2014. Further information can be found at www.avma.org.

NOMENCLATURE DESCRIBING VETERINARY PERSONNEL

The AVMA recognizes the value of veterinary technicians as an integral component of veterinary medicine and urges full utilization of veterinary technicians. The veterinary profession is enhanced through efficient utilization of each member of the veterinary healthcare team by appropriate delegation of tasks and responsibilities to support staff.

AVMA POLICY ON VETERINARY TECHNOLOGY PREAMBLE

The following definitions provide more complete descriptions that encompass the latest developments in the profession from the AVMA. **Veterinary technology** is the science and art of providing professional support to veterinarians. AVMA CVTEA accredits programs in veterinary technology that graduate veterinary technicians and/or veterinary technologists.

A **veterinary technician** is a graduate of an AVMA-accredited program in veterinary technology. In most cases the graduate is granted an associate degree. A veterinary technician's duties are similar to, in human medicine, those of a registered nurse, nurse-anesthetist, operating room technician, dental hygienist, medical laboratory technician, or radiographic technician, all combined into one team member. Professional nursing-related duties that produce income are delegated to a veterinary technician by a licensed DVM in a fee-for-service veterinary practice. Veterinary technicians may also work in research, education, sales, or governmental positions.

A **veterinary technologist** is a graduate of a 4-year, AVMA CVTEA-accredited program who holds a baccalaureate degree from veterinary technician study; or a graduate veterinary technician with a bachelor of science (B.S.) degree in another program with studies in supervision, leadership, management, or a scientific area. Duties of veterinary technologists include veterinary technician duties, often in combination with personnel or hospital management. They may be employed as teachers, research associates, group leaders, sales managers, or clinical technologists in a specialty practice.

Both technicians and technologists, by veterinary practice law, are unable to diagnose, prescribe medications, or perform surgery.

A **veterinary assistant** is a person with less education and training than that required of a veterinary technician. Veterinary assistants can be compared with nurses' aides in human medicine. Generally veterinary assistants are trained on the job (OTJ), but some short-term training programs exist. While accreditation of veterinary assistant programs is not required, NAVTA has a process whereby veterinary assistant programs can be approved. Individuals that complete NAVTA-approved veterinary assistant programs are eligible to take the "approved veterinary assistant" examination. Duties of assistants may include restraining, feeding, and exercising patients, cleaning hospital and boarding premises, and other clinical support tasks. These aides may also be described by the terms clinical, hospital, technician, ward, or veterinary combined with aide, attendant, caretaker, or assistant. They are most appropriately called technician assistants or clinical aides, rather than veterinary assistants. Confusion occurs when comparing duties to a physician's assistant (PA in human medicine) who has more training and requires less supervision than a registered nurse, in contrast with the clinical aide (nurse's aide).

A **veterinarian** is a doctor of veterinary medicine. A veterinarian is a graduate of a 4-year AVMA-accredited veterinary college program. There are presently 30 AVMA-accredited veterinary schools in the US, as well as 5 in Canada and 14 in other countries that are also AVMA accredited. To practice veterinary medicine, veterinarians must pass a licensure examination in the states or provinces in which they wish to practice. Most veterinarians graduating today have 4 years of preveterinary studies, with a B.A. or B.S. degree, in addition to 4 years of study at a veterinary university, culminating in a Doctor of Veterinary Medicine degree (DVM or VMD).

A **veterinary team** is a combination of doctors, paraprofessionals (veterinary technicians and/or technologists), and support staff (receptionists, managers, technician assistants, and caretakers).

The AVMA encourages schools, organizations, and regulatory authorities to use the standard terminology described above.

SCOPE OF VETERINARY TECHNICIAN'S DUTIES

Through recent campaigns by national and state organizations, the general public is becoming more aware of the role of veterinary technicians and the compassionate, skilled care they provide to family pets, companion animals, and livestock. Continued support and improved management practices will leverage the role of veterinary technicians. In the past, veterinary management was doctor centered. Now as well-managed practices become client centered, benchmark standards are achieved and team efficiency improves. These advancements allow for increased employee satisfaction, retention, and salaries. Veterinary schools are teaching veterinary students to view themselves as the "delegators" and not necessarily the "doers." With advanced practice management understanding, veterinary students learn team delivery systems and understand how tasks are delegated to the appropriate employee within the hospital. When practice owners, typically veterinarians, delegate duties to educated, certified managers, veterinary hospitals reach new heights in productivity and human resource potential. Because of the increased awareness and high demand for educated veterinary technicians, students graduating with a degree in veterinary technology have the choice of well-managed practices offering salaries high enough to keep them in the profession. Technicians who are unhappy with their current job conditions must take a good look at all their options. There are veterinary clinics offering benefits, appropriate compensation, career advancement, vacation time, continuing education, and retirement plans.

Veterinary technicians are now assuming a major role in practice by performing medical and surgical nursing procedures, laboratory testing, anesthesia induction and maintenance, monitoring during recovery, management, team training, and other clinical procedures. Veterinarians delegate many income-producing procedures to veterinary technicians and managers empower their teams to excel. This enables the veterinarian to concentrate on prescribing medications, diagnosing, and surgery, increasing his or her productivity (Box 1-1).

For many years consultants have urged veterinarians to delegate technical tasks to technicians; now that advice is being passed on to practice managers and administrators. NAVTA considers delegating tasks to technicians a cornerstone in the effective delivery of veterinary medicine. Table 1-1 contains an example to demonstrate practice revenue when a veterinary technician performs a skill versus the same skill performed by the veterinarian. In the calculation example, the task identified was for a blood draw, taking 10 minutes at a charge of $10, performed 80 times a week. In the equation, a technician is paid $15 an hour and the veterinarian is paid $50 an hour. Simply stated it is in a veterinarian's best interest to delegate appropriate tasks to the appropriate employee. Imagine how valuable the technical staff are when they are fully empowered and leveraged. Apply this tool to producing radiographs, calculating anesthesia and induction, taking a complete history, and completing diagnostic testing.

BOX 1-1 Scope of Veterinary Technician's Duties

Caring for the Hospitalized Patient
Administration of medication
Sample collection
Physical therapy
Specialized intensive nursing care
Bandage/dressing application
Nutritional management

Clinical Pathology
Specimen collection
Hematology procedures
Microbiology techniques
Parasite evaluations
Biochemical analysis
Cytology examinations
Urinalysis

Outpatient/Field Service
Physical examination
History taking
Client education
Administration of medication
Administration of vaccines
Specimen collections

Radiology
Patient preparation and positioning
Radiation calculations and exposure
Radiation safety
Radiographic film developing
Maintenance of equipment

Anesthesiology
Preanesthetic evaluation
Administration of local anesthetics
Administration of general anesthetics
Monitoring
Patient recovery

Dental Prophylaxis
Examination of oral cavity
Cleaning and polishing teeth

Surgical Assisting
Patient preparation
Instrument/equipment sterilization
Surgical suite preparation and maintenance
Assistance during surgical procedures
Postoperative patient care
Wound management

Office/Hospital Management
Medical supplies inventory control
Bookkeeping and practice management
Supervision of hospital personnel
Training of hospital personnel
Reception duties and client education

Biomedical Research
In addition to the above areas of responsibility, veterinary technicians in research may also:
- Supervise operations in research colonies and biomedical facilities
- Assist in design and implementation of research projects

TABLE 1-1 How Delegation Can Raise Income for the Procedure: Blood Draw

FRACTION OF TASK PERFORMED BY TECHNICAL STAFF	INCOME ESTIMATE PER WEEK	INCOME ESTIMATE PER YEAR
0.00%		
10.00%	$ 180.00	$ 9360.00
20.00%	$ 226.67	$ 11,786.67
30.00%	$ 273.33	$ 14,213.33
40.00%	$ 320.00	$ 16,640.00
50.00%	$ 366.67	$ 19,066.67
60.00%	$ 413.33	$ 21,493.33
70.00%	$ 460.00	$ 23,920.00
80.00%	$ 506.67	$ 26,346.67
90.00%	$ 553.33	$ 28,773.33
100.00%	$ 600.00	$ 31,200.00

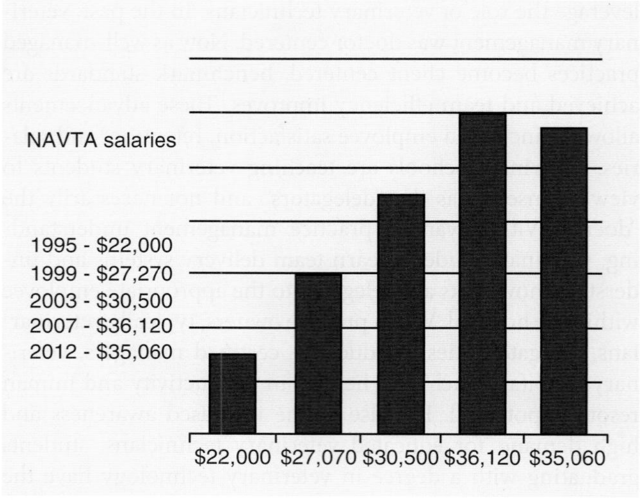

FIGURE 1-1 Historic figures with average salaries for veterinary technicians.

CAREER OPPORTUNITIES FOR VETERINARY TECHNICIANS

NAVTA has coordinated several national surveys, conducting the survey every 4 years. In the last survey (completed in spring of 2012), the average respondent had more than 12.8 years of experience, worked at the same hospital for 7.2 years, and was a 40-year-old woman. Ninety-five percent of respondents were women. The average yearly salary was $35,060 (Fig. 1-1) with part-time workers making an average of $16.80 per hour.

TECHNICIAN NOTE You can easily track the average salary in your surrounding area or in a location you are considering moving to by researching information found on www.salaryexpert.com. Search the title Veterinary Technician, place in the zip code, answer a few questions, and receive a free report. Use this information when discussing a raise with your manager.

NAVTA's 2012 survey results did not provide specific salary averages for various sectors. However, according to the NAVTA 2007 survey, 84% of career positions for veterinary technicians are in veterinary practices. Technicians in mixed-animal practices were making the lowest yearly salary at $28,960. Technicians in specialty and food animal practices were making more than $39,000 a year (Fig. 1-2).

Nonpractice career opportunities include veterinary technician education, university/college, diagnostic/research, not-for-profit organizations, working for the government, and industry. Professional technicians working in industry were making $51,510. Those in diagnostic/research facilities brought home $45,060 (Fig. 1-3).

Other facts to consider related to the 2007 NAVTA survey:

1. Since 1995 the largest jump in salaries was in food animals.
2. 26% of those working part-time were receiving $12 to $14.99 an hour.
3. NAVTA member benefits were significantly higher than their nonmember counterparts.
5. Seventy-seven percent of respondents had an associate degree, 34.2% had a baccalaureate degree, and 4.4% had a graduate degree.

SALARY RANGES FOR VETERINARY TECHNICIANS

It is clear that veterinary technicians can make varied salaries depending upon their career path. Technicians choosing to work in a small, rural, mixed-animal practice may make $14.50 an hour. A technician working for a progressive, well-managed specialty practice may make $20 an hour. A technician may choose to take on management tasks and be promoted to head technician. Along with that promotion comes more responsibilities and $19 an hour (according to an AAHA survey completed in 2007). Another option is working for a corporation as a sales representative getting both a commission on sales and $26 an hour. The choices are numerous, the salaries varied, the responsibilities differ, and skill sets have transformed to meet the growing demand.

A great tool at your fingertips is www.salaryexpert.com. When viewing their site you can enter Veterinary Technician as the title, select a zip code or city you wish to research, answer a few general questions, and request a free salary report. You will be able to determine what the average hourly wage is for technicians in that region along with a few cost-of-living expenses.

Recent research on NAVTA's career center in conjunction with the Veterinary Career Network (VCN) revealed the following job openings for veterinary technicians:

- 222 Private Practice
- 11 Nonprofit/Association
- 8 Academia/Research
- 10 Other
- 3 Industry
- 1 Government/Military

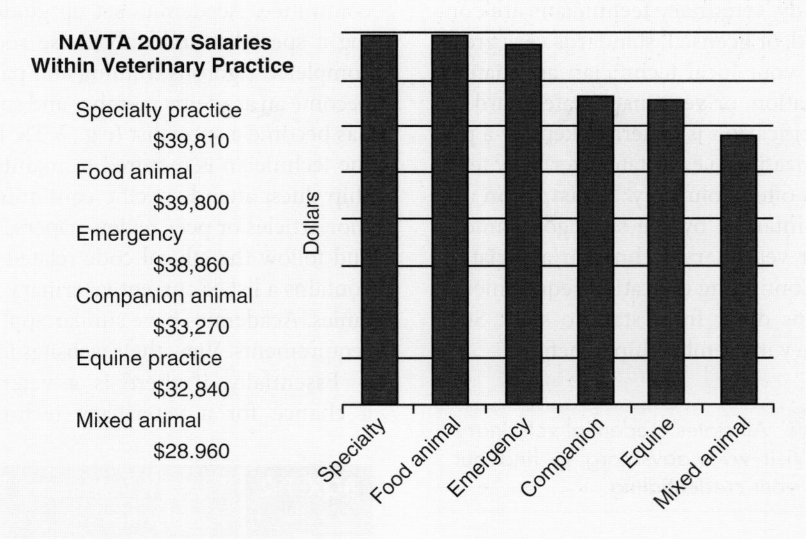

FIGURE 1-2 Historic figures with average salaries for veterinary technicians in private practice.

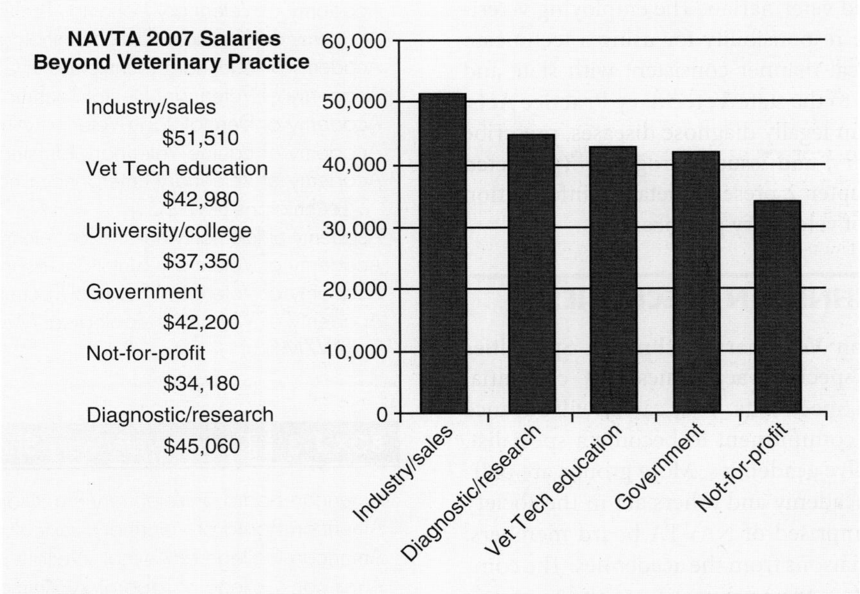

FIGURE 1-3 Historic figures with average salaries for veterinary technicians outside of private practice.

There are hundreds of career-oriented sites allowing you to post your resume and search available positions. View career opportunities and increase your networking.

CREDENTIALED VETERINARY TECHNICIANS: CERTIFICATION, REGISTRATION, AND LICENSING

Upon graduating from an accredited AVMA program, veterinary technicians are eligible to take the Veterinary Technician National Exam (VTNE). The Veterinary Technician Testing Committee (VTTC) of the American Association of Veterinary State Boards (AAVSB) is a committee of veterinarians and technicians appointed by various professional organizations to validate the VTNE. The AAVSB owns and administers the test. View their site to find out exactly who gives the test in each state, www.aavsb.org. Under the veterinary technician section of the AAVSB website, you will find contact information for the program administrator who can answer more of your questions. VTNE scores may be transferred to other states through the AAVSB Technician Information Verifying Agency (TIVA).

> TECHNICIAN NOTE Upon graduating from an AVMA-accredited program, you are eligible to take the VTNE. To learn more, visit www.aavsb.org.

All technicians who maintain their certification, registration, or license after passing the VTNE are referred to as **credentialed veterinary technicians.** Depending on the state and type of governing body, veterinary technicians are considered certified, registered, or licensed; standards vary greatly among states. Contact your local technician association, veterinary medical association, or veterinary state board for further information. **Certification** is generally kept by a private or professional organization (i.e., a state veterinary technician association) and is often voluntary. **Registration** and **licensure** are usually maintained by the state government, veterinary state board, or veterinary technician association and may be mandatory. Continuing education requirements, dues fees, and applications differ from state to state. State technician associations vary in membership benefits.

> *TECHNICIAN NOTE* All states credential veterinary technicians differently. Visit www.aavsb.org to find out which agency maintains your credentialing.

Veterinary technicians are educated to follow specific ethical and legal guidelines while working under the direction and supervision of a licensed veterinarian. The employing veterinarian has the ultimate responsibility for using a technician in an appropriate, ethical manner consistent with state and federal laws. According to the state **Veterinary Practice Acts**, only the veterinarian can legally diagnose diseases, prescribe therapy, perform surgery, and issue a prognosis (predicted medical outcome). Chapter 2 presents detailed information on the laws and ethics of veterinary practice.

VETERINARY TECHNICIAN SPECIALTIES

NAVTA's Committee on Veterinary Technician Specialties (CVTS) oversees the specialty academies that credential **Veterinary Technician Specialists.** Your career will advance when you take on the commitment to become a specialist. There are currently twelve academies. More groups are petitioning to become an academy and others are in the society stage. The CVTS is comprised of NAVTA board members, general members, and liaisons from the academies. The committee meets regularly to review new petitions and to review annual reports. View www.navta.net for more information.

> *TECHNICIAN NOTE* Your national association oversees the guidelines and reviews veterinary technician specialties. Research your options at www.navta.net. Align your passions; set a goal; take your skills to the next highest level, become a VTS.

In most cases a **society** is created by individuals with a common interest in a veterinary technician discipline; there are bylaws, dues, relationships built with allied groups, and leadership opportunities. Once a society has an established foundation of members and primary focus (e.g., Emergency and Critical Care Society), there is a survey completed indicating a need for the specialty; then there is a petition sent to the CVTS to create an academy. An **academy** has its own bylaws, leaders, application committee, testing committee, and credentialing committee. Academies set up guidelines and ethics for testing a specialist and only those society members who have completed rigorous training and passed the specialty test can become an academy member and specialist. Once a technician has become a specialist (e.g., VTS; Emergency Critical Care), the technician is required to maintain professional membership dues, attend specific continuing education courses, author articles or peer review papers, present technical lectures, and follow the ethical code related to that specialty. Box 1-2 contains a list of current veterinary technician specialty academies. Academies have similar applications and credentialing requirements. View their websites for complete information.

Essentially, if there is a veterinary specialty, there is a chance for a veterinary technician specialty. Box 1-3

BOX 1-2 Current Veterinary Technician Specialty Academies

Academy of Veterinary Technicians in Anesthesia and Analgesia (AVTAA)
Academy of Veterinary Behavior Technicians (AVBT)
Academy of Veterinary Clinical Pathology Technicians (AVCPT)
Academy of Veterinary Technicians in Clinical Practice (AVTCP)
Academy of Veterinary Dental Technicians (AVDT)
Academy of Dermatology Veterinary Technicians (ADVT)
Academy of Equine Veterinary Nursing Technicians (AEVNT)
Academy of Veterinary Emergency and Critical Care Technicians (AVECCT)
Academy of Internal Medicine for Veterinary Technicians (AIMVT)
Academy of Veterinary Nutrition Technicians (AVNT)
Academy of Veterinary Surgical Technicians (AVST)
Academy of Veterinary Zoological Medicine Technicians (AVZMT)

BOX 1-3 Current Veterinary Specialties

American Board of Veterinary Practitioners
American Board of Veterinary Toxicology
American College of Animal Welfare
American College of Laboratory Animal Medicine
American College of Poultry Veterinarians
American College of Theriogenologists
American College of Veterinary Anesthesia and Analgesia
American College of Veterinary Behaviorists
American College of Veterinary Clinical Pharmacology
American College of Veterinary Dermatology
American College of Veterinary Emergency and Critical Care
American College of Veterinary Internal Medicine
American College of Veterinary Microbiologists
American College of Veterinary Nutrition
American College of Veterinary Ophthalmologists
American College of Veterinary Pathologists
American College of Veterinary Preventive Medicine
American College of Veterinary Radiology
American College of Veterinary Sports Medicine and Rehabilitation
American College of Veterinary Surgeons
American College of Zoological Medicine
American Veterinary Dental College

contains a list of current veterinary specialty colleges. Veterinarians who complete additional specialized training and pass a certifying examination are referred to as Diplomates of their respective veterinary specialty college.

The veterinary specialty colleges, in the past, have been very supportive of the technician counterpart. These relationships are extremely important and affirm the working relationships that have grown through the decades between veterinarians and their technicians. Veterinarians and technicians taking their careers to the specialty realm receive many benefits: credibility, respect, and typically an increase in salary. Patients and clients are best served by specialists, and the perceived value is much higher.

> TECHNICIAN NOTE Join your local or state veterinary technician association. Benefits include networking, personal and professional growth, camaraderie, and more. You will reap the most benefits when you actively participate, sit on a committee, attend meetings, become a leader, and step outside of your comfort zone.

THE FUTURE OF VETERINARY TECHNOLOGY

For veterinary technology to advance as a profession, veterinary technicians must join state, specialty, national, and professional organizations to advance the cause for better utilization of veterinary technicians, attain greater professional recognition, develop more effective continuing education programs, and generally represent its members in political, legal, and other related matters. Well-managed veterinary hospitals embrace, empower, retain, and support their veterinary technicians. Future advancements in utilization of veterinary technicians depend on the collective efforts of veterinary technicians and allied organizations, to include veterinary hospital managers, veterinary medical associations, and specialty academies. Your involvement is crucial. Your career is what you make of it. No longer can technicians blame the veterinarians for low pay and dissatisfaction. There are veterinary hospitals and career options that can fulfill all your needs, financially, professionally, and emotionally.

> TECHNICIAN NOTE Your national association is only as good as the number of active members. For you to receive the most benefits of membership, you must be engaged. Become a member at www.navta.net.

Trends in veterinary technology will likely be in veterinary technician specialties, alternative medicine to include animal massage and acupuncture, large animal procedures, pet hospice care, relief veterinary technician services, management, and industry's increased awareness of the role veterinary technicians can play in corporations. Veterinary pet health insurance will have more policy holders, hence the need for veterinary teams to learn about and recommend third-party payments. More veterinary technicians will become practice owners, expanding their career options and the opportunity for veterinarians to sell their practices. (Check your state laws to see who can be a veterinary practice owner.) There may be a trend toward a title change to veterinary medical technician or even veterinary nurse. This demand may be initiated by the public and not necessarily the veterinary profession. And yet one more trend may be toward certification of technician assistants. We will see what the next decade brings.

VETERINARY TECHNICIAN PROFESSIONAL ORGANIZATIONS AND RESOURCES

> TECHNICIAN NOTE As a veterinary technician, your responsibilities are threefold: to care for the animals you tend to, work in harmony with your veterinary team, and build strong relationships with your clientele. Professionalism is imperative to your success, through proper communications with your veterinarians, co-workers, and pet owners.

Your career will reach new heights when you actively participate in professional organizations. Professionalism, effective communication, networking, and outstanding technical skills in your career choice will make you stand out above the rest. There are numerous groups to choose from that will elevate your status and the choices are growing at a rapid rate. When you join you increase the membership base, open many doors for networking, and amazing synergy grows. Each state association has its own mission, vision, and values. National organizations also have defined purposes and goals. Research the many organizations that align with your values and support your career. Box 1-4 lists a few of the national groups, organizations, and sites that support veterinary technicians and a brief synopsis of the benefits to members.

BOX 1-4 Groups, Organizations, and Sites that Support Veterinary Technicians

NAVTA
The National Association of Veterinary Technicians in America was created in 1981 to be the national voice of the veterinary technician. Currently there are approximately 28,000 members. It is their goal to influence the future of NAVTA members' professional goals, foster high standards of veterinary care, and promote the veterinary healthcare team. Their website offers a career center, continuing education, state representative contacts, specialty section, quarterly journal (TNJ), information on student chapters (SCNAVTA) and National Veterinary Technician Week (NVTW), and more. www.navta.net

AVMA
Created in 1863, the American Veterinary Association currently has more than 86,000 members. They have a committee that accredits veterinary technician programs around the United States and Canada (CVTEA). The AVMA acts as the collective voice for the veterinary profession. It lists all of the state VMAs and may help you find your state VTA. www.avma.org

(Continued)

BOX 1-4 Groups, Organizations, and Sites that Support Veterinary Technicians—cont'd

RVTTC
The Registered Veterinary Technologists and Technicians of Canada has a career center, VTNE study guide, a list of technician programs, continuing education, and more. www.rvttcanada.ca

CVMA
The Canadian Veterinary Medical Association has a list of accredited programs, career center, and more. http://canadianveterinarians.net/

IVNTA
The International Veterinary Nurses and Technicians Association consists of member countries that seek to foster and promote links with Veterinary Nursing/Veterinary Technician staff worldwide by communication and cooperation. www.ivnta.org

AVTE
The Association of Veterinary Technician Educators offers a biennial symposium, continuing education, career links, a professional journal, recommended review materials for the VTNE, and newsletters. www.avte.net

VHMA
Created in 1981, the membership of Veterinary Hospital Managers Association, currently 1500, includes a number of veterinary technicians. In fact, 25% of certified veterinary practice managers (CVPM) are veterinary technicians. This organization offers continuing education courses, maintains certification for practice managers, conducts surveys, generates a monthly newsletter, and is rapidly growing. www.vhma.org

VetPartners
VetPartners is a resource for veterinary consultants. Members consist of veterinarians, veterinary technicians, practice managers, industry leaders, lawyers, business associates, and more. Review their site if you wish to become a consultant, want to network with consultants, or need to hire a consultant. www.vetpartners.org

AAVSB
The American Association of Veterinary State Boards recently became the owner of the Veterinary Technician National Exam (VTNE). The exam is offered during three examination periods each year. This organization will help you transfer your scores, offers mock exams, lists state technician associations, and has a list of preparation reading resources for the exam. www.aavsb.org

AAHA
Created in 1933, the American Animal Hospital Association accredits nearly 14% of veterinary hospitals serving approximately 6000 practice teams. The standards of excellence expected in both veterinary medicine and practice management are quite high. Students and veterinary technicians can also become a member of AAHA, even if the veterinary hospital where you work is not a member. Continuing education, career center, and bookstore discounts are but a few of the benefits of membership. www.aahanet.org

VSPN
The Veterinary Support Personnel Network has been going strong since 1996 and is fully supported by Veterinary Information Network (VIN). Membership is free. They offer online continuing education (since 2001), live chats, surveys, a bookstore, and more. www.vspn.org

VetMedTeam
Created as the first site offering continuing education to the entire healthcare team, VetMedTeam offers VTNE reviews, membership polls, advanced course studies, and practice management and assistant classes. www.vetmedteam.com

WhereTechsConnect
The largest career center for veterinary technicians and staff, this site was created in 2001. Simply post your resume, review career tips, view hospitals seeking technicians, and participate on their discussion board; all services free for veterinary technicians. Continuing education is also posted. www.wheretechsconnect.com

MyVeterinaryCareer
Created in 2007, this company provides personal career management and recruitment. Through their personalized approach, individual preference review, and your identified values, their team will help match you to a veterinary hospital that aligns with your personal mission, goals, and values. www.myveterinarycareer.com

DVM360
Site offering access to numerous magazine articles, such as *Firstline, Veterinary Economics, DVM Newsmagazine*, and *Veterinary Medicine*. www.dvm360.com

VetFolio
Site offering access to numerous journals, conference proceedings, continuing education courses, and more. www.vetfolio.com

NetVet
Veterinary resource site for veterinary professionals and animal owners. http://netvet.wustl.edu/

BLS.GOV
The Bureau of Labor Statistics provides information about average technician salaries, projections, and more. www.bls.gov

SafetyVet
Created by a veterinary technician in 1998, this site will help you find information on OSHA requirements, safety procedures, your rights as an employee, team training, controlled substance logging, radiation exposure, pregnancy precautions, and more. www.safetyvet.com

SalaryExpert
Site allows for geographical research of veterinary professional salaries. www.salaryexpert.com

Financial Simulator Program
Originally created for veterinary students, the website provides access to an exceptionally valuable personal budget program that resides at this University of Minnesota website. It was created by the Hospital Director at this veterinary school, David Lee, DVM, MBA with James F. Wilson, DVM, JD's editorial oversight. The various elements of this budget program can be used by technicians and students to establish their personal budgets, make plans to repay educational and/or other loans, purchase or lease vehicles, buy homes, plan for retirement, and much more. www.finsim.umn.edu

REVIEW QUESTIONS

Matching

Match the team member with the description.

______**1.** Veterinary Assistant	**A.** a person who has graduated from a 2-year AVMA-accredited program
______**2.** Veterinary Technician	**B.** a person who has graduated from a 4-year CVTEA-accredited program
______**3.** Veterinary Technologist	**C.** a clinical aide with less training than that required of a veterinary technician
______**4.** Veterinary Technician Specialist	**D.** a person who has graduated from a 4-year AVMA-accredited program receiving a Doctor of Veterinary Medicine degree
______**5.** Veterinarian	**E.** credentialed technician who meets requirements established by an academy

Fill in the Blank

Fill in the blanks using the answer choices provided.

1. Upon graduation from an AVMA accredited veterinary technology program, candidate veterinary technicians are eligible to take the ______________________________.

2. The ______________________________ owns and administers the VTNE.

3. Duties of the ______________________ may include restraining, feeding, and exercising patients, cleaning the hospital and boarding premises, and other clinical support tasks.

4. In most cases, graduates of AVMA-accredited programs in veterinary technology are granted an ________________ degree.

5. Veterinary technicians and technologists, by veterinary practice law, are unable to diagnose, ______________________, or perform surgery.

Veterinary Technician National Examination (VTNE)
American Association of Veterinary State Boards (AAVSB)
Veterinary Assistant
Associate
Prescribe

Choose the Best Response

Choose the best answer to the following questions.

1. How many years of college do most veterinarians attend to become eligible for a veterinary license?
  a. 2
  b. 4
  c. 6
  d. 8

2. How many years of college do most veterinary technicians attend to become eligible for credentialing as a veterinary technician?
  a. 2
  b. 4
  c. 6
  d. 8

3. What is the title used when a veterinarian completes additional specialized training and passes a certifying examination?
  a. diplomate
  b. VTS
  c. DVMS
  d. boarded

4. What is the title used when a veterinary technician completes additional specialized training and passes a certifying examination?
  a. diplomate
  b. VTS
  c. DVMS
  d. boarded

5. What organization accredits college programs for educating veterinarians and veterinary technicians?
  a. VHMA
  b. AVMA
  c. NAVTA
  d. NAVLE

RECOMMENDED READING

Felstead K: The truth about the technician shortage, *Firstline*, August 2008. www.dvm360.com.

Rose R, Smith C: *Career choices for veterinary technicians: opportunities for animal lovers*, AAHA Press, books and publications, March 2009. www.aahanet.org.

Smith C: *Team satisfaction pays: organizational development for practice success*, Peshastin, WA, 2008, Smith Veterinary Consulting and Publishing, exercises for team development and personal assessment. www.smithvet.com.

Technicians will weather the economic storm, report says, *Firstline*, February 23, 2009. http://veterinaryteam.dvm360.com/firstline/article/articleDetail.jsp?id=583003.

The NAVTA Journal, www.navta.net.

Veterinary Economics, www.dvm360.com.

2 Ethical, Legal, and Safety Issues in Veterinary Medicine

OUTLINE

LEARNING OBJECTIVES

After reviewing this chapter, the reader will be able to:

1. Discuss ethical issues and guidelines relevant to the veterinary profession.
2. Describe the veterinary technician Code of Ethics.
3. List and describe general categories of laws relevant to the veterinary profession.
4. Define laws protecting veterinary employees against physical injury, sexual harassment, and discrimination.
5. Explain laws relating to ensuring quality veterinary service.
6. Define laws regulating the biomedical industry and Occupational Health Safety related to research.
7. Identify mechanisms to avoid hazards in the veterinary workplace.
8. Identify primary zoonotic diseases that pose a danger to veterinary personnel.
9. Describe procedures to minimize exposure to ionizing radiation and compressed gases.
10. Describe methods to prevent the spread of infectious diseases.
11. Discuss the content and uses of Material Safety Data Sheets.
12. Identify four biosafety hazard levels and precautions for each.

KEY TERMS

American Association for Laboratory Animal Science (AALAS)
American Veterinary Medical Association/Professional Liability Insurance Trust
Animal Welfare Act
Board of Veterinary Medical Examiners
Centers for Disease Control and Prevention (CDC)
Comprehensive Drug Abuse Prevention and Control Act
Controlled Substance Act (CSA)
Department of Labor
Dosimetry badge
Drug Enforcement Agency (DEA)
Employee handbook
Equal Employment Opportunity
Ethics
Ethylene oxide
Federal law
Formaldehyde/Formalin
Hazardous materials plan
Human-animal bond
Malpractice/professional negligence
Material Safety Data Sheet
Negligence
Nonexempt employee
Occupational Safety and Health Act (OSHA)
Personal Protective Equipment (PPE)
Respondeat superior
Right to Know Law
Scavenging system
Secondary container labeling
Standard Operating Procedure (SOP)
State law
Veterinary Medical Association
Veterinary Technician Association
Veterinary State Practice Act
Zoonotic hazards

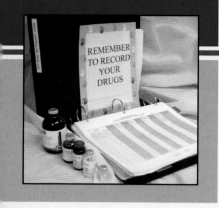

ETHICS

Our lives are governed by rules and laws. As children we are taught the differences between acceptable and unacceptable behavior. We quickly learn the standards by which to judge the actions of others and ourselves, and easily recognize negative behavior when we encounter it. As adults we intuitively know what is right, what is fair, and what is honest.

Our society sets specific standards for proper living. An ethical person lives by these standards. Laws set the maximum limits from which we can deviate from the acceptable norm, established by the people, for the people, and made law through legislation. When someone does something unethical, is it something illegal? Not necessarily. Ethics are usually based on higher principles than the minimal requirements of the law, and as a member of a profession we are expected to adhere to ethical standards above those acceptable for the populace. **Ethics** can be defined as the system of moral principles that determines appropriate behavior and actions within a specific group. Members of the medical profession are expected to adhere to the highest ethical standards. The public accepts, without question, the decisions and judgments made by medical professionals because of their education and expertise.

This text was written for individuals who work within the veterinary profession. We serve the public and the animal kingdom. A veterinary technician should have a profound commitment to honesty, compassion, proficiency, and hard work. Individuals with high ethical standards fit perfectly into the veterinary community. The Veterinary Technician Code of Ethics can be found on NAVTA's website. The NAVTA Ethics Committee created, reviews, and periodically updates the Code. NAVTA also publishes the veterinary technicians oath (Fig. 2-1).

Veterinary Technician's Oath

I solemnly dedicate myself
to aiding animals and society
by providing excellent care
and services for animals,
by alleviating animal suffering,
and by promoting public health.

I accept my obligations to practice
my profession conscientiously
and with sensitivity, adhering to
the profession's Code of Ethics,
and furthering my knowledge
and competence through a
commitment to lifelong learning.

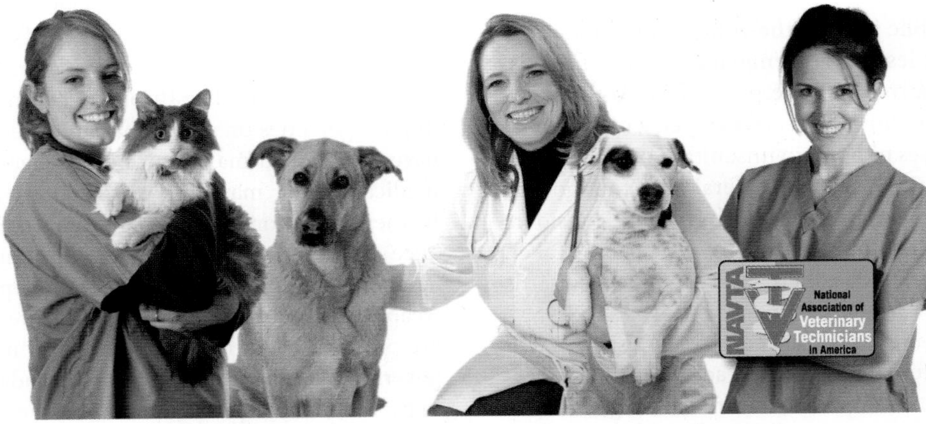

FIGURE 2-1 The veterinary technicians oath. (Courtesy of NAVTA)

ETHICS OF WORKING WITH ANIMALS

The use and abuse of animals has been well documented throughout history. Practices such as rat baiting, dog and cockfights, and the pointless slaughter of animals for sport have passed from commonplace to criminal acts. The American Society for the Prevention of Cruelty to Animals (ASPCA) was created in 1866 and anticruelty laws were passed the same year.

Our culture demands that we treat animals with kindness, respect, and compassion. Animals once thought to exist only for our use and pleasure are now considered as individuals with the ability to feel pain and experience stress. Nowhere is this concept more important than in the veterinary profession. The **human-animal bond,** a very real and maturing concept, defines the special, healthy relationship between people and their pets.

> **TECHNICIAN NOTE** Try these websites to learn more about the human-animal bond:
> - Human Animal Bond Trust, www.humananimalbondtrust.org
> - Human Animal Bond, www.humananimalbond.org
> - The Center for the Human-Animal Bond, www.vet.purdue.edu/chab

A veterinary technician is assumed to be an individual with a strong commitment to the care and welfare of animals. Technicians must make a personal determination concerning the status of the animals with which they share the world. There are many ways to look at this complex relationship.

Some people ask if the rights of an animal should be the same as for humans; they believe that animals should not be used for any purpose. People, they maintain, are merely the highest form of animal life, and all life is important and equal. If you would not do something to a person, they argue, then it should not be done to an animal.

Animal rights activists question the use of animals for food, clothing, entertainment, and biomedical research. Some even question the keeping of animals as pets. They question whether owning a pet is the same as slavery in people. The majority of Americans believe in regulated forms of animal use as long as it is compassionate, humane, and not of trivial importance.

Although the public accepts the concept of animal use, it demands nothing less than exemplary care for animals. This is shown in many ways. The public has no tolerance for a dog owner who criminally starves a pet, a commercial puppy mill that houses puppies in unsanitary conditions, or a biomedical facility that violates federal laws that govern the care and use of animals in research. Society considers it a privilege to own an animal. This privilege can be taken away if the owner does not adhere to acceptable standards of animal care.

The standards for animal care are continually rising, as well they should. Just as humans have made advances in other aspects of life, our relationship with the animal kingdom continually improves. The veterinary profession can take credit for many positive changes that have benefited animals, and it will continue to strive for greater advances in the future.

As your career evolves, you may experience unsatisfactory care and abuse of an animal. Know and understand your state's laws regarding your obligation as a veterinary professional to report animal abuse to the authorities. There is well-documented evidence that links animal abuse and family violence. The presence of animal cruelty in a household often indicates abuse of other family members. If a veterinary technician is suspicious that an animal has been abused, speak promptly with your veterinarian and official authorities. To learn more, contact your local law enforcement agencies, humane society, or veterinary medical association for proper training.

> **TECHNICIAN NOTE** View the Humane Society Veterinary Medical Association's site at www.hsvma.org for details regarding state laws. Many states have statutes and regulations that provide immunity from civil and criminal penalties for veterinarians in connection with reporting animal abuse or neglect.

Ethics of the Veterinary Profession

Questions of ethics within the veterinary community tend to fall into several major categories. We will look at some of these more closely to better understand the ethical challenges that can occur within the veterinary profession.

PROFESSIONAL ETHICS

Medicine will always be an art as well as a science. Professional judgment is the freedom given to all veterinarians to treat a case in a manner that they think best. Sometimes the choices made by the professional are not those that others in the profession would commonly choose. There may be a fine line between freedom and standard of care. Who decides the difference?

Each state government has created laws for the veterinary profession written in the **Veterinary State Practice Act.** The **Board of Veterinary Medical Examiners,** made up of a combination of veterinary professionals and nonveterinarians, is responsible for interpreting the law and the standards of care offered to veterinary patients. The Board's mission is to protect the consumer and review cases brought against a licensed professional. It is the Board's job to determine if there was medical negligence or malpractice. The Board of Examiners, in existence through government funding, may impose penalties on a veterinarian or technician when they have determined malpractice or negligence. The veterinary medical board may impose penalties and fines, require further education in record keeping, send letters of guidance or admonition, or mandate retraining to avoid future complaints. Suspension of a license to practice is the final weapon that a state board uses to ensure that all individuals are practicing to a high standard. You may view your state government website to review past agendas, upcoming meetings, and current professionals who have revoked licenses. In some states, the Veterinary Board of Examiner meetings are opened to the public. You will find attending a meeting is very enlightening. By sitting quietly and listening to the examiners review the cases, you will learn how to avoid revocation of a professional license, whether yours or your veterinarian's.

TECHNICIAN NOTE To locate the laws governing your profession, visit your state or provincial government site to download and read the practice act.

State and national **Veterinary Medical Associations** work closely with their membership to promote and ensure professionalism among their organization. State and national **Veterinary Technician Associations** are trying to increase membership and awareness of the profession. A genuine effort is made, within the professions, to correct deficiencies in individuals whose methods and choices are unacceptable. Licensed veterinarians and technicians may lose their licensing privilege as a result of a chemical substance abuse challenge. Some associations offer peer assistance to help a recovering addict.

As an employee, you have an ethical obligation to discuss any matter concerning animal care that troubles you with the veterinarian. Keep an open mind. Often what may appear as inappropriate action by the veterinarian may be satisfactorily explained with a frank dialogue. In most cases honest discussion will resolve the problem. In extreme cases technicians may have to address their concerns with another veterinarian or the Board of Veterinary Medical Examiners. Cases brought to the Board are critiqued objectively and fairly. Accurate records, documentation of conversations, dates, times, and witnesses are needed to create a solid complaint. Technicians working in the biomedical industry are able to report any suspected acts of animal neglect or abuse to review boards without fear of reprisals.

Record keeping is the single biggest defense against a complaint. When writing in a medical record, follow the information outlined in Chapter 3. Properly identified radiographs, documentation of declined services, and itemized invoices can be reviewed in a case. All entries must be dated, initialed, and legible. Medical records can make or break a person's professional career. Always consider that when documenting laboratory reports, treatments, conversations, history, postsurgical release forms and filling prescriptions.

ETHICS OF SERVICE TO THE PUBLIC

People who work within the veterinary profession are obligated to serve the public, and in doing so to provide medical care and treatment at a level consistent with the standards of the profession. Members of the profession are morally compelled to report abuses inflicted on animals and legally responsible for reporting public health problems.

It is well understood that the public pays veterinarians and their staff for their services. In essence, the veterinary hospital enters into a contract with the pet owner, wherein for a certain amount of money, specific services are rendered. The owner is legally responsible for paying the bill. What are the obligations of the veterinary hospital? Aside from legal obligations of the hospital to competently render the service, the hospital is also morally responsible for treating the animal with care and compassion.

Should the presence or absence of a fee determine if a sick animal is treated? Ethically, the veterinarian and the supporting staff are obligated to provide at least basic lifesaving treatment and pain relief whenever possible to any animal in its care. This may include performing euthanasia on a badly injured stray in obvious pain.

Veterinary professionals also act as teachers. There is an obligation to communicate with the public in clear, easy-to-understand language. The subjects may be as diverse as the care of an animal with diabetes, the correct use of dispensed medication, or nutritional tips. We are obligated to communicate and inform. Consent forms can be used as an educational tool and help define the veterinarian-client-patient relationship. Because of concerns regarding this special relationship, the American Veterinary Medical Association (AVMA) has defined the relationship for the use of dispensing prescribed medications and establishing treatment plans.

BIOMEDICAL RESEARCH

In the field of biomedical research, the veterinary profession is guided by the concept of the "Three *Rs*." The concept was developed by William Russell and Rex Burch in 1959. The Three *Rs* stand for Replacement, Reduction, and Refinement. The public has empowered the veterinary profession to ensure that research strictly follows these principles. Because of the Three *Rs*, animals are only used when there are no viable nonanimal models, the number of animals used is kept to a minimum, and the comfort of the animal becomes of paramount importance. Every research facility that uses animals must have ongoing veterinary care to ensure that the Three *R* principles are applied to all animal research.

OBLIGATIONS TO THE ANIMAL KINGDOM

The primary function of the veterinary profession is to protect the health and welfare of the animals in our care. We are concerned with the treatment of the sick, the prevention of disease, and the general well-being of all animal life. We have become the animal's advocate in society. We care, and are proud of our concern. Moreover, we are not hesitant to insist that anyone with animal contact show the proper respect for that living creature. We demand that pain and discomfort always be minimized if not completely eliminated. We understand the bond between animals and humans and foster that bond whenever possible. It is our mission and our duty.

LAW

In the daily practice of veterinary medicine, the veterinarian and veterinary technician are confronted with a wide variety of legal issues that affect their professional or business decisions. Bodies of law governing daily practices occurring within a veterinary clinic often overlap and fall into one of four categories: federal law, state law, local/municipal law, or common law. **Federal, state,** and local/municipal laws constitute legislative or written laws. Relevant governmental authorities and agencies enforce these laws, and violations may be punishable by fines and/or jail sentences. In contrast, common law is a body of unwritten law (legal interpretation) that has evolved from use and customs and by judicial decisions establishing precedential case law. Government authorities or agencies do not enforce common law in the same way as legislative laws. Common law is enforced by the judicial system when citizens who may have been injured by a violation of the law file civil lawsuits against the violators.

The laws affecting a veterinary practice can be divided into two groups: (1) laws that ensure the quality of veterinary service to patients and (2) laws that provide a nonhostile and safe environment for employees, clients, and the public.

LAWS THAT ENSURE THE QUALITY OF VETERINARY SERVICE

Practice Acts

The Veterinary Practice Act of each state and province is the law defining which persons may practice veterinary medicine and surgery in the state, and under which conditions. Although Practice Acts vary in different states and provinces, they generally define the practice of veterinary medicine and make it illegal to practice without a license, stating the qualifications for receiving a license, stating the conditions under which a license can be revoked, and establishing penalties for violating the Act.

The Practice Acts define the practice of veterinary medicine and surgery as diagnosing, treating, prescribing, operating on, testing for the presence of animal disease, and holding oneself out as a licensed practitioner. Embryo transfer; dentistry; and alternative forms of therapy, such as acupuncture, massage, chiropractic medicine, and holistic medicine, are often regarded within this definition of veterinary medicine and surgery, although this may vary in different locations.

Allowing only licensed veterinarians to legally practice veterinary medicine may raise questions about the duties performed by veterinary technicians or veterinary assistants. After all, many of the procedures performed routinely by technicians (or assistants) fall within the scope of the practice of veterinary medicine and surgery, such as inserting an intravenous catheter, inducing general anesthesia, and extracting teeth (outlined in some practice acts). However, as long as the technician is under the direction and responsible supervision of a licensed veterinarian and the technician does not make decisions requiring a veterinary license, the licensed veterinarian and not the technician is practicing veterinary medicine in such instances. Read your governing body's practice. Inquiry is your best bet; ask that your governing board enlighten you to your duties and responsibilities with updated literature.

Whether a technician is under the direction and responsible supervision of a licensed veterinarian is a subjective determination that takes into account the degree of experience and competence of the technician, the task being performed, and the risks to the patient involved with performing the task. Regardless of how experienced the technician may be, in some states the veterinarian must be on the premises or reachable by telephone or two-way radio communication during and for a reasonable time after any veterinary procedure.

Common Law Malpractice

When a veterinarian agrees to treat a client's animal, common law automatically imposes on that veterinarian a legal duty to provide medical or surgical care to that client's animal in accordance with that of a reasonably prudent veterinary practitioner of comparable training under the same or similar circumstances.

A veterinarian's failure to live up to this particular duty constitutes **negligence,** which may also be referred to as **malpractice** or **professional negligence.**

For malpractice to be subject to litigation, the plaintiff must prove three elements: (1) the veterinarian agreed to treat the patient, (2) the veterinarian failed to exercise the necessary legal obligation of skill and diligence in treating the patient (negligence), and (3) the negligence caused injury to the patient.

Veterinarians can be found negligent and guilty of malpractice for the injurious actions of a technician or assistant under the common law doctrine of **respondeat superior.** For example, if a technician mistakenly gave twice the recommended dosage of anesthesia to a patient and this doubled dose caused the death of the animal, the veterinarian may be found negligent and guilty of malpractice as if the veterinarian had given the wrong dosage. If the technician is licensed in the state, the license may also be revoked.

LAWS THAT PROVIDE A SAFE BUSINESS ENVIRONMENT

Federal, state, and common laws exist to help ensure safe and nonhostile working conditions for employees of a veterinary practice, as well as safe conditions for the public.

Occupational Safety and Health Act

Every employer with one or more employees must operate in compliance with the **Occupational Safety and Health Act (OSHA)** of 1970. OSHA regulations are designed to provide a safe workplace for all persons working in any business affecting commerce. The broad judicial interpretation of commerce includes the business of practicing veterinary medicine and surgery. OSHA requires that all employers "shall furnish to each of his employees employment and a place of employment which are free from recognized hazards that are causing or are likely to cause death or serious physical harm to his employees."

To view the official site, go to www.osha.gov. A complete manual is easily downloaded. Material Safety Data Sheets, training, state rules and regulations, fines, and reporting can be located on the site. As an example, information regarding the 2009 H1N1 influenza guidelines can be readily downloaded.

Common Law Ordinary Negligence

Common law establishes for every business owner a legal duty to provide a reasonably safe work environment for employees, as well as a reasonably safe place for clients. Failure to provide this safe environment may constitute ordinary negligence on the part of the veterinarian/business owner. This ordinary negligence is distinguished from malpractice, which is negligence associated with the rendering of professional veterinary medical services. As with malpractice, however, ordinary negligence is not subject to legal action unless it causes injury to a client or employee. For example, if a practice owner provides poor ventilation in a surgical suite and an employee becomes drowsy from anesthetic gases, the employee could not sue and recover damages from the veterinarian unless he or she experiences injury as a consequence (for example, faints and hits his or her head on the countertop).

In meeting the obligation to provide a safe environment for employees and clients, a veterinarian has a common-law duty to supervise proper restraint of any animal within the veterinarian's control. When a client's animal is being examined and the client restrains the animal, it is the veterinarian and not the client who is primarily responsible for proper restraint of that animal. A veterinarian may be found guilty of ordinary negligence if he or she fails to use reasonable care to avoid foreseeable harm to the restrainer or to other people in the vicinity. The definition of reasonable care or foreseeable harm varies, depending on the experience or training of the veterinarian and the animal handler, as well as the procedure done on the animal. Veterinarians have been sued by clients because the client restrained his or her own animal during a procedure and the animal bit the client. To avoid a possible lawsuit, do not allow an owner to restrain his or her own animal within a veterinary hospital.

Medical Waste Management Laws

Veterinarians who own or operate a veterinary practice may be subject to the requirements of state law governing management and disposal of medical wastes (Fig. 2-2). Local laws may impose additional restrictions on what types of waste transporters and disposal facilities may be acceptable. Typical waste included under these acts are discarded needles and syringes, vials containing attenuated or live vaccines, culture plates, and animal carcasses exposed or infected with pathogens infectious to humans or euthanized with a barbiturate. State and local law may extend these categories of regulated veterinary medical waste to include all carcasses, animal blood, bedding, and pathology waste.

Review your state and county's regulations to determine what requirements govern your veterinary hospital. Companies specializing in the disposal of medical waste can also provide accurate information. Added cost of proper disposal must be addressed as overhead generally increases because of the direct cost of the regulation. Hospital policy manuals may outline how to identify hazardous waste and how to properly dispose of it.

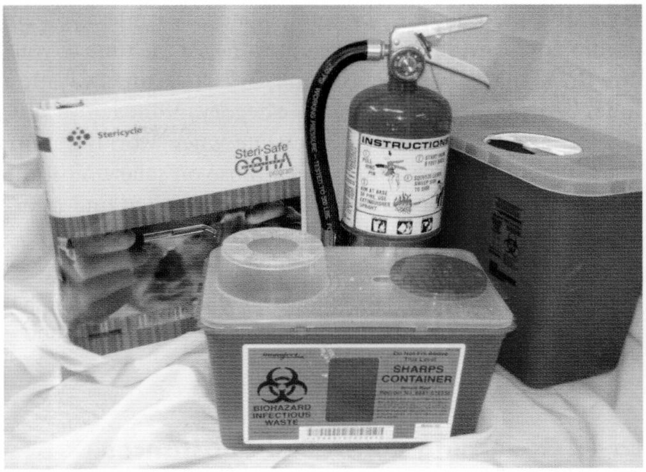

FIGURE 2-2 Syringes and needles must be discarded in a sharps container.

Laws That Maintain a Nonhostile Working Environment

There is a body of federal, state, and common law that restricts a veterinarian, as the owner of a business, from engaging in hiring or firing practices that wrongfully discriminate against individuals. Firing an individual for discriminatory reasons constitutes a violation of the federal or state **Equal Employment Opportunity (EEO)** laws and may provide a basis for the terminated employee to sue the employer under common law for wrongful termination of employment.

According to federal EEO laws, an employer of 15 or more employees may not discriminate against employees in hiring or firing practices (or in any practice, for that matter) on the basis of race, color, religion, sex, or national origin. Sexual harassment and discrimination on the basis of pregnancy or childbirth are forms of sex discrimination made illegal under federal law. Employers also cannot discriminate against individuals in hiring and firing of employees on the basis of age between 40 and 70 years or on the basis of disabilities, including AIDS and rehabilitated drug abuse. At time of hire a manager and new employee may review the **Employee Handbook** together, discussing the hospital's philosophies and policies. An acknowledgment of receipt may be signed and placed in the new employee's file.

Common law also protects employees because it prohibits an employer from terminating that employee for discriminatory reasons or other reasons violating public policy. Under the common law tort of wrongful termination, an employee can directly sue an employer for firing the employee on the basis of sex, race, or religious discrimination, or on the basis that the employee is a whistle-blower (i.e., has complained of sexual harassment or other violations of the law).

Laws That Govern Labor

The Fair Labor Standard Act (FLSA) establishes minimum wage, overtime, record keeping, and youth employment standards for employees working in the private sector and in government. As a veterinary technician or technologist you generally fall under the nonexempt category (unless you are promoted to an administrative position). At the time of your hire the manager will discuss time cards, overtime, vacation time, benefits, and employment category. **Nonexempt employees** are entitled to paid overtime when working more than 40 hours in a workweek, even those on salary. Visit the **Department of Labor** website at www.dol.gov to find information related to technicians and technologists.

> **TECHNICIAN NOTE** View www.dol.gov to research laws governing labor, wages, benefits, exempt status, and more.

Laws Governing Controlled Substances

Controlled substances are drugs that may be subject to abuse by team members, clients, and people who burglarize a veterinary hospital. Federal and state laws have been adopted to govern their manufacture, sale, and distribution. In 1970 the US Congress passed the **Comprehensive Drug Abuse Prevention and Control Act,** regulating the manufacturing, distribution, dispensing, and delivery of certain drugs that have the potential for abuse. Title 2, known as the **Controlled Substance Act (CSA),** is the section most applicable to the veterinary community. The **Drug Enforcement Agency (DEA)** is the primary federal law enforcement agency responsible for combating the abuse of controlled drugs. State and provincial laws differ regarding the regulations of controlled substances. Identify the laws governing veterinary hospitals and controlled drugs in the state or province where you work.

Classifications of Controlled Substances are outlined in Chapter 11. Carefully follow all record keeping, storage, and ordering guidelines related to controlled substances (Fig. 2-3). Report possible abuse or tampering with controlled drugs to your supervisor, hospital manager, or veterinarian.

FIGURE 2-3 The Controlled Substances Act describes record keeping requirements for certain medications.

LAWS THAT CONTROL THE BIOMEDICAL INDUSTRY

During the past century, the biomedical industry has changed our lives. Every antibiotic we use and every vaccine administered to animals and humans can trace its roots to animal research. The life expectancy of humans and their pets is constantly rising. We are living longer, with a higher quality of life, because of the accomplishments of the biomedical industry. These advances have been achieved at the expense of animal life; something that troubles most caring people.

Everyone hopes that the day will come when animals are no longer used as research subjects. The reality of the present is that animal research still represents the best hope of mankind to solve its medical problems.

The vast majority of our population understands this need and also demands that animal research be performed under strict rules and regulations that ensure the maximum welfare of animals. Hence, laws have been written to ensure that animal research is conducted to the highest standards.

Almost all federal laws on the care and use of animals within the biomedical industry originate from two sources: the **Animal Welfare Act (AWA),** under the direction of the Secretary of the US Department of Agriculture (USDA), and the Health Research Extension Act, directed by the Secretary of Health and Human Services. The National Institutes of Health (NIH), a division of Health and Human Services, conducts and supports medical research. The NIH has a branch called the Office of Laboratory Animal Welfare that publishes the Public Health Services (PHS) Policy on Humane Care and Use of Laboratory Animals. The National Research Council publishes The Guide for the Care and Use of Laboratory Animals, which establishes standards for animal care and use. Both the USDA and the NIH require that research institutions conform to the regulations found in that publication.

In very specialized situations other laws and agencies come into play. Research sometimes requires the capture of animals from the wild. In such cases other agencies including the US Fish and Wildlife Service and the Department of the Interior must be used. Some of the laws enforced by these agencies include the Endangered Species Act, the Lacy Act, and the Marine Mammal Protection Act. International treaties intended to protect endangered species and migratory birds are also invoked to enforce specific requirements in certain research projects.

The Animal Welfare Act and the Health Research Extension Act set specific guidelines concerning review of all animal activities by an Institutional Animal Care and Use Committee (IACUC). The laws empower the IACUC to address every aspect of animal use, including a review of the specific research that will be conducted, housing of the animals, specific enrichment plans, pain management, and training of research personnel. Because there is great variation in research projects, each institution is allowed to develop its own Animal Care Policy based on its specific needs and the federal legal requirements. In all cases, the IACUC includes a veterinarian and at least one outside member, a nonscientist with no affiliation with the institution. In this way, the

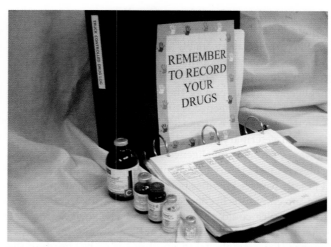

law ensures that the IACUC addresses the needs of the animals and the concerns of the general public. Many veterinary technician education programs fall under the direct laws and regulations of AWA. Visit www.iacuc.org, produced by the American Association for Laboratory Animal Science (AALAS), for more information.

SAFETY

OCCUPATIONAL HEALTH AND SAFETY IN THE BIOMEDICAL INDUSTRY

A small percentage of veterinary technician graduates are employed by the biomedical industry in various capacities. Specific positions offered to graduates of veterinary technician programs vary with the type of institution, but the majority of technicians function as animal caretakers and are generally responsible for the health, comfort, and safety of the animals used in scientific research. Others work in management, product development, product testing, regulatory control, and teaching.

The types of biomedical companies and institutions that employ veterinary technicians are as follows:

- Drug and pharmaceutical manufacturers
- Private and public teaching institutions, colleges, and universities
- Manufacturers of animal support equipment and animal feeds
- Breeders and distributors of research animals
- Private research foundations
- Government agencies

Occupational Health and Safety Programs

Every institution that is considered a part of the biomedical industry should have a written Occupational Health and Safety Program (OHSP) in place to protect the employees who work with animals. The OHSP must be carefully written for the activities and the functions of each specific institution.

A successful program requires the coordination of management, administration, scientists, and workers to ensure that the program adequately covers the complete scope of activities performed at the facility, and all pertinent personnel. Moreover, the program must be flexible enough to adjust to changes that take place in the institution. For example, if a university institutes a new study on tuberculosis, which represents a health hazard not previously encountered, the program must be amended to accommodate the added risk factors. The program must be a dynamic plan that changes as needs change. Specific risks within the institution must be carefully evaluated when writing the Occupational Health and Safety Program. For example, if a facility works with nonhuman primates, the OHSP must address special risks to people exposed to these animals. A facility that will never house nonhuman primates does not have to include such precautions in its program.

A successful program includes a complete medical history of each employee, a preventative medicine section, including a vaccination program suitable for the work performed, a system of ongoing medical evaluation, and a clear and standard policy for emergency situations. The program must also evaluate individual risk factors such as degree of exposure for each person employed at the facility. A person who cleans the research facility hallway for 1 hour per day is handled differently from an attendant who handles animals 6 hours per day.

Standard Operating Procedures

Administrative and health professionals in a research facility carefully list all the different activities performed on a regular basis by all employees. Then each aspect of the procedure is written in a sequential form, taking into consideration all safety precautions. A Standard Operating Procedure (SOP) is an official detailed description of how each important procedure should be performed at the facility. All employees are expected to adhere to the SOP when performing each activity. Once the SOP has been read and understood by a research employee, an administrator or other responsible official of the facility signs the document. A copy of the SOP should be readily available at the work site.

BIOSAFETY HAZARD CONSIDERATIONS IN BIOMEDICAL LABORATORIES

Special considerations must be given to hazards that are unique to the biomedical industry.

The Centers for Disease Control and Prevention (CDC) has established specific guidelines for the safe handling and management of infectious agents in the biomedical industry. Biosafety levels are graded as I, II, III, and IV. The higher the number, the greater the risk. The following is a brief summary of the precautions for each biosafety level. It should be noted that the requirements for each level increase and that requirements for lower levels are automatically included in higher levels.

Biosafety Level I

The agents in biosafety level I are those that ordinarily do not cause disease in humans. It should be noted, however, that these otherwise harmless substances may affect individuals with immune deficiency.

Examples of products and organisms found in biosafety level I include vaccines administered to animals, nonpathogenic strains of bacteria, and infectious diseases that are species-specific, such as canine infectious hepatitis virus.

There are no specific requirements for the handling or disposal of biosafety level I materials other than the normal sanitation that would be used in a home kitchen. This always includes complete washing of counters, equipment, and hands.

Biosafety Level II

The agents in biosafety level II are those that have the potential to cause human disease if handled incorrectly. At this level, specific precautions are taken to avoid problems. The hazards in this level include mucous membrane exposure, possible oral ingestion, and puncture of the skin. Examples of organisms in this level are those that cause toxoplasmosis and salmonellosis. Generally substances in this group have a low potential for aerosol contamination.

Although precautions will vary with the specific substances, these are the general requirements for biosafety level II.

- Limited access to the area, including signs that warn of biohazards
- Wearing of gloves, laboratory coats, gowns, face shields, and use of Class I or Class II biosafety cabinets to protect against splash potential or aerosol contamination
- Appropriate use of sharps containers
- Specific instruction for the disposal and/or decontamination of equipment and potentially dangerous materials, including monitoring and reporting of contamination problems
- Physical containment devices and autoclaves, if needed

Biosafety Level III

Agents in biosafety level III are substances that can cause serious and potentially lethal disease. The potential for aerosol respiratory transmission is high. An example of an organism in this category is *Mycobacterium tuberculosis*.

At this level, primary and secondary barriers are required to protect personnel. General requirements at this level are as follows.

- Controlled access
- Decontamination of waste
- Decontamination of cages, clothing, and other equipment
- Testing of personnel to evaluate possible exposure
- Use of Class I or Class II biosafety cabinets or other physical containment devices during all procedures
- Use of personal protective gear for all personnel

Biosafety Level IV

It is unlikely that persons with limited experience in handing biohazards will ever encounter substances that are included in biosafety level IV. Agents found in this category pose a high risk of causing life-threatening diseases. Included in this level are Ebola and Marburg viruses and other dangerous and exotic agents. Facilities that handle these substances exercise maximum containment. Personnel shower-in and shower-out and dress in full body suits equipped with a positive air supply. Individuals who plan to work in these facilities will undergo extensive training to ensure safety.

OCCUPATIONAL HEALTH AND SAFETY IN VETERINARY PRACTICE

As a veterinary technician, you may be exposed to many hazards in your day-to-day routine and in the performance of nonroutine functions. Hazards can include exposure to pathogenic microorganisms, chemicals, or radiation, in addition to the obvious physical dangers. When properly identified, however, these hazards can be controlled and your risk of injury minimized. Your veterinary hospital will offer training specific to the exposure in your workplace. At time of hire, be sure you discuss personnel protective equipment, evacuation routes and gathering place, safety meetings and emergency contacts, as outlined in the Employee Handbook. The American Veterinary Medical Association's Professional Liability Insurance Trust (AVMAPLIT) (www.avmaplit.com) has safety and training resources for veterinary hospitals. In every state an employee can be legally disciplined, including being terminated, for failure to follow safety rules for the workplace.

> **TECHNICIAN NOTE** The website at www.safetyvet.com was created by Phil Seibert, CVT, and is dedicated to issues related to safety within the veterinary hospital.

Machinery and Moving Parts

Equipment such as fans, chutes, and dryers have moving parts that can cause severe injury. Never operate machinery or equipment without all the proper guards in place. Long hair should be tied back to prevent it from getting caught in fans or other moving objects. Avoid wearing excessive jewelry, very loose-fitting clothing, or open-toe shoes. If you become aware of an unsafe condition, report it to your supervisor immediately.

Slips and Falls

You can reduce the chance of personal injury from slips and falls by wearing slip-proof shoes and using nonslip mats or strips in wet areas. Be especially cautious when walking on uneven or wet floors. Never run inside the hospital or on uneven flooring.

Lifting

When lifting patients, supplies, or equipment, remember to keep your back straight and lift with your legs. Never bend over to lift an object; squat and use your knees when lifting objects. If a motorized lift table is not available, recruit help when lifting patients weighing more than 40 pounds. Remember to follow sound ergonomic principles when positioning or restraining, especially when working with horses or food animals.

Storing Supplies

Store heavy supplies or equipment on the lower shelves to prevent unnecessary strains. Never use stairways as storage areas. Do not overload shelves or cabinets. Store liquids in containers with tight-fitting lids. When possible, store chemicals on shelves at or below eye level. Never climb on cabinets, shelves, chairs, buckets, or comparable items to reach high locations; use an appropriate ladder or stepstool.

Toxic Substances

Eat or drink only in areas free of toxic and biologically harmful substances as outlined in the Employee Handbook. Keep the staff coffee pot and utensils well away from sources of possible contamination, such as the laboratory or the treatment/bathing tub. Ensure that the cabinets above a coffee or food area contain no hazardous chemicals or supplies that could spill on the area. Store food, drinks, condiments, and snacks in a refrigerator free from biological or chemical hazards; vaccines, drugs, and laboratory samples are all potential contamination sources. It is best to have a minimum of two refrigerators; one for biologics and one for employee food.

Heating Devices

When using equipment such as autoclaves, microwave ovens, cautery irons, or other heating devices, take time to learn the rules for safe operation. Burns, especially from steam, are painful and serious and almost always can be prevented. Autoclaves also present a danger from the pressure that is used for proper sterilization. When opening an autoclave, first release the pressure with the vent device and let the steam rise completely before opening the door fully. Always assume cautery devices and branding irons are hot, and use the insulated handle whenever you handle them. Never place heated irons on any surface where they could overheat and start a fire or where someone could accidentally touch them. Microwave ovens should be installed at eye level or below to avoid serious injuries.

Eye Safety

Familiarize yourself with the locations and use of eyewash stations. Always use safety glasses and other personal protective equipment when required. An employer is required by law to provide this equipment when appropriate.

Be sure you know where the eyewash device is before you need to use it. If you splash a chemical in your eyes, do not rub your eyes with your hands. Immediately call for help. With a co-worker's assistance, go to the eyewash station and flush both eyes, even if only one eye is affected. Avoid using the spray attachments for tubs and sinks because the water pressure is unregulated and the streams of water from these devices can be fine enough to lacerate the cornea.

Hazards of Animal Handling

The most important rule to follow: Do not allow clients to restrain their own animals.

The second rule to follow when working around animals is to stay alert. Sudden noises, movements, or even light can cause an animal to react. If you are the primary restraint person, focus your attention on the animal's reactions and not on the procedure being performed. Learn the correct restraint positions for each species you handle regularly.

Chutes and Enclosures. Large animals, such as horses and cattle, can severely injure or even kill you when they try to escape restraint. Never place your hand, leg, or any other body part between the animal and the side of the enclosure, stock, or chute; use a hook or pole to pass ropes or belts through the chute. If you must enter a stall or paddock containing a large animal, stay on the side of the animal nearer the door or gate so that you can escape if the situation becomes hazardous. Temple Grandin, PhD, has written numerous books on the behaviors of both horses and cattle. Her techniques and strategies have aided in the proper handling and understanding of farm animals.

Protective Gear. Your employer is obligated to provide you with **Personal Protective Equipment (PPE)** (Fig. 2-4). Some hazards you may be exposed to when working within a veterinary hospital and the required PPE are listed in Table 2-1.

Make use of any available capture/restraint equipment: cages, snares, cat bags, and poles. Wear latex examination gloves and a surgical mask when handling a stray, wild, or unvaccinated animal. Maintain an appropriate distance from the work area or animal; for example, do not place your face very close to the mouth of the animal (see Zoonotic Hazards section). Wear protective leather gloves when handling a fractious animal.

Barking dogs can be a threat to hearing, especially in indoor kennels. Noise levels in canine wards can reach 110 deci-

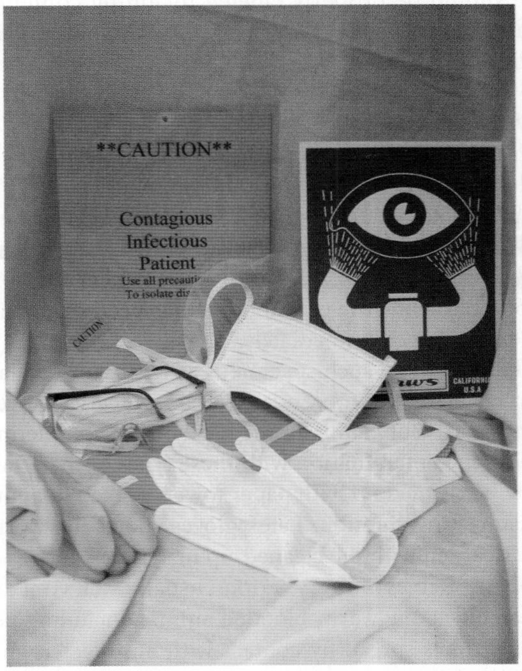

FIGURE 2-4 Personal Protective Equipment includes gloves, masks, and goggles.

TABLE 2-1 Hazards and Personal Protective Equipment

POTENTIAL HAZARDS	PROTECTIVE EQUIPMENT
Radiation exposure while taking radiographs	Lead aprons, gloves, thyroid collars
Bites and scratches	Leashes, muzzles, bags, towels
Bacterial exposure	Safety glasses, eye shields
Exposure to hazardous chemical fumes	Masks
Exposure to hazardous, caustic solutions	Exam gloves, rubber gloves
Loud noises	Ear plugs
Burns	Oven mitts and hot pads

bels (dB). Exposure to these noise levels for a short time, such as going into the kennel to retrieve a patient, poses no serious damage to your hearing, but excessive or long-term exposure can contribute to hearing loss. When working in noisy areas for extended periods (e.g., when cleaning cages), always wear personal hearing protectors rated to filter the noise by at least 20 dB. (The package label indicates the rating.)

Hazards of Bathing and Dipping

Ventilation. Always use the ventilation fan when bathing or dipping. This will keep fumes from shampoos and dips at a safe level. Be sure to wear appropriate protective gear to include safety glasses, gloves, and apron.

Chemical Storage. Chemicals used for bathing and dipping animals can be harmful and must be stored properly. Bottles of dips, shampoos, and parasiticides should be stored in a cabinet at or below eye level. The bottle should be properly labeled including contents and any appropriate hazard warning (see Chemical Hazards section).

Zoonotic Hazards

When treating patients with diseases that are infectious to people (**zoonotic hazards**) or other animals, wear a protective apron, latex exam gloves, face mask, and eye protection. Thoroughly wash your hands with a disinfecting agent, such as chlorhexidine or povidone-iodine scrub, at the completion of treatment. Any clothing that has been contaminated should be changed immediately.

When handling such specimens as fecal samples, laboratory samples, or wound exudates, wear protective gloves and always wash your hands immediately after completing the procedure. Contamination with these types of materials can usually be cleaned up with paper towels soaked in appropriate disinfecting solution. Latex gloves should be worn and then discarded with the cleaned-up materials.

Rabies. Rabies is a very serious, usually fatal viral disease that can affect any warm-blooded animal, including people. Rabies virus is spread by contact with an infected animal's saliva. Usually an uninfected animal becomes infected through the bite of a rabid (infected) animal. The disease has also been transmitted by saliva (even the residue left on a dog's bowl after eating) that contaminates an open wound or contacts the mucous membranes.

The primary barrier to the spread of rabies from the wild animal population to humans is vaccination of pets and other domestic animals. When you must handle an unvaccinated, wild, or stray animal, always wear protective latex gloves and perhaps even protective gown and goggles. A safe and effective human vaccine is available for people who work with animals. Ask your administrator about the hospital's policy on rabies vaccination and employee exposure.

Bacterial Infections. Bacterial infections are certainly possible in the veterinary environment. Aside from the common bacteria that all animals harbor naturally, injury and disease in veterinary patients can expose you to such serious pathogens as *Pasteurella, E. coli,* and *Pseudomonas.* Bacteria are most commonly transferred by direct contact with the animal or its excretions, especially if you have cuts or open sores. Some bacteria are easily aerosolized or released into the air, where they can be inhaled and absorbed through your mucous membranes. The best protection from exposure to bacteria is good personal hygiene and washing your hands after exposure.

Fungal Infections. Ringworm is a superficial skin infection caused by the fungus *Microsporum canis,* among others. Ringworm is very easily transmitted from animals to humans. The most effective protection from ringworm is to wear latex gloves when handling or treating animals with ringworm and to practice good personal hygiene by washing your hands after exposure.

Parasitism. When the eggs of common internal parasites, such as roundworms and hookworms, infect humans, they usually do not mature to adult parasites but they can cause other problems. Some species of roundworm larvae can migrate to virtually any organ in the body and cause a condition known as visceral larva migrans. If this condition develops in a vital organ, such as the eye or brain, severe problems can result. The Companion Animal Parasite Council (www.capcvet.org) offers literature for veterinary professionals including articles on internal and external parasites.

Hookworms can cause a condition known as cutaneous larva migrans. This condition particularly affects children who play in areas where pets defecate frequently, such as a sandbox. Unlike the visceral cysts caused by roundworm larvae, the lesions of cutaneous larva migrans are relatively easy to visualize. These usually appear as red, serpentine lines on the skin of the feet or lower legs.

Borreliosis or Lyme disease, a bacterial infection transmitted by ticks, has become a serious concern for pets and people. When an infected deer tick bites a host (animal or person) during feeding, the bacterium *Borrelia burgdorferi* is transferred to the host. Lyme disease in humans is characterized by joint pain, fever, and other flulike symptoms. The best defense against borreliosis is to check your body for ticks after venturing outdoors and remove them promptly.

Mites causing sarcoptic mange can easily infest people. When treating animals with sarcoptic mange, always wear gloves and a protective gown, and wash your hands thoroughly with disinfecting soap immediately after the procedure.

The coccidian parasite *Toxoplasma gondii* can infect cats and people. Although it is usually not harmful to healthy humans, it might cause serious problems to the fetus of pregnant women. Toxoplasmosis is spread from cats to people usually by ingestion of the infectious oocysts in cat feces, but most humans contract the disease by eating undercooked meat. Pregnant women should avoid cleaning cat litter pans.

Biologics. Vials containing biologics, such as vaccines and bacterins, usually are not considered hazardous unless the agent can infect humans. For example, vials containing such agents as canine distemper virus or feline calicivirus are not usually considered a danger to humans, but vials containing biologically hazardous agents, such as brucellosis bacterins, must be treated as potentially infectious during and after use. Read manufacturer's insert on proper sterilization and disposal of brucellosis bacterins.

Radiation Hazards

Infrequent exposure to small amounts of radiation, such as routine thoracic or dental radiographs, poses little threat to your overall health. However, long-term exposure to small doses of radiation has been linked to genetic, cutaneous, glandular, and other disorders. Exposure to large doses of radiation can cause skin changes, cell damage, and gastrointestinal and bone marrow disorders that can be fatal.

Radiation Safety. When using radiographic equipment, never place any part of your body in the primary beam, even a hand wearing a lead-lined glove. Always wear the appropriate protective equipment, such as lead-lined aprons, thyroid collar, and lead gloves. Lead-impregnated glasses are also recommended. Always use the collimator to restrict the primary beam to an area smaller than the size of the cassette, creating a clear border around all four sides of the film. Digital radiographs add safety protection in that fewer radiographs are taken because the film can be digitally enhanced or altered. However, proper exposure techniques are still necessary to provide diagnostic quality images and reduce exposure to radiation.

Portable x-ray machines, such as those used in large animal and mobile practices, can be particularly dangerous because the primary beam of these machines can be aimed in any direction. When using a portable machine, always be sure there is no human body part in the path of the primary beam, even at a distance. Never hold a cassette, whether wearing lead-lined gloves or not; always use a cassette-holding pole. Also, wear a lead-lined apron, thyroid collar, and gloves.

Everyone involved with radiography must wear a **dosimetry badge.** This badge must always be worn during radiographic procedures to measure any scatter radiation you may receive during the procedure. Your supervisor or hospital administrator will regularly advise you of the readings from your personal dosimetry badge. These reports, required by law, are designed as a warning system to alert you and your supervisor if your exposure to radiation reaches a hazardous level. Your dosimetry badge number follows you wherever you are employed; therefore it gives an accurate lifetime exposure reading. Follow the manufacturer's directions regarding placement of dosimeter and transferring of your badge number to another hospital.

Developing Chemicals. Radiographic developing chemicals (developer and fixer) can be very corrosive to materials and human tissues. Take extreme care when mixing, transferring, agitating, or transporting these chemicals, and do this only in a well-ventilated area. Always turn on the exhaust fan when you are in a darkroom. Use protective gloves and goggles when mixing or pouring chemicals. For manual processing tanks, stir chemicals with care and avoid splashing. After handling radiographic developing chemicals, always wash your hands. See Chapter 6 for detailed information on radiation safety.

Anesthetic Hazards

Long-term exposure to waste anesthetic gases has been linked to congenital abnormalities in children, spontaneous abortions, and liver and kidney damage. OSHA has set the safe exposure limit for halogenated anesthetic agents (e.g., isoflurane) at 2 parts per million.

According to some sources, as much as 90% of the anesthetic gas levels found in the surgery room during a procedure can be attributed to leaks in anesthesia machines. For this reason, always check for leaks in the hoses and anesthetic machine before use. Use hoses and rebreathing bags that are the correct size. Start the flow of anesthetic gas after connecting the patient to the machine. Before disconnecting the patient, continue oxygen flow until the remaining anesthesia gas has been flushed through the scavenging system. Have anesthetic machines professionally serviced on an annual basis.

A well-designed **scavenging system** captures excess gases directly at the source and transports them to a safe exhaust port, usually outside the building. This is the most effective means of reducing exposure of waste anesthetic gases in the workplace. Scavenger units (canisters) can be purchased and used on machines.

When refilling the anesthetic machine vaporizer, move the machine to a well-ventilated area. Use a pouring funnel and avoid overfilling the vaporizer or spilling the liquid anesthetic. If you accidentally break a bottle of liquid anesthetic, immediately evacuate all people from the area. Open the window and turn on the exhaust fans. Control the liquid with a spill kit absorbent or a generous amount of kitty litter. Pick up the contaminated absorbent or kitty litter with a dustpan, and place it in a plastic trash bag.

Some procedures, such as mask or tank induction, defy collection of waste gases. In such instances, be sure the room is well ventilated. Exhaust fans for evacuating room air to the outside are recommended. Air-handling systems that recirculate the air can expose others in the hospital. Induction chambers can be connected to the scavenging system or absorption canister to reduce levels of escaping gases.

When changing the soda lime (carbon dioxide absorbent) in anesthetic machines, wear latex gloves. When the soda lime is wet, as it often is from humidity in the patient's breath, it can be very caustic to tissues and some metals. Place used soda lime granules in a plastic trash bag and dispose of it in the regular trash. Read manufacturer's instructions to determine when to change soda lime.

If you are a woman and become pregnant, discuss the anesthetic exposure risk with your physician as soon as possible and notify your supervisor immediately. Follow established policies regarding safety precautions while pregnant in your place of employment.

Hazards of Compressed Gases

Store cylinders of compressed gas (e.g., oxygen) in a dry, cool place, away from potential heat sources, such as furnaces, water heaters, and direct sunlight. Always secure the tanks in an upright position by means of a chain or strap (including small tanks). Transportation carts and floor-mounting collars are also acceptable methods of securing compressed gas cylinders. If the cylinder is equipped with a protective cap (usually the large ones are), it must be firmly screwed in place when the cylinder is not in use. If you must move a large cylinder, do not roll or drag it; always use a hand truck, dolly, or cart, and strap the tank to the cart before moving. Always wear impact-resistant protective goggles when connecting or disconnecting tanks, because air escaping from tanks can cause trauma to the cornea of your eyes.

More details on safety issues related to anesthetic procedures are located in Chapter 14.

Hazards of Sharp Objects

The most serious hazard of sharp objects (sharps) in a veterinary environment is from the physical trauma and possible bacterial infection caused by a puncture or laceration. To prevent accidents from punctures or lacerations, always keep needles, scalpel blades, and other sharps capped or sheathed until ready for use. When practical, place the sharp in a red sharps container immediately after use. Do not attempt to recap the needle unless the physical danger from sticks or lacerations cannot be avoided by any other means.

When necessary, needles may be recapped using the one-handed method. Place the cap on a flat surface (table or counter). With one hand, thread the needle into the cap. The cap may then be firmly seated using both hands. The needle should not be removed from the syringe, but the entire unit should be disposed of in the red sharps container. When full, the sharps container must be sealed and disposed of following the hospital's prescribed policy.

Ordinary plastic milk containers are not appropriate sharps collection containers; a 22-gauge needle can easily penetrate them. The containers made for this specific purpose (usually red and labeled with a biohazard symbol) are the most effective and are usually very economical. State and local laws may prevent your hospital from using inappropriate sharps containers and fines may be levied against the hospital if they do not meet established standards.

Cutting off the ends of needles before disposal increases the potential for aerosolization of the liquid involved. Collecting sharps in a smaller container and transferring them to a larger container for disposal places someone at an increased risk of exposure. Neither of these practices is recommended.

Never throw needles or other sharps directly into regular trash containers, regardless of whether or not they are capped. Never open a used sharps container. Never insert your fingers into a sharps container for any reason.

> **TECHNICIAN NOTE** You can download numerous documents, posters, and brochures from the official Occupational Safety and Health Administration (OSHA) site. View www.osha.gov to print off regulations, standards, fact sheets, forms, chemical labeling, and small business handbook.

Chemical Hazards

Many products you use every day can be hazardous. Every chemical, even common ones such as cleaning supplies, can cause harm. Some chemicals can contribute to health problems, whereas others may be flammable and pose a fire threat. The most common chemicals used in the veterinary workplace are insecticides, medications, and cleaning agents.

Veterinary hospitals must follow the guidelines of OSHA's **Right to Know Law.** This law requires that you be informed about all chemicals you may be exposed to while doing your job. The Right to Know Law also requires you to wear all safety equipment that is prescribed by the manufacturer when handling a chemical. The safety equipment must be provided by the employer at no cost to you. It is not optional; you must wear what is prescribed.

Hazardous Materials Plan. A strategic component of the Right to Know Law is the **hazardous materials plan.** This plan describes the details of the practice's **Material Safety Data Sheet (MSDS)** filing system and the **secondary container labeling** system (Fig. 2-5). The plan also lists the person responsible for ensuring that all employees have received the necessary safety training. You have a right to review any of these materials, so ask your supervisor where your plan is located.

Part of the planning process includes knowing exactly what chemicals are present in the workplace. There must be an up-to-date list of chemicals known to be on the hospital premises. It surprises some people to learn that the average veterinary hospital has over 200 hazardous chemicals present at any time.

> **TECHNICIAN NOTE** Use this website to search millions of MSDS documents. It's easy to use and can simplify compliance. www.MSDSonline.com

Material Safety Data Sheets. More detailed information about every chemical can be found on the

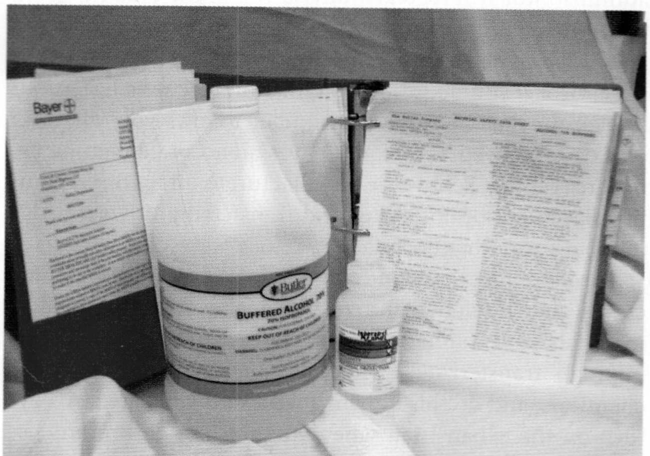

FIGURE 2-5 Material Safety Data Sheets and secondary container labels are important components of the Right to Know Law.

MSDS. At the time of hire your manager will inform you where the MSDS log is kept. When OSHA does their inspection, they will ask where the MSDS log is kept. MSDS documents may look complicated at first glance, but the information that is important to you is easy to find.

Container Labels. When you receive a supply of chemicals from the distributor, every bottle is identified with a label containing directions and any appropriate warnings. Always read, understand, and follow these directions and warnings printed on the label. When possible, keep this label intact and readable. Sometimes it is necessary to dilute a chemical or pour it into smaller bottles for use. These smaller bottles are known as secondary containers. All secondary containers must have a label that indicates the contents and appropriate safety warnings.

Container Caps. Always remember to replace the cap on a chemical bottle after use. Bottles of chemicals should always have tight-fitting, screw-on lids. Always store chemical bottles at or below eye level in a closed cabinet. Never store or use chemicals near food or beverages.

Mixing Chemicals. Be cautious when mixing or diluting chemicals. Always wear latex gloves and protective goggles. Never mix any chemicals unless you know it is safe to do so according to the label or MSDS. Mixing often creates a new, sometimes very dangerous chemical. When making dilute solutions from a concentrate, always start with the correct quantity of water and then add the concentrate. Never add the water to the concentrate, because the chemical may splash or may not react as you expect.

Chemical Spills. Minor spills of most chemicals can be cleaned up with paper towels or absorbent, such as kitty litter, and disposed of in the trash or sanitary sewer. However, some very dangerous chemicals, such as formaldehyde or ethylene oxide, require special procedures. Before you use a chemical with which you are unfamiliar, review the MSDS and learn the procedures you must follow for cleaning up a spill. When cleaning up any spill, always wear latex gloves and any other protective equipment specified on the MSDS. Unless prohibited by the instructions on the MSDS, wash the spill site and any contaminated equipment with a detergent soap and water.

Handling Ethylene Oxide. Some hospitals use **ethylene oxide** gas to sterilize items that would be damaged by other sterilization procedures. Ethylene oxide is a potent human carcinogen. Take the following precautions when handling or using ethylene oxide:

- Carefully read the MSDS for ethylene oxide.
- Store the ethylene oxide in a safe place.
- Use only approved devices to perform ethylene oxide sterilization.
- Read, understand, and follow all written procedures and safety precautions.
- Know the emergency procedures.
- Be aware of monitoring levels.
- Keep ethylene oxide away from flames and sparks, because it is highly flammable.

Handling Formalin.

- Liquid or gaseous **formaldehyde** and **formalin** are serious health hazards in veterinary hospitals. Because formaldehyde is a known human carcinogen, OSHA monitors its use.
- Carefully read the MSDS for formaldehyde/formalin.
- Store formalin containers safely, including specimen jars.
- Use formalin only with good ventilation; avoid breathing vapors.
- Wear goggles and latex gloves; avoid skin and eye contact.

Exposure to formalin can be minimized by use of premixed, premeasured vials of formalin for specimens. Veterinary hospitals that still use bulk formalin for diagnostic laboratory tests (e.g., Knott's test) should consider switching to a newer, less-hazardous method of testing.

Electrical Hazards. Do not remove light switch or electrical outlet covers. Always keep circuit breaker boxes closed. Only persons trained to perform maintenance duties should repair electrical outlets, switches, fixtures, or breakers. If you must use a portable dryer or other electrical equipment in a wet area, it must be properly grounded and plugged into only a ground-fault circuit interruption (GFCI) type of outlet.

Extension cords should be used only for temporary supply applications and should always be of the three-conductor, grounded type. Never run extension cords through windows or doors that could close and damage the wires. Never run extension cords across aisles or floors, which create a tripping hazard. When an extension cord is necessary, it should be adequate for the electrical load. Generally, extension cords longer than 4 feet should not be used for loads greater than 6 amps at 120 volts AC or 3 amps at 240 volts AC.

Equipment with grounded plugs must never be used with adapters or nongrounded extension cords. Never alter or remove the ground terminals on plugs. Appliances or equipment with defective ground terminals or plugs should not be used until repaired.

Fire and Evacuation. At time of hire, review fire safety and locate fire extinguishers with your manager. Read hospital policy on emergency evacuations in your employee handbook. Safety training may include fire or chemical spill drills. Discuss personal safety, emergency evacuation protocols, and animal safety with the hospital administrator.

Always store flammables properly. Materials such as gasoline, paint thinner, and ether should never be stored inside the hospital, except in an approved storage cabinet designed for flammables. Some components of specialty dental and large animal acrylic repair kits are also very flammable. Very small amounts of these components can usually be safely stored in an area with good ventilation free from flames or sparks.

Be alert for situations that could cause a fire. Flammable items, particularly newspapers, boxes, and cleaning chemicals, must always be stored at least 3 feet away from any ignition source, such as a water heater, furnace, or stove. Always use extra care when using portable heaters. Never leave portable heaters unattended, and always be sure they are placed no closer than 3 feet from any wall, furniture, or other flammable material.

Know the location of all fire extinguishers on the premises and how to use them. Before you decide to use a fire extinguisher, be sure the fire alarm has been sounded, everyone has left the building (or is in the process of leaving), and the fire department has been called. The National Fire Protection Association (NFPA) recommends that you never attempt to fight a fire if any of the following conditions apply:

- The fire is spreading beyond the immediate area where it started or has already become a large fire.
- The fire could block your escape route.
- You are unsure of the proper operation of the extinguisher.
- You doubt that the extinguisher is designed for the type of fire at hand or is large enough to suppress the fire.

Know where the designated emergency exits are. Make sure emergency exits are always unlocked and free from obstructions. If you must work in a building during nonoperational hours (when security warrants that the doors are locked), be sure you have at least two clear exits from the building that can be opened without a key.

Personal Safety

Workers in emergency or 24-hour practices should use the barriers that are usually available. Use the buzzer to control access through the front door and one-way locks on the remaining doors. (This lets you out in case of an emergency but keeps the door locked from the outside.) These personal safety techniques are essential in these environments.

In any practice, the potential for robbery is always present. In any situation where someone demands money or drugs while threatening your personal safety, do not attempt to withhold the things they demand. Cooperate with the demands, but do not go with the person, even to the parking lot. Attempt to remember every detail of the person's appearance and demeanor. This greatly increases the likelihood that the police will locate the person. As soon as safely possible, let everyone else know of the situation. Attempt to contact the police if this can be done safely without the intruder's knowledge; otherwise, do it immediately after the intruder has left the premises.

REVIEW QUESTIONS

Matching

Match the following terms with their description or definition:

_____ **1.** Human-Animal Bond
_____ **2.** Drug Enforcement Agency
_____ **3.** Collimator
_____ **4.** Biosafety Level III Agents
_____ **5.** Ringworm
_____ **6.** National Institutes of Health
_____ **7.** Laws
_____ **8.** Fair Labor Standards Act
_____ **9.** Standard Operating Procedure
_____ **10.** Biosafety Level IV Agents
_____ **11.** Ethics
_____ **12.** Common Law
_____ **13.** Biosafety Level II Agents
_____ **14.** Dosimetry Badge
_____ **15.** Biosafety Level I Agents

A. maximum limits from which we can deviate from the acceptable norm
B. system of moral principles that determine behavior
C. a body of unwritten law, evolved from use, custom, and by judge-made decisions establishing precedential case law
D. enforces federal law on the care and use of animals within the biomedical industry
E. ordinarily do not cause disease in humans, but may affect individuals with immune deficiency
F. have potential to cause human disease if handled incorrectly; low potential for aerosol transmission
G. can cause serious and potentially lethal disease; potential for aerosol respiratory transmission is high
H. pose a high risk of causing life-threatening disease
I. superficial skin infection caused by a fungus; easily transmitted from animals to humans
J. radiation safety device found on the x-ray machine; restricts size of primary x-ray beam
K. radiation safety device; measures personal scatter radiation exposure
L. concept defining the special, healthy relationship between people and pets
M. establishes minimum wage, overtime, record keeping, and youth employment standards
N. primary federal law enforcement agency responsible for combating the abuse of controlled drugs
O. an official detailed description of how each important procedure should be performed at a research facility

Choose the Best Response

Choose the best answer to the following questions.

1. Which federal agency is responsible for developing and enforcing regulations to ensure a safe working environment?
   a. DEA
   b. USDA
   c. OSHA
   d. CSA
2. Which federal agency is responsible for enforcing regulations related to controlled drugs?
   a. DEA
   b. USDA
   c. OSHA
   d. CSA
3. Which law regulates the practice of veterinary medicine in a state?
   a. CSA
   b. Practice Act
   c. BVME law
   d. DAVECC
4. Where can detailed information regarding a specific hazardous chemical, its composition, requirements for storage, handling, use, and need for personal protective equipment be found?
   a. the OSHA website
   b. the chemical container label
   c. the MSDS
   d. the practice safety manual
5. Which statement concerning controlled substances log book records is most accurate?
   a. By law, records must be made available to the OSHA inspector.
   b. Only state laws apply to controlled substances.
   c. All veterinary practice personnel can access the records.
   d. All records must be maintained for at least 5 years.

RECOMMENDED READING

American Animal Hospital Association: The link between abuse and domestic violence, *Pet Care Library*, 2009. www.healthypet.com.

American Veterinary Medical Association, www.avma.org/KB/Resources/Reference/human-animal-bond/Pages/Human-Animal-Bond-AVMA.aspx.

King LJ: *Veterinary medicine and public health at CDC*, www.cdc.gov, 2006.

Jack D: Another primer on informed consent (CVC Proceedings), *Veterinary Healthcare*, 2000. www.dvm360.com.

National Research Council, Committee on Occupational Safety and Health in Research Animal Facilities, Institute of Laboratory Animal Resources, and Commission on Life Sciences: *Occupational health and safety in the care and use of research animals*, Washington, DC, 1997, National Academy Press.

National Research Council: *Guide for the care and use of laboratory animals*, Washington, DC, 2004, Diane Pub Co., National Academy Press.

Office of Laboratory Animal Welfare, National Institutes of Health: *Institutional Animal Care and Use Committee Guidebook*, ed 2, Bethesda, MD, 2002, National Institutes of Health.

Repa BK: *Your rights in the workplace*, ed 8, Berkeley, CA, 2007, NOLO.

Seibert PJ Jr: *The complete veterinary practice regulatory manual*, ed 6, Calhoun, TN, Philip J. Seibert, Jr.

US Department of Health and Human Services: *Biosafety in microbiological and biomedical laboratories*, ed 4, Washington, DC, 1999, US Government Printing Office.

Wilson JF: *Law and ethics of the veterinary profession*, Yardley, PA, 1993, Priority Press.

Wilson J, Lacroix C: *Legal consent forms for veterinary practices*, Lakewood, CO, 2001, AAHA Press.

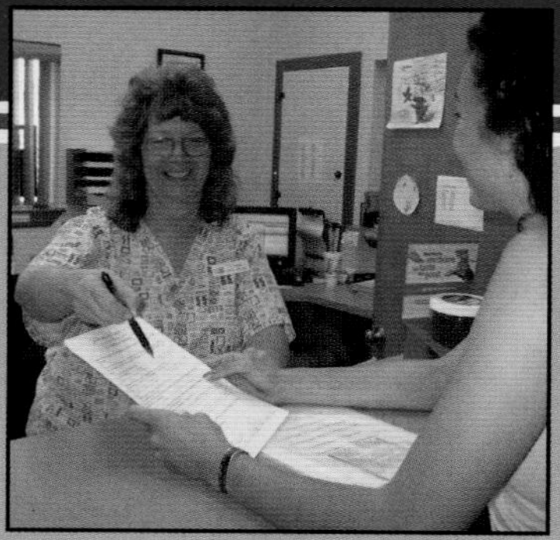

3 Practice Management

OUTLINE

LEARNING OBJECTIVES

After reviewing this chapter, the reader will be able to:

1. Identify common forms used in veterinary practice.
2. Describe the importance of informed consent.
3. Clarify admitting and discharge instructions.
4. Identify effective and professional discharge sheets.
5. Describe procedures used to collect outstanding accounts.
6. Define and educate clients regarding Pet Health Insurance.
7. Define AAHA guidelines and Accreditation Procedures.
8. Describe and comply with the Fair Labor and Standards Act
9. Identify a completed medical record.
10. Identify and use POMR and SOAP record formats.
11. Identify methods used to accurately and efficiently maintain inventory.
12. Calculate inventory markup and cost of services.
13. Identify areas of and decrease loss of inventory.
14. Record controlled substances in appropriate log books.
15. Develop a disaster and recovery plan for a practice.

KEY TERMS

American Animal Hospital Association
Controlled Substance Act of 1970
Controlled substances
Co-pay
Deductible
Direct marketing
Dispensing fee
Economic order quantity
External marketing
Fair Debt Collection Practices Act
Fair Labor Standards Act
Indemnity insurance
Indirect marketing
Informed consent
Internal marketing
Inventory turns per year
Markup
Minimum prescription fee
Outstanding accounts
Overtime
POMR
Premium
Reorder point
Shrinkage
SOAP
SOP

Managing a practice encompasses a variety of tasks. A manager oversees the production of the entire team and is often responsible for the practice's financial well-being. Managers must learn to delegate and empower team members in order to have an efficient, mature organization. Delegation and empowerment can lead to effective teamwork, employee retention, and satisfied employees. Satisfied team members increase client satisfaction, client retention, and client education.

Managing not only includes team member hiring, training, and discipline, it also involves the daily process of the practice. Clients must receive proper education, materials, and superior patient care. In order to provide these essentials, the practice must be able to operate efficiently and seamlessly. Equipment must be purchased, maintained, and replaced when needed. Team members must be trained how to properly operate equipment, which greatly extends the life of the capital.

Inventory must operate at a superior level. A manager must keep products in stock at the right level, preventing **shrinkage,** expiration, or shortage. Economic reorder quantities should be developed for each product, preventing the purchase of excess materials. Under- or overpurchasing of products can produce a tremendous loss for the practice.

Manufacturer and distributor representatives can provide a wealth of information for the entire team. Not only do they provide sales information and product promotion, they can provide the team with education. Most manufacturers have developed presentations to help enhance team member's knowledge of certain diseases. Heartworm disease, for example, should be fully understood by every team member, including the kennel assistants. Dinners and luncheons are often provided to team members during presentations regarding the science and mechanisms of such diseases and products, which ultimately increases client and team satisfaction.

Purchasing computers and software can be an intense project; however, it is very rewarding for the team when the appropriate materials have been selected. Computers and software can streamline the tasks of the employees, creating an efficient, well-organized team. Research should be completed to determine the wants and needs of the practice. Planning, organizing, and training can make the project a success.

> TECHNICIAN NOTE Investing in veterinary software provides one of the best returns on investment (ROI) in veterinary practice.

Practice managers must continue to stimulate the interests of the team, including their own. Challenging skills, continuing education, and certifications can improve every practice manager. The Veterinary Hospital Managers Association (VHMA) provides quality continuing education throughout the year and releases many studies that can enhance management quality. Practice managers can become a Certified Veterinary Practice Manager (CVPM) through VHMA once certain criteria have been met. A CVPM can add value to every practice.

FRONT OFFICE PROCEDURES

Many practices and policies come into play with the receptionist and technicians in the front office. Clients must receive a warm welcome and be able to comfortably approach team members (Fig. 3-1).

Clients should feel that they can ask questions, regardless of the topic. The reception team makes the first impression on every client, which often begins with the phone call. If clients feel they are rushed on the phone, they may feel that the practice does not have time for them. Team members should be able to turn each phone call into an appointment, while being able to schedule the appointment correctly and efficiently.

A client's experience starts with the first impression, and ends when the practice has followed up with the visit. A client may call a practice for the first time to make an appointment, establishing the first impression. The client may choose to make an appointment or call another practice based on the information received. If the client has made an appointment, the second impression begins when they enter the practice. They should be greeted by a warm, sincere individual who has a genuine concern for them and their pet. A negative impression may be developed if they are ignored, have to wait an excessive amount of time, or if the practice exhibits a dirty appearance. The next impression will be set with the technician and veterinary team. If laboratory samples were submitted, a follow-up call would be expected from the veterinarian. If the client has to call the practice to receive results, another negative impression may be made. A team member has the ability to make all of the above situations a positive experience for the client and should strive to do so for each and every client.

> TECHNICIAN NOTE Clients must be greeted and acknowledged when they enter the practice.

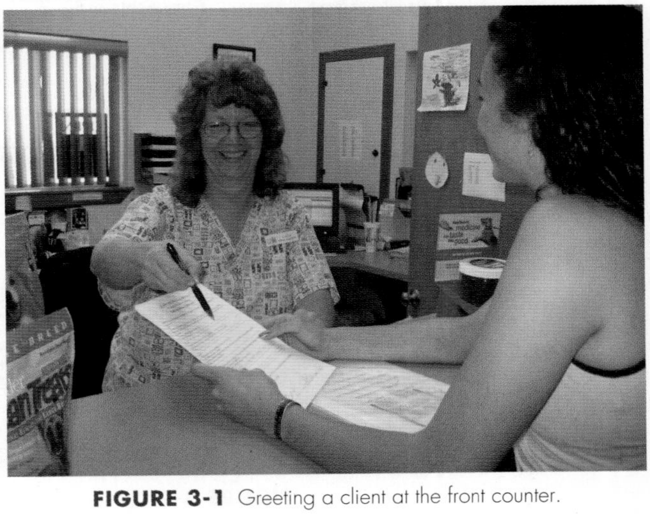

FIGURE 3-1 Greeting a client at the front counter.

Teamwork helps to facilitate positive experiences for clients and employees. Clients perceive a positive atmosphere in a practice when a team works together. Teams can be developed to work in harmony and efficiently. These teams satisfy client needs and wants with relative ease.

PHONE ETIQUETTE

Every telephone call must be handled as if it was the client's first call. The receptionist should answer the phone within three rings; if the receptionist team is busy, another member of the team should receive the phone call. A friendly, helpful tone of voice when answering relays a positive, friendly atmosphere. The receptionist should speak slowly and clearly, with the correct enunciation. Excellent verbal skills will facilitate client retention, education, and compliance.

If a client asks a question that the receptionist cannot answer, the client should be placed on hold, allowing the correct answer to be determined. If the answer will take time to receive, the client can be called back. Clients should never be told, "I don't know" or given an incorrect answer. The practice may lose a client if the information is not provided and can be held liable for incorrect information given over the phone.

Many times, clients call for advice over the phone and do not want to bring a pet in; unfortunately, in today's society any information can be misinterpreted. A pet's condition cannot be diagnosed over the phone, and team members cannot recommend treatments to clients without diagnosing a disease or condition. If a client is concerned enough to place a call to the practice, he or she should be advised to bring in the pet to be examined by the veterinarian. If the wrong treatment is advised to the client, the practice can be held liable. If a recommendation is given to the client, it must be documented in the medical record.

> **TECHNICIAN NOTE** Smiling while answering the phone relays a positive tone of voice to the client.

When clients call to ask questions regarding healthcare, the receptionist should always end the call by scheduling an appointment. Many clients may be price shopping for services. With correct client education, an appointment can be made.

SCHEDULING APPOINTMENTS

Many factors contribute to appointment scheduling. Many computer systems have a template that has already been created to accommodate the schedule the practice has deemed appropriate (Fig. 3-2). If paper schedules are used, appropriate lunch break and surgery schedules must be entered.

Appointment schedules should be developed to maximize production, while minimizing client wait time. A client wait time of 5 minutes can seem to be 15 minutes of wait time for a client. The client's time is just as valuable as the practice time and should be understood as such. If the appointment schedule is running behind, clients should be notified immediately. If enough time permits, clients can be called to notify of the delay; clients who have already arrived at the practice should be updated frequently.

The length of time of appointments should depend on the reason for the appointment. An orthopedic appointment (e.g., limping dog) will likely take longer for the examination and radiographs than a yearly examination with vacci-

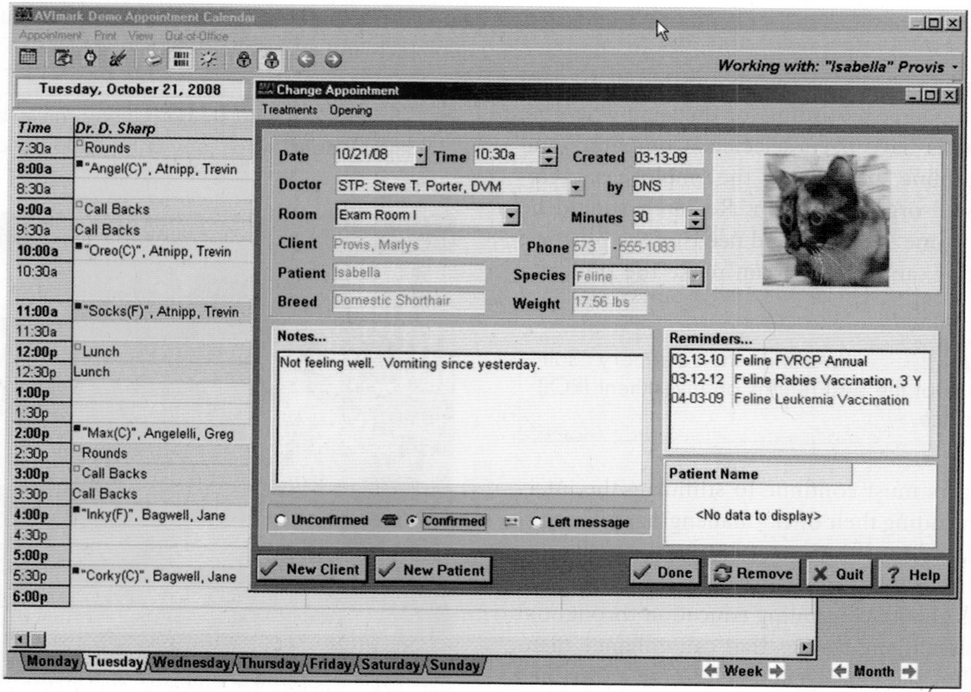

FIGURE 3-2 Computer screen shot; Avimark appointment scheduler.

nations. A senior wellness exam may take more time than a standard regular examination because recommendations for laboratory diagnostics may be made. The practice should develop acceptable time frames for the most common conditions seen in the exam room.

> **TECHNICIAN NOTE** Veterinary Technician appointments can be made for nail trims, anal gland expressions, laboratory diagnostics, and client education.

Appointments for client education, nail trims, and anal gland expressions can be made with veterinary technicians, allowing the veterinarian(s) to see cases that need to be diagnosed. Technicians are an essential tool, allowing the appointment schedule to run on time. The experience and education that credentialed technicians possess is an asset to every practice and maximum utilization of skills enhances practice efficiency.

Many items are needed when an appointment is made for a client. If a paper schedule is used, more information will need to be requested. Computer appointment schedulers will automatically populate the information for current clients. The client's first and last name, pet's name, and the reason for the appointment will be required for both systems. The computer will populate the species, age, and client phone number. Client phone numbers should be verified, allowing the practice to call in case of emergency or a change in the schedule.

All appointments and surgeries should be called and reminded of their appointment one day prior. This allows the team members to remind clients of special instructions, such as no food or water, before surgery. Many practices will recommend that clients bring a fresh fecal or urine sample, and team members can kindly remind clients of this service.

If a recheck, follow-up appointment, or booster vaccination is required, the appointment should be made for the clients before they leave the practice. Clients will return for appointments that have been made, but less frequently return calls to make appointments. If a practice has a high number of clients who wish to call back to make an appointment, then teams may want to keep a running list and call those clients who have not done so or returned for their follow-up examination. A reminder and recall system can also be used with computer software systems that will print reports of noncompliant clients.

> **TECHNICIAN NOTE** Follow-up appointments should be scheduled for clients before they leave the practice.

Many times appointment slots fill up and clients are unable to obtain the appointment that they desire. In order to fulfill clients' expectations, they may be asked to drop off their pets. This allows the patient to be worked in between existing appointments. If additional diagnostics are required, the client can be called, given an estimate, and asked to approve additional testing. When the pet is ready, the owners can be called, and the case can be discussed on the phone or once they arrive. Dropping off patients allows clients to have their pet seen, preventing the frustration of waiting an excess amount of time or delaying the appointment schedule. Technicians must ensure that an accurate history is obtained before the client leaves, as well as an authorization of any treatments or anesthesia that may be required.

GREETING CLIENTS

Clients must always be acknowledged when they arrive to the practice. A client greeter is an excellent resource and one who can help clients with their pets. Not all practices can have the luxury of a client greeter; therefore the receptionist team must greet the clients as they enter. If a receptionist is on the phone, a wave and a smile lets the client know they have been recognized and that a team member will help them shortly. This also applies to team members who are assisting other clients; a quick greeting notifies clients that they have been recognized, without interrupting the initial client.

CLEANLINESS

The receptionist team is responsible for maintaining the reception area. The team should either notify another team member of a soiled reception area or clean the area immediately. Bowel movements, urination, and anal gland odors quickly spread, which can damage a client's first impression of the facility. Hair and dirt should also be swept up immediately. Sweeping and mopping of the reception floor should occur more than once a day, as odors will penetrate the walls and disseminate though the practice rapidly.

Products, shelves, and pictures must be dusted regularly, along with ceiling fan blades, blinds, and window sills. Walls should be washed on a regular basis and chairs cleaned each night. Team members should take a few minutes out of each day to sit in the reception and exam room chairs and look around the room; dirty objects, walls, and items that need to be cleaned can be easily identified.

COMMONLY USED FORMS

Clients will be asked to fill out forms when they arrive at the practice for the first visit. A client form requesting the name, contact information, and driver's license number should be filled out and signed by the client. Most forms include a statement indicating that the client is financially responsible for the patient and understands that all services must be paid for once they are rendered (Fig. 3-3). The receptionist must make sure this form is completed; the phone number is important, allowing client communication, as is the driver's license number in case the client must be turned over to a collections agency for nonpayment of services.

> **TECHNICIAN NOTE** Contact information and driver's license numbers are essential pieces of information on client/patient forms.

ABC Animal Clinic
555 Uptown Circle
Anytown, MN 89000
314-134-4431

Please print clearly

Date: ________

Name ________

Mailing Address ________ Zip Code ________

Street Address ________ Zip Code ________

Home Phone ________ Work Phone ________

Drivers License # ________ State ________

Animals:

Name	Date of Birth	Species	Breed	Color	Gender	Spayed or Neutered?

I understand that payment is required in full on the same date that services are rendered.

____
Signature

FIGURE 3-3 Client and patient form.

Arroyo Vista Animal Clinic
2303 Inspiration Lane

Owners Name ________ Spouse ________

Address ________

Home Telephone ________ Work telephone ________

Employers Name and Address ________

Spouses Employer and Address ________

Best time to call regarding your pet ________ Phone Number ________

In case of emergency, please call ________

WRITTEN ESTIMATES ARE AVAILABLE UPON REQUEST. Please ask the receptionist if an estimate is needed. **ALL FEES ARE DUE AT THE TIME SERVICES ARE RENDERED.** If you plan to pay with check or credit card, please complete the following:

MC Visa Exp Date ________

Drivers License Number ________ State ____ Expires ________

How did you hear of Arroyo Vista Animal Clinic?

Yellow Pages ________ Referral (Name) ________ Other ________

Number and Type of Pets in your household? ________

Pets Origin: Humane Society Pet Shop Kennel Breeder Friend Stray Other

Please see back of sheet for more information

	Pet #1	Pet #2	Pet #3
Name			
Species (Dog, Cat)			
Breed			
Color			
Age			
Date of Birth			
Sex			
Length of time owned			
Spayed or Neutered			
Vitamins? (type)			
Diet (Kind of Food)			
Type of Grooming Products			
Inside or Outside?			
Last Rabies vaccine?			
Last DHLP vaccine? (Dog)			
Last Parvo vaccine? (Dog)			
Last FVRCP vaccine? (Cat)			
Last FeLV vaccine? (Cat)			
Last Leukemia test? (Cat)			
Last Heartworm Test? (dog)			
Heartworm Prevention?			
Last Fecal Exam?			
Last Dental?			
Prior Illness?			
Prior Surgery?			

FIGURE 3-4 Patient history form.

Patient history forms are critical for new patients. Each new patient form should include the name of the client, the patient's name, age, breed, gender, if the pet has been altered, and a medical history, including current medications that the pet is receiving. Clients may become frustrated completing forms; however, a complete history is imperative for quality medicine (Fig. 3-4).

Practices that are not paperless will use paper records that are generally kept in an 8 ½ × 11 file folder with patient separators. Each client has a file folder, and patients are separated with index cards or colored paper (see Medical Records section below). Each patient medical record must include the client's name, contact information, and patient information, including the pet's name, species, breed, gender, and age (Figs. 3-5 and 3-6). Each entry should be dated and initialed by the author making the entry.

Clients must sign release forms for any treatment or procedure that is authorized. Anesthesia consent forms, treatment forms, and euthanasia forms are a few examples of forms clients must sign. A signed **informed consent** form (Fig. 3-7) is defined as a form signed by the client after all information regarding the procedure has been provided and the client has had the opportunity to ask questions. Information that must be documented for clients includes any risks of the procedure (including death, if that is a risk); the potential outcomes of the procedure; and any alternative procedures that are available, along with an estimate of the costs associated with those

Patient Medical Record

Client Name__________ Telephone Number__________

Address__________ Client Number __________

Pet Name__________ Breed __________ Color __________

Sex_____ Altered _____ DOB _____ Age_____ Species __________

Date		Charges

FIGURE 3-5 Medical record.

Arroyo Vista Animal Clinic

2303 Inspiration Lane

Owners Name__________ Patients Name__________

Breed______ Color______ Sex______ Species______

Date	SOAP	

FIGURE 3-6 SOAP format medical record.

ABC Veterinary Clinic

Surgery, Anesthesia and Treatment Consent Form

Client Name__________ Patient Name__________

Date______ Procedure__________ Male / Female

Your pet has been scheduled for a procedure requiring sedation or anesthesia. By signing this form, you authorize ABC Veterinary Clinic and its agents to administer tranquilizers, anesthetics and analgesia medication that are deemed appropriate. Please be aware that all drugs have a potential for adverse side effects in any particular animal. The chances of such occurrence are extremely small; however, death can result in any anesthetized patient.

Owner Initials______ Tech Initials______

In an effort to insure your pets safety and to anticipate any problems before they occur, we advise pre-anesthetic blood work and electrocardiogram prior to anesthesia. Blood work will determine the kidney and liver functions, which participate in the metabolism of anesthesia. An electrocardiogram can detect abnormal arrhythmias, heart rate and conductivity.

I Accept/Decline blood work I Accept/Decline an electrocardiogram

Owner Initials______ Tech Initials______

IV Fluids are advised for all patients undergoing anesthesia. IV Fluids help maintain blood pressure of the patient, while offering support for the kidney's to metabolize the medications. Pets may take longer to recover without IV Fluids.

I Accept/Decline IV Fluids

Owner Initials______ Tech Initials______

Heartworm tests are recommended for our canine companions over 6 months of age. Heartworm disease can cause anesthetic complications. We advise FeLV/FIV test for our feline companions. FeLV or FIV infection can delay healing of any surgical site.

I Accept/Decline Heartworm Test I Accept/Decline FeLV/FIV Test

Owner Initials______ Tech Initials______

Vaccinations are important for disease prevention in your pet. We advise that pets be current on vaccines. Rabies is required by law; every pet must have a rabies vaccine.

Vaccines due: DHPP FVRCP FeLV Rabies

Owner Initials______ Tech Initials______

Booster?

Did pet eat this morning?	Yes	No
Has pet had any allergies or vaccine reactions in the past?	Yes	No
Are we declawing the pet?	Yes	No
Are we removing dewclaws?	Yes	No
Does the pet have 2 testicles?	Yes	No
If the pet is pregnant can we continue with surgery?	Yes	No
Does the pet have an umbilical hernia?	Yes	No
May we repair?	Yes	No
Does the pet have retained teeth?	Yes	No
May we remove?	Yes	No
Does the pet need an e-collar?	Yes	No
Dentals: OK to extract teeth?	Yes	No
OK to take Dental Radiographs if indicated?	Yes	No
OK to apply Doxirobe if indicated?	Yes	No
Is pet currently on antibiotics?	Yes	No
When was last dose?__________		
How many pills are left?__________		
Growth Removal: Histopath?	Yes	No
Location of growths:		

You may contact me TODAY at:__________

Alternative contact phone number: __________

I understand that anesthesia is a risk and authorize the above procedures. I understand that I will be contacted first if any changes in our discussed protocol occur.

Client Signature__________

FIGURE 3-7 Informed consent form.

procedures. Once the client has been informed of all of the above, the client can sign the form. Blanket consent (Fig. 3-8) forms are defined as a consent form that authorizes any procedure, yet does not include the risks, benefits, outcomes, or estimates. Blanket consent forms are not recommended in practice, but are often the sole source of consent forms used. All consent forms must state the client's name, patient's name, name of the procedure, and date.

TECHNICIAN NOTE Blanket consent forms should be replaced with informed consent forms.

ABC Veterinary Clinic

Surgery/Anesthesia Consent Form

Client Name ________________ Date ________________

Pet's Name ________________

Your pet has been scheduled for a procedure requiring sedation or anesthesia. By signing this form, you authorize ABC Veterinary Clinic and it's agents to administer tranquilizers, anesthetics and/or analgesics that are deemed appropriate for your pet. Please be aware that all drugs have the potential for adverse side affects in any particular animal. The chances of such occurrence are extremely small.

I am aware that staff is not on premises after hours, and I agree to indemnify ABC Veterinary Clinic and its agents harmless from and against any and all liability arising from the care that is provided.

In an effort to insure your pet's safety, and to anticipate any problems before they may occur, we have available pre-anesthetic electrocardiogram and blood testing capabilities to detect hidden heart, liver, kidney or other problems which may increase the risk to your pet. The testing is available for an additional charge. If abnormalities are detected, we will attempt to notify you, and the anesthetic procedure may be delayed or modified. Please verify the procedures being performed and indicate your wishes concerning the option of pre-anesthetic testing. If you have any questions, please ask BEFORE signing this form.

Procedures scheduled: ________________

Routine surgical procedures are painful. We recommend post operative pain medication for each procedure. Pain medication is automatically dispensed for each patient. If YOU DECLINE POST OPERATIVE PAIN MEDICATION, PLEASE SIGN HERE

____

How may we contact you TODAY?

Home phone ________________ Work phone ________________

Cell phone/pager ________________ Client signature ________________

FIGURE 3-8 Blanket consent form.

Just as with other consent forms, euthanasia forms must be signed by the owner of the patient. The consent form must state that the pet's death will result. If a necropsy is granted by the pet's owner, the consent form may include the appropriate information, as well as the request for the disposal of the body (Fig. 3-9).

Rabies certificates are most often computer generated (Fig. 3-10); however, those without computer systems must manually complete the certificates (Fig. 3-11). Rabies certificates include the client's name, contact information, patient's name, species, breed, gender, and age. The vaccination information, including the manufacturer of the vaccine, vaccination expiration date, lot number, and tag number are also included. The veterinarian administering the vaccination must sign the certificate. Often a stamp is used in place of the original signature.

Health certificates are issued by the state and the US Department of Agriculture (USDA). Small animals flying within the United States may require an Interstate Health Certificate, whereas those traveling outside the United States will be required to have an International Health Certificate. Different countries have different requirements for animal importation, and each country should be researched for their rules and regulations. Most current regulations can be found on the USDA's website. Large animals (horses and cattle) may be required to have transportation papers, depending on each state's livestock regulations. Horses are required to have a current negative status for Coggins disease (equine infectious anemia) to travel between states.

INVOICING CLIENTS

Invoicing clients can become a difficult situation for clients who cannot afford the medical care that is recommended. Estimates should always be given to clients (whether on the phone or in the hospital) for every procedure. This prevents clients from becoming surprised at the time of collection and prevents clients from arguing the total cost, while informing them that the total amount will be due at the time the service is rendered.

TECHNICIAN NOTE Every client should receive an estimate for procedures, and sign a copy for the medical record.

Euthanasia Release

I, the undersigned, do hereby certify that I am the owner of the animal, and hereby give ABC Veterinary Clinic full and complete authority to euthanize the animal in whatever manner the doctor shall deem fit. I hereby release the doctors and staff from any and all liabilities for euthanizing said animal. I understand that euthanasia results in death.

I do also certify that the said animal has not bitten any person or animal during the last 15 days and to the best of my knowledge has not been exposed to Rabies.

Date ________________ Signature of owner ________________

FIGURE 3-9 Euthanasia form.

RABIES VACCINATION CERTIFICATE *NASPHV FORM 51 (Revised 2007)*					RABIES TAG NUMBER 2590
Owner's Name & Address	Print Clearly				MICROCHIP NUMBER 4944047932
LAST Montoya	FIRST Teresa		M.I.		TELEPHONE (575)526-7170
NO STREET 4364 Lost Lane		CITY Las Cruces	STATE NM		ZIP 88007
SPECIES Dog ☒ Cat ☐ Other ☐ (Specify)	SEX Male ☒ Female ☐ Neuter ☒	AGE 6 Months ☐ Years ☒	SIZE Under 20 lbs ☐ 20 - 50 lbs ☐ Over 50 lbs ☒	PREDOMINANT BREED Labrador Ret Mix; NAME Blue	PREDOMINANT COLORS/MARKINGS Yellow
	Animal Control License ☐ 1 Yr ☐ 3 Yr ☐ Other____				
DATE VACCINATED 10/24/2008	PRODUCT NAME			Veterinarian: Frances S. Bowling License No:	
NEXT VACCINATION DUE BY: 10/24/2011	MANUFACTURER (First 3 Letters) P F I; ☐ 1 yr USDA Licensed Vaccine; ☒ 3 yr USDA Licensed Vaccine; ☐ 4 yr USDA Licensed Vaccine; ☐ Initial dose ☐ Booster dose; Vacc. Serial (Lot) No.			Veterinarian's Signature; Address Jomada Veterinary Clinic 2399 Saturn Circle Las Cruces, NM 88012	

FIGURE 3-10 Rabies certificate, computer generated.

OWNER'S COPY **RABIES VACCINATION CERTIFICATE** *NASPHV Form #51*					Rabies Tag Number
Owner's Name and Address	**Print - use ball point pen or type**				
PRINT - Last		First	M.I.		Telephone
No. Street		City	State		Zip
Species: Dog ☐ Cat ☐ Other: ☐ (Specify)	Sex: Male ☐ Female ☐ Neutered ☐	Age: 3 mo to 12 mo ☐ 12 mo or older ☐ Actual Age____	Size: Under 20 lbs. ☐ 20 - 50 lbs. ☐ Over 50 lbs. ☐ Actual____lbs.	Predominant Breed: ____ Name:	Colors:
DATE VACCINATED: ____ Month Day Year; VACCINATION EXPIRED: ____ Month Day Year	Producer: (First 3 letters); ☐ 1 yr. Lic./Vacc.; ☐ 3 yr. Lic./Vacc.; ____ Other; Vacc. Serial (lot) no.			Veterinarian's: # ____ (License No.); (Signature); Address:	

FIGURE 3-11 Rabies certificate, hand written.

Invoices should be detailed for clients. A client will not perceive the value of the service if a total amount is presented to them without explanation. For example, many clients perceive that a DHLPP injection has only one component because it is only one injection. Invoices should list all five vaccine components of the injection (distemper, hepatitis, leptospirosis, parainfluenza, parvovirus), allowing the client to comprehend the value of such an injection. Once the receptionist can detail the entire invoice for the client, the client will understand the total value of the visit.

Because of the number of **outstanding accounts** in veterinary medicine, extending credit to clients should no longer be allowed. Accounts receivable totals should never exceed 2% to 3% of the total gross revenue amount (Box 3-1). Many veterinarians want to be able to extend the offer of credit to clients. Unfortunately, a majority of clients do not extend the courtesy of repayment to the veterinarian.

Payments made on an account can be made with a variety of methods. Most practices accept cash, checks, and credit cards. Credit cards may include Visa, MasterCard, Discover, or American Express. The credit cards that practices wish to

BOX 3-1 Example of 2% of Gross Revenue

Gross revenue for the fiscal year 2008 = $998,945.98
$998,945.98 x 2% = $19,978.92
Accounts receivable should never exceed $19,978.92 for this practice.

accept are up to the practice. Businesses must pay a percentage of the total month's charges of each credit card accepted to the credit card agency. This is considered a hidden overhead expense that the practice must recover.

TECHNICIAN NOTE All credit card and check transactions should be verified with a driver's license or picture ID.

Team members must verify client identification when they accept either credit cards or checks. Fraud is increasing across the United States, and it is up to the practice to prevent it. Many times driver's license numbers must be written on checks in order to be accepted. This allows district attorney's offices to prosecute hot check writers if needed. If a check verification process is used, a driver's license number must match the checking account information, or the check may be declined.

Credit card machines and check verification systems are an excellent asset to veterinary medicine. They are easy to use and help prevent fraud and hot checks. Both systems use electronic funds transfer (EFT), in which the total amount is deducted from the client's account at the time of the service. The amount is then deposited into the practice's account.

Care Credit is a type of third party payment system used exclusively for medical expenses. Clients must fill out an application in the practice and team members must verify identification before application acceptance. Once the application is complete, a team member can either call in the application or enter the information online. Credit decisions are generally received within 15 minutes of submission.

Monthly Statements

For the few accounts that are allowed to charge, monthly statements must be sent. Monthly statements should include a statement charge, which covers the time required for the team to print and send statements. A minimum of five dollars should be charged (Fig. 3-12). Many practices may also institute a finance charge, which charges the client a percentage of the total amount due. Regulations vary regarding finance fees; therefore regulations must be confirmed before the institution of such fees. Notice of such fees must also be clearly posted for clients to see, as well as notifying them in the statement.

Outstanding Debt Collection

Accounts that are allowed to age to 30, 60, or 90 days post service can become difficult to collect. The longer the invoice ages, the less likely the invoice will be collected. Team members must be diligent when trying to collect accounts and must be most active in the early age process (less than 45 days). Those responsible for collecting accounts should become familiar with the **Fair Debt Collection Practices Act,** which prevents unruly methods when trying to collect accounts. Phone calls cannot be made before 8 AM or after 9 PM in the evening, and the account balance cannot be discussed with any person other than the individual themselves (Box 3-2).

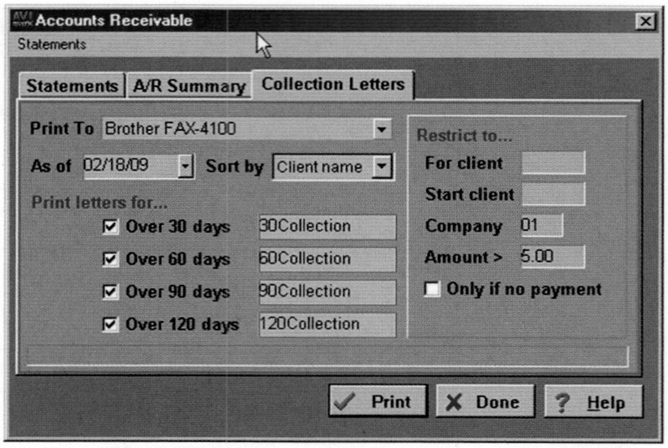

FIGURE 3-12 Avimark collections screen shot.

BOX 3-2 Fair Debt Rules

- Debtors cannot be subjected to harassment, oppressive tactics, or abusive treatment.
- The law prohibits the collector from making any false statements to the client, such as claiming to be a lawyer or government agency.
- Clients may not be called at work if the employer or client objects, or be called at inconvenient times or places, such as before 8 AM and after 9 PM.
- Delinquent payments can only be discussed with the client themselves.

Accounts that cannot be collected by team members must be turned over to a collections agency. These agents are occasionally able to collect accounts that team members have not had success with, because clients do not want their credit scores negatively affected. A report to collections agencies can remain on a client's credit report for 7 years; therefore they are willing to pay the debt. The sooner the overdue amount is turned in to a collections agent, the easier they can collect the account. Many times client addresses and phone numbers change; however, if a collections agency has the driver's license number of the client, an infraction can be reported to the credit bureau. This is why it is critical to have a driver's license number on the client/patient information form.

THE OFFICE VISIT

The office visit for a client begins when they enter the practice. After clients have been greeted by the receptionist team, they are generally placed in an exam room. Usually an

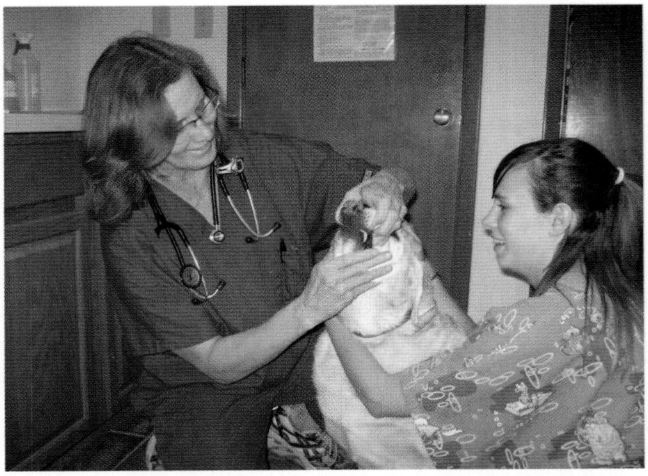

FIGURE 3-13 Veterinarian examining a patient.

BOX 3-3 Education Topics for Puppies, Kittens, Adults, and Seniors

- Vaccine schedule
- Vaccination reactions
- Intestinal parasites
- Nutrition
- Dental disease prevention
- Heartworm prevention
- Flea and tick diseases and prevention
- Spay or neuter procedure
- Obesity prevention or management
- Dental disease
- The aging process and laboratory diagnostics

assistant or technician will take a medical history of the patient. A medical history includes a weight and the vital signs of each patient. Vital signs include a temperature, pulse, and heart and respiratory rate. If any laboratory samples will be needed, a technician may confirm the proper sampling technique, equipment, or products needed and ask the veterinarian for authorization to obtain the samples.

The office visit is the perfect time for technicians to educate clients. Puppy and kitten owners should be informed of vaccination schedules, heartworm and intestinal worm prevention, flea and tick disease and prevention, dental disease, and nutrition (Fig. 3-13). Because vaccine boosters must be given, topics can be spread over several visits. The goal of each visit is not to overwhelm the client with too much information, but provide enough that they perceive the value of their money spent.

Clients with adult patients arriving for yearly exams must be reminded of heartworm disease and prevention, flea and tick preventative, nutrition guidance, and dental disease prevention. Clients look to the veterinary team for guidance and education, and the team must take the time to educate the clients throughout each visit. Box 3-3 provides client education topics that can be covered during office visits. Additional information on the office visit and obtaining the medical history and physical examination is located in Chapter 22.

ADMITTING PATIENTS

If patients will need to be admitted to the hospital for treatment, team members should follow a protocol that helps develop consistency for clients and patients. As previously discussed, a treatment consent form must be given to the owner to sign. The client must be informed of risks, prognosis, and alternative treatments that are available. An estimate should also be provided for the client, highlighting all possible treatments, procedures, medications, or services that are recommended for the owner. Once the client has been informed, she or he can sign the consent form and estimate, indicating the services that the client authorizes.

If a patient is being admitted for boarding, a separate form should be available for clients to complete (Fig. 3-14). Forms should include emergency and alternative contact information, as well as any pertinent information regarding the pet. This information should include current diet, the amount fed per feeding, when the pet is fed, what medications the pet receives, and at what time those medications are administered. If a blanket, toy, collars, or leashes are left, a clear description should be indicated on the admitting sheet.

Clients may also be asked if they would prefer any additional services or treatments to be performed on their pet while in the boarding facility. Often dental prophylaxis, bathing, dipping, or grooming are services clients elect for their pets.

DISCHARGING PATIENTS

Patients that are discharged from the hospital must be released with written instructions (Fig. 3-15). Verbal instructions are not acceptable. Many times clients are given too much information when they arrive to pick up their pets, and they forget a majority of the information. Distractions, such as other pets, clients, and team members, prevent clients from paying attention to the release information; therefore discharge instructions may not be followed.

Invoices and discharge instructions should be detailed with clients before receiving their pet. Please refer to the section below regarding collection and payment. Once a pet has been brought to the owner, the owner is more interested in the pet than the release instructions.

TECHNICIAN NOTE Written discharge instructions should be sent home with every patient.

Discharge instructions must include any recommended restrictions for food, activity, or therapy, and should indicate when to start medication. Doses and instructions for medications should also be included. If a pet has been diagnosed with a particular disease or condition, the client should also be given written materials regarding the diagnosis. The more information that is given to clients, the more satisfied they will be following the recommendations of the team.

Arroyo Vista Animal Clinic
2303 Inspiration Lane, Anywhere, USA
Dr. Larsen, Dr. Cooke and Dr. Thompson
Boarding Admission Form

Owner__________ Date__________
Address__________ Phone__________
City__________ In case of Emergency, please call__________

Pets Name__________ Breed__________ Sex______ Age______ Color______
Date of last vaccine:__________ Please circle which vaccine: DHPP FVRCP FeLV
Date of last Rabies__________ Date of last Bordetella__________
Medications while boarding__________
Belongings__________

Pets Name__________ Breed__________ Sex______ Age______ Color______
Date of last vaccine:__________ Please circle which vaccine: DHPP FVRCP FeLV
Date of last Rabies__________ Date of last Bordetella__________
Medications while boarding__________
Belongings__________

Pets Name__________ Breed__________ Sex______ Age______ Color______
Date of last vaccine:__________ Please circle which vaccine: DHPP FVRCP FeLV
Date of last Rabies__________ Date of last Bordetella__________
Medications while boarding__________
Belongings__________

While boarding, please perform the following procedures:

Physical Exam ______ Vaccinations __________

Heartworm Test ______ Bath ______ Dip ______ Nail Trim______

Other: 1: __________

2: __________

3: __________

4: __________

All animals entering the hospital must be up to date on vaccination and free of external parasites (fleas, ticks) or they will be treated upon admission at the owners' expense.

I authorize Arroyo Vista Animal Clinic to treat my pet(s) in case an emergency situation should arise.

Pets are released only during the regular office hours. It is my responsibility to inform the hospital if I will be delayed in picking up my pets; I will assume all costs associated with an extended stay.

Owner's signature__________ Date__________

FIGURE 3-14 Boarding form.

ABC Veterinary Clinic
123-456-7890
Dr. Roe, Dr. Morton, Dr. Larsen
Post Anesthesia release sheet

Please provide clean, dry bedding and a quiet place for your pet to recuperate. Please notify the hospital with any concerns
DIET:
( ) Wait a few hours after arriving home to offer your pet water. Please give only a small amount. If no vomiting occurs, you may offer more water about an hour later. You may feed a small amount (1/4 normal amount) if water stays down.
( ) You may continue to feed your pet normally.
( ) Special diet instructions __________
ACTIVITY:
( ) Restrict exercise for 1 day. NO RUNNING, JUMPING, CLIMBING OR BATHING.
( ) Restrict exercise for 7 days. NO RUNNING, JUMPING, CLIMBING OR BATHING.
( ) Other __________
OTHER:
( ) Please use paper strips or pinto beans in place of litter for 7 days
( ) Please booster vaccines in 3-4 weeks
( ) Your pets metabolism may permanently decrease after surgery. You may need to decrease the amount of food you feed in order to prevent obesity.
INCISION:
( ) Watch for swelling, redness or drainage. Prevent scratching, rubbing and licking of the incision. Please ask for an E-collar if you think your pet will lick the site.
( ) Ice incision for 5 minutes, 3 to 4 times daily for the first 72 hours.
MEDICATION:
( ) Give pain medication __________
( ) Give antibiotics__________
( ) Give other medication __________
( ) Start medication __________
FOLLOW UP VISITS:
( ) Recheck in ______ days.
( ) There is no need to return for suture removal; the skin was closed with absorbable suture or tissue adhesive.
( ) Not necessary unless you feel there is a problem
Comments:

Doctor__________ Tech______ Client______ Date______

FIGURE 3-15 Discharge instructions.

BOX 3-4 Guidelines for Developing Client Handouts

- Use professional appearance.
- Name, address, phone number, and doctors of the practice should be on the handout.
- Use clear and concise terms that clients can understand.
- Pictures should be used to help the client visualize.
- All client handouts should be typed, not handwritten.

Many computer programs include client education handouts. When selected, they will print the owner's name, patient's name, and doctor on each handout. If a computer handout is not available, a practice manager may create a client handout of the most common diseases and conditions. Literature must appear professional, be mistake free, and be written in a client-oriented manner. Clients must be able to understand the information presented to them; therefore copies of information from veterinary books are often too advanced and can overwhelm the client. Box 3-4 provides guidelines for developing client handouts.

PET HEALTH INSURANCE

Pet health insurance has been available for over 20 years, but has not been a popular choice among owners until recently. Insurance is a method by which pet owners can manage the risks of expensive health care. Accidents and diseases are an unexpected cost for owners, and insurance allows them to provide the best treatment available. Many pet owners are forced to make treatment decisions based on cost alone. Insurance allows owners the financial resource they may need to provide lifesaving treatments they would otherwise not consider.

The National Commission on Veterinary Economic Issues (NCVEI) was a coalition of veterinary associations that analyzed specific business and economic aspects of the veterinary industry. In 1999, NCVEI released a study that indicated that the increased use of veterinary pet health insurance could increase the demand for service, therefore decreasing the euthanasia rate in the United States. Studies indicate that pet owners look to their veterinarians for education regarding pet health and insurance for their pets. It is imperative that the entire staff understand the concept of pet insurance and offer it to all clients.

Clients should be made aware of the various companies that offer pet health insurance. Plans and companies vary in different regions; therefore each policy should be reviewed carefully. Terms that should be considered include whether hereditary conditions are covered and if benefit schedules or exclusions are listed in the policy. Some benefit schedules only cover a small percentage of what would be considered a reasonable expense for a condition. Some companies may not use a benefit schedule and set payout limits instead, regardless of illness or condition. Most pet insurance companies set high dollar amounts "for reasonable expenses"; they do not want to set prices for veterinary practices, nor do they want to dissuade owners from purchasing packages.

Indemnity insurance offers compensation for treatment of injured and sick pets. Owners purchase a policy directly from a pet health insurance company and are eligible for compensation based on the care provided and policy terms. Policies are available for comprehensive illness, standard care, and accident coverage and may cover species ranging from dogs and cats to exotics and birds.

A **premium** is defined as the amount an owner pays monthly or annually to maintain an insurance policy for a pet. Premium amounts are affected by a number of factors, including the deductible, co-pay, and per-incident, annual, or lifetime limit payout. The species and breed of the animal also affects the cost of the premium, as well as if the pet is spayed or neutered, the age of the pet, and the geographical location of the owner in the United States.

> *TECHNICIAN NOTE* Pet health insurance can increase client compliance and retention.

A **deductible** is the amount an owner must pay before the insurance company will offer compensation. Insurance companies vary, and offer either a per-incident deductible or annual deductible. Per incident deductibles refer to the owner paying the chosen deductible amount each time an incident occurs with the pet. An annual deductible refers to an owner paying the chosen deductible one time annually. Once the annual deductible amount has been met, the owner does not have to pay a deductible until the following year. A **co-pay** is the percentage that the owner is responsible for after the deductible has been met. Lower co-pays increase the amount of the premium and generally range from 10% to 20%.

Some insurance companies offer clients a choice of an annual policy or per-incident limit; others offer one or the other. "Annual limits" refers to the maximum amount that the insurance company will pay for a condition or illness during the policy term. "Per-incident limits" refers to the maximum amount an insurance company will pay each time a new problem or disease occurs. "Lifetime limits" refers to the maximum amount an insurance company will pay during the pet's life.

A preexisting health condition is defined as any accident or illness contracted, manifested, or incurred before the policy effective date. The pet may be enrolled; however, any preexisting condition will be excluded from coverage. It is highly recommended to enroll puppies and kittens before any conditions arise.

Purebred pets that are known to have congenital and hereditary conditions may also be excluded from an insurance plan based on company policy. A congenital condition is generally referred to as an abnormality present at birth, whether apparent or not, that can cause illness or disease. A hereditary condition is an abnormality that is transmitted by genes from the parent to the offspring, whether apparent or not, that can cause disease or illness. Some companies may also argue that some congenital defects are hereditary, therefore excluding coverage of the condition. A portosystemic shunt may be an example of such a condition. Policies must be reviewed carefully for such exemptions.

Many companies have a list of exclusions—diseases, conditions, or treatments that are excluded from policies. Many times behavior counseling and medications are not covered, along with compounded medications, nutraceuticals, or diets. Exclusions should be carefully reviewed before choosing a policy.

AAHA AND ACCREDITATION

The **American Animal Hospital Association (AAHA)** strives to set standards for veterinary medicine and is the only organization that accredits veterinary hospitals in North America. Practices that wish to meet the requirements of accreditation are tested to meet more than 900 quality standards that encompass all aspects of animal care, ranging from patient care and pain management to team training and medical record keeping. The AAHA standards are continuously updated to keep accredited practices at the forefront of veterinary medicine and advanced business practices.

> *TECHNICIAN NOTE* AAHA is the only organization that accredits veterinary hospitals in North America.

Approximately 3500 veterinary clinics hold AAHA accreditation designation. AAHA accreditation ensures that a veterinary practice is operating at the highest standards of excellence in animal care. AAHA emphasizes a team approach to veterinary health care and offers resources for the entire staff (Box 3-5).

The process to become AAHA accredited can take approximately one year to accomplish. First, a hospital must become a nonaccredited AAHA member, whereby a practice consultant is assigned to the practice along with an accreditation coordinator. The practice consultant will walk through the practice and determine policies, procedures, and tasks that must be completed in order to pass the 900 standards that have been defined. Once the practice feels they are ready for accreditation, a 4- to 5-hour inspection will occur. Patient admitting, discharge, and hospitalization procedures will be reviewed by the practice consultant. Should the practice not satisfactorily complete all 900 tasks, then the consultant will review changes that need to be made, provide resources to make those changes, and set a date in the future for follow up. Once the practice has met the standards, the accreditation designation will be granted (Fig. 3-16).

For those that become accredited, the AAHA offers staff training programs and continuing education, client newsletters, practice consultants, and the use of the AAHA-accredited logo. Practice consultants follow up with practices on a regular basis and help review policies and procedures, ensuring the practice is providing high-quality medicine and outstanding customer service.

BOX 3-5 Reasons to Become AAHA Accredited

- Increases safety of team members and clients
- Improves communication of team members and clients
- Promotes team building
- Provides practice consultants for each practice, year round
- Challenges everyone to raise the bar in veterinary medicine
- Increases team members' effectiveness
- Provides benchmarks

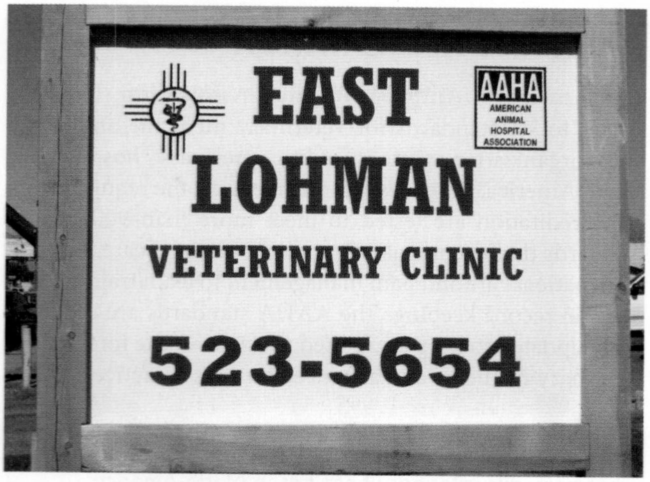

FIGURE 3-16 AAHA practice and logo.

PRACTICE OPERATIONS

Efficiency and organization is the key to a successful practice. Team members must enjoy their job and remain satisfied in order to decrease employee turnover rate. The best team should be hired and trained in order to help promote the practice's missions and goals. All team members should share the same philosophy, enjoy educating owners, and put forth their best effort at all times. When all facets are met, veterinary healthcare is a very rewarding career.

Leading a team is essential to the success of the practice. One does not want to micromanage, because this can inhibit the independence of team members. Rather, delegating and empowering allows teams to use their skills, working together to problem-solve tasks and issues. Allowing teams to problem-solve together creates a successful team environment.

> *TECHNICIAN NOTE* Empowering and delegating team members increases employee retention.

Practice and office managers must become familiar with human relations, laws, and policies in order to protect the hospital and its team. The **Fair Labor Standards Act** was created to protect employees from unfair labor standards. Specific questions cannot be addressed in an interview or the employer could be at risk for a discrimination lawsuit. Various employee records must be retained for a period of time; state and federal regulations vary depending on the record or information in question.

TEAM MEMBERS

It takes a team to make a practice work. If each individual brings an outstanding task or asset to the table, the entire team benefits. One team member may excel at client education and receive compliments and requests from clients. This team member may not be as diligent at cleaning walls when they are soiled as another. However, another team member may not have the exceptional bedside manner of the first team member.

It is imperative that practice managers determine the strong and weak qualities of team members and work to develop the weaker while using the strongest qualities to the maximum potential. It must be remembered that a positive attitude reflects on others and is contagious. When a team member enjoys her or his job, they will pass that attitude on to other team members.

Hiring Team Members

A practice manager can hire an awesome team; however, it can take time to develop that team. One can develop skills with training and continuing education, but one cannot teach work ethic. Hiring employees with a strong work ethic will benefit a practice more than hiring an individual with skill and a poor work ethic. A perfect employee would possess a strong work ethic and excellent veterinary nursing skills. Choosing the right team member to hire is important. The cost of hiring and training a new employee to become a dependable daily contributor to the practice can equal at least one year's salary. Selecting an inappropriate person means turnover and a loss of thousands of dollars to the practice. Staff selection must include a focus on team players. All employees who are team players readily offer help to others when they need it and are equally willing to accept help when needed. This attitude, combined with appropriate cross-training, prepares the team to be responsive to peaks in client demand and patient caseload. It also prepares staff to cover during staff illnesses, vacations, and other absences.

Good hiring practices include using standardized employment application forms, using good interviewing skills, asking for resumes, and checking references. Applications may be purchased, or the practice can devise a personalized form. An attorney should review any forms developed in-house, ensuring that the forms do not contain unlawful questions.

TECHNICIAN NOTE Potential employees cannot be asked about their marital or military status.

Interviewing prospective employees should also follow a standardized format. This is less likely to lead to any discrimination charges. Applicants may be screened with telephone interviews first, and the most likely candidates can then be scheduled for an interview in person. Enough time for each interview should be allowed (usually 30-60 minutes) so that the interviewer will not be interrupted. Questions asked should pertain only to the job. Using a job description will give the prospective employee a good picture of what is really required. Never ask personal questions unrelated to the job position. Box 3-6 lists sample interview questions that can be asked of candidates.

BOX 3-6 Asking the Right Questions

- Are you currently employed? Why or why not?
- How long have you been employed at your current job?
- Why would you want to leave your current position?
- Describe a typical day at your last job.
- What did you enjoy about your past job?
- What position do you expect to fill?
- If you joined our team, what would you bring?
- Describe your summer employment.
- What do you feel are your outstanding qualities?
- What was the least enjoyable aspect of your last job?
- What are some areas you feel you need improvement in?
- Are you able to work a weekend schedule?
- When would you be available to begin work?
- What is your salary requirement?

Training Team Members

Setting expectations and training is crucial. Many new team members are slow to succeed because expectations are not clearly communicated. All positions should have a written job description. This description may include the actual list of duties, as well as the overall hospital philosophy. Training employees in phases can prevent them from becoming overwhelmed the first week of their new job. This can be a number one factor for those not returning after their first few days on the job. Once a phase has been completed, the manager or supervisor should test the team member and then allow the next phase to begin.

Team Leadership

Team leaders must define, teach, and periodically measure skill levels. Good performance must be recognized and rewarded. All staff members need assurance that their jobs are important and recognize that they must perform well in their positions to enjoy both personal and professional success. Rewards and recognition should be made as publicly as possible, such as during staff meetings, with a posted announcement, or published in newsletters. Performance appraisals may be done quarterly or every 6 months. These evaluations let team members know how they are doing while setting new goals for the coming months. Ideally there are no surprises during this process, because consistent employee feedback should let them know how well they are performing.

TECHNICIAN NOTE Performance reviews should be a positive experience, allowing goals to be set for the future.

Reprimands or corrections should be handled privately. Nothing can be gained by pointing out a person's shortcomings in public. Such embarrassment undermines trust, erodes confidence, and weakens team bonds.

Team Member Work Schedules

Practices vary by location, as does the talent that is available by location. Practices located in college towns or larger cities may have a wide application pool, as students with dreams of becoming a veterinarian may be high in number. These students want to learn and excel, earning recommendations from the veterinarian(s). Students generally work part time; therefore the practice may employ a majority of part-time employees. If a practice is located in a smaller town, the choice may be to hire a majority of full-time employees with a few part-time team members to assist during the busy times. Many practices now have extended hours, requiring many hours to be filled by team members, and both part- and full-time members must be employed.

If many students are employed, then the work schedule of employees may change each semester. Part-time employees can also provide assistance when full-time members leave the practice for vacation. Shifts must be covered whenever a team member is on vacation so the team is not shorthanded. Ultimately the patients suffer when a practice is shorthanded; they do not receive the care or diagnostics that they do when the team is fully staffed.

Many practices have instituted a policy that allows team members to have time off, provided their shift is covered before leaving for vacation. If the shift is not covered, alternative methods must be discussed with management. Team members should be able to take time off when they need it; preventing them from doing so builds resentment, which ultimately leads to unhappy employees.

Vacations allow team members to return to the practice rejuvenated. It is widely known that team members in a veterinary practice are very dedicated. They often work extended hours, put forth great effort, and receive very little in return. Vacation is the least that can be offered to these employees, guilt free.

Payroll and Overtime

Team members must be paid an hourly rate. The Fair Labor Standards Act (FLSA) states that every employee must receive an hourly rate. Two exemptions from an hourly pay rate exist: a professional holding a specialized degree or an administrative assistant. These two exceptions (veterinarians qualify) are the only members of a staff who can be paid as a salary basis. Therefore all technicians, assistants, and receptionists must be paid hourly.

> TECHNICIAN NOTE Only veterinarians and administrative assistants are exempt from overtime rules and regulations.

The Fair Labor Standards Act was created to establish minimum wage and overtime pay standards, as well as regulate the employment of minors. State minimum wage may be more or less than the Federal minimum wage; whichever is higher supersedes the other. Minimum wage changes periodically and managers should be aware of changes. Any employee working more than 40 hours within one work week must be paid overtime at 1½ times the regular rate of pay. The FLSA makes reference to a workweek as seven consecutive, regularly recurring, 24-hour periods totaling 168 hours. For the first 40 hours worked in any given workweek, each employee must be paid at least minimum wage. **Overtime** pay must be paid for any hours worked above 40 in a given week, at the stated overtime wage.

Employee Record Keeping

Employee records include a number of documents. The resume, interview questions and answers, references, and background checks must be kept in the employee's personnel file. The new team member must fill out a number of documents, including a W-2 that is to be sent to the payroll department, an I-9 to verify US citizenship, and either the enrollment or decline of insurance, retirement, or any other benefits the practice may offer. Should the employee require any medical attention because of an injury on the job, Workers Compensation (WC) paperwork must be filed with the practice's WC carrier as well as the state labor department. This varies from state to state, so regulations and procedures should be verified. The above documents should also be placed in the employee's personnel file.

All training, reviews, promotions, demotions, or raises that the team member receives must also be documented and kept in the employee's record. It is advised that the practice keep this, and all information listed in the preceding section, on hand for at least 7 years after the employee has left the practice. Future employers or government agencies may call to verify team member information. All paperwork should be kept in a locked file cabinet.

All employee records are strictly confidential information. The owner, practice manager, and the employee the records pertain to are the only members of the team allowed to handle the information. Team member phone numbers, addresses, or other information should never be given to clients or those who call in requesting the information. The team member's safety and security could be jeopardized should this information be given out.

MEDICAL RECORDS

Medical records are a major component of the veterinary practice. A medical record is a legal document that must be complete, legible, and made available to clients at their request. Inactive client records must be maintained for 3 years. As a practical matter, most practices maintain medical records for a much longer period, often for years after a client relationship is terminated or after the patient dies.

> TECHNICIAN NOTE Medical records must be complete and legible.

Completed records must include the client contact information, patient name and information, and the date that the service(s) were rendered. The person who has made entries in the medical record must initial each entry. Written medical records must be legible; any person must be able to decipher abbreviations and/or words. Illegible records may lead to incorrect treatments, incorrect client diagnosis, or incorrect client education. If a record must be presented in a court of law and a judge cannot read the record, the practice may be at fault and held liable for the presenting claim. Cases that are referred to a veterinary specialist may suffer from communication and diagnostic errors if the record is not legible.

Medical records are legal property of the practice; however, clients may request to have copies for themselves, a referral, or for a new veterinarian. It is illegal to prevent clients from receiving their records. The practice is permitted to

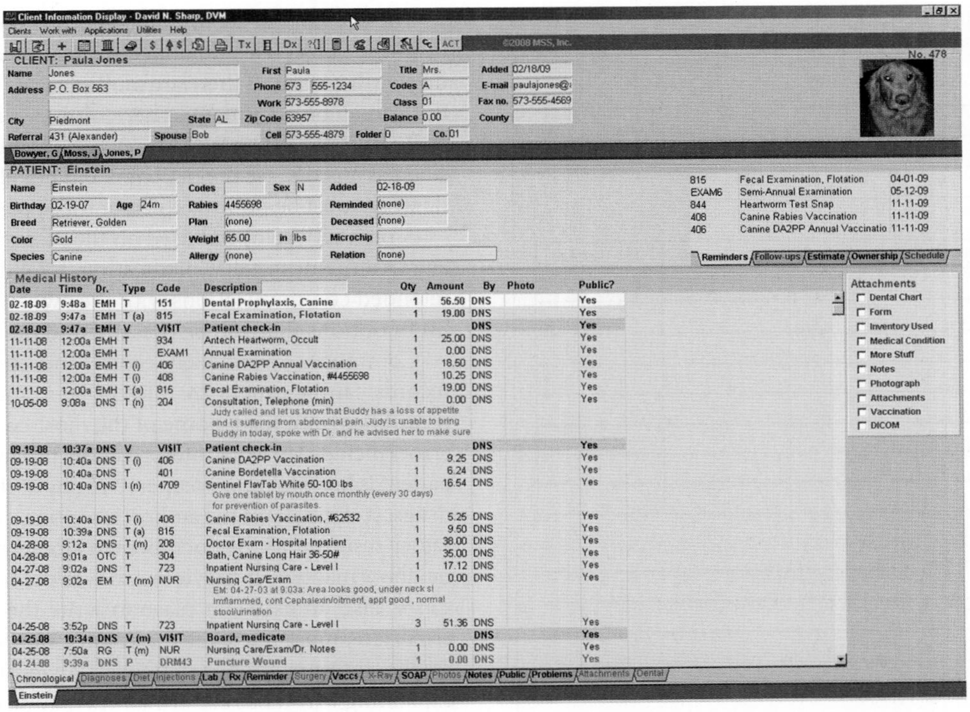

FIGURE 3-17 Avimark medical records screen shot.

charge a fee to cover the cost of creating duplicate records. Medical records and client/patient information is also confidential; cases should never be discussed by name and client information should never be released to any person other than the pet owner.

Should medical records need to be copied for a referral veterinarian, the technician must copy laboratory results that are pertinent to the case as well as a copy of the records. If radiographs are requested and a digital radiograph machine is used, a CD or DVD of the radiographs can be given to the owner or referring veterinarian. If a standard radiograph machine is used, then the radiographs must be checked out to the owner or referral veterinarian. A log should clearly indicate the date, who took the radiographs (the owner or if they were mailed to the referral veterinarian), and the technician assisting the case. Once the radiographs are returned, they can be crossed off the log with a single line strike. This allows the practice to track radiographs if they cannot be located in the practice. Many times owners or referral veterinarians fail to return radiographs, and this allows protection of the general practice.

Medical records may be written, or a practice may be paperless. Paperless medical records must also be complete, and initialed by the author (Fig. 3-17). Many programs will automatically time stamp entries when they are made, along with the team members' initials. Software programs must ensure record safety, preventing record alteration. Some programs can be programmed with a lockout period, preventing record alteration after a 12- or 24-hour period. If any changes need to be made, a second entry can be made, indicating the change.

All entries in written medical records must be in permanent ink and cannot be altered. If a mistake is made, it should be crossed out with a one-line strike. White-Out must never be used in a medical record. Mistakes should be initialed and dated, with the change to follow (Fig. 3-18). This allows an observer to note the nature of the error and to be assured that important evidence has not been destroyed.

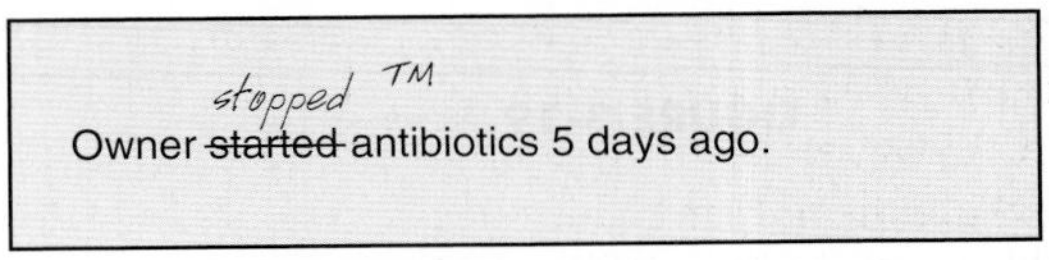

FIGURE 3-18 Example of strike.

Master lists are often used to summarize patient histories. An individual patient record should include a master sheet listing species, gender, breed, age, diet, allergies, unique behaviors, and annual vaccination/parasite control documentation. The master sheet should include a major problem and drug list for which refills are indicated. The master sheet chronologically lists visits, treatments, and client communications (Fig. 3-19).

Record Format

Written medical records are generally held in a clasp-type 8½ × 11 file folder. Each client has one folder, and all patients owned by that client are clipped within the folder. Patients are separated with color-coded tabs. Clinics often find a smaller paper size to be inadequate and may have incomplete records. Other hospitals maintain an entirely computerized medical and financial record for each client. Regardless of the format, the record must be accurate, complete, and secure. Storage and retrieval must be convenient and well organized. Various design formats are commercially

Master Problem List

Client Name__________ Telephone Number__________

Address__________ Client Number__________

Pet Name__________ Breed __________ Color __________

Sex_____ Altered_____ DOB__________ Age__________

	Date Received	Date Received	Date Received	Date Recieved
DHLPP				
FVRCP				
FeLV				
Rabies				
HWT				
FeLV/FIV				

Chronic Diseases/Date of Onset: __________

Current Medications and Directions: __________

FIGURE 3-19 Master sheet.

available to minimize misfiling by incorporating color-coded tabs. If computerized records are used, meticulous accuracy is necessary for all data entry; incorrectly entered computer records may never be retrieved.

POMR and SOAP

Completed medical records must follow a format, especially those with AAHA accreditation. A Problem Oriented Medical Record (POMR) is the most commonly used format that is followed by veterinary healthcare teams. Each entry follows a distinct format: the defined database, the problem list (also referred to as master list), the plan, and the progress section. Within the progress section, a standard SOAP format is followed.

SOAP is defined as Subjective, Objective, Assessment, and Plan. Subjective is the most important element for the reception staff, veterinary technicians, and assistants. Subjective information includes reason for the office visit, history taking, and observations made by the client. Most subjective information is the opinion(s) and perception(s) of the client (Fig. 3-20).

> **TECHNICIAN NOTE** AAHA-accredited hospitals must use POMR/SOAP medical records format.

Objective information is gathered directly from the patient; the physical exam, diagnostic workup, and interpretation are included in this section of the medical record. Objective information is factual information.

The assessment section includes any conclusions reached from the Subjective and Objective section and includes a definitive diagnosis. If there are multiple or a tentative diagnosis, this can all be documented here, along with a list of Rule-Ins or Rule-Outs (R/I or R/O, respectively). Rule-Ins can be classified as any disease the patient could possibly have. Diagnostic work must be done to rule out those particular diseases.

A plan is developed based on the assessment and includes any treatment, surgery, medication, intended diagnostics, or intended communications with the owner. This can also be a list of options that will be presented to the client.

Commonly overlooked errors and incomplete medical records can be caught by diligent team members before the record has been filed. Some of the most common incomplete errors include lab work interpretation, progress notes while the patient is hospitalized, preoperative physical exams, anesthetic drugs, and initials of the author(s) writing in the record. Laboratory results must be documented along with any comments on abnormalities. If previous lab work is being compared to, this is also an excellent place to write the comparison. Veterinarians must interpret the results, not just document the results. Interpretation is defined as analyzing the results and explaining why those abnormalities may be present. The list of R/I and R/O can be completed with the analysis of pending lab work. Animals should have a daily physical exam while they are hospitalized. Results of the physical exam, any medications administered, as well as any urination, bowel movements, or vomiting must be documented in the progress notes. Hospitalization sheets should be used to help keep track of patient status while patients are hospitalized (Fig. 3-21).

Surgical patients must be examined within 12 hours of anesthesia and the exam must be documented in the medical record. Anesthetic drugs, details of the procedure, and the patient's response and/or complications to the procedure must also be documented. The most common error made is not documenting the communication with the owner regarding the prognosis of the patient. The medical record must clearly state if the prognosis is poor, guarded, fair, or excellent.

Medication names, strength, and route given must be accurately written in the medical records. For example, 0.2 mL Cefazolin IV would be incorrect. This description does not indicate how many milligrams (mg) were given. The entry should read: 0.2 ml Cefazolin (100 mg/mL) given IV, or it may read 20 mg Cefazolin, given IV. Many drugs come in different strengths, and it is important to identify and document the correct strength of medication. The same drug can also be administered by different routes. Some drugs will have a different dose, depending on the route administered. It is therefore important to document the route by which the medication was administered.

> **TECHNICIAN NOTE** Patient hospital sheets increase patient care and team member communication.

If the legibility and completeness of the medical record is a problem in practice, labels may be used. Labels can be used for examinations, dental prophylaxis, or surgeries, and be

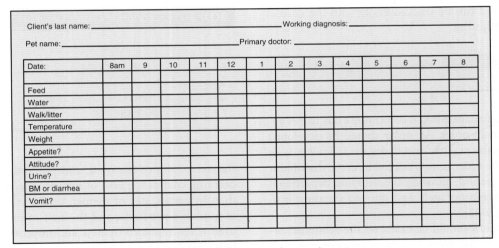

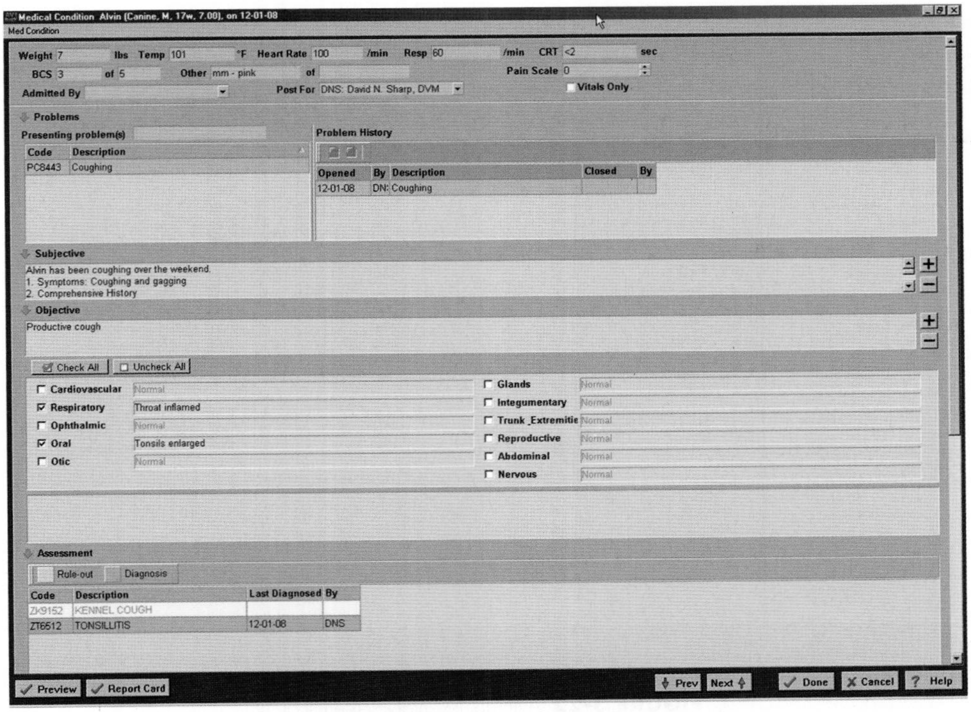

FIGURE 3-20 Avimark SOAP screen shot.

Client's last name: __________ Working diagnosis: __________

Pet name: __________ Primary doctor: __________

Date:	8am	9	10	11	12	1	2	3	4	5	6	7	8
Feed													
Water													
Walk/litter													
Temperature													
Weight													
Appetite?													
Attitude?													
Urine?													
BM or diarrhea													
Vomit?													

FIGURE 3-21 Hospitalization sheet.

developed by the practice manager or ordered from standard office supply and label catalogs.

Standard Operating Procedures (SOP)

SOP descriptions may be written for all standardized procedures used in the practice, and a loose-leaf binder may be used to store SOP sheets in a central location. SOP descriptions may also be used for front office staff, including what kind of questions may be answered by staff, check-in and release procedures, and front office record-keeping procedures. Annual reviews and updates of SOP descriptions are important. Once the SOP binder is in place, one may reference all standardized procedures by "procedure name, SOP" as the patient medical records are completed.

INVENTORY MANAGEMENT

Inventory is one of the largest expenses of the practice. The ultimate goal should be to maintain inventory costs between 12% and 15% of the overall income of the practice. It is imperative that an inventory manager be well organized, motivated, and willing to make changes and improvements on a routine basis. A large amount of money can be lost in inventoried products through shrinkage, product expiration, or missed charges. **Shrinkage** is defined as the loss of product without explanation. Shrinkage may result from employee theft. Products that expire are a large loss. If a bottle has not been opened, some manufacturers may exchange the product; others will not and the practice must take the loss. Missed charges account for a large portion

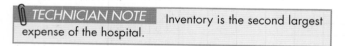

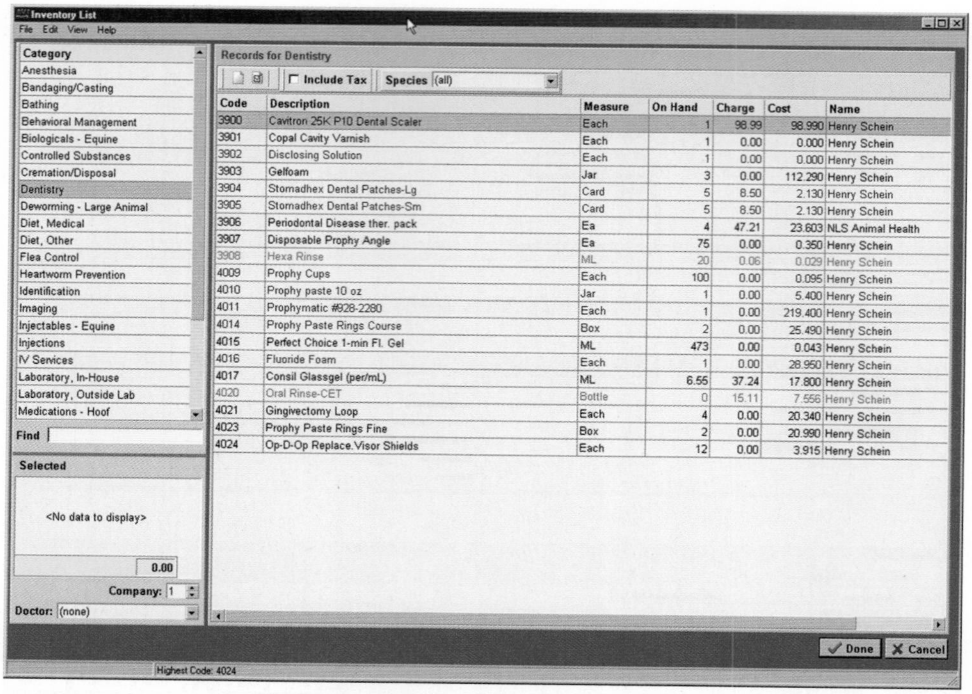

Code	Description	Measure	On Hand	Charge	Cost	Name
3900	Cavitron 25K P10 Dental Scaler	Each	1	98.99	98.990	Henry Schein
3901	Copal Cavity Varnish	Each	1	0.00	0.000	Henry Schein
3902	Disclosing Solution	Each	1	0.00	0.000	Henry Schein
3903	Gelfoam	Jar	3	0.00	112.290	Henry Schein
3904	Stomadhex Dental Patches-Lg	Card	5	8.50	2.130	Henry Schein
3905	Stomadhex Dental Patches-Sm	Card	5	8.50	2.130	Henry Schein
3906	Periodontal Disease ther. pack	Ea	4	47.21	23.603	NLS Animal Health
3907	Disposable Prophy Angle	Ea	75	0.00	0.350	Henry Schein
3908	Hexa Rinse	ML	20	0.06	0.029	Henry Schein
4009	Prophy Cups	Each	100	0.00	0.095	Henry Schein
4010	Prophy paste 10 oz	Jar	1	0.00	5.400	Henry Schein
4011	Prophymatic #928-2280	Each	1	0.00	219.400	Henry Schein
4014	Prophy Paste Rings Course	Box	2	0.00	25.490	Henry Schein
4015	Perfect Choice 1-min Fl. Gel	ML	473	0.00	0.043	Henry Schein
4016	Fluoride Foam	Each	1	0.00	28.950	Henry Schein
4017	Consil Glassgel (per/mL)	ML	6.55	37.24	17.800	Henry Schein
4020	Oral Rinse-CET	Bottle	0	15.11	7.556	Henry Schein
4021	Gingivectomy Loop	Each	4	0.00	20.340	Henry Schein
4023	Prophy Paste Rings Fine	Box	2	0.00	20.990	Henry Schein
4024	Op-D-Op Replace.Visor Shields	Each	12	0.00	3.915	Henry Schein

FIGURE 3-22 Avimark inventory screen shot.

of lost revenue and can be tracked easily with the correct training and monitoring.

> **TECHNICIAN NOTE** Inventory is the second largest expense of the hospital.

The inventory manager should determine a day that is appropriate to place an order. An order should be developed that encompasses the practice's needs for the following 1- or 2-week period. The order must be called in to the distributor before the cutoff period, allowing the shipping department to pack the order appropriately and ship via the most economic route (Fig. 3-22).

Ordering products should be based on the economic order quantity, the reorder point, and the number of inventory turns the product takes within a year. The combination of all three factors will help control inventory, which is commonly a place of missed charges and shrinkage. One must manage inventory well to prevent such losses.

Economic Order Quantity (EOQ)

Inventory should be purchased based on an **Economic Order Quantity (EOQ)**, not on impulse buying or daily ordering techniques. An impulse buyer normally purchases more product than the practice is going to use before the product expires. If an inventory manager purchases products as a daily routine, the practice will likely rack up shipping charges from distributors and manufacturers. The EOQ is an effective, efficient model for determining the quantity of product to order (Box 3-7). The letters in the calculation represent the costs related to ordering the item, sales of the item, and purchase price. Consider carrying cost as the cost of investing in inventory (rather than in certificates of deposit or the stock market), cost of outdated products, and the cost of products no longer used when replaced by new and improved products. The EOQ method should be used for all products that are frequently used on a fairly constant (nonseasonal) basis. Do not use the EOQ formula for ordering infrequently used products, such as chemotherapeutic agents, or seasonally used products, such as flea products. Box 3-8 contains a sample EOQ calculation.

> **BOX 3-7 Economic Order Quantity (EOQ) Equation**
>
> $$\text{EOQ} = \sqrt{2FS} \div (C)(P)$$
>
> F = fixed cost of placing/receiving/pricing/storing an order,
> S = annual sales of the item in units,
> C = carrying cost (usually 25%), and
> P = purchase price per unit.

Reorder Point

A **reorder point** is defined as the point a stock level reaches before reordering. The average shelf life of an item should not exceed 3 months. Anything greater than 3 months decreases the profits of the veterinary hospital and increases the risk of the product expiring, as well as theft or damage to the product. A sales history and EOQ of a product should be examined when determining a reorder point and quantity.

Practices may wish to keep as little inventory on hand as possible. This can be an advantage, as it can lower holding

BOX 3-8 Sample Calculation of EOQ

$$EOQ = \sqrt{2FS} \div CP$$

F = fixed cost of placing/receiving/pricing/storing one order, e.g., $15
S = annual sales of the item in units, e.g., 3000 units of vaccine
C = carrying cost, e.g., 25%
P = purchase price per unit, e.g., $2.75 per dose
The square root of (2)(15)(3000) ÷ (25%)(2.75) = 995 units
The 995 units should be rounded to the nearest convenient unit. Therefore 1000 units should be ordered at one time.

BOX 3-9 Inventory Turns per Year

The average value and inventory turnover is calculated as follows:
Average value of product in stock = beginning physical inventory + year-end physical inventory ÷ 2:
Inventory turnover = total value of product purchased annually ÷ average value of product in stock

costs (costs associated with holding product on the shelf, such as taxes and insurance) and prevent shrinkage (unexplained loss of inventory). However, it can contribute to product shortage (losing clients and money because the product is unavailable for resale).

Inventory Turns per Year

Optimizing **inventory turns per year** is a goal every inventory manager should set. Turns per year is defined as the number of times inventory turns over in a practice, in a specified time. This helps determine correct reorder quantities and points. Each practice should set a goal of 8 to 12 turns per year. This increases profits of the practice, and decreases expired product, shrinkage, holding, and ordering costs. To determine the inventory turns per year, the beginning inventory is subtracted from the ending inventory and divided by 2. This results in the average inventory per year (Box 3-9). The total amount of product purchased during that period divided by the average yields the number of turns per year for that product (Box 3-10). Taking the equation one step further, dividing the number of days in the year (365) by the number of turns per year produces the average shelf life of the item.

TECHNICIAN NOTE Inventory products should turn every 1 to 1½ months.

If a product is used infrequently and expires before the entire amount can be dispensed, the practice may want to consider writing a prescription for the medication. It is less costly to prescribe certain products than for the practice to continue losing profits to satisfy a few clients. Clients will appreciate the lower cost of purchasing the product elsewhere versus incurring the cost of the loss the practice would normally experience.

Computer systems are extremely efficient at aiding in inventory management, production of reports, and decreasing loss. However, physical inventory must be taken at the beginning or ending of each year, as well as spot checks throughout the year. It is also advised to spot check when placing orders to verify quantities on the shelf, in case of error in the inventory system.

Items should be checked when they are received. Expiration dates, correct product, strength, and count should all be verified against the order book and invoice. Items that are received with a short expiration should be returned unless they will be used immediately. Short-dated bottles should not be opened. Most inventory products must be returned unopened and free of tampering in order to be eligible for replacement or credit.

BOX 3-10 Inventory Turns per Year Example

January 1 Inventory = 21,000
December 31 Inventory = 19,000
Total expenditures = $115,000
21,000 + 19,000 ÷ 2 = 20,000
$115,000 ÷ 20,000 = 5.75
5.75 turns occur per year for this product.

BOX 3-11 Example of Prescription Product Markup

28 Cephalexin capsules cost 0.40 each.
Product Markup is 200%
Dispensing Fee is $11.95
0.40 × 200% = .80
(0.80 × 28) + $11.95 = $22.40 + $11.95 = $34.35

Developing an Effective Product Markup

The **markup** of a product is defined as the cost of the product multiplied by a percentage in order to recover hidden costs associated with inventory management. Many practices will mark products up by 100% to 200%. A product markup must be at least 40% in order to break even.

Practices may add a product **dispensing fee** as well as a minimum prescription charge. The average dispensing fee ranges from $6.00 to $14.00 to cover the cost of the label, pill vial, and the time used to count the medication. If a bottle of shampoo or a full bottle of medication is dispensed, the average dispensing fee ranges from $3.00 to $5.00. Many practices initiate a **minimum prescription fee** of $11.00 to $13.00 to help recover hidden pharmacy costs (Box 3-11).

Hidden pharmacy costs include costs associated with expired medications, ordering and shipping costs, as well as insurance and taxes on products and supplies. These costs can increase rapidly and must be recovered.

Pricing for items (such as injections or single-dose items) that are used in the hospital or administered to patients while in the exam room must also be considered. Common methods include charging a flat fee for injections (e.g., $12 per injection) or adding a surcharge for very expensive drugs, such as some postoperative analgesics. In-hospital tablet administration frequently is priced to include drug, labor, and record-keeping costs, such as $3 per administration.

Over-the-counter (OTC) products do not require a prescription and can be sold to clients without a client/patient relationship. A prescription product can only be sold on the order of a veterinarian wherein a current client/patient relationship exists. State practice acts may define the term and dictate how long a client/patient/veterinary relationship exists after the last examination. A client/patient relationship is defined as the relationship shared by the veterinarian, client, and patient. The veterinarian must be familiar with case, patient, and client. It is illegal to sell a prescription product when a current relationship does not exist. Veterinarians can receive heavy fines and license revocation for failure to comply.

> **TECHNICIAN NOTE** A valid client-patient relationship must exist for a veterinarian to dispense prescription products.

Manufacturers may dictate that some products are not prescription products but can only be sold through a veterinarian wherein a client/patient relationship exists. Examples of such products include Frontline, Frontline Plus, and therapeutic diets such as Purina NF, Waltham S/O, and Hills K/D.

Decreasing Loss

Inventory is the second largest liability to a practice, following payroll. A large amount of money is invested into this segment and all areas must be managed well, making changes when necessary to decrease loss. Several methods can be used to decrease the loss of inventoried items and maintain team member accountability: use of travel sheets, appropriate setting of fees, and a structured inventory system. Travel sheets must be used by each team member and double checked by others that all charges have been circled or highlighted. A good policy to instill into team members is that the one who performs the procedure should circle the code. For example, when a veterinarian performs an exam, the veterinarian circles the exam code. If a technician completes a heartworm test, the technician circles the heartworm test code. If an assistant prepares medication, then the assistant circles the medication on the travel sheet (Fig. 3-23). Once the receptionist team receives the record and travel sheet, they can compare the travel sheet to the record, looking for any missed charges.

Tracking inventory and implementing measures to decrease loss through theft is important. A team member taking one box of heartworm preventative adds up when each member takes one box.

Labeling Prescription Items

Every item that is a prescription product must have a label before it leaves the practice. Labels must include the practice name, address, and phone number; doctor's name and date of the prescription; client's last name and patient name; name of the drug; strength of the drug (mg or g); number of items dispensed (tablets, capsules, or mL); and the expiration date of the product. Last, and most important, the directions of the product must be clear. "Give 1 capsule by mouth every 8 hours for 7 days" clearly states that one capsule should be given in the mouth, every 8 hours for 7 days. A label that reads "Give 1 capsule every 8 hours" can be interpreted as: 1 capsule can be placed on the open wound, can be placed over food, or in the water. Clients may also feel that because the presenting symptoms have visually cleared they do not need to continue giving the antibiotic until it is gone. Directions must be detailed and specific.

> **TECHNICIAN NOTE** Prescription labels must include the drug, strength, and expiration date.

DEVELOPING EFFECTIVE COST OF SERVICE

When developing a pricing structure, fees should be divided into two categories: shopped services and in-hospital fees. Shopped fees include vaccinations, heartworm tests, routine surgeries, etc. These fees can be competitively priced with other practices in the community. The fees should cover the cost of the product, the cost of the items needed to complete that service, and the time of the technician or veterinarian to complete the service. For example, a heartworm test should include the cost of the test itself, the syringe and needle needed to draw the blood for the test, and the technician's time to draw the blood and run the test. A percentage needs to be added on top to contribute to the hidden overhead costs of the practice. Practices may forget to add the cost of the items needed to complete the service, as well as the use of the technician's time.

Once shopped service fees have been set, in-hospital fees can be determined. To determine how much a service costs a practice to produce, several key points must be known:

- Fixed costs of hospital per minute
- Direct costs used to produce the service (inventory)
- Staff costs per minute
- Veterinary costs per minute
- Number of staff minutes used to complete the service
- Number of doctor minutes used to complete the service
- Desired profit

The following equation can be used to calculate service pricing:

$$(\text{Fixed costs/minute} + \text{Staff costs/minute}) \times \begin{pmatrix}\text{length of}\\ \text{procedure in}\\ \text{staff minutes}\end{pmatrix} + (\text{DVM costs/minute}) \times \begin{pmatrix}\text{length of procedure}\\ \text{in DVM minutes}\end{pmatrix} + (\text{Direct costs} \times 2) + \text{Profit}$$

Client Number________ Client Name________________ Pet__________ Doctor__________

DISCOUNTS
0107 Monthly Special
0108 Senior Wellness
Senior Citizen

OFFICE CALL
0214 Brief Office Call
0216 Regular Office Call
0219 Well K-9/Fe Exam
0222 Exotics Exam-Reg
0220 Exotics Exam-Brief
226 Exam w/ vaccines
0228 Pre-Op Exam
0232 Recheck N/C
0234 Recheck
0109 Health Certificate
0106 Int'l Health Certificate
0104 Duplicate Rabies Tag

FELINE VACCINES
0608 FVRCP Booster
0612 FVRCP 1 year
0609 FVRCP 3 year
0613 FELV Booster
0610 FELV 1 year
0611 FVRCP/FELV
0607 Rabies Only Fe -1 yr
0618 Rabies Feline 1 year
0605 Feline Yearly Exam
0621 Feline Sr Wellness

PET WEIGHT________

CANINE VACCINES
0603 Parvo
0615 Bordetella
0616 DHPP Booster
0602 DHPP 1 year
0617 DHPP 3 year
0604 Rabies Canine 1 year
0601 Rabies 3 year
0690 Canine Yearly Exam
0620 Canine Sr Wellness
0606 Rattlesnake Vaccine
0619 Lepto

ANESTHESIA
0302 Anesthesia
0304 Extended
0306 Short
0308 Local
0310 Tranquilization
0316 Geriatric Anesthesia

GROOMING
0506 Beak Trim- Small
0508 Beak Trim- Large
0510 Nail Trim
0512 Nail Trim- Exotic
0514 Wing Trim- Small
0516 Wing Trim- Large
0520 Trim Teeth
0518 Pluck ears
0502 Medicated Bath
0501 Shave Cat

DENTAL
0702 Sm Normal Prophy
0704 Lg Normal Prophy
0701 Feline Normal Prophy
0706 Severe Periodontal Dz
0710 Follow-Up
0714 Tooth Ext. Minimum
0716 Tooth Ext. Moderate
0718 Tooth Ext. Extensive
0712 Dental Sutures

HOSPITALIZATION
0902 Board-Canine
0904 Board-Feline
0903 Overnight Board, Sx
0906 Day Board/Obsvtn
907 Hospital Day
0908 Hospital Overnight
909 Hospital Day w/ IV
0910 Hospital Weekend
0912 Hospital Exotic
911 O2 Therepy Half Day
0914 O2 Therepy Full Day
0916 IV Care Daily
0918 IV Care Intensive
0920 IV Catheter
0922 IV Catheter, 2nd
0924 IV Fluids per Liter
0926 IV Fluids One time
0928 Fluid Additives
0925 IV Fluids Hetastarch
0930 SQ Fluids Once
0932 SQ Fluids Per Day
0934 SQ Fluids Exotic
0936 SQ Fluids Disp.
938 SQ Fluids No Tech/Dr.

RADIOLOGY
4125 Radiographs
4126 Radiographs-dental

LAB SERVICES
3505 ACTH Stim
3515 Automimmune Profile
3520 Avian Comp Profile
3526 Avian Post Purchase
3535 Bile Acids
3611 BIPS
3621 Blood Pressure
3560 CBC/Diff
3580 Coagulation Profile
3770 Chemistry #1
3775 Chemistry >2
3590 Culture and Sensitivity
3605 Cytology In house
3593 Cytology-Lab
3610 DTM
3615 Ear Mite Check
3620 Ear Smear
3631 Electrolytes
3603 EKG
3626 EKG >1 per day
3628 EKG Senior Wellness
3630 EKG Repeat
3641 Ehrlicia Canis PCR
3655 Fecal-Direct
3660 Fecal Flotation/Smear
3665 Fecal Recheck
3675 FELV Snap Test
3685 FELV/FIV Snap Test
4081 Fine Needle Aspirate
3695 Fungal Serology
3815 General Health Profile
3710 Heartworm SNAP
3715 Heartworm Difil
3705 HCT/TP
3720 Histopath
3725 Histopath Additional
3730 Histopath Derm
3731 Histopath-Bone Decal
3527 Mammalian Comp Prof
0438 Necropsy In house
0436 Necropsy NMDL
0441 Necropsy Avian-NMDL
3745 Parvovirus Snap Test
3750 Phenobarb Levels
3749 Platelet Count
3601 Pre-Op EKG
3755 Pre-Op Profile
3785 Reptile Std. Profile
3786 Reptile Comp Profile
3795 Schirmer Tear Test
3805 Skin Scrape

LAB SERVICES
3821 T-4 Equilibrum Dialysis
3820 T-4 Dogs
3822 T-4 Cats
3830 Tick Born Dz Panal
4141 Tonopen
3850 Urinalysis- In house
3855 Urinalysis-Lab
3880 Urinalysis-SG
3854 Urinalysis Sediment
3853 Urinalysis-Stick
3852 Urinalysis- Yearly Exam
3860 Vaginal Smear

CLINICAL PROCEDURES
4005 Abdominocentesis
4010 Anal Sac Expression
4015 Anal Sac recheck
4020 Artifical Insemination
4025 Bandage Wound Sm
4030 Bandage Wound Med
4035 Bandage Wound Lg
3085 Cast
4050 Clean Ears
4055 Clip/Clean Wound Sm
4060 Clip/Clean Wound Med
4065 Clip/Clean Wound Lg
4070 Corneal Stain (1)
4071 Corneal Stain (2)
4080 Enema
4083 Flush Anal Glands
4085 Flush ears (1)
4090 Flush ears (2)
4095 Flush Nasal Duct
4105 Home Again Implant
4110 Pass Stomach Tube
4130 Semen Collection/Eval
7002 Splint-Small
5126 Re-Splint Small
7001 Splint-Medium
5131 Re-Splint Medium
7000 Splint-Large
5136 Re-Splint-Large
4140 Thoracocentesis
4145 Transtracheal Wash
4150 Urinary Catheter

EUTHANASIA
WT ________
Dog ________ Cat ________
Mass Cremation
Private Cremation
402 Exotic

SURGICAL PROCEDURES
4205 Abscess Debride
4210 Amputate Limb Sm
4215 Amputate Limb Lg
4220 Amputate Digit
4225 Amputate Tail
4235 Ant. Cruc. Repair
4240 Aural Hematoma-K-9
4341 Aural Hematome-Fe
4245 Biopsy - Wedge
4250 Biopsy - Punch
4246 Biopsy - Bone
4260 C-Section
4265 C-Section w/ OVH
4270 Canine Neuter <50
4275 Canine Neuter >50
4285 Canine OVH <50
4290 Canine OVH 50-99
4272 Canine OVH >100
4295 Canine OVH/Heat
4305 Canine OVH/Preg
4236 Cranial Cruc. SM (1)
4238 Cranial Cruc. LG (1)
4237 Cranial Cruc. SM (2)
4239 Cranial Cruc. LG (2)
4315 Cherry Eye Repair 1
4320 Cherry Eye Repair 2
4325 Cryptorchid Fe-Flank
4330 Cryptorchid Fe-Abdm
4345 Cryptorchid K-9 Abdm
4340 Cryptorchid K-9 Flank
4350 Cystotomy
4355 Debride wound
4360 Declaw/Tendonectomy
4365 Dewclaw Unjointed #1
4370 Declaw Jointed #1
4375 Drain Placement
4385 Entropion per lid
4390 Exploratory
4395 Eye Enucleation
4405 Feline Neuter
4410 Feline Neuter/Declaw
4420 Feline OVH
4425 Feline OVH In heat
4430 Feline OVH Pregnant
4435 Feline OVH Declaw
4441 FHO Feline
4442 FHO Canine
4455 Growth Removal SM
4460 Growth Removal MED
4465 Growth Removal LG
4470 Growth Removal >1
4480 Hernia Repair Inguinal
4485 Hernia Repair Abdom
4490 Hernia Repair Diaphm.
4495 Hernia Repair Umbil.
4505 Patellar Luxation #1
4510 Patellar Luxation #2
4511 Prostatic Wash
4515 Puppy Dewclaws Each
4520 Puppy Tail Docks Each
4525 Pyometra w/ OVH
4530 Rabbit Neuter
4535 Rabbit OVH
4540 Staple Wound per staple
4545 Stenotic Nares Repair
4550 Suture Wound SM
4555 Suture Wound MED
4560 Suture Wound LG
4575 Third Eyelid Flap

CONSULTS
202 Cardiology
213 Repeat EKG
204 Internal Medicine
206 Miscellaneous
208 OFA
210 Radiology
212 Shipping

HEARTWORM MEDICATION
HG Small # ________
HG Medium # ________
HG Large # ________
HG Feline 0-5# #6
HG Feline 5-15# #6

Revolution Feline
Revolution Canine

Frontline Feline
Frontline Canine
Frontline In Hosp Use

POST OP PAIN MEDS
Rimadyl 25mg
Rimadyl 75mg
Rimadyl 100mg
Metacam
Buprinex
Tramadol

INJECTIONS
\# of ML ________

1220 Amiglyde #1
1225 Amiglyde >1
1256 Baytril 100mg/ml
1255 Baytril 22.7mg/ml
1265 Cephazolin
1270 Cephazolin >1
1281 Cortrosyn
1289 Dexameth 2mg/ml
1290 Dexameth 4mg/ml
1305 Diphenhydramine
Ivomec
1335 Immiticide
1390 Methyl Pred Acetate
1410 Pred Acetate
1417 Solu-delta Cortef 100mg
1418 Solu-delta Cortef 500mg
1430 Torbugesic

E-COLLAR

N/C ITEMS
818 HG SM
822 HG M
826 HG LG
2790 Strongid
510 Nail Trim

FIGURE 3-23 Travel sheet.

Overhead costs can be determined from the previous year's financial statements and include every cost except veterinarian compensation and drug and supply costs. Most overhead costs range from $1.50 to $2.00 per minute. Direct costs include all materials used for any given procedure. Once all direct costs have been calculated, double the total to include the costs of ordering, shipping, and unpacking the products. If practices only charge the true direct costs, income will be lost.

Return on doctor time covers how much it costs to pay a doctor for his or her skills. The average small animal veterinarian return is $180 per hour for in-house medical procedures, $2 to $3 per minute for soft tissue surgery, and $3 to $4 per minute for orthopedic surgery. These figures can be used to create a baseline fee for any in-hospital procedure. This formula is essential to setting fair, profitable fees and helps the team understand how and why charges are set.

CONTROLLED SUBSTANCES

Controlled substances are those drugs which have a high percentage of addiction and abuse. The **Controlled Substance Act of 1970** was passed to reduce drug abuse by classifying certain substances as having high abuse potential. The act was established and is controlled by the Drug Enforcement Agency (DEA) and provides approved means for proper manufacturing, distribution, dispensing, and use through licensed handlers.

A controlled substance will have a "C" written in red on the bottle, with a Roman numeral indicating the schedule next to it. Drugs are classified into five schedules, based on their abuse potential. Controlled substances include opiates (narcotics), barbiturates, hallucinogens (Ketamine), amphetamines, and other addictive and habituating drugs. Class I has the highest abuse potential, therefore medical use of these substances is not allowed in the United Sates. Drugs such as LSD and heroin are examples of controlled substances in Class I. Class II drugs produce severe psychic and physical dependencies and include drugs such as morphine, oxymorphone, and pentobarbital. Classes III, IV, and V are less abusive, yet are still controlled. Table 3-1 shows examples of various classes of controlled substances. Fig. 3-24 displays the level of control on various substances. Telazol is CIII, Morphine is CII, and Butorphanol is CIV.

Controlled-substance (CS) products must be continuously locked up in a cabinet or safe that is secured to the wall or ground; it cannot be movable. Only a few members of the team should have access to the drugs, and each drug removed from the cabinet must be logged. Fig. 3-25 gives an example of a controlled substance log.

Any veterinarian dispensing a controlled substance must have a CS license within the state she or he is practicing. Licenses must be on display at all times. Drugs must be logged and inventoried on a regular basis. All drugs must be accounted for and available for inspection at any time by any state or federal licensing board. Those in violation can receive severe penalty and the removal of their license. Any loss greater than 3% per year of drug must be immediately reported to the police department, State Veterinary and/or Pharmacy Board and the DEA (DEA form 106 is used to report losses).

When ordering CS in either class I or II, DEA form 222 must be used and mailed to the distributor. Classes III, IV, and V can be ordered as long as the veterinarian's CS number is on file with the vendor.

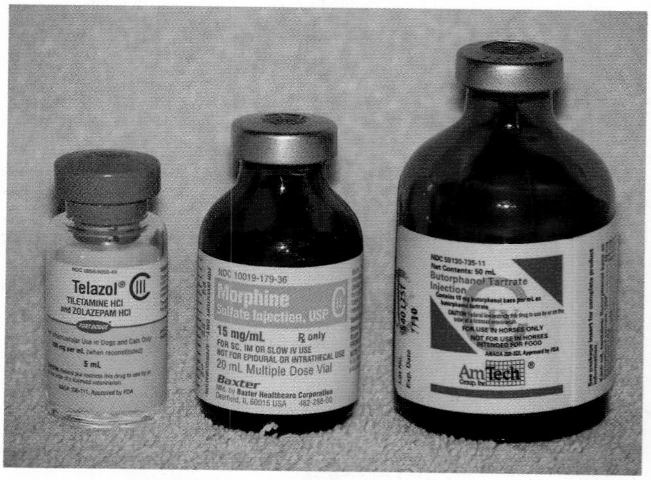

FIGURE 3-24 Controlled substance bottles.

TABLE 3-1 Examples of Controlled Drugs

SCHEDULE	ABUSE POTENTIAL	DISPENSING LIMITS	RESTRICTIONS	EXAMPLES
I	Highest	Research only	DEA 222 required	LSD, Heroin
II	High	Written prescription	DEA 222 required	Oxymorphone, Morphine
		No refills		Pentobarbital, Fentanyl
III	Less than II	Written prescription	DEA Number	Hycodan, Codeine
				Buprenex, Hydrocodone
				Ketamine, Telazol
		Can refill 5 times		Anabolic steroids
IV	Low	Written prescription	DEA Number	Diazepam, Phenobarbital
		Can refill 5 times		Alprazolam, Butorphanol
				Midazolam
V	Low	No DEA Limits	DEA Number	Lomotil, Robitussin AC

Bottle #	Date	Time	Owners Name	Animal Name	Initial Amount	Amt Used	Balance	Initials
1	4-Aug	8:00am	Slatery	Waldo	10 mL	3	7	CS
	4-Aug	8:00am	Garcia	Baby	7	0.5	6.5	NS
	4-Aug	8:15am	Jones	Prancer	6.5	1	5.5	CS
	4-Aug	8:15am	Loving	Tootsie	5.5	0.8	4.7	CS
	5-Aug	8:15am	Pinto	Wonder	4.7	0.4	4.3	NS
	5-Aug	9:15am	Adams	Wendy	4.3	2	2.3	NS
	5-Aug	9:30am	Howard	Bobo	2.3	0.3	2	NS
	6-Aug	8:15am	Bush	Tristen	2	2	0	CS
2	7-Aug	8:00am	Evans	Ashley	10	0.6	9.4	NS
	7-Aug	8:00am	Langford	Bobby	9.4	0.7	8.7	CS
	7-Aug	8:15am	Smith	Capser	8.7	6	2.7	CS
	8-Aug	8:15am	Howard	Wimpy	2.7	2	0.7	NS
			MIA	MIA		0.7	0	CS
3	8-Aug	9:30am	Brown	Blackie	10	1	9	NS
	9-Aug	8:15am	Hyatt	Lawrence	9	2	7	CS
	9-Aug	8:30am	Ralph	Ariel	7	2.5	4.5	CS
	9-Aug	9:00am	Jameson	Taylor	4.5	0.5	4	HP
	9-Aug	10:15am	Lee	Wheeler	4	1	3	HP
	9-Aug	10:30am	West	Katie	3	3	0	SM

Year 2010 Ketamine 100 mg/mL, 10mL

FIGURE 3-25 Controlled substance log.

COMPUTER AND SOFTWARE MANAGEMENT

Computers are an excellent asset to every veterinary practice. Most practices use computers to an extent but may not be using them to their fullest potential. Computers can greatly increase the efficiency of every team member, decrease missed charges, provide professional-appearing client education materials, maintain inventory and accounts receivable, and provide paperless medical records.

Computers and software can be a great expense, but the reward far exceeds the cost of the equipment. Team members should brainstorm and determine the best location for computer terminals in the practice. Many practices use computers in exam rooms, laboratory areas, pharmacy counters, doctor's office, and the reception area. This allows data to be entered in multiple locations of the practice. Pharmacy labels can be generated at any terminal and printed in the pharmacy area. Invoices can also be generated at any location, printing at the receptionist desk.

Team members should also determine what software applications would meet the expectations of team members. In addition to the features listed above, veterinary software can aid in invoice development, client education, practice management, or digital radiology. Veterinary software manufacturers and distributors should provide the team with demonstrations and/or practice modules, allowing the team to determine which software will meet the needs of the practice.

TECHNICIAN NOTE Computers can increase the efficiency and professionalism of every practice.

BOX 3-12 Veterinary Software Companies

Avimark	www.avimark.net
Animal Intelligence	www.animalintelligence.com
CornerStone-Idexx	www.idexx.com/small-animal-health/products-and-services/cornerstone-software.html
DVM Manager	www.dvmmgr.com
DVM Max	www.dvmax.com
Impromed	www.impromed.com
Intravet	www.intravet.com
VetTech Software	www.vet-software.com

Team members should remember to choose a reputable company that has been in the industry for many years, offering continuous updates and new programs. Advanced software companies strive to answer the requests from practices, including safety and security of information. Box 3-12 gives a list of some companies that market veterinary software, and Box 3-13 provides a list of features that may be available.

Advanced software technology must use advanced computers. One cannot expect to run new software on old computers. Software has been developed to run fast and efficiently, and new computers with large amounts of RAM, memory, and storage must be purchased. Many software companies will not guarantee their products without installation on new computers.

Once the decision to purchase new equipment and software has been made, the team must receive training. Team members must become comfortable with the program and

BOX 3-13 Veterinary Computer Software Features

- Financial information (and tracking it)
- Invoices for services rendered
- Reminders and recall notices
- Monthly statements
- Client instructions linked to procedures, vaccination certificates, and prescription labels
- Mailing lists for newsletter, promotional, or informational mailings
- Management data, such as reports on individual and profit center production, trends related to growth or decline of income from various services (e.g., dentistry and hospitalization), cash flow, budgeting, growth or decline in client and/or patient numbers, and owner compliance with wellness recommendations.
- Drug and supply inventory management—calculating turnover rates and generating product orders helps reduce inventory costs.
- Complete patient medical record keeping
- Bookkeeping (general ledger, accounts payable, accounts receivable, payroll processing)
- Medical database references
- E-mail, network access, Internet access, hospital website
- Word processing (letters) and desktop publishing (newsletter)
- E-mail communication with clients, receiving appointment and boarding requests via e-mail, and sending e-newsletters
- Real-time video of boarding pets
- Staff training with CD-ROM programs or Internet classes
- Telemedicine technology, digital cameras, and computerized records that allow for a second opinion with a specialist without leaving the office
- Human resource management—maintaining employee time logs, payroll records, etc.

learn how to best use the equipment to prevent frustration. If teams do not know how to use the software to its fullest potential, money has been wasted. Practice managers should strive to attend continuing education provided by software manufactures to remain updated regarding new features to the software, which can benefit every practice.

As with every situation, a backup plan must exist with computers. Fire, theft, or natural disasters can destroy a practice in a matter of minutes, as can computer viruses or a hacked computer system. It is imperative that security measures be taken to prevent a virus from entering the system. Internet access should be limited to a few individuals and policies should be instituted regarding Internet sites.

Computer systems should be backed up nightly, both on and off premises. On-premises system back up may include a rewritable disk or zip drive. Off-premises system backups can be done through the veterinary software website or another location. Backing up documents off site prevents a thief from stealing the most current copy of data from the practice if they are removing all of the computer equipment. Should a fire or natural disaster occur, the data are also protected.

Computers will not survive a lifetime. Many computers only function optimally for five or six years and then need to be replaced. Computers often give signals as they are slowly fading. At this point, management must locate a backup computer so the day the computer fails, an alternative computer is ready to take its place. This prevents team members from panicking when the system is temporarily unavailable. If it is the main computer that needs to be replaced, the backup data from the previous evening can be uploaded, bringing the system back up and allowing the team to move forward.

FACILITY MAINTENANCE

Practice management must also encompass facility maintenance. It is often the manager who ensures each piece of equipment is functioning optimally, receives monthly maintenance, verifies that appropriate controls and quality testing has been performed on in-house laboratory equipment, and ensures the roof of the practice is not leaking during rainy periods.

Anesthetic machines must be maintained on a regular basis. Soda lime granules must be changed after 6 to 8 hours of use, and if a charcoal canister is used as a scavenger unit, it must be changed after the gain of 20 g in weight. Other scavenger systems must be inspected for leaks, ensuring the system is working properly. Improperly working scavenger systems can pose great safety risks for both the team and the patient. Anesthetic machines should be regularly inspected by a professional anesthetic machine company for cracked hoses, leaks, and proper pressure. Vaporizers should be inspected yearly, and calibrated if necessary.

Autoclaves should be maintained on a weekly basis; cleaning the tanks will ensure that the equipment lasts longer and proper sterilization of surgical materials.

Radiograph machines must be inspected to ensure the proper amount of radiation is being released when exposing a radiograph. Excess radiation can pose risks to the team; environmental inspections are generally performed by the state on a yearly or biannual period.

Microscopes, laboratory machines, and any other equipment should receive maintenance as recommended by the user manual. Quality control checks should be performed on laboratory machines regularly, ensuring the proper machine function. Dates, control results, and maintenance schedules should be recorded and stored for future review.

Building maintenance is absolutely critical. Outside lighting and signage must perform optimally at all times, for safety and to deter crime. Cracks in the building's exterior should be repaired as soon as they are visualized. Once moisture begins to penetrate the building, permanent and expensive damage can occur. The outside of the building should remain clean and free of animal debris and trash. A neat and clean appearance of the practice is essential to positive client perception.

TECHNICIAN NOTE Building inspections should occur every 6 months to look for damages that must be repaired.

Skilled craftspeople must complete some repairs. A list of maintenance and repair personnel should be readily available so that a professional can be quickly summoned in case of an urgent need. This list should include a plumber, electrician, carpenter, lawn service, pest controller, computer supplier, telephone company, and utility suppliers. A supplemental list may include suppliers of major pieces of equipment (e.g., x-ray machine, furnace, air conditioner, blood chemistry analyzer) or systems (telephone or computer system), their telephone numbers, and the model or serial number of the equipment.

MARKETING

There are many facets to marketing; this section will simply summarize the more common methods used in veterinary practice. **Direct** and **external marketing** are aimed at potential clients; yellow pages and newspaper advertising are just a few examples. **Internal marketing** targets existing clients, which promotes and strengthens the bond with clients. Puppy and kitten kits or dental kits are examples of internal marketing. Newsletters, reminders, and recalls can also fall into this category. Indirect marketing is the result of in-house marketing that many team members don't realize is occurring. Client education, clean facilities, and genuine service are all forms of **indirect marketing.**

Many team members market the practice without trying. Excellent client service is the number one tool that team members can use to promote the practice. High-quality veterinary medicine, honesty, and timeliness are important to clients; those who are satisfied will recommend the services of the practice to friends and family.

BROCHURES

A practice brochure can easily be developed and designed by a graphics artist for a professional appearance. Brochures are essential marketing tools that advertise the services the practice offers; many clients do not realize what services are offered in a veterinary hospital. Practices may also want to include information on their doctors, credentialed veterinary technicians, office hours, a map, and details of any specialty items or services offered.

VALUE ADDED SERVICES

A practice can add services to increase value; however, a manager must ensure that all levels of communication, education, and service are being met. Without these factors, a practice will struggle financially, as well as in fulfilling the requirements and satisfaction of the team.

Clients appreciate receiving copies of laboratory results, along with an explanation of interpretation of those results. Clients must receive a phone call from the veterinary health care team before receiving results, allowing them to ask questions that may arise regarding treatment options. After clients receive results, they may research information and call the practice to ask more questions. The team should be prepared to answer questions that arise and appreciate that clients have this interest.

If a practice uses digital radiography or dental digital radiography, a copy of the radiograph should be made for the client. Clients love to have a copy to show their friends and family. The practice name and address should be printed on the copy, which is an excellent source of internal and external marketing.

Websites can offer a variety of valuable information; they can also offer false information. Therefore practices should strive to provide the information to their clients with only one click. Websites can promote practice programs, services, and procedures. Many clients do not realize all the services that are offered in veterinary hospitals, including radiology or dental services.

Websites can be developed in-house or through a web development agency. Whichever the practice chooses, the manager should be able to control the information that is posted and be able to make changes as needed. Medicine, protocols, and promotions change frequently, and the website should be able to accommodate such changes.

Puppy classes are an excellent asset to practices. Not only do they promote the veterinary practice itself, they help owners develop a lasting relationship with their pets. The most common reason for euthanasia in the United States is behavior problems. Therefore the practice can become proactive and prevent these problems before they become issues in the client household.

As a form of internal marketing and value added services, clients appreciate phone calls checking on their pets 24 to 48 hours postoperatively. Clients with patients that were presented for illness should also be called, and the conversation should be documented in the record. Recalls are essential to client satisfaction.

SOCIAL MEDIA

Social media is another form of internal marketing and targets many generations of clients. Educating clients via social media foundations is low cost but requires planning. The term social media is used to apply to many platforms, which change over time. Facebook, Twitter, Pinterest, Google+, and YouTube are top platforms at press time, but could change within a few years. Practices can positively influence clients with informative facts, fun trivia, and behind-the-scenes footage of the hospital. If clients like the information they are receiving, they will share it with their friends and family. In addition to sharing information, clients tend to make recommendations on social media sites. These words are recommendations and serve as referrals for the practice. These referrals are much more powerful than an advertisement could ever be (and they are free!).

A social media plan should encompass the overall marketing plan a practice wishes to implement. For example, if the practice wishes to focus on implementing wellness plans during the first quarter of 2015, the social media platform should support it.

A social media policy is a must for both clients and patients. If any pictures are taken of client or team member pets, a social media release must be signed indicating the approval for use of the photo. The term social media must be used (rather than specific current platforms, such as Facebook, Twitter, Google+) because the face of social media will change over the years, and the general term, social media, is needed to encompass all platforms.

Team member social media policies are a little more complicated than the client's simple approval for use of pictures. Managers and owners cannot dictate what team members post on their personal social media site; however, professional guidelines can be established, and if violated, implications can occur. Managers can, however, mandate that pictures for the hospital's social media platforms be taken on practice-approved cameras (never on personal cell phones) and uploaded by approved team members only. This can prevent the wrong person from uploading embarrassing or incorrect information.

TECHNICIAN NOTE Value added services increase client compliance.

DISASTER PLANNING

It is imperative to plan for disasters. A natural disaster may occur in any part of the nation or world; the location simply changes the possible disasters that may occur. Tornadoes, hurricanes, earthquakes, floods, and fire are a few disasters for which veterinary practices must prepare. A team member should be assigned to oversee the disaster and recovery plans; however, the entire team should prepare the plans together. Allowing multiple team members to develop plans allows different perspectives and thoughts to be included, with the goal of not forgetting important details.

Once a team member has been assigned to oversee the plans, individual team members may be responsible for tasks to complete each plan. Compiling information for emergency phone numbers, facility information, lifesaving procedures, evacuation procedures, hazardous material, and emergency communications can be assigned to individuals or a team. The recovery preparation, including documentation of property assets and important contacts, can be assigned to another. All information should be placed in a binder, in a central location, within the practice. A hard copy should be kept in a fireproof safe. All documents and plans must be reviewed at least annually.

EMERGENCY PHONE NUMBERS

Emergency phone numbers must include the fire department, police department, hospital names and addresses, and all utility companies. Utilities include the electric, water, sewer, gas, and telephone. If a building is rented, then the building owners and maintenance company should be included in the emergency list.

FACILITY INFORMATION

Information regarding the facility must be readily available in every emergency. Critical shut-off valves/switches for gas, water, and electricity must be located. If any keys, tools, or wrenches are required, they should be located at or near the shut-off valve. Instructions to shut off the valves should be placed with the keys or wrenches.

Flashlights should be readily available for each team member. Extra batteries should be kept with the flashlights; batteries should also be rotated before expiration. Team members may wish to consult with local electrical companies or electricians regarding power generators, uninterruptible power supplies, emergency lighting capabilities, and surge protection for large pieces of equipment.

Facility floor plans should be developed and placed in a location that police and fire departments can easily locate to determine what is inside the building before they enter. Hallways, offices, surgical suites, and hazardous chemicals should all be listed on the floor plan.

A team should think of every disaster that could strike and how the practice can be secured. What if there was a fire (Box 3-14)? earthquake (Box 3-15)? hurricane (Box 3-16)? flood (Box 3-17)? An armed intruder? Chemical hazard (Box 3-18)? What if the windows are knocked out? An evacuation plan must be developed for each.

EVACUATION PLAN

An evacuation plan should be developed for both clients and team members. A team member should be designated as the evacuation captain, who will then create an evacuation plan. The captain should train other team members in CPR, first aid, fire extinguishers, and blood-borne pathogens. Plans should be developed for hurricanes, tornadoes, floods, and fire.

To create an evacuation plan, team members must be familiar with exits. A primary evacuation route should be established, followed by a secondary in case the primary is involved in the emergency situation. Team members should be prepared that a client may have a disability and will need assistance to evacuate. Training and role playing will allow team members to become comfortable with the evacuation procedure. The captain should be the last team member to leave the building, and once outside, should account for all employees and clients who were on premises.

BOX 3-14 Fire Safety Checklist

- Provide adequate number of fire extinguishers and service them yearly.
- Train employees how to use fire extinguishers.
- Train employees how to respond to fire.
- Ensure exit signs are lit and readily visible.
- Post emergency evacuation plans.
- Keep all stairwells, aisles, and exits clear. Do not block with furniture, boxes, or other items.
- Store materials no closer than 36 inches from the ceiling.
- Ensure electrical outlets are not overloaded.
- Store hazardous chemicals properly and away from heat sources.

BOX 3-15 Earthquake Safety Checklist

- Train all employees in earthquake awareness and preparedness.
- Establish interior and exterior assembly areas and give employees at least two routes to get there.
- Store earthquake supplies and equipment including lights, search and rescue equipment, medical supplies, food, and water in case employees or clients need to stay overnight because of highway closures.
- Train employees in First Aid, CPR, and Blood Borne Pathogen procedures and ensure first aid supplies are available for their use.
- Preestablish communication systems and test equipment periodically.
- Be aware that earthquakes can create other emergencies such as fires, floods, hazardous materials spills, and other first aid problems.
- Strap down large file cabinets, computers, and shelves to prevent objects from moving and falling on team members.

BOX 3-16 Hurricane Safety Checklist

- Obtain a radio to receive weather reports.
- Establish facility shut-down procedures.
- Establish early warning and evacuation procedures.
- Plan to assist team members and clients who may need transportation.
- Make plans to communicate with employees before and after the hurricane.
- Make plans to protect outside structures, equipment, and windows.
- Prepare to protect, back up, or move vital records (both data and paper records).
- Give team members enough time to get home to protect their families and home.
- Prepare to evacuate.

Employees should remember to maintain calmness in the event of an emergency. Running and screaming only heightens the stress levels of all involved. If it is safe to do so, team members should try to secure the safety of patients, documents, or instruments. In case of a hurricane, team members should have enough time to evacuate the premises of all clients, patients, and team members. Alternative hospitalization plans must be implemented for patients. In the case of tornadoes, time may or may not permit securing the safety of patients. Team members and clients must first be evacuated to a safe area. In the case of fire, team members must evacuate immediately, only returning for patients if it is safe.

TECHNICIAN NOTE Emergency plans should be reevaluated at least annually.

BOX 3-17 Flood Safety Checklist

- Shut off water valves, if safe to do so.
- Shut off power.
- Contact local water and electrical companies.
- Notify building management, if needed.
- If flood warning is issued, move furniture, materials, records and equipment away from area of concern (i.e., doorways, windows, ground level, or basement).
- Shut down and move electrical equipment, if possible.
- Turn off gas to any appliance or equipment that uses gas.

After the Flood

- Watch out for live electrical wires.
- Pump out water slowly to minimize further structural damage.
- Dry out premises and furnishings. Mold, bacteria, and mildew need to be removed from ductwork.
- Secure the property.

BOX 3-18 Hazardous Materials Safety Checklist

Before the Problem Occurs

- Identify type, use, and storage of materials.
- Use seismic restraint, supports, and anchors on equipment, shelving, containers, and tanks storing hazardous materials.
- Inform employees of the danger and post decontamination instructions.
- Develop procedures for immediate cessation of processes that could threaten public health.
- Develop procedures for neutralizing, removing, and containing hazardous materials.
- List agencies prepared to deal with hazardous emergencies.
- Inform the local fire department of hazardous materials and storage locations.
- Coordinate planning efforts with the local fire department.

If Hazardous Material Release Occurs

- Leave the danger area immediately.
- Confine the area by closing doors and windows if applicable.
- Shut off ignition sources if the spill is flammable.
- Call 911.
- Remove clothing and shoes from exposed team members and properly dispose.
- Seek medical care immediately if needed.

When evacuating clients with disabilities, one must always consult with the client as to the best way to move them to a safe location. Wheelchairs should not be taken down stairs; therefore, the client may need to be carried. One must use caution moving extremities because of pain, catheters, braces, etc. Clients who are visually disabled may request the guidance of team members. Explanation of the emergency and the location of the safe zone are imperative; once the location has been reached, the client should be asked if they need any further assistance. They should not be left to guide themselves. Hearing-impaired clients may need explanation if they are not able to hear the alarm system. A note may need to be written (if time and safety allow) explaining the emergency and the location of the safe area.

EMERGENCY COMMUNICATION

Communication is vital in the time of emergency, and the phone system may be overloaded with calls during such situation. Calls made to 911 should only be to report an emergency, not to receive information regarding the emergency. Some phone calls may become automatically blocked by the telephone company to prevent the system from becoming overloaded; in such case, phone calls are diverted to recordings. Out of area calls may be connected quicker than those within the disaster area. One call should be placed to a family or friend, who can than notify others of the disaster and can coordinate efforts if needed. This will allow telephone lines to be available in the disaster areas if needed.

Should the media arrive to the location of the disaster and make unsolicited interviews with team members or clients, team captains may wish to instruct all to decline the interview. A media spokesperson should be appointed to handle the media, as a second disaster may be created if it is not handled appropriately.

STAYING OPEN FOR BUSINESS AFTER A DISASTER

It is important to include "after the disaster plans" in the planning process. Businesses that are prepared can return to normal business more quickly and more efficiently than those that are not prepared. In order to develop a plan, one should determine the essential or critical functions that are necessary for business and list them in order of priority. Critical team members who are required for the practice to function must be identified. Supplies and equipment that will be needed must be listed, and a method of delivery or stage should be identified. Phone lines are essential for business, and one may work with a telephone company to have the lines forwarded to an alternative phone or cellular number.

> **TECHNICIAN NOTE** Planning for the recovery stage of a disaster can increase the rate and efficiency of repairs and help return the business to normalcy.

If medical or financial records were moved off premises, the return of documents must be planned, or if the business will be moving to a temporary location, the movement of such documents must be initiated. Computer systems should have been backed up before the emergency (if it was safe), allowing temporary computers to be uploaded with current information. A mutual aid agreement with neighboring businesses or organizations may aid the temporary relocation of a business.

A method to contact employees after the disaster should be implemented, along with a communications plan for essential and nonessential employees. Employees are the most valuable resource in the event of an emergency; therefore, managers and owners may develop an Employee Assistance Program to aid in the support of the team.

Relationships with trusted vendors should be developed to help replace supplies and products as soon as possible. Vendor contracts may also need to be established for cleanup, salvage, and restoration. This can be a vulnerable time for a business that has just suffered severe damage, and contracts must be established for the protection of the business.

DOCUMENTATION

Documentation of such emergencies is vital—before, during, and after the cleanup procedure. Property assets should be documented and kept on and off premises. Equipment should be listed along with the vendor, purchase price and date, and model and serial numbers. Photographs of major equipment should be taken and stored offsite. Attorneys and insurance adjustors should be consulted as to what information should be gathered and stored.

A log of critical events that occurred during the emergency should be kept. A photograph or video should be taken of the facility before the cleanup begins, and all expenditures must be logged as they are made. An explanation should accompany all receipts, purchase orders, and repairs made. Police and fire reports, scope of work and repairs, and labor and equipment rates should all be kept together. Should any new equipment be purchased after the emergency, vendors, purchase price, model, and serial numbers should be kept in a secure location. Any damage should be documented as required by disaster assistance programs and taxes.

Veterinary technicians and team members who wish to become certified in disaster aid can contact the Humane Society of the United States for more information on Disaster Animal Response Team (DART) training, or visit http://www.ndart.org. Training can be completed by team members, allowing a smoother recovery service for local and state organizations.

REVIEW QUESTIONS

Short Answer

Fill in the blanks.

1. A goal for the inventory manager is to not exceed the average shelf life of an item, which is _____ months.
2. The number of times inventory turns over in a practice in a specified time is referred to as __________ /__________.
3. Employee records should be kept for at least __________ years after the employee has left the practice.
4. A medical record is a legal document that must be maintained for _____ years if the client has not returned to the practice.
5. When ordering a controlled substance in either Class I or Class II, DEA form __________ must be filled out and mailed to the distributor.

Choose the Best Response

Choose the best answer to the following questions.

1. High inventory turnover indicates:
   a. that you are ordering drugs in quantities that are too small and have to reorder too often
   b. that you are ordering too many drugs; they are becoming outdated before they can be used and must be discarded and replaced
   c. an efficient and well-run pharmacy
   d. that too much space and capital are tied up in inventory
2. The veterinarian prescribes a drug at the dose rate of 2 × 100-mg tablets twice per day for 5 days. Each tablet costs 2 cents; there is a markup of 100% on that item; the dispensing fee is $5.00; and there is a minimum tablet cost of 10 cents each. What is the cost to the client for this prescription?
   a. $7.80
   b. $7.00
   c. $5.80
   d. $9.00
3. What is the markup on a tablet that costs 5 cents and is sold for 20 cents?
   a. 25%
   b. 50%
   c. 200%
   d. 300%
4. The most economical amount of a particular product to order, calculated by factoring in fixed costs, carrying cost, and purchase price, is known as the:
   a. restocking cost
   b. economic order quantity
   c. rollover quantity
   d. cost-reversal quotient
5. Dividing the total annual purchases of an item by the average value of that item on hand yields that item's:
   a. rolling average inventory value
   b. inventory turnover
   c. return on investment
   d. profit ratio

RECOMMENDED READING

Ackerman L, Stowe JD: *Blackwell's five minute veterinary practice management consult, Section 6.11*, Ames, IA, 2007, Blackwell.

Heinke MM: *Practice made perfect: a guide to veterinary practice management*, Lakewood, CO, 2001, AAHA Press.

Opperman M: *The art of veterinary practice management*, Lenexa, KS, 1999, Veterinary Medicine Publishing Group.

Prendergast H: *Front office management for the veterinary team*, ed 2, St Louis, 2011, Elsevier.

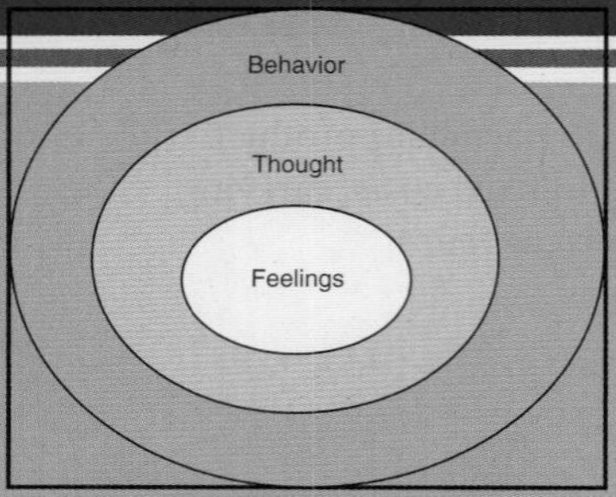

4 Effective Communication in Veterinary Practice

OUTLINE

LEARNING OBJECTIVES

After reviewing this chapter, the reader will be able to:

1. Discuss methods to implement effective communication skills in the veterinary clinic.
2. Identify barriers that prevent successful communication exchanges.
3. Implement effective listening skills to enhance clinical expertise.
4. Implement assertive communication techniques to replace ineffective speech habits and solve conflict situations more successfully.
5. Review techniques to reduce conflict and manage difficult situations with team members.
6. Describe the stages of grief.
7. Explain the importance of the human-animal bond to client and co-worker interaction.
8. Describe appropriate ways to counsel clients on loss of a companion animal.

KEY TERMS

Assertive communication
Body language
Nonverbal communication
Receiver
Sender

As a veterinary technician your success in practice will not be based solely on technical expertise, but to a larger degree on the ability to communicate professionally, effectively, and assertively with the entire veterinary health-care team and clients. The advantage of mastering communication skills lies not just in improved client interactions, but also on a host of personal and professional aspects as well (Box 4-1). Eighty percent of failure in the workplace is based on poor communication. Fortunately, with the implementation of simple yet effective communication techniques, it is possible to dramatically reduce the effects of poor communication in your work environment (Box 4-2). Mastering these skills provides a solid foundation that will enable your flourishing career to develop and benefit you personally as well.

THE COMMUNICATION PROCESS

If you have ever uttered the words, "this would be a great job if I could just work with the patients and not the people," you are not alone. It's quite likely that you are similar to most veterinary technicians; it's easy to apply your technical knowledge and expertise, but the challenging part of your career is interacting with clients and team members. Realistically, the majority of your time will be spent communicating with others. The ability to interrelate professionally defines your level of success. Your expertise is most valuable when it can be expressed in a way that is understood; you actively listen to the needs of clients and understand how to serve them, as well as have the ability to build working relationships in cooperation with other team members.

BOX 4-1 Benefits of Effective Communication in Veterinary Practice

- Enhances understanding of employer work expectations
- Decreases team conflict
- Improves career satisfaction
- Strengthens client education and recommendation abilities
- Encourages other team members to improve communication patterns
- Reduces errors that occur because of poor communication

BOX 4-2 Seven Essential Communication Skills That Veterinary Technicians Should Master

1. Use active listening skills.
2. Identify and eliminate communication barriers.
3. Use assertive communication and be understood.
4. Implement conflict reduction techniques.
5. Incorporate problem-solving methods.
6. Use collaborative problem-solving skills.
7. Assure that written as well as verbal skills are developed.

Effective communication between team members entails a **receiver** and a **sender** of a message. The receiver is the person listening to the message, whereas the sender is the one who is talking and giving the message. Ideal conversations entail having an interaction that allows all team members involved the ability to be both a sender and a receiver. All too often conversations are about individuals trying to do both tasks at the same time. In these conditions a true exchange of information is severely limited.

The goal of communication is to exchange thoughts and ideas in a flowing two-way manner. Anything that interrupts this flow will diminish the outcome. Communication occurs through four primary methods: listening, speaking, reading, and writing (Fig. 4-1). Computerization is increasing the reading and writing component through e-mail, furthering the need to be clearly understood in writing. But live person to person contact is still the most common form of communication interaction.

TECHNICIAN NOTE Communication occurs through listening, speaking, reading, and writing.

Whether you are interacting with clients, supervisors, or co-workers, the more of your senses that you use in a positive way, the more likely you will inspire a positive interaction with another person. Communication has several dimensions and occurs on many levels simultaneously. In the workplace you can use your senses of sight, touch, hearing, and smell to create favorable surroundings, promote positive interaction, and accomplish your tasks. Using more of the different elements in combination will increase the powerful impact when communicating with others. People communicate by verbal (spoken and written) and nonverbal means. Contrary to what most people think, nonverbal communication is more persuasive than verbal communication and is a substantial part of interactions with others.

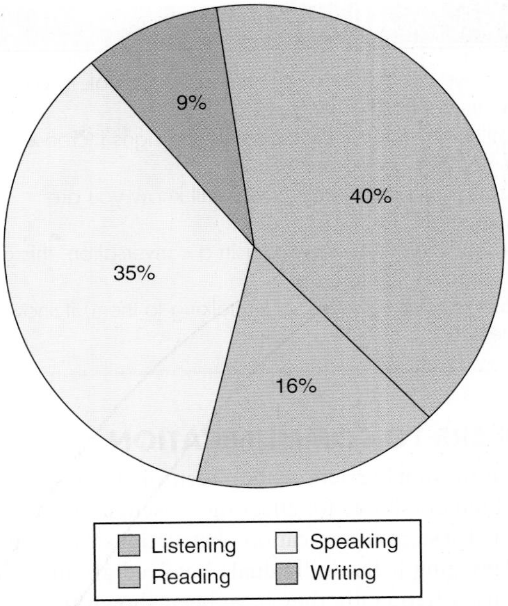

FIGURE 4-1 The communication process.

More than 70% of communication is nonverbal. **Nonverbal communication** involves emotions, which alter the interpretation of the message. It also signals your social and professional position within the workplace (how you relate to supervisors, peers, and subordinates). Nonverbal communication can be likened to the way in which wolves communicate their social position within the pack, using displays of submissive or dominant behavior (e.g., posture, tail carriage, eye contact).

Nonverbal communication is also often demonstrated in **body language.** Body language is a subcategory of nonverbal communication. It is the use of the eyes, gestures, and body in conveying a message. The true essence of a message is either supported or unsupported by body language, and this message is often without thought by the person. Body language can be automatic, given without thought. Ever try to shake your head yes while you were saying the word no? The mind and body seeks to have verbal and nonverbal messages agree. That is why when they don't agree, the communicator may seem uncomfortable or unwilling to make eye contact. Understand that your team members and your clients look at your body language to assure you are professional, knowledgeable, and caring (Box 4-3).

The ultimate goal, regardless of the process, is to be understood. To achieve this ultimate goal is not a minor talent, as most people are not well informed on how to communicate either as sender of information or as a receiver. Most communication patterns are based on habit and often result in the use of barriers. These barriers diminish understanding the message and the chance that an accurate and honest discussion will occur. According to estimates, these barriers are used up to 90% of the time in daily conversation.

BOX 4-3 Positive Body Language

- Use eye contact; it invites someone to speak to you. Not too much; that's staring.
- Smile with eye contact; together the signs increase immediacy of conversation.
- Use facial expressions; others will know you are interested.
- Do not let your eyes wander in a conversation; this can be seen as indifference.
- Face toward someone when talking to them; it shows interest.

BOX 4-4 Common Communication Barriers

- Ordering
- Excessive questioning
- Labeling (name calling)
- Falsely praising
- Excessive logical argumentation
- Advising
- Threatening
- Excessive reassuring
- Diagnosing
- Moralizing

BARRIERS TO COMMUNICATION

Communication barriers are best identified as responses that hold a high possibility for affecting a discussion in a negative manner. These communication obstructions can be particularly damaging if the individuals involved are under stress. When used frequently they have been shown to lower self-esteem and increase defensiveness. On reviewing the list of common communication barriers in Box 4-4, they appear to be quite harmless and without any negative connotations. So, how can they be so damaging to communication? These barriers have been shown to increase the chance that collaboration will not occur and that a greater distance can exist between the individuals. This is only heightened when emotions are running high or the stress level is elevated. This does not mean that any time these barriers are used a negative condition will result; it only suggests that if not considered, a negative result can occur.

These barriers can be placed into three primary categories: (1) solution sending, (2) judging, and (3) failure to respond to concerns. Although we all use these barriers from time to time, it is essential to fully comprehend their potential in damaging your goal to achieve mutual understanding. In the veterinary practice any element that detracts from optimal communication must be assessed and controlled to ensure the highest quality of medicine is practiced for the patient and superior service is maintained for the client.

Awareness of communication barriers is the first important step in reducing their impact. It is also important to take into perspective that these elements are assumptions based on what you believe about someone. The only assumption that should be made in professional communication is to believe that other people mean well. Review a recent conversation that occurred between you and a client and consider if any of these barriers were used and how they might have influenced your ability to gain mutual understanding. Now as you build your awareness, the next step is to enhance your listening skills. This will help you to better understand others, avoid making assumptions, and build **assertive communication** patterns. It will help you to replace ineffective speech habits and solve conflict situations more successfully. The use of these barriers will decrease over time.

BUILD EFFECTIVE LISTENING SKILLS

Wisdom is the reward that you get for a lifetime of listening when you would have preferred to talk.

DOUG LARSON

In the fast-paced environment of the veterinary practice, veterinary technicians will be faced with a great need to understand and retain information coming from many directions—the client, the practice owner, the sales representative, the practice manager, and the other health care team members (Box 4-5). Are you really listening? A recent study demonstrated that around 75% of oral communication is ignored. Hearing and listening are very different. Hearing is the physiological action of capturing auditory waves, whereas listening includes engaging the psychological process to evaluate and consider the message of another person.

Active listening requires focus and engagement. The message you are sending to that client or your peer is that what they are saying is important and you want to understand their need (Box 4-6). How do you feel when someone really listens to you? Satisfied, cared about, and rewarded are common outcomes from active listening experiences. Clients who know that someone truly has taken the time and made the effort to accurately understand their needs and concerns have a stronger relationship with the practice and are more likely to recommend the practice to other pet owners. Active listening is not just a good idea; it is a critical tool to a veterinary technician's success in the practice.

The entire message is not just in words but in the tone of voice and the body language as well. Body language and tone of voice are particularly effective in conveying the total message of the words spoken. This means that on a telephone conversation with a client, it is even more important to tune into what is being said as the other clues through body language are not available.

TECHNICIAN NOTE Active listening is a skill that can be learned and practiced.

To adapt better listening skills, it is vital to understand the three stages of listening and to take a proactive position

BOX 4-5 Benefits of Effective Listening

- Demonstrates respect
- Enables stronger working relationships
- Diminishes conflict
- Decreases miscommunication
- Demonstrates empathy
- Positions individuals for greater understanding of one another
- Essential to veterinary technician career success

BOX 4-6 Active Listening Traits

- Strong eye contact
- Positive head nodding
- Thoughtful silence
- Appropriate environment
- Paraphrasing ("What you are saying is ...")
- Meaningful reflection ("If I understand you ...")
- Avoid distracting behavior
- Leaned/faced toward speaker

BOX 4-7 3 Steps to Active Listening

1. **Receive the message**—Listen and look for the total visual and auditory message. Listen for the entire message; if you are thinking about what to say, you are not actively listening.
2. **Process the message**—Evaluate and analyze; ask yourself, "What does the speaker want me to know?" This takes concentration and focus. As emotions escalate, this becomes even more essential.
3. **Respond to the message**—Let the speaker know you have not only heard, but you understand the visual message as well. Be sure to avoid responses that are based on communication barriers (Box 4-4).

to build this skill over time (Box 4-7). This breakdown of the listening stages may appear very elementary, but unfortunately all too often in clinics this process is not followed. Messages are missed; frustration continues to grow; clients become dissatisfied when their needs are not met; and team members find themselves in stressful situations that could have been avoided.

The active listener is most often the controller of the conversation. Listening skills such as direct eye contact and focused attention convey interest and a desire to understand. They nourish the feeling that the speaker is not merely being listened to, but deeply understood. This is an advanced level of listening that not only lessens the chance of misunderstanding but also increases the chance that additional information will be shared (Box 4-8). Remember the last time someone interrupted you when you were speaking. Your intention was to share your thoughts and ideas. The person interrupted, possibly making barrier-creating remarks or stating unimportant opinions. Suddenly, what you were about to say was lessened and decreased in importance so the chances of you continuing to try and share your message is virtually eliminated. This situation is an excellent example of what commonly occurs, the damage that can happen, and the valuable information that is left unsaid.

BOX 4-8 Implementing Active Listening Skills

- Focus on what is being said, not what you want to say.
- Listen carefully for things that clients share; don't just listen to them.
- Listen twice as much as you speak and speak less than half the time in a conversation.
- Decide that listening is your key to success in the practice.
- Use short responses when someone is expressing something important to them; let them get the message out.
- Identify if the speaker is talking to you about feelings or facts; this helps to determine your response.
- Nod your head, or give positive facial expressions to someone when they are sharing information and you do not know how to respond.
- Recognize what you have missed before implementing active listening skills.

Each individual has a goal in listening. Development of listening skills is topically very elementary, yet their application can be very complex if not a bit uncomfortable. As these skills are used over time, the advantage becomes evident and the ability to use them assumes the form of habit.

Along with effective listening skills is the development of empathetic listening; a critical skill, particularly in the veterinary practice. Clients are faced with a broad spectrum of emotions surrounding the serious illness or loss of their pet and empathetic listening is a less intimidating way to establish a respectful and understanding environment. Judgment must be eliminated in communication with clients in these emotional situations. A judgmental type of response will most often cause alienation at a time when common understanding is vital to assist the client. Ms. Jones may say, "I can't believe Rascal is gone, I don't know what we will do without him." The empathetic listener would be able to respond, "Your family is going to miss Rascal and it is hard to be without him." The exchange is free from judgment; it demonstrates focused listening, caring, understanding, and empathy.

The implementation of valuable listening skills will facilitate strong communication to occur consistently in the workplace with clients, co-workers, and employers. As these skills are developed, they create the foundation to expand and improve oral communication expertise. Your effective interaction with clients and co-workers radically expands your ability to triumph in the veterinary clinic, develop strong business and client relationships, and reduce conflict. Listening will always remain the cornerstone of successful communication skills.

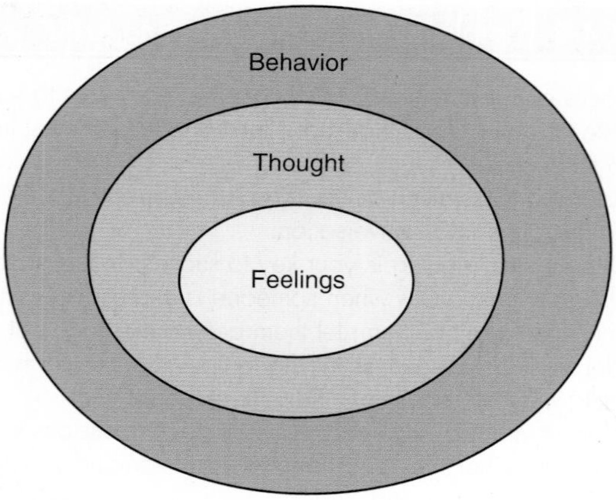

FIGURE 4-2 The speaker's "secret code." Behavior is visible; the emotions and thoughts are not as easily observed.

ASSERTIVE COMMUNICATION STRATEGIES

Words by themselves are imprecise. Often in the veterinary clinic what we want to express does not fit into words and sentences very well. This lack of precision requires skilled communicators to gain an understanding of the speaker's "secret code." As we have spent a lifetime developing our own code, it is just as important to realize that this is true for our team members and clients. We can see the behavior of a speaker; it's the visible representation, whereas the emotions and thoughts are not as easily observed (Fig. 4-2). A client's or co-worker's thoughts are not effortlessly understood and even less often are the feelings identifiable. **Assertive communication** is a proven method to increase the understanding of thoughts and feelings and help break the secret code of others, among other benefits (Box 4-9). This style of communication also influences how others receive and interpret your messages as well. Focus in this style is placed on speaking in a positive, proactive manner and sharing your concepts and issues in the most effective way possible.

There is an 8-step process to follow to integrate assertiveness into your communication style; it is called the DISCOVER Method (Box 4-10).

Decide What You Want

Before you get what you want, you must first know what you want. Accuracy in conveying thoughts, ideas, and concerns is based on having a goal and an innate understanding of what is the end point. What do you want? Without close consideration of what the goal is, there can be a continual problem and no solution. How to proceed and what to say will be dependent on what is the desired outcome of a conversation, business relationship, or situation.

Identify Negative Tendencies

With 70% of daily thoughts being negatively based, it is easy to understand how these thoughts can influence the outcome of a conversation or situation. Remember when you had a disagreement with a co-worker that resulted in tension between you? Now you want to try and resolve this issue and all your thoughts are, "Why does this always happen to me?" "I just know they will never be nice to me again," or "Things never change, so why try?" Soon these repetitive thoughts defeat the belief that a situation can change. To change this process, you must first be aware of the statement's negativity and the barricade they represent to meeting your goals.

BOX 4-9 Benefits of Assertive Communication

- Expresses your needs and ideas more clearly
- Enhances self-esteem
- Improves confidence level
- Increases respect for others' points of view
- Enhances your character
- Decreases sense of guilt or anxiety
- Enables you to be direct without being blunt
- Increases constructive over destructive communication patterns
- Identifies how to be positive without sugar-coating messages
- Emphasizes what you can do, not what you can't do

BOX 4-10 The DISCOVER Method

- Decide what you want.
- Identify negative statements.
- Substitute positive thoughts.
- Choose a technique.
- Own the changes.
- Victory celebrated.
- Evaluate the experience.
- Remember it in the future.

Substitute Positive Thoughts

It's time to challenge and replace those statements. When you realize that this negative monologue is occurring, exchange those thoughts with "It's fortunate that I have the skills now to resolve this situation" or "If it is to be, it's up to me." Studies show that relationships are actually stronger after resolving a conflict situation than if the conflict never occurred. This is a daunting challenge to change these thoughts; they are a lifetime habit for most people. By identifying the thoughts, replacing them, and reinforcing your choices the habit is broken.

Choose a Technique

After you have replaced the negative statements, it is time to determine how to establish assertive communication with the other individual that meets your goal. In most situations using the tips and techniques in Box 4-11 will work well. In situations where conflict, emotion, or stress is at high levels, it's advisable to role play with a friend what you want to say. Write out your most important points to use during the exchange. Practice what you want to say into a mirror to check your expression and body language along with what you say to ensure an assertive, positive position.

BOX 4-11 Tips and Techniques to Be Assertive

1. Use tact; express emotions verbally and not nonverbally.
2. Give other people the opportunity to respond.
3. Respect everyone. You don't have to agree with what is said, but respect their right to say it.
4. Use "I" instead of you. Reduce the inference of blame.
5. Stay assertive. Passivity creates frustration and can allow problems to build.
6. Deal with situations as they arise except if you need to "cool off" before speaking.
7. Remember your goals.
8. Minimize negative inner thoughts.
9. Express your thoughts, ideas, and feelings directly.
10. Encourage others by example.

Own the Changes

Let's say that Mr. Johnson is coming in to pick up his pet, Casey. The medical record indicates that the pet needs to have a teeth cleaning. Dr. Anders has asked that you speak with the client about the procedure. Ownership of the situation means that you determine what needs to be said, set your goal, and take the initiative to make the interaction. Maintain an assertive style. When you speak with Mr. Johnson, after shaking hands and making strong eye contact, your opening statement is, "It was a pleasure boarding Casey with us while you were away Mr. Johnson. Dr. Anders noticed that Casey has advanced dental disease and here is what is recommended …" The speaker is respectful, positive, direct, assertive, and owns the exchange. Even when a client declines a recommendation, assertive communication maintains a positive note and leaves the door open to future opportunities.

Victory Celebration

It doesn't matter if your implementation of assertive communication was a total triumph or a miserable failure. The victory is in taking the risk, challenging yourself to use a different approach, and developing your skills. Remember how good it feels to take action and learn from an experience. Pat yourself on the back. Do a victory dance and revel in the feeling of being in control of your communication future.

Evaluate the Experience

After celebrating your success, review what happened and what you can learn from this interaction. Perhaps, if appropriate, ask the other person for feedback on your communication style. Consider what you would do differently and what you will continue to do in the future.

Remember It in the Future

Be kind to yourself; having adapted this process to your style, your communication training will most likely exceed the training of 90% of your team members. Although no one makes these types of changes overnight, it is plausible to achieve a smooth, positive, and effective assertive communication style over time with continued implementation, close examination, and demonstrated mutual respect.

BOX 4-12 Benefits of Conflict Resolution

- Builds personal development
- Strengthens work relationships
- Reminds about "different" not being "bad"
- Enhances self-esteem
- Lessens stress level
- Heightens job satisfaction
- Improves ability to look at different perspectives
- Gains appreciation of others

CONFLICT MANAGEMENT

The single most common reason that you will leave your job at the veterinary practice is conflict. The idea of conflict to many team members in a clinic brings to mind angry words, heated exchanges, name calling, tension, and hurt feelings. With all of those potentially damaging elements to the workplace environment, it is hard to understand why little formal training is given to new employees about how to manage and reduce conflict situations. How co-workers respond to conflict situations can ultimately define their success in the veterinary practice. Sadly, it is all too often that the hardest working and most caring individuals in the clinic will become the first casualties when conflict runs rampant through the workplace.

Happily, it is no longer obligatory to feel powerless in a cycle of heated outbursts, damaged business relationships, and unbearable tension. By facing and managing conflict directly, it is possible to eliminate tension and angry emotions along with strengthening co-worker relationships (Box 4-12). Conflict is based on different perspectives in a situation. The listener supposes that the individual speaking has greater value than what is actually being presented. Remember, the emotional reaction of what is occurring supersedes and escalates the situation. If an angry co-worker shouts something at you and you feel this is for no reason at all, your position may be one of outrage and anger at having been treated in this manner. It's not what was said but what is perceived to have occurred. Perception becomes reality. This is an important point to remember, e.g., on that occasion when a client is explaining what she thought she heard about how to administer the medication that was prescribed. How many times has a client called and offered to start giving a medication that was intended to be given until gone. Their perception is reality.

Conflict is everywhere, and early in our work experiences we learn that it is best avoided. Although it is a positive strategy to reduce the occasions of conflict, it is not realistic to believe that avoiding conflict is a successful way to deal with this issue. The foundation of conflict resolution is to accept the idea that discord is not always negative but can be positive, perhaps even enlightening if effectively handled with easily learned skills and techniques. Once the aversion to conflict has been resolved, it is time to master the skills of conflict management. As you review this process, think of a conflict situation you faced in the past that did not end well.

BOX 4-13 Inflammatory Statements/Phrases

Avoid the following when resolving conflict:

- "You never/always ..." This is an extreme statement; things are rarely all or none.
- "But ..." Can be read as negating everything said before "but"; try to substitute "and" instead.
- "You make me so ..." Blame placing.
- "You should ..." Blame placing.
- "I can't ..." May be read as unwilling to cooperate.

Consider how you could have used these steps to change that outcome.

Day after day veterinary health care teams face situations that exhaust their energy, create stress, and lessen their job satisfaction. These situations don't usually involve patient care, but team interactions and conflict. On Saturday Mary shouted "If I have to work one more Saturday because Sarah can't get her butt out of bed on time, I swear I am going to quit!" A statement such as this nearly guarantees that there will be a conflict between Mary and Sarah at some point. Let's decide that we are going to counsel Mary on how to manage this issue for a positive, successful result. Choosing what that desired outcome is for Mary and having a plan on how to resolve the situation will dramatically improve the level of success. As a follow up to the initial step, it is equally important to recognize potential barriers that will hinder the plan. Usually the biggest obstacle is the use of inflammatory remarks or statements. Any phrase that will likely impart a negative response needs to be avoided. Review the barriers to communication seen earlier in this chapter along with Box 4-13 to identify potential barriers. Avoidance of these common phrases and barriers will allow the discussion between Mary and Sarah to focus on the issues at hand and strengthen their understanding of one another. Full use of active listening skills is also an essential part of the resolution strategy. Keep in mind, "Your ears protect your mouth from your feet."

Explore and understand the perception of the other person to bridge the gap. It is the perception that is the reality to this individual. Emotions and feelings can run high. Although we want to believe that we always maintain our composure and listening skills in disagreements, the evidence is often just the opposite. Most commonly in situations involving heightened emotions our mind engages what we want to say while the other person is speaking. If you are thinking about what to say, you are not listening. This action almost ensures you will miss the important information that is being shared, and the chance to grasp an understanding of the other person's position is lost. To eliminate this issue, incorporate the 3-second rule. Before replying to the other person, wait 3 seconds after they have stopped speaking. Use that time to create your response. It is even a good idea to let the other person know that you are listening carefully to what they say, and to best understand their feelings you will be hesitating before responding. This sets a foundation of focusing on resolving an issue and not escalating a conflict.

The mindset to consider listening as an attitude to be used in all team interactions has been shown to reduce misunderstandings and develops a greater appreciation for the perspective of co-workers. With the mindset of listening, your ability to reduce and resolve conflict has improved dramatically with just this single step. Now let's explore a 5-step plan that will work out the majority of conflict circumstances in the veterinary practice.

Case Example

Janet and Shawn have worked on the same veterinary health care team at Golden Veterinary Center. Janet is the head receptionist and Shawn is the surgery technician. For the last few months tension has been increasing between the receptionists and the technicians regarding the scheduling of surgeries. Several technicians have told Shawn that they are "sick and tired" of the way those people at the front desk over-schedule and never get the schedule correct. Shawn decided to speak with Janet about the situation. Unfortunately, the conversation ended with Janet accusing the technicians of being lazy and Shawn accusing the receptionists of being poorly trained. Since that meeting the tension has continued to escalate to the point where the only exchange between the receptionists and technicians is along the lines of angry stares and rolling eyes. What can be done to resolve this situation?

Build a Solution

Before initiating the 5-step plan for resolution, it is essential to remember that in these kinds of occasions it is not about who is right and who is wrong; but rather what can be done to help return the team to a working, cohesive group. Each step of the plan must be completed to its fullest potential before moving forward to the next step to obtain the most desirable results. Failure to resolve a situation is most often a reflection of having not fully completed a step before moving forward. It is not unusual for these situations to appear to worsen at the early stages of resolution. This is comparable to when a small erosion appears around a dog's tooth and in further examination, the tooth and gingival are far more damaged below the gumline than what appears topically. We must look farther and deeper to understand issues of conflict and to resolve them effectively.

Step 1: Create a Solution Setting. In the rush to try and correct a conflict it is easy to disregard the importance of having the right environment where resolution can flourish. Building the right solution environment will also reduce the chance of recurrence of the issue as well. Where would be a good location to speak with someone regarding a problem? It is inappropriate to speak with someone about a problem in front of other co-workers. Choosing the correct time is also of consideration. Friday night at 5:30 PM after a grueling day of back to back appointments and a full hospital ward is not conducive for individuals to calmly air their issues. Choose a time and place that is comfortable, agreeable to all people involved, and allows the amount of time necessary to come to a common agreement (Box 4-14). It may be best to choose a location outside the office to reduce interruptions

BOX 4-14 Create the Right Environment for Resolution

- Pick the right time.
- Pick the right place.
- Choose to listen.
- Point out the goal, the benefits of resolution.
- Make it private.
- Reduce interruptions.
- Focus on the issues, not the personality.

and distractions. Although this may not always be possible, remember that the primary issue why you will leave your job is conflict, so resolution to conflict is a very important matter.

To create the right environment for Janet and Shawn, they decided to go out to lunch together on Wednesday. They discussed the need for privacy and lack of distraction with their practice manager and she agreed that an extended lunch was a good idea. The practice manager also stressed that although the situation was certainly stressful for everyone involved, the resolution to the situation would benefit everyone in the clinic. They also agreed that they would spend an hour on the issue and then set another meeting if they were unable to reach an agreement. Engaging in a marathon resolution session will increase the stress and decrease the ability to stay on the topic at hand. Bear in mind that it may take a few meetings to come to a favorable conclusion. Even during this process, individuals can see that the problem is being resolved and the tension will reduce in the work setting.

A positive resolution environment is created by the location, the time, and the demonstration of commitment by all parties involved. The individuals need to show their interest in resolving the situation and to look at the problem from many perspectives outside of their own. This may not always be possible. The person who has assumed the leadership role to manage the conflict must make it known that the focus will be on fixing the problem, not the person.

TECHNICIAN NOTE Effective conflict resolution requires a positive environment.

Step 2: And the Problem Is .... Our attitudes come from a lifetime of experiences, learning, and expectations. These attitudes directly influence our perceptions and as such give us an often unique perspective on events. Now, take this point and remember that everyone involved has this same base of experience and will likely draw on their personal knowledge to view the conflict. Difference is not bad, and understanding those different perspectives will identify the core of the problem. People will have dissimilar points of view in a situation coupled with an array of emotions. Clarification of each person's views will begin the process by identifying the problem. Be sure to first understand their view of the problem before proceeding. Ask questions to verify you are correct in understanding their point of view and to encourage them to focus on the problem and not on the emotion. Individuals involved in conflict often feel it influences all aspects of the professional relationship they have with co-workers. Even though a pet may have an ear infection, it does not mean that the pet's overall health is poor. Let co-workers know that conflict is just a component of the total work relationship and not the entire team connection.

The process of understanding the different perceptions about the situation has also highlighted all of the parts of the issue as well and allowed for identifying what needs to happen to see resolution. Clarification and acknowledgement of each person's frustration, miscommunication, and feelings is essential in verifying that each point of view is completely understood. The co-workers involved also know now that they are valued and considered in developing a plan to end the problem.

Janet and Shawn each expressed their thoughts and issues about the problem. They both used active listening and did not try to dispute the feelings of the other. They both looked for what they had in common in the situation. Both of them were very unhappy about the tension and the backbiting that had been occurring among the team members. They felt this common ground would assist them in ending this unpleasant situation.

Step 3: Develop Your Plan. Focus needs to be placed on the present. An agreement must be reached that the past experiences will be let go for a true and lasting resolution to occur. From the past, we can learn what might have been possible to have prevented the current problem but it will not assist in providing an overall end to the issue. Evaluate all possible ways to resolve the situation. Start with brainstorming, by asking the co-workers to create a list of all of the pieces of a resolution plan. Encourage all ideas to be expressed. Agree that while building this list, no ideas will be evaluated, just put on the list. There are no wrong or right ideas, merely ones to stimulate the group to focus on resolution.

Everyone is encouraged to participate. When the list contains all of the ideas from the co-workers, begin to identify the top ideas that they believe can be developed to resolve the situation. When the top ideas have been identified, the next phase is to build action steps to implement the idea. Action steps are created by listing what exactly must happen to complete the idea (Box 4-15). Lists of all the action steps form the plan. The group must now decide a timeline for the implementation of these steps as well as who on the team will be working to complete these tasks. Everyone should be involved in the resolution because this builds commitment and ownership to the plan.

After discussing their perceptions and concerns, Janet and Shawn decided to brainstorm to identify ways to resolve this problem and reduce the possibility of it happening in the future. The steps they created included each of them discussing the situation with their team, highlighting that no one wants to continue with the current tension and

BOX 4-15 Effective Action Steps

- Are measurable; you know when each is completed
- Have action; are described with verbs: "We will develop ..." "Create a ..."
- Illustrate an understanding of the team's needs and desired outcome
- Are time bound; when will the step be completed?
- Are neutral and do not favor one team member over another
- Encourage everyone to contribute
- Build a partnership for resolution

that they were working together to help resolve the situation. The receptionists and technicians would each rotate through the other's area on a regular basis to better understand what it was like to do the other's position. There would be cross training as well to better understand the needs of each position. It was also brought up that the receptionists were often understaffed and that newly hired people may have unknowingly contributed to the situation. The team would work together to build a point system for the surgeries. Each type of surgery would be given a point value and then a certain amount of points would be allotted for each day. In the future Janet and Shawn would work more closely together to address any issues as soon as they occurred. Emphasis would be placed on remembering that the team works together to provide the best veterinary health care for their patients and communication was the key to their success.

Step 4: Implement the Plan. The steps are placed into a logical order, clearly defined, and methodically implemented. The action steps are assigned to team members for implementation and given dates for completion. Communication on how steps are progressing and any issues that arise are essential in ensuring the plan moves forward. Be sure to keep everyone informed on your progress. Sometimes it appears that the list of action steps is huge and the movement forward is very slow. Emphasize the outcome and the benefits the team will see by reducing the recurrence of the problem and the skills that are being learned during the journey toward resolution.

Janet and Shawn built a graph that showed progress on the different steps of their plan. They communicated back to their co-workers and their practice manager the strides that were being made by the team. The communication between Janet and Shawn improved considerably, enabling the handling of concerns to occur quickly and completely.

Step 5: Celebrate. The resolution of the conflict is ample reason to celebrate. It is essential to emphasize the successful actions of the team to realize the issues, act to correct the problems, and work together to create a pleasant, effective work environment. The skills learned in these situations enable team members to become more effective in their positions and less likely to leave their jobs because of frustration and inability to change undesirable issues in their career.

When everyone had cycled through the cross-training process, Janet and Shawn had a surprise breakfast for all of the team to celebrate their success and to highlight the benefits. Each group was given an opportunity to discuss the information that they had learned from the experience. The team showed remarkable progress. Although there was still some residual animosity, the positive changes were quite visible. The tension in bringing the two groups together was dramatically lowered. They also noticed that the incidence of receptionists' quitting had also decreased.

THE HUMAN-ANIMAL BOND

Over the past century, veterinary medicine has evolved from a focus predominantly on food animals to a companion animal orientation. Pets have moved from the backyard to the house to the bedroom and are perceived as members of the family. Client expectations are changing as medicine changes and more is learned about the human-animal bond.

TECHNICIAN NOTE Many clients consider their pets to be members of the family.

Clients who are not well informed about the human-animal bond may not take into account the impact on household members when making decisions about veterinary care. If there is little bond with the animal, decisions may be influenced more by financial considerations. This is particularly troubling when the decision maker is not as bonded to the pet as other household members. It has been reported that children who are left out of life and death pet care decisions or who are not told the truth by their parents hold lifelong resentment. It is therefore critical for the veterinary team to help the decision maker understand the impact of the human-animal bond and how it may affect household members. It is equally important to involve household members in decisions about pet care. Hospitals should continuously document the relationships and bonds within the household in client records so that all members of the veterinary team can use this knowledge to assist clients and animals.

During a patient's health care crisis, it is a delicate matter to help clients who face difficult decisions. Clients are best served if they consider the human-animal bond in their decisions, but they must not be made to feel guilty or inadequate if financial realities keep them from doing everything that can be offered. The veterinary team's responsibility is to help the animal and prevent suffering, as well as serve the client. This points out the benefit of prevention; by educating clients about the human-animal bond long before there is a crisis, and by encouraging them to have pet health insurance, you help ease the difficult passages.

The opposite extreme from clients who have little appreciation for the human-animal bond is clients who are extremely bonded. These clients are well aware of this bond. They may seek or demand services that have never been requested and that the hospital is not prepared to deliver. Clients such as these actually lead the profession to offer new levels of service and veterinary care. The services that your veterinary team performs only for this special client today will be the norm in a few years. Examples are home care by assistants or technicians, respite care, hospice care, and high-technology services such as CT scans and MRI.

Clients consider companion animals to be members of the family or household, in a role very comparable to children. They are perceived as helpless innocents who are dependent on the adult people in the house for nurturing and protection. Your goal is to be a partner with the client in helping maintain the bond between them. Part of nurturing the bond is to help clients have realistic expectations of behavior in relation to the species and breed of pet. In addition, you must help clients understand animal behavior and learn to communicate with the animal. Of pets relinquished to animal shelters, the largest number are there because of behavior problems. These problems are mostly preventable or treatable with client education and animal training. Behavior that went uncorrected for too long either prevented the human-animal bond from forming or broke the bond and resulted in the pet being given up. An important service you can provide to clients and pets is to be a knowledgeable resource on behavior and training. Recognizing and correcting problem behaviors early in a relationship can literally be lifesaving for the pet.

It is important to recognize and honor the bond between the client and pet by treating the pet as an individual, not as an example of a particular species or breed. You should try to build on the bond the pet has already established with the client and form your own bond with the animal. This can be challenging, because animals are often stressed just by coming to the hospital and can be more interested in avoiding you than bonding with you. Animals are not all equally lovable and friendly, but as a professional you have an obligation to try to give them all your best care. Remember that the way the animal interacts with the client at home may be completely different from the way it interacts with you in the hospital. The careful use of gentle but firm physical restraint, and chemical restraint when needed, will protect you and the animal. It will also reassure the client that the pet is precious to you as well.

Assistance animals such as guide dogs and hearing ear dogs require special care on the part of the veterinary team in recognition of both the dependency of the client on the animal and the very deep bond between them. You must ask the human companion to direct you and be forthright about any questions or concerns. You must be prepared to alter some of your routine policies and procedures to best serve assistance animals. Avoid separating the person and the animal if at all possible. You must also discuss in great detail any procedure that may temporarily incapacitate the assistance animal and prevent it from working. Sedation or tranquilization of any kind will make it unsafe for the animal to work until it has fully recovered.

Hospitalization, which is a routine to people who work in animal hospitals, is stressful to clients who are highly bonded to their pets. They not only miss their pet's companionship, but also worry about them just as parents worry and are distressed by having a child in the hospital. The veterinary team can relieve this strain on both the patient and the client by making patient visits possible and convenient. Frequent calls to give progress reports also help ease the client's mind.

As pets approach the end of life, clients may begin to recognize how strongly they are bonded and anticipate the loss they will experience when the pet dies. This realization makes the pet's remaining days more precious than ever. The mission of the veterinary team is to prevent suffering and support the highest quality of life possible during this time before the pet dies or is euthanized. Human hospice offers a model of how to achieve these goals. Hospice endeavors to keep patients in their homes, surrounded by family and friends, pain free, with their symptoms controlled, so that their last days can be good ones. The patient and family are supported with skilled nursing, respite care for caregivers, as well as spiritual, psychosocial, and bereavement support. Veterinary hospitals can offer these services by having staff provide home care under the direction of the veterinarian, and by finding credentialed psychosocial and spiritual counselors to offer services as needed.

> **TECHNICIAN NOTE** Assist clients in the bereavement process by suggesting ways to memorialize their pet.

Clients can be assisted in the bereavement process by suggesting ways to memorialize and honor the unique individual and the special relationship with it. Funeral and burial ceremonies, donations, clay paw prints, pictures, and plantings are all ways of recognizing a special and meaningful relationship. Clients who are most bonded with their animals are at risk of suffering the most grief over their loss. These clients will not get new animals until their grief is resolved, and these are exactly the clients who will provide the best homes for animals and the best veterinary care. It is in the best interest of the client, the animal, and the veterinarian to help clients through their bereavement and become ready to welcome another animal into their homes.

GRIEF COUNSELING

Clients anticipating or experiencing loss of a companion animal are emotionally vulnerable. The hospital is also vulnerable. What you do or say to a client while he or she is experiencing the loss of a companion animal can encourage or discourage his or her future relationship with the practice. At such a time you have the opportunity to provide the best service your hospital has to offer.

The bonds people form with their pets may be as deep or deeper than those formed with friends or family members. Pets make us feel better when we are ill, comfort us when we are lonely, accept us when we have made a mistake, and love us unconditionally. This human-animal bond can be broken in many ways. The pet may die of natural causes, run away or be stolen, killed accidentally, or euthanized. Clients with a deep emotional attachment to their pets can expect to grieve when they lose them.

It is important to respect the feelings of clients experiencing such loss. To do this, you must first understand the stages of grief and determine the significance of the loss to the client. Elizabeth Kübler-Ross, MD, was the first to outline predictable stages of the process of grieving in her book, *On Death and Dying*. Although she wrote about human loss, the stages can be applied to the loss of pets as well.

Loss of a pet elicits a wide range of emotions in clients; these can be associated with certain stages of the grieving process. You can assist the client's smooth transition from one stage to another. The grieving process is not a steady, linear ascent from depression to joy; rather, it can be likened to a roller coaster ride, with ups and downs at every turn. At the end of the ride is a state of resolution and acceptance, in which the client is at peace with what went before.

By familiarizing yourself with the characteristics of each stage, you will recognize at what point your client is in this process and be able to shape your responses appropriately. These responses can facilitate the smooth transition from one stage to the next in the process of grieving.

STAGES OF GRIEF

The stages of grief include denial, bargaining, anger, guilt, sorrow, and resolution. These stages frequently occur in this order, but they can occur in other sequences. Some stages may be repeated.

Denial

Denial, the first stage of grief, may be played out during the first 24 hours if the animal's death is sudden, or for several days if a terminal illness has been diagnosed. Denial is a coping mechanism that cushions the mind against the shock it has received.

Bargaining

Clients may bargain with God or another higher entity for the life of a pet, or bargain with the pet itself, trying to make it live. They may offer the pet vitamins, tempt it with its favorite foods, and promise never to scold or neglect it again. Bargaining is a way of keeping hope alive and buying time to fully accept the outcome of the situation. When bargaining does not yield the desired results, anger is a natural response.

Anger

When faced with the loss of a treasured pet, clients may become angry with the veterinarian, technician, office staff, family, friends, and themselves. The veterinarian who has failed to "save" the pet, or who has made the diagnosis, may be the initial recipient of the wrath. More often it is the reception staff members who bear the brunt of the anger, either directly or indirectly. Clients may be fearful of alienating the practitioner on whom they have come to rely. If clients are angry with themselves for overlooking clinical signs or waiting too long to seek care, this self-directed anger, once dissipated, gives way to guilt.

Guilt

Guilt is an unproductive, debilitating emotion that often inhibits progress toward resolution of the loss. It is the enemy of healing and closure and, if excessive, may require the attention of a mental health professional. When guilt subsides, it opens the door for sorrow.

Sorrow

Sorrow, or deep sadness, is the core of the grieving process. Though it can be kept at bay during the early stages through the intensity of denial, anger, and guilt, sorrow eventually settles in and permeates all aspects of life.

Sorrow is, in fact, a healing emotion. This is the time when tears flow freely. Clients feel relief and release from the pent-up emotions of previous days or weeks. Tears may come at work, in the supermarket, or while driving down the freeway. Clients may report sleep and appetite disturbances at this time. The practitioner may want to remind them, soon after a terminal illness is diagnosed, that adequate rest and nutrition are important. With time, sorrow dissipates, and everyday tasks begin to dominate awareness. Tears no longer break through into daily activities but can surface at more convenient times, such as in the evening after work. Clients then feel more in control and are able to see an end to the intense pain that is true sorrow.

Resolution

In the resolution phase of grieving, clients realize that the pet is gone, that no amount of wishing will make it different, and that they will survive the loss that previously seemed engulfing. Now they can look at photographs of the pet and smile rather than cry; they can remember walks in the park in the summer, instead of anxious trips to the veterinarian; anniversaries and holidays can be recalled with tenderness rather than despair. During this stage of grief, clients may consider sharing life with another pet for the sheer pleasure of having something warm and furry to hug again.

Loneliness

Regardless of how a loss occurs and how well prepared a client is, all clients feel their lives touched by loneliness. This can occur in the presence of family and friends, as well as in the company of remaining pets at home. The client shared a relationship with the departed pet that was special and separate from other relationships. Although other pets, family members, and friends can provide company and comfort, they cannot fill the space left by the departed pet. Loneliness arises from this space, and the space fills slowly as the grief process unfolds. Clients may express anger at losing this particular pet while others to whom they are less attached are healthy and well.

An appropriate response from the staff or veterinarian may be, "Even though you have other pets at home, you may still be lonely for Taffy. While you are healing from this loss, your other pets will still be there to love you."

REPLACEMENT

The decision to replace a deceased pet with a new one should be left solely to the individual experiencing the loss. The veterinary staff should not influence the decision in any way. Some pet owners choose to bond with new pets before their elderly pets die. Others decide that the presence of a new pet in their home would be stressful for the older pet and decide to wait. Some clients may never again adopt new pets. Everyone involved must consider the client's needs, as well as the needs of the current pet. It is important to try to not "fix" the client's loss by suggesting replacement.

If a client is trying to avoid the experience of loss by finding a replacement for the pet, bonding with the new pet usually does not occur. The new pet is not accepted as a unique being if the owner wants it to be just like the deceased pet. Often these new pets are given away or neglected. Owners may comment that the new Max is nothing like the old Max. Occasionally a client who had taken good care of a previous pet brings in a pet that has been neglected. This client probably has not bonded successfully with the new pet and may need support in deciding whether to keep it or find a new home for it. The client may not have resolved the loss of the previous pet and may need to see a counselor or support group that deals with pet loss issues.

ASSISTING BEREAVED PET OWNERS

Clients grieve in a variety of ways. Some demonstrate their emotions openly, whereas others may show little if any feeling in your presence. Do not assume that a stoic display means the client is not grieving.

Assess your client's feelings to determine how much support you should provide. When clients show reluctance to accept concerned overtures from you, take a minute to let them know that you care about their well-being. By acknowledging their sadness, you open the door for them to experience their emotions, giving the simple message that it is acceptable to grieve.

Veterinary staff members are in a position to encourage healthy coping skills in their clients. Clients look to the veterinary staff for support, assurance, understanding, and validation when facing a loss. If you can assist your clients in this way, you are building the foundation for natural resolution of the loss. In doing so, you continue to maintain their respect and solidify your working relationship. Recognizing the different stages of grief assists you in providing your clients with the type of support they need.

ACKNOWLEDGING THE LOSS

What a client needs and values most from the staff is their time and presence. In being present with clients during a loss, you help to legitimize the grief reaction and give them permission to verbalize their feelings. Many pet owners go to great lengths to appear stoic in the presence of others. In our society, death is often dealt with through denial, so it is vital that you validate the client's loss. The most beneficial thing a veterinary staff member can do for their clients is to let them know that grieving for the loss of a pet is perfectly normal.

Sending a card, personal note, or flowers to the client are all ways of expressing condolences. What clients will remember the most is how they were cared for during their loss. Being cared for and acknowledged is something a client will remember long after the flowers have wilted and the note or card has been discarded.

Veterinary staff members may feel uncomfortable in attending a grieving client. Some pet owners attribute unrealistic powers of control over life and death to their veterinarians. This is especially true for "last hope practitioners," veterinarians who are specialists in their fields. A client whose pet has cancer and who has been referred to an internist for treatment may have a strong need to believe that this doctor with specialized skills will be able to help the pet. This can place the veterinarian in the difficult position of conveying the limitations of treatment to the client.

Being with a client who is very tearful or angry can be an uncomfortable experience. You may worry that you will do or say the wrong thing. You may find it easier to hide behind the professional role and keep the client emotionally at a distance. This often leaves the client feeling neglected and abandoned. A client is less likely to return to an emotionally nonsupportive veterinary facility, even if the very best treatment was provided for the terminally ill pet.

Your responsibility is not to work in the capacity of a therapist or counselor. However, learning and using a variety of counseling and communication skills can enhance your relationships with your clients. By communicating effectively with your clients, you help them to accept and resolve their losses sooner than pet owners whose losses have not been properly acknowledged.

Useful skills and techniques that can be used to assist your clients include attending, effective listening, reflection, and validation.

Some clients are easier to help than others, and you must make an extra effort to support the more difficult ones. Demonstrate that you are attempting to understand what the clients are expressing by responding at appropriate intervals to their comments. Avoid using clichés or telling them that you know exactly how they feel; you don't.

Try saying, "What I hear you saying is …" Let the client tell you what the loss means to her. Ask the client, "How can I help you? What things have you done in the past that have supported you through a difficult time?"

Reflection

Summarizing what the client is expressing is called reflection. When you reflect their underlying concerns, clients feel that you understand what they are saying. In addition, you can reframe the experience of loss and hopelessness into one of hope and possibility.

By establishing open communication, you will be in a position to offer the kind of help that clients need. Some clients may only need to hear that they did the right thing and want to be informed of disposing of the remains. Others need emotional support and may be referred to a group or private therapist.

Validating the Loss

When your clients tell you what the loss means to them, it is important to let them know that you understand the relationship they have shared with the pet. In validating the loss, you will discover that a pet can fulfill many needs of pet owners. Be alert for key comments, such as, "We never had any children. Kelsey was like our child," "Buttons was my whole life," or "How will I ever feel safe alone at night without Cole?" A pet may have served as a child to some, a best friend to others, or even as a bridge to the past. It may have accompanied the owner from college to career, to marriage, and on through other important life stages. It may have been a source of comfort during a stressful time: a divorce, loss of a loved one, a move, or a change in jobs.

Attending

Without realizing it, you can make it difficult for clients to express their feelings and concerns. The way you sit, stand, look at, or speak with them can inhibit or enhance communication.

An open posture with uncrossed arms and legs demonstrates to your clients that you are available and ready to listen. Facing them directly while maintaining comfortable eye contact sends the message that you are interested in what they have to say. Avoid standing behind the counter, desk, or exam table when clients are expressing their feelings about their pet to you.

Effective Listening

Listening effectively is much more than hearing what a client is saying. Listening effectively means giving your complete attention and allowing time for the client to ramble, cry, and show anger. You should learn to tolerate periods of silence from the client. You may feel a strong desire to fill in the silence with words; refrain from doing so. The client needs you to be there silently.

By recognizing the different components of grief, you can accept a client's expressions of anger and denial and be empathetic about the guilt and deep sadness. Whether the client's initial reaction is overt despair or quiet shock, your interactions set the stage for the grieving process that follows.

The current loss can trigger remembrance of past losses, particularly for the elderly client. This compound effect may threaten to overwhelm the client. Clients can be reminded that this is a common reaction to loss of a pet.

Use your own words to convey messages of understanding and empathy toward your clients. The idea is to listen and then respond to clients by expressing the core significance of the loss. Validating the loss helps the client feel special and cared for by the veterinarian and the hospital staff.

Achieving Closure

The perfect way to end a conversation with a grieving client is to give a directive. For example, "I would like you to go home, get some rest, and then think about the options we discussed." Or you can inform the client about a support group in your area for bereaved pet owners. For example, "There is a place you can go and meet with other pet owners who are sharing similar feelings to yours." You can give the client a brochure or offer to make an appointment for him to talk with the support group leader.

Make clients take comfort in thinking about ways in which to honor their pets. For example, clients can donate to a charity in honor of a pet, plant a rosebush near the burial site, or create a scrapbook of memories shared with the pet.

The following suggestions may be helpful in assisting your clients:

- Provide facial tissues.
- Schedule appointment times to allow additional time to be spent with a bereaved pet owner or one whose pet is seriously ill.
- Create a brochure that includes all available support information (pet loss support groups, private therapists, hotlines, burial information, literature on pet loss, etc.). Make the brochure available to clients anticipating a loss as well as to those experiencing one.
- Send a sympathy card or flowers immediately after the loss. Late arrivals can be painful reminders for clients.
- Collect any fees owed before the euthanasia procedure is performed. A client will find it awkward to have to regain composure and pay a bill after the emotional experience of saying goodbye to a beloved pet.
- Let clients know that you and the rest of the staff are available to assist them, before and after the loss of a pet. Most pet owners have questions regarding their pets' illness and need reassurance that they did the right thing.
- If possible, maintain a private area in which clients can say goodbye to the pet, grieve, or regain composure. If such an area is not available, consider allowing extra time in the examination room before or after the loss.
- When attending to the patient, make certain that the owner can tell that the pet is comfortable and cared for. A simple gesture, such as placing a towel on a cold examination table, can demonstrate your compassion for the patient. If you send a final bill to the client, make sure it does not arrive on the same day as the sympathy card or flowers.

EFFECTS OF PATIENT LOSS ON STAFF

As difficult as the loss of a pet may be for a client, the loss of a patient may be difficult for the staff and veterinarian as well. Because euthanasia is an acceptable and legal means of terminating an animal's life, veterinary practitioners and their staff face a stress that is unknown to most other medical practitioners.

Each member of the staff has a personal set of beliefs and feelings regarding the issue of loss. Some may feel awkward attending a grieving client. Others may have unresolved feelings about pets they have lost themselves. Most people in the veterinary field have a love for animals and want to help them. Few consider the effect of the loss of a patient on themselves.

When assisting bereaved pet owners, staff members may feel emotions comparable to those the client experiences. Learn how to empathize and assist in a caring manner while still maintaining emotional distance.

The following steps will help you in this process:

- Take a team approach to cases in which euthanasia is an option. This can alleviate some of the feelings of failure and grief regarding loss of a patient.

- Create and participate in a support group for veterinary staff. This is a forum for airing private feelings and receiving feedback from peers.
- Refer pet owners to a pet loss support group. This provides clients with a safe place to share feelings and validates the fact that loss of a patient is a real and important consideration for everyone involved.
- Encourage open communication among staff members, confrontation of personal feelings and beliefs surrounding death, and self-examination regarding the emotional reaction to loss of a patient.

When a client is facing the crisis of losing a treasured pet, you can play a positive role in guiding the client through an emotionally difficult time, thereby solidifying your working relationship with the pet owner. Clients who respect the veterinarian and staff will speak highly of them to others, refer other pet owners to the practice, and return with new pets. Pet loss is an opportunity for everyone concerned to grow emotionally and to solidify working relationships.

COMPOUNDED LOSS

When faced with loss of a pet, the owner is often reminded of losses from the past, both human and animal. A compound loss can feel so overpowering that a client may respond in a way that seems out of proportion to the current facts. When this occurs, you might say, "I can see that you are troubled and concerned about Woody. Have you had other experience with loss?"

Sometimes an invitation to talk about a previous pet loss elicits information regarding past loss of family and friends, the demise of a relationship, or loss of a job. If the information is forthcoming, you can tell the client, "I know that when faced with the loss of a pet that you love, you can be reminded of other previous losses, and this can hurt more than if you were dealing with a single loss. Don't be surprised if you are suddenly recalling sad times from the past. Just know that it is very natural, at a time like this, to remember family and friends who are no longer with you. Try talking things over with a close friend, or, if you'd like, I can give you some referrals for counseling that might help you get through this difficult time."

Recognizing and Responding to Signals

A client may convey feelings of deep despair either verbally or through body language. Such statements as, "Muffin is the only friend I have in the world. I don't know how I can face another day without her by my side," or "Nothing matters now that Jake is dying. It will kill me to bring him in for euthanasia. I might as well be dead, too," should alert you to the need for outside professional evaluation and treatment.

You must determine if these clients have a reliable, concerned friend or relative who can stay with them, particularly if you have doubts about their safety if left alone. Make appropriate referrals and offer to call for an appointment before they leave the office. Do this openly to encourage trust and open communication. Knowing that an appointment has been arranged can have a calming and reassuring effect. Make every effort to secure the first appointment available and, if possible, telephone the client the next day for a "welfare check" and reminder of the appointment date and time. Extract a promise from the client that he or she will contact the crisis intervention hotline if he or she experiences overwhelming loneliness and sadness. Make certain you know the telephone number and that the client leaves your office with it.

If the client refuses any referrals or assistance and you sense that the client is a danger to himself or herself, you may need to resort to police escort of this client to a local psychiatric clinic for evaluation and treatment. This may be an extreme measure, but it could save a life. Let the veterinarian know about any concerns you may have regarding a client. Develop a protocol for clients experiencing emotional problems surrounding the death or illness of a pet. You might say to the client, "I know that you do not want to accept a referral for help, but I am so concerned about you that I will notify the police for assistance in getting you the help you need. I really do care about you and don't want anything bad to happen to you." Remember that extreme actions displayed by a client sometimes call for extreme reactions by the staff.

> **TECHNICIAN NOTE** Contact your local mental health department for assistance in compiling a list of mental health professionals and support groups.

Referring to Mental Health Professionals

Clients experiencing intense anger, despair, and guilt often benefit from professional intervention outside of your office. Maintain a list of counselors and support groups for referral of clients experiencing grief associated with pet loss. A pet loss support group can provide a client with a safe place to express his or her feelings. It offers clients the opportunity to meet with like-minded pet owners with whom to share their fears, tears, memories, and finally, smiles.

When making referrals for group or individual counseling services, you might say something like, "I know you are very sad about Mitzi's ailing health. Here is some information about a support group for people who are struggling with the loss of a pet. This may help you to sort out some of your feelings."

Your local mental health department can assist you in compiling a list of mental health professionals and support groups. The Delta Society in Bellevue, WA, maintains a list of pet loss support counselors and groups throughout the country. It also can provide you with additional books and videotapes on grief counseling. Assembling a community referral file for your clients takes time and effort, but this special service conveys the hospital staff's concern for their safety and well-being.

SUMMARY

Communication is a fundamental element in the success of veterinary technicians in practice today. It is no longer effective to have merely technical expertise; communication skills must also be present. The well-being of patients, superior service to clients, and the happiness of the team are all benefits to the practice that nurtures and develops the communication proficiency of the healthcare team.

REVIEW QUESTIONS

Multiple Choice

1. When a person has folded arms, it generally indicates that he or she is
   a. angry
   b. defensive
   c. uncomfortable
   d. superior
2. Body language accounts for almost ___% of communication.
   a. 70
   b. 50
   c. 20
   d. 10
3. A body posture that may reflect lack of confidence is
   a. head down, shoulders in
   b. back straight, shoulders back
   c. arms folded, head up
   d. straight back, head down
4. To demonstrate that you are interested in what another person is saying, you should
   a. maintain eye contact
   b. stare at them
   c. cross your arms
   d. fold your hands
5. When educating clients about their pet's health, what should you always use?
   a. proper medical terminology
   b. models and handouts
   c. a loud commanding tone of voice
   d. their pet to show them what is wrong
6. Owners that are well bonded to their pets are more likely to
   a. request euthanasia so their pet doesn't suffer
   b. become angry with the practice staff
   c. get a new pet as soon as one dies
   d. recognize signs of illness in their pets
7. Which method is effective at helping to strengthen the human-animal bond?
   a. choosing an active pet
   b. recommending puppy/kitten socialization class and obedience training
   c. getting a new pet as soon as one dies
   d. choosing a sedentary pet
8. What percentage of the households in the US that own at least one pet indicate that their bond with their pet is "very strong"?
   a. 10%
   b. 30%
   c. 50%
   d. 80%
9. Empathetic listening:
   a. demonstrates focused listening and understanding
   b. is intimidating to the speaker
   c. causes a judgmental type of response
   d. will alienate clients
10. Assertive communication helps to increase understanding of:
   a. thoughts and feelings
   b. behavior and body language
   c. people and their communication styles
   d. people's love of their pets

Matching

Match each stage of grief with its description.

___1. Denial
___2. Bargaining
___3. Anger
___4. Guilt
___5. Sorrow
___6. Resolution

A. blame directed at the veterinarian, staff members, or client themselves
B. sadness, and perhaps release of days or weeks of pent-up emotions
C. a coping mechanism that cushions the mind against the shock it has received
D. realization that the pet is gone, nothing will change that, and client will survive this loss
E. unproductive, unreasonable feeling of responsibility that may inhibit progress toward resolution of the loss
F. a way of keeping hope alive and buying time to fully accept the outcome of the situation

Match the following terms with their definition.

_____1. Compounded Loss
_____2. Action Steps
_____3. Empathetic Listening
_____4. Body Language
_____5. Assertive Communication

A. communicating without judgment, demonstrating caring and understanding
B. communication with focus on speaking in a positive and proactive manner
C. use of eyes, gestures, and body in conveying a message
D. a list version of exactly what must occur to resolve a conflict
E. situation where a client facing the loss of a pet is reminded of losses from the past

RECOMMENDED READING

Adler M: *How to speak, how to listen*, New York, 1997, Collier Books.

Allessandra T, Hunsaker P: *Communicating at work*, New York, 1993, Simon and Schuster.

Bacal R: *Complete idiot's guide to dealing with difficult employees*, Madison, WI, 2000, CWL Publishing.

Bordeaux D: *12 Steps to personal and professional development*, Mill Valley, CA, 1993, Wildflower Press.

Deep S, Sussman L: *What to say to get what you want*, Reading, MA, 1992, Addison-Wesley.

Fuller G: *The workplace survival guide*, Englewood Cliffs, NJ, 1996, Prentice Hall.

Griffin J: *How to say it at work*, ed 2, New York, 2008, Prentice Hall.

Guntzelman J, Reiger M: Helping pet owners with the euthanasia decision, *Vet Med* 88:26–34, 1993.

Guntzelman J, Reiger M: Supporting clients who are grieving the death of a pet, *Vet Med* 88:35–41, 1993.

Hart LA, Hart BL: Grief and stress from so many animal deaths, *Companion Animal Practice* 1:20–21, 1987.

Kübler-Ross E: *On death and dying*, New York, 1968, Collier Books.

Siress R: *Working woman's communication survival guide*, Englewood Cliffs, NJ, 1994, Prentice Hall.

Tingley JC: *Say what you mean, get what you want*, New York, 1996, American Management Association.

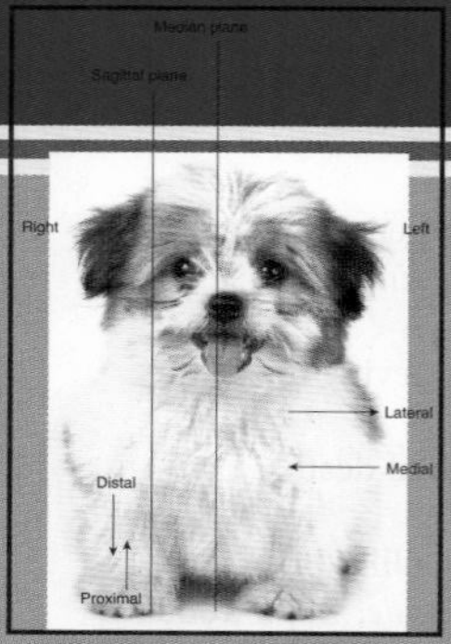

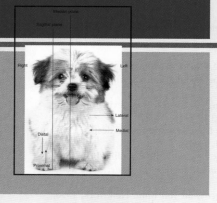

5 Medical Terminology

OUTLINE

LEARNING OBJECTIVES

After reviewing this chapter, the reader will be able to:

1. Construct medical terms from word parts.
2. Describe how to construct medical terms.
3. Define the meanings of common prefixes and suffixes used in medical terms.
4. List combining forms used to refer to various body parts.
5. Discuss terms for direction, position, and movement.
6. Define terms used for common surgical procedures, diseases, instruments, procedures, and dentistry.
7. Name the types of cells and tissues that make up the animal body.
8. Name the types of bones and muscles that make up the animal body.
9. List and describe the components of the integument.

KEY TERMS

Abduction
Adduction
Caudal
Combining form
Combining vowel
Compound word
Cranial
Distal
Dorsal
Extension
Flexion
Lateral
Medial
Oblique
Palmar
Peripheral
Plantar
Prefix
Proximal
Recumbent
Root word
Rostral
Suffix
Superficial
Supine
Ventral

Veterinary medical terminology is the "language" of the veterinary profession. This language is used in everyday speech, recorded in medical records, and used in journal articles and published textbooks for veterinary technicians and veterinarians. The most important part of this chapter is to learn correct pronunciation and proper spelling of medical terms. Next you will learn to memorize word parts and their meanings. Then you will be able to recognize and use medical words correctly. To assist with correct pronunciation, accented syllables are printed in UPPERCASE LETTERS. Syllables that are not accented are in lowercase letters. In multisyllabic words with primary and secondary accents, the syllable with the primary accent is in **BOLDFACE UPPERCASE LETTERS,** and the syllable with the secondary accent is in UPPERCASE LETTERS. Unaccented syllables are in lowercase letters. Words of one syllable are in lowercase letters. Multisyllabic words, in which all syllables receive equal stress, are in lowercase letters.

INTRODUCTION TO WORD PARTS

PREFIX

A prefix is a syllable, a group of syllables, or a word joined to the beginning of another word to alter its meaning or create a new word. The prefix may provide position, time, amount, color, or direction to a root word. A prefix is not often used as a word alone unless a hyphen is inserted between it and the following word.

Example: *Pre-* is a prefix meaning "before, in space or in time." When joined to the root word *natal,* meaning "birth," the result becomes the medical word: *PREnatal.* Prenatal means "before birth." The prefix *pre* used alone means nothing to the reader.

ROOT WORD

A root word is the subject part of the word consisting of a syllable, group of syllables, or word that is the basis (or word base) for the meaning of the medical word.

Example: *CARdi-* is a root word meaning "heart." The root word used alone means nothing to the reader, as shown in the following example.

Example: The patient was diagnosed with *CARdi.* Now add the suffix *itis* (meaning "inflammation") to the end of the root word. The sentence begins to make sense with this addition: The patient was diagnosed with carDItis, or inflammation of the heart.

COMBINING FORM

A combining form is a word or root word that may or may not use the connecting vowel *o* when it is used as an element in a medical word formation. The combining form is the combination of the root word and the combining vowel. It is generally written in the following manner:

Example: CARdi/*o*: the combining form for the heart (root word plus combining vowel)

See *combining vowel.*

COMBINING VOWEL

A combining vowel is a vowel, usually an *o,* used to connect a word or root word to the appropriate suffix or to another root word.

COMBINING VOWEL ADDED TO A SUFFIX

A suffix is a syllable, a group of syllables, or a word added at the end of a root word to change its meaning, give it grammatical function, or form a new word. Suffixes normally do not stand alone as words. When they are used alone, a hyphen is used preceding and attached to the suffix.

Example: *-gram* is a suffix meaning "a recording by an instrument." A cardiogram is a recording of heart movement made by an instrument.

COMPOUND WORD

A compound word is two or more words or root words combined to make a new word.

Example: *Horse* and *fly* combine to form the word *HORSEfly.*

TECHNICIAN NOTE Prefixes, root words, and suffixes can be combined to form medical terms.

USING WORD PARTS TO FORM WORDS

USE OF THE PREFIX

A prefix is attached to the beginning of a root word to form a new word.

Example: Prefix + Root Word = New Word

Prefix	Root word	Combined	Definition
de-	horn	DEhorn	To remove the horns
semi-	PERme-able	semiPER-meable	Allowing only certain elements or liquids to pass through a membrane

SUFFIX

A suffix is attached to the end of a root word to form a new word.

Example: Root Word + Suffix = New Word

Root word	Suffix	Combined	Definition
TONsil	-itis	TONsilItis	Inflammation of the tonsils
THYroid	-ectomy	THYroid-**EC**tomy	Removal of the thyroid gland

COMPOUND WORD

Two words are joined together to form a new word.

Example: Root Word 1 + Root Word 2 = New Word

Word 1	Word 2	Combined	Definition
lock	jaw	LOCKjaw	Common name for the disease tetanus
blood	worms	BLOOD-worms	Worms (nematodes) that inhabit a main artery of the intestines in horses

There are certain rules peculiar to the use of combining forms and the combining vowel *o.* These rules are as follows:

- If a suffix begins with a consonant, use the combining vowel *o* with the root word (the combining form), to which the suffix will be added.

Example: *CARdi/o* (combining form for heart) plus the suffix *megaly* (meaning "enlargement of") forms *CARdio-**MEG**aly,* meaning "enlargement of the heart." Note the combining vowel *o* is retained.

- Do not use the combining vowel *o* when a suffix begins with a vowel.

Example: *HEPat/o* (combining form for liver) plus the suffix *osis* (meaning "a condition, disease, or morbid process"), combine to form *HEPa**TO**sis,* meaning "a disease occurring in the liver." Note the combining vowel *o* is not used.

- If the suffix begins with the same vowel with which the combining form ends (minus the combining vowel *o*), do not repeat the vowel when forming the new word.

Example: *CARdi/o* minus *o* is *CARdi-*. *CARdi-* plus *-itis* (meaning "inflammation of") combines to form *carDItis,* meaning "inflammation of the heart." Note, as the rule states, this word may have only a single *i* as the medical root word joins the suffix.

Combining forms	Suffix	Combined	Definitions
cardi/o	-logy	CARdiOLogy	Study of heart diseases
mast/o	-itis	masTItis	Inflammation of the mammary glands

PREFIX AND SUFFIX

In this situation, no root word is used. The prefix is added directly to the suffix.

Prefix	Suffix	Combined	Definition
dys-	-uria	dysUria	Trouble urinating
POLy-	-phagia	POLyPHAgia	Eating to excess

PREFIX, ROOT WORD, AND SUFFIX

Words are formed by adding both the prefix and suffix to the root word.

Prefix	Root word	Suffix	Combined	Definition
un-	sound	-ness	unSOUNDness	A form of physical dysfunction
PERi-	cardi-	-al	PERiCARdial	In the area surrounding the heart

DEFINING MEDICAL TERMS USING WORD ANALYSIS

Analyzing words teaches you to think logically and makes words easier to remember. The process of word analysis is the reverse of word construction. When analyzing a word, start at the end of the word (the suffix) and work toward the beginning (prefix). Analyze the components in sequence.

> TECHNICIAN NOTE Analyze medical terms by defining each word component in sequence starting at the suffix.

Example: oVARioHYSter**EC**tomy =
ovari/o/hyster/ectomy
4 3 2 1

1. The suffix *-ectomy* means to surgically remove.
2. The root word *hyster* refers to the uterus.
3. The *o* is the combining vowel for the previous root word.
4. The root word *ovari* refers to the ovaries.

Thus, *ovariohysterectomy* means "excision (surgical removal) of the uterus and ovaries." Note that steps 3 and 4 may be combined into one step, using the combining form *ovari/o,* which refers to the ovaries.

COMBINING FORMS FOR BODY PARTS AND ANATOMY

Following is a list of body parts and their respective combining forms. This is not a complete list of combining forms, but it represents some used often in veterinary terminology. To learn these words and their meaning requires memorization. Students should use handheld flash cards with the combining form on one side and the meaning or body part on the other.

Combining Form	Body Part
abdomin/o	abdomen
aden/o	gland
adren/o	adrenal gland
angi/o	vessel
arteri/o	artery
arthr/o	joint
atri/o	atrium
blephar/o	eyelid, eyelash
bronch/o	bronchus
cardi/o	heart
cephel/o	head
cerebell/o	cerebellum
cerebr/o	cerebrum
cervic/o	cervix or neck of an organ
cheil/o	lip
chol/o, chole-	bile
cholecyst/o	gallbladder
chondr/o	cartilage
cili/o	eyelid, eyelash
col/o	colon
colp/o	vagina
cost/o	rib
crani/o	cranium, skull
cyst/o	bladder
cyt/o	cell
dactyl/o	digit, toe
dent/o	tooth, teeth
derm/o, dermat/o	skin
duoden/o	duodenum
encephal/o	brain
enter/o	intestines
epididym/o	epididymis
epis/o, episi/o	vulva
esophag/o	esophagus
faci/o	face
fibr/o	fibers
gastr/o	stomach
gingiv/o	gums
gloss/o	tongue
gnath/o	jaw
hem/o, hemat/o	blood
hepa-, hepat/o	liver

Combining Form	Body Part
hist/o	tissue
hyster/o	uterus
ile/o	ileum (of intestine)
ili/o	ilium (of pelvis)
jejun/o	jejunum
kerat/o	cornea or horny tissue
labi/o	lip
lapar/o	flank, abdomen
laryng/o	larynx
lip/o	fat
lymph/o	lymph
mast/o, mamm/o	mammary glands
mening/o	meninges
metr/o	uterus (special reference to inner lining)
muscul/o, my/o, myos-	muscle
myel/o	bone marrow or spinal cord
nephr/o	kidney, nephron
neur/o	nerve
occipit/o	back of head
ocul/o	eye
odont/o	tooth, teeth
onych/o	claw, hoof
ophthalm/o	eye
orchi/o, orchid/o	testes
or/o	mouth
oste/o, oss/eo, oss/i	bone
ot/o	ear
ovari/o	ovary
palat/o	palate
peritone/o	peritoneum
pharyng/o	pharynx
phleb/o	vein
pil/o	hair
pneum/o	lung, air, breath
pod/o	foot
proct/o	rectum
pulmo-, pulmon/o	lung
pyel/o	pelvis of kidney
rect/o	rectum
ren/o	renal (kidney)
rhin/o	nose
splen/o	spleen
spondyl/o	vertebra, spinal column
steth/o	chest
stomat/o	mouth
tars/o	ankle
ten/o, tend/o	tendon
thorac/o	thorax
thym/o	thymus gland
thyr/o, thyroid-	thyroid gland
tonsill/o	tonsil
trache/o	trachea
trich/o	hair
tympan/o	tympanum (middle ear), tympanic membrane, eardrum
ureter/o	ureter
urethr/o	urethra
ur/o	urine
uter/o	uterus
vagin/o	vagina
vas/o	vessel or duct
ven/o	vein
ventricul/o	ventricle
vertebr/o	vertebra
vulv/o	vulva

Remember, words for some body parts have more than one combining form. Examples from the previous list are the following:

mouth = or/o, stomat/o

teeth = dent/o, odont/o

There are no general rules for when one or the other is used. This must be learned by listening and reading to be aware of how these combining forms are used. You already know some of them. For instance, you know that there is oral medication, not stomatal medication. Often the different combining forms refer to a specific part of a structure or a specific use of the structure. *Or/o* often refers to the mouth as the first part of the digestive system, whereas *stomat/o* refers to the lining of the oral cavity or the opening to the oral cavity (e.g., stomatitis, stomatoplasty).

SUFFIXES FOR SURGICAL PROCEDURES

Following is a list of suffixes for surgical procedures. Using the rules for word construction, you can form words to describe a variety of surgical procedures on various body parts or define these words using the word analysis technique previously described.

Suffix	Meaning	Example and definition
-centesis	to puncture, perforate, or tap—permitting withdrawal of fluid, air, etc.	AbDOMinocenTEsis = surgical puncture of the abdomen to remove fluid from the peritoneal cavity
-ectomy	to excise or surgically remove	CHOLecysTECtomy = surgical removal of the gallbladder
-ize	use, subject to	An**ES**theTIZE = subject to anesthesia
-pexy	fixation or suturing (a stabilizing type of repair)	GAStroPEXy = fixation of the stomach to the body wall
-plasty	to shape, the surgical formation of, or plastic surgery (meaning "to improve function, to relieve pain, or for cosmetic reasons")	CHEIloPLASty = plastic repair of the lips (to improve looks and function)

Suffix	Meaning	Example and definition
-rrhaphy	to surgically repair by joining in a seam or by suturing together	HERniORRhaphy = surgical repair of a hernia
-stomy	to make a new, artificial opening in a hollow organ (to the outside of the body), or to make a new opening between two hollow organs	CoLOStomy = surgical creation of a new opening between the colon and the outside of the bodyGAStroDUodeNOStomy = to create a new opening between the stomach and the duodenum
-tomy	to incise or cut into (making an incision)	LAPaROTomy = surgical incision into the abdomen

SUFFIXES FOR DISEASES OR CONDITIONS

The same rules and procedures used to form and analyze surgical words can be used with suffixes that refer to diseases or conditions to describe a problem affecting a particular organ or body part. Following is a list of these suffixes.

Suffix	Meaning	Example and definition
-algia	pain	MyALgia = muscular pain
-emesis	vomit	HemateMEsis = vomiting blood
-emia	blood condition	AnEmia = lack of blood
-esis, -iasis, -asis	infestation or infection with, a condition characterized by	ParEsis = partial paralysis LithIasis = condition characterized by formation of calculi
-genesis	development, origin	CarCINo**GEN**esis = development of cancer
-ism	a state or condition, a fact of being, result of a process	HyperCORtiSONism = condition resulting from excessive cortisone
-itis	inflammation of	TONsilItis = inflammation of the tonsils
-megaly	enlarged	HePAto**MEG**aly = enlarged liver
-oma	tumor	LEIomyOMa = tumor of smooth muscles
-osis	abnormal condition or process of degeneration	NePHROsis = degenerative disease of the kidneys
-path, -pathy	disease	pathogenic = disease causing
-penia	deficiency or lack of	LEUko**PEN**ia = deficiency of white blood cells
-phage, -phagy	eating	COproPHAgy = eating feces
-phobia	abnormal fear or intolerance of	PHOto**PHO**bia = intolerance of light
-plasia, -plastic, -plasty	forming, growing, changing	ANa**PLA**sia = changing structure of cells**RHI**no-PLASty = surgical change to the nose
-pnea	breathing	DYSpnea = difficulty breathing
-rrhea	flow or discharge	DIar**RHE**a = discharge of feces

PREFIXES FOR DISEASES OR CONDITIONS

Following is a list of prefixes used to create words indicating a specific problem within the body or a body system.

Prefix	Meaning	Example and definition
a-, an-	without or not having	aNEmia = not having enough red blood cells
anti-	against	AntibiOTic = drug that acts against bacteria
brachy-	short	BRAchycePHALic = short head
brady-	slow	BRAdy**CAR**dia = excessively slow heart rate
cata-	down, under, lower, against	CaTAbolism = breaking down
contra-	against, opposed	CONtra**IN**diCAted = something that is not indicated
crypt/o	hidden	CryptORCHidism = hidden or undescended testis
de-	remove, take away, loss of	deHYdrated = excessive loss of body water
dis-	apart from, free from	DISin**FEC**tion = to free from infection
dolich/o-	long	DOlichocePHALic = long head
dys-	difficult, painful, abnormal	DysPHAgia = difficulty eating or swallowing
e-, ec-, ex-	out of, from, away from	ecTOPic = out of place
eu-	normal, good, true, healthy	EUthan**A**sia = inducing death painlessly

Prefix	Meaning	Example and definition
glyc/o-, gluc/o-	sugar, sweet	HyperglycEMia = a condition of excessive sugar in the blood
hem/a-, hemat/o-, hem/o-	blood	HEmat**UR**ia = blood in the urine
hemi-	half	hemiPLEgia = paralysis of one side of the body
hydr/o-	water, fluid	HYdro**CEPH**alus = fluid in the brain
hyper-	high, excessive	HYper**THER**mia = body temperature higher than normal
hypo-	low, insufficient	HYpo**THY**roidism = deficiency of thyroid activity
macro-	large	MAcrocyte = large cell
mal-	bad, poor	MALoc**CLU**sion = poor fit of upper and lower teeth when jaws close
meg/a-, meg/alo-	large, oversized	**ME**gaCOLon = abnormally enlarged colon
micro-	small	MIcroph**THAL**mos = abnormally small eye
necr/o-	death	NEcropsy = examination of dead animal
neo-	new	NeoPLAStic = new tissue growth
olig/o-	few, little	OLig**UR**ia = scant urine production
pan-	all, entire	PanzoOtic = throughout an animal population
poly-	many, much	POLy**PHA**gia = excessive eating
pseudo-	false	PSEUdocy**E**sis = false pregnancy
py/o-	pus	PYo**ME**tra = pus in the uterus
tachy-	fast, rapid	TACHy**CAR**dia = excessively fast heart rate
ur/e-, ur/ea-, ur/eo-, ur/in-, ur/ino, ur/o	urine or urea	GlucosURia = sugar in the urine UrEMia = urea in the blood

PLURAL ENDINGS

It is important to understand the methods for converting singular forms of medical words to their plural forms, and vice versa. Following is a list of common singular endings and their corresponding plural endings.

Singular	Plural	Example
-a	-ae	VERtebra, VERtebrae
-anx	-anges	PHAlanx, phaLANges
-en	-ina	LUmen, LUmina
-ex, -ix	-ices	Apex, Apices; CERvix, CERvices
-is	-es	TEStis, TEStes
-inx	-inges	MENinx, meNINges
-ma	-mata or -mas	ENema, ENeMAta or ENemas
-um	-a	Ovum, Ova
-ur	-ora	FEMur, FEMora
-us	-i	Uterus, Uteri

SUFFIXES FOR INSTRUMENTS, PROCEDURES, AND MACHINES

Below is a list of suffixes that, when added to a combining form of a body part, form a word pertaining to an instrument, procedure, or a machine that looks into, cuts, or measures a body part.

Suffix	Meaning	Example and definition
-gram	product, written record, "picture," or graph produced	ELECtro**CAR**diogram (ECG, EKG) = graphic tracing of the electrical currents flowing through the beating heart
-graph	instrument or machine that writes or records	ELECtro**CAR**diograph = machine that records electrical impulses produced by the beating heart
-graphy	procedure of using an instrument or machine to record	ELECtroCARdi**O**Graphy = procedure of using an electrocardiograph to produce an electrocardiogram
-meter	instrument or machine that measures or counts	TherMOmeter = instrument used to measure body temperature
-metry -imetry	procedure of measuring	doSIMetry = act of determining the amount, rate, and distribution of ionizing radiation
-scope	instrument for examining, viewing, or listening	OtoSCOPE = instrument for looking into the ears
-scopy	act of examining or using the scope	LAPa**ROS**copy = procedure of using a laparoscope to view the abdominal cavity

Suffix	Meaning	Example and definition
-tome	instrument for cutting, such as into smaller or thinner sections	MicroTOME = instrument for cutting tissues into microthin slices or sections

TERMS FOR DIRECTION, POSITION, AND MOVEMENT

TECHNICIAN NOTE Anatomic terms of direction are used when describing locations of lesions on an animal's body and for positioning animals for radiography.

Following is a list of words used to describe direction or the position of a body part relative to other body parts.

CRAnial: Pertaining to the cranium or head end of the body, or denoting a position more toward the cranium or head end of the body than another reference point (body part) (Figs. 5-1 to 5-3). Example: The head is **cranial** to the tail.

CAUdal: Pertaining to the tail end of the body, or denoting a position more toward the tail or rear of the body than another reference point (body part) (Figs. 5-1 to 5-3). Example: The tail is **caudal** to the head.

ROStral: Pertaining to the nose end of the head or body, or toward the nose (Figs. 5-1 to 5-3). Example: The nose is **rostral** to the eyes.

MEdial: Denoting a position closer to the median plane of the body or a structure, toward the middle or median plane, or pertaining to the middle or a position closer to the median plane of the body or a structure (Figs. 5-1 to 5-3). Example: The **medial** surface of the leg is the "inside" surface.

LATeral: Denoting a position farther from the median plane of the body or a structure, on the side or toward the side away from the median plane, or pertaining to the side of the body or of a structure (Figs. 5-1 to 5-3). Example: The **lateral** surface of the leg is the "outside" surface.

DORsal: Pertaining to the back area of a quadruped (animal with four legs), or denoting a position more toward the spine than another reference point (body part) (Figs. 5-1 to 5-3). Example: The vertebral column is **dorsal** to the abdomen.

VENtral: Pertaining to the underside of a quadruped, or denoting a position more toward the abdomen than another reference point (body part) (Figs. 5-1 to 5-3). Example: The intestines are **ventral** to the vertebral column.

peRIPHeral: Pertaining to or situated near the periphery, the outermost part, or surface of an organ or part. Example: The enamel of a tooth is **peripheral** to the dentin and central root canal.

CENtral: Pertaining to or situated near the more **proximal** areas of the body or a structure; opposite of peripheral. Example: The spinal cord is central to the sciatic nerve.

SUperFIcial: Situated near the surface of the body or a structure; opposite of deep. Example: The skin is **superficial** to the muscles.

deep: Situated away from the surface of the body or a structure; opposite of superficial. Example: The muscles are deep to the skin.

adJAcent: Next to, adjoining, or close. Example: The tongue is adjacent to the teeth.

PROXimal: Nearer to the center of the body, relative to another body part, or a location on a body part relative to another, more distant, location (Figs. 5-1 to 5-3). Example: The humerus is **proximal** to the radius.

DIStal: Farther from the center of the body, relative to another body part or a location on a body part relative to another closer location (Figs. 5-1 to 5-3). Example: The tibia is **distal** to the femur.

obLIQUE: At an angle, or pertaining to an angle. Example: The vein crosses **obliquely** from the dorsal left side to the ventral right side.

reCUMbent: Lying down; a modifying term is needed to describe the surface on which the animal is lying. Example: An animal in dorsal **recumbency** is lying on its dorsum (back), face up.

SUpine, SUpinNAtion: Lying face up, in dorsal recumbency. **Supination** is the act of turning the body or a leg so that the ventral aspect is uppermost.

prone, proNAtion: Lying face down, in ventral recumbency. Pronation is the act of turning the body or a leg so the ventral aspect is down.

PALmar: **Palmar** pertains to the caudal surface of the front foot distal to the antebrachiocarpal joint; also pertains to the undersurface of the front foot (Figs. 5-1 to 5-3).

PLANtar: **Plantar** pertains to the caudal surface of the back foot distal to the tarsocrural joint; also pertains to the undersurface of the rear foot (Figs. 5-1 to 5-3).

abDUCtion: Movement of a limb or part away from the median line or middle of the body (Fig. 5-4).

adDUCtion: Movement of a limb or part toward the median line or middle of the body (Fig. 5-4).

FLEXion: The act of bending, such as a joint (Fig. 5-5).

exTENsion: The act of straightening, such as a joint; also, the act of pulling two component parts apart to lengthen the whole part (Fig. 5-5).

DENTAL TERMINOLOGY

The teeth have their own set of positional terms listed below.

ocCLUsal: The chewing or biting surface of teeth; toward the plane between the mandibular and maxillary teeth (Fig. 5-6).

BUccal: Toward the cheek; tooth surface toward the cheek (Fig. 5-6).

LINGual: Pertaining to the tongue; tooth surface toward the tongue (Fig. 5-6).

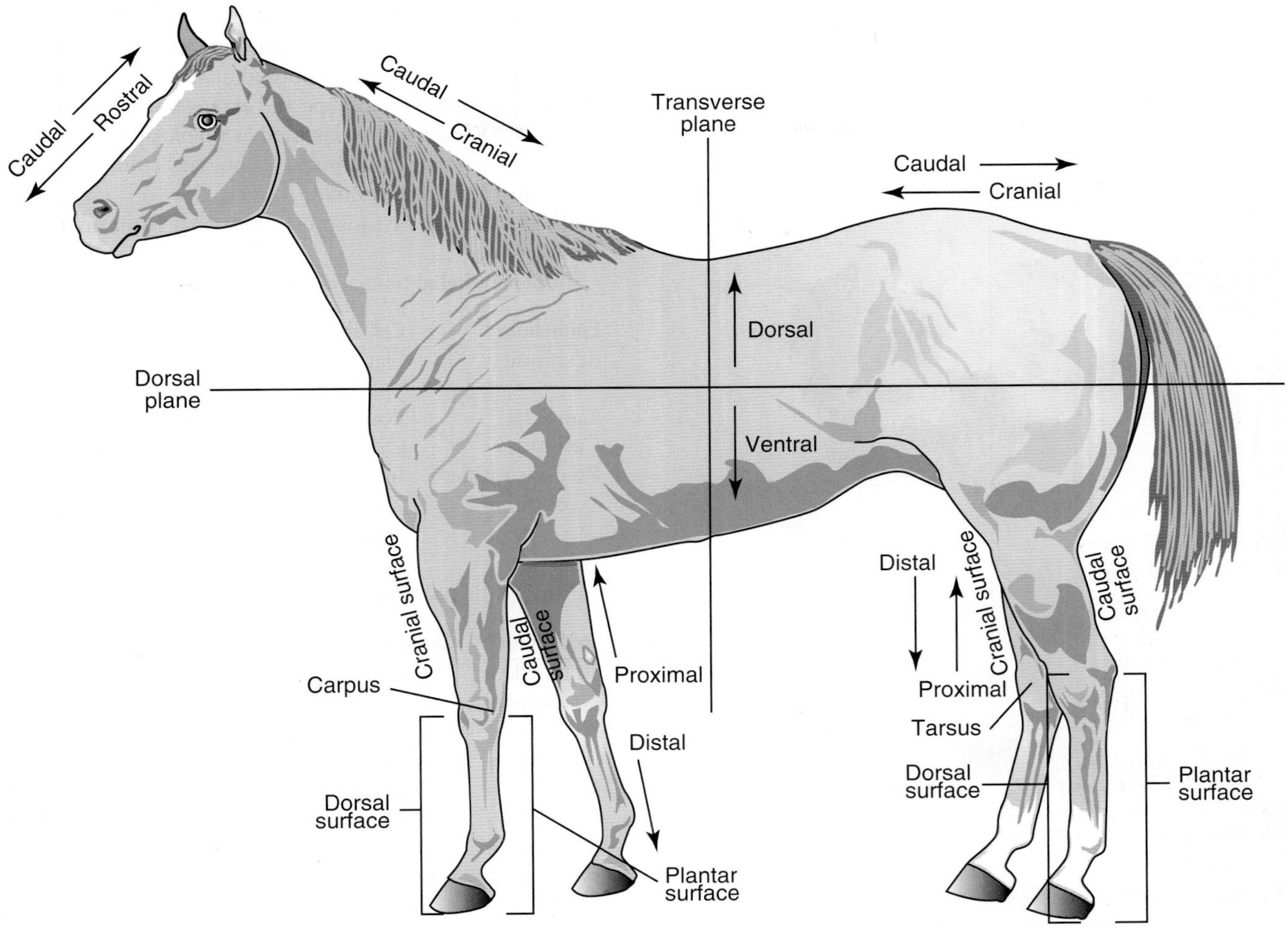

FIGURE 5-1 Anatomical planes and directional terms. Horse. (From Colville T, Bassert JM: *Clinical anatomy and physiology laboratory manual for veterinary technicians*, St Louis, 2009, Mosby.)

CONtact: Tooth surface facing an adjacent or opposing tooth (Fig. 5-6).

MEsial: Tooth surface closest to the midline of the dental arcade.

SPECIFIC TERMINOLOGY OF ANATOMY AND PHYSIOLOGY

CELLS

Unlike single-celled animals, complex (multicelled) organisms have specialized cells that allow the whole body to operate. Groups of specialized cells make up tissues. Four basic types of tissues make up the animal body: epithelial tissue, connective tissue, muscle tissue, and nervous tissue. Functional groupings of tissues make up organs, such as the kidneys, that contain elements of all four basic tissues. Systems are groups of organs that are involved in a common activity. For example, the salivary glands, esophagus, stomach, pancreas, liver, and intestines are all parts of the digestive system.

> TECHNICIAN NOTE The four basic types of tissues are epithelial tissue, connective tissue, muscle tissue, and nervous tissue.

EPITHELIAL TISSUE

Epithelial tissue covers the interior and exterior surfaces of the body, lines body cavities, and forms glands. Its function includes protection from physical wear and tear as well as penetration by foreign invaders, selective absorption of substances (e.g., by the intestinal lining), and secretion of various substances. All epithelial tissues share three common features:

- They consist entirely of cells.
- They do not contain blood vessels. Epithelial cells derive nourishment from blood vessels in the connective tissues beneath them.
- At least some epithelial cells are capable of reproducing. Epithelial tissue cells must be capable of compensating for wear and tear, as well as injuries.

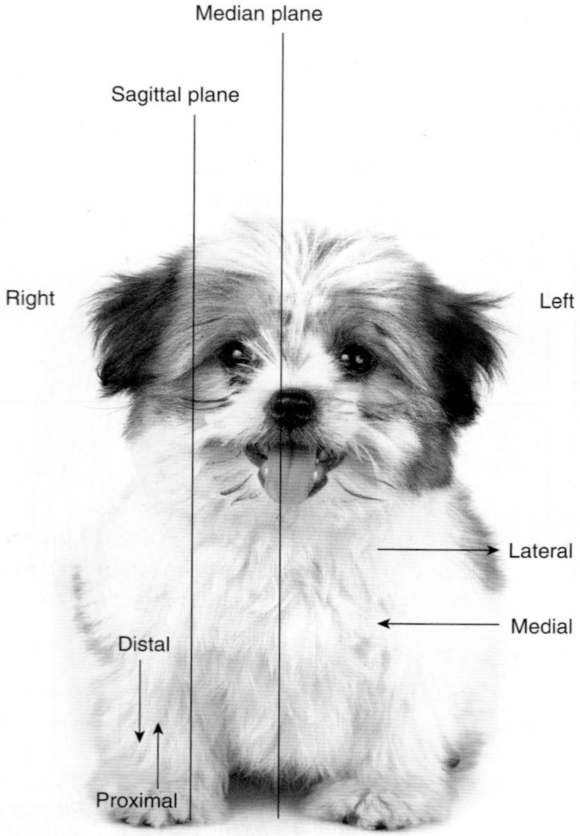

FIGURE 5-2 Anatomical planes and directional terms. Dog. (From iStock.com/Portogas-D-Ace.)

The covering and lining of epithelial tissue can be either simple (one cell-layer thick) or stratified (more than one cell-layer thick), and it can be composed of several different cell types. Depending on the shape and arrangement of cells, the epithelial tissue is further classified as *simple* or *stratified:*

Simple epithelium: squamous, cuboidal, columnar, and pseudostratified columnar

Stratified epithelium: squamous, cuboidal, columnar, and transitional

Simple epithelial tissues are the following:

Epithelium	Cell shape	Example
Squamous	Flat, platelike	Blood vessel lining
Cuboidal	Round or cuboidal	Kidney tubules
Columnar	Cylindrical	Intestinal lining
Pseudostratified columnar	Irregular; nuclei not uniform in position	Upper respiratory tract lining

Stratified epithelial tissues are the following:

Epithelium	Characteristics	Example
Stratified squamous	Thick and tough. Deepest cells reproduce, pushing daughter cells toward the surface. They gradually die and assume a flattened shape as they move farther from their nutrient source in the underlying connective tissue	Skin

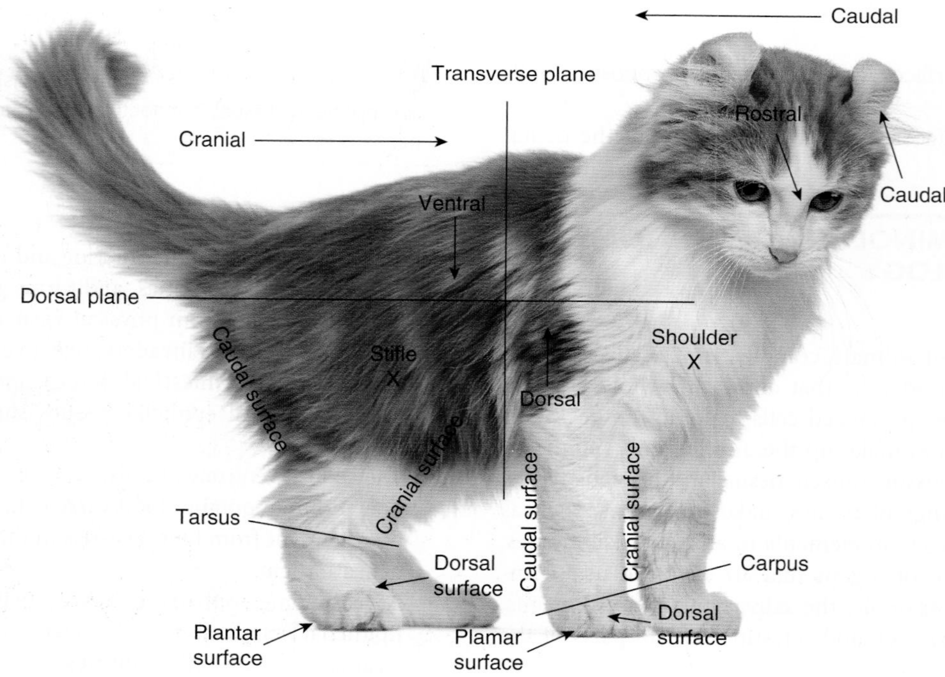

FIGURE 5-3 Anatomical planes and directional terms. Cat. (From iStock.com/Eric Isselée.)

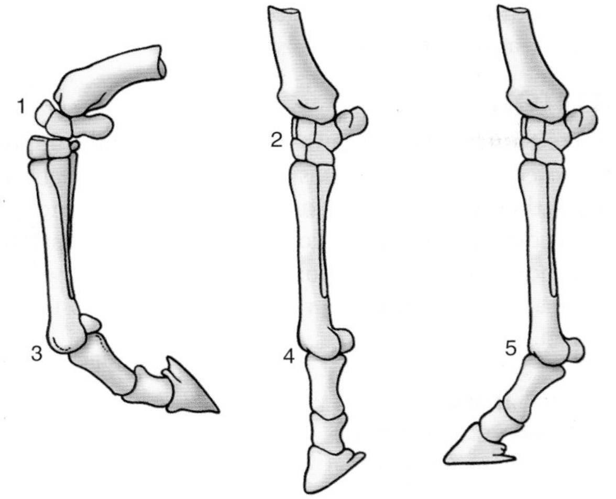

FIGURE 5-4 Terms denoting limb movement: flexion and extension. (From Dyce K, Wensing C, Sack W: *Textbook of veterinary anatomy,* ed 4, St Louis, 2009, Elsevier.)

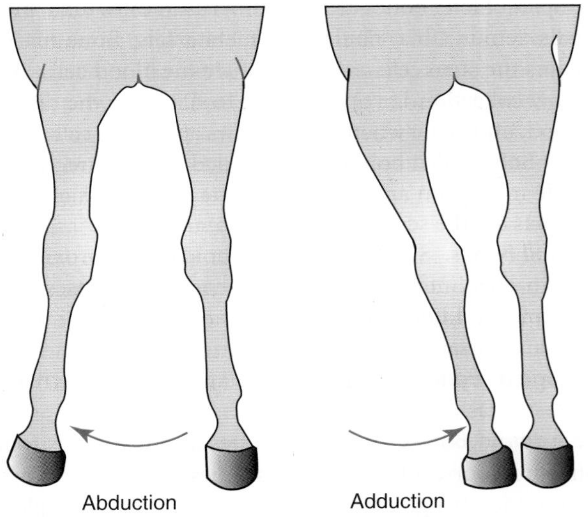

FIGURE 5-5 Terms denoting limb movement: adduction and abduction. (From Colville T, Bassert JM: *Clinical anatomy and physiology for veterinary technicians,* ed 2, St Louis, 2008, Mosby.)

Epithelium	Characteristics	Example
Stratified cuboidal	Rare in the body	Ducts of sweat glands
Stratified columnar	Rare in the body and usually seen where one type of epithelium is blending into another type of epithelium	Junction of oropharynx and nasopharynx
Transitional	Capable of considerable stretching	Urinary bladder lining

Glandular epithelium cells are specialized cells that secrete substances directly into the bloodstream or out onto a body surface. The ductless glands that secrete directly into the bloodstream are the endocrine glands (e.g., pituitary gland, thyroid, testes, ovaries, and adrenal gland). They produce hormones. Exocrine glands secrete substances through ducts. They can be simple, with a single duct (e.g., sweat glands), or compound, with a branching duct system (e.g., mammary glands).

CONNECTIVE TISSUE

Connective tissue holds the different tissues together and provides support. It contains few cells and more fibers as compared with epithelial tissue. If the body consisted entirely of cells, it would lie like a puddle of gelatin on the ground. Cells are very soft in consistency. Firmer connective tissue is necessary to support the cells and allow the body to assume an efficient shape and overall structure.

The cells of most connective tissues produce nonliving, intercellular substances that connect and give support to other cells and tissues. These intercellular substances range from various types of fibers to the firm, mineralized matrix of bone.

> TECHNICIAN NOTE Six main types of connective tissues are present in the body: adipose connective tissue, loose connective tissue, dense connective tissue, elastic connective tissue, cartilage, and bone.

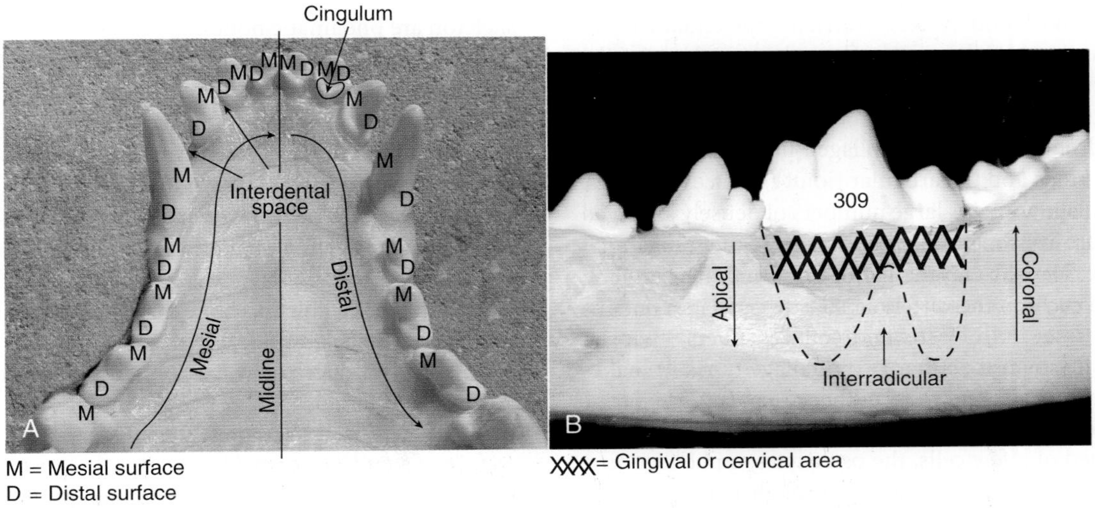

FIGURE 5-6 Positional terms pertaining to the teeth. (From Bassert JM, McCurnin, DM: *McCurnin's clinical textbook for veterinary technicians,* ed 7, St Louis, 2010, Saunders.)

Six main types of connective tissues are present in the body: adipose connective tissue, loose connective tissue, dense connective tissue, elastic connective tissue, cartilage, and bone. Blood is also a connective tissue; it will be discussed with the rest of the blood vascular system.

Adipose connective tissue consists of collections of lipid-storing cells, what we commonly refer to as fat. It represents the body's storage supply of excess nutrients. When the dietary intake of nutrients exceeds the body's needs, adipose connective tissue proliferates. In leaner times, when the dietary nutrient intake is insufficient, the lipid stored in the adipose connective tissue can be mobilized to meet the body's nutritional needs.

Loose connective tissue is found throughout the body wherever cushioning and flexibility are needed. It is commonly found beneath the skin and around blood vessels, nerves, and muscles. Its main components are fiber-producing cells, fibroblasts, and three types of fibers (collagen fibers, reticular fibers, and elastic fibers). Collagen fibers are predominant and are very strong to provide strength to the organs. Reticular fibers form a supportive framework. Elastic fibers are a minor component and provide some degree of elasticity. Both sets of fibers are intertwined in a loose mesh that provides cushioning and flexibility in virtually all directions.

Dense connective tissue has the same components as loose connective tissue but is much more densely packed. One variety of dense connective tissue has the fibers arranged in parallel bundles. This type of tissue is regularly arranged. It makes up tendons, which attach muscles to bones, and ligaments, which attach bones to other bones. The other type of tissue is irregularly arranged. It is like a densely compacted version of loose connective tissue. It is found in the capsules that surround and protect many soft internal organs.

Cartilage consists of a few cells, called chondrocytes, and various types and amounts of fibers embedded in a thick gelatinous intercellular substance, the matrix. Cartilage is firmer than fibrous tissue, but not as hard as bone, and contains no blood vessels. Nutrients for chondrocytes must diffuse through the matrix from the periphery of the cartilage. This limits how thick cartilage can become. Hyaline cartilage is smooth and glossy in appearance. It contains more chondrocytes and a few collagen fibers. It is found in the tracheal rings and the articular (joint) surfaces of bones. Fibrous cartilage contains large numbers of densely arranged collagen fibers in its matrix and few chondrocytes, making it very durable. It makes up the majority of the intervertebral disks, which cushion the vertebrae. Elastic cartilage contains large numbers of both elastic and collagen fibers, giving it more flexibility than the other two cartilage types. It makes up parts of the larynx and most of the earflap (pinna).

Bone is second only to the enamel of teeth in its hardness. It is composed of a few cells, the osteocytes, embedded in a matrix that has become mineralized through a process called ossification. It is important to note that, despite its hard, dead appearance, bone is living tissue with an excellent capacity for regeneration and remodeling.

SKELETON

The skeleton is the framework of bones that supports and protects the soft tissues of the body. Some bones, such as the bones of the skull, which enclose and protect the delicate brain, surround sensitive tissues. Most of the bones of the skeleton, however, form the scaffolding around which the rest of the body tissues are arranged.

Types of Bones

Long Bones. Long bones have two extremities (epiphysis) and a shaft (diaphysis). A small portion of long bone between epiphysis and diaphysis at both ends is metaphysis, which contains a hyaline cartilage or growth plate. It is the part where bone grows in length on both extremities. A long bone contains a medullary cavity filled with a bone marrow. Examples of long bones are the humerus, radius, ulna, metacarpals, femur, tibia, fibula, and metatarsals. Bone marrow contains the stem cells, which produce the blood cells. Bone marrow collection is very valuable to diagnose the diseases of blood, especially when blood shows abnormal cells.

Flat Bones. Flat bones are expanded in two directions to provide maximum area for muscle attachment. Examples of flat bones are the scapula, skull bones, and pelvis.

Small Bones. Small bones are cuboidal or approximately equal in all dimensions located at complex joints such as the carpus and hock joint. Examples of small bones are the carpal and tarsal bones.

Irregular Bones. Irregular bones are bones with irregular shape, such as the vertebrae.

Sesamoid Bones. Sesamoid bones are tiny bones found along the course of the tendons. These bones reduce the friction and change the direction of a tendon. Examples of sesamoid bones are the patella and fabellae. The patella, or kneecap, is the largest sesamoid bone.

Pneumatic Bones. Pneumatic bones contain air spaces to make the skeleton lighter. Most of the bones of a bird's skeleton are pneumatic bones.

Common Bone Features

- An *articular surface* is a surface in which a bone forms a joint with another bone. It is usually very smooth and is often covered with a layer of hyaline cartilage.
- A *condyle* is a large, convex articular surface usually found on the distal ends of the long bones that make up the limbs.
- A *foramen* is a hole in a bone through which blood vessels and nerves usually pass.
- A *fossa* is a depression in a bone usually occupied by a muscle or tendon.
- A *facet* is a flat and smooth articular area, such as the surface of a tarsal or carpal bone.
- A *bone head* is a spherical articular projection usually found on the proximal ends of some limb bones.

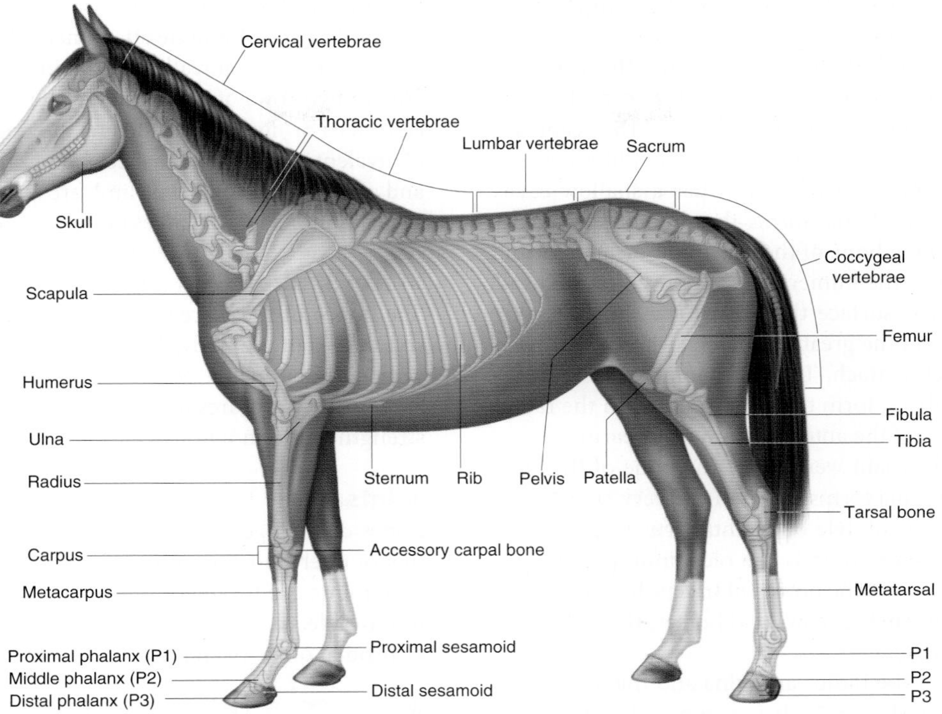

FIGURE 5-7 Skeleton of a horse. (From Aspinall V: *The complete textbook of veterinary nursing,* ed 2, St Louis, 2011, Elsevier.)

- The *neck of a bone* is the often-narrowed area that connects a bone head with the rest of the bone.
- A *process, tuber, tubercle, tuberosity,* or *trochanter* is a lump or bump on the surface of a bone. It is usually the site where the tendon of a muscle attaches to a bone. The larger the process, the more powerful the muscle that attaches at the site.

Axial Skeleton

The axial skeleton is composed of the bones located on the axis or midline of the body. It is composed of the bones of the skull, the spinal column, the ribs, and the sternum (Fig. 5-7).

The skull is composed of many bones, most of which are held together by immovable joints called sutures. The skull bones can be divided into the bones of the cranium and the bones of the face (which extend in a rostral direction from the cranium). The bones of the cranium house and protect the brain, and the bones of the face house mainly digestive and respiratory structures.

The spinal column is composed of a series of individual bones called vertebrae. The vertebrae form a long, flexible tube called the vertebral canal. The vertebral canal houses and protects the spinal cord. The vertebrae are divided into five groups, and each vertebra is numbered within each group from cranial to caudal (Fig. 5-7). The *cervical* vertebrae (C) are in the neck region. The first cervical vertebra (C1) is the atlas that forms a joint with the skull. The *thoracic vertebrae* (T) are dorsal to the chest region and form joints with the dorsal ends of the ribs. The *lumbar vertebrae* (L), which are dorsal to the abdominal region, are fairly large and heavy because they serve as the site of attachment for the large sling muscles that support the abdomen. The *sacral vertebrae* (S) in the pelvic region are fused together into a solid structure called the *sacrum,* which forms a joint with the pelvis. The caudalmost vertebrae, the *coccygeal vertebrae* (Cy), form the tail. The number of vertebrae in each region varies with species. Following is the vertebral formula of different species:

Dog: C 7, T 13, L 7, S 3, Cy 20-23
Cow: C 7, T 13, L 6, S 5, Cy 18-20
Horse: C 7, T 18, L 6, S 5, Cy 15-20

The ribs support and help form the lateral walls of the thorax or chest (Fig. 5-7). Their number varies with the species, but the number of rib pairs is usually the same as the number of thoracic vertebrae. They form joints with the thoracic vertebrae dorsally and are continued ventrally by rods of hyaline cartilage, the costal cartilages. The costal cartilages of ribs at the cranial end of the thorax are connected directly to the sternum at their ventral end. The costal cartilages of the caudal ribs do not reach the sternum; they connect to the costal cartilage cranial to them. The spaces between ribs are referred to as *intercostal spaces.*

The sternum forms the ventral portion of the thorax (Fig. 5-7). It is composed of a series of rodlike bones called *sternebrae.* The manubrium sterni is the first (cranialmost) sternebra, and the xiphoid process is the last (caudalmost). These two bones are often used as external landmarks on the animal.

Appendicular Skeleton

The appendicular skeleton is composed of the bones of the limbs (appendages). The forelimb is referred to anatomically as the thoracic limb, and the hind limb is termed the pelvic limb.

From proximal to distal, the bones of the thoracic limb are the scapula, humerus, radius and ulna, carpal bones, metacarpal bones, and phalanges (Fig. 5-7). The scapula is the shoulder blade. It is a flat bone with a shelflike spine on its lateral surface. At its distal end, it has a shallow cavity called the *glenoid cavity* that forms the shoulder joint with the humerus (the long bone of the brachium or upper arm.) The proximal end of the humerus is composed of the head, the smooth articular surface that forms the shoulder joint with the scapula, and the greater tubercle, where the powerful shoulder muscles attach. The distal joint surfaces of the humerus, the condyles, form the elbow joint with the radius and ulna, the bones of the antebrachium or forearm.

The radius is the main weight-bearing bone of the antebrachium, and the ulna forms much of the very snug-fitting elbow joint with the condyle of the humerus (Fig. 5-7). At the proximal end of the ulna is the olecranon process, the point of the elbow where the powerful triceps brachii muscle attaches. In animals such as cows and horses, the radius and ulna are fused together.

Located between the radius and ulna and the metacarpal bones is the carpus (Fig. 5-7). It is composed of two rows of short bones and is equivalent to the human wrist. Just distal to the carpus are the metacarpal bones, equivalent to the bones of the human hand between wrist and fingers. The phalanges are the bones of the digits, equivalent to human fingers. Dogs and cats have five digits (toes) in each forelimb. Cows, sheep, and goats have two digits (split hooves), and horses have one digit. Each digit is composed of either two phalanges (proximal and distal), as in the human thumb, or three phalanges (proximal, middle, and distal), as in human fingers.

The bones of the pelvic limb, from proximal to distal, are the pelvis, femur, patella, tibia and fibula, tarsal bones, metatarsal bones, and phalanges (Fig. 5-7). The pelvis is composed of three pairs of bones that are fused in the adult animal: the ilium, the ischium, and the pubis. The cranial part of the ilium is the iliac crest, which is one of the sites to aspirate bone marrow. At the junction of the three bones on each side is a deep cavity, the acetabulum, which is the socket portion of the ball-and-socket hip joint.

The femur is the long bone of the thigh region (Fig. 5-7). The head of the femur forms the ball portion of the hip joint, and the greater trochanter is the site of attachment for the powerful gluteal (rump) muscles. At its distal end are the condyles, which form the stifle joint with the tibia, and the trochlear groove, in which the patella rides.

The patella, or kneecap, is the largest sesamoid bone in the body. Sesamoid bones are located in tendons that change direction sharply at joints. The patella helps distribute the force of the quadriceps femoris muscle, the main extensor muscle of the stifle joint.

The tibia is the main weight-bearing bone of the distal leg. The fibula is thin and runs along the entire length of the tibia in dogs and cats. In other species, such as cows and horses, the fibula is a very small, sometimes incomplete bone that is primarily a site of muscle attachment (Fig. 5-7).

The tarsus is equivalent to the human ankle, and it consists of two rows of short bones. The tuberosity of the large calcaneus or fibular tarsal forms the point of the hock joint, equivalent to the human heel bone. The metatarsal bones and phalanges of the pelvic limb are comparable to the metacarpal bones and phalanges of the thoracic limb.

Visceral Skeleton

The bones of the visceral skeleton, when present, occur in soft tissues of the body. The *os penis* of the dog is a well-developed bone in the penis. The *os cordis* forms part of the supporting structures in the heart of cattle. The *os rostri* helps strengthen the snout of swine.

Joints

Bones come together at joints. Our usual image of joints is that of freely movable joints, such as the elbow or hip. However, joints can be any of three main types: fibrous joints are immovable, cartilaginous joints are slightly movable, and diarthrodial or synovial joints are freely movable.

> **TECHNICIAN NOTE** Joints are classified as one of three main types: fibrous joints, cartilaginous joints, and diarthrodial or synovial joints.

Fibrous joints hold bones together but do not allow movement at the joint site. The sutures that hold many of the skull bones together are immovable joints. Cartilaginous joints allow a slight rocking movement. The cartilaginous intervertebral discs and the symphysis that unites the pubic bones of the pelvis allow a slight amount of movement.

Synovial joints are what people usually think of when they think of joints. They allow free movement between bones in several directions. Synovial joints usually have smooth articular surfaces covered by articular cartilage, and a fibrous joint capsule. The inner side of the joint capsule is lined by synovial membrane, which secretes the synovial fluid that is oily in nature and covers and protects the articular cartilages from wearing against each other. The normal synovial fluid is clear, sticky, slippery, and viscous. When the joint is inflamed, the fluid becomes thin and less slippery and cannot protect the cartilage anymore. Many joints also have fibrous ligaments that hold bones together. Most ligaments are *extracapsular* (located outside the fibrous joint capsule), such as collateral ligaments. Some ligaments are *intracapsular* (located inside the joint cavity), such as cruciate ligaments that connect the distal end of the femur to the proximal end of the tibia.

Synovial joints allow some combination of six potential joint movements: **flexion, extension, adduction, abduction,** rotation, and circumduction. Flexion decreases the angle between two bones; extension increases the angle. Adduction moves the extremity toward the median plane, and abduction moves it away from the median plane. Rotation is a twisting movement of a part on its own axis. The shaking of the head of a wet dog is a rotation movement. Circumduction is a movement in which the distal end of an extremity describes a circle.

INTEGUMENT

The integument is the outer covering of the body. It consists primarily of the skin, hair, claws, or hooves and horns. In nonmammalian species, it also includes such structures as feathers and scales. In addition to its obvious protective role, the integument has several other important functions. Its multitude of sensory receptors makes it one of the most important parts of an animal's sensory system. Integument also helps in regulating body temperature through its ability to adjust blood flow to the skin, adjust the position of hairs, and secrete sweat. The integument also produces vitamin D and secretes and excretes a number of substances through various types of skin glands.

Skin

The skin is the largest body organ. It consists of two main layers: the superficial epithelial layer (epidermis), and the deep connective tissue layer (dermis).

The epidermis is composed of keratinized stratified squamous epithelium. The surface layer of the epidermis dries out and is converted to a tough, horny substance called keratin, which also makes up the bulk of hair, claws or hooves, and horns (antlers).

Within the deepest layers of the epidermis of most animals are melanocytes, cells that produce granules of the dark pigment *melanin*. This pigment gives color to the skin, hair, and other integumentary structures. An albino animal has a total lack of melanin, resulting in pale, white skin and hair, and unpigmented irises in the eyes.

The dermis layer of skin is composed of collagen, elastic, and reticular fibers. It contains hair follicles, sebaceous glands, sudoriferous glands, and arrector pili muscles. In addition, this layer also contains various sensitive nerve endings and blood vessels. The sebaceous glands are the oil glands of the skin. They secrete oily sebum, which helps waterproof the skin and keep it soft and pliable. Sebum is secreted directly onto the shafts of hairs in the hair follicles. Sudoriferous glands are the sweat glands, which primarily help cool the body. Some animals, such as horses, have sudoriferous glands spread over their entire body. Others, such as dogs and cats, have only a few, clustered in the footpad and nose areas.

The hypodermis or subcutis is a layer of loose connective tissue just below the dermis, which connects the skin to underlying muscles. It also contains some fat cells. The subcutaneous injection is administered in this layer by lifting a fold of skin.

> **TECHNICIAN NOTE** The skin consists of two main layers: the superficial epithelial layer (epidermis) and the deep connective tissue layer (dermis).

Hair

Hair covers most of the body surface of most animals. Hair is composed of densely compacted keratinized cells and produced in glandlike structures called hair follicles. Hairs are constantly shed and replaced. The visible part of each hair is referred to as the hair shaft. The portion within the skin is called the hair root. The color of hair results from granules of melanin that are incorporated into the hairs during the course of their development. At the base of some hair roots, a tiny muscle, the arrector pili muscle, attaches. When it contracts, it pulls the hair into a more upright position. This produces "goose bumps" or "raised hackles." The purpose of erecting the hair generally is to retain heat when an animal is cold by fluffing up the haircoat or to make the animal look larger and more fearsome as a part of the sympathetic nervous system "fight or flight" response.

Claws and Hooves

Claws and hooves are horny structures that cover the distal ends of the digits. They are composed of parallel bundles of keratinized cells organized into an outer wall and a bottom sole.

Horns

Like claws and hooves, horns are composed of bundles of keratinized cells. They are organized around bony "horn cores," outgrowths of the frontal bones of the skull.

MUSCULAR SYSTEM

The general function of muscle is to move the body, both internally and externally. The nervous system gives the orders, and the muscular system is among the most important systems that carry them out. There are three distinctly different kinds of muscle in the body: skeletal muscle, cardiac muscle, and smooth muscle. All these muscles have the property to contract and relax, which help them to perform various functions.

> **TECHNICIAN NOTE** There are three types of muscle in the body: skeletal muscle, cardiac muscle, and smooth muscle.

Skeletal Muscle

Skeletal muscle derives its name from the fact that it moves the skeleton. It is also known as voluntary striated muscle because it is under conscious control, and its cells, at the microscopic level, have a striped or striated appearance.

Skeletal muscle cells (myocytes) are shaped like long cylinders or fibers. These very large cells usually have multiple nuclei. Most of their mass is composed of smaller myofibrils composed of smaller protein filaments. The net effect is an intricate arrangement of filaments that can slide over each other, shortening the muscle cell when it contracts.

Skeletal muscle fibers respond to impulses delivered by nerves. The "connection" of a nerve fiber with a skeletal muscle fiber is called the neuromuscular junction. Each nerve fiber supplies more than one muscle fiber. A motor unit is composed of a nerve fiber and all of the muscle fibers it supplies. If there are small numbers of muscle fibers per nerve fiber, fine, delicate movements are possible. The muscles that move the eyeball fall into this category. On the other hand, muscles that must make very large, powerful movements, such as the leg muscles, have a large number of muscle fibers supplied by each nerve fiber.

Skeletal muscles are usually attached to bones at both ends by tendons. The more stable of the muscle's attachments is called its origin. The more movable of the attachments is called the *insertion.*

Cardiac Muscle

Cardiac muscle is found only in the heart. It is also known as involuntary striated muscle because it is not under conscious control and its cells are striped, or striated.

Cardiac muscle cells have no characteristic shape. Rather, they form an intricate branching network in the heart. They are firmly attached to each other, which allows considerable force to be generated as they contract.

Cardiac muscle cells each have an innate contractile rhythm that does not require an external nerve supply. The rhythmic contractions of the heart chambers are coordinated by a system of specialized cardiac muscle cells. The heart does have an autonomic nerve supply, but it does not initiate contractions of the muscle cells: it serves to modify them. Sympathetic stimulation increases the rate and force of cardiac muscle contractions. This is part of the fight or flight response. Parasympathetic stimulation has the opposite effect; it decreases the rate and force of contraction. Through this autonomic stimulation, the rate and force of cardiac contractions can be adjusted according to the body's needs.

Smooth Muscle

Smooth muscle is found mainly in internal organs. It is called smooth because its cells do not show any stripes or striations under magnification. It is involuntary muscle because it is not under conscious control.

Cells of smooth muscle are spindle-shaped, being wide in the middle and tapered at the ends. Depending on their location, they may be short and thick or long and fiberlike. Two types of smooth muscle are found in the body: visceral smooth muscle, found in hollow abdominal organs, and multiunit smooth muscle, found where fine contractions are needed.

Visceral smooth muscle occurs in large sheets in the walls of the gastrointestinal tract, uterus, and urinary bladder. These muscle cells are linked, so entire areas of cells act as a large unit. Nerve supply is autonomic and serves mainly to modify contractions. Sympathetic stimulation (fight or flight) decreases activity, whereas parasympathetic stimulation (rest, rejuvenation) increases visceral smooth muscle activity.

Multiunit smooth muscle consists of individual muscle units that each require specific nerve stimulation to contract. Unlike visceral smooth muscle cells, these muscle cells are not linked, so their contractions are localized and discrete. Multiunit smooth muscle is found where fine, though involuntary, movements are needed, such as in the iris and ciliary body of the eye, the walls of blood vessels, and the walls of tiny air passageways in the lungs.

REVIEW QUESTIONS

Matching

Match the prefix/suffix with its meaning.

_____**1.** -megaly	**A.** against
_____**2.** ante-	**B.** inflammation
_____**3.** intra-	**C.** between
_____**4.** para-	**D.** state or condition
_____**5.** -crine	**E.** beside, apart from
_____**6.** anti-	**F.** before
_____**7.** -ize	**G.** within
_____**8.** -itis	**H.** secrete
_____**9.** inter-	**I.** around, surrounding
_____**10.** -osis	**J.** use, subject to
_____**11.** peri-	**K.** enlarged
_____**12.** sym-	**L.** with

Choose the Best Response

Choose the best answer to the following questions.

1. The term for toward the midline is:
- **a.** medial
- **b.** lateral
- **c.** proximal
- **d.** distal

2. The paw is _______ to the shoulder.
- **a.** cranial
- **b.** caudal
- **c.** distal
- **d.** proximal

3. Another term for growth plate is:
- **a.** physis
- **b.** shaft
- **c.** diaphysis
- **d.** trophic

4. The part of the small intestine is the:
- **a.** ileum
- **b.** ilium

5. Gastroplasty contains the suffix that means:
- **a.** excision
- **b.** forming an opening
- **c.** surgical repair
- **d.** incision

6. An incision into the duodenum is a:
- **a.** duodenectomy
- **b.** duodenoscopy
- **c.** duodenostomy
- **d.** duodenotomy

7. Which terms pertain to the tongue?
   a. lingual and gingival
   b. lingual and glossal
   c. lingual only
   d. gingival and glossal
8. Enteritis means inflammation of the:
   a. internal organs
   b. peritoneum
   c. small intestine
   d. esophagus
9. Mouth lacerations or cuts would most likely cause:
   a. hematemesis
   b. proteinuria
   c. polydipsia
   d. dysphagia
10. Cystotomy is:
   a. resection of the urinary bladder
   b. incision of the urinary bladder
   c. inflammation of the urinary bladder
   d. herniation of the urinary bladder

RECOMMENDED READING

Christenson D: *Veterinary medical terminology*, ed 2, St Louis, 2008, Saunders.

Cohen BJ: *Medical terminology*, ed 4, Philadelphia, 2003, Lippincott.

Colville J, Oien S: *Clinical veterinary language*, St Louis, 2013, Mosby.

Leonard PC: *Quick and easy medical terminology*, ed 6, St Louis, 2010, Saunders.

McBride DF: *Learning veterinary terminology*, ed 2, St Louis, 2002, Mosby.

Mosby's medical, nursing & allied health dictionary, ed 6, St Louis, 2002, Saunders.

Saunders veterinary terminology flash cards, St Louis, 2009, Saunders.

Shiland BJ: *Mastering health care terminology*, ed 3, St Louis, 2010, Mosby.

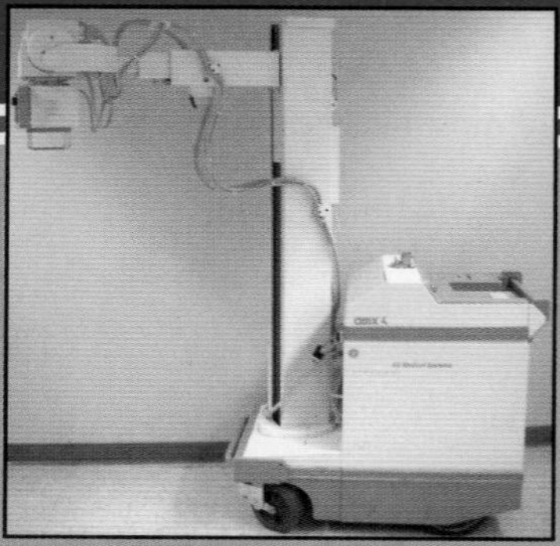

6 Diagnostic Imaging

OUTLINE

LEARNING OBJECTIVES

After reviewing this chapter, the reader will be able to:

1. Describe the components of the x-ray machine and the function of each part.
2. Explain how x-rays are produced.
3. Discuss the factors that affect radiographic quality.
4. Describe techniques and devices used to optimize radiographic quality.
5. Discuss the dangers of radiation and methods to avoid radiation injury.
6. Describe the procedures used to develop radiographs.
7. Explain proper positioning of animals for various radiographic studies.
8. Describe the basic physics of ultrasound.
9. List the components of ultrasound machines and the function of each part.
10. List the non–x-ray imaging modalities and provide an overview of each.

KEY TERMS

ALARA
Anechoic
Annular array
Anode
Bucky
Cathode
Collimators
Contrast
Direct-exposure film
Distance enhancement
Echoic
Fiberoptic
Film focal distance (FFD)
Film latitude
Fluoroscopy
Focused grids
Gain
Heel effect
Hyperechoic
Hypoechoic
Intensifying screens
Isoechoic
Kilovoltage peak (kVp)
Latent image
Linear-array scan
Maximum permissible dose (MPD)
Milliamperage (mA)
Mirror-image
Object film distance (OFD)
Penumbra effect
Power
Radiographic density
Radiolucent
Radiopaque
REM
Sievert (SV)
Slice thickness
Sonolucent
Source image distance (SID)
Time gain compensation
Ultrasonography

Diagnostic imaging is an integral part of the diagnosis and treatment of patients. Radiography and ultrasonography are the two most common modalities available within the clinical setting, with some referral hospitals having state-of-the-art imaging modalities such as computed tomography (CT), magnetic resonance imaging (MRI), and nuclear medicine (NM). Typically, the veterinary technician is responsible for the operation of imaging equipment. A thorough understanding of the physics behind the various imaging modalities is needed to produce diagnostic-quality studies.

X-RAY GENERATION

X-rays are a form of electromagnetic radiation. X-rays are similar to visible light but have a shorter wavelength, higher frequency, and higher energy. It is the higher energy that makes x-rays dangerous. The x-rays are generated when fast-moving electrons (from the cathode) collide with the anode (positive end of x-ray tube). Within the x-ray tube, at the time of the exposure, a stream of electrons is accelerated toward a tungsten anode target. The energy of the electrons interacting with the atoms of the target is converted to heat (99%) and x-rays (1%). Heat generation in the x-ray tube is a limiting factor in the production of x-rays.

X-RAY TUBE ANATOMY

The x-ray tube consists of a **cathode** (−) that contains a tungsten filament where the electrons are generated when heated. This tungsten filament is housed within a focusing cup to focus the beam of electrons on the focal spot of the anode. The **anode** (+) contains a rotating tungsten target wherein x-rays are generated at the focal spot, which is oriented at an angle of 11 to 20 degrees. The x-rays produced are directed downward through the window by this angle. Both the anode and cathode are enclosed in a vacuum glass or metal envelope. A beryllium window in the glass envelope allows x-rays to pass with minimal filtration, which is called inherent filtration (about 1 mm Al equivalent). An aluminum filter is placed outside the window in the collimator housing (typically on top of the mirror) to absorb the low-energy (soft) x-rays, while allowing the more energetic and useful x-rays to form the primary x-ray beam. This is called the added filtration (usually 1.5 mm Al equivalent). By law, any x-ray tube that generates over 70 kVp must have a collimator, because there has to be a total filtration of 2.5 mm Al equivalent. The lower energy x-rays thereby do not enter the patient. If they were allowed to do so, there would be an increased dose to the patient from x-rays that would never make it out of the patient and thereby not contribute to image formation. The entire x-ray tube is surrounded by oil that acts as an electrical barrier while absorbing heat generated by the tube. The tube and oil are encased in a lead housing to prevent damage to the glass envelope from the outside and to absorb stray radiation (Fig. 6-1).

The **heel effect** is the result of unequal distribution of the x-ray beam intensity emitted from the x-ray tube along the cathode-anode axis. Tubes with lower target angles (e.g., 11 degrees) have a distribution of x-ray beam intensity that decreases rapidly on the anode side of the tube (Fig. 6-2) as a result of primary x-ray beam absorption by the anode material. This can be used as an advantage when radiographing areas of unequal thickness, such as

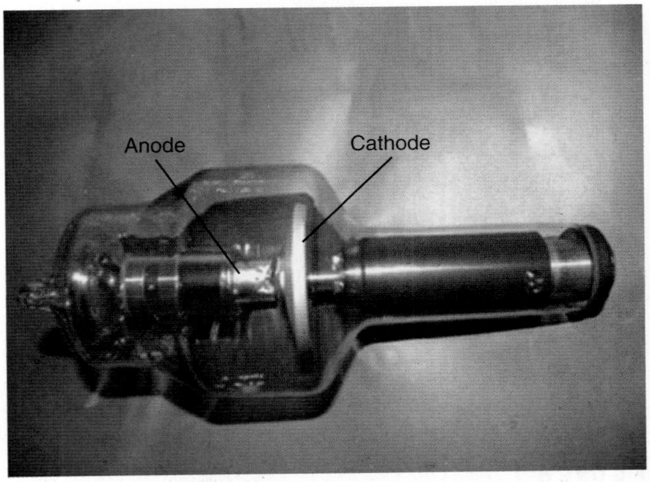

FIGURE 6-1 Anatomy of an x-ray tube.

the thorax or abdomen. By placing the patient's head toward the anode side, the part of the x-ray beam with the higher intensity (cathode side) is directed to the thickest area of the patient, as in this example of radiographing a thorax. This produces a more even film density. The heel effect is most noticeable when using large film sizes, low kVp, and long focal-film distance.

> **TECHNICIAN NOTE** The anode heel effect refers to the unequal distribution of x-ray beam intensity along the cathode-anode axis.

RADIOGRAPHIC IMAGE QUALITY

RADIOGRAPHIC DENSITY

Radiographic density is the degree of blackness on a radiograph. The dark areas are made up of black metallic silver deposits on the finished radiograph. These deposits occur in areas where x-rays have penetrated the patient and exposed the emulsion of the film. Radiographic density can be intensified by increasing the mAs (a product of the milliamperage and time), which is a result of increasing the **mA (milliamperage)** or the exposure time seconds (s). This increases the mAs by either increasing the number (quantity) of x-rays produced as a result of increasing the number of electrons in the electron cloud or the time the electrons are allowed to travel from the cathode to the anode. A higher **kilovoltage peak (kVp)** yields more radiographic density by increasing the penetrating power (quality) of the x-ray beam.

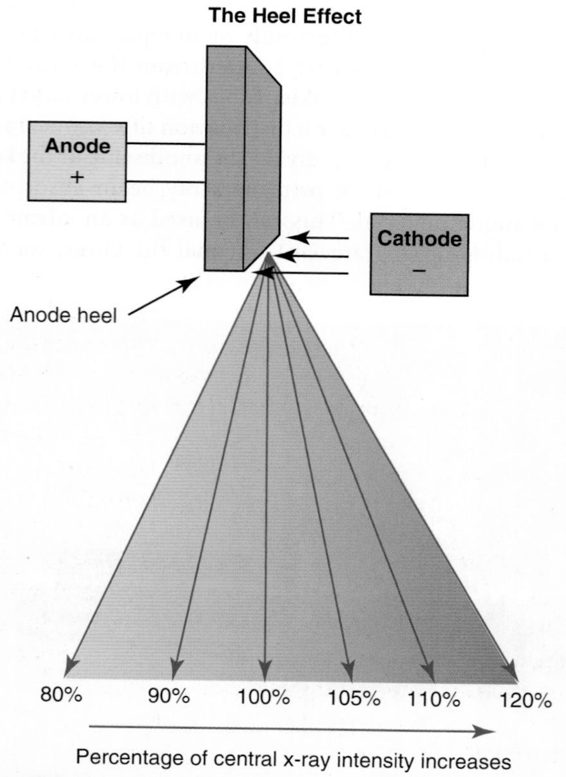

FIGURE 6-2 The anode heel effect. The x-ray beam intensity decreases toward the anode side because of absorption by the target and anode material. *(Courtesy of Jessica Johnson.)*

> **TECHNICIAN NOTE** Radiographic density refers to the degree of blackness of the film, whereas radiographic contrast refers to the varying shades of gray on the film.

RADIOGRAPHIC CONTRAST

Radiographic **contrast** is defined as the differences in radiographic density between adjacent areas on a radiographic image. Radiographs that show a long scale of contrast have a few black-and-white shades, with many shades of gray. A short scale of contrast has black-and-white shades, with only a few shades of gray in between. For most studies, a long scale of contrast is desirable. Obtaining a long scale of radiographic contrast depends on four factors: subject density, kVp level, film contrast, and film fogging.

Subject density is the ability of the different tissue densities to absorb x-rays. The extent to which x-rays penetrate the various tissues depends on the differences in atomic number and thickness.

On radiographs, air or lung tissue will appear **radiolucent** or black, because these allow more of the radiation to pass through. With increasing density, the tissue will appear whiter, or more **radiopaque,** as it absorbs more of the radiation (Fig. 6-3). Bone, containing mainly calcium and phosphorus, has a high average atomic number as compared with muscle, which contains mainly hydrogen and nitrogen. Bone absorbs more x-rays than muscle and appears whiter (radiopaque) on the finished radiograph, whereas air in the thorax will appear more radiolucent in comparison. The thickness of the area also affects the number of x-rays absorbed. If you radiograph an area that ranges from 5 to 20 cm in thickness, the 20-cm-thick area absorbs more x-rays than the 5-cm area.

> **TECHNICIAN NOTE** Denser tissues, such as bone, absorb greater amounts of x-rays and appear white on a radiograph, whereas less dense tissues, such as lung tissue, absorb fewer x-rays and appear black on the finished radiograph.

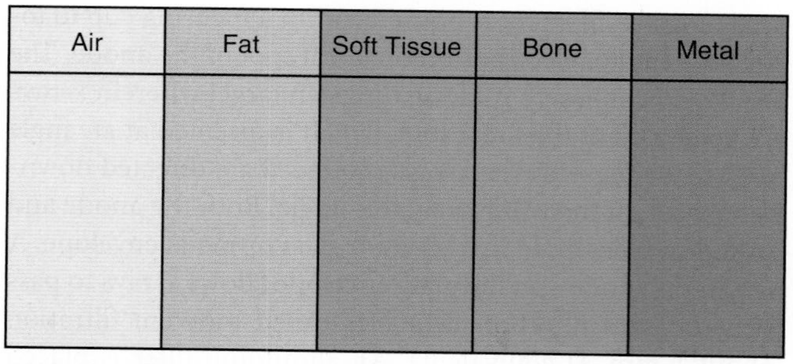

FIGURE 6-3 Various exposed film densities. Air is the least dense (most radiolucent), resulting in film exposure, whereas metal is the most dense (thus the most radiopaque) and absorbs more x-rays, allowing few x-rays to penetrate the film. *(Courtesy of Heidi Anthony.)*

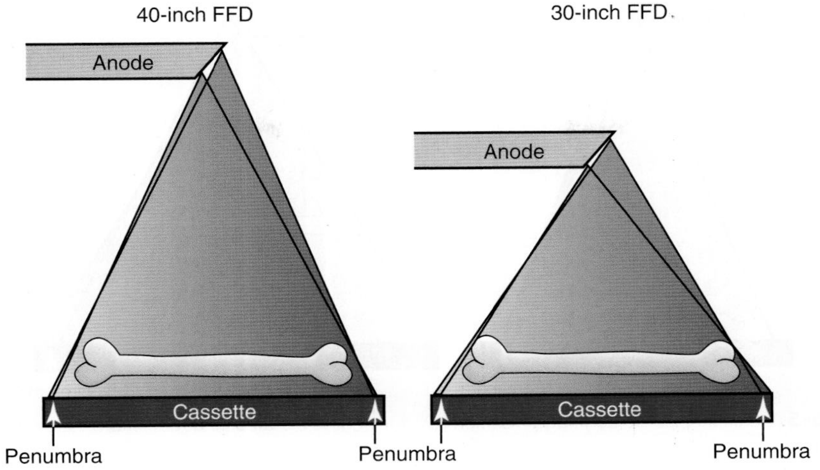

FIGURE 6-4 Increasing the source image distance (SID) decreases the amount of penumbra, increasing the radiographic detail.

The scale of radiographic contrast can be lengthened or shortened by increasing or decreasing the kVp. As kVp increases, the scale of contrast gets longer (more grays can be visualized). Radiographs made with a high kVp have more exposure latitude, allowing minor errors in technique without affecting the diagnostic quality of the radiograph.

Film contrast also affects radiographic contrast. Some types of film can produce a long scale of contrast or long latitude. Long-latitude film allows for more variation in technique while still producing a diagnostic radiograph. The scale of contrast can be shortened by changing the exposure technique when using long-latitude film. However, the scale of contrast cannot be lengthened when using contrast film (film that produces a short scale of contrast).

Film fogging can greatly decrease radiographic contrast by decreasing the differences in densities between two adjacent shadows. Care must be taken in the storage and handling of x-ray film to prevent fogging. Film can become fogged from low-grade light leaks in the darkroom, scatter radiation, heat, and improper processing.

RADIOGRAPHIC DETAIL

A diagnostic radiograph is one with diagnostic radiographic detail. Radiographic detail is considered to be of diagnostic quality when the interfaces between tissues and organs are sharp. Many factors can affect the detail on a radiograph. The most common are patient motion and the **penumbra effect.**

Patient motion causes loss of detail because of blurred interfaces. A blurred image is generally a result of long exposure time combined with motion of the patient. This can be controlled by using the shortest possible exposure. If the image remains blurred, the patient should be sedated.

> **TECHNICIAN NOTE** Patient motion and the penumbra effect have the greatest influence on radiographic detail.

A loss of detail is also caused by the penumbra effect. The x-rays will pass out of the x-ray tube, and the diaphragm allows collimation (limitation) of the x-ray beam. The fuzziness is caused by stray x-rays and is known as penumbra. The smallest focal spot size should be used whenever possible to prevent this effect.

Excessive penumbra causes blurring at the edges of the shadows cast by the x-ray exposure. Three main factors influence the amount of penumbra on a radiograph. Changes in these factors increase or decrease the radiographic detail. The first factor is the size of the focal spot. The larger the focal spot, the more pronounced the penumbra effect. Decreasing the focal spot size decreases the penumbra. However, this cannot be changed on most equipment. Manufacturers design the focal spot as small as possible while maintaining the ability to dissipate heat effectively.

Another factor that affects the amount of penumbra is the source image distance. Source image distance is the distance between the source of the x-ray and the film. The term **source image distance (SID)** is preferred, but **film focal distance (FFD)** and SID are used interchangeably.

The penumbra effect can be decreased by increasing the source image distance (Fig. 6-4). There is a limit to how much the SID can be increased because of what is stated in the inverse square law. The intensity decreases at a rate inverse to the square of the distance. In simpler terms, if the SID is doubled, the mAs must increase four times to maintain the same radiographic density. In most cases this is not practical, because the shortest possible exposure times are necessary to counteract patient motion. An SID of 36 to 40 inches is sufficient to minimize the penumbra effect.

The third factor that affects penumbra is the object-image distance (OID). This is the distance from the object being imaged to the film or image receptor. The penumbra is decreased by keeping the OID as short as possible (Fig. 6-5). Using a combination of these factors, the penumbra can be minimized and good radiographic detail achieved.

Distortion

Foreshortening occurs when the object is not parallel to the recording surface. This distorts size by shortening the length of the object. This occurs mainly when imaging the

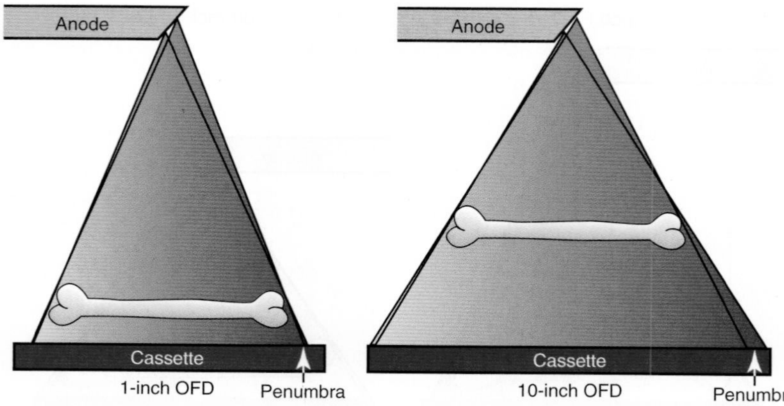

FIGURE 6-5 Increasing the object-image distance (OID) increases the amount of penumbra, decreasing the radiographic detail.

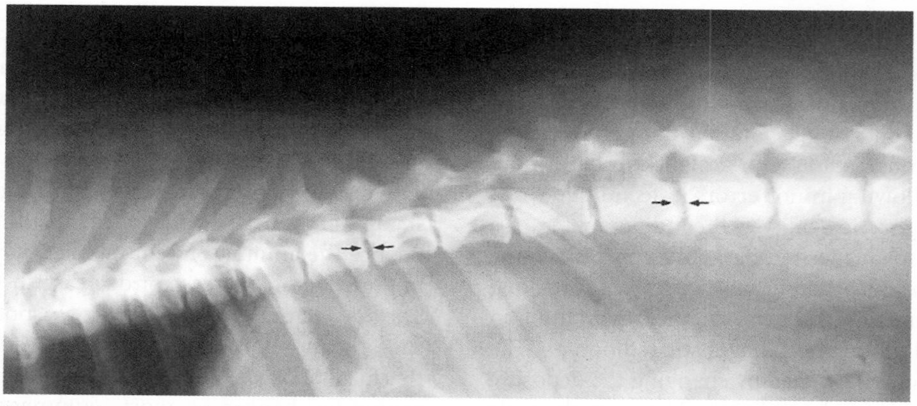

FIGURE 6-6 The intervertebral spaces appear narrow toward the edges of the radiograph *(arrows)* as compared with the spaces in the center of the radiograph.

long bones, such as the humerus or femur. If one end of the bone is farther from the recording surface than the other, the bone appears shorter. The object being radiographed must be parallel to the recording surface and the OID kept as short as possible. Increasing the OID increases the penumbra and greatly magnifies the size of the object. The degree of magnification increases as the distance to the recording surface becomes greater.

It is important to accurately project areas between a series of radiodense and radiolucent objects. The vertebral column is a good example. The vertebrae must be parallel to the recording surface. When radiographing the cervical vertebrae in lateral recumbency, if the patient is allowed to lie naturally, the midcervical vertebrae tend to sag. This produces false narrowing of the intervertebral spaces. A small amount of padding beneath the patient brings the vertebral column parallel to the recording surface. Care must be taken not to use too much padding because this can elevate the spinal column, also producing false narrowing of the intervertebral spaces.

Distortion can also occur when the x-ray beam is not perpendicular to the recording surface. X-rays in the center of the primary beam penetrate perpendicular to the intervertebral spaces. As the distance from the center of the primary beam increases, the x-rays strike the intervertebral spaces at an increasing angle. False narrowing of the intervertebral space occurs because of this increase in distance from the center of the primary beam (Fig. 6-6). To combat such distortion, sometimes it is necessary to make multiple images of the vertebral column, centering the primary beam over multiple areas. This type of distortion is also apparent when radiographing complex joints, such as the stifle and elbow. When imaging these areas, be sure the center of the primary beam is directly over the joint.

TECHNICIAN NOTE Distortion occurs when the x-ray beam is not perpendicular to the recording surface.

Scatter Radiation

When an x-ray photon strikes an object, it can do one of three things. It can pass through the object, be absorbed by the object, or produce scatter radiation (secondary radiation). Scatter radiation fogs the film, greatly decreasing the contrast. It also is a safety hazard to patients and personnel. Scatter radiation is projected in all directions. Exposure techniques that use a high kVp produce more scatter radiation. Body parts measuring 10 cm or more produce enough scatter radiation to significantly decrease detail on the radiograph. Beam-limiting devices are commonly used to decrease scatter radiation by confining the primary beam to the area being examined. Several types of beam-limiting devices are available. Cones are lead cylinders placed over the collimator on the x-ray tube head. This restricts the primary beam to the size of the cone used. These are no longer in common use. Diaphragms are sheets of lead with a rectangular, square, or circular opening that limits the size of the primary beam to the size of the diaphragm used. **Collimators** consist of adjustable lead shutters installed in the tube head of the x-ray machine. Finally, filters are used to absorb the less penetrating or soft x-rays as they leave the tube head. Filters are made of a thin sheet of aluminum and are placed over the tube window.

TECHNICIAN NOTE The collimator in the x-ray tube head is used to limit the size of the primary beam, thus reducing scatter radiation.

Grids. Grids are used to decrease scatter radiation and increase the contrast on the radiograph. As the thickness of the area being imaged increases, the amount of kVp required also increases. As the kVp increases, more scatter radiation is produced. To minimize scatter radiation, grids are necessary when radiographing areas 10 cm or more in thickness.

A grid is a series of thin, linear strips made of alternating radiodense and radiolucent material. The radiodense strips are made of lead, whereas the radiolucent spacers are plastic, aluminum, or fiber. The grid is placed within or under the table between the patient and the imaging receptor. X-rays that penetrate the patient and pass in perfect alignment between the lead strips expose the film. Scatter radiation diverges in all directions and is more likely to be absorbed by one of the lead strips.

The grid also absorbs a portion of the usable x-rays. To compensate for this loss, the number of x-rays generated must be increased by increasing the mAs. Depending on the type of grid used, the increase may be up to 6.6 times the mAs required for the tabletop exposure.

Grids are manufactured with either parallel or focused lead strips arranged in crossed or linear configuration. Parallel grids have the lead strips placed perpendicular to the grid surface. X-rays and scatter radiation that interact with the lead strips are absorbed, whereas the ones that interact with the spacers pass through to expose the film. A disadvantage of a parallel grid is that the x-ray beam diverges at increasing angles and is absorbed at the periphery of the grid. This decreases the number of x-rays reaching the film near the grid edges, commonly called grid cutoff. **Focused grids** have the lead strips placed at progressively increasing angles to match the divergence of the x-ray beam. By angling the lead strips, cutoff of the primary beam is eliminated and radiographic density is uniform. The grid manufacturer supplies a list of distances, called the grid focal distance, and setting the SID out of the grid focal distance results in primary beam cutoff on the periphery of the radiograph (Fig. 6-7). Cutoff of the primary beam also occurs if the grid is not perpendicular to or centered with the x-ray tube (Fig. 6-8).

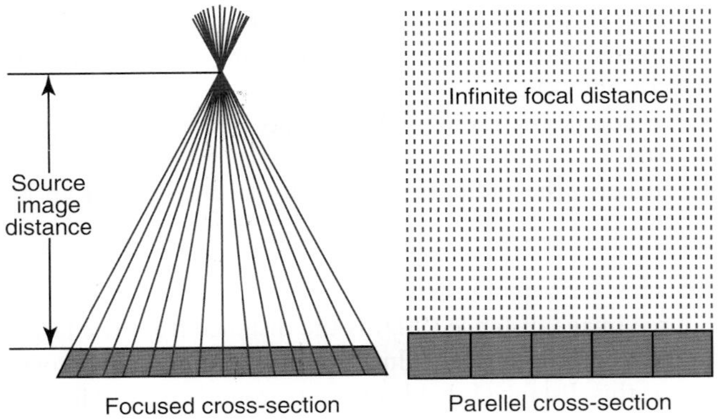

FIGURE 6-7 The focused grid has lead strips angled so that the lines are drawn through each lead strip continuing out of the grid. They will intersect at a grid focus point. The grid is termed *parallel* when strips are not angulated but are instead located at 90 degrees to the grid surface.

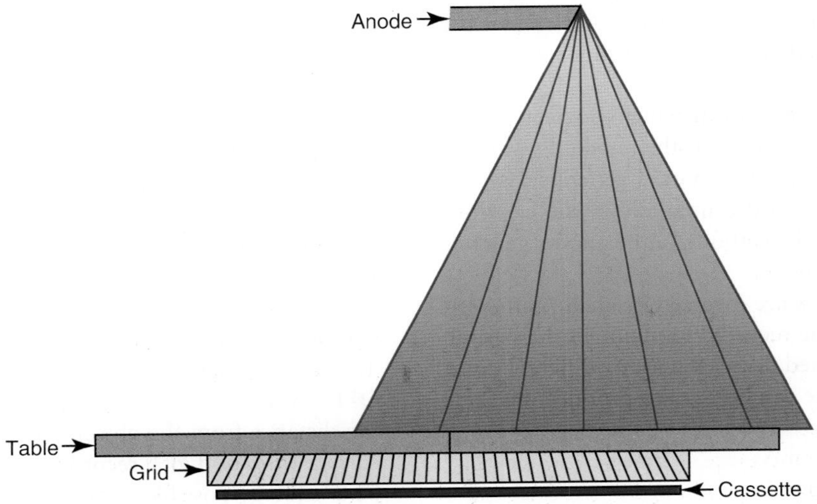

FIGURE 6-8 Grid cutoff. When the grid is not centered with the x-ray tube, grid cutoff occurs. This produces visible grid lines more prominently on one end of the film and an overall decrease in radiographic density.

Grids produce thin white lines on the finished radiograph. Visibility of the grid lines can be decreased in three ways. First, the lead strips can be made as thin as possible while retaining the ability to effectively absorb scatter radiation. The thinner the lead is, the thinner the white line is that it produces on the radiograph.

The second way is to increase the number of grid lines per inch, making the individual lines less visible. To increase the grid lines per inch and keep the thickness of the lead the same, the width of the radiolucent strips must be decreased. This produces a grid with more lead in it, which absorbs more of the primary beam and requires higher mAs. A grid with 80 to 100 lines per inch is sufficient to make the grid lines less visible.

The third way is by using a Potter-Bucky diaphragm, also called a **Bucky**. This device sets the grid in motion as the x-rays are generated, blurring the white grid lines on the radiograph. The Bucky is placed in a cabinet beneath the x-ray table, with a tray to hold the cassette. When a grid is used in combination with a Bucky, fewer lines per inch are necessary. This allows for use of lower mAs. One disadvantage of using a Bucky mechanism in veterinary medicine is the noise and vibration it produces. Some animals may object to this and struggle or move during the x-ray exposure.

EXPOSURE VARIABLES

Four exposure factors control radiographic density, contrast, and detail. These are mAs, kVp, focal-film distance, and object-film distance. Changing one of these factors usually requires adjustments in another factor to maintain the same radiographic density.

mAs

The mAs is a product of the milliamperage and the exposure time. The milliamperage controls the number of electrons in the electron cloud generated at the filament of the cathode. This is done by controlling the temperature of the cathode filament. When the mA is increased, the temperature of the filament is increased, producing more electrons to form the electron cloud. Increasing the mA increases the amount of radiographic density, because more x-rays are generated.

The other factor is the time during which the electrons are allowed to flow from the cathode to the anode. By varying the exposure time, the number of x-rays generated is controlled. Using a longer exposure time allows the electrons more time to cross from the cathode to the anode, generating more x-rays.

Exposure time and mA are inversely related. As mA increases, the exposure time required to maintain the desired number of x-rays generated decreases. Many different combinations of mA and time can be used to produce the same mAs. For example:

300 mA at 1/60 sec = 5 mAs
200 mA at 1/40 sec = 5 mAs
100 mA at 1/20 sec = 5 mAs

When faced with a choice of which mAs to use, always choose the one with the fastest exposure time to allow less movement on the film, which results in the largest mA. The mAs can be used to adjust the radiographic density by following these rules:

- To double the radiographic density, double the mAs.
- To halve the radiographic density, halve the mAs.

Kilovoltage Peak

The kilovoltage peak (kVp) is the voltage applied between the cathode and the anode. It is used to accelerate electrons flowing from the cathode toward the anode side. Increasing the kVp increases the positive charge on the anode. This causes the electrons to move faster, increasing the force of the collision with the target. This produces an x-ray beam with a shorter wavelength and more penetrating power. The correct kVp setting is determined by the thickness of the part being imaged, thus, the thicker the part, the higher the kVp setting, because more penetration is needed. A higher kVp produces a longer scale of contrast and more exposure latitude. Greater exposure latitude allows for more variation in exposure factors, which will still produce a diagnostic radiograph. As with mAs, there are rules when changing the radiographic density with kVp:

- To double the radiographic density, increase the kVp by 20%.
- To halve the radiographic density, decrease the kVp by 16%.

Source Image Distance

Source image distance (SID) is the distance from the target to the recording surface (film). For most radiographic procedures, this distance is held constant, around 36 to 40 inches. In some situations, the SID must be changed. This requires changing one of the other factors to maintain radiographic density. The inverse square law states that the intensity of the x-ray beam is inversely proportioned to the square of the distance from the source of the x-ray. If the SID is doubled, the mAs must be increased four times to maintain radiographic density. The same number of x-rays must diverge to cover an area that is four times as large. Changing the SID does not affect the penetrating power of the beam, so kVp remains constant.

TECHNICIAN NOTE The higher the mA setting on the x-ray machine, the greater the number of x-rays produced. The higher the kVp, the greater the penetrating power of the x-rays.

Object-Image Distance

The object-image distance (OID) (aka: **object film distance, OFD**—with digital imaging, the term OID is being used) is the distance from the object being imaged to the recording surface (film or digital recording plate). This distance should be as short as possible to minimize the penumbra effect and the magnification that occurs with a long OID.

RADIOGRAPHIC FILM

While the number of veterinary practices still using film-based systems is declining, some clinics still utilize this technology. X-ray film consists of three layers: a thin protective layer, an emulsion containing silver halide crystals, and a polyester film base. The first layer is a thin, clear gelatin that acts as a protective coating. This protective material helps protect the sensitive film emulsion. The second layer is the emulsion that contains finely precipitated silver halide crystals in a gelatin base.

The emulsion coats both sides of the film base. This gives the film greater sensitivity, increasing the speed, density, and contrast. By increasing the speed of the film, the exposure required to produce an image can be decreased, thus decreasing exposure of the patient and veterinary personnel. The silver halide emulsion is 90% to 99% silver bromide crystals and 1% to 10% silver iodide crystals. The gelatin that suspends the silver halide crystals is a colloid. It liquefies in high temperatures and remains solid in cool temperatures. When placed in the developing chemicals, the emulsion swells, allowing the chemicals to act on the exposed or sensitized crystals without losing the crystals. Once the emulsion is dry, it hardens again, trapping the black metallic silver. The film base is in the center of the film, giving it support. It does not produce a visible light pattern or absorb the light, although a blue tint has been added to ease eyestrain.

When the silver halide crystals are exposed to electromagnetic radiation, they become more sensitive to chemical change. These sensitized crystals are what make up the **latent image.** When the film is placed into the developer, the latent image is reduced to black metallic silver. The remaining silver halide crystals are removed in the fixer. This produces varying shades of black metallic silver and the clear film base.

Film is sensitive to all types of electromagnetic radiation. These include gamma radiation, particulate radiation (alpha and beta), x-rays, heat, and light. Film is also sensitive to excessive pressure, so care must be taken when handling and storing radiographic film.

> *TECHNICIAN NOTE* X-ray film is sensitive to heat, light, and pressure in addition to x-rays and other forms of radiation.

The two types of film used in veterinary radiography are screen-type film and direct-exposure film. Screen-type film is more sensitive to the light produced by intensifying screens. Two screen-type films are blue-sensitive film and green-sensitive film. Blue-sensitive film is more sensitive to light emitted from screens containing blue-light-emitting phosphors. Calcium tungstate and some rare-earth phosphors are the most common blue-light-emitting phosphors. They emit light in the ultraviolet, violet, and blue-light range. Green-sensitive film is most sensitive to light from green-light-emitting phosphors. Rare-earth phosphors are the most common green-light-emitting phosphors. **Direct-exposure film** is more sensitive to direct x-rays than it is to light. Because it does not use the intensifying effect of the screens, it requires higher mAs than screen film. General anesthesia or heavy sedation may be necessary to prevent patient motion and blurring on the radiograph because of the higher mAs. Direct-exposure film is mainly used to image the extremities or rostral mandible or maxilla, where good detail is needed. It is often used in imaging of exotic animals and in dental radiology studies. It is packaged in a paper folder enclosed in a stout lightproof envelope. Take care when handling this film, because it is protected only by paper. Pressure artifacts can easily occur. Some direct-exposure film can only be manually processed because of the thickness of the emulsion. However, some types of direct-exposure film can be processed in an automatic developer.

Film speeds are rated as high (regular or fast), average (par), and slow (detail). The faster the film, the more sensitive it is and the lower mAs it requires. High-speed film requires less exposure than slow-speed film to produce a given radiographic density. Film speed is changed by increasing the size of the silver halide crystals. High-speed film has larger silver halide crystals than average-speed or slow-speed film. The drawback to using high-speed film is that, with the larger crystal size, the image has a more granular appearance. This decreases the detail considerably. Average-speed (par) film should be used for most veterinary radiography.

Another important feature in x-ray film is **film latitude.** This is the film's inherent ability to produce shades of gray. Film with long or increased latitude can produce images with a long scale of contrast (many shades of gray). Longer-latitude film is desirable, because it allows for greater exposure errors but still produces a diagnostic radiograph.

Proper storage and handling of the film are important to ensure a good diagnostic radiograph. Unexposed film should be stored in a cool, dry place, away from strong chemical fumes. A base fog can develop if film is stored under adverse conditions over a long period. Film is pressure-sensitive, so it should be stored on end and not laid flat on its side.

INTENSIFYING SCREENS

Intensifying screens contain fluorescent crystals bound to a cardboard or plastic base. When exposed to x-rays, they emit foci of light. Placing radiographic film in direct contact with the screens accurately records any x-rays that penetrate the patient. Approximately 95% of the film's radiographic density results from fluorescence of the intensifying screens, and only 5% is the result of direct x-ray exposure. For each x-ray photon the screen absorbs, it emits 1000 light photons, amplifying the photographic effect of the x-rays. The film is sandwiched between two screens mounted inside a light-proof cassette. The cassette holds the film in close uniform contact with the screens (Fig. 6-9).

The screens are supported by a plastic or cardboard base. Next to the base is a thin reflecting layer, which reflects the light back toward the film side or front of the screen. The third is the phosphor layer. The most common phosphor used today consists of rare-earth elements such as lanthanum oxybromide and gadolinium oxysulfide that emit green light. Rare earth screens allow shorter exposure time. Over the phosphor layer

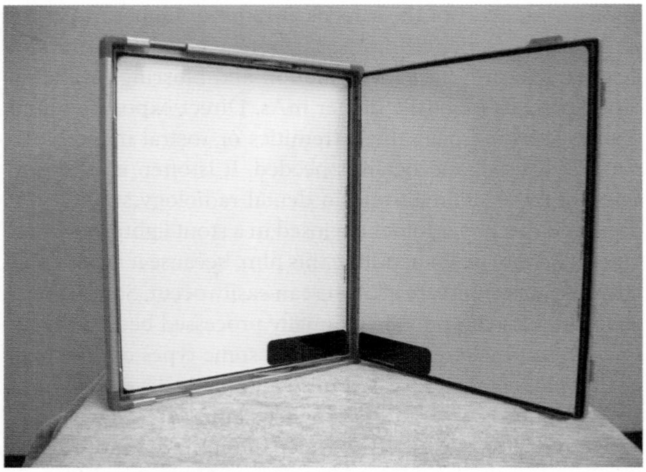

FIGURE 6-9 Cassette with intensifying screens.

is a thin waterproof protective coating that prevents static during cassette loading and unloading. It also provides physical protection and a surface that can be cleaned.

Intensifying screens are available in three different speeds: high (regular), par (medium), and slow (detail or fine). High-speed screens require less exposure time as compared with the par or slow speeds, but detail is decreased. With shorter exposure times, high-speed screens are ideal for imaging soft tissues, such as the thorax and abdomen, which are accompanied by unavoidable movement. Better detail can be achieved with slow-speed screens requiring longer exposure time. When changing from a high-speed screen to a par-speed screen, the mAs must be increased two times. When changing from high speed to slow speed, the mAs must be increased four times to maintain radiographic density.

Proper care of intensifying screens is very important. Routine cleaning is necessary to ensure that the screens are free from dirt and foreign material. Such material can block the light emitted from the screens, leaving parts of the film unexposed. The result is a white area on the film in the likeness of the foreign material. Identifying the cassettes inside on the intensifying screen and also on the outside of the cassette enables the dirty cassette to be retrieved and cleaned. Processing chemicals can cause permanent damage if the screen surface is not promptly cleaned. The screens should be cleaned with a soft, lint-free cloth and screen-cleaning solution. If a commercial cleaner is not available, warm water is acceptable. Do not use denatured alcohol or abrasive products, because they can damage the protective coating and phosphor layer. Be sure to allow the screen to completely dry before reloading.

Cassettes are precision instruments and should be handled that way. Do not drop them or set heavy objects on them. This can result in poor film-screen contact and blurring of one area of the image. To check the film-screen contact of your screens, place paper clips over the surface of the cassette. Use enough to completely cover every area. Expose the cassette using 50 to 60 kVp and half the mAs you would use for non-grid extremity. Process the film and view it dry. Any areas with poor film-screen contact are indicated by a blurred image of the paper clips.

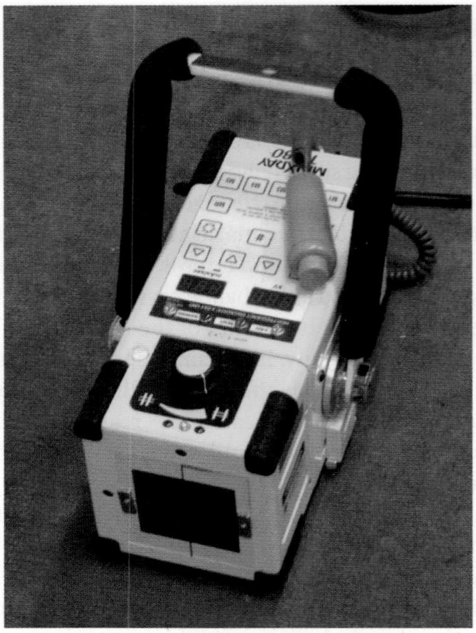

FIGURE 6-10 Portable x-ray unit.

X-RAY EQUIPMENT

There are many factors to consider when choosing x-ray equipment. The needs of individual practices will vary depending on the species to be radiographed, the caseload, and the type of technology desired. There are three basic types of x-ray equipment from which to choose: portable, mobile, and stationary units. A portable unit can be carried to the animal. These machines generally have a fixed mA set by the manufacturer at 15 to 30 mA, a variable kVp ranging from 40 to 90, and exposure times as short as 1/120 second (Fig. 6-10). Portable units are ideal for large-animal extremities but can be used to radiograph some small animals. Because the mA is fixed, the exposure time is changed to increase the radiographic density. For this reason, motion can be a problem for some because of the prolonged exposure times.

The mobile unit can be transported to the patient. However, because of its large size, it is limited to in-hospital use, such as in the treatment room or perhaps in a driveway (Fig. 6-11). These units generally produce a maximum 300 mA, 125 kVp, and 1/120-second exposure. The tube head on a mobile unit can be lowered to the ground for large-animal radiography or suspended above a table for small-animal radiography.

Stationary units are those that are installed in a room with proper leaded wall shielding for radiography. These units have many different exposure capabilities, depending on the quality desired. A general small-animal practice that does mainly routine radiographic examinations may be well-served by a machine with 300 mA, 125 kVp, and at least 1/120-second output (Fig. 6-12). However, practices that

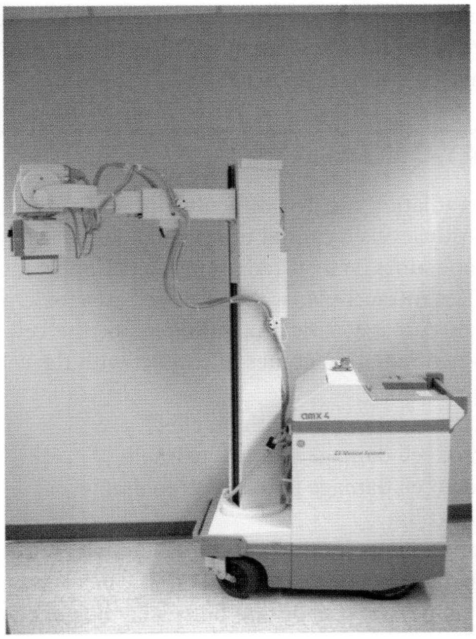

FIGURE 6-11 Mobile x-ray unit.

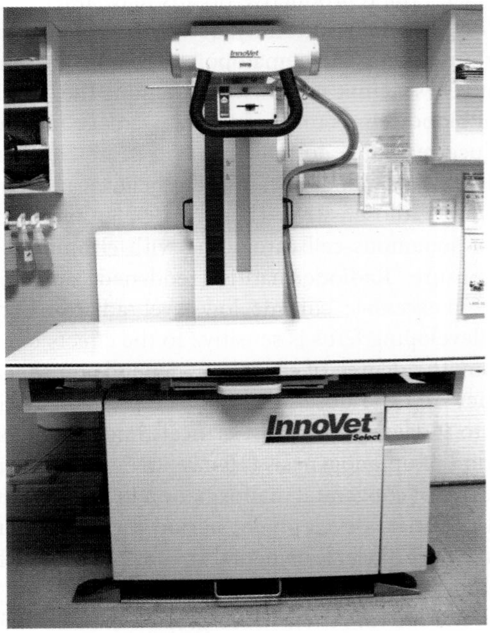

FIGURE 6-12 Standard x-ray unit.

provide specialty services, such as internal medicine or surgery referrals, will require higher-output equipment.

Caseload should be taken into account when choosing x-ray equipment. If a practice has an average of one to two cases requiring radiographs per week, with a majority of large-animal extremities and an occasional small animal film, a portable unit would probably be considered appropriate. If a practice has an average of 3 to 15 radiography cases per week, with a mixture of large and small animals, a mobile unit may be considered. A high-volume practice that radiographs an average of more than 16 cases per week will benefit from a stationary unit.

Accessory equipment used depends on the type of x-ray machine needed. Basic equipment requirements for a stationary x-ray machine include the x-ray generator system, collimator, grid, table, tube stand, and positioning aids. Because most large-animal extremity radiographs are made with portable or low-output x-ray machines, tube stands and cassette holders must be used. These pieces of accessory equipment allow the individuals to be positioned farther from the primary beam, thus decreasing personal exposure. Cassettes and x-ray tubes should never be hand held.

DIGITAL X-RAY IMAGING

The increased availability and affordability of digital radiography has made replacing analog systems much easier. Digital radiography refers to the process whereby images are obtained and displayed on appropriate computer monitors in gray scale digital display. There are three main types of digital systems currently available. These include computed radiography (CR), digital radiography (DR), and charge coupled devices (CCD) technologies. An advantage with digital radiography is that the digitized image can then be enhanced and viewed by using computer software that enables contrast, brightness, zoom, and pan adjustments as well as measurement of various anatomic structures.

> *TECHNICIAN NOTE* Digital radiographic images can be manipulated to enhance contrast and brightness and to allow for enlargement and measurement of anatomic structures.

Other advantages of digital radiography include elimination of the need for film, processing chemicals, and screens. Existing x-ray machines can be retrofitted for DR use or standard CR systems will be accepted without any changes being made to the grid cabinet or Bucky mechanism. With CCD systems, however, a brand new radiology generator and table will need to be purchased. However, the current CCD systems are competitively priced as compared to CR and DR systems. Digital radiography systems may reduce the amount of repeat radiographs needed as a result of inappropriate exposure settings or chemical processing errors.

It should be noted that a hard copy film can still be made from digital radiography. There are multiple manufacturers of dry laser printers for printing images if necessary.

COMPUTED RADIOGRAPHY

Computed radiography (CR) uses a cassette system not unlike conventional film-screen systems. Instead of having two screens and a film within the cassette, there is an imaging plate (IP) that contains a photostimulable phosphor, which can store the radiation level received at each point on the plate. This eliminates the need for film as a medium for viewing radiographs. Instead of chemical processing, the cassette is run through a computer scanner that uses a scanning laser beam. This causes the electrons to relax to a lower energy level, which emits light. These light measurements are proportional to the amount of radiation reaching and being absorbed by the IP in a given area. This light is then measured and the digital image created. The imaging plate is then erased by fluorescent light in the reader and the IP is reloaded into the cassette for re-use. The imaging plate can be re-used thousands of times.

DIGITAL RADIOGRAPHY

Digital radiography (DR) also uses an imaging plate comprising an array of detectors. These detectors translate or convert the x-rays into an electrical signal or pulse that is then digitalized by the computer to an image. This imaging plate is connected directly to a computer that is dedicated to that function, thereby eliminating the need for a cassette such as that which is used in a CR system. This plate can be permanently placed in an x-ray table or be portable depending on the user's needs.

DIGITAL RADIOGRAPHY STORAGE

Digital radiography (and other modalities such as CT, MRI, ultrasound, and nuclear medicine) uses a DICOM (digital imaging and communications in medicine) format, which is the universally accepted format for the dispersion and storing of medical information. Each DICOM file includes the pertinent information associated with the patient such as modality, date and time of examination, and patient identification and number. DICOM files are encrypted so that patient and image data are kept secure and tamper proof.

> *TECHNICIAN NOTE* Digital radiographs, CT, MRI, and ultrasound images are stored using a universally accepted format known as DICOM.

Storage of these DICOM files can be as simple as archiving to a compact disc (CD), digital video discs (DVD), magnetic optical disks (MOD), or managed through a picture archival computing system (PACS). This greatly reduces the amount of space needed for storage. A PACS has the advantage of storing multiple patients and making images available to multiple computers within a hospital or a network of hospitals. It is capable of handling multiple modalities and enhances communication between clinicians. A typical setup for PACS is a dedicated computer workstation, monitor, and server. **Fluoroscopy** is used for those patients in which the visualization of dynamic structures is of importance. Using an x-ray tube, a beam is directed through a patient onto a fluorescent screen or image intensifier to form an image. This is commonly referred to as "real-time" because it is a continual stream of images. The image is then transferred to a monitor and can be recorded on spot film, videotape, or digitalized by computer. Fluoroscopy is generally used for gastrointestinal studies (such as barium studies, gastrograms, and upper GI studies), angiography (cardiac catheterizations), and myelography. Fluoroscopy is not a commonly used modality in the general clinical setting because of economic limitations. However, referral clinics and most university veterinary hospitals have one or have access to one.

RADIATION SAFETY

Ionizing radiation can be a difficult concept to grasp, because at diagnostic levels it cannot be seen, felt, or heard by the patient or operators. Why is radiation safety important? Radiation ionizes intracellular water. This releases toxic products, which can damage critical components of the cell, such as DNA. When radiation comes in contact with the cells of living tissue, it can:

- Pass through the cells with no effect
- Produce cell damage that is repairable
- Produce cell damage that is not repairable
- Kill the cells

Radiation damages the body in several ways. It may have carcinogenic effects, which means that cancer may develop in body tissues. Effects on the body may be genetic, occurring in future generations. Tissues that are most sensitive to ionizing radiation are those with rapidly growing or reproducing cells. The reproductive organs may suffer from temporary or permanent infertility, decreased hormone production, or mutations. The hematopoietic (blood-forming) cells are relatively sensitive to ionizing radiation. The lymphocytic series of blood cells is most sensitive. Damage to blood cells can reduce resistance to infection and cause clotting disorders. The thyroid gland, intestinal epithelium, and lens of the eye are also radiosensitive. There may be an increased incidence of squamous-cell carcinoma with chronic, low-level skin exposure. Radiodermatitis (reddened, dry skin) can result from excessive, chronic, low-level radiation exposure.

The developing fetus is sensitive to the effects of ionizing radiation. The degree of sensitivity depends on the stage of pregnancy and the dose received. The preimplantation period (0 to 9 days) is the most critical time for the embryo. The period of organogenesis (10 days to 6 weeks) carries the greatest risk of congenital malformation in the fetus, because this is the critical development period for fetal organs. The fetus may have skeletal or dental malformations. Other abnormalities include microphthalmia (small eyes) and overall growth retardation. A fetal dose greater than 25 rads (0.25 Gray) is recognized as the threshold for significant damage to the fetus (for an explanation of these units of measure, see the Terminology section). The fetal period (6 weeks to term) is the least sensitive time for the fetus; however, growth may be affected and mental retardation may still occur. Irradiation after 30 weeks is less likely to cause abnormalities because the sensitivity of the fetus approaches that of the adult.

TERMINOLOGY

REM stands for roentgen equivalent man. REM are used to express the dose equivalent that results from exposure to ionizing radiation. REM takes into account the quality of radiation, so doses of different kinds of radiation can be compared. **Sievert (SV)** is the current terminology used to define a REM

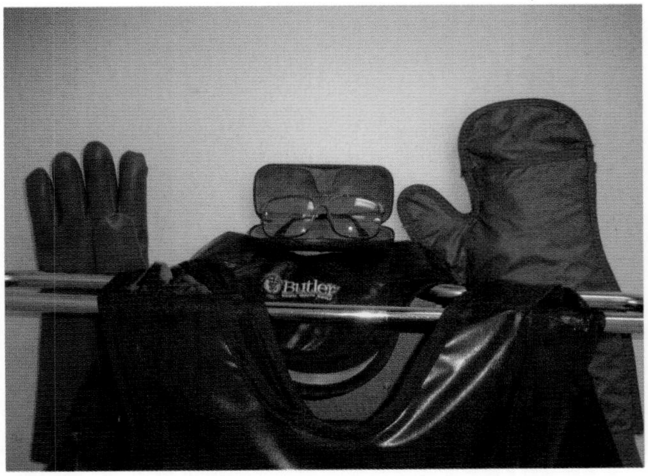

FIGURE 6-13 Lead gloves, gowns, thyroid shield, and lead-based glasses must be properly used and stored.

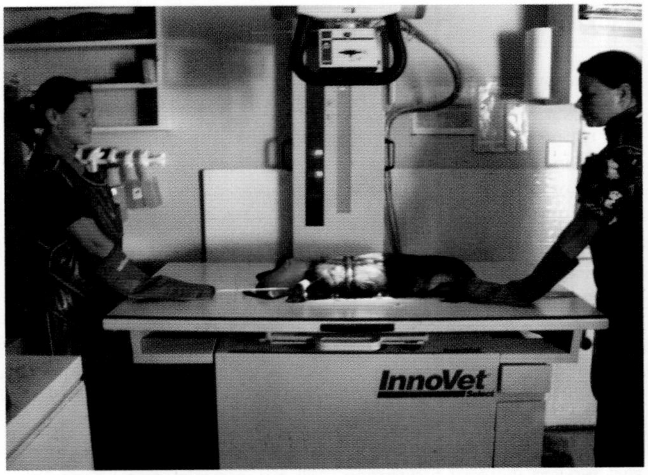

FIGURE 6-14 The restrainers have increased their distance from the primary beam by using mechanical devices (sand bags and tape) and are wearing the proper protective gear.

(1 SV = 100 REM). A millirem (MREM) is equal to 0.001 REM or 1/1000 REM. A rad is the Radiation Absorbed Dose. Current terminology is Gray (GY) (1 GY = 100 rad). This chapter concerns x-rays only and not other types of radiation, so rads can be considered equivalent to REMs. Other types of radiation must have a quality factor figured in to determine the dose. MPD is the **maximum permissible dose.** The National Council on Radiation Protection and Measurements recommends that the dose for occupationally exposed persons not exceed 5 REM per year. An occupationally exposed individual is one who normally performs his or her work in a restricted access area and has duties that involve exposure to radiation. **ALARA** stands for As Low As Reasonably Attainable. The MPD for nonoccupational persons is 10% of the MPD for occupationally exposed persons, or 0.5 REM per year. This is known as the ALARA MPD. Also, a fetus should not receive more than 0.5 REM during the entire gestation period. A pregnant employee who chooses to continue working around radiation-producing devices should wear an additional badge at waist level, underneath the lead gown, to monitor the fetal dose. This badge should not exceed 0.05 REM per month.

There are three important ways to minimize occupational exposure to radiation. The first is lead shielding. Lead shielding should be a requirement for all personnel remaining in the room while an exposure is made. Lead gowns, gloves, and thyroid shields (Fig. 6-13) should all contain at least 0.5 mm of lead. Lead-based glasses can also be worn to protect the lens of the eye.

Lead apparel is expensive, so it should be handled appropriately. Lead aprons should be draped over a rounded surface, without folds or wrinkles, to prevent cracks in the lead. Lead gloves can be stored with open-ended soup cans inserted to prevent cracks and to provide air circulation to the liners. Lead gloves should be radiographed every 6 months to check for damaged areas. Lead gowns should be checked every 12 months to screen for holes and cracks in the lead. Check gloves and gowns for damage by radiographing them using 5 mAs and 80 kVp. This can be adjusted as needed to attain the proper density in the radiographs.

Another method for decreasing personnel exposure is by increasing the distance from the primary beam. If the animal cannot be sedated or anesthetized, personnel restraining the animal should try to remain as far as possible from the x-ray source during exposure. During exposure, if restraining, one should use tape and sandbags and/or many other varieties of mechanical restraints to extend the distance of the gloved hands from the collimated area (Fig. 6-14). Employees should take care to wear lead apparel properly to obtain full protection. Placing a glove on top of a hand for protection does not protect the hand from scatter radiation. The scatter can come from any direction, including from under the tabletop.

Using the fastest film-screen combinations allows reduced exposure time for the patient and personnel by using less mAs. Proper darkroom practices and technique charts allow for consistent production of high-quality films, which reduces the number of repeated radiographs. It is very important to collimate the primary beam down to the area of interest, because this reduces exposure of personnel to scatter (secondary) radiation. A 2-mm aluminum filter is used at the tube window to filter out soft rays that are too weak to penetrate the patient. If these rays are not filtered out, they scatter about the room, fogging the film and striking personnel.

Each clinic should have a radiation protection supervisor. A veterinary technician can fill this role. Responsibilities include educating personnel on radiation safety, monitoring safety practices, and maintaining a radiologic badge system. The supervisor also maintains x-ray equipment, darkroom facilities, and radiographic records. A good radiation control program consists of safe x-ray equipment, low-exposure techniques, use of positioning aids, proper measuring of patients, proper positioning methods, shielding, and monitoring personal radiation exposure (Box 6-1). The x-ray equipment is usually under control of the state government (e.g., State Board of Health). Regulations vary between states, so check with your state government about their policy regarding radiation-producing devices.

BOX 6-1 General Radiation Safety Rules

- Always wear lead gloves and apron as well as lead thyroid shield when remaining in the room during radiography or fluoroscopy. Lead protective shielding *must* be worn by all individuals involved in restraint of the animal.
- Always wear a radiation monitoring device on your collar *outside* the apron or on the edge of the glove when working around x-ray equipment. *Note:* Badges should not be exposed to sunlight, dampness, or extreme temperatures. This could cause falsely high readings.
- Never allow any part of your body to be exposed to the primary beam. Lead clothing does not protect against primary beam exposure.
- Wear lead-based glasses to protect the lens of the eye.
- Using mechanical restraints such as tape and sandbags, as well as increased distance, will aid in minimizing exposure.
- Use alternative methods of restraint (drugs, tape, sandbags, etc.) when using high-exposure radiographic techniques.
- Pregnant women and persons under the age of 18 years should not be involved in radiographic procedures. Use proper safety precautions.
- Only the people required for restraint should remain in the room when an exposure is made.

TECHNICIAN NOTE **Methods to reduce occupational exposure to ionizing radiation include the use of lead shielding and proper use of patient positioning aids.**

DARKROOM TECHNIQUES

Along with a good technique chart, proper darkroom techniques should be followed to ensure consistent production of high-quality radiographs. Properly exposed radiographs can quickly become non-diagnostic with poor film handling and darkroom techniques.

DARKROOM SETUP

For most veterinary practices, the darkroom does not need to be large or fancy, as long as the layout is designed for efficiency. The room must be just large enough to provide a "dry bench" area away from the "wet bench" area (Fig. 6-15). The dry bench area is for unloading and loading cassettes and film storage. The wet bench area is for film processing and drying. These areas must be separated to prevent processing chemical splashes from damaging the dry films or sensitive intensifying screens. In a small room this can be achieved by placing a partition between the two areas. Sufficient electrical outlets should be available to power the safelights, viewboxes, and labeling equipment.

The most important feature of a darkroom is that it be light tight. White light that leaks around the door, through a blackened window, or around ventilation fans can fog the film. Film is more sensitive after it has been exposed to x-rays, so even low-grade light leaks decrease the quality of the finished radiograph. When checking for light leaks, stand in the darkroom for at least 5 minutes to allow your eyes to adjust to the darkness. Look around the door frame, ventilation fan, or blackened windows for any signs of white light. When performing this test, vary the intensity of light outside the door. Because work in the darkroom is done with a limited amount of light, painting the walls and ceiling a light color that reflects the available light helps greatly.

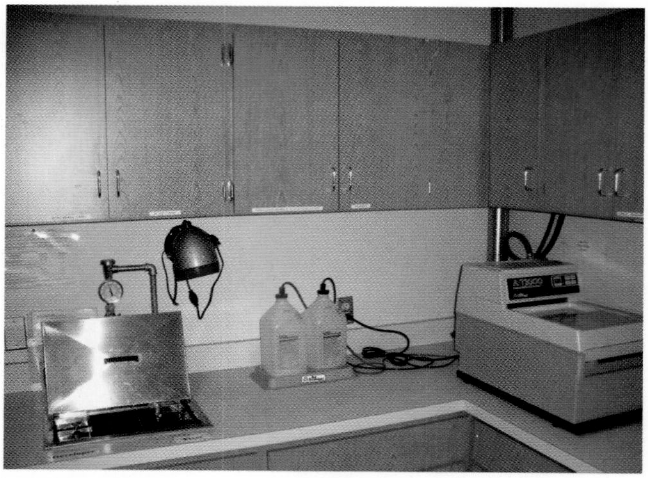

FIGURE 6-15 Darkroom processing area. Note the dry and wet prep areas are well separated.

The darkroom should have adequate ventilation to prevent volatile chemical fumes from accumulating in the room. These fumes can cause fogging of the film, damage to electrical equipment, and health problems for personnel. A light-tight ventilation fan installed in the ceiling helps remove the fumes and also controls the temperature and humidity in the room. The exhaust from automatic processors and film dryers should also be vented away from the darkroom, because they contain volatile chemical fumes.

Cleanliness is important in the darkroom, because intensifying screens and the film are handled in this area. Dirt and hair on countertops can fall into cassettes, causing white artifacts on subsequent radiographs from that cassette. Chemical spills also cause artifacts on the radiographs and damage the intensifying screens. Keeping both wet and dry areas of the darkroom clean prevents these problems. Film hangers for manual processing should also be cleaned regularly. Chemicals that remain on the hanger clips could drip down the next film to be processed, causing an artifact.

FILM IDENTIFICATION

Permanent labeling is necessary for all radiographs. Each film must be identified before the film is processed for legal purposes and for certification organizations. The labeling can be done during the exposure or after the exposure, but it must be done before the film is processed. The label should include the clinic name, date, owner's name, address, patient's name, and some patient data, such as age and breed.

There are several methods for film identification (Fig. 6-16). One method is the photo labeler. This uses a cassette containing a leaded window that protects the area during exposure. During identification, the window slides back from the protected area to expose the information on a card. This forms a latent image of the information on the film. Manual printers

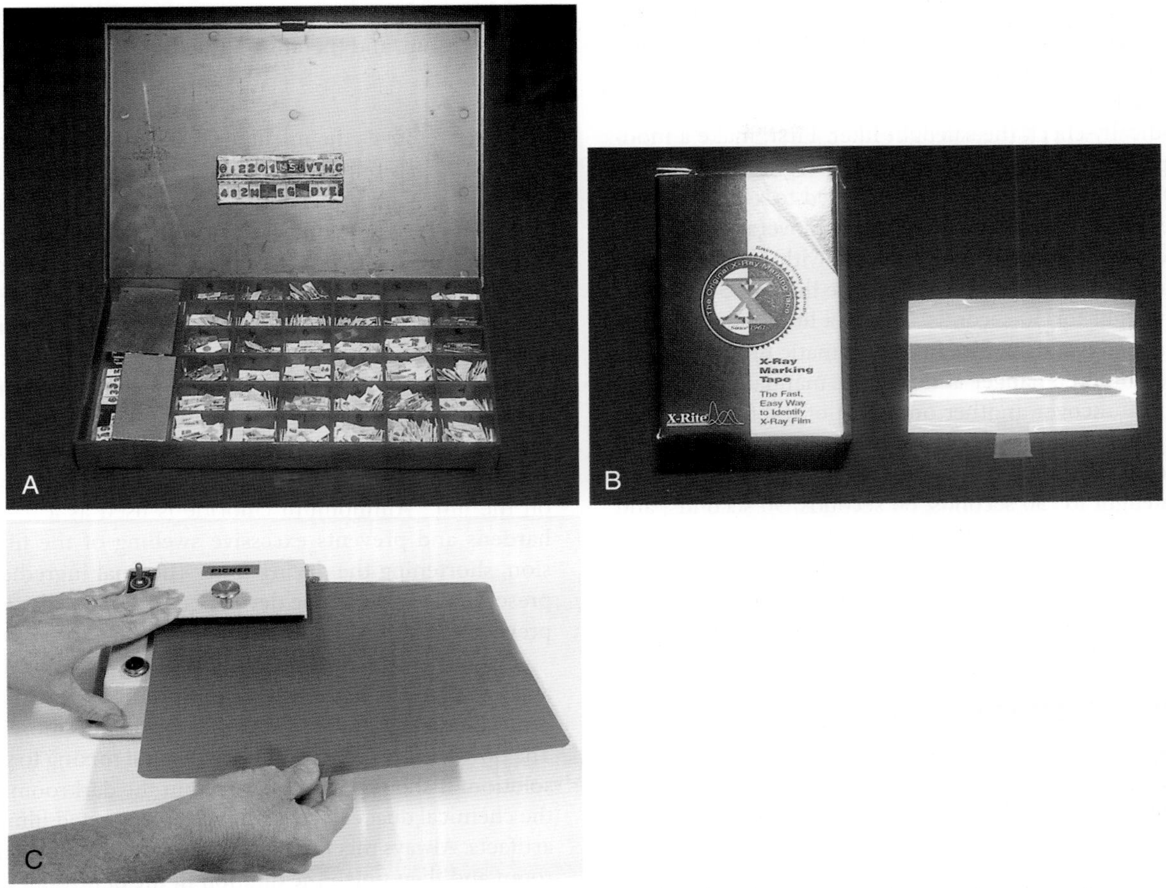

FIGURE 6-16 Film labeling. **A,** Leaded letters and numbers placed on the cassette at the time of exposure. **B,** Radiographic label tape. **C,** Light flasher. Patient information is printed onto a radiograph with an identification printer. (A and B from Figure 16-1, C from Figure 16-2, in Bassert J, Thomas J: *McCurnin's Clinical Textbook for Veterinary Technicians*, ed 8, St Louis, 2014, Saunders.)

are similar to photo labelers, except they use a flash of light through an information card to produce a latent image on the film. The manual printer is placed in the darkroom, and the film is taken out of the cassette to be identified. Another method uses lead letters or radiopaque tape. These are placed on the cassette during exposure of the radiograph.

> *TECHNICIAN NOTE* X-rays must be labeled with the clinic name and location, date the x-ray was taken, owner's name, and patient's name.

SAFELIGHTS

Safelight illuminators are important for darkroom processing. A safelight provides sufficient light to work in the room but does not cause fogging of the film. Safelights can be mounted to provide light directly or indirectly. With direct lighting, the safelight is mounted at least 48 inches above the workbench and directed toward the workbench. Indirect lighting has the safelight directed toward the ceiling and uses the reflected light to illuminate the room. With indirect lighting, the safelight can be mounted closer to the bench but should be as high as possible (Fig. 6-17).

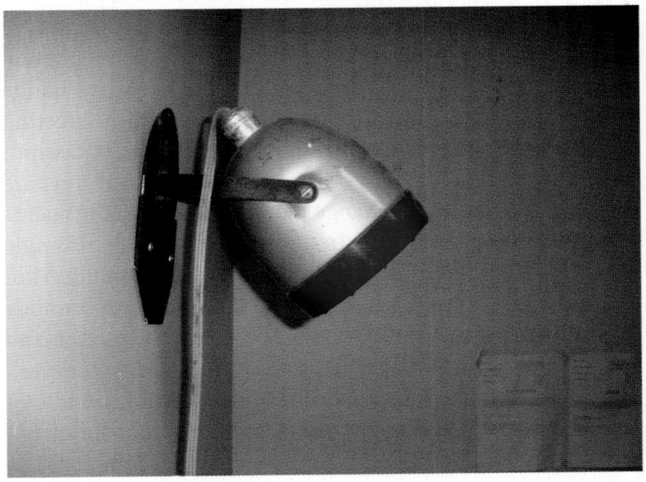

FIGURE 6-17 Direct safelight illumination.

Many types of safelight filters are available to filter out light in different areas of the light spectrum. The type of film used dictates which filter is necessary. Film that is blue-light-sensitive requires a safelight that filters out blue and ultraviolet light. Film that is green-light-sensitive requires a safelight to filter both green and blue light. This filter can also be used with blue-light-sensitive film. A red light bulb should never be used to replace a safelight filter. It does not filter the light; it only colors it. A white frosted 7½- to 10-watt bulb is recommended for most safelight filters.

Periodically check the safelight filter. First, make a moderate exposure on a film using approximately 1 to 2 mAs and 40 to 50 kVp. Film that has been exposed to x-rays is more sensitive to low-grade light, producing an overall fogged appearance. Cover two thirds of the film with black paper or cardboard, and allow the remaining one third to be exposed to the safelight for 30 seconds. This is a little longer than it should take to place the film in an automatic processor or to place the film on a hanger and into the manual tanks. After 30 seconds, uncover another one third of the film and wait 30 more seconds. Repeat the process for the final one third, and develop the film. This test exposes portions of the film to the safelight for 30 seconds, 60 seconds, 90 seconds, and then it is processed. When the film is dry, look for areas of increased film density. If an increase in density is detected, a close check of the darkroom is necessary. Improper safelight distance, a cracked safelight filter, and light leaking around the filter can all cause film fogging.

FILM PROCESSING CHEMISTRY

Developer

The developer's main function is to convert the sensitized silver halide crystals into black metallic silver. Sensitized silver halide crystals are those that have been exposed to electromagnetic radiation, making them susceptible to chemical change. The developer contains five ingredients: a solvent, reducing agents, restrainer, activator, and a preservative.

Water is used as the solvent to keep all the ingredients in solution. It also causes the film emulsion to swell so that the reducing agents can penetrate the sensitized crystals. Reducing agents change the sensitized silver halide crystals into black metallic silver. The most common reducing agents are a combination of hydroquinone and p-methyl aminophenol. Restrainers are used to protect the unexposed silver halide crystals by preventing the reducing agents from affecting the unsensitized crystals. Potassium bromide and potassium iodide are the most common restrainers. Bromide ions are produced during the exchange between the reducing agents and the sensitized crystals. In a fresh solution, the bromide ions are not available. They are added as a starter solution but are not placed in replenishing solutions. Excessive bromide ions inhibit the reducing agents. Activators help soften and swell the film's emulsion so that the reducing agents can work effectively. Reducing agents cannot function in an acidic or neutral solution. The activators, usually a carbonate or hydroxide of sodium or potassium, provide an alkaline pH in the range of 9.8 to 11.4. Preservatives prevent the solution from rapidly oxidizing. Sodium and potassium sulfite are the most commonly used preservatives.

Developing chemicals are manufactured in two forms: liquid and powder. The liquid form requires dilution with water. The powder form should never be mixed in the darkroom, because the chemical dust contaminates unprotected film, causing artifacts. Always mix the powder in a bucket outside the darkroom, and then finish the dilution in the darkroom.

Fixer

The fixer removes the unchanged silver halide crystals from the film emulsion, leaving the black metallic silver. It also hardens the film emulsion, decreasing the susceptibility to scratches. The fixer contains five ingredients: a solvent, a fixing agent, an acidifier, a hardener, and a preservative.

As with the developer, the solvent for the fixer is water. It keeps the ingredients in solution and causes the film emulsion to swell, allowing the fixing agents to reach the unexposed crystals. The fixing agent is sodium or ammonium thiosulfate. This clears the remaining silver halide crystals from the film emulsion. The acidifier is acetic or sulfuric acid and is used to neutralize any alkaline developer remaining on the film. Ammonium chloride is used as a hardener. It hardens and prevents excessive swelling of the film emulsion, shortening the drying time. The final ingredient is the preservative. As with the developer, sodium sulfite is used to prevent decomposition of the fixing agents.

Fixer chemicals are manufactured in two forms: liquid and powder. The liquid form requires dilution with water. It is more expensive than the powder form but is more efficient. The powder form requires dissolving and mixing to get it into solution. It should never be mixed in the darkroom, because the chemical dust can contaminate unprotected film, causing artifacts. Always mix the powder in a bucket outside the darkroom and then finish the dilution in the darkroom. Also, the powder requires a longer clearing time than the liquid form.

FILM PROCESSING EQUIPMENT

Manual Processing

With the ready availability of reasonably priced automatic processors, few veterinary clinics now use manual methods. However, there are still some locations where these are present. Manual processing is sometimes used for dental radiographs and some other non-screen films used for exotic animal radiography. Manual processing tanks are usually made from stainless steel and are large enough to accept 14-by-17-inch film hangers. Tanks with 5-gallon capacity are sufficient. Plastic or wooden lids are needed to cover the developer and fixer tanks. This reduces the rate of evaporation and oxidation of the chemicals. Separate stirring rods for the developer and fixer are used to mix the chemicals before processing. Also, an accurate timer and a floating thermometer should be available.

Developing x-ray film is a chemical process that depends on the duration of immersion in the chemicals and the temperature of the chemicals. The recommended time for development is 5 minutes. This allows just enough time for the reducing agents to convert the sensitized silver halide crystals. The temperature of the chemicals is also important. The warmer the temperature, the more the emulsion swells and the faster the chemicals work. Cold temperatures also affect the chemicals by decreasing their ability to penetrate the film emulsion. Manufacturers generally recommend a temperature for the chemicals they produce. Most use 68° F (20° C), with 5 minutes of developing time. For some cases this may not be possible, so the time can be adjusted to compensate for the increase or decrease in temperature. The time can be decreased by 30 seconds for every 2° increase in developer temperature or the time can be increased by 30 seconds for every 2° decrease in developer temperature. This applies only between 65° F (18° C) and 74° F (23° C).

The rinse bath removes developer from the film, preventing carryover into the fixer tank. Agitating the film in the running water bath for 30 seconds adequately removes the developer. The rinse water should be continually exchanged to prevent accumulation of developer. The temperature of the incoming rinse water can often be used to regulate the temperature of the developer and fixer tanks.

The fixing process is also dependent on immersion time and temperature of the chemicals. The standard temperature is 68° F (20° C), and the fixing time is double the developing time. The temperature affects the time the film is left in the fixer. The warmer the chemicals are, the shorter the fixing time will be. The film can be removed from the fixer after 30 seconds and viewed with white light. However, it must be placed back into the fixer for the remainder of the time. The clearing time increases as the thickness of the emulsion increases. Direct-exposure film has a thicker emulsion and requires a longer time in the fixer.

The final wash rinses away the processing chemicals. Failure to rinse the film completely results in a film that eventually becomes faded and brown. This is caused by oxidation of the chemicals remaining in the film emulsion. The wash tank should have fresh circulating water to decrease the time needed for the final wash. Generally the wash time is at least 30 minutes. Procedure 6-1 shows the steps for manual processing.

PROCEDURE 6-1 Procedure for Manual Processing of X-Ray Film

1. Check chemical temperature (optimal chemical temperature is 68° F (20° C).
2. Check chemical levels and stir both chemical tanks.
3. Clean countertops.
4. Turn on water to the wash tank.
5. Turn on the safelight and turn off the white lights.
6. Unload the cassette and place the film on the appropriate size film hanger.
7. Immerse the film in the developer. The optimal time is 5 minutes at 68° F (20° C).
8. Gently agitate the film to dislodge any air bubbles that may cling to the film's surface.
9. After 5 minutes of developing time, place the film in the wash tank and agitate for 30 seconds.
10. Lift the film out of the wash tank, allowing the excess water to drain back into wash tank.
11. Place the film into the fixer tank and agitate gently to dislodge air bubbles that cling to the surface. Leave the film in the fixer tank for 10 minutes.
12. Place the film in the wash tank for at least 30 minutes.
13. After washing the film, let the film hang until dry.

Maintenance. There are two methods for maintaining manual processing tanks. The first is the exhausted method. With this method, allow the chemicals to drain back into their respective tanks and not into the wash tank. This permits the exhausted chemicals to remain in the tank, maintaining the chemical levels. The second method is the replenishing method. Do not allow the chemicals to drain back into their respective tanks, but place them in the wash tank. The chemical levels are maintained with replenishing chemicals that are more concentrated than the initial solutions. In this way, the potency and levels of the chemicals can be preserved. With either method, the chemicals should be changed every 3 months.

Automatic Processing

Use of an automatic processor has some advantages over manual processing. Automatic processors can develop film more quickly. They can process and dry a film in 90 to 120 seconds. Also, automatic processors consistently provide high-quality radiographs. This eliminates the need for repeat radiographs because of processing errors.

Automatic processors move the film through the developer, fixer wash bath, and dryers at a uniform rate of speed. Chemicals and film are specially manufactured to withstand the high temperatures involved in automatic processing. The chemicals are kept at temperatures around 95° F (35° C), depending on the type of film and equipment used. The emulsion on film designed for automatic processing is harder than on film designed for manual processing, preventing scratches from the roller. This film can also be manually processed in case of mechanical problems with the automatic processor.

Maintenance. Small tabletop automatic processors are easily maintained in most veterinary practices. The equipment should be completely cleaned every 3 months. This includes draining and cleaning the tanks. A 1:32 solution of laundry bleach (e.g., Clorox) helps to reduce algae and remove chemical buildup. The rollers can be cleaned with a mild detergent and soft sponge. When any cleaning solution is applied to the tanks or rollers, they should be rinsed thoroughly before replacing the chemicals. Also, check the springs and gears for signs of wear and replace if necessary. Wipe the feed tray and top rollers with a clean soft sponge every day. This helps remove dirt, debris, and chemical residue between episodes of routine maintenance.

Silver Recovery

When an exposed film is placed in the developer, the exposed silver halide crystals are converted to black metallic silver. The remaining silver halide crystals are removed from the film in the fixer. Over time, the fixer solution becomes rich with silver that can be reclaimed. Silver recovery systems can be attached to automatic processors to filter and store the silver that would normally be discarded down the drain. The black metallic silver in the radiographs can also be recovered.

The manual processing fixer solution, silver recovery systems, and old radiographs can be sold to companies that reclaim the silver. These companies are usually listed in the Yellow Pages under the headings "Gold and Silver Refiners and Dealers."

RADIOGRAPHIC ARTIFACTS

An artifact is any unwanted density in the form of blemishes arising from improper handling, exposure, processing, or housekeeping. Artifacts can mimic or mask a disease process or distract from the overall quality of the film.

Before radiographing an animal, check for external debris, wet hair, or any lumps or bumps on the patient. Remove any dirt or mats from the coat. If the coat is wet, dry it as much as possible. Remove any collars, leashes, or halters. Bandage material is visible on radiographs, so remove it if feasible. Boxes 6-2 and 6-3 list common artifact problems.

BOX 6-2 Causes of Common Radiographic Artifacts That Occur Before Processing

Fogged Film

- Film exposed to excessive scatter radiation. A grid is necessary when radiographing areas measuring 10 cm or more. (overall gray appearance)
- Film exposed to radiation during storage
- Film stored in an area that was too hot or humid
- Film exposed to a safelight filter that was cracked or inappropriate for the type of film used
- Film exposed to a low-grade light leak in a darkroom
- Film expired

Black Crescents or Lines

- Rough handling of film before or after exposure (Figure 1)

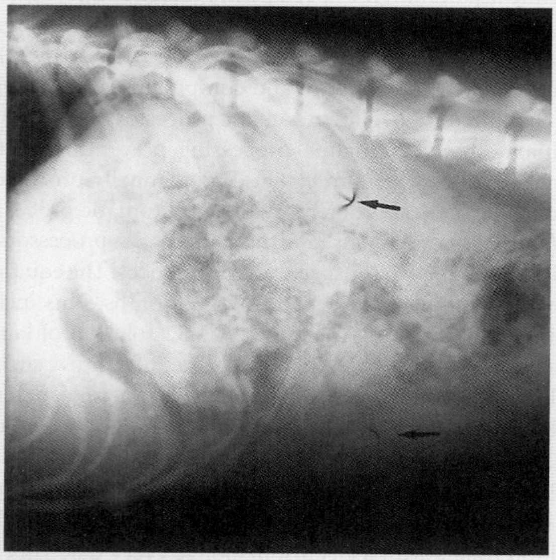

FIGURE 1 Black crescent from rough handling of the film before or after exposure.

- Static electricity caused by low humidity
- Scratched film surface before or after exposure
- Fingerprints from excessive pressure before or after exposure

Black Areas

- Black irregular border on one end of film caused by light exposure while still in the box or film bin
- Black irregular border on multiple sides of the film caused by felt damage in the cassette

White Areas

- Foreign material between the film and screen (Figure 2)

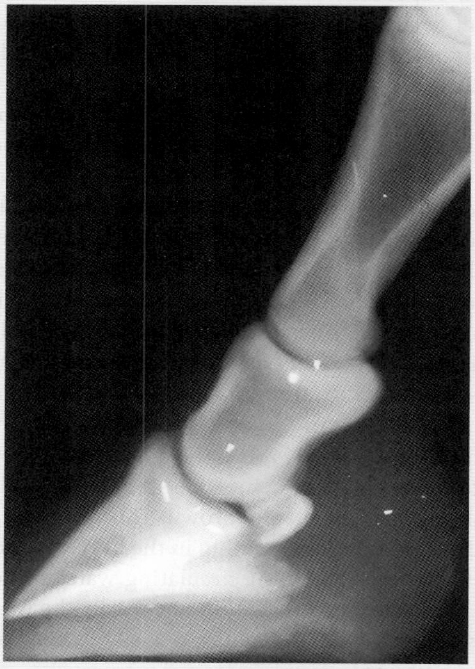

FIGURE 2 Foreign material between the film and screen blocks light from exposing the film, creating white areas.

- Chemical spill on the screen, causing permanent damage to the phosphor layer
- Contrast medium on the patient, table, or cassette
- White fingerprints on film from oil or fixer on fingers before processing

Visible Gridlines

- Grid lines on the entire film from focal-film distance outside the range of the grid's focus
- Grid lines more visible on one end of the film and an overall decrease in radiographic density caused by the grid's not being centered in the primary beam
- Grid lines on the entire film caused by the grid's not being perpendicular to the center of the primary beam
- Grid lines more visible in some areas than others from grid damage

Decreased Detail

- Patient motion
- Poor film-screen contact
- Increased object-film distance
- Decreased focal-film distance

BOX 6-3 Causes of Common Radiographic Artifacts That Occur During Manual or Automatic Processing

Increased Radiographic Density With Poor Contrast
- Film overdeveloped (longer than manufacturer recommendation)
- Film developed in hot chemicals. Correct temperature for manual tanks is 68° F (20° C); for automatic processors, it is 95° F (35° C)
- Film overexposed

Decreased Radiographic Density With Poor Contrast
- Film underdeveloped (shorter than manufacturer recommendation)
- Film developed in cold chemicals. Correct temperature for manual tanks is 68° F (20° C), for automatic processors, it is 95° F (35° C)
- Film processed in old or exhausted chemicals
- Film underexposed

Uneven Development
- Lack of stirring allowing chemicals to settle to tank bottom
- Repeated withdrawal of the film from the tank to check on development results
- Uneven chemical levels

Black Areas, Spots, or Streaks
- Identical black areas on two films processed together from films stuck to one another in the fixer and not cleared properly
- Black area on only one film from film sticking to side of tank
- Well-defined spots or streaks from developer splash before processing
- Black lines along the full length of the film and equal distance apart from pressure of rollers in the processor

Defined Areas of Decreased Radiographic Density
- Identical light areas on two films processed together from sticking together in the developer
- Light area on one film from film sticking to the side of the tank during development (Figure 1)
- Air bubbles clinging to the film during development
- Well-defined spots or streaks from fixer splash before processing

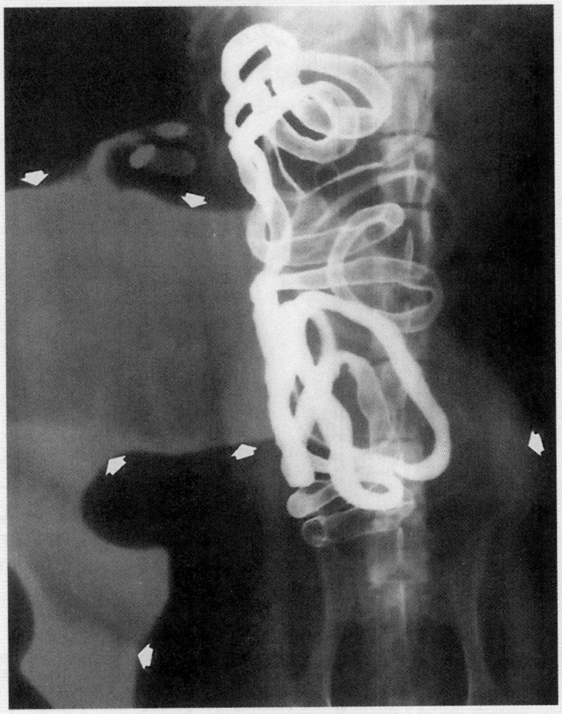

FIGURE 1 This radiograph stuck to the side of the manual tank while in the developer. The arrows outline the artifact. A light image can still be seen, because the file has emulsion on both sides of the film base. One side developed normally.

Clear Areas or Spots
- Streaks where emulsion scratched away
- Large clear areas from leaving film in final wash too long and emulsion sliding off film base

Entire Film Clear
- No exposure
- Film placed in fixer before developer

Film Turns Brown
- Improper final wash

RADIOGRAPHIC POSITIONING AND TERMINOLOGY

Proper patient positioning is as important as the radiograph itself. Misinterpretations can result from inaccurate positioning. A basic knowledge of directional terminology is essential when describing radiographic projections. The American College of Veterinary Radiology (ACVR) has standardized the nomenclature for radiographic projections by using currently accepted veterinary anatomic terms. The projections are described by the direction the central ray enters and exits the part being imaged (see Fig. 6-18).

- *Ventral (V):* Body area situated toward the underside of quadrupeds.
- *Dorsal (D):* Body area situated toward the back or topline of quadrupeds. Opposite of ventral.
- *Medial (M):* Body area situated toward the median plane or midline.
- *Lateral (L):* Body area situated away from the median plane or midline.
- *Cranial (Cr):* Structures or areas situated toward the head (formerly anterior).
- *Caudal (Cd):* Structures or areas situated toward the tail (formerly posterior).
- *Rostral (R):* Areas on the head situated toward the nose.
- *Palmar (Pa):* Situated on the caudal aspect of the front limb, distal to the antebrachiocarpal joint.

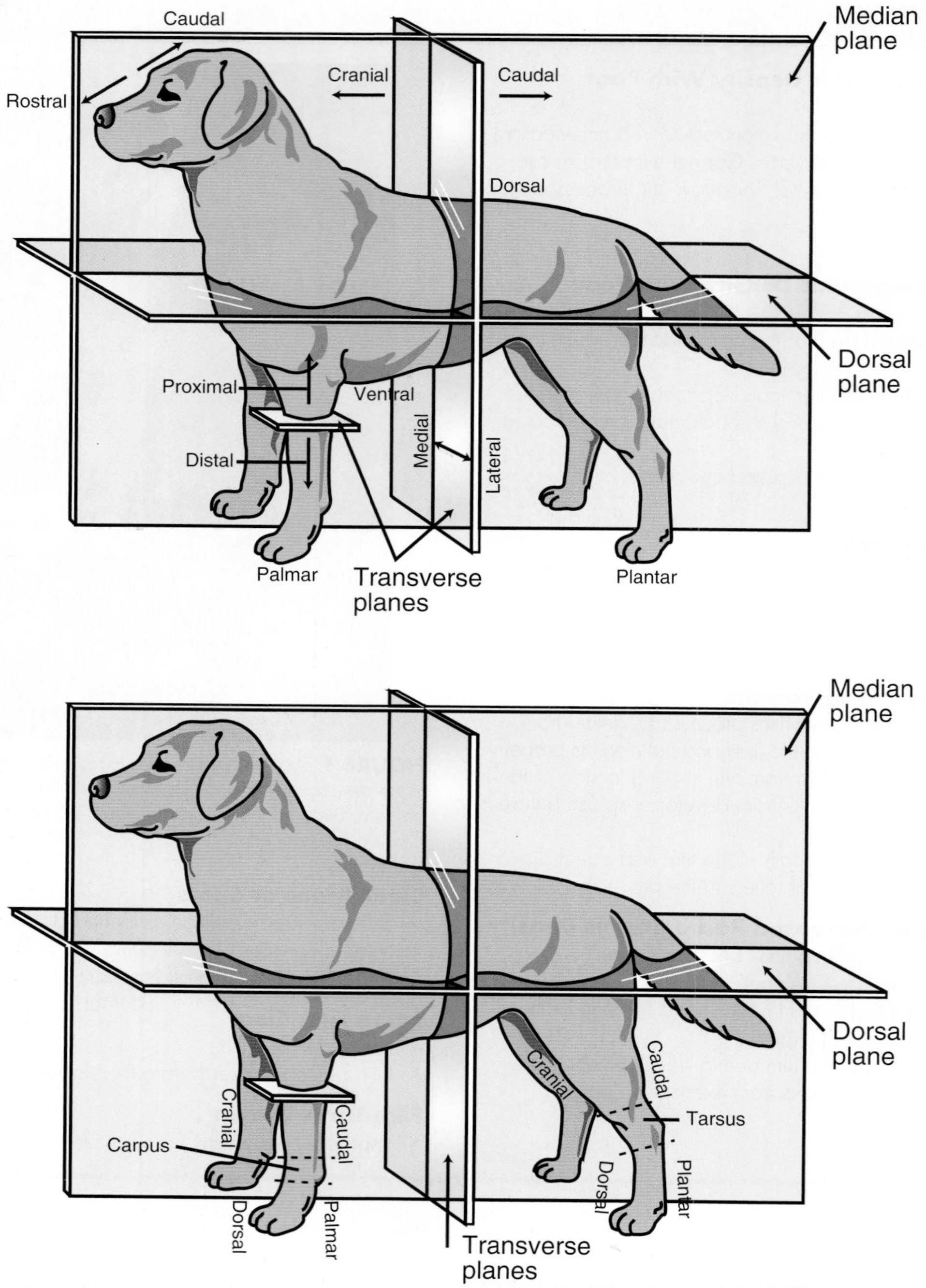

FIGURE 6-18 Anatomical planes of reference and directional terms. (From Colville TP, Bassert JM: *Clinical anatomy and physiology for veterinary technicians*, ed 2, St Louis, 2008, Mosby.)

- *Plantar (Pl):* Situated on the caudal aspect of the rear limb, distal to the tarsocrural joint.
- *Proximal (Pr):* Situated closer to the point of attachment or origin.
- *Distal (Di):* Situated away from the point of attachment or origin.

OBLIQUE PROJECTIONS

Oblique projections are used to set off an area that normally would be superimposed over another area. Some rules should be followed when deciding what type of oblique projection is needed and how it is identified.

- The area of interest should be as close to the cassette as possible. This decreases magnification and increases detail.
- Place a marker on the cassette or near the anatomy within the primary beam during exposure to indicate the direction of entry and exit of the primary beam.

Table 6-1 shows the landmarks used to produce radiographs of various body parts.

TABLE 6-1 Diagnostic Imaging
Landmarks Used in Producing Radiographs of Various Body Areas

BODY PART	CRANIAL OR PROXIMAL LANDMARK	CAUDAL OR DISTAL LANDMARK	CENTER LANDMARK	COMMENTS
Thorax	Manubrium sterni	Halfway between xiphoid and last rib	Caudal border of the scapula	Expose at peak inspiration
Abdomen	Halfway between the xiphoid and the caudal border of the scapula	Greater trochanter	Last rib	Expose at peak expiration
Shoulder	Midbody scapula	Midshaft humerus	Over joint space	
Humerus	Shoulder joint	Elbow joint	Midshaft	
Elbow	Midshaft humerus	Midshaft radius	Over joint space	
Radius/Ulna	Elbow joint	Carpal joint	Midshaft	
Carpus	Midshaft radius	Midshaft metacarpus	Over joint space	
Metacarpus	Carpal joint	Include digits	Midshaft	
Pelvis	Wings of ilium	Ischium		
Pelvis VD, flexed	Wings of ilium	Ischium		Pushes stifles cranially
Pelvis VD, extended	Wings of ilium	Stifle joint		Femora parallel to each other and table
Femur	Coxofemoral joint	Stifle joint	Midshaft	
Stifle	Midshaft femur	Midshaft tibia	Over joint space	
Tibia/fibula	Stifle joint	Tarsal joint	Midshaft	
Tarsus	Midshaft tibia	Midshaft metatarsal	Over joint space	
Metatarsus	Tarsal joint	Include digits	Midshaft	
Cervical Vertebrae	Base of skull	Spine of scapula		Extend front limbs caudally; collimate width of beam to increase detail
Thoracic Vertebrae	Spine of scapula		Halfway between xiphoid and last rib	Collimate width of beam to increase detail
Thoracolumbar vertebrae			Halfway between to increase detail	Collimate width of beam xiphoid and last rib
Lumbar vertebrae	Halfway between xiphoid and last rib	Wings of ilium		Collimate width of beam to increase detail

CONTRAST STUDIES

The purpose of a contrast study is to delineate an organ or area against surrounding soft tissues. They are useful in determining the size, shape, position, location, and function of an organ. The information obtained from a contrast study complements or confirms findings of the survey radiographs. A contrast study should never replace survey radiographs.

With contrast studies, tissues of interest appear either radiopaque or radiolucent on the finished radiograph. Areas that are radiopaque appear white. Positive-contrast agents are radiopaque on a radiograph. Radiolucent areas on the finished radiograph appear black. Negative-contrast agents produce radiolucencies on a radiograph.

Obtaining survey radiographs before doing a contrast study establishes proper exposure technique and proper patient preparation. In addition, a diagnosis may be achieved from survey radiographs, eliminating the need for the contrast study. Because most contrast studies require multiple images, it is very important to label each film with the time and sequence. Always record the amount, type, and administration route of the contrast agent.

POSITIVE-CONTRAST MEDIA

Positive-contrast media contain elements with a high atomic number. Elements with a high atomic number absorb more x-rays. Thus fewer x-rays penetrate the patient and expose the film, making a white area on the radiograph. Two common types of positive-contrast agents are barium sulfate and water-soluble organic iodides (Fig. 6-19). Barium sulfate is commonly used for positive-contrast studies of the gastrointestinal tract. It is insoluble and not affected by gastric secretions. Therefore it provides good mucosal detail on the radiograph. Barium sulfate preparations are relatively inexpensive and are manufactured in the form of powders, colloid suspensions, pastes, or as barium-impregnated polyurethane spheres (BIPS). One disadvantage of using barium sulfate is that it can take 3 or more hours to travel from the stomach to the colon. Also, it can be harmful to the peritoneum, so it should never be used when gastrointestinal perforations are

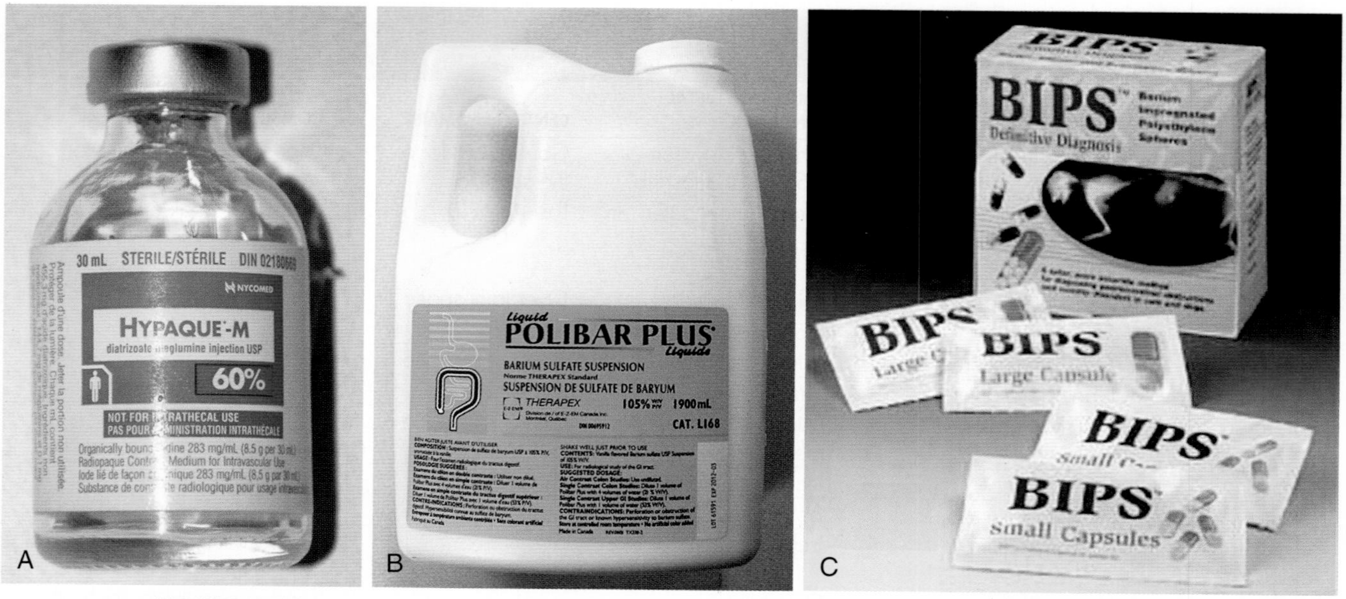

FIGURE 6-19 Positive contrast media. **A,** Iodine. **B,** Barium. **C,** Barium-impregnated polyurethane spheres (BIPS). (From Figure 25-1 in Brown M, Brown L: *Lavin's Radiography for Veterinary Technicians,* ed 5, St Louis, 2014, W.B. Saunders.)

suspected. Barium is insoluble and the body cannot eliminate it, resulting in granulomatous reactions in the abdominal cavity. While administering barium orally, take care to prevent the patient from aspirating barium into the lungs. Aspiration of large amounts can be fatal. Barium sulfate may also aggravate an already obstructed bowel by causing further impactions.

Water-soluble organic iodides in ionic form are also used for positive-contrast procedures. Different forms of the water-soluble organic iodides can be administered intravenously, orally, or by infusion into a hollow organ or into the subarachnoid space. Because they are water-soluble, they are absorbed into the bloodstream and excreted by the kidneys.

A commonly used oral form of ionic water-soluble organic iodide is a solution of meglumine and sodium diatrizoate. It is used to perform contrast studies of the gastrointestinal tract when perforation is suspected. When this agent is administered orally, transit through the gastrointestinal system is rapid, usually within 48 to 60 minutes. However, the hypertonic solution draws fluid into the bowel lumen. Thus the contrast medium is diluted, decreasing the quality of the study. Fluid loss may further complicate hypovolemia in a dehydrated animal. Water-soluble organic iodides should never be used in place of barium sulfate and should be used only when perforations are suspected.

Ionic water-soluble organic iodides for intravenous use are prepared in various combinations of meglumine and sodium diatrizoate. Diatrizoate can also be infused into hollow organs, such as the urinary bladder, or into fistulous tracts. Sodium diatrizoate is commonly used for excretory urography because it provides better opacification of the kidneys. Nausea, vomiting, or decreased blood pressure can occur when a large bolus of contrast medium is injected intravenously. Ionic water-soluble organic iodides cannot be used for myelography, because they are irritating to the brain and spinal cord.

Nonionic water-soluble organic iodides are used for myelography. Because of their low osmolarity and chemical nature, they cause fewer adverse effects when placed in the subarachnoid space. Two commonly used media are iopamidol and iohexol. Nonionic water-soluble organic iodides are suitable for myelography and can also be used intravenously.

NEGATIVE-CONTRAST MEDIA

Negative-contrast agents include air, oxygen, and carbon dioxide. They all have a low atomic number, appearing radiolucent on the finished radiograph. Oxygen and carbon dioxide are more soluble than water. Care must be taken not to overinflate the organs, such as the bladder. Air embolism can occur when air enters ulcerative lesions, causing cardiac arrest.

DOUBLE-CONTRAST PROCEDURE

Double-contrast procedures use both positive- and negative-contrast media to image an organ or area. The most common organs imaged with double-contrast are the urinary bladder, stomach, and colon. In most cases, the negative-contrast medium is added first, then the positive-contrast medium. Mixing negative-contrast medium with positive-contrast medium can cause air bubbles to form, which might be misinterpreted as lesions.

DIAGNOSTIC ULTRASOUND

Diagnostic ultrasound (**ultrasonography**) is a noninvasive method of imaging soft tissues. A transducer sends low-intensity, high-frequency sound waves into the soft tissues, where they interact with tissue interfaces. Some of the sound waves are reflected back to the transducer and some are transmitted into deeper tissues. The sound waves that are reflected back to the transducer (echoes) are then analyzed by the computer to produce a gray-scale image. Use of ultrasound in conjunction with radiography gives the veterinarian an excellent diagnostic tool. Radiographs demonstrate the size, shape, and position of the organs. Ultrasound displays the findings found on the radiographs as well as the soft tissue textures and the dynamics of some organs (e.g., motility of the bowel).

> TECHNICIAN NOTE Ultrasound imaging is ideal for displaying the characteristics of soft tissues.

TRANSDUCERS

Ultrasound transducers emit a series of sound pulses and receive the returning echoes. A weak electrical current applied to the piezoelectric crystals incorporated in the transducer causes the crystals to vibrate and produce sound waves. After sending a series of pulses, the crystals are dampened to stop further vibrations. When struck by the returning echoes, the crystals vibrate again, and convert these echoes into electrical energy.

Transducers are available in different configurations, which are mechanical or electronic. The scan plane can either be a sector scan (pie-shaped image) or a **linear-array scan** (rectangular image). A mechanically driven sector scan can be produced by a belt and pulley used to wobble a single crystal or rotate multiple crystals across a scan plane. Another method of producing a sector scan is with use of phased-array or annular-array configurations. With phased-array configuration, the crystals are pulsed sequentially with a built-in delay to create a "pseudo-sector" scan plane. **Annular array** arranges the crystals in concentric rings. By using electronic phasing of the many crystals, annular-array transducers produce a two-dimensional image by steering the entire array through a sector arc.

Sector scanners are useful when imaging areas limited by ribs, gas-filled bowels, or lungs. The narrow near field and wide far field enable the transducer scan plane to be positioned between or around these structures. Linear-array scanners produce a scan plane by alternately firing groups of crystals in sequence. The pulsing of each group of crystals occurs so rapidly that individual pulses cannot be observed by the human eye. Linear-array scanners are useful in areas with unrestricted window size. The rectangular scan plane is ideal for equine tendons or large or small animal transrectal imaging.

The frequency of the transducer determines the amount of detail or resolution of the image. As frequency increases, the wavelength gets shorter. The shorter the wavelength is, the better the resolution of the image will be.

Transducers are expensive and the most fragile part of ultrasound equipment. Care must be taken when handling them. Avoid hard impacts that can severely damage the sensitive crystals. Prevent exposure to extreme temperature changes. Some transducers are sensitive to certain types of cleaning agents. Always refer to manufacturer's instructions for appropriate cleaning products.

DISPLAY MODES

There are three different display modes: A-mode (amplitude mode), B-mode (brightness mode), and M-mode (motion mode).

A-mode

A-mode is the earliest form of ultrasound and is the simplest as far as computer software. With A-mode, the returning echoes are displayed as a series of peaks on a graph. As the intensity of the returning sound increases, the peak at that tissue depth increases. A-mode is not used to show tissue motion or anatomy. The main use in veterinary medicine was to measure the amount of subcutaneous fat in pigs.

B-mode

B-mode uses bright pixels or dots on a screen, whereas A-mode uses peaks on a graph. A dot on the monitor screen corresponds to the depth at which the echo was formed. The degree of brightness is proportional to the intensity of the returning echo. As intensity increases, the brightness of the dot increases. The image that is generated is a two-dimensional anatomic slice that is continually updated. This mode is currently used for diagnostic applications.

M-mode

M-mode is the continuous display of a thin slice of an organ over time. M-mode projects the echoes from a thin beam of sound over a time-oriented baseline. The main use is with echocardiography to assess the size of the heart chambers and the motion of the heart valves and walls.

TERMINOLOGY DESCRIBING ECHOTEXTURE

The terminology used to describe tissue texture within an ultrasound image is simple. Echogenic or **echoic** means that most of the sound is reflected back to the transducer. Echogenic areas appear white on the screen. **Sonolucent** means that most of the sound is transmitted to the deeper tissues, with only a few echoes reflected back to the transducer. Sonolucent areas appear dark on the screen. **Anechoic** is used to describe tissue that transmits all of the sound through to deeper tissues, reflecting none of the sound back to the transducer. Anechoic areas appear black on the screen and are generally fluid-filled structures.

Soft tissues are represented not only as black or white but also as many shades of gray. Additional terminology has been established to describe these areas. **Hyperechoic** is used to describe tissues that reflect more sound back to the transducer than surrounding tissues. Hyperechoic areas appear brighter than surrounding tissues. **Hypoechoic** is used to describe tissues that reflect less sound back to the transducer than surrounding tissues. Hypoechoic areas appear darker

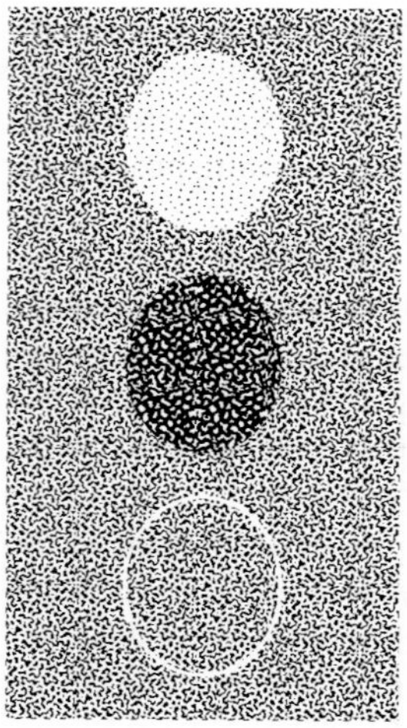

FIGURE 6-20 Hyperechoic, hypoechoic, and isoechoic areas. An area within an organ or the whole organ that is brighter than the surrounding tissue is described as hyperechoic. Areas that are darker than the surrounding tissue are described as hypoechoic. Areas that are the same as the surrounding tissue are described as isoechoic.

than surrounding tissues. **Isoechoic** is used to describe tissue that appears to have the same echotexture on the screen as surrounding tissues (Fig. 6-20).

Terminology has been established to describe areas displayed on the monitor screen. The screen is divided into nine zones, with each zone having its own label. In this way, the sonographer can verbally indicate the area of interest, such as mid field right or near field left.

PATIENT PREPARATION

To achieve an optimal acoustic window and produce the best-quality image, the transducer head must be placed in close contact with the skin. The animal's hair must be clipped and in some cases shaved before the study. Occasionally thin-coated animals can be imaged with minimal preparation. An acoustic coupling gel is used to eliminate the air interface and to improve the acoustic window. Before applying the acoustic coupling gel, wipe the area with alcohol or generous amounts of soapy water to remove any loose hairs, dirt, and skin oils.

Fasting of small animals before abdominal ultrasound examination is recommended. Ingesta and gas in the bowel decrease the amount of the abdomen that can be visualized.

INSTRUMENT CONTROLS

Ultrasound equipment has many controls for adjusting the quality of the image. Improper adjustment of any of these can greatly decrease the quality of the image.

Brightness and Contrast

The monitor has controls to adjust the brightness and contrast for the image being displayed. If the brightness has been adjusted too high or too low on the monitor, compensating with any other control cannot correct the brightness or darkness. Most machines have a gray bar that displays the gray-scale capability. This capability varies from 16 to 128 shades of gray. The brightness and contrast should be adjusted so that black, white, and all the intermediate shades of gray can be seen.

Depth

The depth control allows for adjustment of the amount of tissue being displayed on the monitor. The depth from the surface of the transducer is measured in centimeters. The area of interest (e.g., kidney, heart) should cover at least two thirds of the screen. Decreasing the amount of depth being displayed causes the area in the near field to become larger.

Gain and Power

The **gain** (overall) and **power** (output) controls can affect the overall brightness of the image. Gain and power compensate for attenuation of the sound beam as it travels through the tissues. Increasing the gain increases the sensitivity of the transducer to receiving the returning echoes. This can be compared with the volume on a hearing aid; thus, turning the volume up increases the hearing aid's ability to hear incoming sounds. The power controls the intensity of the sound generated by the transducer. Increasing the power increases the intensity of the sound wave leaving the transducer. The sound is attenuated at the same rate, but a higher-intensity sound wave transmitted into the tissues produces a higher-intensity echo returning to the transducer.

Time Gain Compensation

The controls that make up the **time gain compensation** (TGC) are the most important and most often improperly set. The purpose of the TGC is to make like tissues look alike. The intensity of the sound decreases progressively as it returns from deeper tissues. For example, when imaging the liver, three similar reflectors located at 4 cm, 6 cm, and 8 cm of depth should have the same brightness on the monitor. However, because of the attenuation of the echoes returning from the deeper tissues, the brightness gradually decreases. To compensate for the loss of energy, TGC adds increasing amounts of electronic gain to the returning echoes. The three echoes returning from different depths then have the same brightness on the monitor.

The typical controls that make up the TGC are near field gain and far field gain. The near field gain controls the amount of electronic gain added to the sound returning from the near field. This should be set so that the echoes blend uniformly with those displayed in the mid field. The far field gain controls the amount of electronic gain added to the echoes returning from the far field. With some of the new ultrasound equipment, the TGC is in the form of multiple slide pods. The pods at the top control the near field gain, whereas the pods closer to the bottom control the mid field and far field.

If proper brightness cannot be achieved, verify the following items. First, check the brightness and contrast controls on the monitor. If the brightness and contrast controls are incorrectly set, changing the TGC cannot compensate for this

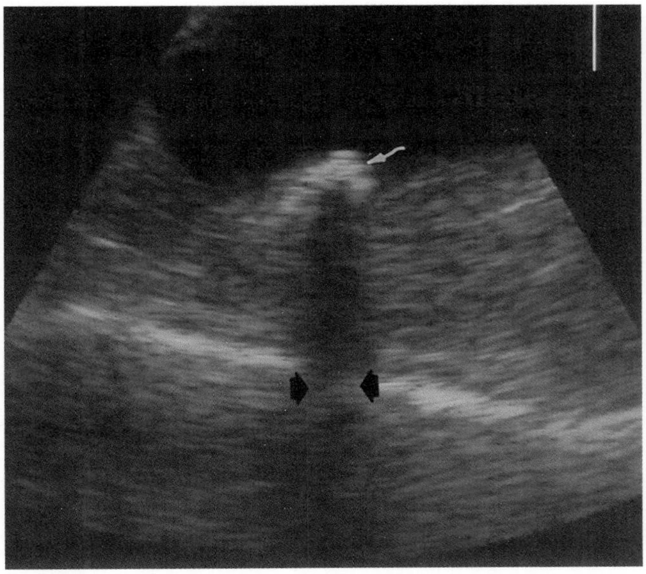

FIGURE 6-21 Acoustic shadowing from a calculus in the urinary bladder. The highly reflective surface of the calculus is shown *(white arrow)*. Shadowing caused by the calculus is also shown *(black arrow)*.

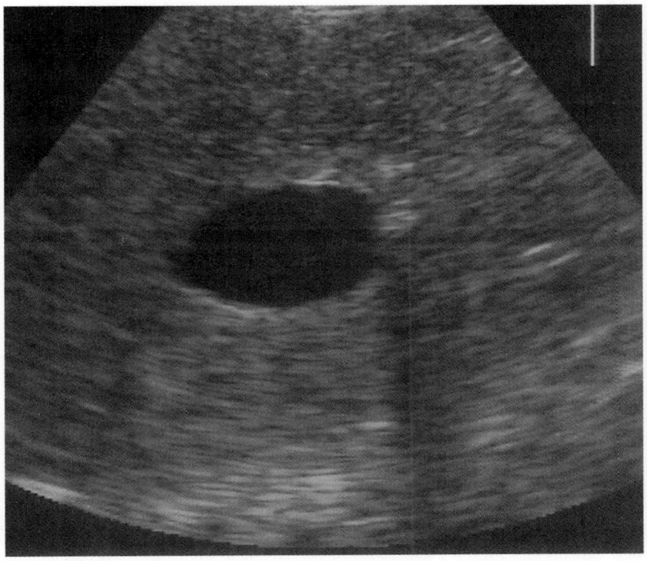

FIGURE 6-22 Distance enhancement. In the liver this is caused by sound waves passing through the fluid-filled gallbladder.

error. Next, check the power setting to make sure it is not too low. If all controls are set correctly, attempt to improve the acoustic contact with the skin by applying more coupling gel or shaving the clipped area with a razor. If none of these adjustments are productive, change to a lower-frequency transducer. Some resolution is lost, but it is a necessary trade-off when brightness cannot be achieved.

ARTIFACTS

Artifacts can occur during any ultrasound study. Proper identification of these artifacts is important to prevent confusion or misinterpretation. Some artifacts are beneficial in making a diagnosis. Two such artifacts include acoustic shadowing and **distance enhancement.** Others, if not readily identified, can be confused as part of the anatomy or a disease process.

Acoustic shadowing occurs when the sound is attenuated or reflected at an acoustic interface (Fig. 6-21). This prevents the sound from being transmitted to the deeper tissues, resulting in no echoes or fewer echoes returning from those areas. Structures that can cause acoustic shadowing include bone, calculi, mineralized tissues, and occasionally fat. For acoustic shadowing to occur, the interface must be in the focal zone of the transducer. If not, the shadowed area may be in with echoes from surrounding tissues as the sound beam diverges. This artifact is more pronounced with higher-frequency transducers.

Distance enhancement occurs when the sound beam traverses a cystic structure (Fig. 6-22). Tissues deep to the cystic structure appear brighter than surrounding tissues. The enhancement occurs because the sound that travels through the fluid-filled areas is less attenuated than in surrounding tissues. This artifact is useful in establishing that an anechoic or hypoechoic structure is in fact fluid-filled.

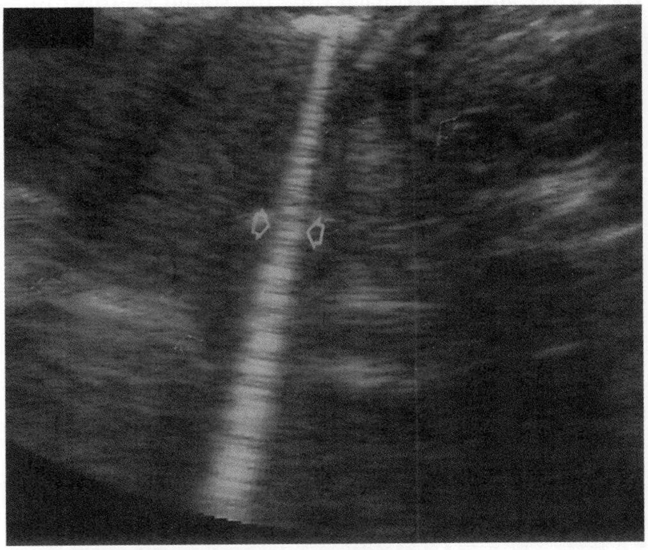

FIGURE 6-23 Reverberation artifact caused by gas in the small intestine of a dog. Notice the equally spaced echoic lines *(white arrows)* trailing from the highly reflective interface created by the gas.

Many artifacts have no diagnostic use, though if not identified as artifacts they can lead to confusion. One of these includes the **slice thickness** artifact. This artifact occurs when imaging an anechoic or hypoechoic structure. Echoes are added when the transducer receives echoes with different amplitudes from the same area at the same depth. The computer then averages these amplitudes and incorporates them in the two-dimensional image. Decreasing the overall gain can minimize this artifact; however, it does not totally eliminate it. Reverberation occurs when sound is reflected off a highly reflective interface (e.g., soft tissues to air or soft tissues to bone/metal) and then reflected back into the tissues by the surface of the transducer (Fig. 6-23). This bouncing back and forth can continue until the sound energy has

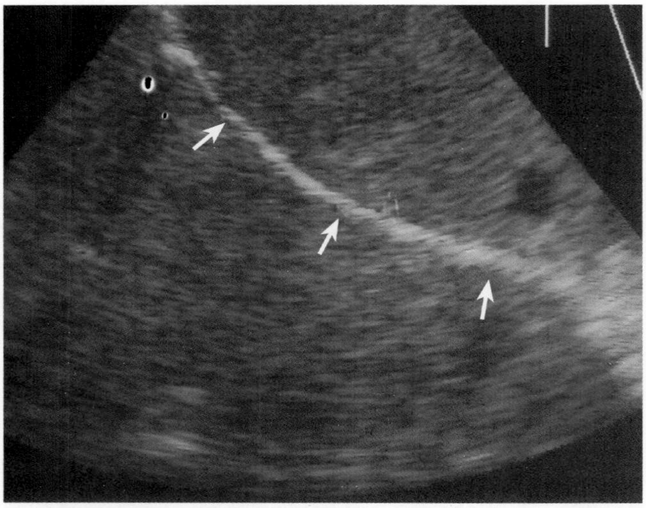

FIGURE 6-24 Mirror-image artifact. The arrows indicate the liver/diaphragm to lung interface. The actual liver is in the near field *(top right)*. The far field *(bottom left)* represents the mirror image of the liver.

completely attenuated. Each time the sound returns to the transducer, it produces an image at a location on the screen that is proportional to the time of travel between the transducer and the reflective interface. This creates a series of lines per equal distance apart on the screen.

The **mirror-image** artifact creates the illusion of liver on the thoracic side of the diaphragm or the appearance of a second heart beyond the lung interface (Fig. 6-24). This artifact can be produced in areas with strongly reflective interfaces. Sound transmitted into the liver is reflected off the diaphragm. Some of those echoes are not reflected directly toward the transducer but back into the liver. In the liver, some of the misdirected echoes are reflected back to the diaphragm and then to the transducer. The computer sees the misdirected echoes as being reflected from the other side of the diaphragm. One way this artifact can be minimized is by decreasing the depth to include only the area of interest.

ENDOSCOPY

Endoscopy is an essential tool for diagnosing many conditions and diseases. The opportunity to examine and obtain tissue samples without the invasiveness of surgery makes endoscopy one of the best methods of evaluating the digestive system. Responsibilities of veterinary technicians assisting with endoscopy include selection, care, and maintenance of the endoscopes, and care and positioning of the patient.

TECHNICIAN NOTE Endoscopic imaging can be used to diagnose disease as well as collect tissue samples for analysis.

TYPES OF ENDOSCOPES

Rigid endoscopes are commonly used for rhinoscopy, female cystoscopy, laparoscopy, arthroscopy, vaginoscopy, and thoroscopy. Flexible endoscopes are used for gastrointestinal endoscopy, male cystoscopy, and bronchoscopy exams. Flexible endoscopes are also used for percutaneous placement of gastrostomy tubes in small animals (Fig. 6-25).

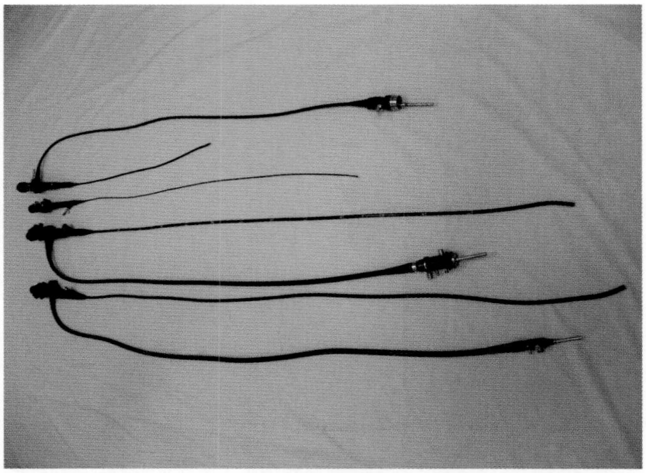

FIGURE 6-25 Variety of endoscopes. *Top to bottom:* Storz, Olympus, Cystoscope, and Bronchoscope.

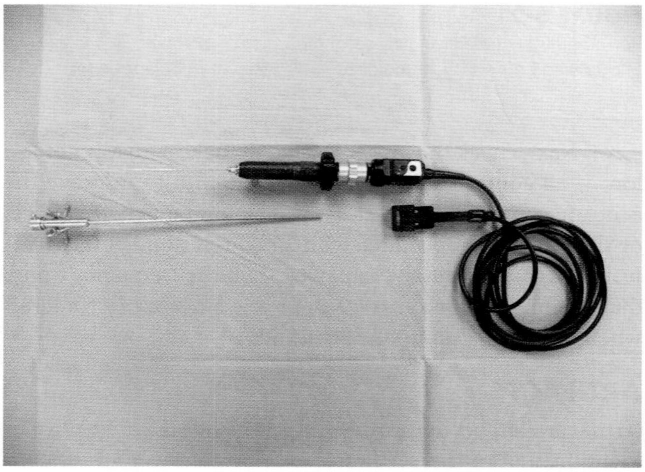

FIGURE 6-26 Rigid endoscope with camera.

Rigid Endoscopes

Rigid endoscopes are composed of a metal tube, lenses, and glass rods (Fig. 6-26). They vary in size and characteristics; however, all are composed of a hollow tube containing no fiber bundles. Rigid endoscopes tend to be less expensive than flexible endoscopes, but their uses tend to be limited to that for which they were designed.

Rigid endoscopes should be held by the eyepiece and *not* by the rod. Even slight bending of the rod section could change the angle of deflection, decreasing the degree of visualization. Rigid endoscopes should never be handled in bunches or piled on top of one another.

Flexible Endoscopes

There are two types of flexible endoscopes: fiberoptic and video. **Fiberoptic** endoscopes use glass fiber bundles for transmission of images. These bundles transmit light from the light source to the distal tip of the endoscope. Fiberoptic glass fiber bundles are very fragile and can be damaged easily. Broken fibers show up on the monitor screen as black dots. Too many of these black dots (many broken fiber bundles) can significantly reduce the field of view. For this reason, fiberoptic endoscopes must be handled very carefully and never bent at a sharp angle.

Video endoscopes contain a microchip located at the distal end of the endoscope that records and transmits the image to a computer and then to a monitor screen. The image can be recorded on a VCR, and pictures can be recorded to show the owner and be included in the patient's record. Many operators find the video endoscope more ergonomically pleasing, because the controls are held at the waist and not near the face.

PURCHASING AN ENDOSCOPE

Although the cost of an endoscope may be a substantial initial investment, many years of use and its value as a diagnostic tool will make the endoscope more than just a convenience to the veterinary hospital. The endoscope should pay for itself in the first year. The endoscope's life expectancy is generally 5 to 10 years but the life of cystoscopes tends to be shorter because of their delicate nature and small size. The life of the cystoscopes is generally 1 to 5 years. Commonly associated costs include the intravenous catheter, preprocedure enemas, preanesthetic blood studies and evaluation, the endoscopist's time, anesthesia, and laboratory fees. Skilled technical time involved in the preparation and cleaning of the endoscope must also be considered.

An endoscope of poor quality will rarely be used, so the veterinary team must decide which endoscope is appropriate for the hospital. A good-quality fiberoptic endoscope can be used for many purposes including gastrointestinal endoscopy, colonoscopy, and respiratory procedures in large dogs. For most small-animal practice situations, a 110-cm gastroscope/duodenal flexible endoscope should provide sufficient length for dogs and cats.

The diameter of the endoscope is also an important factor. Most human endoscopes are appropriate for endoscopic examination of large dogs; however, a human pediatric endoscope (insertion tube diameter 7.9 to 9 mm) is ideal. Larger endoscopes are difficult to pass into the pyloric canal to the duodenum in small dogs and cats. The endoscopes for most rhinoscopy and cystoscopy procedures, however, require a smaller diameter size. A 4.8 mm pediatrics bronchoscope and 2.5 mm cystoscope are better equipped for bronchoscopy and cystoscopy exams concurrently.

Some important characteristics that an endoscope should possess include four-way deflection capability, 180-degree upward deflection tip, water flush, air insufflations, and suction. Many models can be completely immersed, allowing thorough cleaning and disinfection.

One can easily locate a good-quality, low-cost, used endoscope through a human hospital. These hospitals are constantly updating their equipment and are often willing to sell their relatively new equipment at a reduced price. If you are considering a used endoscope, be sure to check for holes, cracks, or scratches on the insertion tube that might promote leakage of fluids into the endoscope. Look through the eyepiece and check for broken fibers, which appear as small black dots. A few fiber bundles can be expected to break over time, but an excessive number of broken bundles will inhibit visualization. Also check the intensity of the light by attaching the endoscope to the light source. If you purchase a used endoscope from a human hospital, be sure to ask for the operator's manual or other information that accompanies the endoscope. If no information is available, call the manufacturer of the endoscope and request a new operator's manual.

THE ENDOSCOPY ROOM

In an ideal situation, all endoscopic examinations are performed in the same room. This room should preferably be out of the way of hospital traffic. Because the lights are usually dimmed during endoscopic examination to reduce glare on the viewing monitor, a room with curtains or shades is ideal. The room should never be so dark, however, that proper anesthetic monitoring is inhibited.

A sturdy cart with three or four shelves can conveniently store the light source, suction unit, endoscope, and any accessory equipment until ready for use. All necessary equipment should be located near this endoscopy unit so that it can be reached quickly if needed during endoscopy. These items should be meticulously organized. The assisting staff must be able to locate any necessary equipment quickly during a procedure.

To avoid complications and delays, the procedure room should be well stocked before the endoscopic examination begins. All anesthetic equipment must be ready before the procedure begins. Procedure cards or checklists are excellent ways to ensure that each type of endoscopic examination starts with the proper equipment.

ACCESSORY INSTRUMENTS

Accessory instruments can be passed through the working channel of the flexible endoscope and directed to a specific area. The most basic instruments include biopsy forceps, foreign body removal forceps, and a cytology brush (Fig. 6-27).

Endoscopes are fragile and expensive, so personnel must be instructed in their proper care, use, and maintenance before endoscope use. Before each endoscopic examination, be sure each piece of ancillary equipment is functioning properly, and anticipate the need for these pieces of equipment. They should be cleaned as soon as possible after use or the jaws of the forceps may become locked in the closed position. If this occurs, soaking the tip of the biopsy forceps in warm water for 10 to 15 minutes helps to loosen the debris around the jaws.

All personnel involved with endoscopic procedures should wear latex examination gloves. This protects the animal from contamination and also protects the clinician and technician. The endoscope should not be allowed to directly

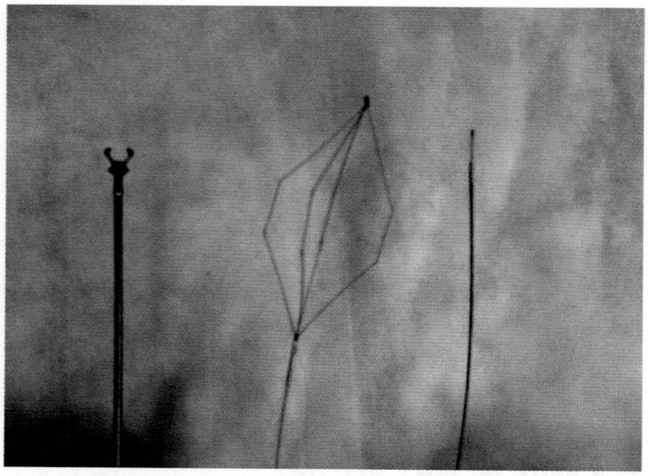

FIGURE 6-27 Accessory equipment. *Left to right:* Rat tooth forceps, basket foreign-body retrieval forceps, and cytology brush.

contact the video accessories or any other potentially conductive object; wearing latex gloves offers an added protection against electrical shock.

CLEANING A FLEXIBLE ENDOSCOPE

All endoscopy equipment should be thoroughly cleaned as soon as possible after the procedure. The manufacturer's specific cleaning instructions should be carefully followed. Endoscopes must be handled carefully during cleaning and never placed where they could fall or be bumped. It is also a good idea for the person cleaning the endoscope to wear latex examination gloves. Gather the following supplies:

- Latex examination gloves
- Cleaning solution
- Two large basins for cleaning solution and distilled water
- Distilled water
- Methyl alcohol
- Lint-free gauze pads
- Cotton-tipped applicators
- Channel-cleaning brush

Immediately after the procedure, flush water and then air through the air-water channel of the flexible endoscope. Gently wipe off the insertion tube with a soft gauze or cloth that has been soaked in an approved detergent solution. Do not squeeze the flexible section. Place the distal end of the endoscope in detergent water and suction a small amount through. Alternately suction water and then air a few times. Remove the air-water valve, suction valve, and biopsy cap, and place them in a small amount of cleaning solution to soak. Pass the channel-cleaning brush through the biopsy channel, and suction the channel repeatedly until the brush comes out clean. Clean the brush each time it is passed through the channel.

If the endoscope has a suction cleaning tube, it should then be placed on the biopsy port. Place the end of the suction cleaning tube and the end of the endoscope into a mixture of detergent and water. Cover the suction valve hole with your finger and suction soapy water, then distilled water, and then air to dry the endoscope. Remove the suction cleaning tube, and carefully clean the valve holes with a cotton-tipped swab. Clean and rinse the air-water valve, suction valve, and biopsy cap, and replace them on the endoscope.

It is a good preventive measure to lightly lubricate the air-water and suction valves periodically to prevent cracking. Wipe off the outside of the endoscope with an alcohol-soaked gauze pad. Clean the lenses with an approved lens cleaner by applying some lens cleaner onto a soft gauze pad and rubbing the lens; then rub with a clean gauze pad. Replace any lens caps, light source insertion bar covers, and ethylene oxide sterilization caps before placing the endoscope back into the cabinet. For proper drying of the biopsy channel, leave the biopsy port in an open position.

Biopsy instruments should be immersed in soapy water, brushed carefully with a cleaning brush, and then rinsed. Check to be sure that the jaws of biopsy instruments are not sticking by carefully opening and then closing them.

STORING AN ENDOSCOPE

The ideal way to store a flexible endoscope is in a hanging position in a well-ventilated cabinet. This allows the endoscope to drain completely after cleaning and permits better air movement through the channels. The padded case in which the endoscope was supplied by the manufacturer is another possible storage area; however, little air circulates in these containers and moisture in the channels of the endoscope offers an environment for bacterial growth. Rigid endoscopes are best stored in their original carrying case.

GASTROINTESTINAL ENDOSCOPY

Flexible endoscopes are most commonly used to examine the gastrointestinal tract, including the esophagus. Gastrointestinal endoscopy allows visualization of the upper and lower digestive tract, including its contents.

Patient Preparation

The patient should be fasted for 12 to 24 hours. A longer period of fasting may be required in patients with delayed gastric emptying. An intravenous catheter should be placed and fluid administration started. There are various opinions as to which drugs may impair passage of the endoscope into the duodenum; however, a combination of atropine and morphine is known to make endoscope passage more difficult. Use of these drugs together should be avoided for gastrointestinal endoscopy. Endotracheal intubation and proper endotracheal tube cuff inflation are needed to avoid aspiration of gastric contents in the event of regurgitation.

Place the patient in left lateral recumbency, with a mouth speculum placed to prevent damage to the endoscope from biting (Fig. 6-28). Raise the table to a height that does not require excessive bending of the endoscope near the hand piece. Lubricate the insertion tube with a water-soluble lubricant, such as K-Y Jelly, avoiding the distal end of the endoscope. Use of petroleum-based lubricants, such as Vaseline, is not advised because over time they cause stretching and deterioration of the rubber components of the endoscope.

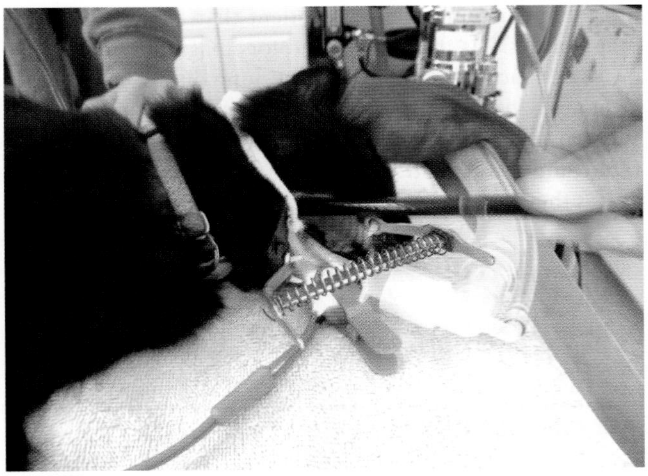

FIGURE 6-28 Endoscopic procedure. Patient is in lateral recumbency using mouth speculum.

As the endoscope is introduced into the patient's mouth, avoid scraping the endoscope against the teeth in the back of the mouth. Air insufflation is usually needed to facilitate visualization; however, over-insufflation may cause over-distention of the stomach or abdomen and can interfere with ventilation.

Obtaining Samples

Tissue samples are obtained by grasping the mucosa with biopsy forceps. The biopsy forceps are passed down the operating channel of the endoscope with the forceps jaws in a closed position. Care must be taken to not open or close the forceps too forcefully, as they can become locked or broken. Also, make sure the jaws of the biopsy forceps are in the closed position before bringing them back out through the biopsy channel of the endoscope; otherwise the accessory equipment and the endoscope may be damaged.

Once a tissue sample is obtained, the specimen is gently teased out of the forceps with a 25-gauge needle or flushed directly from the biopsy forceps into a vial of preservative or biopsy cassette using sterile saline. Upon completion of the gastroscopic examination, the stomach and esophagus are suctioned with the endoscope using gentle external pressure on the abdomen to remove fluids, debris, and excess air.

The endotracheal tube cuff should remain partially inflated when extubating to bring out any remaining material.

COLONOSCOPY

Flexible colonoscopy allows examination of the transverse and ascending colon, cecum, ileocolic valve, and ileum.

Ideally, all feces should be removed from the colon before endoscopic examination; however, this is not always possible. Food should be withheld from the patient for at least 36 hours. Several different colonic cleansing protocols can be used, depending on how cooperative the patient is and the amount of help available. For rigid colonoscopy, a warm-water enema (10 to 20 ml/kg) the evening before the procedure, another enema the following morning, and a final enema 1 hour before the examination usually provide enough cleansing.

To successfully observe the entire colon with a flexible endoscope, the bowel must be completely cleansed before the examination. Colon electrolyte lavage solutions, such as Golytely (Braintree Laboratories, Braintree, MA) or Colyte (Endlaw Preparations, Farmingdale, NY), are administered orally by stomach tube, usually the day before the procedure. Often a repeat dose is given the morning of the examination. These commercial solutions are superior to traditional soapy water enemas. Rigid colonoscopy can be performed using heavy sedation, but a light plane of anesthesia is usually preferred. The patient is placed in right lateral recumbency, with the table slightly tilted so that any residual material drains away from the endoscopist.

Anesthesia is necessary for flexible colonoscopy. The patient is placed in left lateral recumbency to assist passage of the endoscope into the transverse and ascending colon. Colonic insufflation is used to facilitate passage of the endoscope, and often air escapes through the anal sphincter. If this occurs, manual pressure around the anus by a gloved assistant helps to prevent this escape of air.

BRONCHOSCOPY

Airway endoscopy (bronchoscopy) allows visualization of the trachea and bronchi. It is most useful when diagnosing a collapsed trachea, collapsed main stem bronchi, airway parasitism, lower airway infections and inflammatory diseases, and foreign bodies. Tissue samples may also be obtained through the endoscope for histopathologic, cytologic, and microbiologic examinations.

The most common endoscope used for medium-size or large dogs is a small-diameter gastrointestinal endoscope. For smaller dogs and cats, a flexible human pediatric bronchoscope is required. Because bronchoscopes have a smaller working channel, any biopsies obtained are smaller. Before use for lower airway endoscopy, the endoscope must be sterilized according to the manufacturer's guidelines.

General anesthesia is required for lower airway endoscopy. In medium-size to large dogs, the endoscope is passed through a shortened sterile endotracheal tube. Oxygen and/or anesthetic gases can also be delivered to the patient using a bronchoscope tube adapter. The patient must be closely monitored for proper oxygenation and anesthetic depth. A mouth speculum is necessary to prevent damage to the endoscope.

In cats and small dogs, the bronchoscope is passed down the trachea without an endotracheal tube in place. Great care must be taken to evaluate the patient before the procedure, because the patient's airway is occluded by the endoscope. It may become necessary to stop the endoscopy for some time while the patient is oxygenated. Oxygen can also be delivered through the suction channel of the bronchoscope to help prevent hypoxemia.

CYSTOSCOPY

Cystoscopy can allow visualization of the vagina in female dogs, urethra, urinary bladder, and ureteral locations. It is most useful in diagnosing urethral neoplasia, urethral inflammatory diseases, ectopic ureters, bladder wall defects and it can help locate stones not visualized with ultrasounds or radiographic exams. For female patients a rigid endoscope is best used, whereas flexible cystoscope is required for male patients. Both scopes should be sterilized by the manufacturer's recommendations before use, and sterile gloves should be worn during the exam to decrease the risk of introducing infection. This procedure can be performed in most dogs but not in cats because of limitations in scope size.

General anesthesia is required for this procedure. Female patients are positioned in sternal recumbency with their hind end propped up with a towel or other padding and their hind end slightly past the table edge to allow easier access by the endoscopist. Male patients are positioned in lateral recumbency of the endoscopist's preference. The tail is clipped to the side to keep it out of the way. The vaginal area or tip of the penis is clipped and prepped sterilely. Biopsy instruments can be passed through the biopsy channel to collect samples.

RHINOSCOPY

Rhinoscopy allows visualization of the nasopharynx and nasal passages. This aids in diagnosing upper respiratory diseases such as tumors, polyps, infections (fungal and bacterial), foreign bodies, and inflammatory diseases such as chronic active rhinitis. General anesthesia is required for this exam and patients should be positioned in sternal recumbency with their heads elevated slightly with towels or padding. A mouth gag should be placed to make sure the animal does not bite down on the scope. Care should also be taken that the scope is not scraped past the teeth while introducing it into the mouth to avoid trauma and tearing into the scope.

The nasopharyngeal exam is accomplished using a flexible small diameter bronchoscope where the scope is passed into the mouth and retroflexed around the soft palate. At this point the choanal openings and nasopharynx can be fully visualized. To visualize the nasal passages, a cystoscope is required to visualize the fine turbinate structures of the nose. Fluids are liberally run through the biopsy channel during this portion of the scoping procedure to help clear away blood and mucous material. Samples of tissue can be collected through the biopsy channels.

COMPUTED TOMOGRAPHY

Using x-rays and a bank of detectors, a computed tomography (CT) scan provides a cross-sectional image of all tissue types of the body region scanned based on the physical density of the tissue compared to water. Within the CT scanner, there is an x-ray tube and multiple detectors on a slip ring device that allows the tube to freely move in a circular motion around a patient. The patient is stationary on a table that is passed through the rotating x-ray beam. The images are then reconstructed into thin slices through the patient, like a slice from a loaf of bread. The raw data from the image acquisition can be reprocessed using a dedicated computer for soft tissue or edge enhanced display or reformatted into other imaging planes, such as dorsal and sagittal planes from the original data that was acquired in a transverse plane. This form of imaging, tomography, provides the radiologist much more information about the patient than conventional radiography. CT is frequently used for imaging many disease processes such as cancer, fractures, lung disease, and vascular anomalies. CT also provides invaluable information for surgical and radiation treatment planning. Unlike radiography and ultrasound, tomographic imaging frequently requires the patient to be anesthetized for the examination.

> *TECHNICIAN NOTE* A CT scanner produces cross-sectional images by placing the patient on a table that is passed through a rotating x-ray beam.

MAGNETIC RESONANCE IMAGING

Magnetic resonance imaging (MRI) uses a high-strength external magnetic field, a variety of radiofrequency excitation pulses, and the natural resonance (normal circular motion of the atom) of protons (hydrogen ions) in the body to visualize the structure and function of organs. MRI is primarily used to examine the internal organs and is noninvasive and superior to other modalities for imaging soft tissues. The primary examinations performed using MRI include imaging of the brain, spinal cord and intervertebral disc areas, tumor localization and extension within soft tissues, tendon and muscle injury, vascular and arterial anomalies or disease, and thoracic and abdominal organs. The principles of MRI imaging are very complex. Many types of magnets are used, but they can be summarized as being low and high field strengths depending on the strength of the magnetic field, which is measured in tesla (T). Low-strength magnets are 0.4 T or less and high field is 0.6 T and higher. The patient is placed in this external, strong magnetic field, and the magnetic field is then manipulated by small increments as specific radiofrequencies (RF) are transmitted into the patient to cause certain changes in the orientation and speed with which the protons resonate. All of the protons then relax, based on the immediate interactions of the protons as well as the type of tissue of which the protons are a part. This relaxation produces weak radiofrequency signals, which are then detected by coils surrounding the area of interest of the patient. These signals are then processed through a computer and converted into images of the patient.

Depending on the MRI scan performed, contrast medium may or may not be administered. Gadolinium is the most common contrast medium agent used for enhancement of tissues in MRI. Given intravenously, it enhances or brightens tissues such as vessels and tumors.

Serious safety concerns apply when housing and operating an MRI unit. It is prudent to remember that for superconducting magnets of high field strength, the magnet is always on. No ferromagnetic object can be taken into the room where the magnet resides. The magnet will forcibly pull any ferromagnetic objects into the magnet. This could cause serious damage to the MRI machine, the patient, or the operator who might be within its path. A few examples of ferrous objects include: gas anesthesia machines, collars, watches, glasses, hairpins, ink pens, clipboards, intravenous

(IV) poles, and cell phones. Certain metallic surgical implants may also be of concern. It is necessary to know what type of implant and the manufacturer to make sure that there is no ferromagnetic component within it. Microchips do not seem to cause any issues other than magnetic susceptibility artifacts in the image. Keep a small magnet outside the room and test objects for their magnetism when there is any doubt. Because general anesthesia is required for MRI, the use of intravenous injectables is the most common route of anesthesia. However, there are MRI-compatible gas anesthetic machines and monitoring equipment available. Although MRI units are uncommon in the general veterinary practices, most university veterinary hospitals and referral hospitals have MRI units or access to one for diagnostic imaging.

> *TECHNICIAN NOTE* Nuclear scintigraphy and MRI imaging modalities are commonly performed at veterinary teaching hospitals and some large veterinary referral practices.

NUCLEAR MEDICINE

Nuclear medicine, also called scintigraphy, is an imaging modality that uses radionuclides and a gamma camera for the detection of decay of gamma radiation that is emitted from the radionuclide within the patient. This allows for imaging of anatomic, physiologic, or metabolic processes that occur within the patient. The most common radionuclide used for imaging is technetium-99m (^{99m}Tc). ^{99m}Tc has a low-energy gamma ray (140 keV) with a short physical half-life of 6 hours. ^{99m}Tc is typically bound to a specific pharmaceutical that then targets the organ of interest after being administered intravenously. The most common nuclear medicine studies performed in veterinary medicine are thyroid scans, bone scans, renal function testing with GFR calculation, and hepatobiliary scans. The most common therapeutic nuclear medicine application in veterinary medicine is radioactive iodine (^{131}I). Iodine-131 is used for the treatment of hyperthyroidism and thyroid tumors.

Because of the potential for radioactive contamination, latex gloves and lab coats are worn at all times when handling any radionuclide or radioactive patient. Special housing considerations are a factor for the radioactive patient after the study, because the excretion of technetium is primarily within the urine and feces. Each state or locality has strict release criteria for patients that are imaged with radionuclides. Special holding areas are required to isolate the radioactive patient to prevent contamination of other areas of the hospital and personnel. Radioactive iodine patients require an isolated and well ventilated area because of the potential for aerosolization of iodine. Radioactive iodine may be excreted in saliva, feces, and urine. As the I-131 has a longer physical half-life (2.82 days), patients are required to stay in the area of isolation longer than the patients undergoing a ^{99m}Tc-radiopharmaceutical study.

REVIEW QUESTIONS

Matching—Terms Associated With Radiographic Quality

Match the term associated with radiographic quality with its definition.

_____1. Anode heel effect
_____2. Radiographic density
_____3. Radiographic contrast
_____4. Subject density
_____5. Radiographic detail
_____6. Artifacts
_____7. Penumbra

A. loss of detail due to geometric unsharpness
B. unwanted density in the form of blemishes
C. the sharp interfaces between tissues and organs
D. unequal distribution of the x-ray beam intensity
E. differences in radiographic density between adjacent areas on a radiographic image
F. degree of blackness on a radiograph
G. the ability of the different tissue densities to absorb x-rays

Matching—Terms Associated With Radiographic Positioning

Match the term associated with radiographic positioning with its definition.

_____1. Ventral (V)
_____2. Dorsal (D)
_____3. Medial (M)
_____4. Lateral (L)
_____5. Cranial (Cr)
_____6. Caudal (Cd)
_____7. Rostral (R)
_____8. Palmar (Pa)
_____9. Plantar (Pl)
_____10. Proximal (Pr)
_____11. Distal (Di)

A. situated closer to the point of attachment or origin
B. situated on the caudal aspect of the rear limb, distal to the tarsus
C. areas on the head situated toward the nose
D. body area situated toward the median plane or midline
E. situated away from the point of attachment or origin
F. structures or areas situated toward the head
G. body area situated toward the underside of quadrupeds
H. structures or areas situated toward the tail
I. situated on the caudal aspect of the front limb, distal to the carpus
J body area situated toward the back or topline of quadrupeds
K. body area situated away from the median plane or midline

Choose the Best Response

Choose the best answer to the following questions.

1. You are doing a safelight quality control test with an initial moderate exposure. There is no area of increased density. This means that:
   - **a.** There is no problem with the safelight or light leaking around the door.
   - **b.** You need to get a brand new safelight as you will always have fogging.
   - **c.** You have less than 30 seconds to get the film in the processing solutions.
   - **d.** You must have completed the test incorrectly.
2. There is an interesting correlation between kVp and electromagnetic radiation. Generally as the:
   - **a.** kVp is increased, the penetration is increased
   - **b.** kVp is increased, the penetration is decreased
   - **c.** kVp is decreased, the penetration is increased
   - **d.** kVp is decreased, the penetration is decreased
3. In terms of subject density, the order of least dense to most dense would be:
   - **a.** metal, bone, water, fat, gas
   - **b.** fat, water, gas, bone, metal
   - **c.** water, gas, fat, bone, metal
   - **d.** gas, fat, water, bone, metal
4. The quality of the beam refers to:
   - **a.** kVp
   - **b.** mAs
   - **c.** rectification that is required
   - **d.** darkness of the radiograph
5. Scatter will be more noticeable if there is a thicker patient and:
   - **a.** lower kVp and larger field size
   - **b.** lower kVp and smaller field size
   - **c.** higher kVp and smaller field size
   - **d.** higher kVp and larger field size

RECOMMENDED READINGS

Barr F: *Diagnostic ultrasound in the dog and cat*, London, 1990, Blackwell Scientific.

Brearley MJ, et al.: *A colour atlas of small animal endoscopy*, St Louis, 1991, Mosby.

Brown M, Brown L: *Lavin's radiography for veterinary technicians*, ed 5, St Louis, 2014, Saunders.

Burk RL, Ackerman N: *Small animal radiology and ultrasonography*, ed 3, St Louis, 2003, Saunders.

Curry TS, et al.: *Christensen's physics of diagnostic radiology*, ed 4, Philadelphia, 1990, Lea & Febiger.

Han CM, Hurd CD: *Practical diagnostic imaging for the veterinary technician*, ed 3, St Louis, 2000, Mosby.

Nyland TG, Mattoon JS: *Small animal diagnostic ultrasound*, ed 3, St Louis, 2014, Saunders.

Sirois M, Anthony E: *Handbook of radiographic positioning for veterinary technicians*, Clifton Park NY, 2010, Delmar Cengage.

Tams T: *Small animal endoscopy*, ed 3, St Louis, 2010, Mosby.

Thrall DE: *Textbook of veterinary diagnostic radiology*, ed 6, St Louis, 2013, Saunders.

Traub-Dargatz JL, Brown CM: *Equine endoscopy*, ed 2, St Louis, 1997, Mosby.

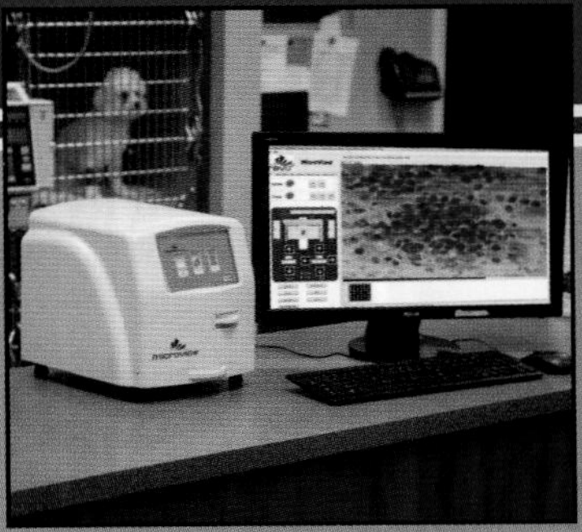

7 Hematology and Hemostasis

OUTLINE

LEARNING OBJECTIVES

After reviewing this chapter, the reader will be able to:

1. Describe methods used to collect blood samples for laboratory examination.
2. Describe preparation of diagnostic samples for laboratory examination.
3. List and describe common procedures used for hematologic examinations.
4. Describe characteristics of normal and common abnormal cells in peripheral blood.
5. Discuss methods used to maintain accuracy of laboratory test results.
6. List and describe methods for evaluation of hemostasis in domestic animals.

KEY TERMS

Absolute value
Accuracy
Activated clotting time
Agranulocyte
Anemia
Band cell
Basophilia
Buffy coat
DIC
Differential cell count
Eosinophilia
Erythrocyte indices

KEY TERMS—cont'd

Granulocyte
Hemolysis
Hemostasis
Heterophil
Icterus
Left shift
Leukopenia
Leukemia
Leukocytosis
Lipemia
M:E ratio
Megakaryocyte
Neutropenia
Neutrophilia
Packed cell volume
Pancytopenia
Polychromasia
Polycythemia
Precision
Preprandial samples
Refractometer
Reticulocyte
Schistocyte
Target cells
Thrombocyte
Thrombocytopenia

Hematologic examination, or the analysis of blood, is a very powerful diagnostic tool. Veterinary technicians provide a valuable service by acquiring the skills necessary to perform this analysis. Only through practice and attention to detail can the veterinary technician develop the confidence and proficiency to perform these procedures.

Hematologic procedures include collecting and handling blood samples, performing a CBC, assisting with bone marrow examination, and performing routine blood coagulation tests. The recent focus on economic health of the veterinary clinic has also provided an opportunity for veterinary technicians to perform additional diagnostic testing, improve overall animal care, and provide an additional source of revenue for the clinic.

LABORATORY INSTRUMENTATION AND EQUIPMENT

A variety of types of equipment are needed for the in-house hematology laboratory. One of the most important items is the microscope. Ideally, each practice laboratory will have at least two microscopes. One should be designated solely for use with blood smears and cytology preparations. The other can be used for examination of parasitology and urine specimens. This will help to maintain the microscopes in the best working order, because the corrosive fluids sometimes used in parasitology testing can damage the microscope. Examination of blood smears requires a high-quality binocular microscope, preferably with planachromatic (flat-field) lenses and a focusable substage condenser (Fig. 7-1). Centrifuges are also required for clinical testing. The centrifuge is used to prepare blood samples for chemical testing and for completion of the packed cell volume test that is part of the complete blood count (CBC). There are thousands of types of centrifuges available for the clinic laboratory. Several centrifuges are now available that allow the use of small volumes of sample (Fig. 7-2). Other equipment and supplies that may be needed for the veterinary practice laboratory include:

- Refractometer
- Pipettes
- Differential cell counter
- Hand tally counter
- Automated or manual cell-counting equipment
- Water bath or heat block

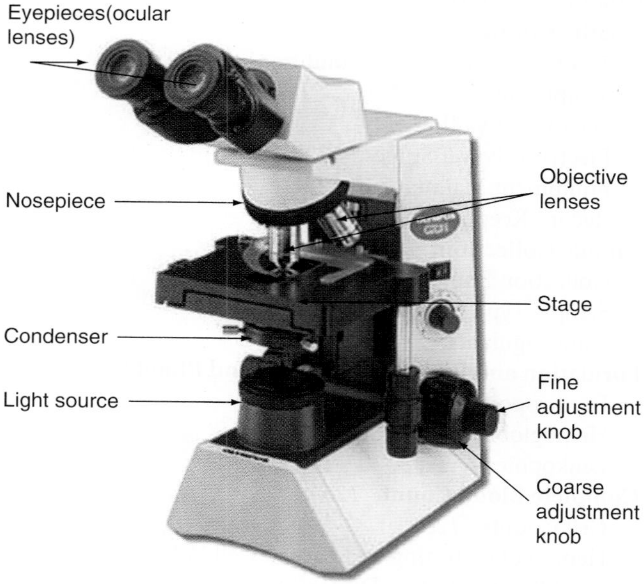

FIGURE 7-1 A binocular microscope for use in the veterinary clinical laboratory.

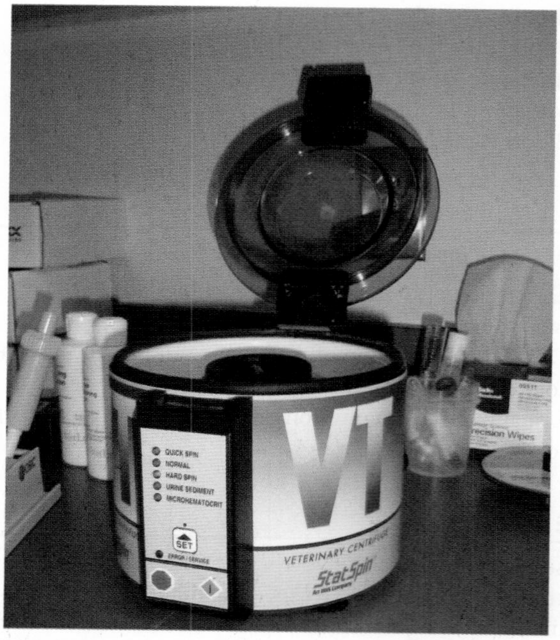

FIGURE 7-2 The StatSpin centrifuge. This angled-head centrifuge is specifically designed for small sample volumes.

TECHNICIAN NOTE A high-quality binocular microscope is needed for proper performance of hematology testing.

LABORATORY SAFETY

The veterinary practice laboratory has the potential to be a safety hazard if specific policies and procedures are not in place to ensure safe working conditions. A sample laboratory safety policy can be found in Box 7-1. For example, individuals who wear contact lenses should be required to remove them when working in the laboratory. Contact lenses block fluids used to flush the eyes in an emergency, and most individuals are too disoriented to be capable of removing them during an emergency. Assuring that all chemicals are stored properly and that the laboratory has adequate ventilation can minimize chemical hazard from volatile fumes. Specific recommendations for chemical safety are contained in the material safety data sheet (MSDS) provided by each chemical manufacturer. MSDSs contain storage concerns, requirements for personal protective equipment use, and emergency procedures that may be needed. All personnel in the clinic must be made aware of the hazards associated with working in the veterinary practice laboratory and the procedures to be used in emergencies. Even when the clinic has an appropriate written safety policy, safety concerns may arise unless the policies are followed and enforced by everyone in the clinic. There are also laws that require specific safety procedures. Additional safety concerns also relate to quality control. In particular, proper maintenance of equipment is essential. Some laboratory equipment can be hazardous if not properly maintained (e.g., centrifuges). This maintenance requirement affects the operation of the equipment and the accuracy of results obtained from its use. Additional safety concerns applicable to veterinary practice can be found in Chapter 2.

QUALITY CONTROL

Veterinarians expect veterinary technicians to present them with dependable analytic results. Through a well-planned and carefully controlled quality-control program, veterinary technicians can provide veterinarians with accurate laboratory results. Quality control (also called quality assurance) is a series of steps and procedures to ensure that the analytic results from a laboratory represent the state of the animal from which a sample was taken. If these in vitro results are to be of any value to a veterinarian, they must match as closely as possible the in vivo values of the animal at the time the sample was obtained.

BOX 7-1 Sample Laboratory Safety Policy

The safety procedures contained in this document are designed to minimize any potential source of injury to employees of this facility. All employees are required to adhere to these policies to ensure a safe workplace for everyone.

The clinical lab is equipped with the following safety equipment: fume hood, eye wash station, electrical surge and dropout extension, first aid kit, pipettors, chemical spill cleanup kit, fire extinguisher, and fire blanket.

All employees are required to familiarize themselves with these devices and be able to use and operate them effectively.

General Rules

1. Smoking, eating, or drinking is prohibited in the lab.
2. No foods or beverages may be stored in the lab refrigerator or general lab area.
3. Lab coats must be worn at all times.
4. Long hair must be confined while in the lab.
5. Shoes must be worn in the lab; open-toe or canvas shoes are prohibited.
6. No pipetting of materials by mouth!
7. All employees are responsible for safe and proper operation of equipment. Read the operator's manual and be familiar with the operation of any instrument before attempting its use.

Lab Housekeeping

1. All glassware must be washed immediately after use. Cracked or chipped glassware must be discarded at once.
2. All work surfaces must be cleaned with a 10% bleach solution at the end of the work period.
3. Lab work areas must be kept clear of personal belongings.
4. Employees must wash hands thoroughly before leaving the lab.

Reagents

1. Fume hood must be used for dispensing reagents with potentially hazardous fumes.
2. All reagents will be stored properly in designated areas.
3. Carrying reagents must be done cautiously, using unbreakable containers whenever possible.
4. All reagent, stock, and dispensing containers MUST be labeled with identity, date, and initials of individual preparing reagent and MUST contain proper hazard warning labels.

Biologicals

1. All biologicals (blood, urine, body fluid, control materials) must be treated as potentially infectious.
2. Disposable latex gloves MUST be worn at all times when handling or transporting biological materials.
3. Spilled biological material must be cleaned up with 10% bleach solution.

Disposal

1. Reagents suitable for sewage disposal should be poured into running water in the sink.
2. Hazardous reagents will be disposed of in proper central waste containers.
3. All reagent bottles must be thoroughly rinsed before disposal.
4. Biological materials and their containers should be disposed of in biohazard bags.

Unlike human medical office laboratories, there are no laws that require quality control and proficiency programs for veterinary practice laboratories. However, without an appropriate quality control program, the accuracy and precision of test results cannot be assured. **Accuracy** refers to how closely the test result is to the actual patient value. **Precision** refers to the reproducibility of a test result. Inaccurate test results can lead a veterinarian to make an incorrect diagnosis. Based on inaccurate test results, the veterinarian may prescribe medications that are contraindicated or may withhold medications that are essential for recovery. There are a few tests performed in the laboratory that may have a relatively low precision rating simply as a function of the test methodology. For example, manual cell counts have one of the lowest accuracy ratings because there are numerous components of the test that could be faulty. For that reason it is often necessary to repeat the procedure and then calculate a mathematical average of the two test results to report as the patient value. Any test with a low precision rating should be repeated and the results averaged to improve accuracy.

Other factors that affect accuracy and precision include test selection, test conditions, sample quality, technician skill, electrical surges, and equipment maintenance.

TEST SELECTION AND TEST CONDITIONS

Test selection refers to the principle of the test method. Many of the tests used in veterinary laboratories were adapted from human medical laboratory tests. Because the veterinary clinic often sees a diversity of species with very different physiologic parameters, some of these tests may not provide an accurate representation of patient health status. For example, some tests for amylase may be invalid when used with canine samples. This is often because of limitations in the linearity of a test. That is, the test may not be capable of measuring in a range likely to be found in a given species. Additionally, the clinical significance of test results may vary among different species. In addition to assuring that the test method is appropriate, tests should be chosen based on their accuracy. Regardless of the method used, care must be taken to follow the analytical procedure exactly. Any deviation can seriously affect accuracy of results. Some tests can be carried out only under specific conditions of temperature or pH. These tests will be highly inaccurate with even slight variations in test conditions.

SAMPLE QUALITY

Sample quality also greatly affects quality of test results. In veterinary medicine this can be a significant concern. Samples that are lipemic, icteric, or hemolyzed require special handling before use with most clinical analyzers. Collection of blood samples from properly fasted animals using appropriate techniques and equipment will minimize this significant source of error.

> TECHNICIAN NOTE Careful attention to proper sample collection methods will help ensure accurate hematology results.

TECHNICIAN SKILL

Human error is perhaps the most difficult testing parameter to control. Personnel responsible for performance of clinical testing must be appropriately trained in test principles and procedures. Even the use of the wrong type of pipetting device can seriously affect test accuracy. Mechanisms should be in place to provide for the continual education of all clinical laboratory personnel.

ELECTRICAL POWER SURGES

Although not an obvious source of error, electrical power surges and dropouts can significantly alter equipment function. Repeated surges shorten the life of light sources in microscopes and photometric equipment. Changes in the intensity of the light source yield inaccurate test results. All electrical equipment should be connected to a device designed to protect it from surges and electrical dropout.

EQUIPMENT MAINTENANCE

Maintenance of equipment must also be included in quality control programs. A regular, written schedule of equipment maintenance is vital to ensure proper operation. This will allow changes in equipment function to be detected before obvious errors begin to occur. Always follow manufacturer recommendations for routine maintenance of instruments and equipment.

The accuracy of clinical instruments must also be verified on a regular basis by analyzing control materials. Control material contains specific concentrations of blood constituents. Busy practice laboratories should run controls on a daily basis. The equipment manufacturer provides recommendations regarding the frequency of control material analysis. The control is analyzed as if it were a patient sample. The control is designed to function the same as a patient sample would under the same conditions. Control results should be charted and analyzed regularly to help identify any changes in performance of the equipment. Standards are not acceptable as substitutes for controls. Standards are nonbiological substances used to calibrate equipment.

RECORD KEEPING

The results of assays of control samples should be recorded, graphed, and kept in a permanent file. Graphing the control results enables laboratory personnel to detect changes or trends in assay results. Figure 7-3 shows an example of a control serum graph used in a clinical laboratory that assays control serum once a day. If the results of a control assay do not fall within the acceptable range, the sample should be reassayed. If the results are not within the acceptable range for the second assay, the instrument and the technician's technique must be evaluated. When the control sample values continually fall outside the acceptable range, there has been a shift of the mean itself and a systematic error is involved.

Some manufacturers provide a quality-control service in which test samples are sent to many clinical laboratories for assay each month. The results from all the laboratories are

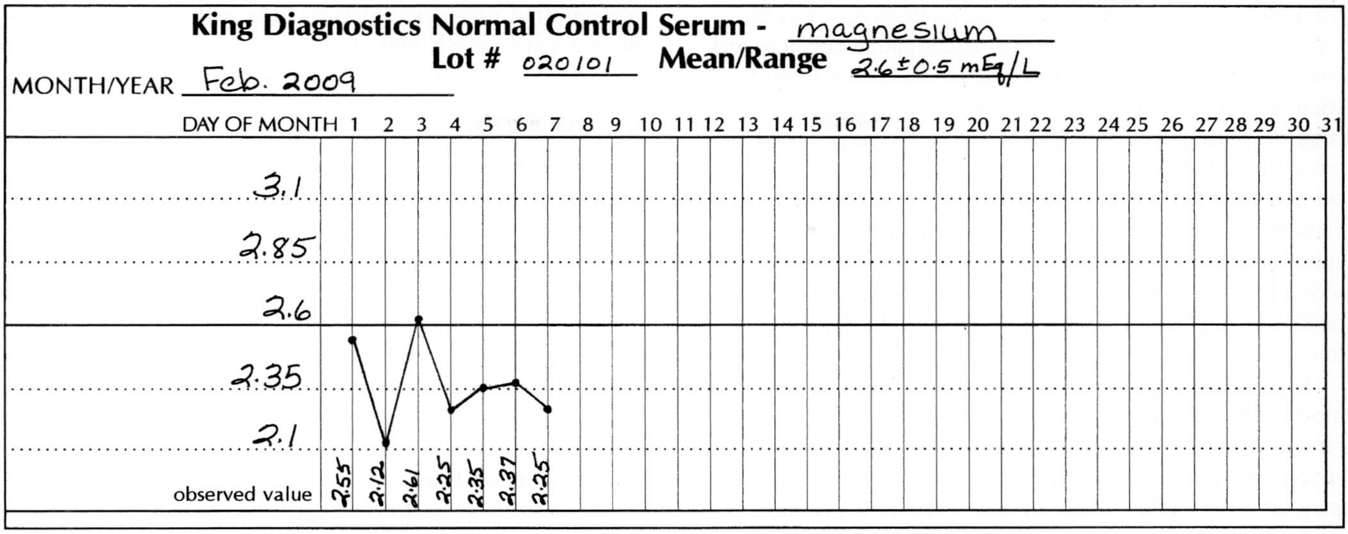

FIGURE 7-3 Example of a graph used to chart control values.

collected and compared. From these results, the manufacturer can identify laboratories with accuracy problems.

SAMPLE COLLECTION

Sample quality has a significant impact on test accuracy. Careful attention to collection procedures will minimize these problems. When preparing to collect blood, the technician should first determine what specific test procedures will be needed. This will determine, in part, the equipment and supplies needed and the choice of a particular blood vessel from which to collect the sample. Unless the purpose of the test is to monitor therapy, always collect the blood sample before any treatment is given. It is important to remember that treatments, such as fluid therapy, may affect results. Certain test methods cannot be accurately performed once the patient has received certain pharmaceutical therapies. **Preprandial samples**, or samples from an animal that has not eaten for some time, are ideal. Postprandial samples, or samples collected after the animal has eaten, may produce many erroneous results. Increased amounts of lipid (**lipemia**) may also be present in postprandial blood samples. Lipemia also increases the likelihood of hemolysis in the sample, and further complicates analyses.

Improper handling of blood may render a blood sample unusable for analysis or result in inaccurate results. The methods and sites of blood collection depend on the species, the amount of blood needed, and personal preference.

Venous blood is preferred for use in hematologic testing and is easily accessible in most species. The cephalic vein is the preferred site in dogs and cats when relatively small volumes of blood are needed. The femoral vein (lateral in the dog, medial in the cat) is a reasonable substitute, especially in fractious cats. Jugular venipuncture is an efficient way to collect a large volume of blood. It is the preferred site in large domestic animals (Table 7-1). The brachial vein is the preferred site in birds. The auricular vein in rabbits works well for blood collection. The tail vein, infraorbital sinus, and cardiac puncture can be used in some laboratory animals. Collection from the infraorbital sinus or heart requires that the animals be anesthetized.

TABLE 7-1 Commonly Used Blood Collection Sites

ANIMAL	VEIN
Dogs	Cephalic vein Jugular vein Femoral vein
Cats	Cephalic vein Jugular vein
Horses	Jugular vein
Cattle	Coccygeal vein Subcutaneous abdominal vein Jugular vein
Birds	Brachial vein
Rabbits	Auricular vein
Rodents	Tail vein Cardiac puncture

Ideally, you should clip the collection site to remove hair. Clean the site with alcohol or another suitable antiseptic and allow it to dry before proceeding with the venipuncture. Take care not to stress the animal during blood collection. Use only the amount of restraint necessary to immobilize the animal. Excitement and stress can cause splenic contraction, which can alter the results of tests performed on red blood cells (RBCs). Results of several white blood cell (WBC) tests are also affected.

COLLECTION EQUIPMENT

A variety of collection equipment is available for use with veterinary patients. Blood may be collected in a syringe or specialized vacuum device, such as the Vacutainer system (Becton-Dickinson, Rutherford, NJ). When the needle/syringe method is used, the needle chosen should always be the largest one that the animal can comfortably accommodate. For most small animals, 20- to 25-gauge needles work well. In large animals, 16- to 20-gauge needles are routinely used. The syringe chosen should be one that is closest to the required sample volume. Use of a larger syringe could collapse the patient's vein. Using a large syringe with a small-bore needle can result in **hemolysis** (rupture of red blood cells) when the syringe plunger is pulled back with great speed and force. Remove the needle before expelling the blood into the collection tube. Erythrocytes (red blood cells, or RBCs) may hemolyze (rupture) if forced back through the needle.

Vacutainers are useful for multiple samples and when blood can be collected from a larger vessel, such as the cephalic or jugular vein. The Vacutainer system consists of a special needle, a needle holder, and vacuum-filled tubes that may be empty (clot tubes) or may contain a premeasured amount of anticoagulant (Fig. 7-4). Draw a fixed amount of blood into the tube, based on tube size and amount of vacuum in the tube. Collapse of veins, especially in smaller animals, may occur because of excessive negative pressure exerted by the vacuum. Using small vacuum tubes may remedy this problem.

> *TECHNICIAN NOTE* Always fill blood collection tubes properly to ensure the correct ratio of blood to anticoagulant.

Fill collection tubes with the proper amount of blood, regardless of the method used to collect the sample. Unless otherwise directed, fill the tube about ⅔ to ¾ full. This ensures a proper blood-to-anticoagulant ratio. Mix the blood adequately by inverting the tube gently for 10 to 20 seconds after transferring the blood. It is important to try for a precise venipuncture to prevent formation of blood clots in the sample resulting from platelet activation after multiple attempts at venipuncture. Serious errors may result if a sample is not labeled immediately after it has been collected. Label the tube with the date and time of collection, owner's name, patient's name, and patient's clinic identification number.

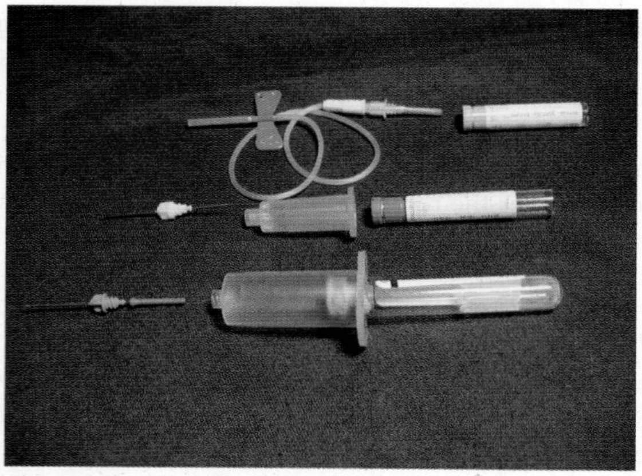

FIGURE 7-4 The Vacutainer blood collection system consists of a needle, holder, and collection tube. Several types of systems are available.

If submitted to a laboratory, include with the sample a request form that includes all necessary sample identification and a clear indication of which tests are requested.

SAMPLE TYPE

Whole Blood

Whole blood is composed of cellular elements (erythrocytes, leukocytes, and platelets), and a fluid called plasma. To collect a whole blood sample, place the appropriate amount of blood into a container with the proper anticoagulant and gently mix the sample by inverting the tube multiple times. Whole blood may be refrigerated if analysis is to be delayed, but it should never be frozen unless the plasma has been separated from the cellular elements. If the blood has been refrigerated, warm the sample to room temperature and mix gently before analysis.

Plasma

To obtain a plasma sample, collect the appropriate amount of blood in a container with the proper anticoagulant and gently mix well. Centrifuge the closed container for 10 minutes at 2000 to 3000 rpm to separate the fluid from the cells. After the sample is centrifuged, remove the plasma from the cells, being careful not to contaminate the plasma with any pelleted cells, and transfer the plasma into another appropriately labeled container. Separate plasma from the cellular elements as soon as possible after collection to minimize any artifactual changes. Plasma can be refrigerated or frozen until analysis is performed, depending on the specific requirements of the desired test(s).

ANTICOAGULANTS

Anticoagulants are used when whole blood or plasma samples are needed. The choice of a particular anticoagulant should be based on the tests needed. Some anticoagulants can interfere with certain test methods. The most commonly used anticoagulant for hematology studies is ethylenediaminetetraacetic acid (EDTA). Tubes that contain EDTA have a lavender or purple rubber stopper.

EDTA functions as an anticoagulant by binding calcium, which is necessary for clotting to occur. It is preferred for routine hematologic studies because it preserves cell morphology better than other anticoagulants. Even if collected in an EDTA tube, blood should be analyzed as quickly as possible, preferably within 2 hours after collection. Blood preserved in EDTA stays fresh for several hours or even overnight if stored in a refrigerator at 4° C. However, morphologic changes in the cells, such as cytoplasmic vacuolation, irregular cell membranes, and crenation (shrinkage of RBCs), may occur in stored samples, especially when the ratio of blood to anticoagulant is incorrect. This can make interpretation of observations difficult and result in inaccuracies.

> *TECHNICIAN NOTE* EDTA is the preferred anticoagulant for hematology testing.

It is for this reason that blood smears are best made immediately with fresh blood or within 1 hour after collection in an EDTA tube. If there is any delay in examining the blood, it is important to gently remix the blood by inverting it several times before making a blood smear. Crenation may occur if the tubes are not sufficiently filled, causing a relative excess of EDTA in the sample.

Heparin functions as an anticoagulant by activation of antithrombin III, which prevents conversion of prothrombin to thrombin. Heparin is not a permanent anticoagulant; it inhibits coagulation for only 8 to 12 hours. Tubes containing heparin (green-top tubes) may be used if tests run on whole blood are done promptly. Heparin may cause cells to clump and stain poorly. Heparin tubes may be a good choice for storing small blood samples from birds, because you can use the whole blood for hematologic tests and then collect plasma after spinning the sample.

Sodium citrate (blue-top tubes) anticoagulant is used for coagulation tests. However, it is generally not suitable for routine hematologic studies because it can cause distortion in cell morphology.

FORMATION AND FUNCTIONS OF BLOOD AND BLOOD CELLS

Blood is composed of plasma and cells. Blood plasma is more than 90% water. The remainder of plasma consists of proteins, hormones, vitamins, and similar substances. The cells contained in plasma make up about 45% of the total blood volume and include erythrocytes (red blood cells), leukocytes (white blood cells), and platelets.

The formation of blood cells is called hematopoiesis. In the adult animal, blood cell formation occurs in the bone marrow. In the prenatal animal, blood cell formation occurs in multiple organ sites such as the liver and spleen. Other organs play a role in blood cell formation, both in the adult and prenatal animal.

ERYTHROPOIESIS

The formation of erythrocytes is called erythropoiesis. This process is stimulated by the hormone erythropoietin. Cells in the kidney monitor the oxygen levels in tissues and stimulate the release of the hormone in response to tissue hypoxia. Erythropoietin stimulates the erythrocyte stem cell, the hemocytoblast (located in the bone marrow), to differentiate into a rubriblast. Mitosis of erythrocyte precursor cells continues in the bone marrow as the cells continue to mature. Once the cell reaches the **reticulocyte** stage, it may be released from the bone marrow into peripheral circulation. Reticulocytes can continue their maturation in circulation. Younger cells within the maturation series are not capable of further development once released from the bone marrow.

HEMOGLOBIN SYNTHESIS

Hemoglobin is a protein that comprises approximately 30% of the volume of an erythrocyte. The remainder of the cell consists of about 65% water and 5% organelles, enzymes, and salts. Hemoglobin functions to bind oxygen and thus allow the erythrocyte to carry oxygen to the body tissues. It also binds carbon dioxide and removes it from the tissues. Hemoglobin formation begins during the rubricyte stage of erythrocyte maturation and ends during the metarubricyte stage. Because mature erythrocytes do not contain a nucleus, they cannot synthesize cellular proteins. Cellular enzymes needed to provide energy to the cell are synthesized as the cell matures in the bone marrow. This limitation in the amount of available enzymes is responsible for the relatively short life span of an erythrocyte. This life span is variable among different species (Table 7-2).

An increase in the numbers of circulating erythrocytes is termed **polycythemia.** Polycythemia may be pathologic, physiologic, or apparent. Apparent polycythemias are seen in dehydrated patients. Physiologic polycythemia results when an animal is stressed during blood collection. Stress causes splenic contraction and releases vast numbers of red blood cells into circulation. **Anemia** refers to a decrease in the oxygen-carrying ability of the blood. This may be caused by decreased production of erythrocytes, increased destruction of erythrocytes, or decrease in hemoglobin concentration of the erythrocytes. Hemoglobin testing, **packed cell volume** (PCV), and RBC indices are used to differentiate the specific cause of anemia. Evaluation of erythrocyte morphology on the blood smear also provides diagnostic information useful in classification of anemia.

TECHNICIAN NOTE Hemoglobin and PCV testing and RBC indices help determine the cause of anemia.

LEUKOPOIESIS

The formation of white blood cells (leukocytes) is called leukopoiesis. Leukocyte maturation occurs primarily in the bone marrow, although other organs are also involved. Leukocytes are classified as either granulocytes or agranulocytes, and the formation and maturation of these two groups of leukocytes differs considerably. Leukocytes perform their function within the tissues and not in the blood. Therefore most leukocytes remain in circulation only a few hours. Some leukocytes continue maturation once in tissue spaces. The granulocytes (neutrophils, eosinophils, and basophils) develop from a stem cell known as a myeloblast. Maturation then proceeds through a promyelocyte, myelocyte,

TABLE 7-2 Erythrocyte Life Span

SPECIES	LIFE SPAN (DAYS)
Bovine (adult)	160
(3 mos)	55
Equine	140-150
Porcine	62
Canine	107-115
Feline	68
Ovine	70-153
Caprine	125

metamyelocyte, band, and segmented stage. Production of specific granules occurs during the myelocyte stage. In most veterinary species, the band and segmented stages are commonly found in peripheral circulation. Agranulocytes (lymphocytes and monocytes) have diverse patterns of development and maturation. The monocyte seen in peripheral circulation is one stage in the development of the tissue macrophage. Monocytes, therefore, do not perform their functions in circulation. Lymphocytes show extreme diversity in maturation, function, and appearance. Their primary functions relate to production of antibody and regulation of the immune system.

An increase in the numbers of circulating leukocytes is termed leukocytosis. Leukocytosis is often the result of viral or bacterial inflammation. Leukopenia is the term used to describe a decrease in circulating leukocytes. Neutropenia refers specifically to a decrease in circulating neutrophils and neutrophilia to an increase in circulating neutrophils.

Hematopoietic tumors (neoplasia of blood-forming tissues) are common in domestic animals. These disorders are broadly classified as either lymphoproliferative or myeloproliferative, depending on the type of cell or cells from which the tumor originates. Lymphoproliferative disorders originate from lymphocytes or plasma cells (a tissue cell of lymphoid origin). Myeloproliferative disorders arise from nonlymphoid cells that originate in the bone marrow. Neoplasms of red blood cell and megakaryocyte origin are also included in this group. These tumors are called leukemias if the neoplastic cells originate in the bone marrow.

Hematopoietic disorders are often diagnosed by finding specific early stages (blast forms) of cell types in peripheral blood and/or bone marrow. Lymphoblastic leukemia may be diagnosed by finding lymphoblasts in the blood and/or bone marrow. If neoplastic cells are found in the peripheral blood, the term leukemic blood profile is often used.

COMPLETE BLOOD COUNT

The CBC is a cost-effective way to obtain valuable hematologic information on a patient. With practice and attention to detail, you can perform a CBC quickly, easily, and accurately in any veterinary hospital. CBCs are indicated for diagnostic evaluation of disease states, well-animal screening (e.g., geriatric), and as a screening tool before surgery. A CBC includes total erythrocyte and leukocyte counts, packed cell volume, hemoglobin concentration, and RBC indices. Additional tests that should be included at the time of the CBC are:

- Measurement of total solids
- Evaluation of serum color and clarity
- Buffy coat evaluation
- Platelet estimate
- Platelet assessment

Most components of the CBC are performed with automated analyzers. Manual methods are rarely performed in clinical practice. Automated analyzers can provide accurate and cost-effective results. However, care should be taken in choosing the most appropriate instrument for your clinic.

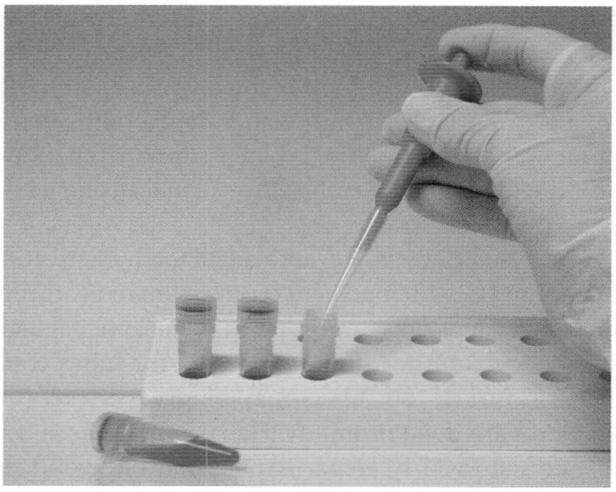

FIGURE 7-5 The Leukopet system used for counting of avian WBCs.

Hematology analyzers for veterinary use employ impedance methods, buffy coat analysis, or laser methods when evaluating a sample. Some analyzers may incorporate a combination of methods. Each method has specific advantages and disadvantages. Regardless of which analyzer you use, an understanding of the test principles used with your analyzer is essential. Knowing the limitations of the analytical system enhances the validity of your test results. Regular quality control is also essential for assuring the accuracy of your test results.

CELL COUNTS

Counting of erythrocytes and leukocytes is a routine part of the CBC. Cell counts are not generally performed with manual methods except in avian and exotic animal practice. Manual white blood cell count methods for exotic animal samples can be performed using the Leukopet system (Fig. 7-5). This system includes a pipette that holds a predetermined amount of blood and a reservoir that contains a diluting and lysing agent. Procedure 7-1 describes the method for counting of avian leukocytes cells using the Leukopet system.

The Leukopet system uses a premeasured volume of phloxine as a diluent. Once filled with the appropriate volume of blood and mixed, a small amount of the blood-diluent mixture is placed on a hemocytometer. The hemocytometer contains an optical-quality cover glass and measured grid that contains a specific volume.

Hemacytometers are counting chambers used to determine the number of cells per microliter (μl, mm^3) of blood. Several models are available, but the most common type used has two identical sets of fine grids of parallel and perpendicular etched lines called Neubauer rulings (Fig. 7-6). Each grid is divided into 9 large squares. The 4 corner squares are divided into 16 smaller squares and the center square is divided into 400 tiny squares (25 groups of 16 each). The area of each grid (Neubauer ruling) is designed to hold a precise amount of sample (0.9 μl). Knowing the number of cells in set parts of the grid and the amount of sample in that area is the basis for calculating the number of cells per microliter of blood. Mechanical counters are available to manually keep track of the number of cells observed.

PROCEDURE 7-1 Avian White Blood Counts with the Leukopet System and Hemacytometer

1. Attach a clean, unused disposable pipet tip to the 25 µl pipetter.
2. Unscrew the cap of one of the prefilled phloxine tubes and place in a tube rack.
3. Using the pipetter, aspirate 25 µl of freshly drawn anticoagulated blood. Carefully wipe excess sample from the outside of the pipette.
4. Dispense the blood sample into the tube of phloxine and rinse the pipet tip **thoroughly** by aspirating and dispensing the phloxine/blood solution at least six times. It is critical that all of the blood be rinsed from the pipet tip to ensure a proper dilution. Depending on the viscosity of the sample, this may require additional rinsing of the tip.
5. Cap the tube and mix well by inverting several times. Do not shake.
6. Allow tube to incubate for 10 minutes but no longer than 1 hour.
7. Make sure the hemacytometer and its special coverslip are clean and free of dirt and fingerprints. Clean them with lens cleaner and paper.
8. Using the rinsed pipette, aspirate a sample from the tube and charge (fill) each side of the hemacytometer at the etched groove. Do not overfill or underfill the counting chamber. This can cause uneven distribution of cells throughout the Neubauer ruling and contributes to an inaccurate count.
9. Allow to stand for up to 10 minutes for cells to settle.
10. Place the hemacytometer on the microscope stage. Lower the condenser of the microscope to increase contrast so that the cells are easier to see.
11. Using the 10× objective, count the heterophils and eosinophils in both chambers of the Neubauer hemacytometer. Cells that touch the lines between two squares are considered as within that square if they touch the top or the left-center lines. Cells that touch the bottom or right lines are not counted with that square. All squares from each side (grid) of the hemacytometer are counted, and the total number from both sides of the hemacytometer are used to calculate the total leukocyte count as follows:

$$\text{Total WBC}/\mu l = \frac{\begin{array}{c}\text{Total Heterophil} + \text{Eosinophil}\\ \text{(both chambers)} \times 1.1 \times 16 \times 100\end{array}}{\begin{array}{c}\%\ \text{Heterophils} + \%\ \text{Eosinophils}\\ \text{(from differential count)}\end{array}}$$

An estimate of the red blood cell counts may be obtained by dividing the packed cell volume by 6. For example, if the PCV is 36, the estimated RBC count is 36 divided by 6 = 6 million RBCs/µl.

Automated analyzers used for counting blood cells are present in most veterinary clinics. Numerous veterinary analyzers are currently available. CBCs performed in this manner may be cost effective if several CBCs are done each day.

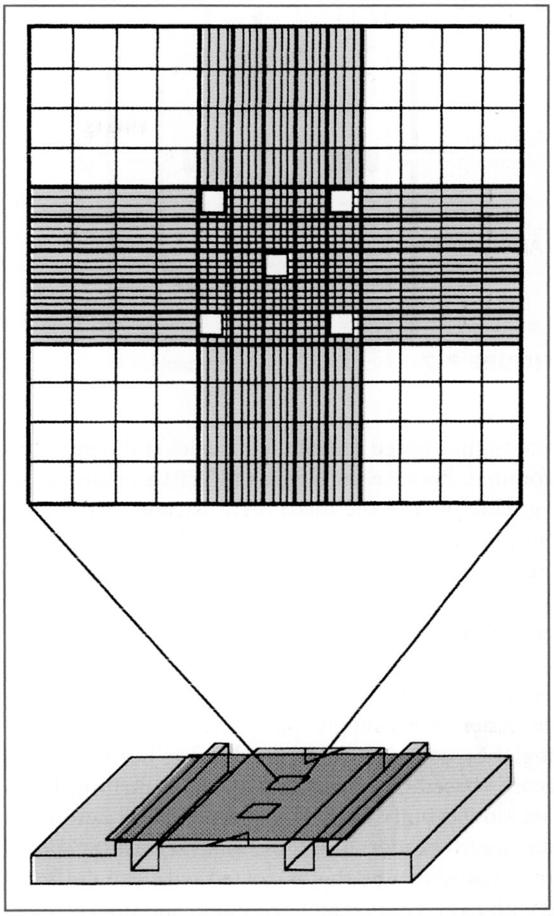

FIGURE 7-6 Neubauer hemacytometer.

Advantages of automation include speed, accuracy, and consistent results. Disadvantages of certain analyzers include the need for regular maintenance and quality control. Automated hematologic examination only partially replaces a manual CBC. The veterinary technician still must perform several aspects of the CBC, usually the **differential cell count** and total protein concentration. Each instrument has a specific protocol for use; therefore, the technician should study the operator's manual or contact the manufacturer before using the equipment. Following is a brief description of the types of automation used in veterinary practice.

Impedance Counters

Impedance counters can rapidly and efficiently count RBCs, WBCs, and platelets. They are based on the idea of counting particles (cells) as they flow past a detection device. The analyzers are designed to count all particles of a specific size that pass through an aperture (Fig. 7-7). The analyzer must be set to the sizes of the blood cells seen in the species being evaluated. A blood sample is placed in an electrolyte solution and then drawn through the aperture. As cells pass through the aperture, a specific amount of the electrolyte solution is displaced. The analyzer counts each of these displacements as a cell. Some units also determine hemoglobin concentration, red cell indices, and provide histograms. These counters

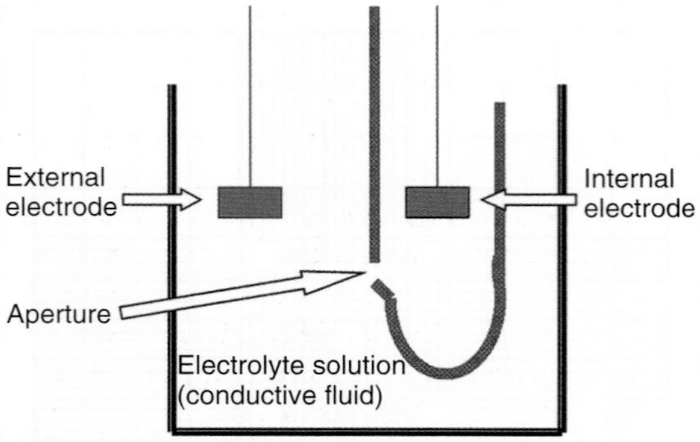

FIGURE 7-7 Principle of impedance analysis for cell counts.

have computer-based settings for species and type of cells being counted. Because the RBCs and WBCs of animal species vary greatly in size, the instrument is calibrated and set for the proper species. Platelet clumps, especially seen in cats, can be erroneously counted as leukocytes by cell counters.

Qualitative Buffy Coat System

Buffy coat analyzers provide an estimate of the cell count rather than a true count. This estimate is then used to calculate other hematologic parameters, such as PCV and hemoglobin concentration. Qualitative buffy coat (QBC) analysis is based on measurement of a centrifuged, stained, and expanded buffy coat by a computerized automatic microhematocrit reader. The QBC analyzer uses a specialized microhematocrit tube that is coated with stain. The tube is filled with EDTA anticoagulated blood and then centrifuged. The centrifuged blood separates into layers based on density of the cells. RBCs are found at the bottom of the tube, as in the manual microhematocrit method. The **buffy coat** is expanded into several layers and is divided into a **granulocyte** (combined neutrophil, eosinophil, basophil) layer, an agranulocyte (combined lymphocyte/monocyte) layer, and a platelet layer. If many reticulocytes or nucleated red blood cells (NRBCs) are present, these may form a layer at the top of the RBC column (below the buffy coat). The tube is then placed in an optical scanning device, which measures the degree of stain fluorescence in each cell layer. The analyzer provides a report for different hematologic values and a graph illustrating cell numbers and fluorescence for each cell layer. These values include hematocrit, hemoglobin, mean corpuscular hemoglobin concentration (MCHC), total WBC count, granulocyte count (percentage and absolute count), lymphocyte/monocyte count (percentage and absolute count), and platelet count. The QBC performs only a partial white blood cell differential and cannot replace blood smear evaluation. It is especially important to examine the blood smear if findings are abnormal. Total protein concentration can be measured on plasma separated in the specialized tube.

Laser Flow Cytometry

Laser-based analyzers are the most accurate of the hematology analyzers. They also tend to be the most expensive type of in-house analyzer. A focused laser beam is used, and the relative size and density of the cells differentiates the various cell types. This method also allows for a fairly accurate differential blood cell analysis and a reticulocyte count. Rapid test performance and built-in quality control procedures are characteristic of laser-based analyzers. Most analyzers of this type also provide a histogram, which can provide a more accurate representation of the cell types present.

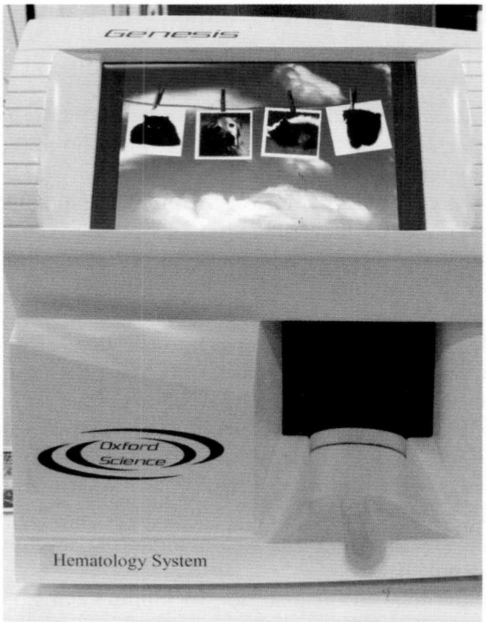

FIGURE 7-8 The Genesis hematology analyzer (Oxford Science, Oxford, CT) combines impedance and laser-based methods. (From Figure 8-1 in Sirois M: *Laboratory procedures for veterinary technicians*, ed 6, St Louis, 2015, Mosby.)

Combination Methods

A number of analyzers are available that combine some of the previously mentioned methods. One of the most common types is designed so that impedance methods are used to obtain accurate cell counts while laser flow cytometry is used to obtain the differential blood cell analysis (Fig. 7-8).

HEMOGLOBIN TESTING AND PACKED CELL VOLUME

A variety of methods are used to measure hemoglobin concentration. These require that the red blood cells be lysed to release the hemoglobin from the cells. Once that step is accomplished, the hemoglobin measurement may use a color-matching method or a photometric method. Color-matching methods tend to be the least accurate analyses and are not commonly used. A color standard is used to compare the color of the lysed blood sample and equate it to a specific hemoglobin concentration. Automated and semiautomated methods are available that use this technology. Photometric analysis of hemoglobin concentration is more accurate than color-matching methods. The photometric technique requires mixing the lysed blood sample with a specific reagent and measuring the resulting colored-complex with a photometer. The light absorbance of the colored complex equates to a specific hemoglobin

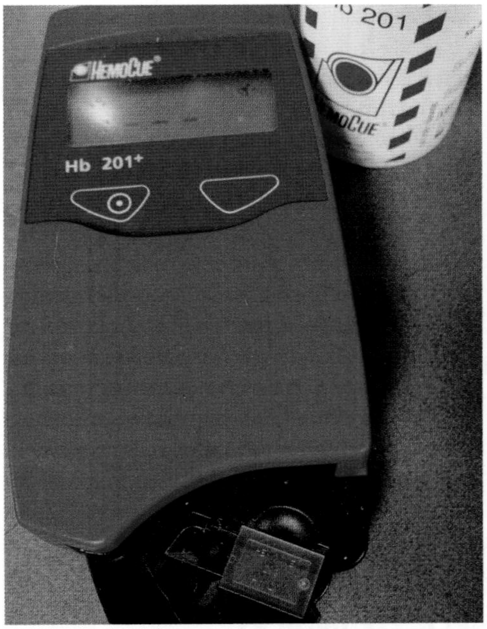

FIGURE 7-9 The HemoCue is a type of photometer that is used to measure hemoglobin concentration. (From Figure 9-10 in Sirois M: *Laboratory procedures for veterinary technicians*, ed 6, St Louis, 2015, Mosby.)

concentration. Unlike color-matching methods, photometric methods are capable of measuring all forms of hemoglobin. Most color-matching methods only provide the concentration of oxyhemoglobin. A variety of handheld analyzers are available that measure hemoglobin (Fig. 7-9).

TECHNICIAN NOTE The PCV is a measure of the percentage of the blood that is occupied by red blood cells.

The PCV is another vital part of the CBC. The PCV, also known as the hematocrit (Hct), is an expression of the percentage of whole blood occupied by RBCs. PCV can be performed with either a macrohematocrit or microhematocrit technique. The microhematocrit method, abbreviated mHct, is the most commonly performed PCV test in veterinary practice (Procedure 7-2). A blood-filled capillary tube is centrifuged for 2 to 5 minutes, depending on the type of centrifuge. The blood separates into a plasma layer, a white buffy coat composed of WBCs and platelets, and a layer of packed red cells (Fig. 7-10). Measuring the RBC layer in the capillary tube determines the PCV. The precision of a PCV is approximately 1%, making it a very accurate test.

A low PCV may indicate anemia. There are many causes of anemia, including blood loss, neoplasia, parasitism, and chronic infection. An increased PCV also has several possible causes, including dehydration and splenic contraction in an excited animal.

PCV values may be erroneously high because of clots in the sample, failure to adequately mix the EDTA and blood, and insufficient centrifugation time.

PROCEDURE 7-2 Microhematocrit Procedure

1. Fill two microhematocrit tubes about three fourths full with whole blood. Wipe the excess blood from the outside of the tube. Use plain (anticoagulant-free) microhematocrit tubes with anticoagulated blood. Use heparinized tubes when collecting blood from a venipuncture site.
2. Push sealing clay into one end of each microhematocrit tube. Rotate each tube as it is pressed into the clay to ensure a tight seal.
3. Put the tubes in a microhematocrit centrifuge, with the clay seal to the *outside*. Centrifuge for 2 to 5 minutes, depending on the model of the centrifuge used.
4. Determine the PCV for each tube by measuring the length of the column of RBCs using a microhematocrit tube reader. Average the two readings.

PCV values may be erroneously low if the microhematocrit tube contains excessive plasma because of inadequate mixing of the sample. Sample dilution because of low blood-to-anticoagulant ratio may also cause a spurious decrease in PCV.

After determining the PCV, evaluate the plasma for turbidity and color (Box 7-2). An icteric, or yellow, plasma layer may occur with liver disease or hemolytic anemia. Normal adult ruminants and horses may have yellow plasma resulting from carotenes in the blood. A hemolytic, or red, sample can occur from improper sample collection and handling or with hemolytic anemia. Sometimes the buffy coat is red tinged, especially in very sick animals or if there is an increased number of immature RBCs in the circulation. Lipemic plasma appears cloudy (turbid) and white, indicating excessive lipids in the blood. This can occur if blood was collected from an animal that was not fasted, or it may be pathologic. **Icterus**, hemolysis, and lipemia may be quantified as slight, moderate, or marked. The width of the buffy coat should be assessed. With experience, you may be able to generally assess the WBC count from buffy coat width, if the total WBC count is very high or low. This is not an accurate method, but can signal the technician to be on the lookout for an abnormal WBC count.

Microfilariae in heartworm-positive dogs also may be observable at the buffy coat/plasma interface. The interface should be examined with a microscope at low power (100× magnification). The wiggling movement of the microfilariae displaces the plasma.

In certain situations, it may be valuable to microscopically examine the buffy coat for infectious agents and cell types, including cancer cells. The procedure can be performed using a standard microhematocrit tube centrifuged for a PCV. After centrifugation, snap the tube just below the buffy coat layer. Transfer the buffy coat and a small portion of the plasma to a clean slide. A compression smear is then made and the smear air-dried. (See Chapter 9 for details on preparing compression smears.) The slide can be sent to a commercial laboratory for special staining and analysis (i.e., immunoassays). The slide may also be stained and

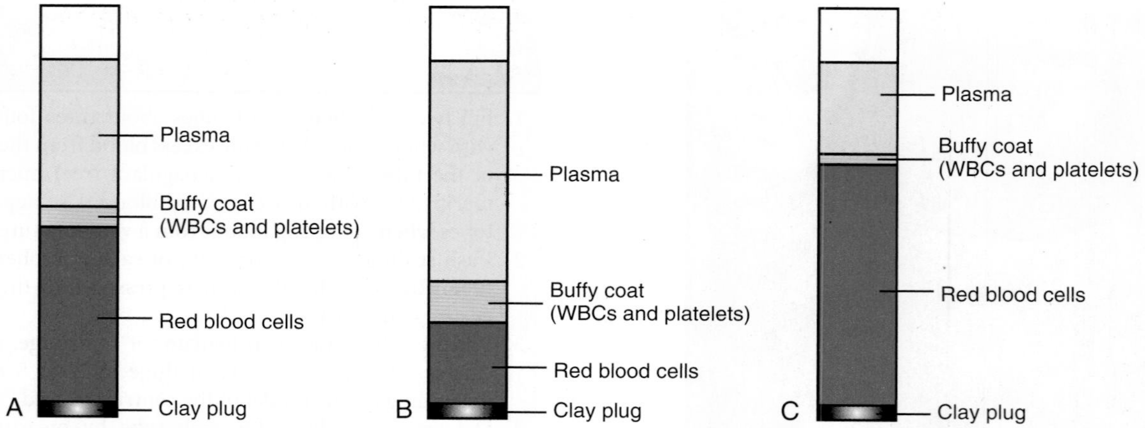

FIGURE 7-10 Separated layers in a centrifuged hematocrit tube. (From Colville T, Bassert JM: *Clinical anatomy and physiology for veterinary technicians*, ed 2, St Louis, 2008, Mosby.)

BOX 7-2 Visual Assessment of Plasma Turbidity and Color

Normal:	Clear and colorless to light straw yellow
Icterus:	Clear and yellow
Hemolysis:	Clear and red
Lipemia:	Turbid and white

examined for neoplastic cells or infectious agents as well as for performing differential cell counts on patients with low WBC counts.

TOTAL PLASMA PROTEIN DETERMINATION

The serum or plasma total protein level can be rapidly and reliably measured using a handheld **refractometer** (Procedure 7-3). Several types of refractometers are available. Those encountered in practice have built-in scales that you can view by looking through a viewfinder at one end of the refractometer. Most refractometers have a scale to measure both protein and specific gravity. The protein value is read directly from the scale in g/dl. Calibration of the refractometer should be verified periodically as part of routine quality-control procedures. This involves taking a reading on distilled water at an ambient temperature of 21 to 29° C (70 to 85° F). The reading should be at 1.000 on the urine specific gravity scale. If it is not, adjust the reading by turning the zero-set screw on the instrument. Refer to the manufacturer's manual for details.

Accurate plasma protein determination is difficult in lipemic samples, because the turbidity produces an indistinct line of demarcation on the scale. Hemoglobinemia caused by hemolysis can falsely increase plasma protein values because of the presence of the heme portion of hemoglobin. The yellow color of an icteric sample does not interfere with refractometry.

Common causes of increased plasma protein levels include dehydration and increased production of globulins associated with inflammation. Plasma protein values decrease with overhydration, renal disease, gastrointestinal losses, and reduced protein production by a diseased liver.

ERYTHROCYTE INDICES

Erythrocyte indices are calculated values that use the RBC count, hemoglobin measurement, and PCV. The erythrocyte indices include the mean corpuscular volume (MCV), mean corpuscular hemoglobin (MCH), and mean corpuscular hemoglobin concentration (MCHC). The term *corpuscular* is an old term used to describe red blood cells. These measurements provide data on the overall size of the red blood cells as well as the relative amount of hemoglobin within the individual red blood cells. The equations used to calculate the RBC indices are in Table 7-3.

Of the three RBC indices, the MCHC is considered the most accurate because the tests used to calculate the ratio (PCV and hemoglobin) are more accurate than cell counts. The most useful of the indices is the MCV because it represents the average volume of a single erythrocyte. The MCV varies greatly depending on species. RBC indices should be confirmed by evaluating the morphology of the erythrocytes on the blood smear.

TECHNICIAN NOTE Abnormalities in erythrocyte indices should be confirmed by evaluating the morphology of the erythrocytes on the blood smear.

HISTOGRAMS

A histogram is a graph that provides a visual report of the sizes (on the x-axis) and numbers (on the y-axis) of the various cellular components. The histogram can be used to verify results of the blood smear and provide an indication of any problem with test results. For example, when megathrombocytes or platelet aggregates are present, the WBC count performed on most automated analyzers will be falsely elevated because those large platelets are usually counted as leukocytes. The histogram can provide evidence of this anomaly because the WBC curve on the histogram will be altered.

PROCEDURE 7-3 Plasma Protein Determination

1. After centrifuging a filled microhematocrit tube, carefully break the tube just above the buffy coat/plasma interface.
2. Transfer plasma to the refractometer by allowing the sample to fill the space between the cover plate and glass surface by capillary action. You need only a very small amount of the sample. Use a syringe and needle to force the plasma onto the surface of an open refractometer. Do not tap the sample out of the tube, because this can scratch the surface of the refractometer.
3. Hold the refractometer horizontally, allowing the overhead light to reach the top of the instrument.
4. Look through the viewfinder and focus the scale by turning the eyepiece.
5. Read the protein value in g/dl at the interface of the light and shaded area. Record the value. Readings may vary slightly when different people read values on a refractometer (Fig. 1). This results from a slight variation in an individual's perception of where the shaded line is read.
6. Clean the instrument with water and a soft, lint-free cloth or lens paper.

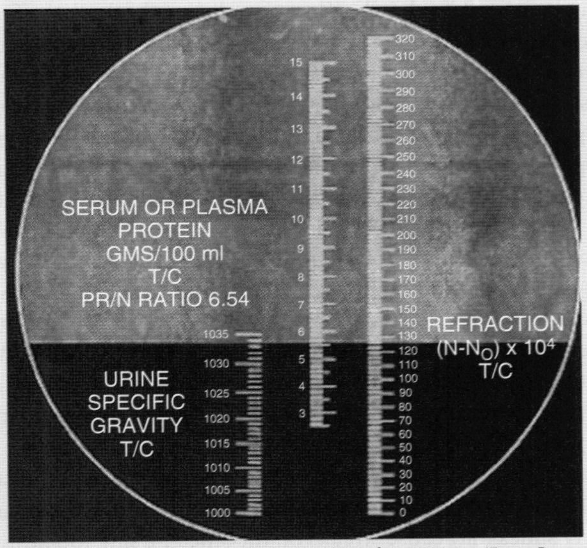

FIGURE 1 The reading scale within the refractometer. (From Bassert JM, McCurnin DM: *McCurnin's clinical textbook for veterinary technicians*, ed 7, St Louis, 2010, Saunders.)

TABLE 7-3 Equations Used to Calculate RBC Indices

PARAMETER	EQUATION	UNITS
MCV	$\frac{PCV \times 10}{RBC\ count}$	Femtoliter
MCH	$\frac{Hb \times 100}{RBC\ count}$	Picogram
MCHC	$\frac{Hb \times 10}{PCV}$	Percent

DIFFERENTIAL BLOOD CELL COUNT

Although most veterinary hematology analyzers provide at least a partial differential white blood cell count, a blood smear must still be prepared and evaluated. There are a large number of abnormalities that are not routinely reported by automated analyzers. These include:

- Nucleated red blood cells
- Megathrombocytes
- Heinz bodies
- Bacteria
- Lymphoblasts
- Basophils
- Neoplastic cells
- Cellular inclusions (e.g., parasites, viral materials)
- Toxic granulation
- Platelet clumps
- Polychromasia
- Target cells
- Hemoparasites
- Left shift
- Hypersegmentation

EVALUATING THE BLOOD SMEAR

The CBC must include a differential blood cell count that enumerates various types of white blood cells present and also describes morphology of both red and white blood cells and platelets. A platelet estimate is also performed on the blood smear. In addition to reporting the morphologic changes, a rating system is used to characterize the relative numbers of abnormal cells seen on the blood smear.

Patience and practice are required to develop the skills necessary to prepare and evaluate blood smears (Procedure 7-4). Only one drop of blood is needed to make a smear. It is best to use blood from the tip of the needle immediately after the blood is collected. This prevents development of artifacts related to the presence of anticoagulant. If you cannot make a smear immediately, make the smear as soon as possible after collection. Automated systems that smear and stain the blood smear are also available for use in the veterinary practice (Fig. 7-11).

TECHNICIAN NOTE The preferred sample for preparation of the differential blood cell smear is the blood drop on the tip of the needle immediately after the blood is collected.

The two methods of preparing blood smears are the wedge (glass slide) method and the coverslip method. Always use precleaned, glass microscope slides and coverslips and always hold slides by their edges to avoid smudging with grease or fingerprints. Even precleaned slides need to be cleaned, because they have a thin film that aids in preventing them from sticking to one another that also inhibits the blood cells from adhering to the glass slide or coverslip.

PROCEDURE 7-4 Making a Wedge Smear

1. Place a small drop of blood at the end of a clean glass slide using a microhematocrit tube or the end of a wooden applicator stick. Place this slide on a flat surface or suspend in midair between the thumb and forefinger.
2. Hold a second slide (the spreader slide) at a 30-degree angle and pull back into contact with the drop of blood, spreading blood along the edge of the spreader slide. Push the spreader slide forward in a rapid, steady, even motion to produce a blood smear that is thick at one end and tapers to a thin, feathered edge at the other (Fig. 1). The blood smear should cover about three-quarters of the length of the slide.

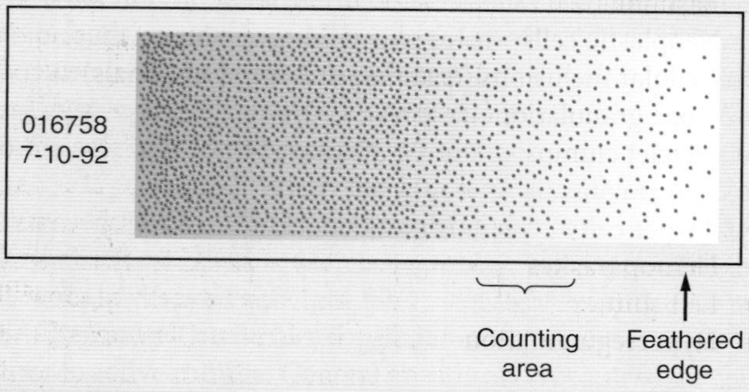

FIGURE 1 Blood smear showing the label area, monolayer counting area, and feathered edge.

3. Air-dry the smear by waving the slide in the air. This fixes the cells to the slide so that they are not dislodged during staining.
4. Label the slide at the thick end of the smear. If the slide has a frosted edge, this may be written on.
5. After drying, stain the smear with Wright stain or a Romanowsky-type stain, available in commercial kits (e.g., Wright Dip Stat3; Medi-Chem, Santa Monica, CA). These kits contain an alcohol fixative, a methylene blue mixture to stain cell nuclei and certain organelles bluish-purple, and eosin to stain hemoglobin and some WBC granules reddish-orange. Follow the directions packaged with the staining kit. Smears typically must be immersed in each solution for 5 to 10 seconds.
6. After staining, rinse the slide with distilled water. Allow the slide to dry upright with the feathered edge pointed upward. This allows the water to drip off the slide away from the smear.

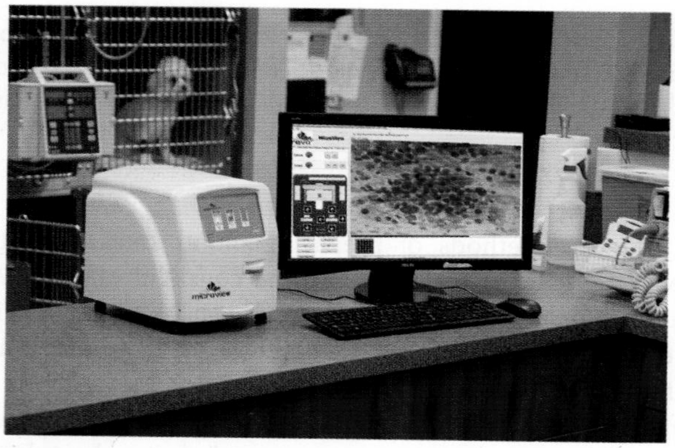

FIGURE 7-11 The MicroView automated system for preparation and evaluation of blood smears.

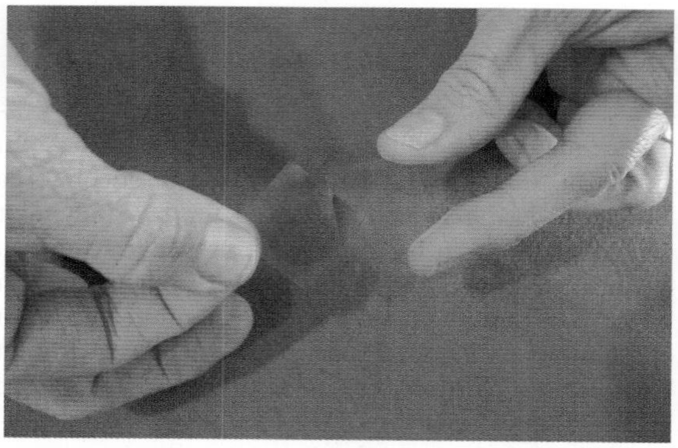

FIGURE 7-12 Preparing a blood smear by the coverslip method.

Clean the slides with alcohol and allow them to dry before making the blood smear. Charged slides (also known as positively charged slides) have a special adhesive coating that allow the specimen to easily adhere to them and do not need to be precleaned though they are considerably more expensive.

The wedge method is the most common type of smear used for routine hematology. The coverslip method is often preferred for avian blood smears because it renders a thinner smear, which facilitates cell identification. It is also less traumatic on fragile avian blood cells. The coverslip method allows for a more even distribution of blood cells and is more representative of the peripheral blood, whereas the wedge smear method results in the larger cells being "pushed" out to the feathered edge. In either method, it is important to develop a systematic approach of evaluating the blood smear to complete the differential count, cellular morphology, and platelet assessment.

Coverslip smears are made by putting one small drop of blood in the center of a clean, square coverslip (Fig. 7-12). Place a second clean coverslip diagonally on top of the first, causing the blood to spread evenly between the two surfaces. Then pull the coverslips apart horizontally in a single smooth motion just as the blood has completely spread. Wave the smears in the air to promote drying and stain them in a similar manner as described in Procedure 7-4 for making wedge smears.

Improper technique and inappropriate staining can result in inferior or useless blood smears. Jerky movements and dirty slides may cause streaks on the smear. Using too little or too much blood results in improper smear length. Clots or fat in the blood can cause small holes in the smear and an uneven feathered edge. If the blood is from an anemic patient (decreased PCV), increase the spreader slide angle to about 45 degrees. Conversely, the angle should be decreased to about 20 degrees if the blood is concentrated (increased PCV). Increasing the spreader slide angle makes a thicker smear, whereas decreasing it makes a thinner smear (Fig. 7-13).

Table 7-4 lists problems related to staining. Cells appear dark if overstained, whereas extensive rinsing may cause them to look faded. Changing stains regularly is necessary for consistent results and preventing stain precipitation on the smear. Refractile artifacts on RBCs are another common problem. These are usually caused by moisture in the fixative solution. Take care not to confuse these artifacts with cellular abnormalities.

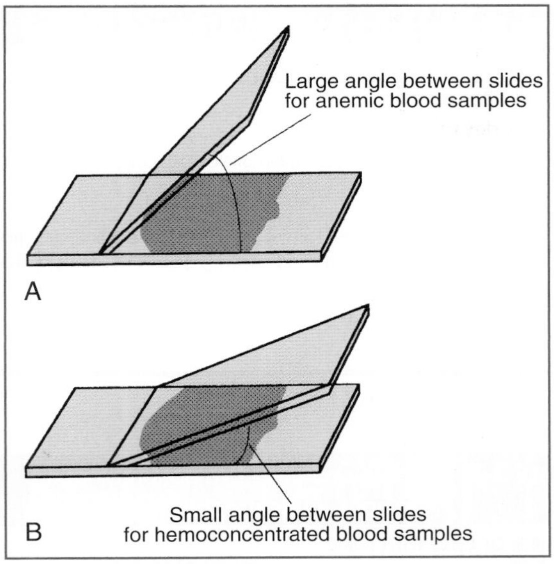

FIGURE 7-13 Difference in slide angle necessary for making blood smears from anemic or hemoconcentrated blood. **A,** Large angle for anemic blood. **B,** Small angle for hemoconcentrated blood.

PERFORMING THE DIFFERENTIAL

Place the slide on the microscope stage and examine the blood smear in a systematic manner. It is important to examine slides the same way each time to avoid making mistakes in counting cells or missing important observations (Fig. 7-14). Scan the smear at low power (100× magnification) to assess overall cell numbers and distribution. With practice, you can quickly estimate the total WBC count as either too high or low. The WBC estimate formula is:

$$\text{Estimated WBC Count} = (\text{Avg. no. WBC [on LPF from } 5-10 \text{ fields]} \div 4) \times 1000/\text{mm}^3$$

i.e., if 178 WBC were seen in 5 fields; average would be 35.6

$$35.6 \div 4 = 8.9 \times 1000/\text{mm}^3 = 8900/\text{mm}^3$$

Platelet clumps (aggregates) and blood parasites (e.g., microfilariae) are sometimes found at the feathered edge and must be noted on the hematology report.

TABLE 7-4 Some Possible Solutions to Problems Seen with Common Romanowsky-Type Stains

PROBLEM	SOLUTION
Excessive Blue Staining (RBCS May be Blue-Green)	
Prolonged stain contact	Decrease staining time
Inadequate wash	Wash longer
Specimen too thick	Make thinner smears, if possible
Stain, diluent, buffer, or wash water too alkaline	Check with pH paper and correct pH
Exposure to formalin vapors	Store and ship cytologic preps separate from formalin containers
Wet fixation in ethanol or formalin	Air dry smears before fixation
Delayed fixation	Fix smears sooner, if possible
Surface of the slide was alkaline	Use new slides
Excessive Pink Staining	
Insufficient staining time	Increase staining time
Prolonged washing	Decrease duration of wash
Stain or diluent too acidic	Check with pH paper and correct pH; fresh methanol may be needed
Excessive time in red stain solution	Decrease time in red stain solution
Inadequate time in blue stain solution	Increase time in blue stain solution
Mounting coverslip before preparation is dry	Allow preparation to dry completely before mounting coverslip
Weak Staining	
Insufficient contact with one or more of the stain solutions	Increase staining time
Fatigued (old) stains	Change stains
Another slide covered specimen during staining	Keep slides separate
Uneven Staining	
Variation of pH in different areas of slide surface (may be due to slide surface being touched or slide being poorly cleaned)	Use new slides, and avoid touching their surfaces before and after preparation
Water allowed to stand on some areas of the slide after staining and washing	Tilt slides close to vertical to drain water from the surface or dry with a fan
Inadequate mixing of stain and buffer	Mix stain and buffer thoroughly
Precipitate on Preparation	
Inadequate stain filtration	Filter or change the stain(s)

Continued

TABLE 7-4 Some Possible Solutions to Problems Seen with Common Romanowsky-Type Stains—cont'd

PROBLEM	SOLUTION
Inadequate washing of slide after staining	Rinse slides well after staining
Dirty slides used	Use clean new slides
Stain solution dries during staining	Use sufficient stain, and do not leave it on slide too long
Miscellaneous	
Overstained preparations	Destain with 95% methanol and restain; Diff-Quik-stained smears may have to be destained in the red Diff-Quik stain solution to remove the blue color; however, this damages the red stain solution
Refractile artifact on RBC with Diff-Quik stain (usually due to moisture in fixative)	Change the fixative

From Cowell RL, et al: *Diagnostic cytology and hematology of the dog and cat*, ed 3, St Louis, 2008, Mosby.

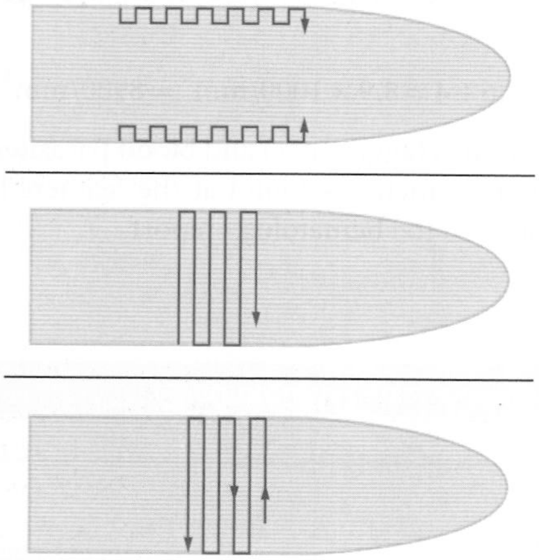

FIGURE 7-14 Scanning patterns used for performing a differential WBC count.

A monolayer (single layer of blood cells) is located adjacent to the feathered edge. The cells should have even distribution and not be overlapping. It is here, using the oil-immersion objective (1000× magnification), that the differential WBC count takes place. The procedure requires that 100 WBCs be counted, identified, and recorded. Because 100 WBCs are counted, the number of each WBC type observed is recorded as a percentage. This is called the relative WBC count. Various counting devices are available to aid the differential WBC count. Once the relative percentages of each cell type have been determined, the **absolute value** of each cell type must be calculated. This is accomplished by multiplying the total white blood cell count by the percentage of each cell type.

$$\text{Total WBC count} = 6000/\mu l\text{, with } 80\% \text{ neutrophils observed}$$

$$6000 \times 80\,\% = 4800 \text{ neutrophils}/\,\mu l \text{ of blood}$$

TECHNICIAN NOTE All morphologic abnormalities noted on the blood smear must be semiquantified.

TABLE 7-5 Semiquantitative Evaluation of Toxic Changes in Neutrophils by Amount

NUMBER OF CELLS WITH TOXIC CHANGE	PERCENTAGE (%)*
Few	5-10
Moderate	11-30
Many	>30
Observed Change	Severity of toxic change
Döhle bodies	Slight
Cytoplasmic basophilia	Slight to marked, depending on intensity
Cytoplasmic vacuolization (Foamy cytoplasm)	Moderate to marked, depending on amount
Indistinct nuclear membrane	Marked
Severe cell degeneration	

*If toxic changes occur in fewer than 5% of neutrophils, they are not reported.

The morphology of RBCs and WBCs is then assessed and recorded. The presence of any abnormal cells or toxic changes should be semiquantified (Table 7-5). A platelet estimate and evaluation is also performed (see Platelet Assessment Methods section).

ERYTHROCYTE MORPHOLOGY

VARIATIONS IN ERYTHROCYTE MORPHOLOGY

Normal erythrocyte morphology varies greatly among different species (Table 7-6). Unlike the RBCs of mammals, avian RBCs are nucleated. Veterinary technicians should be able to identify normal as well as abnormal RBC morphology. Morphology is evaluated using the oil-immersion objective (1000× magnification) in the monolayer portion of the smear.

Changes in the appearance of erythrocytes occur in a variety of conditions. In general these changes fall into one or more of the following categories: (1) changes in size, (2) changes in shape, (3) changes in color, (4) changes in cell behavior, and (5) appearance of inclusions. Box 7-3 contains the terms used to describe variations in erythrocytes on the blood smear.

TABLE 7-6 Characteristics of Normal Red Blood Cells in Animals

SPECIES	DIAMETER	ROULEAUX	CENTRAL PALLOR	ANISOCYTOSIS	POIKILOCYTES	BASOPHILIC STIPPLING IN REGENERATIVE RESPONSE	RETICULOCYTES (NORMAL PCV)
Dogs	7.0 m	+	++++	—	—	—	±1.0%
Pigs	6.0 m	++	±	+	++ ++	—	±1.0%
Cats	5.8 m	++	+	±	—	±	±0.5%
Horses	5.7 m	++ ++	±	±	—	—	0% (will not increase in response to anemia)
Cattle	5.5 m	—	+	++	—	+++	0% (will increase in response to anemia)
Sheep	4.5 m	±	+	+	—	+++	0% (will increase)
Goats	3.2 m	—	—	±	++ (in young)	++	0% (will increase)

Number of plus (+) signs indicates degree of characteristic; number of minus (–) signs indicates degree of absence of characteristic.

When five or more nucleated red blood cells are seen on the blood smear, it is necessary to correct the total white blood cell count because these cells would likely have been counted as leukocytes with either manual or automated analysis of leukocytes. The equation used to calculate the corrected WBC count is:

$$\frac{\text{Observed WBCs} \times 100}{100 + \text{no. NRBCs}} = \text{Corrected WBC Count}$$

For example, if the total WBC count is 9300/μl and 16 NRBCs are observed per 100 WBCs, the corrected WBC count is 9300/μl × 100 ÷ 100 + 16 = 8017/μl (round up or down to a whole number). Note that the corrected total WBC count is always *lower* than the original WBC count. The corrected total WBC count is then used to calculate the absolute count for each type of WBC.

BLOOD PARASITES

A variety of blood parasites can be seen on a peripheral blood smear. The majority of these are found on or within erythrocytes. Parasites may also be found free of cells and within leukocytes and platelets. Box 7-4 contains a summary of parasites commonly encountered on a blood smear.

LEUKOCYTE MORPHOLOGY

Segmented neutrophils, also known as segs or polymorphonuclear (PMN) cells, are mature WBCs that function mainly as phagocytes and are involved in inflammation. They have an irregular nucleus that is dark and dense and segmented into three to five lobes. Their cytoplasm is usually colorless to pale pink in most species. Bovine neutrophils have pink to orange cytoplasm. The cytoplasm may contain very fine, diffuse, dark granules. They are the most common type of WBC found in most mammalian species. Blood cells from exotic species can be difficult to classify and identify as abnormal. **Heterophils** are the functional equivalent of neutrophils in rabbits, rodents, birds, reptiles, and amphibians. They have a segmented nucleus and variably sized red-brown granules. In most birds, the granules are oval- or needle-shaped. Heterophils may exhibit cytoplasmic **basophilia** and vacuolization as toxic changes.

LYMPHOCYTES

Lymphocytes have a round to slightly indented nucleus that almost completely fills the cell. The cytoplasm is light blue and may contain a few purple granules, especially in ruminants. Lymphocytes vary in size. Small lymphocytes are mature and have a thin rim of cytoplasm. Large lymphocytes (less mature) have larger nuclei and abundant cytoplasm. Lymphocytes are the predominant WBC type in ruminants. Some bovine lymphocytes may be quite large, with nuclei that contain nucleolar rings, causing the lymphocytes to resemble neoplastic lymphoblasts (atypical lymphocytes).

MONOCYTES

Monocytes are very large WBCs with diffuse, less dense nuclear chromatin. The nucleus may vary in shape, including oval, kidney bean, amoeboid, bilobed, trilobed, and horseshoe shapes. The cytoplasm of monocytes is blue-gray and abundant. Vacuoles and/or fine granules may be present. Monocytes may be difficult to distinguish from toxic band neutrophils or earlier stages. Identifying an obvious band and noting its color is helpful. The cytoplasm of monocytes is usually darker than that of bands. The cell in question is most likely a monocyte if a **left shift** is not present.

EOSINOPHILS

Eosinophils have a lobulated nucleus and red-orange (eosinophilic) granules in their cytoplasm. Canine eosinophils contain round granules that vary greatly in size and number. They usually stain the same color as RBCs. The eosinophils of sighthounds (e.g., Greyhounds) may be difficult to identify because a colorless area often replaces the granules. Feline eosinophils contain numerous, small, rod-shaped granules.

BOX 7-3 Morphology of Erythrocytes

Normocytes
In canine, anucleate, biconcave discocytes with central pallor in canine. Anucleate round cells in feline.

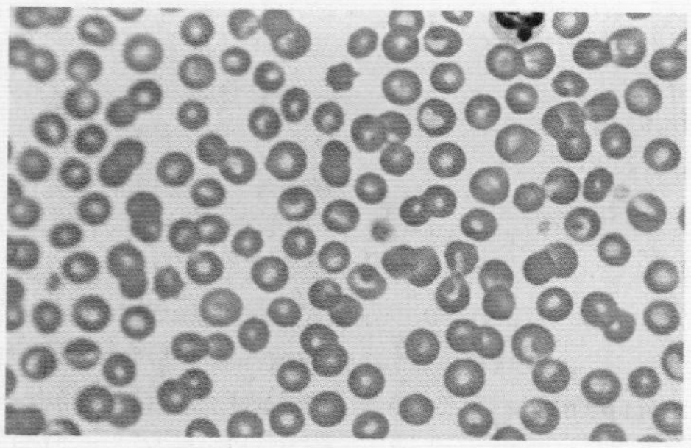

Normal canine red blood cells and platelets. (Courtesy Dr. E. Lassen.)

Morphologic Variation in Size

Anisocytes
Cells that vary in size. This variation is seen in splenic or liver disorders and is a sign of the regeneration of anemia

Macrocytes
Cells that are larger than normal. This variation represents immature cells. Macrocytes usually appear as reticulocytes with an NMB stain.

Microcytes
Cells that are smaller than normal. This variation is often seen in iron deficiency.

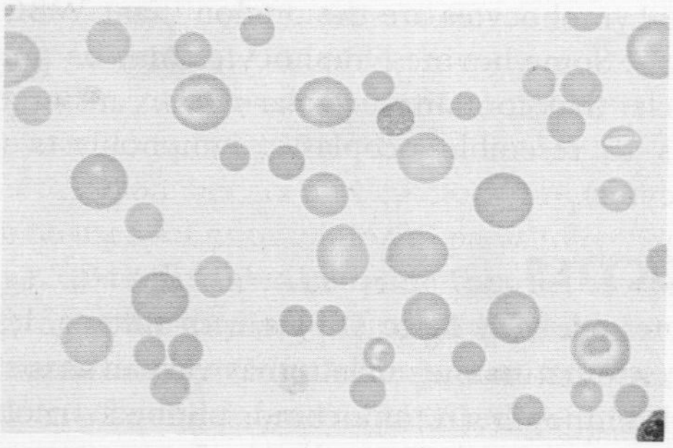

Mixed anisocytosis in a canine blood smear. Several target cells are also present. (From Cowell RL et al: *Diagnostic cytology and hematology of the dog and cat*, ed 3, St Louis, 2008, Mosby.)

Morphologic Variation in Shape

Poikilocytes
Generic name for any abnormally shaped cell. The specific abnormality should be further characterized as appropriate.

Schistocytes (schizocytes)
Fragmented cells. This variation is caused by mechanical trauma. Schistocytes are seen in disseminated intravascular coagulation (DIC), neoplasia, and other disorders.

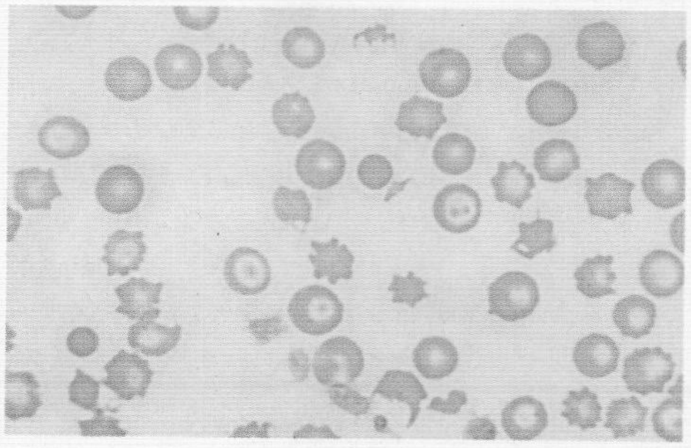

Schistocytes in a smear from a dog with iron deficiency. Target cells and red cells with other membrane abnormalities (keratocytes) are also present. (Courtesy Dr. Mary Anna Thrall.)

Acanthocytes
Cells with long, irregular surface projections

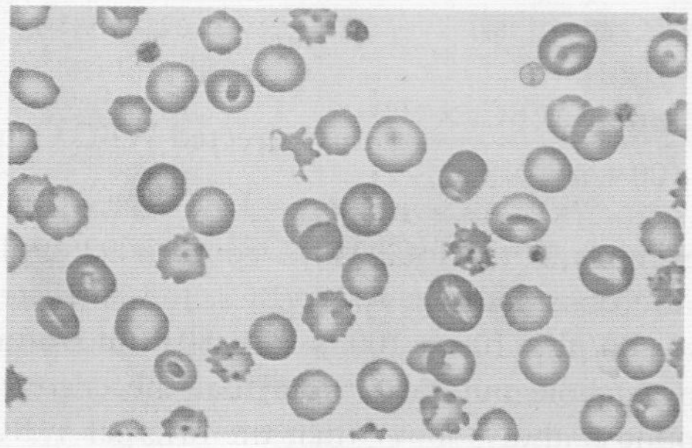

The large bluish-staining red cells in this smear of canine blood are polychromatophils. Also present are leptocytes (folded cells and target cells) and acanthocytes (spur cells). (Courtesy Dr. Mary Anna Thrall.)

Anulocytes
Bowl-shaped erythrocytes that form as a result of loss of membrane flexibility that does not allow the cell to return to a normal shape after passing through a capillary. These cells may be seen in any acute disease.

Dacryocytes
Teardrop-shaped cells seen in certain myeloproliferative diseases. These may be produced as an artifact but can be identified by the direction of the elongated tail. Dacryocytes produced as artifact have their tails pointing in the same direction.

BOX 7-3 Morphology of Erythrocytes—cont'd

Keratocyte

Commonly referred to as "helmet cells," "blister cells," or "bite cells." Associated with hemangiosarcoma, neoplasia, glomerulonephritis, and various hepatic diseases.

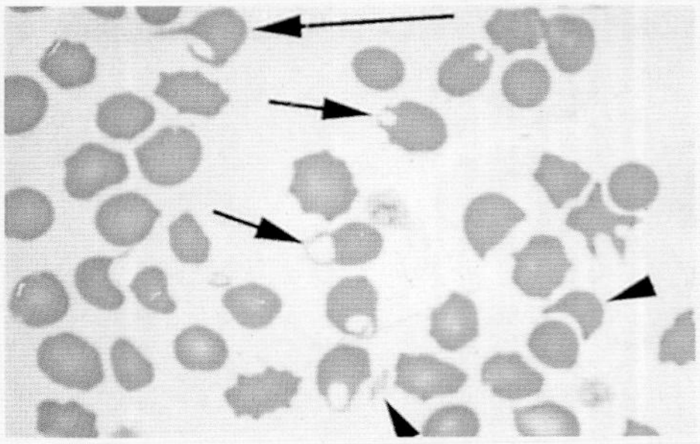

Numerous keratocytes *(arrows)* and a schistocyte *(arrowhead)* are present in this blood smear from a cat with iron-deficiency anemia.

Echinocytes

Cells with regular cytoplasmic projections around the periphery giving the cell the appearance of a scalloped border.

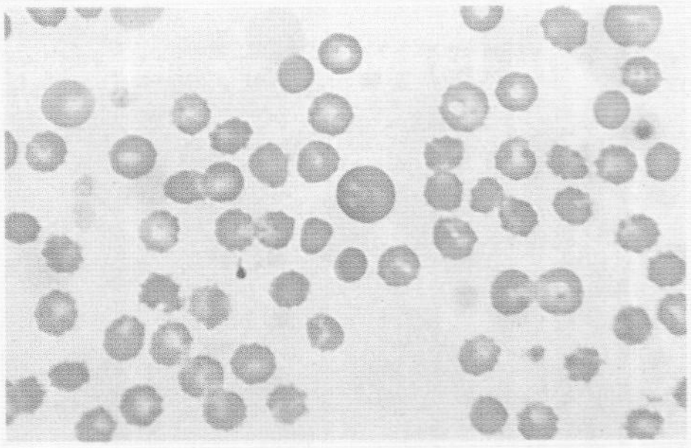

Echinocytes in a canine blood smear. Note the polychromatophil in the center.

Spherocytes

Small dense cells with no area of central pallor.

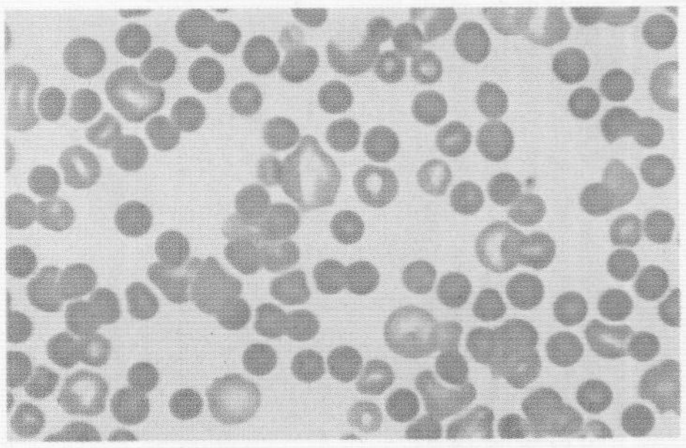

Most of the red blood cells in this smear from a dog with immune-mediated hemolytic anemia are spherocytes, lacking central pallor. (Courtesy Dr. Mary Anna Thrall.)

Stomatocytes

Cells with a slitlike center opening.

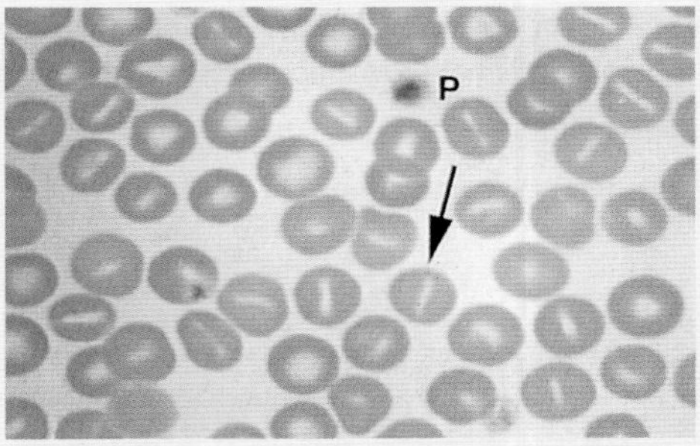

Folded cells and stomatocytes *(arrow)* and a platelet *(P)* on a canine blood smear.

Leptocytes

Also referred to as codocytes or target cells; cell has an increase in membrane surface relative to cell volume.

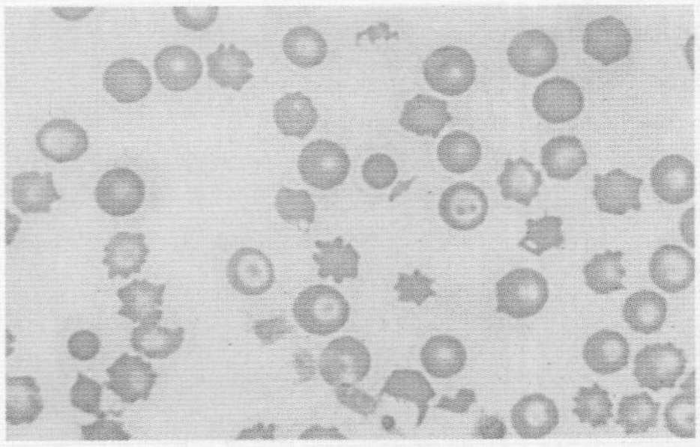

Schistocytes in a smear from a dog with iron deficiency. Target cells and red cells with other membrane abnormalities (keratocytes) are also present. (Courtesy Dr. Mary Anna Thrall.)

Morphologic Variation in Color

Polychromasia

Cells that exhibit a bluish (basophilic) tint.

Hypochromasia

Cells with an increase in the area of central pallor.

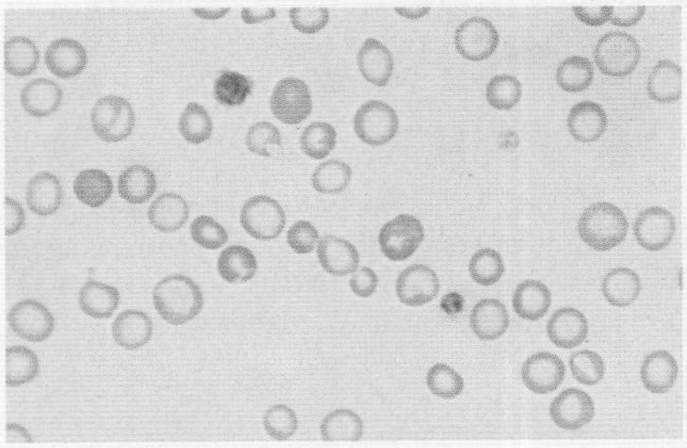

Hypochromasia in a smear from a dog with iron deficiency. Note the increased central pallor. Several polychromatophils are also present. (Courtesy Dr. Mary Anna Thrall.)

Hyperchromic or Hyperchromatophilic

Cells that appear darker than normal. These are often microcytic spherocytes.

Continued

BOX 7-3 Morphology of Erythrocytes—cont'd

Variation in Cell Behavior

Rouleaux

Cells appear to be stacked on top of one another. These cells are normal in equine blood. This variation is seen as an artifact if a sample is held too long before making the blood smear.

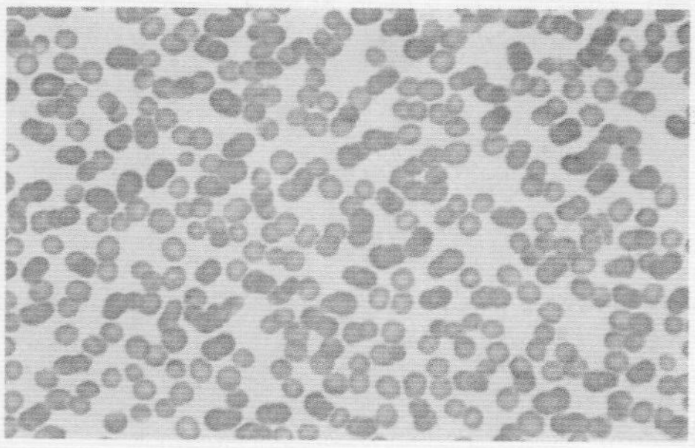

Normal equine red blood cells with rouleaux formation. (Courtesy Dr. E. Lassen.)

Autoagglutination

Three-dimensional clumps of cells. This variation is seen in immune-mediated hemolytic anemia.

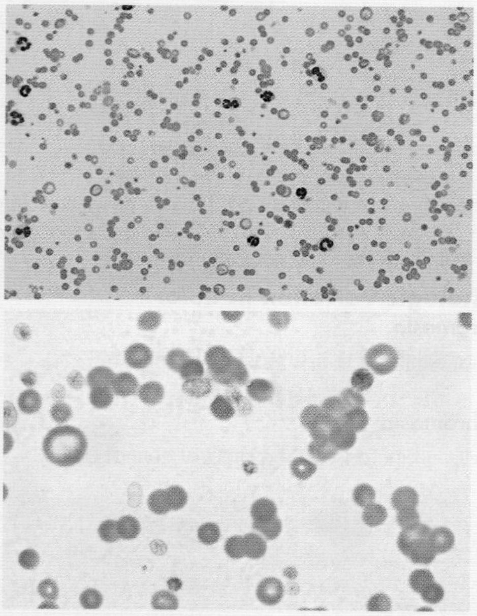

Low-power view *(top)*, high-power view *(bottom)* of agglutinated red blood cells in a smear from a dog with immune-mediated hemolytic anemia. (Courtesy Dr. Mary Anna Thrall.)

Inclusions and Other Abnormalities

Basophilic stippling

Characterized by bluish granular bodies on the surface of an RBC. This abnormality is seen in regenerative anemia in ruminants and is diagnostic for lead poisoning in small animals.

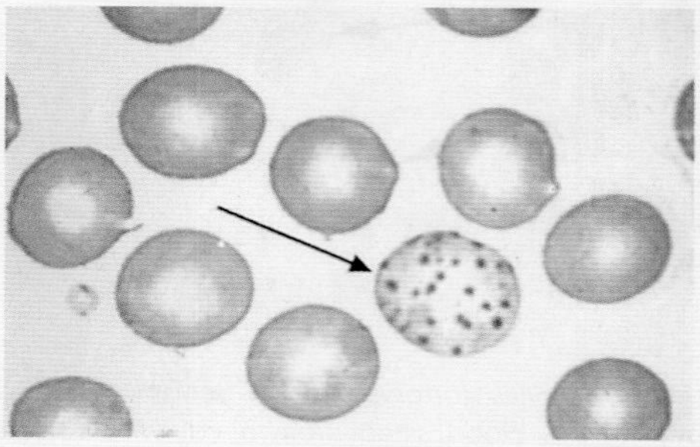

Howell-Jolly bodies and basophilic stippling in feline red blood cells. (Courtesy Dr. E. Lassen.)

Heinz bodies

Round structures within the cell that represent denatured hemoglobin. A small number may be normally present in feline.

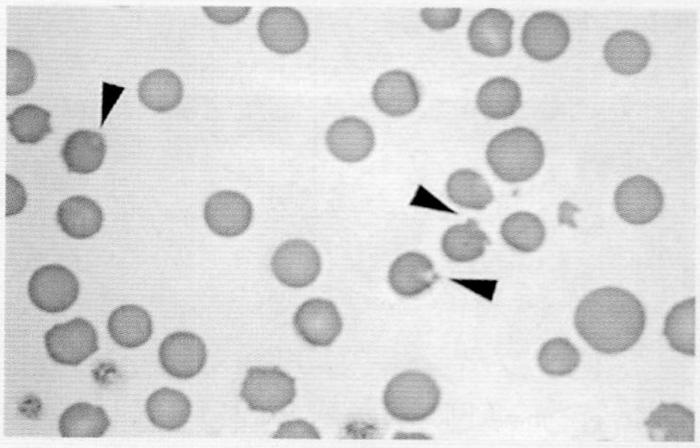

Heinz bodies *(arrowheads)* on a feline blood smear stained with Wright's stain.

BOX 7-3 Morphology of Erythrocytes—cont'd

Howell-Jolly bodies

Basophilic nuclear remnants in the RBC. This abnormality is common in feline regenerative anemias.

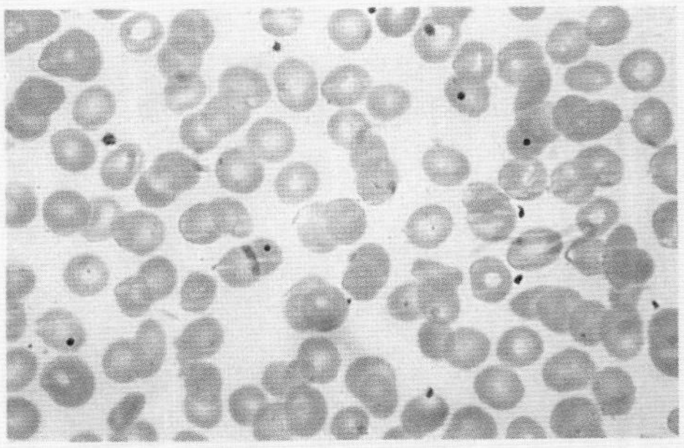

Howell-Jolly bodies on a canine blood smear.

Nucleated RBCs

Immature erythrocytes released from the bone marrow before extrusion of the nucleus. Seen in regenerative anemias, lead poisoning, extramedullary hematopoiesis, and bone marrow disease.

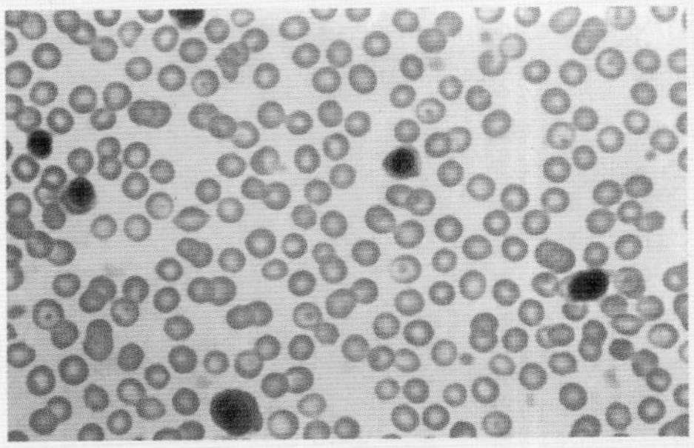

Nucleated red blood cells in a smear from a dog with lead poisoning. (Courtesy Dr. E. Lassen.)

Eosinophilic granules in horses are very large and round, and stain bright orange. The granules in swine and ruminants are uniformly small and round, and they stain pinkish-red. Increased eosinophil numbers (**eosinophilia**) may occur with parasitic disease or allergies.

BASOPHILS

Basophils have a lobulated nucleus and numerous dark purple (basophilic) granules in the cytoplasm. Canine basophils usually have few basophilic granules. They may occasionally be seen degranulated and appear as if vacuoles are present. Feline basophils have many round granules that stain lavender (grayish-purple). Equine and ruminant basophils are usually packed with granules and stain dark blue. Basophil numbers are often increased in allergies and some metabolic disorders and will be seen with an accompanying eosinophilia.

Box 7-5 contains a summary of morphologic characteristics of leukocytes.

VARIATIONS IN LEUKOCYTE MORPHOLOGY

Changes in the appearance of leukocytes generally occur as a result of disease processes that affect the appearance and/or function of the cell. These changes can also occur as normal reactions to a disease process and may be nonpathologic. Leukocyte changes may affect the cell nucleus, cytoplasm, or both. Additional abnormalities include the appearance of juvenile cells and parasites. The following sections contain terms used to describe variations in leukocytes on the blood smear. Box 7-6 contains a summary of common morphologic abnormalities in leukocytes.

PLATELETS

Platelets are sometimes referred to as **thrombocytes.** In mammals, they are derived from the bone marrow cell called a **megakaryocyte.** Mammalian platelets are fragments of the cytoplasm of this bone marrow cell. In other animal species, the platelets are actual cells with a different bone marrow precursor. Platelets function to provide an initiating coagulation factor. They are also capable of plugging small ruptures in small blood vessels.

PLATELET ASSESSMENT METHODS

A platelet estimate is performed by counting the number of platelets seen on the blood smear as averaged over 10 oil-immersion fields. The presence of an average of 8 to 12 platelets is reported as adequate. To get an indirect measure of platelet number, count the number of platelets seen per 100 white blood cells on the blood smear. This number is then used to calculate the platelet estimate using the following equation:

$$\text{Platelet Estimate} = \text{Avg. no. Platelets} \times 20,000/\text{mm}^3$$

TECHNICIAN NOTE To perform a platelet estimate, count the number of platelets seen on the blood smear in 10 oil-immersion fields.

Automated analyzers may also provide a platelet count. Morphologic changes in platelets include aggregation and giant platelets. These abnormalities will not be evident with automated analyzers and must therefore be detected using the blood smear.

BOX 7-4 Blood Parasites

Mycoplasma

Small, round, or rod-shaped structures that stain darkly with Wright or Romanowsky-type stain. They are often found as single organisms or pairs on the periphery of an RBC. They may also appear as chains or rings on an RBC.
Common parasite of feline RBCs; formerly referred to as *Hemobartonella* and the disease is commonly known as feline infectious anemia (FIA) or hemobartonellosis.

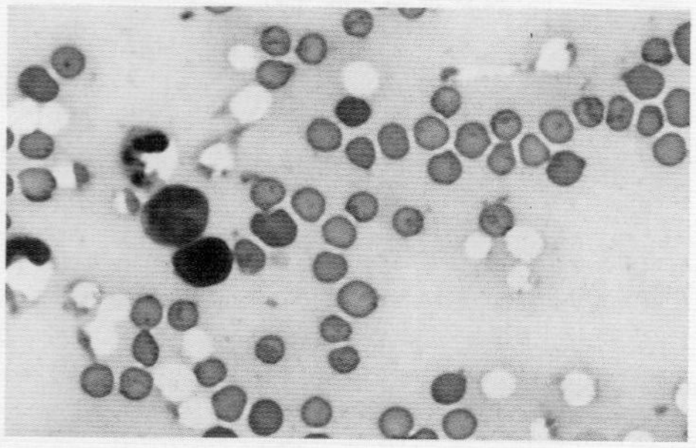

Mycoplasma felis in feline red blood cells (new methylene blue, counterstained with Wright stain). (Courtesy Dr. E. Lassen.)

Eperythrozoon

Rod and ring forms are found on the RBC surface. The ring form is the most common. Occurs in cattle, sheep, and swine.

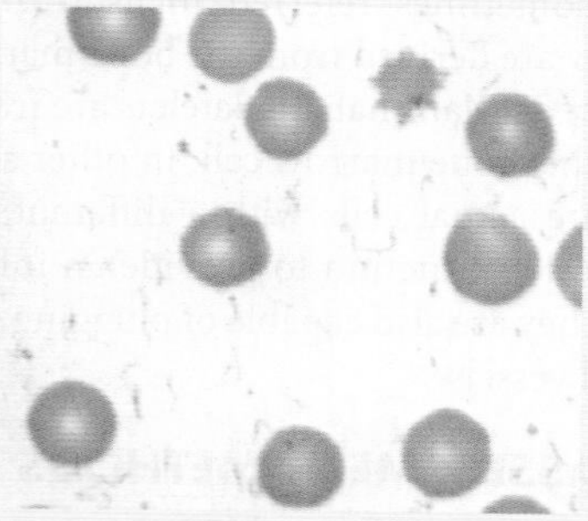

Eperythrozoon organisms in a blood smear of a heifer. (From Divers, TJ: *Rebhun's Diseases of Dairy Cattle*, ed 2, St Louis, 2007, Saunders.)

Cytauxzoon felis

An irregular ring form within RBCs.
Very rare parasite found in cats. Macrophages in the bone marrow may also contain the organism.

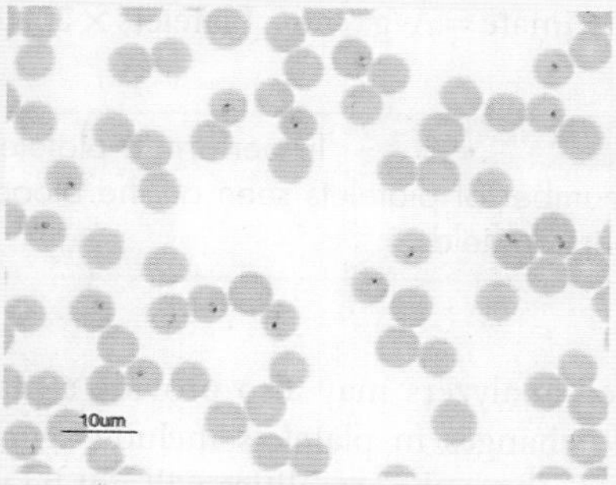

Ring form of *Cytauxzoon felis*. (From August JR: *Consultations in feline internal medicine*, vol 5, St Louis, 2007, Saunders.)

Babesia

Large, round, oval, or teardrop-shaped bodies. They can occur singly, in pairs, or in multiples of two. Infected RBCs are often seen at the feathered edge of a blood smear. Found in many species.

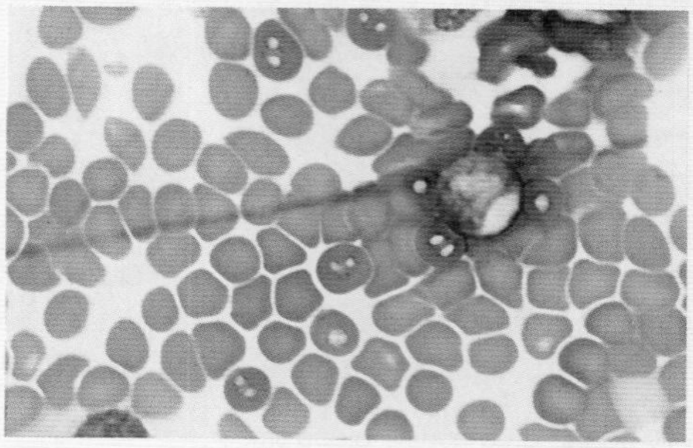

Babesia canis in a canine blood smear. (Courtesy Dr. Mary Anna Thrall.)

Dirofilaria immitis

Microfilariae of *Dirofilaria immitis* can sometimes be found near the feathered edge of a blood smear. A microfilaria is about the width of an RBC.

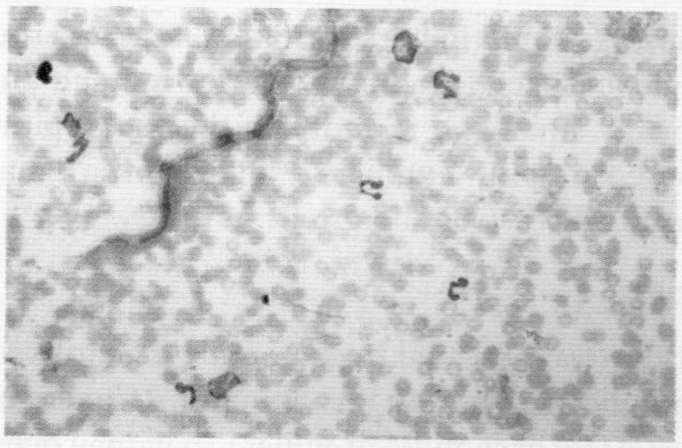

Microfilaria of *Dirofilaria immitis* in a canine blood smear.

Ehrlichia

Group of parasites containing a variety of species; some infect leukocytes, some infect platelets.

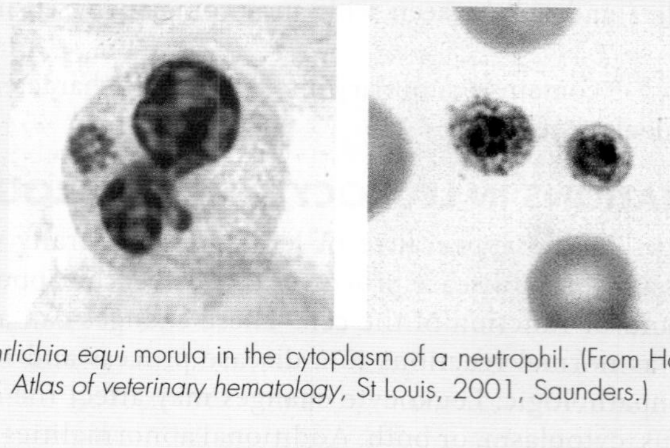

Ehrlichia equi morula in the cytoplasm of a neutrophil. (From Harvey JE: *Atlas of veterinary hematology*, St Louis, 2001, Saunders.)

BOX 7-5 Morphologic Characteristics of Leukocytes

Neutrophil

Phagocytosis and destruction of foreign agents and cellular debris

Irregular, dense nucleus segmented into three to five lobes

Colorless to pale pink cytoplasm

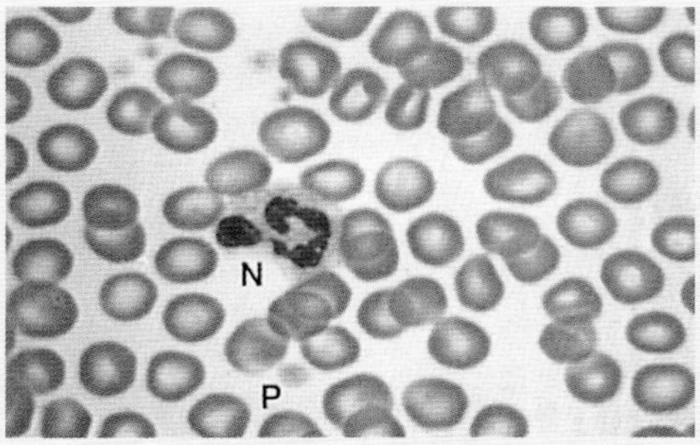

A canine neutrophil *(N)* and platelet *(P)* in a blood smear from a normal patient.

Eosinophil

Allergic reactions, phagocytosis

Lobulated nucleus and red-orange (eosinophilic) granules that vary in appearance in different species

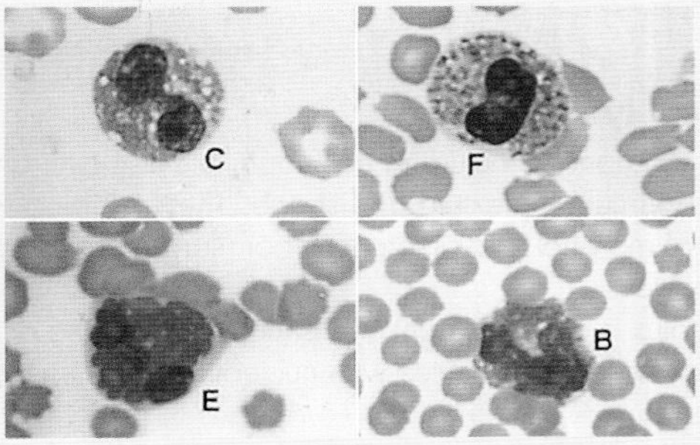

Canine *(C)*, feline *(F)*, equine *(E)*, and bovine *(B)* eosinophils demonstrating the variable size, shape, and color of granules in different species.

Basophil

Initiation and mediation of immune responses and hypersensitivity allergic reactions

May or may not contain blue-staining granules that are fairly homogeneous in appearance

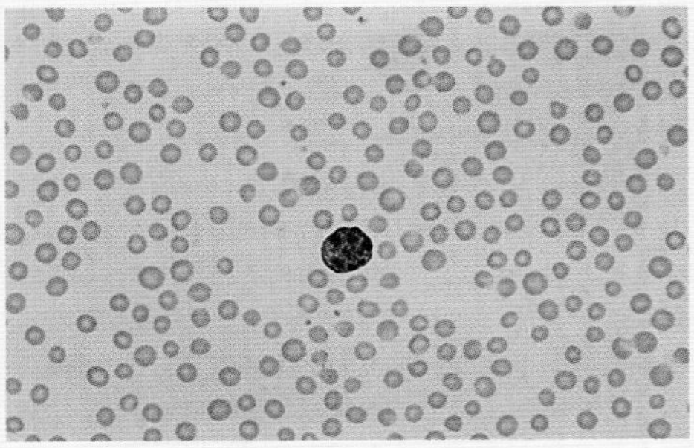

Basophil in a bovine blood smear. (Courtesy Dr. E. Lassen.)

Monocyte

Precursors to tissue macrophage; phagocytosis and processing of antigens

Amoeboid nucleus; few azurophilic granules

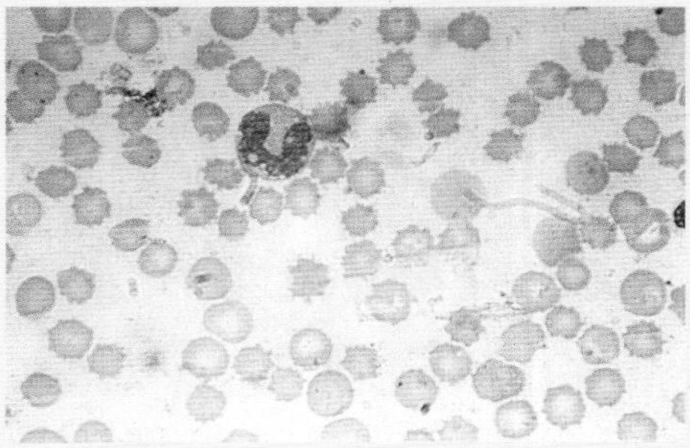

A normal canine monocyte showing the characteristic kidney bean–shaped nucleus and vacuoles.

Lymphocyte

Cytokine production and cell-mediated immune response; antibody production

Round to slightly indented nucleus that almost completely fills the cell. Light blue cytoplasm may contain a few purple granules. Vary in size: small, mature lymphocytes have scant cytoplasm. Large lymphocytes have larger nuclei and abundant cytoplasm.

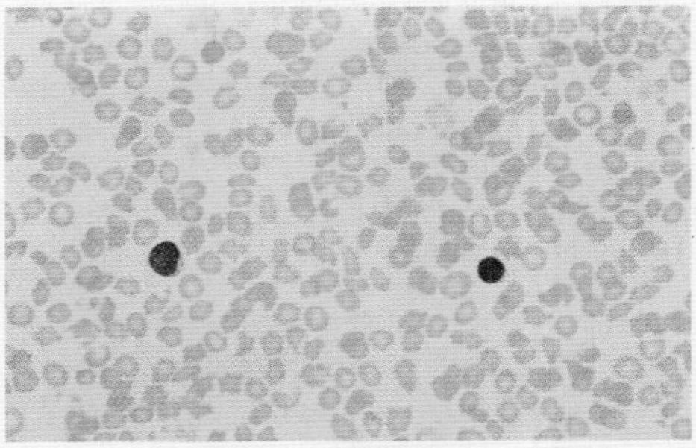

Lymphocytes in a feline blood smear. (Courtesy Dr. E. Lassen.)

BOX 7-6 Morphologic Variation in Leukocytes

Hypersegmentation

Neutrophil nucleus with more than five lobes
Associated with a variety of conditions including chronic infection, pernicious anemia, and steroid use

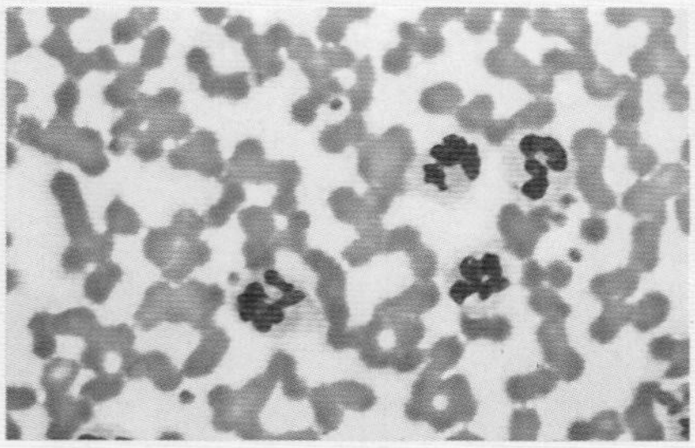

Nuclear hypersegmentation of canine neutrophils. (Courtesy Dr. E. Lassen.)

Karyorrhexis/Karyolysis

A cell containing a nucleus that is lysed, or damaged
In WBCs in peripheral circulation, this is an artifact caused by the use of inappropriate anticoagulants.

Pyknosis

A cell containing a nucleus that is condensed

Döhle bodies

Coarse, irregular, gray to blue cytoplasmic inclusions representing ribosomal material. They often are seen in pairs near the periphery of the cell. When alone, they represent a mild toxic change. Feline neutrophils appear to easily form Döhle bodies.
This variation is common in feline and may be seen with chronic bacterial infection and some viral diseases.

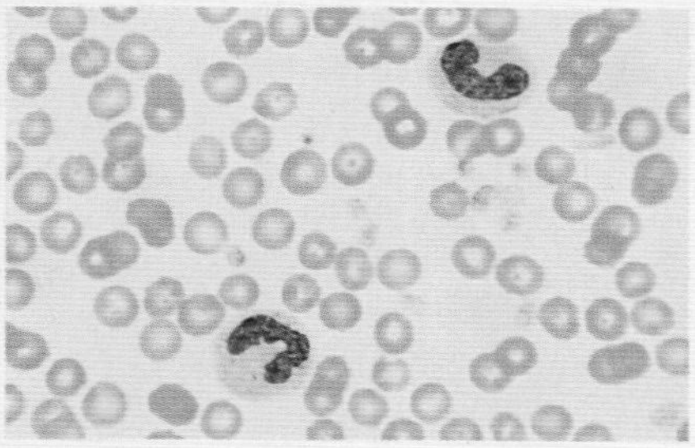

Toxic neutrophils containing Döhle bodies in a canine blood smear. (Courtesy Dr. Mary Anna Thrall.)

Toxic granulation

Appearance of numerous large, prominently stained granules that range in color from dark purple/red to black.
Seen in most infectious diseases. Toxic granulation may be described by number (few, moderate, many) or severity (slight, moderate, marked), as indicated in Table 7-5.
The overall toxicity is based on the most severe change observed. Toxic granulation is a moderate to severe toxic change. It is particularly evident in equine blood.

Myelocytes

Not usually found in peripheral blood unless severe inflammation or infection is present

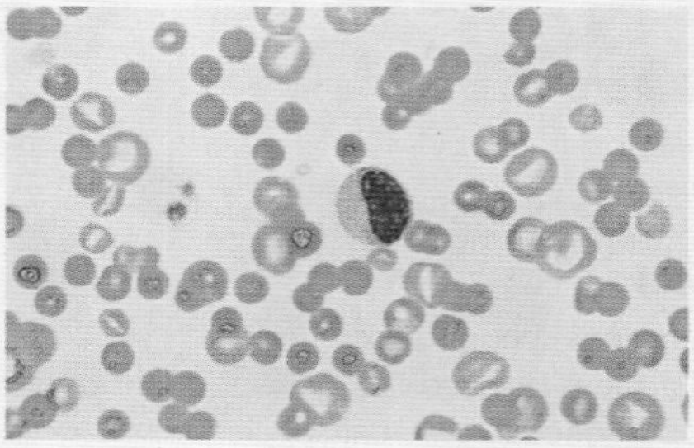

Myelocyte *(center)* in a canine blood smear. (Courtesy Dr. Mary Anna Thrall.)

Atypical lymphocytes

Variety of changes including eosinophilic cytoplasm and changes in nuclear texture and shape. They exhibit a wide variety of morphologic differences from large to classic small lymphocytes.
A nucleolus is a round, light-blue structure within the nucleus.
A few of these lymphocytes with nucleoli may be seen in sick animals.

BOX 7-6 Morphologic Variation in Leukocytes—cont'd

Reactive lymphocytes

Dark blue cytoplasm and a darker nucleus

Reactive lymphocytes (immunocytes) are lymphocytes with a very dense, eccentric, irregular nucleus. Their cytoplasm typically stains intensely royal blue and may have a pale Golgi zone. Reactive lymphocytes may be observed during periods of antigenic stimulation. They are occasionally present in normal animals; report them as a morphologic change only if more than 5% of lymphocytes are of this type. Reactive and atypical lymphocytes are counted along with the other lymphocytes in the differential count. They may be quantified as few—5% to 10% of lymphocytes, moderate—11% to 30%, and many—more than 30%.

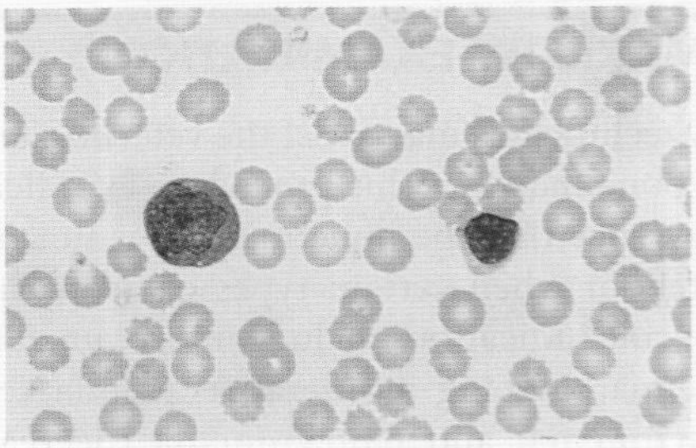

Reactive lymphocyte *(left)* and normal lymphocyte *(right)* in a canine blood smear. (Courtesy Dr. Mary Anna Thrall.)

Lymphoblasts

Large, immature lymphocytes that contain a nucleolus. Large numbers of circulating lymphoblasts suggest a neoplastic disease of lymphocytes (lymphoproliferative disorders). Extreme lymphocytosis (more than 20,000/μl) may be present in these cases.

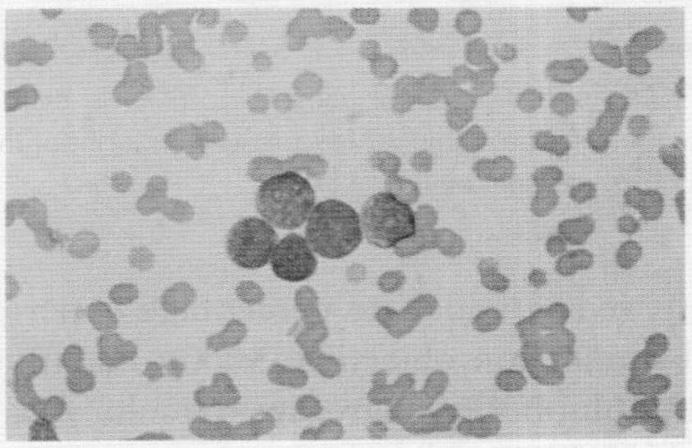

Atypical lymphocytes (lymphoblasts) in a feline blood smear. (Courtesy Dr. E. Lassen.)

Basket cell

Degenerative WBCs that have ruptured. Pale-staining, amorphous bodies of stain.

Also referred to as smudge cells. These may be an artifact if blood is held too long before making the smear. Basket cells are also associated with leukemia. A few smudge cells may be expected; large numbers may indicate excessive cell fragility, which is common in very sick animals.

RETICULOCYTE COUNTS

The presence of increased numbers of basophilic macrocytic cells on a blood smear usually indicates an increase in the number of circulating reticulocytes. Although reticulocytes are capable of completing maturation in the peripheral blood, their oxygen-carrying capacity is less than a mature erythrocyte. An increase in the number of circulating reticulocytes is an indication of regenerative anemia. Reticulocyte counts can be performed using a blood smear stained with a vital stain such as new methylene blue. Vital stain allows for visualization of the intracellular structures found in reticulocytes, specifically iron not yet incorporated into hemoglobin as well as fragments of cellular organelles. Reticulocytes are immature RBCs that contain ribonucleic acid (RNA) that is lost as the cell matures. Reticulocyte numbers increase when the bone marrow is responding to an anemic state. When reticulocytes are stained with a vital stain, such as new methylene blue, their RNA is visible as blue granules or aggregates. These cells correspond to the larger, blue-gray polychromatic RBCs seen in Wright-stained smears.

TECHNICIAN NOTE Cats have both a punctate and an aggregate form of reticulocyte.

Cats have two types of reticulocytes. The aggregate type (0%–0.4% in normal cats) is similar to those found in other species and is the type that is counted in all species (Fig. 7-15). The punctate type has a few small, blue-stained granules (not aggregates). This type of reticulocyte may compose up to 10% of RBCs in healthy animals. Their numbers are increased in regenerative anemia; thus, both types can be reported, though the younger aggregate forms are the only reticulocytes typically recorded.

Reticulocytes do not occur in horses, even with regenerative anemia. They are not found in healthy ruminants but do increase in responding anemias. Reticulocytes are common in healthy suckling pigs. Less than 1% of the RBCs in adult pigs are reticulocytes; reticulocyte numbers increase in regenerative anemias of pigs.

To make a blood smear to examine for reticulocytes, mix a few drops of blood with an equal amount of new methylene blue stain in a test tube and allow it to stand for at least 15 minutes. Make a wedge-type smear with the mixture and allow it to air-dry. Some prefer to counterstain this slide with Wright or Romanowsky-type stain. This will result in a staining pattern in which the RBCs will appear reddish and the aggregate granules prominent blue, making the reticulocytes easier to count as well as being a permanent stain. Counting the reticulocytes allows evaluation of the degree of bone marrow response when anemia is present.

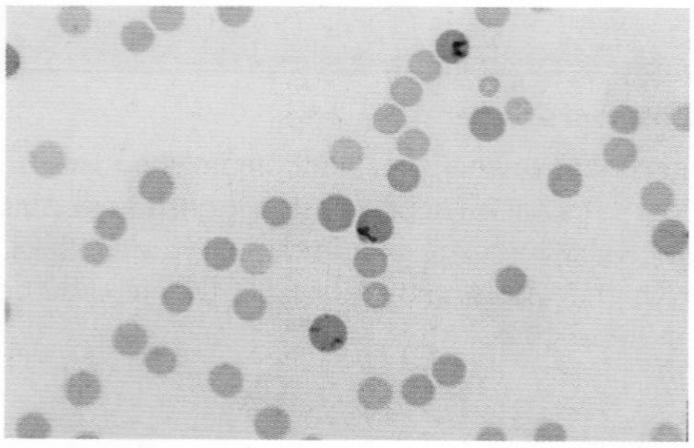

FIGURE 7-15 In this smear of feline blood, three aggregate reticulocytes are evident in the center. Also present throughout the smear are punctate reticulocytes (brilliant cresyl blue).

The observed reticulocyte percentage is performed using the oil-immersion objective (1000× magnification) by counting the number of aggregate reticulocytes among an estimated 1000 RBCs. The observed percentage can easily be calculated by dividing by 10 the number of reticulocytes counted per 1000 RBCs. The observed reticulocyte count is only a relative number and should then be corrected for the degree of anemia. If no RBC value is available the Corrected Reticulocyte Percentage (CRP) should be used. If an RBC count is available, the Absolute Reticulocyte Count is a more accurate number and should be calculated instead.

A CRP is calculated by multiplying the observed percentage by the patient's PCV and dividing by the normal mean PCV (45% in the dog, 37% in the cat). A CRP value above 1% in dogs and above 0.4% in cats indicates a regenerative response to anemia.

If a total RBC count has been performed, you can calculate an absolute reticulocyte count by multiplying the observed reticulocyte percentage by the RBC count. This gives the number of reticulocytes per microliter (μl) of blood. In most animals (except horses), an absolute reticulocyte count above 80,000/μl indicates a regenerative response to anemia. A delay of as much as 4 days is common before significant reticulocytosis is seen.

$$\text{Observed Reticulocyte percentage} = \frac{\text{Observed Retic \#}}{1000} \times 1000\,\%$$

$$\text{Corrected Reticulocyte Percent} = \frac{\text{Observed Retic }\%}{\text{Normal Mean PCV}} \times \text{Patient PCV}$$

$$\text{Absolute Reticulocyte Count} = \text{Observed Retic Percentage} \times \#\text{ of RBCs}$$

For a canine patient, given the values:

- 27 reticulocytes counted
- RBC value = 3.2×10^6

Each formula is calculated as follows:

$$\frac{27}{1000} \times 100\,\% = 2.7\,\% \text{ Observed Reticulocyte Percentage}$$

$$\frac{27}{45\ \%} \times 21\,\% = 1.26\,\% \text{ Corrected Reticulocyte Percentage}$$

$$2.7\,\% \times \left(3.2 \times 10^6/\text{mm}^3\right) = 86,400/\text{mm}^3 \text{ Absolute Reticulocyte Count}$$

ERYTHROCYTE SEDIMENTATION RATE

Erythrocyte sedimentation rate (ESR) is occasionally performed in veterinary medicine. The ESR is a measure of the rate that red blood cells fall in their own plasma under controlled conditions. This rate is affected by a number of factors including membrane defects. Because the total number of RBCs affects the ESR, the observed ESR must be corrected for the PCV. This is accomplished by subtracting the observed ESR from the ESR that would be expected from a normal animal of the same species. For example, a canine with a PCV of 45% would be expected to have an ESR of 5 mm. If the observed ESR is 12 mm, the corrected ESR would be reported as +7 mm.

BONE MARROW EXAMINATION

Veterinary technicians may assist the veterinarian in examination of bone marrow. This procedure is indicated when there is evidence that the bone marrow is not responding appropriately or when certain types of neoplasia are suspected. Specific indications include unexplained nonregenerative anemia, ongoing regenerative anemia, leukopenia, **thrombocytopenia**, and **pancytopenia** (decreased numbers of all cell lines). Bone marrow evaluation is also used to confirm certain infections (e.g., ehrlichiosis) and diagnose hematopoietic neoplasms (e.g., lymphoproliferative disorders).

In small animals bone marrow is aspirated under general anesthesia or using local anesthesia. Local anesthesia is preferred for large animals. It is crucial to follow aseptic technique throughout the procedure. The proximal end of the femur, the craniolateral portion of the humerus, and the iliac crest are common sites of bone marrow aspiration in dogs and cats. The sternum, ribs, and iliac crest are often used in large animals. Special bone marrow needles are preferred, although an 18-gauge needle may be used in cats with thin bones. Bone marrow needles have a stylet to prevent occlusion of the needle with bone and surrounding tissue as it is inserted into the marrow cavity. A syringe is used to aspirate a few drops of bone marrow, filling the hub of the needle. The needle is removed from the bone and the contents immediately used to make slides. Alternatively, the marrow may be mixed with EDTA so smears can be made a short time later or if more time is needed to obtain additional samples.

Bone marrow is thicker than blood and contains particles or spicules. Blood contamination can be minimized by vertically positioning the slide to drain off excess blood before making the smear. Marrow smears can be made in various ways. A preferred method is to place the anticoagulated aspirate in a Petri dish. Then, using a microhematocrit tube, tilt the dish, pick the marrow particles from draining blood using capillary action, and transfer them to make a coverslip smear. Another method is to expel a drop of aspirate (particularly if no anticoagulant is used) directly on a clean slide, which is placed at a 45- to 70-degree tilt to allow the contaminant blood to run off. A compression smear is then made from this residual sample by placing a second clean slide perpendicular to the first one at the top of the slide where the spicules are located. Allow the aspirate to spread then gently pull the top slide horizontally, without exerting any pressure on the slide. (See Chapter 9 for more details on cytology preparations.) With either method, the slide or coverslip is air dried and stained as described previously. You may then examine smears or send them to a commercial laboratory for analysis.

To examine the stained smears, use low-power (100×) to evaluate overall cellularity and megakaryocyte number. In adult animals, cellularity is normal if the particles are composed of about 50% nucleated cells and 50% fat. Describe the marrow as hypercellular or hypocellular, based on the proportion of cells present. There should be 2 to 3 megakaryocytes per low-power field.

At higher magnification, examine erythroid and myeloid cells. Rubricytes and metarubricytes should make up 90% of the nucleated erythroid cells. Metamyelocytes, bands, and segmented myeloid cells should make up 90% of the myeloid cells. Determine the ratio of myeloid to erythroid cells (**M:E ratio**) by counting 500 nucleated cells and classifying them as erythroid or myeloid. Normal M:E ratios should be between 0.75:1.0 and 2.0:1.0. Neoplasia is a possibility if all the cells look alike. Bone marrow status should never be evaluated without the results of a concurrent peripheral hemogram. If histologic examination of marrow is required, a core biopsy can be obtained using a Jamshidi bone marrow needle.

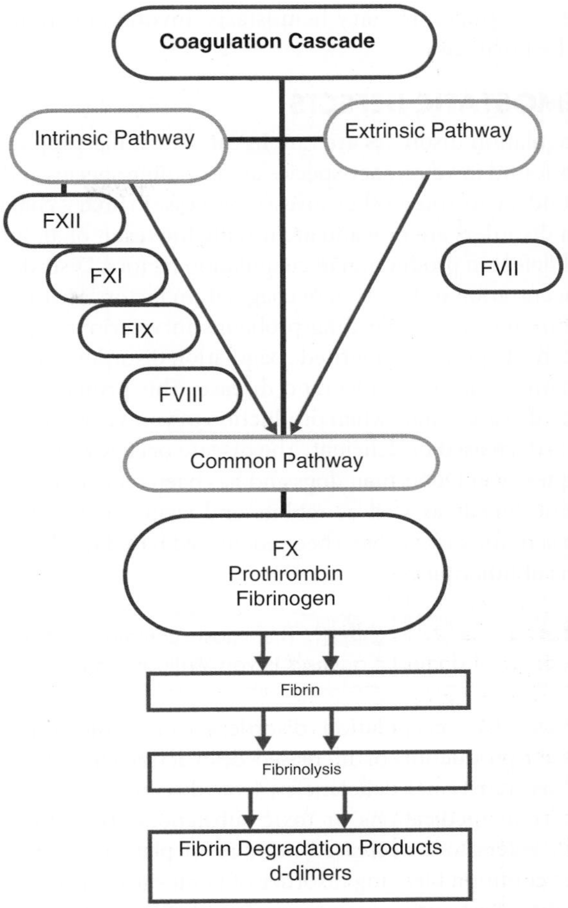

FIGURE 7-16 A summary of the blood coagulation process.

HEMOSTASIS

OVERVIEW OF HEMOSTASIS

Hemostasis refers to the ability of the body systems to maintain the integrity of the blood and blood vessels and is a complex interaction among blood vessel walls, platelets, and coagulation factors.

Primary hemostasis can be initiated when a blood vessel is ruptured or torn or when any tissue is damaged and tissue factor is released. Exposed blood vessel endothelium is a charged surface and platelets are attracted to this surface. As platelets congregate at the site, they undergo morphologic and physiologic changes. These changes cause the platelets to adhere to each other as well as the blood vessel. This also causes platelets to release small vesicles, known as microparticles, from their surface. The surface of the platelets and microparticles contain a coagulation factor (phosphatidylserine) that aids in activation of secondary hemostasis. Secondary hemostasis is a complex series of reactions known as the coagulation cascade. Platelet surfaces and the surface of microvesicles (which are also released from leukocytes and endothelial cells) serve as binding sites for coagulation factors. Many of the components of the secondary systems also serve to recruit and activate additional platelets. Figure 7-16 provides an overview of hemostasis. Table 7-7 lists the coagulation factors and their common synonyms. The coagulation factor complexes amplify the coagulation cascade and generate large amounts of thrombin, which converts fibrinogen to fibrin. Each factor participates in a chemical reaction that serves to initiate the next reaction in the pathway. The coagulation pathways do not operate as independent and redundant pathways. Platelets are essential for secondary hemostasis and thrombin generated by the coagulation cascade recruits and activates additional platelets and inhibits fibrinolysis. The end result of the coagulation cascade is the formation of a mesh of fibrin strands that forms the clot.

TABLE 7-7 Blood Coagulation Factors

DESIGNATION	SYNONYM
Factor I	Fibrinogen
Factor II	Prothrombin
Factor III	Tissue thromboplastin
Factor IV	Calcium
Factor V	Proaccelerin
Factor VII	Proconvertin
Factor VIII	Antihemophilic factor
Factor IX	Christmas factor, Plasma thromboplastin
Factor X	Stuart-Prower factor
Factor XI	Plasma thromboplastin antecedent
Factor XII	Hageman factor
Factor XIII	Fibrin-stabilizing factor

The final phase, tertiary hemostasis, involves degradation of the fibrin clot.

HEMOSTATIC DEFECTS

Coagulation disorders are rare in cats. Most bleeding disorders found in veterinary species are in canine species and are secondary to some other disease process. Primary coagulation disorders are rare and are usually the result of an inherited defect in production of coagulation factors. Disorders in concentration or function of coagulation factors are the least common cause of bleeding problems in veterinary species. The most common inherited coagulation disorder of domestic animals is von Willebrand disease. This primary hemostatic disease results when production of von Willebrand factor is decreased or deficient. The disease occurs with relative frequency in Doberman dogs and has been reported in other canine breeds as well as rabbits and swine. Three distinct forms of the disease have been identified based on their patterns of inheritance.

> TECHNICIAN NOTE The most common inherited disorder of domestic animals is von Willebrand disease.

Secondary coagulation disorders can result from decreased production or increased destruction of platelets as well as nutritional deficiencies, liver disease, and ingestion of certain medications or toxic substances. Thrombocytopenia refers to a decreased number of platelets and is the most common bleeding disorder of hemostasis in veterinary patients. This can occur as a result of bone marrow depression that reduces the production of platelets, or autoimmune disease that increases the rate of platelet destruction. A large number of infectious agents, such as *Ehrlichia*, *Dirofilaria*, and parvovirus, can also affect thrombocyte production and destruction. Because the liver is the site of production of most coagulation factors, any condition that affects liver function can result in a coagulation disorder. Ingestion of toxic substances such as warfarin can also create bleeding disorders. Warfarin is a common component of rodenticides and acts to inhibit vitamin K function. Because vitamin K is required for synthesis of coagulation factors II, VII, IX, and X, ingestion of warfarin can create a deficiency in several necessary components of the coagulation cascade. Ingestion of medications such as aspirin can also cause bleeding disorders.

DISSEMINATED INTRAVASCULAR COAGULATION

Although not a disease entity on its own, disseminated intravascular coagulation (**DIC**) is associated with many pathologic conditions. **DIC** is often seen in trauma cases as well as in a large number of infectious diseases. A large number of events can trigger DIC. The resulting hemostatic disorder may manifest as systemic hemorrhage or microvascular thrombosis. Because the triggering event and the resulting disorder are diverse, the laboratory findings are highly variable. Most patients with DIC have alterations in three or more coagulation tests, including prolonged partial thromboplastin time (APTT) and elevated fibrinogen, as well as significant thrombocytopenia. **Schistocytes** may be seen on the blood smear on DIC patients because of the intravascular destruction of erythrocytes.

> TECHNICIAN NOTE Schistocytes are a common finding on the blood smear in patients with DIC.

Clinical presentation of patients with bleeding disorders include petechia (pinpoint hemorrhage), ecchymoses (superficial hemorrhage of about 1 cm in diameter), purpura (bruising), epistaxis (bleeding from the nares), and prolonged bleeding following trauma or surgery. Patients may exhibit hematuria as a result of bleeding into the urinary bladder, melena as a result of bleeding into the digestive tract, or bleeding into joint cavities.

ASSESSMENT OF COAGULATION AND HEMOSTASIS

Coagulation tests may be appropriate if a bleeding disorder is suspected or as part of a presurgical screening protocol. Coagulation tests are designed to evaluate specific portions of the hemostatic mechanisms. Some tests measure just the mechanical phase (primary hemostasis) of hemostasis. Others can measure specific parts of the chemical phase (secondary hemostasis). All patients should be evaluated for coagulation defects before undergoing surgery. Most coagulation tests can be completed with minimal time and equipment and are relatively inexpensive. Samples for coagulation testing are plasma collected into an appropriate anticoagulant. Tests to determine the concentration and/or function of specific coagulation factors are not routinely performed in veterinary practice.

PRIMARY HEMOSTATIC TESTS

PLATELET COUNTS AND ESTIMATES

Platelet counts are part of all coagulation profiles as well as evaluating the blood smear for platelet morphology and clumping. A platelet estimate is performed by counting the number of platelets seen on the blood smear as averaged over 10 oil-immersion fields and multiplied by 20,000/mm^3. Most automated analyzers provide a platelet count. However, platelet clumping and the presence of giant platelets are fairly common in veterinary species and may lead to inaccurate results. It is important to confirm platelet counts by evaluating a blood smear.

> TECHNICIAN NOTE Always confirm platelet counts by viewing a blood smear.

BUCCAL MUCOSAL BLEEDING TIME

This is a primary assay for the detection of abnormalities in platelet function. The test requires a Simplate I or II spring-loaded lancet, blotting paper or #1 Whatman filter paper, a stopwatch, and a tourniquet. The patient should be anesthetized and placed in lateral recumbency. A strip of gauze

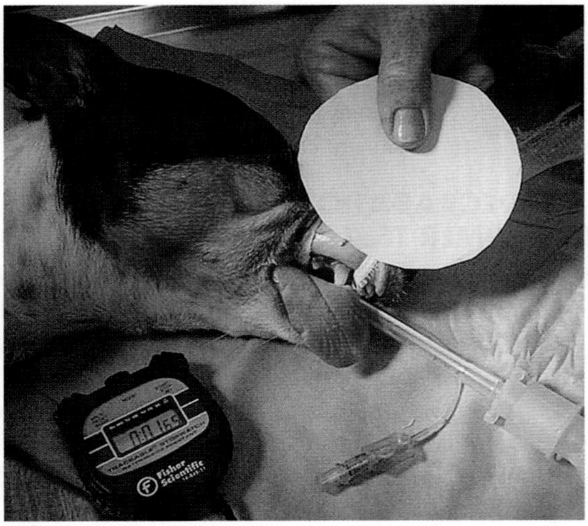

FIGURE 7-17 The buccal mucosa bleeding time test.

is used to tie the upper lip back in order to expose the mucosal surface. A 1-mm-deep incision is made using the Simplate device (Fig. 7-17) and a timer started. Standard blotting paper or #1 Whatman filter paper is used to wick the blood from the area around the incision site. This is performed by lightly touching the paper to the drop of blood, allowing it to absorb, and is repeated every 5 seconds until bleeding has stopped. A prolonged bleeding time (>4-5 minutes) occurs with most platelet dysfunction syndromes. It will also be prolonged in thrombocytopenia so a platelet count must also be performed.

SECONDARY HEMOSTATIC TESTS

ACTIVATED CLOTTING TIME

This test can evaluate every clinically significant clotting factor except Factor VII. Activated clotting time (ACT) is not as sensitive as PTT. Alterations in test results are not generally seen until patient values for coagulation factors are reduced by 90%.

The ACT test uses a preincubated tube that contains a diatomaceous earth material. A clean venipuncture is performed, and 2 ml of blood is collected in the tube. A timer is started as soon as the blood enters the tube. The tube is gently mixed three times and placed in a 37° C incubator or water bath. The tube is observed at 60 seconds and then at 5-second intervals for presence of a clot. The diatomaceous earth tubes are not as widely available as they once were because many practices now use automated coagulation analyzers. Normal references will vary, though they are approximately greater than 120 seconds for dogs and greater than 90 seconds for cats. A 25% increase in time is considered significant.

PROTHROMBIN TIME TEST

The prothrombin time (PT) test is usually performed with automated analyzers (Fig. 7-18). This test evaluates the extrinsic coagulation pathway. Most analyzers require a citrated plasma sample to which tissue thromboplastin reagent is added. A reagent designed to recalcify the sample is then added. Under normal conditions, a clot should form within

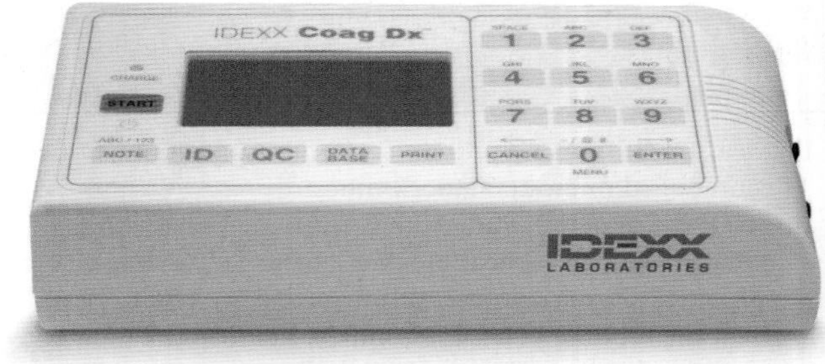

FIGURE 7-18 The Coagulation DX Analyzer provides measurements of prothrombin time and activated partial thromboplastin time.

6 to 20 seconds. Some automated analyzers are available that can use whole-blood samples and provide a rapid and accurate prothrombin time test.

ACTIVATED PARTIAL THROMBOPLASTIN TIME TEST

The activated partial thromboplastin time (APTT) test requires an automated coagulation analyzer. The test evaluates the secondary hemostatic pathways. Older instruments used for these tests were generally not practical for use in veterinary clinics. Several reagents were required, and the tests were difficult to perform accurately. New analyzers for APTT testing are now available that can use whole blood or plasma samples (collected in citrate anticoagulant tubes) and have no requirement for external reagent. The tests are simple, rapid, and provide an accurate evaluation of APTT. APTT increases can occur when any of the coagulation factors are reduced to 30% of normal.

FIBRINOGEN DETERMINATION

Fibrinogen is a protein produced by the liver and is involved in blood coagulation. Fibrinogen synthesis increases when inflammation is present. This is especially apparent in large animals, making fibrinogen a useful indicator of inflammation in large animals. Automated analysis of fibrinogen is complicated and not routinely available for use on in-house laboratory analyzers. One manual method that may be used for fibrinogen determination involves the use of two hematocrit tubes (Procedure 7-5). The tubes are centrifuged as for a PCV, and the total solids determined on one tube with a refractometer. The second tube is then incubated at 58° C for 3 minutes. The second tube is recentrifuged, and the total solids are measured. This test is based on the idea that fibrinogen becomes denatured and precipitates out of plasma heated to 56 to 58° C. This test is rapid and provides a reasonable approximation of plasma fibrinogen levels. Because only a small amount of fibrinogen is normally present in serum, it is more reliable to detect increased levels than decreased levels in plasma.

Normal plasma fibrinogen concentrations are 100 to 700 mg/dl, depending on the species. Severe inflammation cause increases above this value. This test is usually reserved for large animals because increases are a consistent finding in these species. Serial sampling is of value in these situations to find a decrease or increase over a time period.

PROCEDURE 7-5 Plasma Fibrinogen Procedure

1. Measure the plasma protein concentration on one of two centrifuged microhematocrit tubes.
2. Insert the remaining tube into a warm-water bath or an incubated sand-filled heat block at 56° to 58° C. Make sure the entire plasma column is immersed in the water or sand.
3. Heat the tube for at least 3 minutes. Remove the tube and examine the plasma layer for turbidity.
4. Recentrifuge to concentrate the fibrinogen in the top portion of the buffy coat.
5. Carefully break the tube at the plasma/fibrinogen interface and measure the plasma protein concentration. Subtract the second value from the first. The difference is the fibrinogen concentration. This value is measured as g/dl but may also be reported as mg/dl. (To convert from g/dl to mg/dl, move the decimal point three places to the right.)

PIVKA TEST

PIVKA is an acronym that refers to proteins induced (or invoked) by vitamin K absence. Recall that vitamin K is required to activate coagulation factors II, VII, IX, and X. When vitamin K is deficient, the concentration of the precursor proteins of those coagulation factors builds up and can be detected by the PIVKA. The test can be used to differentiate rodenticide toxicity from primary hemophilia when ACT is prolonged. It is more sensitive than PT when there is a depletion of these factors. The APTT test usually does not prolong until 48 hours after exposure. The PIVKA test usually becomes prolonged within 6 hours following ingestion of an anticoagulant rodenticide.

FIBRIN DEGRADATION PRODUCTS AND D-DIMER TESTS

Both of these tests are used to evaluate thrombus formation and fibrinolysis. D-dimers and fibrin degradation products (FDPs) are formed when the protein plasmin acts on fibrin or fibrinogen to dissolve a clot. The clot is broken down into several fragments, some of which can be detected with the FDP test. An increase in the presence of FDPs indicates active fibrinolysis. D-dimers are a type of FDP resulting from the degradation of cross-linked fibrin strands in the clot. This is a common finding in DIC. These tests are therefore useful in identifying the presence of DIC and will also provide diagnostic information in cases of thrombosis, liver failure, trauma, and hemangiosarcoma.

The FDP test requires some special instrumentation but is rapid and easy to perform. Several rapid in-house test kits are now available for detecting canine D-dimers. The kits differ significantly in test principle. They may be based on immunochromatography, latex agglutination, or immunoturbidometric analysis.

REVIEW QUESTIONS

Matching

Match the following cells with their functions.

____**1.** neutrophil
____**2.** eosinophil
____**3.** basophil
____**4.** monocyte
____**5.** lymphocyte

A. allergic reactions, phagocytosis
B. precursors to tissue macrophage; phagocytosis and processing of antigens
C. phagocytosis and destruction of foreign agents and cellular debris
D. cytokine production and cell-mediated immune response; antibody production
E. initiation and mediation of immune responses and hypersensitivity allergic reactions

Choose the Best Response

Choose the best answer to the following questions.

1. The Vacutainer most suitable for collection of blood for hematology is the:
a. red-top
b. purple- or lavender-top
c. green-top
d. blue-top

2. Which of the following causes a false decrease in PCV?
a. shortened centrifuge time
b. icterus
c. low blood-to-anticoagulant ratio
d. clots in the blood sample

3. The normal PCV in dogs is about:
a. 45%
b. 35%
c. 38%
d. 52%

4. Normal plasma protein values are in the range of:
a. 6 to 8 g/dl
b. 5.5 to 7.0 mg/dl
c. 4 to 6 mg/dl
d. 8 to 10 mg/dl

5. When making a blood smear with a sample that is very thick and contains some small clots, you should:
a. increase the spreader slide angle to about 45°
b. decrease the spreader slide angle to about 20°
c. dilute the sample 2:1 with EDTA
d. make the smear from a fresh sample

6. Lead poisoning can cause:
a. basophilic stippling
b. spherocytosis
c. echinocytosis
d. anisocytosis

For the next five questions, select the correct answer from the four options below:

a. Howell-Jolly bodies
b. Heinz bodies
c. rouleaux
d. agglutination

7. Which abnormality is characterized by grapelike clusters of RBCs that do not break up when the sample is diluted with saline?
8. Which RBC abnormality is often seen in healthy horses?
9. Pale or bluish, round areas attached to the RBC membrane, caused by chemical- or drug-induced oxidative injury, are called _____________.
10. Which RBC abnormality is characterized by coinlike stacks of RBCs?
11. Round, basophilic nuclear remnants in the RBCs of animals with regenerative anemia are called ________.
12. When the WBC differential is described as having a left shift, it means there is:
    a. a marked decrease in the number of neutrophils
    b. a shift in the neutrophil-lymphocyte ratio (N:L) in favor of neutrophils
    c. an increase in the number of immature (band) neutrophils
    d. an increase in the number of **hypersegmented,** or old neutrophils
13. Corticosteroids, stress, and excitement can each cause:
    a. neutrophilia
    b. neutropenia
    c. eosinophilia
    d. a left shift
14. Which of the following is a toxic change observed in neutrophils?
    a. Döhle bodies
    b. Howell-Jolly bodies
    c. Heinz bodies
    d. nuclear pyknosis
15. Which test of the coagulation system requires a blood tube containing diatomaceous earth?
    a. activated clotting time
    b. bleeding time
    c. whole blood clotting time
    d. one-stage prothrombin time

RECOMMENDED READING

Cowell RL: *Diagnostic cytology and hematology of the dog and cat*, ed 3, St Louis, 2007, Mosby.

Meyer D: *Veterinary laboratory medicine: interpretation and diagnosis*, ed 3, St Louis, 2006, Saunders.

Sirois M: *Laboratory procedures for veterinary technicians*, ed 6, St Louis, 2014, Mosby.

Sodikoff CH: *Laboratory profiles of small animal disease*, ed 3, St Louis, 2001, Mosby.

Willard MD: *Small animal clinical diagnosis by laboratory methods*, ed 5, St Louis, 2013, Saunders.

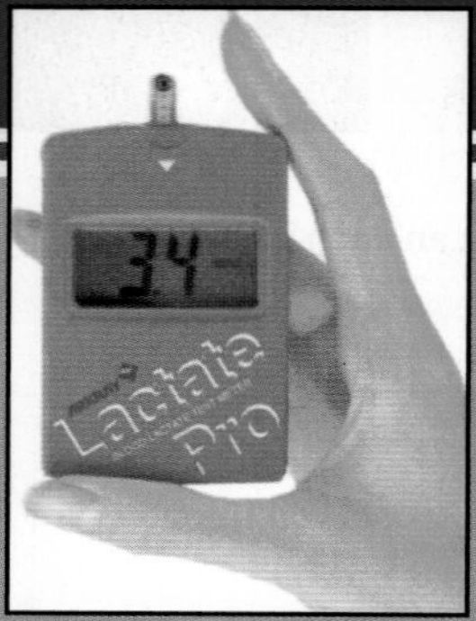

8 Clinical Chemistry and Serology

OUTLINE

LEARNING OBJECTIVES

After reviewing this chapter, the reader will be able to:

1. Describe methods used to collect samples of blood for laboratory examination.
2. Discuss ways in which diagnostic samples are prepared for laboratory examination.
3. Differentiate between serum and plasma.
4. List and describe equipment needed for clinical chemistry and serology testing.
5. State the advantages, disadvantages, and limitations of various models of clinical chemistry analyzers.
6. Describe the principles of operation of various chemistry and electrolyte analyzers.
7. List and describe the indications for and types of tests used in clinical chemistry testing.
8. List and describe the biochemical assays commonly performed to assess liver, kidney, and pancreatic function.
9. List the major intracellular and extracellular electrolytes and describe their roles in mammalian physiology.
10. Describe the roles of the white blood cells in the immune system.
11. List the types of immunologic tests and describe the test principles employed by those tests.
12. Discuss methods used to verify accuracy of laboratory test results.

KEY TERMS

Accuracy
Active immunity
Adaptive immunity
Agglutination
Albumin
Alkaline phosphatases
ALT
Amylase
Anion
Antigen
AST
Autoimmunity
Azotemia
Bile acids
Bilirubin
Cation
Cell-mediated immunity
Cholestasis
Cholesterol
Complement
Control
Coombs test
Creatinine
Electrolyte
ELISA
Fructosamine
Globulin
Glucose
Humoral immunity
Hypersensitivity
Immunodiffusion
Immunoglobulin

KEY TERMS—cont'd

Isoenzymes
Ketoacidosis
Kinetic assay
Lipase
Lipemia
Passive immunity
Polymerase chain reaction
Specificity
Spectrophotometers
Standard
Titer
Urea
Uric acid

Laboratory analysis of blood biochemical constituents is performed for a variety of reasons. A blood sample may be collected from a patient as part of a general wellness screening process, to confirm or rule out a specific disease, as part of management of a clinical case to evaluate the status of a previously diagnosed condition, or as part of emergency medical therapy. Biochemistry profiles, or groups of tests, are routinely performed using serum as the preferred sample type, although heparinized plasma may also be used on some analyzers. Determinations of levels of the various chemical constituents in blood can provide valuable diagnostic information. The chemicals being assayed are usually enzymes associated with particular organ functions or metabolites and metabolic by-products that are processed by certain organs. Serologic testing usually refers to immunodiagnostic testing. These tests are generally performed on the same type of sample as the blood chemistry profile.

TECHNICIAN NOTE Clinical chemistry testing usually requires either a serum or plasma sample.

SAMPLE COLLECTION

Unless the purpose of the test is to monitor therapy, always collect the blood sample before any treatment is given. Administration of certain medications and treatments often affects results of biochemical testing. Preprandial samples, or samples from an animal that has not eaten for 12 hours, are ideal. Postprandial samples, or samples collected after an animal has eaten, may produce erroneous results. For example, after meals, the blood glucose concentration frequently increases. Also, an increased BUN concentration may be present if the meal was high in protein. Increased amounts of lipid (lipemia) are usually present in postprandial blood samples.

BLOOD COLLECTION

Regardless of the method of blood collection, it is vital that the sample be labeled immediately after it has been collected. The tube should be labeled with the date and time of collection, the owner's name, the patient's name, and the patient's clinic identification number. If submitted to a laboratory, include with the sample a request form that includes all necessary sample identification and a clear indication of which tests are requested.

Make venipuncture with the least tissue injury possible to minimize contamination with tissue fluid and to minimize hemolysis. Use of a vacuum tube (Vacutainer, Becton-Dickinson, Rutherford, NJ) or syringe is determined by the size of the animal (and vein) and the quantity of sample desired. All blood samples collected in a tube containing anticoagulant should be gently inverted several times immediately after collection to distribute the anticoagulant. If a Vacutainer is used, fill the tube to capacity to ensure the proper blood-to-anticoagulant ratio. If a syringe and needle are used, remove the needle from the syringe before transferring the blood to the vial, because forcing blood through the needle may result in hemolysis.

Small Animals

In adult dogs and cats, the jugular vein is the preferred site for collection of blood samples. It is relatively easy to locate, and the size of the vein allows adequate quantities of blood to be collected. Alternate sites include the cephalic and femoral veins. Vacutainers may be used with large dogs, but in very small animals the vacuum in the tube can collapse the vein unless a small capacity tube is used. Blood samples from small animals are routinely collected with a calibrated syringe and a needle of appropriate size. If the needle bore is too small or too large, it may cause disruption of erythrocytes (hemolysis). Needles of 20 to 25 gauge work well for collection of samples from dogs and cats.

Large Animals

The jugular vein is a suitable site for collection of blood samples in most large animals. In adult cattle, the subcutaneous abdominal (milk) vein and coccygeal (tail) vein are alternate sites. Alternate sites for sample collection from horses include the cephalic, lateral thoracic, and saphenous veins. Vacutainers work well, but needles and calibrated syringes can also be used. Needle gauges range from 16 to 20, with lengths of 1.5 to 2 inches; 20-gauge needles of 1.5 to 4 inches are used to obtain samples from the cranial vena cava of pigs. Because the blood of goats is easily hemolyzed if collected with a Vacutainer, a syringe and a 20-gauge needle are recommended for collection of caprine blood samples.

SAMPLE TYPE

WHOLE BLOOD

Whole blood is composed of cellular elements (erythrocytes, leukocytes, platelets) and a fluid called plasma. Collect the whole-blood sample by placing the proper amount of blood into a container containing the appropriate anticoagulant and then gently mixing the sample by inverting the tube multiple times. Whole blood may be refrigerated if analysis is to be delayed, but it should never be frozen. If the blood has been refrigerated, warm the sample to room temperature and gently mix by inversion before analysis. Few blood chemistry or serology tests are capable of using whole-blood samples. The majority of those tests are ones that are performed with dedicated instruments that measure a single biochemical constituent, such as glucose or lactate. These primarily use small handheld analyzers.

PLASMA

To obtain a plasma sample, collect the appropriate amount of blood in a container with the proper anticoagulant and gently mix well. Centrifuge the closed container for 10 minutes at 2000 to 3000 rpm to separate the fluid from the cells. After the sample is centrifuged, remove the plasma from the cells, being careful not to contaminate the plasma with any of the pelleted cells, and transfer the plasma into another appropriately labeled container. Separate plasma from the cellular elements as soon as possible after collection to minimize any artifactual changes. Plasma can be refrigerated or frozen until analysis is performed, depending on the specific requirements of the desired test(s).

Plasma collected in tubes containing heparin as the anticoagulant (sodium heparin, potassium heparin, ammonium heparin, or lithium heparin) can be used for most assays included on a routine biochemical profile. However, do not use potassium heparin if electrolyte levels are being measured, because artifactual increases of potassium concentrations can occur. Heparin functions as an anticoagulant by activation of antithrombin III, which prevents conversion of prothrombin to thrombin. Heparin is not a permanent anticoagulant; it inhibits coagulation for only 8 to 12 hours. When biochemical analysis must be performed quickly, as in an emergency situation, collection of a blood sample with a heparin anticoagulant is indicated. The plasma can be harvested immediately after collection and centrifugation, rather than the time delay (necessary for the blood to clot) required to harvest a serum sample.

Plasma collected in tubes containing ethylenediaminetetraacetic acid (EDTA) as the anticoagulant (which is routinely used for complete blood counts) should not be used for serum biochemical analysis, because spurious values for electrolytes, trace elements, and many serum enzymes will result. EDTA functions as an anticoagulant by binding calcium, which is necessary for clotting to occur. Because EDTA binds calcium, any test procedure that requires calcium cannot be performed on samples collected in EDTA. Other anticoagulants, such as potassium oxalate and sodium citrate, also function by binding calcium, and therefore should not be used to collect plasma for biochemical analysis.

SERUM

Serum is plasma that has had the coagulation proteins, such as fibrinogen, removed during the clotting process (Fig. 8-1). A serum sample is obtained by placing blood in a container

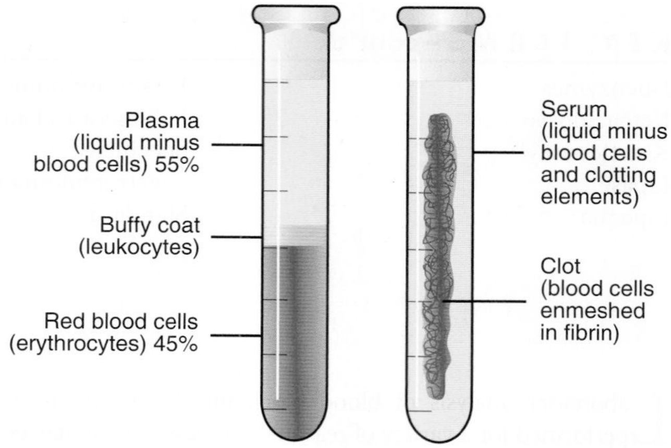

FIGURE 8-1 Difference between blood plasma and blood serum. Plasma is whole blood minus cells; serum is whole blood minus the cells and clotting elements. Plasma is prepared by centrifuging anticoagulated blood; serum is prepared by allowing blood to clot. (From Figure 12-4 in Colville T, Bassert JM: *Clinical anatomy and physiology for veterinary technicians,* ed 3, St Louis, 2016, Mosby.)

with no additives and allowing it to clot at room temperature. Once sufficient time has passed for the clot to form (usually 30 minutes), the closed container is then centrifuged at 2000 to 3000 rpm for 10 minutes, and the serum is harvested. Centrifugation for longer periods can result in hemolysis.

If the serum is not separated from the clot, numerous artifactual changes can result in erroneous laboratory values. An artifactual decrease in glucose concentration can occur because of glucose metabolism by blood cells. Release of inorganic phosphorus from high-energy phosphate bonds results in artifactual increases in serum phosphorus concentrations. Leakage of potassium from red blood cells (RBCs) occurs in large animal species and in some small animal species, resulting in erroneously high potassium concentrations. Artifactual increases of serum enzymes such as aspartate aminotransferase (AST) and alanine aminotransferase (ALT) may also occur. Once harvested, the serum may be refrigerated or frozen. Freezing may affect some test results, so check the test protocol before freezing the sample.

Blood can also be collected in serum tubes containing a gel substance that, during centrifugation, moves into a position between the clot and the serum. Using this type of serum tube, called a serum separator tube, does not necessarily prevent artifactual changes. The benefit of a serum separator tube is that the gel substance facilitates removal of serum without accidental aspiration of cellular elements, which would contaminate the serum sample.

All of the above-mentioned artifactual changes can occur without the problems of hemolysis or lipemia being present. Hemolysis can result from difficult blood collection, mixing too vigorously after sample collection, forcing the sample through a needle when transferring it to a tube, or freezing a whole-blood sample. The syringe must be completely dry before it is used, because water in the syringe can cause hemolysis. Also, it is beneficial to remove the needle from the syringe before transferring the blood into a tube. Cells can be ruptured when blood is forced through the needle. To reduce the chance of hemolysis occurring when transferring blood to a tube, expel the blood slowly from the syringe without causing bubbles to form. Hemolysis may cause errors in testing resulting from direct interference, dilution, and/or release of substances found in high concentrations within erythrocytes.

Hemolysis may not be apparent until after a blood sample has been centrifuged. A trained observer can detect visibly hemolytic serum (slight pink discoloration) at hemoglobin concentrations as low as 20 mg/dl. Mild to moderate hemolysis has minimal effect on most routine serum chemistry assays, but bilirubin and ALT levels are often increased. Also, **lipase** activity is inhibited by hemolysis, resulting in falsely decreased values. If marked hemolysis is present, the results of most assays are likely to be affected, resulting in inaccurate values.

Lipemia also affects the results of serum biochemical assays, resulting in erroneous values. **Lipemia** describes the milky appearance of serum or plasma resulting from increased concentrations of triglyceride-containing lipoproteins. Transient lipemia is common approximately 4 to 6 hours after a meal. Ideally, collect blood samples from an animal that has been fasted for at least 12 hours. This should eliminate any lipemia resulting from ingestion of food. Water need not be withheld. Lipemia can cause erroneous results for all routine clinical chemistries. Light scattering is the most common source of error in testing of lipemic samples. Light scattering may result in falsely increased or decreased values, depending on whether lipemia in the sample results in an increase or decrease in light absorbance measured by the **spectrophotometer.** Endpoint enzymatic assays are generally more severely affected by lipemia than are **kinetic assays.** However, results are invalid in markedly lipemic samples and should be interpreted with caution even in mildly lipemic samples. Lipemia can result in falsely decreased values of electrolytes if a flame photometer is used to measure the electrolytes. If an ion-specific electrode is used to determine electrolyte concentrations, lipemia does not affect results (see Electrolytes section).

LABORATORY SELECTION

There are several choices of where to obtain clinical chemistry results. Veterinary reference laboratories, human hospitals, or in-clinic chemistry analyzers are the most common choices. There are advantages and disadvantages to each choice. Price, service, and quality are the main variables to consider.

The main benefit to choosing a veterinary reference laboratory is that the staff members should be familiar with and have established reference ranges (normal values) for domestic species with the equipment used in that particular laboratory. Some laboratories may have reference ranges for certain exotic animal species as well. In addition to providing chemistry profiles, these laboratories may also offer endocrine testing, microbiology, cytology, and histopathology services. Using a single laboratory for all services can be very convenient. Also, many of these laboratories offer consultations with specialists, such as internists and clinical pathologists. These laboratories are generally available only in larger metropolitan areas. Some reference laboratories may have arrangements with an overnight mailing service so that results are available the next day. Most of these laboratories provide results via telephone, fax, or e-mail, in addition to mailing a printed copy of the results. One disadvantage is that quality assurance standards have not been established for veterinary laboratories, in contrast to the standards that have been established for human laboratories.

Laboratories in human hospitals provide an alternative for obtaining clinical chemistry results. Unlike veterinary reference laboratories, these laboratories must adhere to rigorous quality control standards, and the testing methods are of high quality. Human hospital laboratories are not likely to have established reference ranges for animal species. The cost of having animal samples analyzed at a human hospital may be quite reasonable because of the high volume of human samples assayed. However, some of the assays included in routine chemistry profiles performed at human hospital laboratories are not validated for animal species.

LABORATORY EQUIPMENT

Chemistry machines designed for in-clinic use are improving in quality and becoming more affordable and easier to use. A great advantage of in-clinic chemistry analyzers is that the results can be obtained very quickly. Also, performing these tests in-clinic can be a source of profit. Factors to consider are the initial cost of the machine, cost of the reagents, anticipated use of the machine, and amount of maintenance the machine requires. Quality control procedures are essential for any test that is performed on an in-clinic basis. The machine must be kept calibrated, and regular **control** samples that contain known quantities of a substance or substances must be assayed. If these are not done, the potential for erroneous results is great.

FEATURES AND BENEFITS OF COMMON ANALYZER TYPES

Most in-clinic automated blood chemistry analyzers employ photometric principles. Photometry involves the addition of a reagent to a serum or plasma sample that creates a color change in the system. The degree of color change is then measured with a spectrophotometer (Fig. 8-2). The primary difference between the various photometric analyzers lies in the format of the tests. Several important questions must be answered when determining which type of analyzer to purchase for in-house testing. These include the intended purpose of the testing (i.e., presurgical screening versus tracking disease progress), anticipated test volume, and ease of operation and maintenance. Methods for ensuring quality of results should also be evaluated when choosing an analyzer. Costs associated with various analyzers also vary a great deal. When determining costs, be sure to

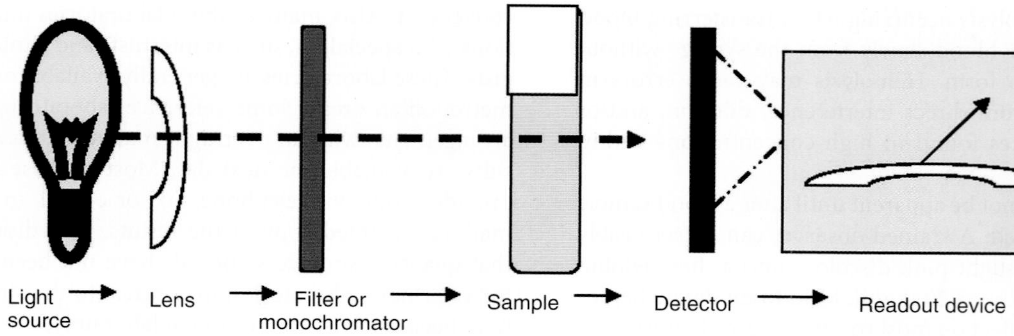

FIGURE 8-2 Principles of spectrophotometry.

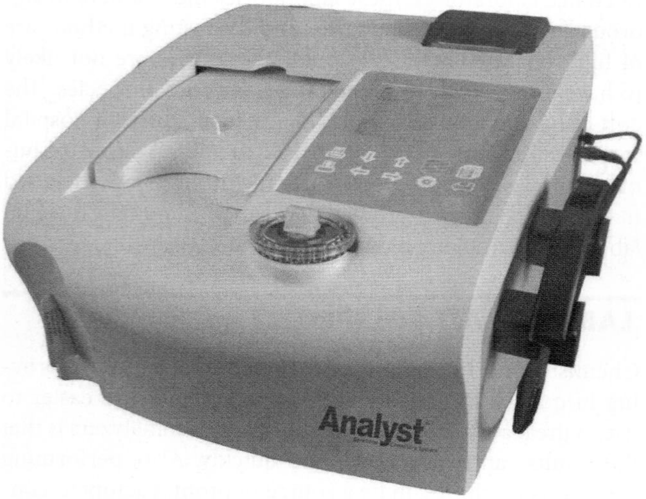

FIGURE 8-3 Analyst blood chemistry analyzer.

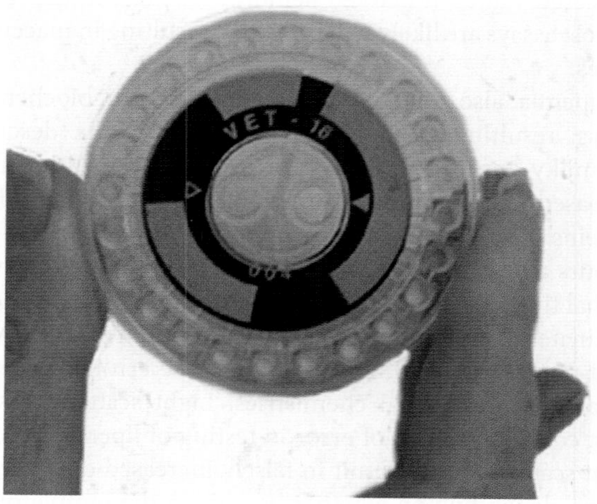

FIGURE 8-4 Reagent rotor for use in the Analyst blood chemistry analyzer.

include technician time to prep and run samples and instrument prep and maintenance time along with the actual costs per test or profile.

Analyzers using "dry" systems include those with reagent-impregnated slides, pads, or cartridges. Most of these use reflectance assays (rather than the absorbance assay of a traditional photometric analyzer). Dry systems tend to have comparatively higher costs associated with them than other analyzer types. Most are not configured for veterinary species and have fairly high incidences of sample rejection with compromised samples or samples from large animals. However, they have the benefit of not requiring reagent handling, and performance of single tests is relatively simple. Running profiles on these types of systems tends to be more time-consuming than most other analyzer types.

Liquid systems include those that use lyophilized reagent or those that provide prepared liquid reagent. The most common type of lyophilized reagent systems for veterinary clinical practice use rotor technology (Fig. 8-3). The rotors consist of individual cuvettes (optical-quality reagent wells) to which sample is added (Fig. 8-4). These systems tend to be quite accurate, although some are not configured for veterinary species. They are usually cost-effective for profiles but some are incapable of running single tests. Other liquid systems in common use include those with unitized reagent cuvettes and those with bulk reagent. The unitized systems have the advantage of not requiring reagent handling but tend to be the most expensive of all the liquid reagent systems. It is also time-consuming to run profiles with these systems, but single testing is simple. Bulk reagent systems may supply reagent either in concentrated form that must be diluted or in working strength. Working strength reagent systems do not usually require any special reagent handling. These analyzers are the most versatile in that they can perform either profiling or single testing with relative ease. Most require little prep time. However, some have extensive maintenance time, in particular with calibration of test parameters.

Samples that are compromised by hemolysis, icterus, or lipemia may yield inaccurate results with many of the automated analyzers (Table 8-1). Most automated blood chemistry analyzers work by passing light in the ultraviolet or visible range of the spectrum through the sample-reagent complex and measuring the amount of light transmitted. Hemolysis, icterus, and lipemia affect the amount of light transmitted through the complex. Chemistry methods that use infrared wavelengths have minimized these problems but are not widely available for veterinary use.

TABLE 8-1 Effects of Sample Compromise

SAMPLE CHARACTERISTIC	EFFECT	RESULT
Lipemia	Light scattering	↑
	Volume displacement	↓
	Hemolysis	↑↓*
Hemolysis/blood substitutes	Release of analytes	↑
	Release of enzymes	↑↓*
	Reaction inhibition	↓
	Increased absorbance	↑
	Release of water	↓
Icterus	Spectral interference	↑
	Chemical interaction	↑
Hyperproteinemia	Hyperviscosity	↓
	Analyte binding	↑↓*
	Volume displacement	↓
Medications	Reaction interference	↑↓*

*Variable effect depending on analyte and test method.

TYPES OF PHOTOMETRIC TESTING

Most photometric analyzers use endpoint readings. The analyzer then uses either a one-point calibration or an internal standard curve to calculate the patient results. Either method requires the use of a standard. A **standard** is a nonbiologic solution of the analyte, usually in distilled water, with a known concentration. For a one-point calibration, the standard is analyzed in the same manner as a patient sample, and the reaction characteristics are mathematically compared with the patient sample. The specific type of calculation varies depending on the analyzer. In general, however, the ratio of the optical density (OD) of the reacted standard is compared with the optical density of the patient sample. An example of this type of calculation is as follows:

$$\text{Patient sample concentration} = \frac{\text{Patient sample OD} \times \text{concentration of standard}}{\text{OD of standard}}$$

The internal standard curve is created when the analyzer is calibrated. To perform a standard curve, serial dilutions are created of the standard solution, and each is analyzed to determine its absorbance or transmittance of light. The results from each dilution are plotted on a graph as a straight line (Fig. 8-5). The concentrations of subsequent patient samples are determined by locating the intersection of the absorbance of the reacted patient sample with the line on the graph. Analyzers that use standard curve methods must be recalibrated each time a new lot number of reagent is purchased.

Some assays use kinetic methods rather than endpoint. These are primarily used for enzyme assays or when the reagent is enzyme-based. Kinetic reactions measure changes in color development over specific periods of time. Fixed-time reactions are similar to kinetic except that the color development is not linear at any prolonged point throughout the reaction. These tests use readings at two points during the reaction, taken at the times when the reaction is closest to linear.

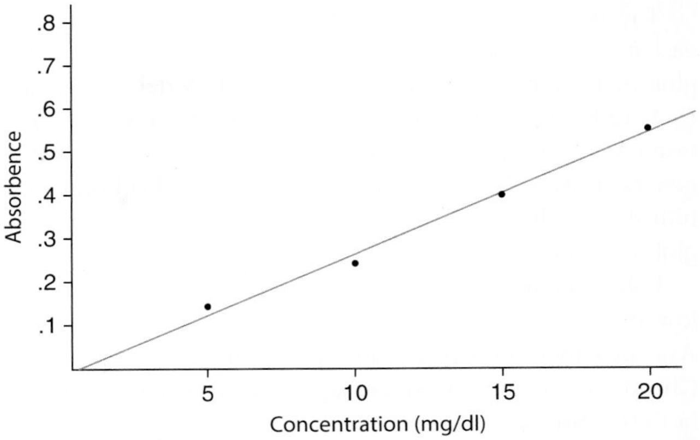

FIGURE 8-5 Completed standard curve for calcium plotting absorbance vs. concentration.

BOX 8-1 Hepatobiliary Function Tests

AST (aspartate aminotransferase)
ALT (alanine aminotransferase)
AP (alkaline phosphatase)
Total serum bilirubin
Direct/conjugated bilirubin
GGT (gamma glutamyl transferase)
Bile acids
Ammonia
Cholesterol
Total serum protein
Serum albumin
Glucose
Plasma fibrinogen

HEPATOBILIARY FUNCTION TESTING

Hepatic cells exhibit extreme diversity of function and are capable of regeneration if damaged. As a result, there are over 100 types of tests to evaluate liver function. The most common tests performed on veterinary species are listed in Box 8-1. In most cases evaluation of several liver function tests is required to assess the overall status of the liver. Liver cells also compartmentalize the work, so damage to one zone of the liver may not affect all liver functions. Liver function tests are often done with serial determinations. Usually liver disease is greatly progressed before clinical signs appear. Liver function tests are designed to measure substances that are produced by the liver (primarily proteins), modified by the liver (e.g., bilirubin), or released when hepatocytes are damaged (primarily liver enzymes). Species variations exist in the concentrations of these components so not every test will provide diagnostic information in every species.

TECHNICIAN NOTE The most commonly performed hepatobiliary tests in small animal practice are ALT, ALP, Bilirubin, and Total Protein.

The most common types of tests for hepatobiliary disease are the leakage enzyme tests, which include ALT, AST, glutamate dehydrogenase (GD), and sorbitol dehydrogenase (SD) tests. The cholestatic tests include alkaline phosphatase (ALP) and gamma glutamyl transferase (GGT). Other general tests of liver function include total bilirubin, direct bilirubin, indirect bilirubin, bile acids, ammonia, albumin, globulin, and cholesterol.

Following liver parenchymal damage, ALT increases, followed by AST. AST returns to normal more rapidly than ALT, provided there is no subsequent muscle tissue damage. Chronic or ongoing liver damage is likely if ALT and AST both remain elevated.

SD and GD indicate acute damage, but these tend to return to normal within a day or two. SD can be used to determine if an AST increase is because of liver or muscle damage. **Cholestasis** can result from impaired bile flow or can be drug-induced. ALP and GGT are normally present in very low concentrations in serum.

Impaired bile flow stimulates production of ALP. This may also be linked to retention of bile acids. Increased ALP may also be caused by excessive glucocorticoid concentration or administration of anticonvulsants or megestrol acetate.

PROTEIN

In the small veterinary practice total protein is usually measured with a refractometer (see Procedure 7-3). This instrument gives a measurement of the refractive index of a substance and is a function of the total amount of material dissolved in the plasma. Proteins represent the primary solid component in plasma or serum. Total plasma protein measurements include fibrinogen values. Total serum protein concentrations include all plasma proteins except fibrinogen and certain other coagulation proteins, which have been removed during the coagulation process. The majority of serum proteins are produced by hepatocytes. Most chemical analyses to measure total protein use the biuret method, which involves the addition of reagent that acts on molecules with multiple peptide bonds. Precipitation (trichloroacetic acid) and dye-binding (Coomassie blue) methods have been used to measure the low levels of protein found in such fluids as cerebrospinal fluid and urine.

Serum protein levels are affected by the rate of protein synthesis in the liver, the rate of protein catabolism in the animal, hydration status, and alterations in distribution of proteins in the body. Dehydrated animals usually have elevated total protein values; overhydrated animals usually have decreased total protein values. Other conditions in which total protein concentrations may be helpful include coagulation (clotting) abnormalities, renal disease, weight loss, diarrhea, edema, and ascites.

Marked hemolysis falsely increases total protein values. Do not use lipemic samples, especially if the refractometric method is used. Moderate icterus has no effect on the refractometric method. Heat, ultraviolet light, surfactant detergents, and chemicals can break down proteins, leading to artificially low results.

Albumin

Albumin is one of the most important proteins in plasma or serum. It makes up approximately 35% to 50% of the total serum protein concentration. Albumin is synthesized by the liver. Severe hepatic insufficiency is a cause of decreased albumin levels. Albumin levels are also influenced by dietary intake, renal disease, and intestinal protein absorption. Albumin functions as a transport and binding protein of the blood and is responsible for maintaining osmotic pressure of plasma.

The most commonly performed test for albumin is the dye-binding assay. The test involves conjugation of albumin to a biological dye (usually bromcresol green) at a specific pH. This test is affected by certain anticoagulants, so plasma samples are not usually used for albumin testing. Hemolysis may increase the apparent albumin level if the bromcresol green method (commonly used in veterinary laboratories) is used. Methods of measurement used in some human laboratories (those that use bromcresol purple) can be unreliable. Check the test protocol for the method used. Keep the sample covered to prevent dehydration, which can falsely elevate protein levels.

Globulin

Globulins are a complex group of proteins that include all of the proteins (plasma or serum) other than albumin and coagulation proteins. The globulins are separated into three major classes by electrophoresis: alpha, beta, and gamma globulins. Most alpha and beta globulins are synthesized by the liver. The proteins in these groups include **complement**, transferrin, ferritin, other acute-phase proteins of inflammation, and lipoproteins. The gamma globulins (**immunoglobulins**) are synthesized by plasma cells and are responsible for the body's immunity provided by antibodies. Immunoglobulins identified in animals include IgG, IgD, IgE, IgA, and IgM.

Direct measurement of globulin is not usually performed. Globulin concentration is calculated by subtracting the albumin concentration from the total serum protein.

Albumin-to-Globulin Ratio

The albumin:globulin (A:G) ratio may be reported on chemistry profiles. The normal A:G ratio is approximately 0.5 to 1.5 across species. An increased A:G ratio may occur with any condition that increases albumin (e.g., dehydration) and/or decreases globulin. A decreased A:G ratio may occur with any condition that decreases albumin and/or increases globulin (e.g., inflammation). Although A:G ratios are frequently reported, they are of little significance without knowledge of the absolute total protein, albumin, and globulin values.

Fibrinogen

Fibrinogen is synthesized by hepatocytes. It is one of the factors necessary for clot formation and is the precursor of fibrin, which is the insoluble protein of blood clots. Clot formation is impaired when fibrinogen concentrations are decreased. Because fibrinogen is removed from plasma when

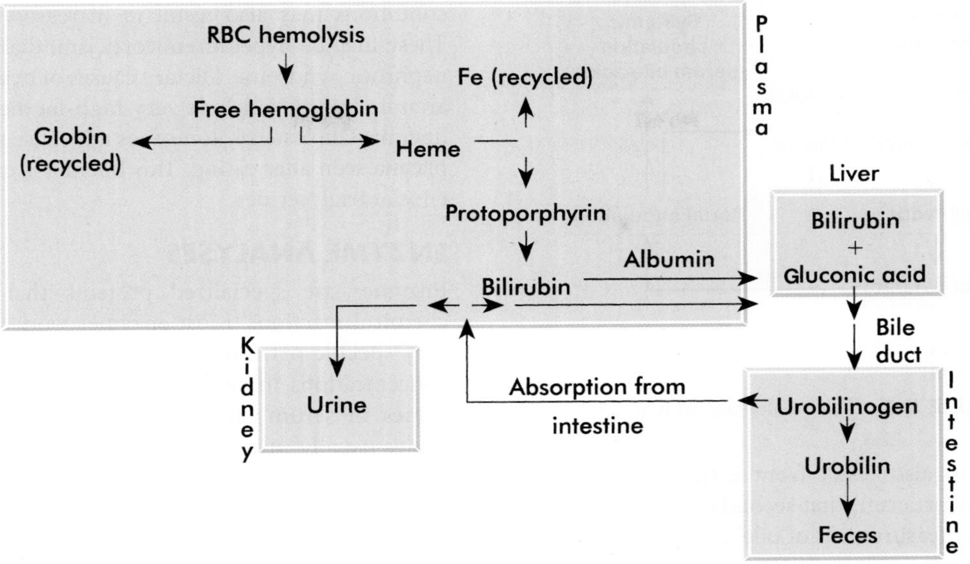

FIGURE 8-6 Bilirubin metabolism.

a blood clot forms, no fibrinogen is present in serum. Acute inflammation or tissue damage can elevate fibrinogen levels.

Fibrinogen concentration can be determined with automated analyzers or estimated as described in Chapter 7.

Bilirubin

Bilirubin is an insoluble molecule derived from the breakdown of hemoglobin in the spleen. The molecule is bound to albumin and transported to the liver. The hepatic cells metabolize and conjugate the bilirubin to the molecule bilirubin glucuronide. This molecule is then secreted from the hepatocytes and becomes a component of bile. Bacteria within the gastrointestinal system act on the bilirubin glucuronide and produce a group of compounds collectively referred to as urobilinogen. Urobilinogen is broken down to urobilin before being excreted in feces. Bilirubin glucuronide and urobilinogen may also be absorbed directly into the blood and excreted via the kidneys (Fig. 8-6).

Measurements of the circulating levels of these various populations of bilirubin can help to pinpoint the cause of jaundice. Differences in the relative solubility of each of these molecules allow them to be quantified individually. In most animals the prehepatic (bound to albumin) bilirubin composes about two thirds of the total bilirubin in serum. Alterations in the ratios of the various bilirubin compounds help determine whether liver damage is present or other conditions (e.g., bile duct obstruction) are contributing to disease. Both unconjugated and conjugated bilirubin are found in plasma (and serum). Assays can directly measure total bilirubin (conjugated plus unconjugated) and conjugated bilirubin. Conjugated bilirubin is also referred to as direct bilirubin, because test methods directly measure the amount of conjugated bilirubin in the sample. Unconjugated bilirubin is also referred to as indirect bilirubin, because it reacts with test substrates only after addition of alcohol (indirect reacting). Measuring the light transmission through the sample before addition of alcohol gives the concentration of conjugated bilirubin (direct reacting); measuring the light transmission through the sample after addition of alcohol gives the concentration of total bilirubin. The concentration of unconjugated (indirect) bilirubin is determined by subtracting the conjugated (direct) bilirubin concentration from the total bilirubin concentration.

Bilirubin is assayed to determine the cause of jaundice (icterus), to evaluate liver function, and to check the patency of bile ducts. Blood levels of conjugated bilirubin are elevated with hepatocellular damage or bile duct injury and/or obstruction. Excessive erythrocyte destruction often results in production of more unconjugated bilirubin than the liver can process. Initially the elevated bilirubin levels in the blood are primarily composed of unconjugated bilirubin; however, with time, more and more conjugated bilirubin appears.

Bile Acids

Bile acids are produced from cholesterol in the liver and serve many functions, including aiding in fat absorption and modulating cholesterol levels. The gallbladder stores bile acids, and they are then released into the intestinal tract. Most bile acids are actively resorbed in the ileum and carried to the liver where they are reconjugated and excreted as part of the enterohepatic circulation of bile acids (Fig. 8-7). This recirculation functions to conserve bile acids and is so efficient that the entire pool of bile acids is generally recirculated three to five times after every meal, with only small amounts being lost in the feces or bypassing the liver into the systemic circulation. Because of this, blood levels of bile acids in normal animals are very low, especially in fasted animals. When functional hepatic mass is reduced, extraction of bile acids from blood is affected. Measurement of bile acid concentration is, therefore, a good indicator of hepatobiliary function. In general, elevated bile acid concentrations are not specific for the type of underlying disease. Increased bile acid

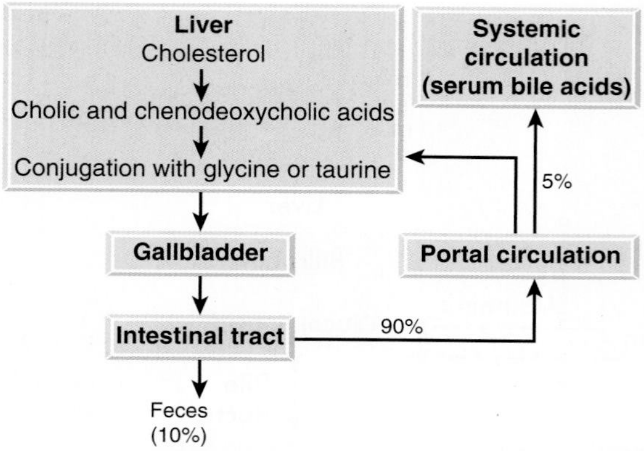

FIGURE 8-7 Circulation of bile acids.

concentrations can also result from extrahepatic diseases (e.g., hyperadrenocorticism) that secondarily affect the liver. In small animals, measurement of bile acids in paired (fasting and 2-hour postprandial) samples is often useful in increasing the overall test sensitivity. **Cholestasis** causes backup of bile acids into blood (along with conjugated bilirubin). Other variables independent of hepatobiliary function affect bile acid concentrations including decreased gastrointestinal transit time or spontaneous gallbladder contraction. Prolonged fasting, intestinal malabsorption, or decreased intestinal transit time through the bowel (e.g., diarrhea) can lower bile acid concentrations. In horses increased bile acid concentrations result from hepatobiliary disease or decreased feed intake. Most horses with hepatobiliary disease have markedly increased bile acid concentrations. The normal bovine has extremely variable serum bile acids concentration, making the test ineffective in detection of disease.

Ammonia

Ammonia is produced in the intestine (primarily in the colon) from the action of bacteria on dietary proteins. Ammonia is absorbed in the intestine and carried in the portal vein to the liver, where it is effectively cleared from the circulation. The hepatocytes convert ammonia to **urea** via the urea cycle. Much like bile acids, blood ammonia levels are increased with reduced hepatic mass and abnormalities in portal circulation. Ammonia levels have been measured in cases of suspected hepatic encephalopathy.

Samples for ammonia determination are not stable and must be stored on ice immediately after collection, centrifuged in a refrigerated centrifuge, separated from the RBCs, and assayed as soon as possible (preferably within 15 minutes). Sample collection must be as smooth as possible, because occlusion of a vein for prolonged periods results in ammonia accumulation.

Cholesterol

Cholesterol is produced in almost every cell in the body and is especially abundant in hepatocytes, adrenal cortex, ovaries, testes, and intestinal epithelium. The liver is the primary site of synthesis in most animals. Cholesterol levels are frequently elevated in animals with hypothyroidism, although other conditions may also result in increased cholesterol levels. These include hyperadrenocorticism, diabetes mellitus, and nephrotic syndrome. Dietary causes of hypercholesterolemia are rare but may include very-high-fat diets or postprandial lipemia. Cholesterol alone does not cause the grossly lipemic plasma seen after eating. This lipemia is caused by the presence of triglycerides.

ENZYME ANALYSES

Enzymes are specialized proteins that catalyze various chemical reactions. Most enzymes work intracellularly at a very specific pH. Enzymes are usually not present in high concentrations in serum. Increased concentrations of enzymes in serum often indicate cellular damage. Enzyme assays usually involve measurement of the outcome of enzyme activity rather than specific measurement of the concentration of the enzyme. Enzymes related to liver function in most mammals include the phosphatases, transaminases, and dehydrogenases.

Phosphatases

Blood contains two major groups of phosphatases. They are the **alkaline phosphatases** (ALPs) and the acid phosphatases (ACPs). Determinations of ACP levels are not commonly done, but may help in diagnosis of certain types of hemolytic anemia. ALPs are **isoenzymes** with multiple organ sources, including the liver, kidney, bone, and intestine. The extent of the increase aids in determining whether the patient has intrahepatic damage or extrahepatic damage. The half-lives of intestinal and renal isoenzymes are extremely short (minutes), as compared with the half-lives of hepatic enzymes (hours to days). Because of this, the intestinal and renal isoenzymes of ALP are not usually found in serum (or plasma) in high concentrations. Special analytic methods in commercial or research laboratories can be used to determine which isoenzyme is increased. Increases in circulating levels of ALPs are almost always the result of liver damage.

ALP is most often used to detect cholestasis in dogs and cats. Production of ALP is induced by increased pressure within the biliary system during any form of cholestasis. The cholestasis may be intrahepatic because of tumors, swelling, inflammation, or anything blocking bile flow, or it may be extrahepatic because of bile duct obstruction. ALP is a sensitive indicator of cholestasis in dogs and cats, but it is not useful in large animals because of the wide variation of ALP concentrations normally found in large animal species.

In dogs certain drugs induce ALP synthesis. The magnitude of increase may be great. The most commonly used drugs that induce ALP synthesis are glucocorticoids, such as prednisone or cortisone. Exogenously administered or endogenous (caused by hyperadrenocorticism) glucocorticoids stimulate this effect. It occurs through induction of a unique isoenzyme of ALP. Anticonvulsants, such as phenobarbital, primidone, and diphenylhydantoin, also induce synthesis of ALP (hepatic isoenzyme). These increases in ALP are caused by drug induction and do not necessarily indicate liver disease.

ALP levels can be increased in young growing animals because of bone remodeling and increases in the bone isoenzyme. Other causes of increased osteoblastic activity, such as primary hyperparathyroidism, fracture healing, and neoplasia, can also result in increased serum ALP activity. Placental ALP is present in mares and queens during pregnancy.

Transferases

This group of enzymes is found primarily in tissues that have high rates of protein metabolism, especially kidney, liver, and muscle. In veterinary medicine, the transferases of clinical significance are gamma glutamyl transferase (GGT), alanine aminotransferase (ALT), and asparate aminotransferase (AST). In dogs and cats, damage to hepatocytes results in release of large amounts of ALT. In other species, ALT levels have little clinical significance. AST assays are used primarily to evaluate the extent of skeletal muscle damage in the equine and may also be used to evaluate cardiac muscle damage in some species.

Alanine Aminotransferase. ALT is a liver-specific enzyme and a good indicator of hepatocellular damage in dogs, cats, and primates because the primary/major source of serum ALT is the hepatocyte. It is not useful in large animal species, such as horses, cattle, sheep, and pigs, because the hepatocytes of these species contain insignificant amounts of ALT.

Aspartate Aminotransferase. Hepatocytes are one source of serum AST, but there are other sources. Skeletal and cardiac muscle both contain significant amounts of AST. Other sources include erythrocytes, kidneys, and pancreas. Increased levels of AST indicate liver or muscle damage. It is important to remember that AST is not considered a liver-specific enzyme. Increased serum AST levels are a result of hepatic injury (as previously discussed), muscle cell injury, or hemolysis. Elevations of AST along with elevations of creatine kinase (CK) suggest muscle damage. Elevations in AST with normal CK levels suggest hepatocellular injury or prior muscle injury in which the CK level has returned to normal.

Gamma Glutamyl Transferase. GGT is similar to ALP in that it is bound to microsomal membranes within the cell. Serum levels of GGT are increased when the cell is stimulated to increase synthesis. GGT is present in most cells but is found in high concentration in liver, pancreatic, and renal tubular cells. GGT from renal tubular cells is released into the urine during renal tubular damage, not into the blood. Pancreatic GGT is apparently secreted into the intestines and also does not cause elevated serum concentrations. Therefore serum GGT is considered a liver-specific enzyme. As with ALP, the major inducer of hepatic GGT is cholestasis. This occurs in all species. GGT is an excellent indicator of cholestasis in horses, ruminants, and swine. GGT can also be used in dogs and cats, and is often evaluated in conjunction with ALP for these species.

Dehydrogenases

This group of enzymes functions in cellular metabolism and includes the lactate dehydrogenases (LD) and the sorbitol dehydrogenases (SD). Any disease characterized by membrane defect will result in release of LD into surrounding tissue. SD is present in a variety of organs, but in most species it has the greatest concentrations in the liver. SD is the preferred assay to evaluate equine liver function.

Sorbitol Dehydrogenase. Sorbitol dehydrogenase (SD) is found in high concentrations in hepatocytes of all species, including large animals, and is considered a liver-specific enzyme. SD is unstable, and serum activity decreases rapidly. Samples should be analyzed within 12 hours of collection.

Glutamate Dehydrogenase. Glutamate dehydrogenase (GD) is highly concentrated in the liver of cattle and sheep, as well as in the liver of other species. Increased serum values of GD indicate hepatic necrosis. GD is considered a liver-specific enzyme.

KIDNEY FUNCTION TESTING

The kidneys have an important role in the homeostatic mechanisms of the body. They function to maintain the volume and composition of extracellular fluid and are involved in excretion of metabolic waste products and other chemicals. The functional unit of the kidney is the nephron, which consists of a network of capillaries (the glomerulus) and tubules that are lined with epithelial cells. Nearly all blood constituents pass through the glomerulus and enter the tubules. In a normally functioning nephron, about 80% of the water and all of the amino acids and glucose that enter the tubules are either reabsorbed or actively transported back into circulation. Ions (primarily sodium, chloride, and bicarbonate) are also selectively reabsorbed. Any constituent not reabsorbed or transported back into circulation is excreted in the urine.

Kidney damage may result in an inability of the glomerulus to retain cells and proteins, or impair the resorptive capability of the tubules. The primary chemical tests of kidney function are urea nitrogen and creatinine.

Urea Nitrogen

Blood urea nitrogen (BUN) is the principal product of protein catabolism. Normally, all urea passes through the glomerulus and about half is reabsorbed by passive diffusion. Azotemia (increase in BUN levels) can occur when blood flow through the kidneys alters the glomerular filtration rate, or when the urinary tract is obstructed. Dehydration will also result in azotemia because urea must be excreted in a large amount of water. Differences in rates of protein catabolism between male and female animals, young and adult animals, different species, and nutritional status will also affect BUN levels. The majority of tests for urea nitrogen are photometric analyses.

Creatinine

Serum creatinine is produced from metabolic breakdown of phosphocreatine in muscle tissue. The day-to-day rate of creatinine production is relatively constant in any animal and is dependent on the animal's total muscle mass. Creatinine is also primarily cleared by the kidney. Glomerular filtration is the primary mode of elimination. Creatinine is minimally resorbed by the tubules, so it is not influenced by the rate of urine flow, as is BUN.

Creatinine is used to evaluate renal function based on the ability of the glomeruli to filter creatinine from the blood and eliminate it in urine. Like BUN, if serum creatinine values are increased because of decreased renal function, this indicates that approximately 75% of the nephrons are nonfunctional.

Creatinine testing is often done in conjunction with urea nitrogen testing. An alteration in the ratio of the concentrations of these two components is a more significant indicator of renal disease than individual measurements of either component. There are a number of photometric procedures available for serum creatinine testing.

TECHNICIAN NOTE The primary chemical tests of kidney function are urea nitrogen and creatinine.

Uric Acid

Uric acid is an end product of catabolism of nucleic acids. It is the primary end product of nitrogen metabolism in avian species, and is actively secreted by the renal tubules. Measurement of plasma or serum uric acid is therefore preferred over urea levels as an indicator of kidney function in birds. In most animals, uric acid is bound to albumin, passes through the glomerulus, and then is reabsorbed. It is usually converted to allantoin and excreted in the urine. In Dalmatian dogs the liver is unable to convert uric acid, so these animals excrete uric acid rather than allantoin. This also predisposes the breed to urate urolithiasis. Photometric analysis of uric acid is a complex procedure not commonly performed in veterinary clinical practice. However, newer methods of chemical analysis using liquid stable reagents can allow for uric acid testing in the veterinary practice laboratory. In birds increases in uric acid concentration can be an artifact seen when samples are collected from a toenail that has fecal urate contamination.

PANCREATIC FUNCTION TESTING

The pancreas functions as both an endocrine and exocrine organ. Exocrine activities of the pancreas involve the production of digestive enzymes (Table 8-2). The endocrine part of the pancreas contains small nodules of endocrine cells, the islets of Langerhans. Two hormones are produced within the islets: insulin and glucagon. Insulin is necessary for the body's cells to use glucose for fuel. It prevents abnormally high blood glucose levels and allows glucose to enter the cells for use. A defect in insulin secretion or action leads to diabetes mellitus, characterized by abnormally high blood glucose levels and many metabolic difficulties. The other pancreatic hormone, glucagon, has the opposite effect, and tends to increase the blood glucose level. Trauma to pancreatic tissue is often associated with pancreatic duct inflammation that results in a backup of digestive enzymes into peripheral circulation. Common tests for evaluation of the endocrine functions of the pancreas are summarized in Box 8-2.

TABLE 8-2 Major Pancreatic Enzymes

ENZYME	DIGESTIVE ACTIVITY
Amylase	Carbohydrates
Lipase	Lipids
Nucleases	Nucleic acids
Chymotrypsinogen	Protein
Trypsinogen	Protein

BOX 8-2 Test to Evaluate the Endocrine Pancreas

Glucose
Serum glucose
Fructosamine
Glycosylated Hemoglobin
β-Hydroxybutyrate
Glucose tolerance tests
Urinalysis; urine glucose and ketones

Amylase

Amylase is produced in a variety of tissues, including the salivary glands, small intestine, and pancreas. Serial determinations of amylase in conjunction with lipase provide the best indication of pancreatic function. Amylase functions in the breakdown of starches and glycogen in sugars to form such sugars as maltose and residual glucose. Increased levels of amylase can occur with acute pancreatitis, flare-ups of chronic pancreatitis, and obstruction of the pancreatic ducts.

Nonpancreatic disease may also increase serum amylase levels. Most commonly, amylase levels are elevated with renal disease. Renal disease can cause amylase levels that are approximately 2.5 times the upper limit of normal. Increased amylase levels have also been reported with certain liver and intestinal diseases (intestinal obstructions).

Amylase levels can be determined by two methods: amyloclastic or saccharogenic. Amyloclastic methods measure the rate of disappearance of starch and should be used for canine serum. Saccharogenic methods, which measure the rate of appearance of reducing sugars and are valid for humans, give falsely elevated results in canine samples because of other enzymes found in canine serum.

TECHNICIAN NOTE Serial determination of both amylase and lipase are commonly performed to diagnose and manage pancreatitis in small animals.

Lipase

Lipase functions to break down the long-chain fatty acids of lipids. In experimental pancreatitis, lipase levels rise rapidly and are elevated for more than a week. However, not all animals with pancreatitis have elevated lipase levels. Lipase activity may also be elevated by nonpancreatic factors, such as chronic renal failure, exploratory surgery, and corticosteroid use.

Nearly all serum lipase is derived from the pancreas. Excess lipase is easily filtered through the kidneys, so lipase levels tend to remain normal in early stages of pancreatic disease. Gradual increases are seen as disease progresses. With chronic, progressive pancreatic disease, damaged pancreatic cells are replaced with connective tissue that cannot produce enzyme. As this occurs, amylase and lipase levels both decrease.

Test methods for determining lipase activity are usually based on hydrolysis of an olive oil emulsion into its constituent fatty acids. The quantity of sodium hydroxide required to neutralize the fatty acids provides a measure of lipase activity. Immunologic testing for canine pancreatic lipase can also be performed and is a rapid and accurate in-house test.

Glucose

A small portion of the pancreas is involved in the production of insulin. Insulin is required to facilitate the uptake of **glucose** by body cells. Blood glucose measurements provide an indicator of the status of pancreatic endocrine activity. However, these can be affected by a variety of factors, including diet and stress. The blood glucose level reflects the net balance between glucose production (dietary intake, conversion from other carbohydrates) and glucose use (energy expended, conversion to other products). It also reflects the balance between blood insulin and glucagon levels.

Glucose use depends on the amount of insulin and glucagon being produced by the pancreas. As the blood insulin level increases, so does the rate of glucose use, resulting in decreased blood glucose levels. Glucagon acts as a stabilizer to prevent blood glucose levels from becoming too low. As the insulin level decreases, so does glucose use, resulting in increased blood glucose concentration. Although excess serum glucose can result from a variety of disease conditions, the highest blood glucose values are seen in diabetes mellitus. This condition results from either decreased or defective production of insulin. Without sufficient insulin, the body cells are unable to take up glucose. Although the nephron normally resorbs blood glucose from the filtrate, excess glucose cannot be effectively resorbed by the nephron. This results in glycosuria (glucose in the urine). Glycosuria alters the solute concentration of the filtrate and causes an increased loss of electrolytes and nitrogen into the urine.

A variety of photometric test methods are available to evaluate blood glucose. Dedicated instruments for blood glucose testing are also readily available. Most of these were initially designed for use in human medicine to allow diabetic patients to monitor their own blood glucose levels (Fig. 8-8). Many of these types of analyzers use whole blood samples and tests must be performed immediately after blood collection. For traditional photometric tests that use serum or plasma, it is vital that the serum or plasma be removed from contact with the erythrocytes immediately after blood collection. If the sample is left in contact with the erythrocytes, the blood glucose levels can drop up to 10% per hour at room temperature. Erythrocytes use glucose for energy. In a blood sample, erythrocytes may decrease the glucose level enough to give false-normal results if the original sample had an elevated glucose level. If the sample originally had a normal glucose level, a falsely low level may result. If the blood sample cannot be centrifuged and the serum or plasma is not separated from the erythrocytes, collect the sample in a sodium fluoride tube. The sodium fluoride tube usually contains a potassium oxalate anticoagulant. Sodium fluoride inhibits use of glucose by erythrocytes and therefore stabilizes glucose levels in the sample. Glucose levels remain stable for 12 hours at room temperature and for 48 hours if the sample is refrigerated. Fill this tube at least halfway with blood; otherwise the fluoride concentration may be high enough to interfere with glucose analysis.

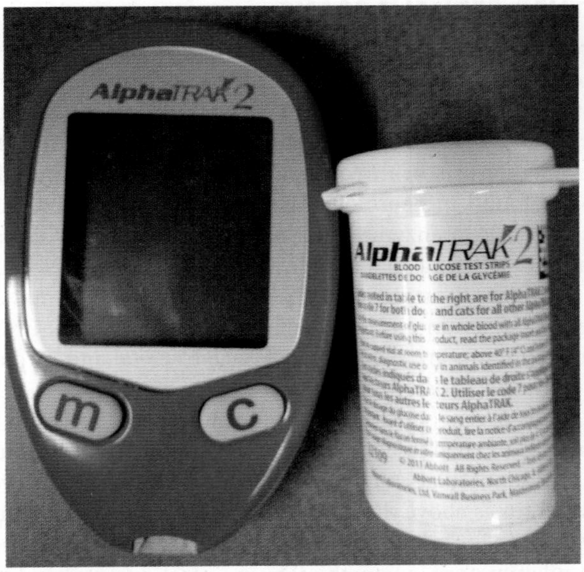

FIGURE 8-8 This dedicated glucose-measuring instrument is available over the counter in many pharmacies. (From Figure 31-10 in Sirois M: *Laboratory procedures for veterinary technicians,* ed 6, 2015, St Louis, 2015, Mosby.)

Refrigeration slows glucose use by erythrocytes. Because eating raises the blood glucose level and fasting decreases it, a 12-hour fast is recommended when possible for all animals except for mature ruminants before the blood sample is collected.

Fructosamine

Fructosamine is a more specific indicator of pancreatic endocrine activity than glucose. Fructosamine is a glycosylated serum protein. The reaction between glucose and the protein is irreversible. It therefore provides an indication of the average glucose levels over the life span of the protein (approximately 1 to 3 weeks). Falsely low fructosamine levels may be present when decreased total protein and/or albumin are also present.

β-Hydroxybutyrate

When cells cannot use glucose for energy, other metabolic pathways are activated. Although the same pathways are used in normal metabolism, cells of the diabetic patient overuse these pathways. This leads to the buildup of abnormal levels of metabolic by-products, such as ketones. Ketones cause decreased body pH and affect all metabolic systems. This condition is known as **ketoacidosis.** The primary ketone produced in ketoacidosis is β-hydroxybutyrate (βHB). A few test kits are now available that allow this testing to be performed in-house.

OTHER SERUM ASSAYS

Creatine Kinase

Creatine kinase (CK), also referred to as creatine phosphokinase (CPK), is a cytoplasmic enzyme that appears in the serum in increased concentrations after cellular injury. This enzyme consists of three isoenzymes: CK_1, CK_2, and CK_3. CK_1 is found in neurologic tissue, cerebrospinal fluid, and viscera. This isoenzyme is not present in serum and/or plasma. CK_2 is found mainly in cardiac muscle. CK_3 is found in skeletal and cardiac muscle. The last two isoenzymes are present in serum and/or plasma. Therefore changes in CK concentrations are specific for muscle (skeletal and cardiac) injury or necrosis.

CK is a very sensitive enzyme, and serum levels can be dramatically increased after relatively minor insults to muscle. Intramuscular injections are enough to raise CK levels several times above the normal range. Other causes of muscle damage include the following:

- Inflammatory myopathies from infectious causes (e.g., *Clostridium*) or noninfectious causes (e.g., immune-mediated, eosinophilic)
- Traumatic myopathies (e.g., accidental, postoperative, downer animals, CNS diseases, seizures)
- Degenerative myopathies (e.g., muscular dystrophy, myotonia, hyperadrenocorticism, hypothyroidism, equine rhabdomyolysis, transport myopathy, malignant hyperthermia, capture myopathy)
- Nutritional myopathies (e.g., vitamin E/selenium deficiency)
- Ischemic myopathies (e.g., bacterial endocarditis, heartworm disease, thrombosis)

Lactate Dehydrogenase

Lactate dehydrogenase (LD) is a serum enzyme that catalyzes the conversion of lactate to pyruvate. Like CK, there are many isoenzymes. Different amounts of isoenzymes are present in different tissues. Almost all tissues have LD, although liver, muscle, and erythrocytes are the major sources of increased blood LD levels. As compared with CK, the magnitude of LD rise is less dramatic following muscle injury.

LD values are frequently included in biochemistry profiles. This enzyme is not considered organ-specific, because it has many sources and the concentrations in each tissue are not high enough to result in significant elevations.

Lactate

Lactate, also referred to as lactic acid, is produced from pyruvate and catalyzed by the enzyme lactate dehydrogenase. Increased levels of lactate are an indication of tissue hypoxia. Lactate values are frequently used to monitor and develop prognostic indicators for critically ill patients. Handheld meters for in-house use are available for lactate testing. Few of these have been validated for veterinary species (Fig. 8-9).

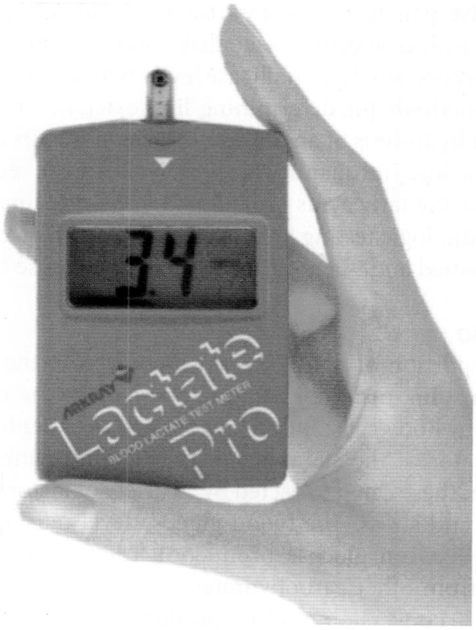

FIGURE 8-9 Handheld lactate meter.

Electrolytes

Electrolytes are minerals that exist as positively charged or negatively charged particles in an aqueous solution. Positively charged particles are called **cations,** and negatively charged particles are called **anions.** These particles play essential roles in processes that are vital to normal physiologic function and life. They function primarily in regulation of acid/base and osmotic balance of the body. There are two commonly used methods of measuring electrolytes: flame photometry and ion-specific electrodes. Flame photometry has been the standard for many years and is still used in some research laboratories. This method measures concentrations of electrolytes relative to the entire plasma volume. Ion-specific electrodes are more widely used and measure the concentration of electrolytes relative to the amount of plasma water. Automated ion-specific instruments are readily available and reasonably priced, so many veterinary practices now have the ability to perform electrolyte testing (Fig. 8-10). Plasma is approximately 93% water, with the remaining percentage composed of lipids and proteins; electrolytes are distributed only in the water phase. Samples that are hyperlipemic or hyperproteinemic may demonstrate reduction in electrolyte activity because of displacement of plasma water by lipids or proteins. Some of the functions of electrolytes include maintenance of water balance and fluid osmotic pressure, normal conduction of nervous impulses, normal contraction of muscles, and maintenance and regulation of body fluid pH. Electrolytes also function as vital cofactors in many enzymatically mediated metabolic reactions.

> **TECHNICIAN NOTE** Electrolyte analyzers used in veterinary practice employ ion-specific electrode methodology.

The electrolytes that are most commonly measured are sodium, potassium, chloride, calcium, inorganic phosphorus, and magnesium. Electrolytes can be measured using serum

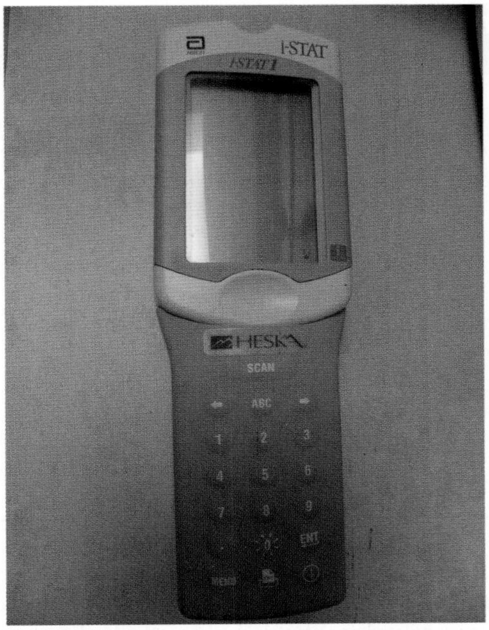

FIGURE 8-10 Electrolyte analyzer for veterinary practice use.

or heparinized plasma. It is important to remember that different salts of heparin are available: sodium heparin, potassium heparin, ammonium heparin, and lithium heparin. When selecting an anticoagulant, do not choose a form of heparin that contains the substance that is being measured.

Sodium

Sodium (Na^+) is the major cation of plasma and interstitial fluid. Plasma and interstitial fluid make up what is known as extracellular fluid. Sodium plays an important role in maintaining extracellular fluid and vascular volume, because it is the most important contributor to effective osmolality. Effective osmolality is a term used to describe the number of particles that cannot easily cross cellular membranes (impermeant particles) in a solution. Effective osmolality is the major factor in determining fluid shifts between intracellular and extracellular fluid. Hyponatremia (decreased sodium) causes hypoosmolality and movement of fluid from the vascular space to the intracellular space. This causes vascular hypovolemia and may result in cellular swelling. Hypernatremia (increased sodium) results in hyperosmolality and movement of intracellular water into the extracellular space, leading to cellular dehydration.

Potassium

Potassium (K^+) is the major intracellular cation. Because potassium is found predominantly intracellularly, the measure of plasma potassium concentration is not necessarily a good indicator of total body potassium. Potassium distribution across the cell membrane is important in normal function of cardiac and neuromuscular tissues. Hypokalemia (decreased potassium) decreases cell excitability, causing weakness and paralysis. Hyperkalemia (increased potassium) increases cell excitability; the most serious manifestation is abnormal cardiac rhythm.

Using potassium heparin as the anticoagulant may result in falsely elevated values. Hemolysis may falsely elevate the results in large animal species (cattle, horses, pigs, some species of sheep) because intraerythrocytic potassium concentrations are higher than potassium concentrations in plasma (or serum). This is not true for cats and most species of dogs. Mild hemolysis in cats and dogs does not affect plasma or serum potassium concentration. One notable exception is the Akita. This breed of dog has high intraerythrocytic potassium concentrations. Platelets and leukocytes have enough intracellular potassium to affect plasma potassium levels only if they are present in markedly increased numbers and the plasma is not separated from the clot quickly.

Chloride

Chloride (Cl^-) is the predominant extracellular anion and is an important component of serum osmolality. It also helps to maintain electroneutrality (equal number of positive and negative charges) for all of the sodium present.

An increase in chloride is termed hyperchloremia; a decrease is termed hypochloremia.

Calcium

Approximately 99% of calcium (Ca^{++}) in the body is found in bones. Only a small percentage of calcium is present in extracellular fluid (including blood), but its presence is essential. Calcium ions are required for preservation of skeletal structure, muscle contraction, blood coagulation, activation of several enzymes, transmission of nerve impulses, and decreasing cell membrane and capillary permeability. Calcium in whole blood is found primarily in plasma (or serum), as erythrocytes contain very little calcium.

An increase in calcium is termed hypercalcemia; a decrease is termed hypocalcemia. Although not a specific indicator of pancreatic function, serum calcium levels are often altered as a result of the acidosis found in many diabetic patients. In normal animals, calcium levels remain fairly constant. Assays for total serum calcium employ photometric methods. Do not use EDTA or oxalate anticoagulants when collecting samples for calcium analysis, because they bind calcium and therefore make it unavailable for assay. Hemolysis may result in a slight decrease because of dilution with erythrocytic fluid.

Inorganic Phosphorus

More than 80% of the phosphorus (P) in the body is found in bones, with less than 20% in extracellular fluids. These extracellular phosphorus ions play an important role in carbohydrate metabolism as metabolic intermediates and high-energy phosphate bonds. Phosphorus is also a component of nucleic acids, phospholipids, nucleotides, and body fluid buffers. Most of the phosphorus in whole blood is found within erythrocytes as organic phosphorus (phosphoric esters). The phosphorus in plasma and serum is inorganic, and it is usually measured in the laboratory.

An increase in phosphorus is termed hyperphosphatemia; a decrease is termed hypophosphatemia.

Magnesium

Magnesium (Mg^{++}) is the fourth most common cation in the body and the second most common intracellular cation. Magnesium is found in all body tissues, although approximately 60% is found in bones. It is an activator (catalyst) for many biological enzymes, and the actions of magnesium extend to all major anabolic and catabolic processes. Magnesium balance is primarily affected by absorption from the gastrointestinal tract and excretion by the kidney. Clinical disorders related to magnesium deficiency are primarily seen in cattle and sheep, although disorders of magnesium metabolism have been reported in cats, horses, and goats.

An increase in magnesium is termed hypermagnesemia; a decrease is termed hypomagnesemia.

BASIC PRINCIPLES OF IMMUNOLOGY

The term immune system refers to a variety of cells, tissues, organs, and organ systems that are involved in the body's defense mechanisms. Some components are present and active in the body at all times. Others are created or activated in response to a foreign substance. Immunity can generally be divided into two types: passive and active. **Passive immunity** includes maternal antibodies from colostrum and physicochemical barriers, such as the skin and mucous membranes. **Active immunity** is developed or acquired and is classified as humoral or cell-mediated immunity. **Humoral immunity** is mediated by production of unique proteins (antibodies), which are responsible for specific recognition and elimination of antigens. Foreign substances that are capable of generating a response from the immune system are referred to as **antigens.** Antigens include bacteria, viruses, parasites, or even the body's own tissues (**autoimmunity**). Specific substances on the surface of the antigen are responsible for the recognition of an antigen by the body's immune system. These substances are usually proteins and act as "markers" for the immune system. Recognition of these markers often results in the formation of antibody by the immune system. When antibodies are produced, the immune system retains a memory of the antigen and can respond more quickly to future attacks by the same antigen. **Cell-mediated immunity** is dependent on cells, in particular lymphocytes. Like antibodies, these lymphocytes recognize specific antigens, such as those of fungi, parasites, intracellular bacteria, or tumor cells, and help remove them from the animal by lysing the infected/cancerous cell or organism (Table 8-3).

Components of the immune system that are present continuously include the skin, mucous membranes, and certain body fluids and cells. These components are collectively referred to as the natural defenses and provide physical and/or chemical barriers to invasion by antigens. The natural defenses generally act in the same manner regardless of which specific antigen is encountered. For example, hydrochloric acid in the stomach or lysozymes in saliva both are capable of destroying bacterial antigens. The action of the hydrochloric acid and lysozymes is similar regardless of the specific bacteria present. Similarly, intact skin acts as a physical barrier to prevent antigens from entering the body.

TABLE 8-3 Humoral Immune Response vs. Cell-Mediated Immune Response

	HUMORAL IMMUNE RESPONSE	CELL-MEDIATED IMMUNE RESPONSE
Cell type involved	B-lymphocyte that transforms into a plasma cell after antigenic stimulation	T-lymphocyte that transforms into a cytotoxic T cell, helper T cell, or suppressor T cell after antigenic stimulation
Substance produced	Immunoglobulins (antibodies)	Lymphokines
Cellular mobility	B-lymphocytes and plasma cells stay in lymphoid tissue; antibodies are released into plasma	T-lymphocytes can enter circulation and travel to the site where an antigen entered the body

Components of the immune system that are involved in reacting to specific antigens include several types of white blood cells and a number of biochemicals. These components are collectively referred to as **adaptive immunity.** The biochemicals are primarily enzyme systems that function in the formation of antibodies. The major enzyme system is known as the complement system. The complement system represents a series of enzymes that must react in a stepwise fashion in order to function. The completion of each step results in generation of additional compounds whose end result will be neutralization or lysis of the antigen. Additional biochemicals are involved in the formation of specific antibodies.

ROLE OF WHITE BLOOD CELLS IN IMMUNITY

Each of the white blood cells (leukocytes) has a specific role within the immune system. Most mammals have two types of white blood cells: granulocytes and agranulocytes.

Granulocytes

Granulocytes play a role in both the natural defenses and the adaptive defenses. Both eosinophils and basophils are involved in the inflammatory response generated when an antigen invades the body. Eosinophils and basophils release specific chemicals to help activate other aspects of the immune system. Neutrophils also play a major role in the immune response. The respiratory, digestive, and urinary systems contain groups of neutrophils, referred to as resident neutrophils, which act as scavengers and function to phagocytize foreign substances. Phagocytosis literally means "cell eating." The neutrophils engulf the antigen and then release chemicals that damage the foreign agent (Fig. 8-11). This phagocytic activity is part of the natural defenses. When these defenses are incapable of fully neutralizing the antigen, the neutrophils become active within the adaptive defenses. Specific neutrophils function in the adaptive defenses by "processing" the antigen and "presenting" it to a cell that is capable of triggering the

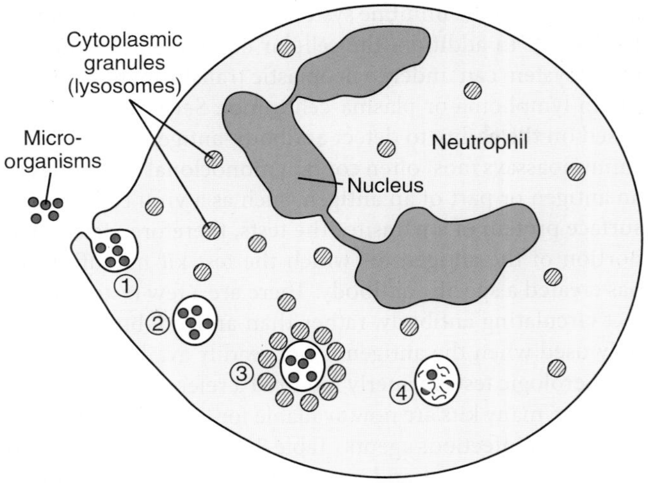

FIGURE 8-11 Phagocytosis and destruction of microorganisms. 1, Neutrophil membrane engulfs microorganisms. 2, Phagocytic vacuole is formed. 3, Cytoplasmic granules (lysosomes) line up around phagocytic vacuole and empty their digestive enzymes into vacuole. 4, Microorganisms are destroyed. (From Colville T, Bassert JM: *Clinical anatomy and physiology for veterinary technicians*, ed 3, St Louis, 2016, Mosby.)

cascade of reactions that result in antibody formation. Antigen processing is a complex process that results in exposure of the surface marker protein on the antigen. This allows for recognition of the antigen as a foreign substance. The neutrophil then interacts with another cell that will respond by triggering additional parts of the adaptive defenses.

Agranulocytes

Monocytes and lymphocytes each have unique roles within the immune system. Monocytes act in a manner similar to phagocytic neutrophils. They are often referred to as tissue macrophages and are capable of phagocytosis, and antigen processing and presentation. Lymphocytes are the primary cellular components of the antibody-producing systems. Specific subpopulations or subgroups of lymphocytes each play a specific role in this process. These subgroups are referred to as T-lymphocytes and B-lymphocytes. Although there are no apparent differences in appearance of the cells in different subgroups, they are biochemically and functionally diverse groups that are derived and matured in different ways and in different locations in the body.

T-lymphocytes are involved in assisting in full activation of B-lymphocytes (although B-lymphocytes can be activated without this interaction). B-lymphocytes are responsible for creation and secretion of antibody that is specific for a certain antigen. The process is triggered when an antigen-presenting cell (e.g., macrophage or neutrophil) presents an antigen to a B-lymphocyte. That specific B-lymphocyte then is sensitized to that particular antigen and begins to synthesize and release antibody. B-lymphocytes have an additional capability of memory. As B-lymphocytes are maturing, they develop with the capability of producing antibody against a specific antigen that has been presented to them during their maturation. When an antigen that has been previously encountered by a B-lymphocyte is encountered again, the B-lymphocyte is able to respond more quickly and begin producing antibody almost immediately. The production of specific antibody is referred to as humoral immunity because the antibody is secreted into the body fluids, or humors. T-lymphocytes, in addition to their role in the activation of B-lymphocytes, are also capable of direct attack on antigens. This is referred to as cellular immunity.

TABLE 8-4 Functions of the Classes of Immunoglobulins

IMMUNOGLOBULIN CLASS	FUNCTION
IgG	Neutralization of microbes and toxins; Opsonization of microbes for phagocytosis by macrophages and neutrophils; Activation of complement; Fetal and neonatal immunity by passive transfer across placenta and in colostrums
IgM	Activation of complement
IgE	Immediate hypersensitivity reactions, such as allergies and anaphylactic shock; Coating of helminth parasites for destruction by eosinophils
IgA	Mucosal immunity; Protection of respiratory, intestinal, and urogenital tracts
IgD	B-lymphocyte surface antigen receptor in some species

Antibodies

The production of a specific antibody is a critical part of the immune system response. Antibodies are protein molecules produced by a certain subgroup of B-lymphocytes when they are presented with a substance that is recognized as foreign (the antigen).

Antibodies are also referred to as immunoglobulins and are present in several forms in the body. Each type is responsible for a specific activity within the immune system (Table 8-4). The five types of antibodies are referred to with the abbreviation Ig (for immunoglobulin) followed by a letter that designates the type of antibody (Fig. 8-12). The five types of antibodies found in most mammalian organisms are IgG, IgM, IgA, IgD, and IgE.

Each antibody is produced at a specific time in the immune system response. Some are also produced when certain types of antigens are involved (e.g., parasites). An immunoassay is any test that uses interactions between antibody and antigen to produce a result. Commercial production of monoclonal antibodies to many different antigens has resulted in a variety of test kits for use in the veterinary laboratory. These specific antibodies to many different antigens can be produced and used in the laboratory for rapid identification of disease-producing organisms. In general these tests are very easy to perform, take minimal time, and are relatively inexpensive.

The antigens are usually present in the blood, so the sample used for immunoassays is often a blood sample. Depending on the test being used, the sample may be whole, anticoagulated blood, serum, or plasma. A few immunoassays

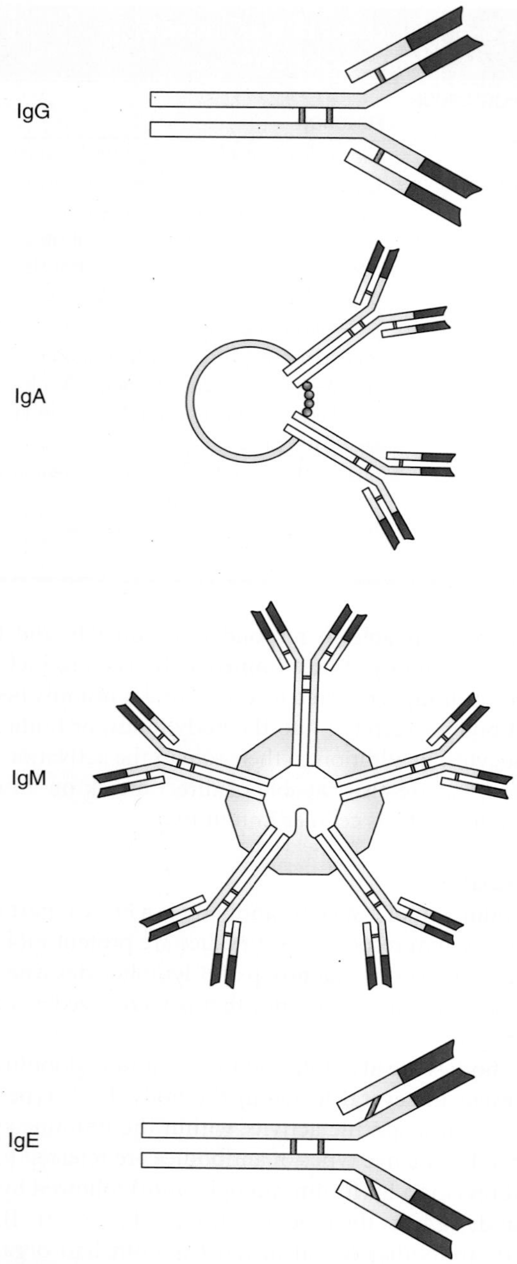

FIGURE 8-12 Schematic representation of IgM (pentamer), IgG and IgE (monomers), and IgA (dimer).

may use urine, feces, or saliva as the sample. With a few exceptions, in-house immunologic test kits use enzyme-linked immunosorbent assay (ELISA) or immunochromatography (ICT) assay methods. It is vital that veterinary technicians understand the principles of these in-house immunologic tests to avoid false results.

TYPES OF IMMUNOLOGIC TESTS

Dysfunction of the immune system can lead to an overactive immune system that produces immune-mediated disease, or an underactive immune system that produces immunodeficiency disorders. These disorders can involve any component of the immune system (passive, humoral, or cell-mediated). In addition, the cellular components of the immune system can undergo neoplastic transformation, resulting in lymphoma or plasma-cell tumor. Serologic testing is based on the ability to detect antibody-antigen interactions. Immunoassays most often contain monoclonal antibodies to an antigen or part of an antigen, such as a viral capsule or a surface protein of a parasite. The tests, therefore, detect that portion of the antigen for which the test kit manufacturer has created a specific antibody. There are a few tests that detect circulating antibody, rather than antigen, but these are only used when the antigen is not readily available for testing. Serologic tests formerly required a reference laboratory; however, many kits are now available for in-house testing for a variety of infectious agents (Table 8-5). Many kits are based on ELISA technology and may detect either antigens (organism) or antibodies (humoral immune response), depending on the kit.

> TECHNICIAN NOTE ELISA tests are the most common immunoassays performed in clinical practice.

ENZYME-LINKED IMMUNOSORBENT ASSAY

ELISA tests are the most common types of immunologic tests performed in veterinary clinics. Every ELISA test has the same basic components:

- solid phase
- conjugate
- chromogen

The solid phase may be a microwell, wand, flow-through membrane, or chromatographic strip. Conjugate reagents are imbedded on the solid phase and usually consist of monoclonal antibodies bound to an enzyme. The chromogen is a photosensitive reagent that produces a color change in the test system. Adding patient sample to the solid phase is the first step in the test. The sample is allowed to incubate. If specific antigen is present in the sample, it will bind to the antibody on the test surface. After the appropriate incubation time, the patient sample is washed away. If antigen has bound to the solid phase, it will not be washed away. Chromogen is then added that can react with the bound enzyme-antigen-antibody complex, if present, and produce a color change in the test system (Fig. 8-13). There are a few ELISA tests that are designed to detect antibodies in the patient samples. In those cases, the antigen is usually what is bound on the solid phase.

ELISA technology has been adapted to detect multiple types of components in serum, including cell surface markers and hormones.

RAPID IMMUNOMIGRATION (RIM)

The rapid immunomigration assay (also known as immunochromatography) is similar to the ELISA method except that gold staining is used to replace the chromogen. This format has become more common in veterinary practice in recent years. In these test formats, also known as lateral flow assays, the conjugate is an antibody bound to colloidal gold or

TABLE 8-5 Commercially Available Immunologic Test Kits

DISEASE/CONDITION	PRODUCT NAME	MANUFACTURER	TYPE OF TEST	USE
Bile acids test	SNAP Bile Acids*†	IDEXX	ELISA	For measurement of serum bile acids
Blood group test	RapidVet-H	DMS Laboratories	Agglutination	To classify dogs as DEA 1 (+) or (-) or cats types A, B, or AB
	RapidVet-H IC	DMS Laboratories	Immunochromatography	To cats as types A, B, or AB
Borreliosis, heartworm, anaplasmosis, and ehrlichiosis	SNAP 4 Dx Plus	IDEXX	ELISA	For detection of heartworm antigen or *Borrelia burgdorferi, Anaplasma phagocytophilum/Anaplasma platys* or *Ehrlichia canis/Ehrlichia ewingii* antibodies
Borreliosis, heartworm, and ehrlichiosis	SNAP 3 Dx Test	IDEXX	ELISA	For detection of *Borrelia burgdorferi* antibodies, heartworm antigens, and *Ehrlichia canis* antibodies in dogs
Bovine viral diarrhea virus	1SNAP BVDV	IDEXX	ELISA	For detection of high levels of bovine viral diarrhea virus antigen in ear-notch and serum samples
Brucellosis	D-Tec CB	Synbiotics	Latex agglutination	For detection of antibodies to *Brucella canis* in dogs
Canine pancreas specific lipase	SNAPcPL	IDEXX	ELISA	For evaluation of the level of pancreas-specific lipase in dogs
Cortisol	SNAP Cortisol*†	IDEXX	ELISA	For evaluation of cortisol level in dogs
Ehrlichiosis	WITNESS Ehrlichia	Synbiotics	Rapid Immunomigration	For detection *Ehrlicia canis* antibody in dogs
Equine infectious anemia	AGID EIA Ab	IDEXX	Agar gel immunodiffusion	For detection of infectious anemia antibodies in horses
	CELISA EIA	IDEXX	CELISA antibody test kit	
Failure of passive transfer	SNAP Foal IgG Test Kit	IDEXX	ELISA	For semiquantitative measurement of IgG levels in equine serum or whole blood
Feline heartworm, leukemia virus, and immunodeficiency virus	SNAP Feline Triple	IDEXX	ELISA	For detection of heartworm antigen, feline leukemia virus antigens and FIV antibodies in cats
Feline infectious peritonitis	Virachek/CV	Synbiotics	ELISA	For detection of antibodies to feline corona virus in cats
Feline leukemia virus	Assure/FeLV	Synbiotics	ELISA	For detection of feline leukemia virus antigens in cats
	SNAP FeLV antigen test kit	IDEXX	ELISA	
	Virachek/FeLV	Synbiotics	ELISA	
	WITNESS FeLV	Synbiotics	Rapid Immunomigration lateral flow immunoassay	
Feline leukemia virus and immunodeficiency virus	SNAP FIV/FELV Combo	IDEXX	ELISA	For detection of feline leukemia virus antigens and FIV antibodies in cats
	WITNESS FeLV-FIV	Synbiotics	Rapid Immunomigration lateral flow immunoassay	
Feline pancreas specific lipase	SNAP fPL	IDEXX	ELISA	For evaluation of the level of pancreas-specific lipase in cats
Giardia	SNAP Giardia	IDEXX	ELISA	For detection of *Giardia lamblia* antigen in dogs and cats

Continued

TABLE 8-5 Commercially Available Immunologic Test Kits—cont'd

DISEASE/CONDITION	PRODUCT NAME	MANUFACTURER	TYPE OF TEST	USE
Heartworm infection	Petchek	IDEXX	ELISA	For detection of heartworm antigens in dogs
	Dirochek	Synbiotics	ELISA	For detection of heartworm antigens in dogs and cats
	Heska Solo Step FH & CH	Heska	Lateral flow immunoassay	For detection of heartworm antibodies in cats and antigens in dogs
	SNAP Heartworm RT Test	IDEXX	ELISA	For detection of heartworm antigens in dogs
	Witness HW	Synbiotics	ELISA	For detection of heartworm antigens in dogs and cats
Leishmaniasis	WITNESS Leishmania	Synbiotics	Rapid Immunomigration lateral flow immunoassay	For detection of *Leishmania infantum* antibodies in dogs
Microalbumin	E.R.D.-Health Screen	Heska	ELISA	For detection of low levels of albumin in urine of dogs and cats
Neospora caninum	Neospora X2 Ab	IDEXX	ELISA	For detection of antibodies to *Neospora caninum* in bovine serum
Newcastle disease	NDV ab	IDEXX	ELISA	For detection of antibodies to Newcastle disease virus in chicken serum
	NDV-T Ab	IDEXX	ELISA	For detection of antibodies to Newcastle disease virus in turkey serum
Ovulation timing	WITNESS-LH	Synbiotics	Rapid Immunomigration lateral flow immunoassay	For the semiquantitative measurement of luteinizing hormone levels in dogs and cats
Paratuberculosis (Johne's disease)	MAP Ab test	IDEXX	ELISA	For detection of antibody to *Mycobacterium avium* subsp. *paratuberculosis* in bovine milk, serum or plasma
Parvovirus infection	SNAP Parvo test	IDEXX	ELISA	For detection of parvovirus antigens in canine feces
	ASSURE/Parvo	Synbiotics	ELISA	
	WITNESS CPV	Synbiotics	Rapid Immunomigration lateral flow immunoassay	
Porcine reproductive and respiratory syndrome	PRRS X3 Ab	IDEXX	ELISA	For detection of PRRS antibodies in porcine serum or plasma samples
Pregnancy, canine	Relaxin	Synbiotics	RIM	For detection of pregnancy by measurement of relaxin
Progesterone	Ovuchek Premate	Synbiotics	ELISA	For the determination of progesterone in canine serum
Pseudorabies	PRV/ADV gB Ab	IDEXX	ELISA	For detection of antibodies to the gB antigen of pseudorabies virus in pig serum
	PRV/ADV gI Ab	IDEXX	ELISA	For detection of antibodies to the gI (gE) antigen of pseudorabies virus in pig serum
Rheumatoid arthritis	Synbiotics CRF (canine rheumatoid factor)	Synbiotics	Latex agglutination	For detection of rheumatoid arthritis factor in canine serum
Salmonellosis	SE Ab test	IDEXX	ELISA	For detection of antibodies to *Salmonella enteritidis* in chicken serum or egg yolk
Thyroxine	SNAP Total T4 Test† SNAP T4*	IDEXX	ELISA	For measurement of total thyroxine in dogs, cats, and horses

*Requires use of the SNAP Reader Analyzer.
†Requires use of the SNAPshot Dx Analyzer.

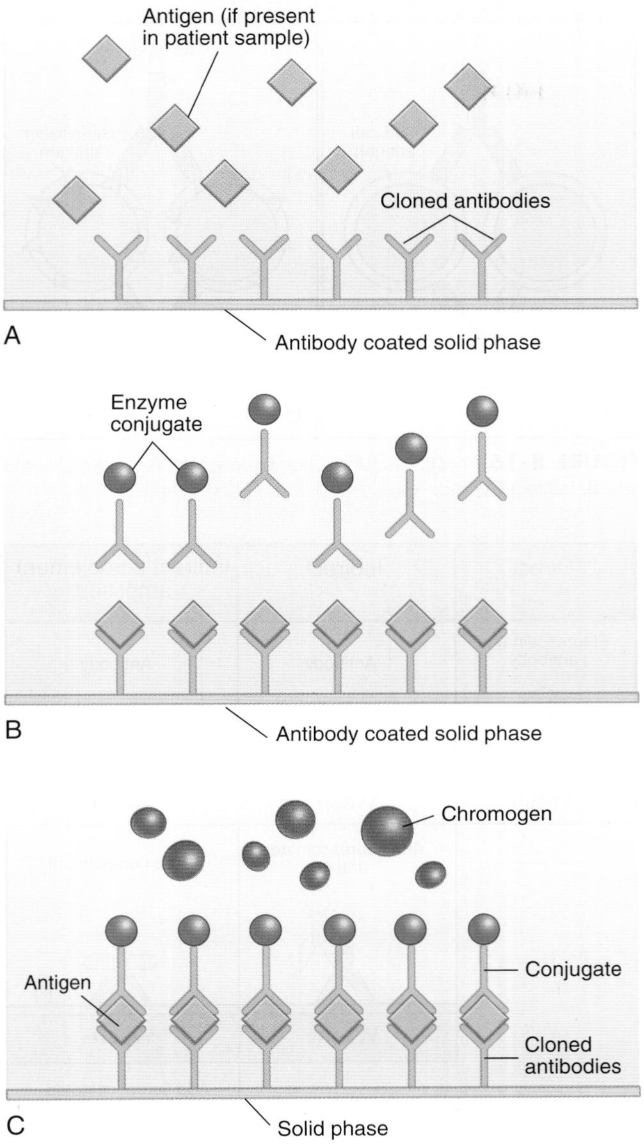

FIGURE 8-13 Principle of ELISA reaction.

latex, instead of an enzyme. The solid phase of a RIM test is a chromatographic strip. Most RIM tests require a flow solution, usually a buffered saline, to aid in the movement of the sample across the chromatographic strip. Some RIM tests do not require flow solution because the sample volume is large enough to flow onto the solid phase without additional steps. The RIM method does not use temperature-sensitive enzymes, so the test kit can be kept at room temperature.

Chromatographic strips have been used for many years in reference laboratories in the performance of certain serum chemistry assays. The RIM test is performed by adding a patient sample to the absorptive pad on the solid phase. The absorptive pad functions to absorb the sample and filter out solid substances, such as blood cells. The conjugate is released as the sample flows onto the solid phase. The sample and conjugate then pass across two test areas. The first test area, known as the patient line, contains antibodies to the

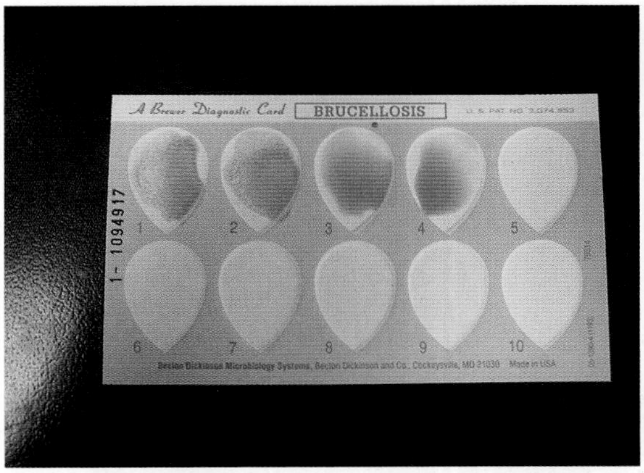

FIGURE 8-14 Clumped latex particles representing antigen-antibody complexes. Samples 1 and 2 indicate a positive reaction. Samples 3 and 4, showing no clumping, indicate a negative reaction.

antigen that the test is designed to detect. If the antigen is present in the sample, it will bind to the antibodies on the patient line. When that occurs, conjugate also reacts and produces a color change on the patient line. The sample and conjugate continue to flow to the second test area. The second area is a control line that contains antibodies to the conjugate. A color change is produced on this line and indicates that the test is functioning correctly.

AGGLUTINATION TEST

Agglutination tests are used for detection of antibodies to large particulate antigens. The test requires adding a specific antigen to the test sample. If the sample contains the antibody for that antigen, **agglutination** (clumping) occurs.

In some agglutination tests, the antigen may be coated with latex beads to induce agglutination reactions. Agglutination tests are usually performed on a slide. Latex agglutination is commonly used to diagnose brucellosis in dogs. Latex particles are coated with *Brucella* antigen. Serum from the patient is added to these particles. If the animal's serum contains antibodies to *Brucella,* they form complexes with the latex particles, causing agglutination (Fig. 8-14). The serum can further be manipulated to detect separate classes (IgG versus IgM) of antibody. Other kits using this methodology include blood typing tests and tests for organisms that cause mastitis and for canine rheumatoid factor.

PRECIPITATION TESTS

There are three major types of precipitation tests: immunodiffusion, radioimmunodiffusion, and immunoelectrophoresis. Several types of electrophoresis procedures are performed. These are primarily performed in reference or referral laboratories, rather than in clinical practice.

Immunodiffusion

The **immunodiffusion** method is used to test for equine infectious anemia. This is commonly referred to as the Coggins test. The test requires an agar plate with wells cut into it. The wells contain patient sample, a positive control, and negative control. If specific antibody is present in the sample,

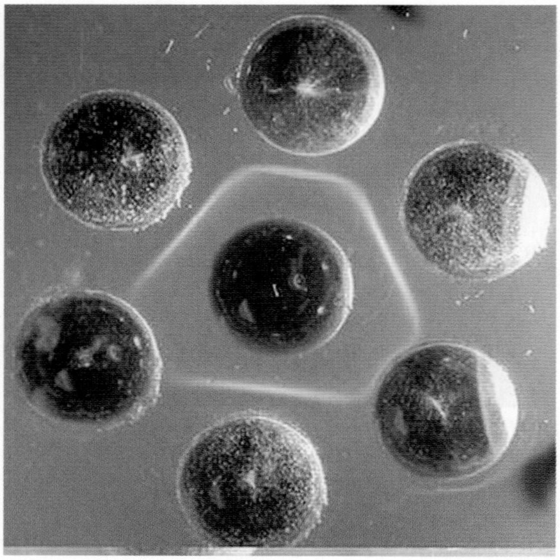

FIGURE 8-15 Agar plate showing lines of precipitation. No lines of precipitation are evident near negative patient wells.

precipitate forms where the diffusing antigen (positive control) and antibody meet (Fig. 8-15).

Radioimmunoassay

The radioimmunoassay is usually performed in research laboratories rather than clinical practice. The principle is similar to ELISA except that a radioisotope is used in place of the conjugate. This procedure can detect either antigen or antibody. The amount of radiation detected equates to a volume of antigen or antibody present in the sample.

COOMBS TEST

The **Coombs test** is used to detect auto-antibodies (antibodies to one's own tissues). The test detects immunoglobulin (IgG or IgM) or complement (C3) bound to the surface of RBCs. There are two types of Coombs tests. The indirect Coombs detects circulating auto-antibodies. The direct Coombs test is used for diagnosis of hemolytic disease. In the direct Coombs test, RBCs from the patient are incubated with a species-specific antiglobulin reagent. The sample is then evaluated for agglutination (irregular clumps of 3 to 5 or more RBCs). Agglutination occurs if the erythrocytes have enough antibody or complement on their surface to allow cross-linking between the cells (Fig. 8-16). Although the Coombs test is fairly simple to perform, the expense of stocking the species-specific Coombs reagent for only occasional tests makes it impractical to run in-house. The tests are usually sent to an outside reference laboratory.

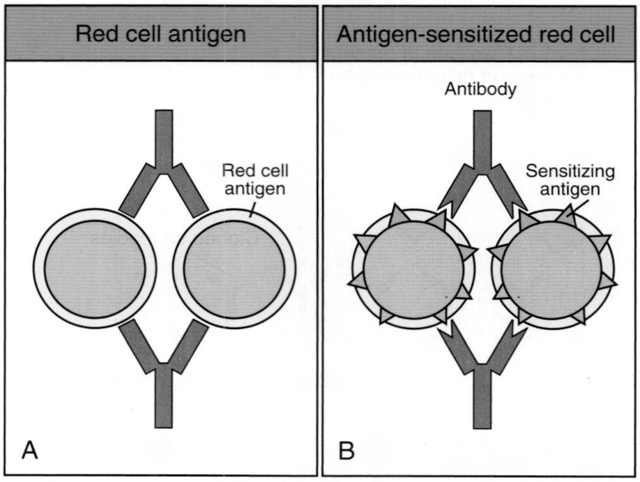

FIGURE 8-16 Principles of the Coombs reaction. **A,** Direct Coombs test. **B,** Indirect Coombs test.

FLUORESCENT ANTIBODY TESTS

Although not commonly performed in veterinary practices, fluorescent testing is available at most veterinary reference laboratories. These test procedures are frequently used to verify a tentative diagnosis made by the veterinarian. Two methods are available—direct and indirect antibody testing—both of which detect the presence of specific antibody or antigen in a sample (Fig. 8-17)

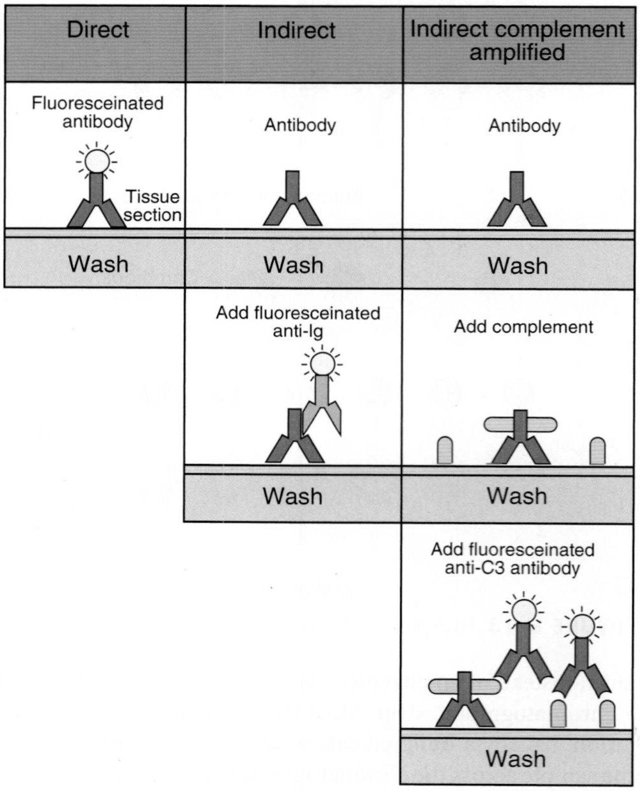

FIGURE 8-17 Fluorescent antibody technique.

INTRADERMAL SKIN TESTING

Patients with allergic skin diseases may be diagnosed with a combination of clinical signs and exclusion of suspected allergens or may require immunologic intradermal testing. Common causes of allergic skin disease include food allergy, contact dermatitis, insect bites and stings, inhalant allergy (e.g., pollen, mold), and atopy. Allergies are mediated by IgE antibody molecules and can be detected by using allergenic extracts of grasses, trees, weed pollens, molds, dust, insects, and other possibly offending antigens. The extracts are injected intradermally, and the injection sites are monitored for allergic reactions. A positive reaction appears as a raised welt, meaning that the animal is allergic to that antigen.

TUBERCULIN SKIN TEST

The tuberculin skin test involves a cell-mediated immune reaction. Animals infected with *Mycobacterium tuberculosis, M. bovis,* and *M. avium* bacteria develop characteristic delayed **hypersensitivity** reactions when exposed to purified derivatives of the organism called tuberculin. In the tuberculin skin test, tuberculin is injected intradermally at a site in the cervical region or in a skin fold at the base of the tail in large animals. A delayed local inflammatory reaction is observed if the animal has been exposed to *Mycobacterium* organisms. The reaction to injection is delayed because a day or more passes before the T-lymphocytes migrate to the foreign antigen injected into the dermis.

ANTIBODY TITERS

Results of some antibody tests may be reported as positive or negative. In other words, the test indicates the presence or absence of antibody to the particular infectious agent in the patient's serum. Results of other antibody tests may be reported as antibody **titers,** or levels. The patient's serum is serially diluted to different concentrations, such as 1:10, 1:40, and 1:160, meaning 1 part serum in 9 parts saline, 1 part serum in 39 parts saline, and 1 part serum in 159 parts saline, respectively. A test to detect antibodies (e.g., hemagglutination test, complement-fixation test, or IFA test) is done on each of these dilutions, and the greatest dilution that tests positive is reported. For example, if 1:10 and 1:40 are positive and 1:160 is negative, the titer is reported as 1:40. If none of the dilutions is positive, the titer may be reported as negative or the test may be repeated at lesser dilutions, such as 1:2, 1:4, or 1:8. A higher titer (positive at greater dilutions) indicates that more antibody is present. More antibody is present in a sample with a titer of 1:160 than in a sample with a titer of 1:40.

Note that antibody titers are conventionally expressed in terms of dilution. It is important to note that when measuring titers of antibodies to infectious agents, they are typically measured in two samples collected over a 2- to 4-week period to assess for a fourfold increase in antibody titer. An antibody titer in a single sample may indicate only that the animal has been previously exposed to an infectious agent; the animal may not currently have an active infection. A rising titer in two or more samples indicates an active infection. Usually it is best to run both titers at the same time to minimize the error in measuring antibody at two different times. This requires that the first sample is drawn, separated, frozen, and stored in such a way that it can be easily retrieved when the second sample is collected.

MOLECULAR DIAGNOSTICS

A large variety of diagnostic tests are now available that use analysis of DNA or RNA. The most widely used type of molecular diagnostic test is the **polymerase chain reaction** (PCR). The PCR test involves identification of a DNA segment, and replication of the segment, followed by separation on electrophoretic gel. The technique can be used to detect the presence of specific antigens in a sample (Table 8-6) but has numerous additional applications in veterinary medicine (Table 8-7).

TABLE 8-6 Molecular Diagnostic Tests for Veterinary Pathogens

ORGANISM	SUGGESTED SAMPLES
Bacillus anthracis	Blood
BVD1, BVD2	Lymph nodes, spleen, serum
Chlamydia spp.	Placenta, liver
Clostridium perfringens	Isolated colony from bacterial culture
Escherichia coli virulence	Isolated colony from bacterial culture typing panel
Leptospira spp.	Urine, liver, kidney
Mycobacterium paratuberculosis	Intestinal mucosa, mesenteric lymph nodes
PPRS virus	Serum, spleen, lung
Salmonella spp.	Intestinal mucosa, feces, other tissues
West Nile virus	Kidney, heart, brain, liver, spleen

BVD, Bovine viral diarrhea virus.
PRRS, Porcine reproductive and respiratory syndrome.

TABLE 8-7 Selected Veterinary DNA Tests

ANIMAL	TEST	TEST SAMPLE
Bird	Bird sexing	Blood or freshly plucked feathers
Dog	DNA banking and profiling	Buccal swab (for animal identification)
Dog	Inherited disease screening	Buccal swab
Dog	Parentage verification	Buccal swab
Horse	DNA banking (for animal identification)	15-20 hairs pulled from mane, including hair root bulbs
Horse	Hyperkalemic periodic paralysis screening	15-20 hairs pulled from mane, including hair root bulbs
Cat	DNA banking and profiling	Buccal swab (for animal identification)
Cat	Parentage verification	Buccal swab
Cat	Polycystic kidney disease	Buccal swab

COMMON ERRORS AND ARTIFACTS

In spite of what may seem like very simplistic technology, the proper performance of the tests is vital to ensuring accurate results. Each test method mentioned has specific advantages and limitations. However, if the test is not performed correctly, a number of other factors can produce false-positive or false-negative results. A false-positive result is a positive test result on a sample from a patient that is in fact negative for the antigen. A false-negative result is a negative test result on a sample from a patient that is in fact positive for the antigen. Many immunoassays incorporate controls that help determine the accuracy of the test results. A visible positive control indicates that the test kit is functional. The most common causes of false results are poor sample quality, inadequate washing (ELISA tests), improper incubation, cross-reacting proteins, or expired or improperly stored kits.

Although it is uncommon, an ELISA test may produce false results when the patient sample contains very high levels of antigen and/or antibody. A patient can be exhibiting a very strong immune response and be producing high levels of antibody. It is possible for these antibodies to bind all the antigen in the sample so that none is available for binding to the solid phase.

SAMPLE QUALITY

Manufacturers of immunoassays usually provide very specific information on the type of sample required for proper test performance. In most cases, the use of hemolyzed or lipemic samples will lead to ambiguous or erroneous test results. Hemolysis and lipemia can interfere with the absorption and flow of sample on an RIM test and can create background color on both RIM and ELISA tests that complicate interpretation of results.

WASHING

Each of the common in-house test methods (ELISA and RIM) function on the premise that conjugate binds to the antigen from the patient sample that has bound to the antibody of the solid phase. At that point in the test, nothing short of a major chemical reaction can break the bond between the antigen-antibody complex.

This is a critical feature of an ELISA test because the next step in the test is usually the wash step. The purpose of the wash step is to remove any unbound sample and conjugate. If any unbound conjugate remains after the wash step, it will react with the chromogen and produce a false-positive result. It is impossible to overwash an ELISA test system. However, underwashing is the most common cause of false-positive results. In addition to the positive control mentioned above, ELISA tests also contain negative controls. No color in the negative control indicates that the wash step was adequate and no known cross-reacting substances are present. A few test kits state that the positive control should merely be of greater color intensity than the negative control. However, any color development in the negative control indicates that the washing step may have been inadequate. Some ELISA tests have the wash step built into the system. The SNAP test is a membrane-ELISA test that contains wash solution within the test unit (Fig. 8-18). The wash solution is released when the test unit is "snapped." This minimizes the possibility of false-positive results from inadequate washing of the test system.

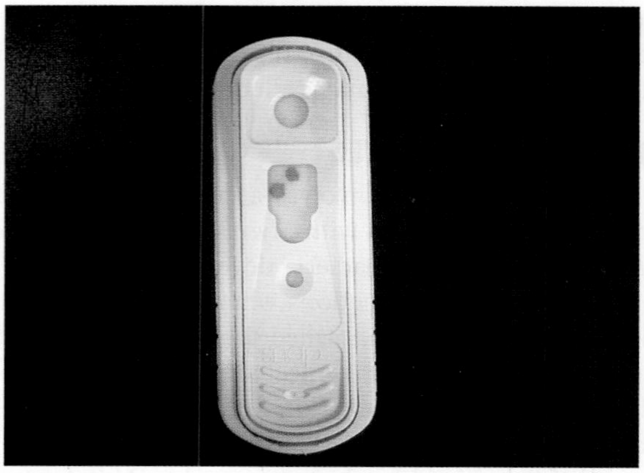

FIGURE 8-18 SNAP Test for *Ehrlichia* antibodies. A positive test result indicated on the ELISA membrane format. A positive control spot is also seen.

INCUBATION

Test incubation times are established to give optimum accuracy. Not waiting the full time may decrease the sensitivity of the test (i.e., the ability to detect positives) and lead to false-negative results. Overincubation may lead to false-positive results. The final incubation period is particularly important. It is possible that very small amounts of chromogen may remain after the wash step. The conjugate can continue to react with the chromogen and generate color after the normal incubation period. A test that is negative at the end of the incubation period and then appears positive even a few minutes later is still considered a negative test result.

STORAGE

The enzyme-conjugate reagent used in ELISA tests requires refrigeration. Improper storage of the kit (i.e., storage at room temperature) can inactivate the reagent and lead to false-negative results. However, it is crucial that the ELISA kit be warmed to room temperature before use. The reaction between the enzyme-conjugate and the chromogen is temperature-dependent. When the enzyme-conjugate is at a lower than normal temperature, the reaction with the chromogen will be delayed and the incubation period will not be sufficient to detect a positive result.

CHOOSING A TEST KIT

There are numerous parameters to consider when choosing a diagnostic test kit. Cost is often a primary factor. Microwell ELISA tests tend to be less expensive and more accurate than other ELISA methods. Membrane ELISA tests are more expensive but somewhat easier to carry out. Test accuracy should also be a primary concern when choosing a test kit. No test is 100% accurate. The test manufacturer provides data on sensitivity and specificity of the test. Sensitivity refers to the ability of the test to yield positive results on a sample that is in fact positive. Specificity refers to the ability to yield negative results on a sample that is in fact negative. Predictive value is a term used to describe the percentage of false-positive and false-negative results that are obtained with a particular test. Predictive value is a function of both test sensitivity and specificity as well as the prevalence of the antigen in the test population. For example, most heartworm antigen tests kits are approximately 95% sensitive and 99% specific. If the prevalence of heartworm disease in dogs is 1% (i.e., 1 in 100 dogs has the antigen), the test is likely to detect the 1 animal in 100 that has the antigen. However, because the specificity is 99%, there is a chance that 1 in 100 animals tested will yield a false-positive result. When the disease prevalence is higher, say 5%, the same test sensitivity and specificity will most likely detect all 5 positive patients in 100. However, the 99% specificity still will likely yield 1 in 100 false-positive results. That is, for every 100 patients tested, 6 positive results will likely be obtained. There will be 5 true positives and 1 false positive. Therefore, as the prevalence of a specific antigen in the population increases, the incidence of false-positive results decreases.

TEST SIGNIFICANCE

The results of immunoassays are only one part of the information the veterinarian considers when making a diagnosis. Physical examination results, patient history, and test results are all part of the diagnostic process. The veterinary technician must be able to provide accurate and reliable test results to aid the veterinarian in determining the diagnosis and prognosis for the patient.

For many years, the only means available for completing immunologic examination in animals was to submit samples to referral and reference laboratories. This often delayed the diagnosis and treatment of the patient. The ready availability of accurate, reliable in-house immunoassays has greatly improved service to our clients and patients.

REVIEW QUESTIONS

Matching

Match each of the following functions with its corresponding immunoglobulin.

______1. Coating of helminth parasites for destruction by eosinophils	A. IgG
______2. Neutralization of microbes and toxins	B. IgM
______3. Fetal and neonatal immunity by passive transfer across placenta and in colostrums	C. IgE
______4. Protection of respiratory, intestinal, and urogenital tracts	D. IgA
______5. Mucosal immunity	E. IgD
______6. Activation of complement	
______7. Immediate hypersensitivity reactions, such as allergies and anaphylactic shock	

Fill in the Blank

Provide answers to complete the following statements.

1. Bile acids are produced from _______in the liver.
2. Conjugated bilirubin is also referred to as _____ *bilirubin.*
3. Urobilinogen is broken down to _______ before being excreted in feces.
4. Globulins are a complex group of proteins that include all of the plasma proteins other than _____ and coagulation proteins.
5. Cholestatic tests include ________________ and gamma glutamyl transferase (GGT).
6. In Dalmatian dogs, the liver is unable to convert ____ to allantoin.
7. Amylase is produced in a variety of tissues, including the ___________, _______ _____________, and ___________.
8. The primary ketone produced in ketoacidosis is ________________.
9. ___________is a serum enzyme that catalyzes the conversion of lactate to pyruvate.
10. ________ values are frequently used to monitor and develop prognostic indicators for critically ill patients.
11. _________ is the major cation of plasma and interstitial fluid.
12. _______is the predominant extracellular anion and is an important component of serum osmolality.
13. The _______ system represents a series of enzymes that must react in a stepwise fashion in order to function.
14. The respiratory, digestive, and urinary systems contain groups of neutrophils, referred to as__________ , which act as scavengers and function to phagocytize foreign substances.
15. _________ are often referred to as *tissue macrophages* and are capable of phagocytosis, and antigen processing and presentation

Choose the Best Response

Choose the best answer to the following questions.

1. Which artifactual change is most likely to occur if the serum is not separated from the clot within about 2 hours of blood collection?
   a. increased chloride concentration
   b. decreased glucose concentration
   c. decreased phosphorus concentration
   d. decreased potassium concentration
2. An elevation in BUN as a result of dehydration is referred to as:
   a. prerenal azotemia
   b. renal azotemia
   c. postrenal azotemia
   d. azoturia
3. Which sample type is best for blood calcium analysis?
   a. EDTA plasma
   b. serum or EDTA plasma
   c. serum or heparinized plasma
   d. serum or oxalated plasma
4. The predominant plasma protein is:
   a. fibrinogen
   b. albumin
   c. IgG
   d. creatinine

5. The Coombs test is used to diagnose:
   a. combined immunodeficiency
   b. immune-mediated hemolytic anemia
   c. systemic lupus erythematosus
   d. feline infectious peritonitis
6. Regarding antibody titers, which statement is most accurate?
   a. Results are reported as either positive or negative.
   b. The higher the dilution, the more antibody is in the sample.
   c. A single, high-dilution titer (1:160 or above) is indicative of an active infection.
   d. The higher the dilution, the harder the immunologist has to look to find antibody in the sample.
7. What effect does an icteric sample have on total plasma protein determination by refractometry?
   a. No effect
   b. Slightly increased value
   c. Decreased value
   d. Markedly increased value
8. Assay for which of the following is used to assess carbohydrate metabolism?
   a. Fibrogen
   b. GGT
   c. Bile acids
   d. Glucose
9. The preferred site for blood collection in animals is:
   a. cephalic vein
   b. jugular vein
   c. saphenous vein
   d. femoral vein
10. Samples collected with heparin anticoagulant are unsuitable for ___ analysis.
   a. electrolyte
   b. glucose
   c. enzyme
   d. urea

RECOMMENDED READING

Abbas AK: *Cellular and molecular immunology*, ed 8, Philadelphia, 2014, Saunders.

Male D: *Immunology*, ed 8, St Louis, 2012, Mosby.

Sirois M: *Laboratory procedures for veterinary technicians*, ed 6, St Louis, 2014, Mosby.

Sodikoff C: *Laboratory profiles of small animal diseases*, ed 3, St Louis, 2001, Mosby.

Tizard IR: *Veterinary immunology: an introduction*, ed 9, Philadelphia, 2013, Saunders.

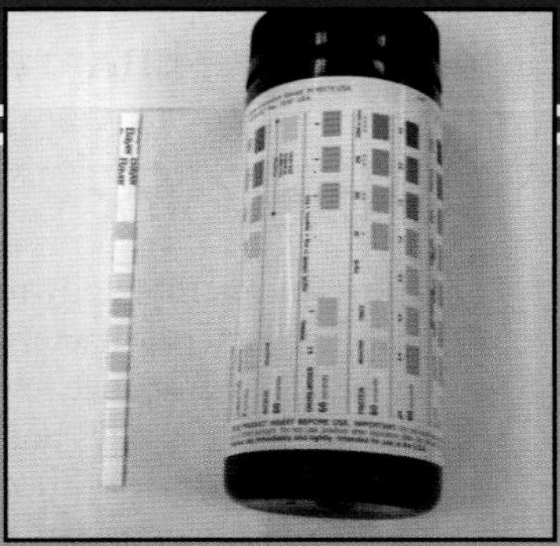

9 Microbiology, Cytology, and Urinalysis

OUTLINE

LEARNING OBJECTIVES

After reviewing this chapter, the reader will be able to:

1. List and describe methods used to collect samples of body tissues and fluids for laboratory examination.
2. Describe methods used to prepare diagnostic samples for laboratory examination.
3. List and describe microbiologic tests commonly performed to identify bacterial, fungal, and viral pathogens.
4. Discuss procedures used in cytologic examination of body tissues and fluids.
5. List tests commonly performed in analyzing urine specimens.
6. Describe techniques of sample collection and processing for cytology and microbiology samples.
7. Identify common normal cells in cytology samples.
8. Identify common abnormal cells in cytology samples.
9. Describe methods for differentiation of inflammatory and neoplastic cytology samples.

KEY TERMS

Acid-fast
Alpha hemolysis
Anuria
Bacilli
Bacteriology
Benign
Beta hemolysis
Biopsy
Blood agar
Capnophilic
Carcinoma
Cast
Catalase
Centesis
Cocci
Dermatophyte
Differential media
Enriched media
Exudate
Granulomatous
Hematuria
Hemoglobinuria
Histopathology
Hyperplasia
Hyphae
Ketonuria
Macrophage
Mast cell
Mesenchymal
Metastasis
Mueller-Hinton media
Mycology
Neoplasia
Oliguria
Oxidase
Proteinuria
Pyogranulomatous
Sarcoma
Selective media
Sensitivity test
Specific gravity
Struvite
Suppurative
Transudate
Urolithiasis

MICROBIOLOGY

The term microbiology refers to the study of microbes, specifically bacteria. Bacteria are small prokaryotic cells that are anuclear and have few cellular organelles. Microbiologic evaluations of tissues and body fluids can be used to determine the presence of specific disease-causing organisms and to aid in managing patient therapy. Samples for microbiologic evaluation can be collected quickly by various methods, including swabbing, scraping, and aspiration. The specific techniques used depend on the type of lesion and its location on the animal's body. Careful attention to aseptic technique is critical to achieving diagnostic quality results.

CHARACTERISTICS OF BACTERIA

Bacteria are variable in size, ranging from 0.2 to 2.0 µm. They can be classified into one of four general categories and can take a variety of arrangements (Fig. 9-1). Although most cellular organelles are absent, bacteria contain cell walls, plasma membranes, and ribosomes. Some contain capsules and flagella, and can develop endospores. These characteristics are often used in the differentiation of specific bacterial pathogens.

> *TECHNICIAN NOTE* Bacteria can be cocci, bacilli, spirals, and palisades shapes and can occur singly, in pairs, tetrads, chains, or clusters.

Most bacteria are chemoheterotrophic. That is, they obtain nutrients from nonliving components of their environment. Growth factors such as vitamins, amino acids, and nucleotides are also essential. Oxygen and temperature requirements vary among different species (Box 9-1). The majority of species require a pH in the range of 6.5 to 7.5. Bacteria reproduce primarily by binary fission, and their numbers grow exponentially until essential nutrients are depleted, toxic waste products accumulate, and/or space becomes limiting. Generation time refers to the time required for bacterial populations to double and is variable with different species and under different environmental conditions (Fig. 9-2).

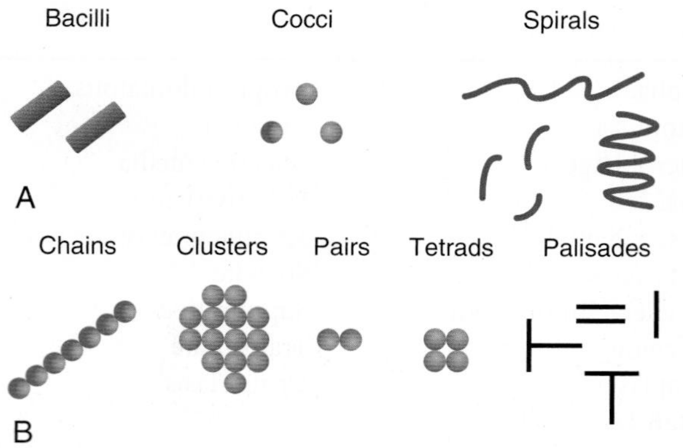

FIGURE 9-1 Bacterial cell shapes and arrangements.

MYCOLOGY

The study of fungi is referred to as **mycology.** Fungi are groups of organisms that are characterized by vegetative structures known as **hyphae.** Hyphae can grow into matted structures known as mycelia. Fungi contain eukaryotic cells with cell walls composed of chitin. The organisms are heterotrophic and may be parasitic or saprophytic. Fungi can be differentiated based on the structure of the hyphae and on the presence of spores. Different groups of fungi produce different types of spores. A variety of fungal organisms can affect veterinary species and cause superficial mycosis or deep mycosis. Table 9-1 summarizes fungal pathogens of veterinary importance, species affected, resultant diseases or lesions, and specimens required for diagnosis.

MATERIALS NEEDED FOR THE IN-HOUSE MICROBIOLOGY LAB

A review of scientific or veterinary supply catalogs will yield hundreds of products used in microbiology and cytology testing. The average small animal practice in-house laboratory

BOX 9-1 Temperature and Oxygen Requirements of Bacteria

Optimum Temperature
- Psychrophiles: 0-30° C
- Mesophiles: 20-40° C
- Thermophiles: 40-80° C

Oxygen Requirements
- Aerobes require oxygen.
- Anaerobes require absence of oxygen.
- Facultative can grow under a variety of conditions.
- Microaerophilic prefer reduced oxygen tension.
- Capnophilic require high levels of carbon dioxide.

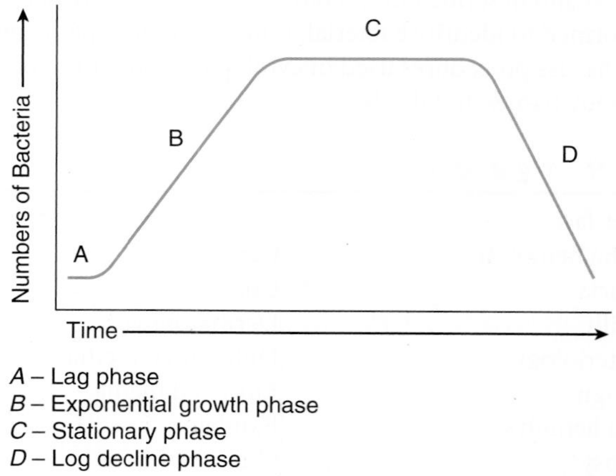

FIGURE 9-2 Generalized bacterial growth curve. *A,* Lag phase (phase of cell enlargement). *B,* Log phase (exponential growth phase). *C,* Maximum growth phase (stationary phase). *D,* Logarithmic decline phase (death phase).

TABLE 9-1 Summary of Pathogenic Fungi, Species Affected, Disease or Lesions Caused, and Specimens for Diagnosis

ORGANISM	SPECIES AFFECTED	DISEASE OR LESION	SPECIMENS
Microsporum			
M. canis	Dogs, cats	Ringworm	Fresh plucked hair and skin scrapings from edges of lesions
M. distortum	Dogs, cats, horses, pigs	Ringworm	
M. gallinae (T. gallinae)	Chickens, turkeys("white comb")	Ringworm	
M. gypseum	Horses, cats, dogs, other species	Ringworm	
M. nanum	Pigs	Ringworm	
M. persicolor	Voles, bats, dogs	Ringworm	
Trichophyton			
T. equinum	Horses, donkeys	Ringworm	
T. erinacei	Hedgehogs, dogs, people	Ringworm	
T. mentagrophytes	Most animal species	Ringworm	
T. rubrum	primarily people, but also dogs, cats	Ringworm	
T. simii	Poultry, monkeys	Ringworm	
T. verrucosum	Primarily cattle	Ringworm	
Candida			
Candida albicans	Chickens, turkeys, other birds	Infection of mouth, crop, esophagus	Fresh affected tissue or scrapings from affected tissue
Other *Candida* spp. (such as *C. tropicalis*) can cause lesions	Dogs	Mycotic stomatitis	Fixed affected tissue
	Cats	Enteritis of kittens	
	Calves, foals	Infections of oral and intestinal mucosae	
	Cattle	Mastitis	
	Horses	Genital infections—both sexes	
	Pigs	Infection of esophagus and stomach	
Malassezia pachydermitis	Dogs	Chronic otitis externa	Fresh ear swabs
Cryptococcus Neoformans	People, dogs, cats(infection frequently affects nervous systems)	Subacute or chronic affected tissue	Fresh nasal discharge, milk
Cryptococcus			
(worldwide distribution)	Cattle	Sporadic cases of mastitis	Fixed affected tissue, brain, lung
Coccidioides Immitis			
(SW USA and South America; occurs in soil)	People, horses, cattle, sheep, dogs, cats, captive feral animals	Disease characterized by granulomas, often in bronchial and mediastinal lymph nodes and lungs; can cause lesions in brain, liver, spleen, kidneys	Fresh and fixed lesions and affected tissue
Histoplasma Capsulatum			
(NE, central, and S central USA; and occurs in soil)	People, dogs, cats, sheep, pigs, horses	Disease that generally affects reticuloendothelial system; dogs, cats: ulcerations of intestinal canal; enlargement of liver, spleen, lymph nodes; TB-like lesions	Fresh and fixed lesions or affected tissue
Histoplasma Farciminosum			
(Mediterranean, Asia, Africa, and part of Russia)	Horses, mules, donkeys	Epizootic lymphangitis, African farcy, or Japanese glanders	Fresh pus and discharges from lesions

Continued

TABLE 9-1 Summary of Pathogenic Fungi, Species Affected, Disease or Lesions Caused, and Specimens for Diagnosis—cont'd

ORGANISM	SPECIES AFFECTED	DISEASE OR LESION	SPECIMENS
Blastomyces Dermatitidis			
(USA, Canada, and Africa; occurs in soil)	People, dogs, cats, sea lions	Granulomatous lesions in lungs and/or skin and subcutis	Fresh and fixed tissue lesions and affected tissue
Sporothrix schenckii	People, horses, dogs, pigs, cattle, fowl, rodents	Subcutaneous nodules or granulomas that eventually discharge pus; can include involvement of bones and visceral organs	Fresh and fixed pus, granulomas
Rhinosporidium Seeberi			
(not yet cultured in vitro)	Horses, dogs, cattle, people	Characterized by polyps on the nasal and ocular mucous membranes	Fresh nasal discharge and polyps; fixed polyps
Aspergillus			
A. fumigatus main pathogen; potentially pathogenic *A. flavus* *A. nidulans* *A. niger*	Many animal species and birds	Fowl: air sac infection; diffuse and nodular forms in lungs "brooder pneumonia" in chicks and poults; cattle: occasional mycotic abortion and mastitis; horses: guttural pouch mycosis; dog: infection of nasal chambers	Fresh deep scrapings or affected tissue Abortions
A. flavus	Ducklings, domestic birds, pigs, dogs	Aflatoxicosis; affects liver and sometimes kidneys	Suspect food product
A. parasiticus			
A. ochraceus			
A. clavatus	Pigs	Hemorrhagic disease; profuse hemorrhage in many tissues, jaundice, and liver lesions	
	Cattle	Trembling syndrome: *A. flavus* and *A. fumigatus* toxins; abortion; toxins of *A.ochraceus* cause fetal death; hyperkeratosis lesions on muzzle and mouth from *A. clavatus* toxins	
Petriellidium Boydii			
(*Allescheria boydii*)			Fresh milk, uterine discharges, affected tissue
	Cattle	Abortion, mastitis	
	Equidae	Abortion, metritis, infertility	
	People, other animals	Mycetoma; progressive disease of subcutis	Fixed affected tissue

requires just a few of these. A high-quality binocular microscope is an essential piece of equipment. Microbiology equipment requirements include a small incubator, autoclave, and a refrigerator for storage of supplies. Consumable supplies needed are those required for sample collection and preparation as well as culture media and stains for microbiology specimens. The specific choice of collection method depends on the location of the lesion on the animal's body as well as the specific type of testing desired. Samples that are to be immediately processed can usually be collected using sterile cotton swabs. However, this is the least suitable method of collection because contamination risk is high and cotton can inhibit microbial growth. Oxygen can also be trapped in the fibers, making recovery of anaerobic bacteria less likely. Should delays in processing the sample be expected, a rayon swab in transport media (e.g., Culturette) must be used to preserve the quality of the sample. Aspirated samples and tissue samples can be collected in a fashion similar to that described later in this chapter for cytology samples.

The following guidelines should be kept in mind for proper specimen collection and handling:

- *Collect the specimen aseptically.* Specimen contamination is the most common cause of diagnostic failure. The importance of aseptic collection of microbiologic specimens cannot be overemphasized. Collect samples as soon as possible following the onset of clinical signs and before initiation of any treatment.
- *Collect tissue samples that are at least 5 to 15 cm² (block or wedge-shaped).* This will allow for processing the sample with a variety of methods if needed.
- *Keep multiple specimens separate from each other to avoid cross-contamination.* This is essential for intestinal specimens because of the normal flora found there. In addition, samples that contain formalin should be stored and/or shipped to outside laboratories in containers that are separate from prepared slides and nonformalinized specimens. Formalin fumes can render samples unsatisfactory for further analysis.
- *Label the specimen container, especially if a zoonotic condition is suspected, such as anthrax, rabies, leptospirosis, brucellosis, or equine encephalitis.* Tissues from animals with suspected zoonoses should be submitted in a sealed, leakproof, unbreakable container.
- *Keep the specimen cool during transport.* Any sample that can be frozen should be frozen (especially in summer). Swabs must be sent in transport medium. Bacteriologic, virologic, and *Mycoplasma* tests require separate swabs for each. Samples for anaerobic culture must be submitted cool or frozen.
- *If shipping involves dry ice, seal the container or swab to prevent entry of CO_2 into the container.* Carbon dioxide released by dry ice may kill bacteria and viruses.
- *Swabs placed in viral transport medium cannot be used for bacterial culture.* Use duplicate bacterial transport medium.
- *If using an outside referral laboratory, send the specimen to the diagnostic laboratory by the fastest possible means.* If the sample will be arriving during a weekend, inform the laboratory ahead of time so that arrangements can be made for pickup.
- *Discuss the results with the veterinarian promptly, in a clear, concise manner.* Failure to do so reflects adversely on both the veterinarian and the laboratory.

Figure 9-3 shows the typical sequence of procedures used in processing microbiologic specimens.

SAMPLE PROCESSING MATERIALS

Preparation of samples for microbiology requires some unique supplies. Glass slides and cover slips are needed when performing Gram stain procedures, and they can be of average quality. Inoculating loops or wires for transfer of specimens to culture media are also needed. A propane (Bunsen) burner or alcohol lamp is required to sterilize the inoculating loops and to flame the mouth of culture tubes before inoculation. When anaerobic or microaerophilic microbes are suspected pathogens, a candle jar or anaerobe jar (Gas Pak) will be required to provide the appropriate environment for microbial growth.

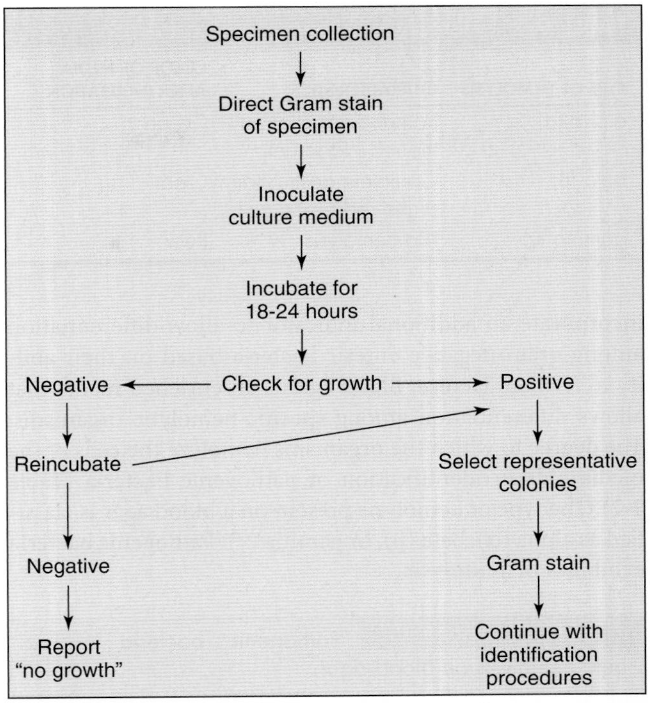

FIGURE 9-3 Typical sequence of procedures used in processing microbiologic specimens.

CULTURE MEDIA

Culture media are available in dozens of formulations. General-purpose nutrient media provides basic requirements for bacterial growth. **Selective media** contain additives that allow certain microorganisms to grow while inhibiting the growth of others. **Enriched media** also promote growth of certain microbes by providing specific growth factors for bacteria with strict nutrient requirements. These types of bacteria are referred to as fastidious. **Differential media** contain additives that detect certain biochemical reactions of the bacteria. Media are also available that incorporate characteristics of more than one type. Most small-animal practice microbiology laboratories will require just a few of these. Media are also supplied as either solid forms on culture plates or in tubes, liquid form in tubes, or in dehydrated form. Dehydrated media are the least expensive. However, they require additional preparation time and must be autoclaved before use. This may not be financially justifiable unless the practice is performing very large numbers of microbiology tests.

> TECHNICIAN NOTE Culture media formulations include selective, enriched, and differential media.

In veterinary practice, the most commonly used solid media in culture plates are **Mueller-Hinton,** Trypticase soy agar with 5% sheep blood (commonly called **blood agar**), and MacConkey or Eosin-Methylene Blue (EMB). Mueller-Hinton is the recommended media for culture and sensitivity testing. MacConkey and EMB are both selective media that support the growth of gram-negative bacteria and

TABLE 9-2 Hemolytic Patterns on Blood Agar

TYPE OF HEMOLYSIS	CHARACTERISTICS	COLOR OF MEDIA AFTER INCUBATION
alpha (α)	Partial destruction of the red blood cells	Green
beta (β)	Complete destruction of the red blood cells	Clear
gamma (γ)	No hemolysis	Red

incorporate an additional indicator to allow differentiation among gram-negative enteric bacteria based on their ability to ferment lactose. Blood agar is an enriched media that allows differentiation among specific hemolytic organisms. The degree to which the organisms hemolyze the cells of the media aids in identification of pathogenic bacteria (Table 9-2). The type of hemolysis present on a blood agar is classified as alpha (α), beta (β), or gamma (γ). Pathogenic bacteria exhibit **beta hemolysis.**

> TECHNICIAN NOTE Pathogenic bacteria exhibit beta hemolysis on blood agar.

Solid media in culture tubes are used primarily for growth of fungi and yeasts. Additional media available in this form include those used for biochemical testing of microbes. The most common types of slant media tubes are Sabauraud Dextrose or Bismuth-Glucose-Glycine Yeast (commonly referred to as "biggy"). The media is usually solidified into a slant-top configuration. Either type is suitable for growth of **dermatophytes** and is usually described as dermatophyte test media (DTM) regardless of which specific media is present. Fungal cultures of solid tissue samples may require the use of a 20% potassium hydroxide reagent for preparation of the sample.

A variety of companies produce culture plates that incorporate several different media within individual compartments on a culture plate. Items such as the Bullseye Veterinary Plate (Fig. 9-4) and the Bacti-Vet Culture System provide five different types of media that can simultaneously select and differentiate microbes as well as provide antibiotic sensitivity data.

Broth media in tubes is necessary for blood cultures and is also available in forms to provide differentiation of gram-negative enteric bacteria. Thioglycollate broth is a general-purpose media that can be used for urine cultures. Specific blood culture tubes are available as evacuated tubes used for blood collection. These contain both anticoagulant and culture media.

Bacteria may often be partially differentiated based on their growth patterns on agar plates. Evaluation of colony characteristics should include form, elevation, margin, texture, and pigmentation (Fig. 9-5). The specific configuration a bacterial colony makes depends on the type of culture media used as well as environmental conditions.

STAINS

Gram stain is an essential component of the microbiology lab. It is available in kit form or can be purchased as individual

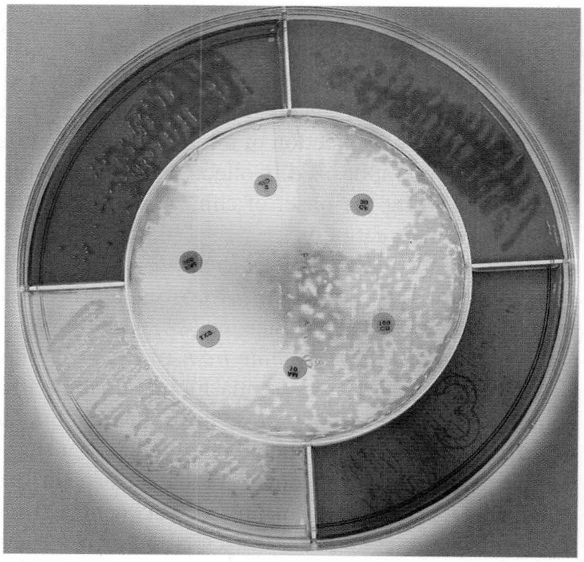

FIGURE 9-4 Bullseye culture media. The center section contains Mueller-Hinton media for performing the antibiotic susceptibility test. (From Figure 38-9 in Sirois M: *Laboratory Procedures for Veterinary Technicians*, ed 6, St Louis, 2015, Mosby.)

solutions. For differentiation of certain types of bacteria, a variety of other stains are also available. Acid-fast stains are useful in the identification of *Mycobacterium*. These involve the addition of an agent such as dimethyl sulfoxide (DMSO) before addition of the primary stain. The agent allows the stain to penetrate the stain-resistant cells of *Mycobacterium*. The subsequent addition of acid alcohol or dilute alcohol removes the stain. If the stain is not removed, the organism is said to be **acid-fast.** The Ziehl-Nelson technique is a modification of this procedure.

> TECHNICIAN NOTE Gram stain is the primary differential stain used in microbiology testing.

Flagella stains, capsule stains, endospore stains, and fluorescent stains are also available but have limited application in the average veterinary microbiology lab. Fluorescent stains tend to be quite expensive and are used primarily for the identification of *Legionella* and *Pseudomonas*. Flagella stain usually contains crystal violet and is used to detect and characterize bacterial motility. These tend to be somewhat expensive for the small veterinary practice laboratory. Other methods that can be used to test motility include the use of concave slides to produce hanging drop preparations or the use of motility test media. Capsule stains are used for detection of pathogenic bacteria. All bacteria that contain capsules are pathogenic. However, not all pathogenic bacteria contain capsules. Capsule stains often require the use of bright-field phase contrast microscopy. Endospore stains are used to detect the presence, location, and shape of spores. These characteristics can aid in differentiation of bacteria. Spores may be centrally located, terminal, or subterminal (Fig. 9-6). Endospore staining is performed on older cultures (>48 hours) because spore formation

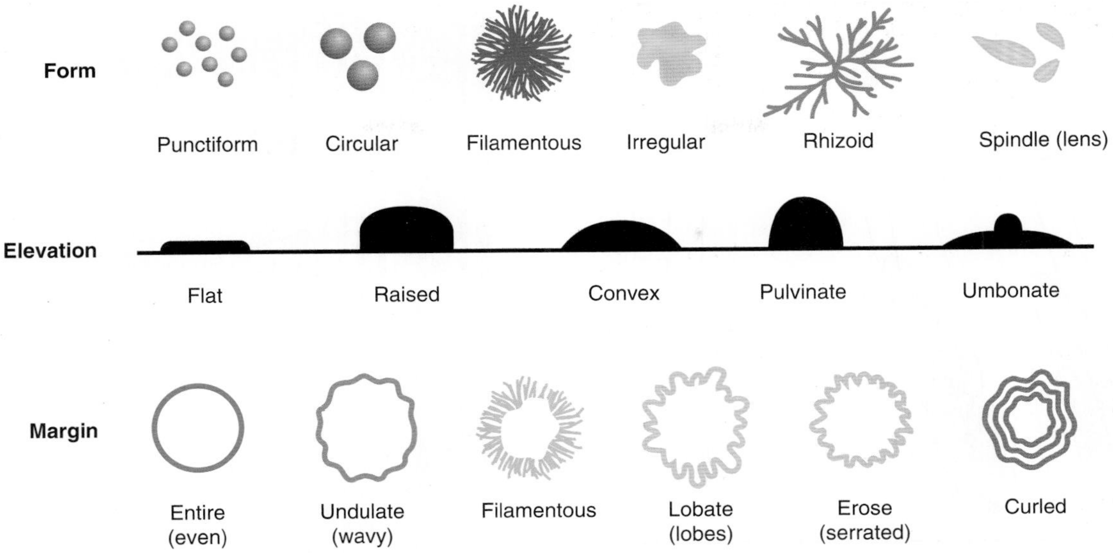

FIGURE 9-5 Bacterial colonies may be described on the basis of their form, elevation, and margins.

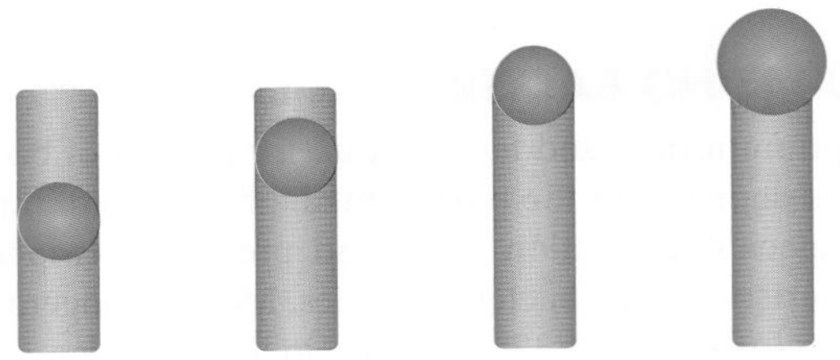

FIGURE 9-6 Bacterial endospores.

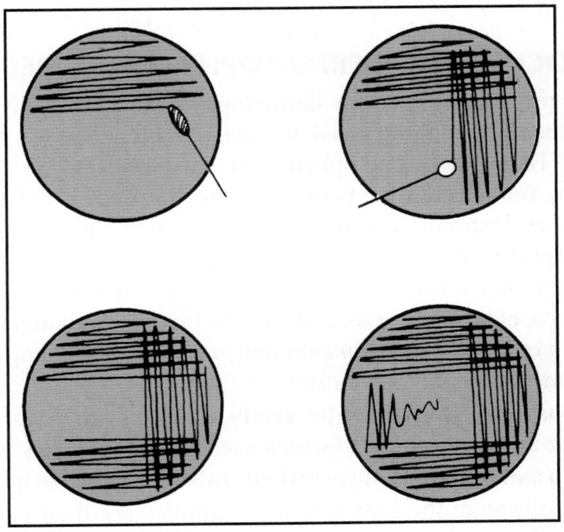

FIGURE 9-7 Quadrant streak method for isolation of bacteria.

occurs during the log decline phase. The procedure involves addition of malachite green to the specimen on the slide and then heating the slide. The slide is washed and counterstained with safranin or basic fuchsin. Spores appear dark blue/green with the remainder of the bacterial cell pink or red. Spores may also be found free from cells. Simple stains, such as crystal violet or methylene blue, are usually used for yeasts. Lactophenol cotton blue stain is often needed to prepare fungal culture samples for analysis and can also be used for cellophane tape preparations of external lesions.

ADDITIONAL MATERIALS

Antimicrobial sensitivity discs are necessary when performing a culture and sensitivity. The specific types of antimicrobial discs purchased depend on the suspected pathogens. Antimicrobial discs are available in a variety of concentrations. These allow more specific determination of therapeutic levels needed, once the antimicrobial is chosen. A 3% potassium hydroxide solution (also used to perform the catalase test) should be available for clarification of results when Gram staining yields ambiguous or variable answers.

INOCULATING CULTURE MEDIA

Aseptic technique is crucial to achieving diagnostic quality results in microbiology. Culture media and processing supplies must be sterile. There are several methods for inoculation of culture media depending on the characteristics of the sample and the type of testing needed. Because many samples contain multiple types of bacteria, the majority of bacterial tests involve an initial step designed to isolate the bacterium of interest. Before inoculating the culture plate, an inoculation loop or wire is passed through a flame and briefly cooled. The loop or wire is lightly touched to the sample and then streaked onto a culture plate using the quadrant method (Fig. 9-7). If the sample was collected using a sterile swab, this can be used directly on the culture plate. The procedure for inoculating agar slants requires a sterile wire. The slant is generally divided into a butt portion and slant surface. The media can be inoculated either on the butt only, the slant only, or both (Fig. 9-8). Motility test media is prepared as an agar slant. Broth media, such as blood culture tubes, are inoculated in a manner similar to that used for agar slants.

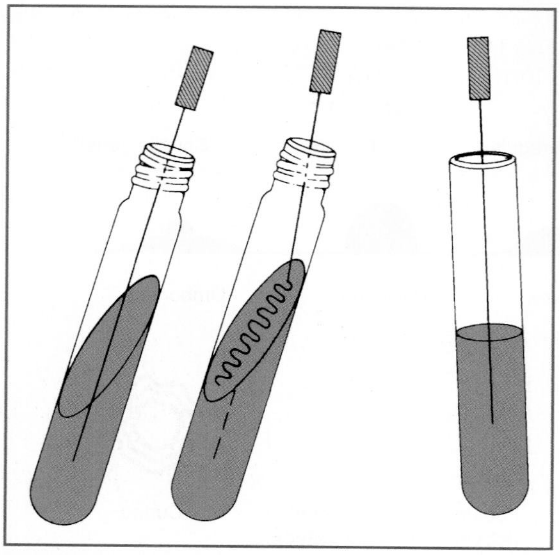

FIGURE 9-8 Inoculation procedure for tube media. *Left,* Inoculation of agar slant and butt, such as triple sugar iron. *Right,* Inoculation of motility test media. (From Bassert JM, McCurnin DM: *McCurnin's Clinical Textbook for Veterinary Technicians,* ed 7, St Louis, 2010, Saunders.)

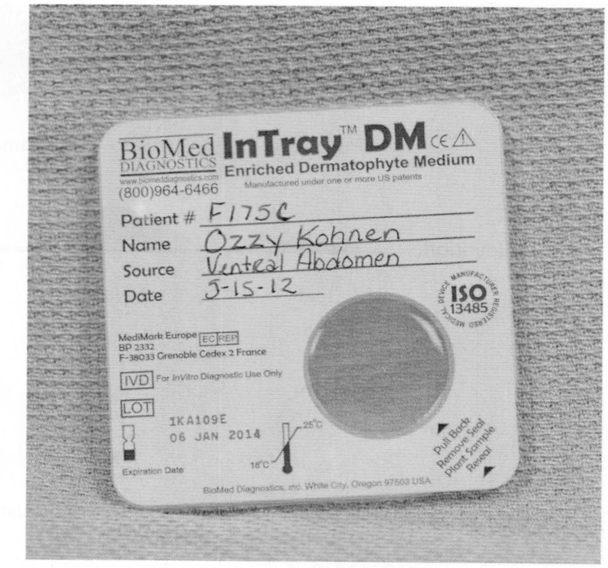

FIGURE 9-9 InTray DM. This is a commonly used dermatophyte test medium. (From Figure 38-13 in Sirois M: *Laboratory Procedures for Veterinary Technicians,* ed 6, St Louis, 2015, Mosby.)

INOCULATING DERMATOPHYTE TEST MEDIA

The procedures used for dermatophyte testing are slightly different than those used for general bacteriology testing. Either a dermatophyte test medium (DTM) or a plain Sabouraud's dextrose agar can be used. DTM usually incorporates an additional reagent that causes a color change in the medium when *Microsporum canis* is present (Fig. 9-9). However, it is important to note that some common contaminants can also induce this color change and some cultures of *M. canis* do not produce color change on the medium.

Suspect lesions may be gently cleaned with soap and water and clean thumb forceps used to remove a few hairs and a small amount of epidermal scales from the periphery of the lesion. The hair and scale samples are then placed onto the surface of the culture medium. A portion of the sample is pressed down into the medium. The culture is loosely covered and placed in a cabinet or drawer at room temperature. Starting at 48 hours after incubation, the inoculated medium must be inspected each day for evidence of color change. A flocculent growth accompanied by color change suggests *M. canis* infection. If no growth occurs after 7 days, the specimen should be redistributed over the medium and the culture procedure repeated. If growth is evident, the material should be stained and examined microscopically. A drop of lactophenol cotton blue stain is placed in the center of a microscope slide. A 2-inch piece of clear (not frosted) cellophane tape or FungiTape (Scientific Device Laboratory) is pressed against the flocculent material observed growing on the media. The tape is lifted and then pressed down into the drop of stain previously placed on the slide. The sample is evaluated microscopically and the characteristics of the organisms used to verify the species present (Fig. 9-10).

INCUBATING BACTERIAL CULTURES

The optimum time and temperature for growth of bacterial cultures depends on the type of media being used, the bacterial species' generation time, and preferred temperature characteristics of the bacterial species. Most pathogenic bacteria are incubated at 37° C. Some incubators also contain mechanisms to read and record biochemical reactions.

Incubators should contain thermostatic controls (temperature and preferably humidity). Some have oxygen and carbon dioxide controls as well.

BIOCHEMICAL TEST MATERIALS

Biochemical tests are often necessary to differentiate specific types of microbes. Figure 9-11 provides an example of how differential staining, biochemical testing, and other criteria are used for primary identification of bacteria. Biochemical testing may involve the use of specific liquid reagents or use media that contain the necessary reagents. The most commonly performed tests in the small veterinary practice laboratory are the oxidase test and catalase tests. Reagents to perform these tests are quite inexpensive and readily available. The catalase test is performed on gram-positive cocci and small gram-positive bacilli. It tests for the enzyme catalase, which acts on hydrogen peroxide to produce water and oxygen. A small amount of a colony from a blood agar plate is placed on a microscope slide and a drop of catalase reagent (3% hydrogen peroxide) is added. If the colony is catalase positive, gas bubbles are produced. No bubble production indicates a negative result.

Many biochemical tests are available in a slide form that contains the necessary reagent impregnated in a pad on the slide. Coagulase testing may sometimes be required and can be performed as either a slide or tube test. Coagulase reagent tends to be relatively expensive. Enterotubes are a type of

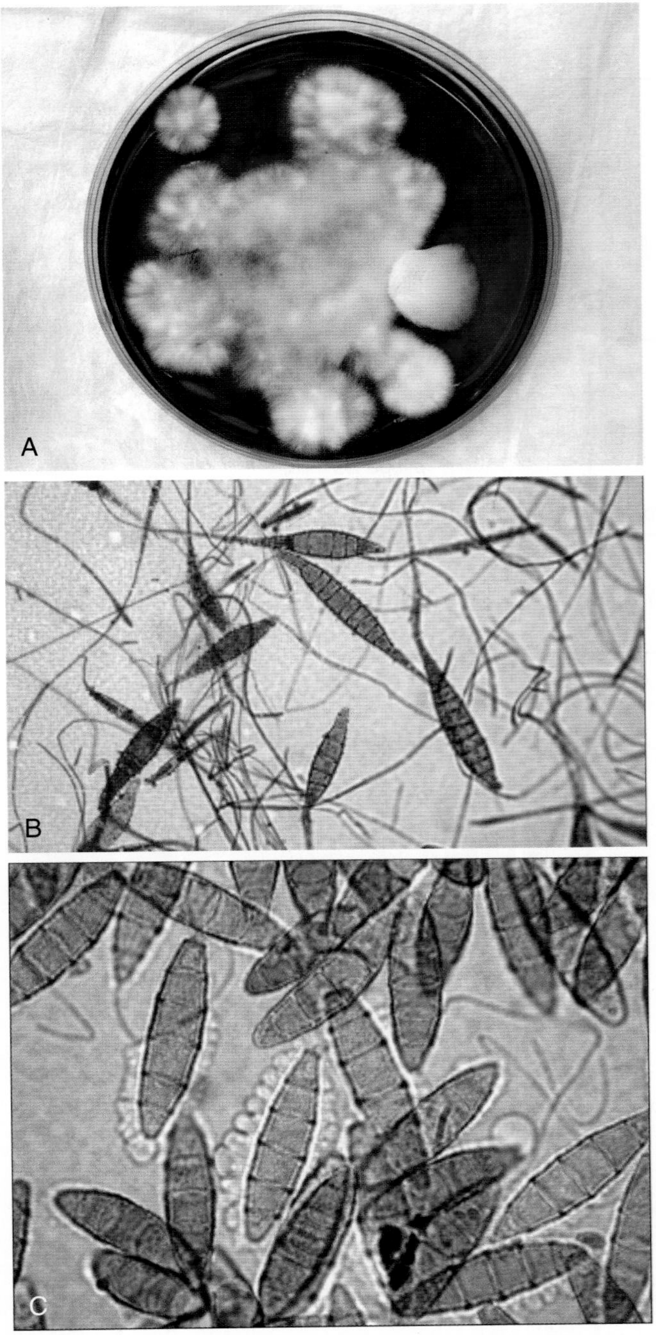

FIGURE 9-10 Dermatophyte test medium (DTM) fungal culture. **A,** *Microsporum canis* demonstrating the typical white, fluffy colony growth and red color change. The red color should develop as soon as colony growth becomes visible. **B,** Microscopic image of *M. canis* organisms, as viewed with a 10× objective. Note the six or more cell divisions. **C,** Microscopic image of *M. gypsum*, as viewed with a 10× objective. Note the six or fewer cell divisions. (From Figure 2-7 in Hnilica KA: *Small Animal Dermatology*, ed 3, St Louis, 2011, W.B. Saunders.)

commercially available microbiology test kit that incorporates multiple types of media designed to provide differentiation of enteric bacteria based on their biochemical reactions on the media. These tend to be relatively expensive and may not be financially justified unless large numbers of microbiology tests are performed on a variety of species. Individual culture media tubes can be purchased that provide many of the same test results as Enterotubes. These may decrease the overall cost of testing when only a few biochemical tests are needed. The most commonly used biochemical tests that use differential media are the Sulfide-Indole-Motility (SIM) media, Simmons' Citrate Media, and Triple Sugar-Iron media. These are all solid media prepared in tubes with slanted surface agar. SIM testing requires the addition of Kovac's reagent following incubation of the sample.

IMMUNOLOGIC TESTING

Because microbes contain compounds that can serve as antigens, immunologic tests can sometimes be used for determination of the presence or absence of specific microbes. The majority of these types of tests require specialized and expensive equipment and reagent that may not be financially justifiable for the small veterinary practice. Immunologic tests using the enzyme-linked-immunosorbent reaction are available for detection of *Brucella* antibodies and are also available for some species of *Salmonella*, and *Staphylococcus*.

Table 9-3 summarizes bacterial pathogens of veterinary importance.

ANTIMICROBIAL SENSITIVITY TESTING

Bacterial samples isolated from patient samples are often processed with the antimicrobial **sensitivity test.** This test indicates which antimicrobial is needed to treat the patient and at which concentrations it should be administered. The test must be performed on a pure, fresh culture taken before the initiation of any treatment. Gram staining is used to determine which antimicrobial discs to use. The most common method for performing antimicrobial sensitivity testing is the agar diffusion method. The test uses paper discs impregnated with antimicrobials that are placed on the surface of the bacterial culture (usually a freshly inoculated Mueller-Hinton agar plate) and allowed to incubate. After the incubation period, usually 18 to 24 hours, the plate is examined for bacterial growth. If the bacterium is sensitive to a particular antimicrobial, a zone around the paper disc will be evident. The diameter of the zone is then measured and interpreted using a standardized comparative chart (Fig. 9-12). A similar method can be used to determine the minimum inhibitory concentration (MIC) of an antimicrobial. This is the smallest concentration of the specific antimicrobial that can inhibit the growth of a given bacteria. Paper discs with varying concentrations of the chosen antimicrobial are placed on a freshly inoculated culture plate and incubated. Measuring the zones of inhibition around each of these discs will aid in choosing an appropriate concentration of medication to be given to the patient.

QUALITY CONTROL CONCERNS

An effective quality control program is vital to achieving accurate and reliable results in any laboratory. Samples for microbiologic analysis are greatly affected by inappropriate or

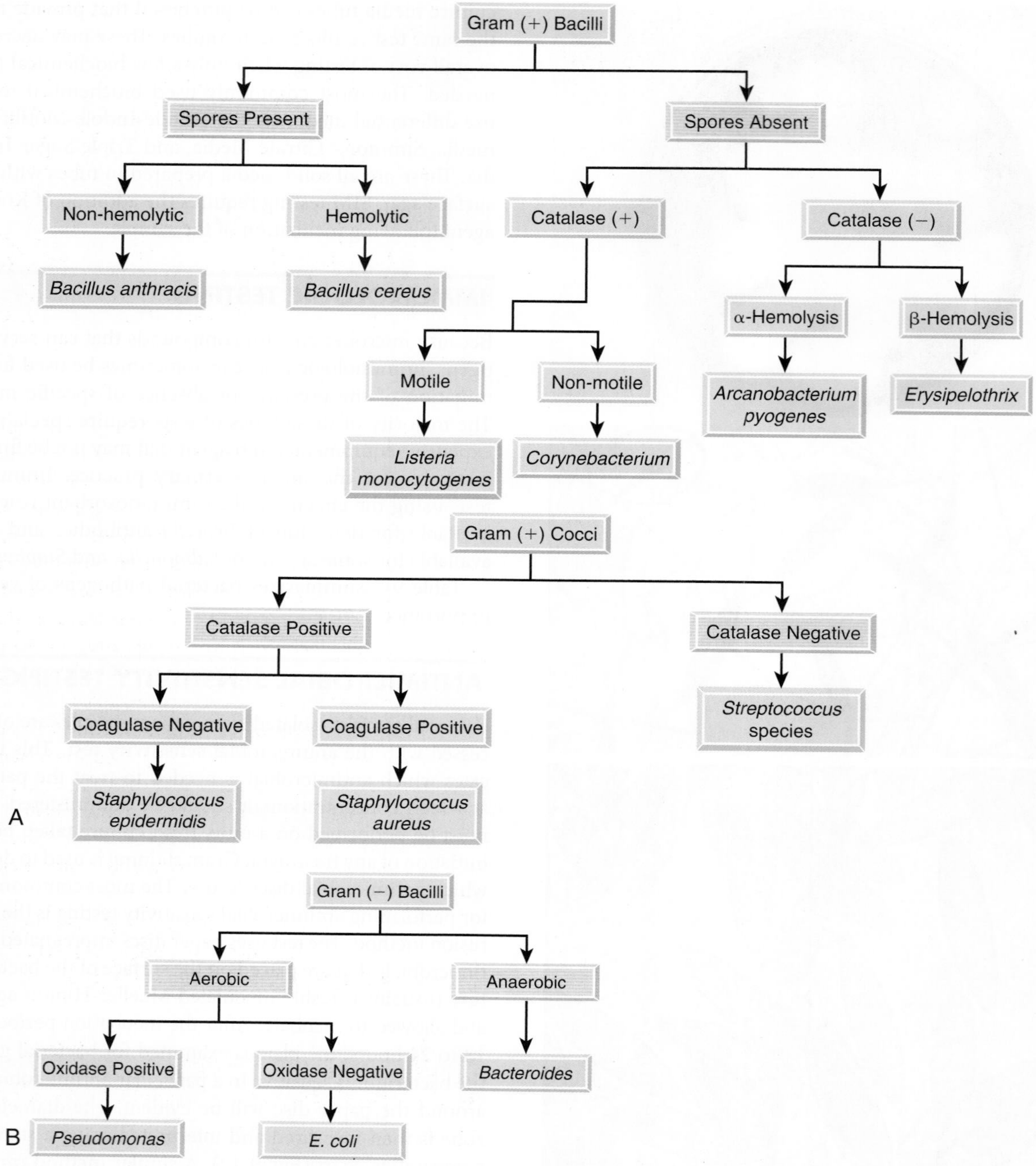

FIGURE 9-11 Examples of flow charts used for differentiation of bacteria.

improperly performed collection methods. Careful attention to aseptic technique is critical. The timing of sample collection and processing must also be considered. Samples that are collected after medical treatment has begun or that are held long periods of time before processing will yield unreliable results. Staining supplies and reagents must be stored and used correctly for maintenance of the integrity of these items. In addition to maintaining the sterility of collection and processing supplies, equipment used in the microbiology laboratory requires regular verification of performance. This includes verification of temperatures in autoclaves and incubators. Such routine quality control must be performed on a regular schedule and the results recorded so that equipment malfunctions can be detected early.

CYTOLOGY

The primary goal of the cytology evaluation is differentiation of inflammation and **neoplasia.** The types and numbers of cells present in a properly collected and prepared cytology specimen can provide rapid diagnostic information to the clinician. Samples for cytology evaluation can be collected quickly and do not generally require specialized materials or equipment for proper evaluation. With careful attention to

TABLE 9-3 Bacterial Pathogens of Veterinary Importance

GROUP	GENERA
Spirochetes	*Leptospira* *Borrelia* *Treponema* *Brachyspira*
Spiral and curved bacteria	*Campylobacter* *Helicobacter*
Gram-negative aerobic bacilli	*Pseudomonas* *Francisella* *Brucella* *Neisseria* *Bordetella*
Gram-negative facultative bacilli	*Escherichia* *Proteus* *Shigella* *Yersinia* *Salmonella* *Citrobacter* *Klebsiella* *Aeromonas* *Enterobacter* *Actinobacillus* *Serratia* *Haemophilus* *Pasteurella*
Gram-negative anaerobic bacilli	*Bacteroides* *Fusobacterium*
Gram-positive bacilli	*Bacillus* *Listeria* *Clostridium* *Erysipelothrix* *Lactobacillus*
Gram-negative pleomorphic	*Rickettsia* *Haemobartonella* *Ehrlichia* *Eperythrozoon* *Anaplasma* *Chlamydia* *Mycoplasma*
Gram-positive cocci	*Staphylococcus* *Streptococcus* *Enterococcus*

appropriate collection, preparation, and staining technique, a high-quality cytology sample can be obtained. Such samples yield valuable results for the clinician and often preclude the need for more invasive procedures to determine diagnosis, treatment, and prognosis for a patient.

Several different preparations are often made from each sample. This allows for additional diagnostic testing without additional collection. Samples may be processed as compression or modified compression preparations, impression smears, line smears, starfish smears, or simple smears. The exact type of preparation depends on the characteristics of the sample. Some samples may also require concentration by centrifugation. Fluid samples often require anticoagulant

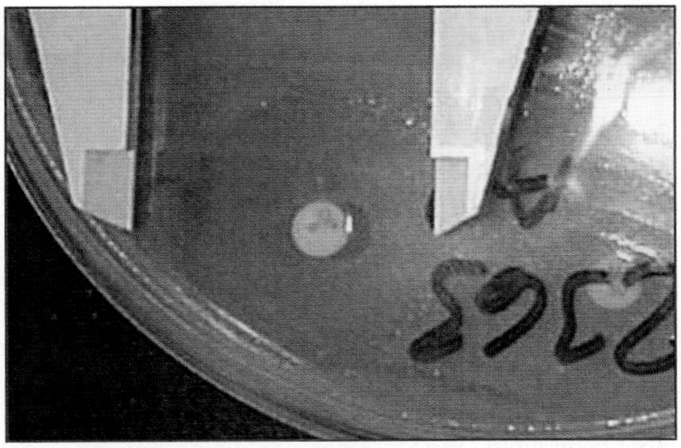

FIGURE 9-12 The use of a caliper to measure zone of inhibition. (Courtesy B. Mitzner, DVM.)

and/or preservatives. A variety of staining techniques are also available for cytology specimens. Some samples will require processing with more than one staining procedure.

Collected and processed correctly, a cytology specimen is characterized as inflammatory, neoplastic, or mixed. The specimen is then described according to the presence of specific cell types. Neoplastic cells are further evaluated for malignant changes. Inflammatory processes are characterized as either **suppurative, pyogranulomatous,** or eosinophilic when specific cell types and numbers of cells are evident on the cytology preparation. In general, samples that are inflammatory are characterized by a predominance of neutrophils and **macrophages** (tissue monocytes). Neoplastic samples are characterized by large numbers of tissue cells. There may be a combination of cell types present. This may indicate a neoplastic disease with secondary inflammation. Box 9-2 contains a list of commonly used supplies for cytology sample collection.

> *TECHNICIAN NOTE* Inflammatory specimens contain primarily neutrophils and macrophages, whereas neoplastic specimens primarily contain tissue cells.

COLLECTION AND PREPARATION OF SAMPLES FROM TISSUES AND MASSES

IMPRESSION SMEARS

Impression smears are prepared from active lesions on an animal's body or from tissues removed during surgical procedures. For impression smears from active lesions, an initial impression is made before cleaning the lesion or initiating treatment. Additional smears are prepared after cleaning the lesion. To prepare the smear, gently touch a clean glass slide to several areas of the lesion. Although this type of sample can be prepared quickly and easily, it tends to yield the fewest number of cells and can also be contaminated by bacteria that may be present because of secondary bacterial infection. Impression smears of tissue samples are made in a similar manner except that a fresh section of the tissue is made and then the tissue is blotted to remove excess blood and tissue fluid. These excess fluids may prevent tissue cells from adhering to the slide (Procedure 9-1).

BOX 9-2 Basic Equipment Used for Cytologic Examination

- Binocular microscope
- Immersion oil
- 20- or 22-gauge, 1.5-inch needles
- 6- and 12-ml syringes
- Glass slides and cover slips
- Stains: Diff-Quik (Scientific Products), Hema-Quik (Curtis Matheson Scientific), Quik Stain II (Scientific Products) new methylene blue, Gram stain
- Coplin staining jars
- Specimen tubes: red-top tubes contain no anticoagulant; lavender-top tubes contain EDTA as anticoagulant
- Forceps, scalpel blades
- Refractometer
- Hemacytometer

PROCEDURE 9-1 Preparing Impression Smears

Materials

- Scalpel
- Forceps
- Paper towels and/or gauze sponges
- Glass slides

Procedure

1. Section the tissue to expose a fresh surface.
2. Hold the tissue fragment with forceps.
3. Blot excess fluid on a paper towel or gauze sponge until the tissue is nearly dry.
4. Gently touch the tissue to the surface of a slide repeatedly down the length of the slide. Reblot as needed.
5. Allow the slide to air dry.

SCRAPINGS

Scrapings can be prepared from either external lesions or from tissues removed during surgical procedures. This type of sample yields a greater number of cells than impression smears. To prepare a scraping, the lesion or tissue must be cleaned and blotted dry. If using tissue samples, a fresh section is cut before obtaining the sample. A dull scalpel blade is held at a 90-degree angle to the lesion or tissue and is gently pulled across the surface. A compression smear is then prepared from the material on the edge of the scalpel blade. The sample can also be smeared across a slide directly from the scalpel blade.

TECHNICIAN NOTE Cytology samples from solid masses are collected using impression smears, swabbing, scraping, or fine needle biopsy.

SWABBINGS

Swab smears can provide valuable diagnostic information for certain types of specimens. This type of sample preparation is most useful for fistulated lesions or collections from the vaginal canal. A sterile cotton swab is moistened with 0.9% saline and lightly swabbed along the surface of the tissue. The swab is then gently rolled across the surface of a clean glass slide.

PROCEDURE 9-2 Fine-Needle Aspiration

Materials

- 20- or 22-gauge, 1.5-inch needles
- 6- to 12-ml syringes
- Glass slides

Procedure

1. Clean the site.
2. Immobilize the mass or lymph node with one hand.
3. Insert the needle into the mass and redirect through the mass several times while aspirating to collect cells.
4. Release pressure from the syringe plunger before removing the needle from the mass.
5. Prepare compression or wedge smears immediately.

FINE NEEDLE BIOPSY

A fine-needle **biopsy** sample can often provide a great amount of information to the clinician and may preclude the need for biopsy of lesions of internal organs. This type of sample preparation may also be preferred for collection of samples from superficial lesions because bacterial contamination can be kept to a minimum. If microbiologic tests are to be performed on a portion of the sample collected or a body cavity (such as peritoneal and thoracic cavities and joints) is to be penetrated, the area of aspiration is surgically prepared. Otherwise preparation is essentially the same as would be required for venipuncture. An alcohol swab may be used to clean the area.

The procedure may be performed using either an aspirate (Procedure 9-2) or nonaspirate technique. For the aspiration biopsy, equipment needed includes a 3- to 20-mL syringe and a 21- to 25-gauge needle. Samples collected from softer tissue require smaller syringes and needles. Firmer tissues require larger syringes and large-bore needles. Collection of samples from solid masses is performed by inserting the needle into the tissue and pulling the plunger about three-fourths of the way out of the barrel. This exerts a negative pressure on the tissue and draws material into the needle. Samples should be collected from several areas of the tissue by releasing the pressure on the syringe and redirecting the needle into another location. The nonaspirate procedure can be used to collect samples from solid masses. To perform this procedure, attach a 22-gauge needle to a 10-ml syringe that has the plunger removed (Fig. 9-13) or a needle with no attached syringe. Introduce the needle into the mass, and move the needle rapidly back and forth through the mass. Shearing and capillary action force cells into the needle. Once removed from the mass, the material is expelled onto a clean glass slide by rapidly or forcefully pressing the plunger of the syringe.

PREPARATION TECHNIQUES FOR SOLID SAMPLES

Samples collected from organs and masses can be prepared in several ways. Regardless of preparation method chosen,

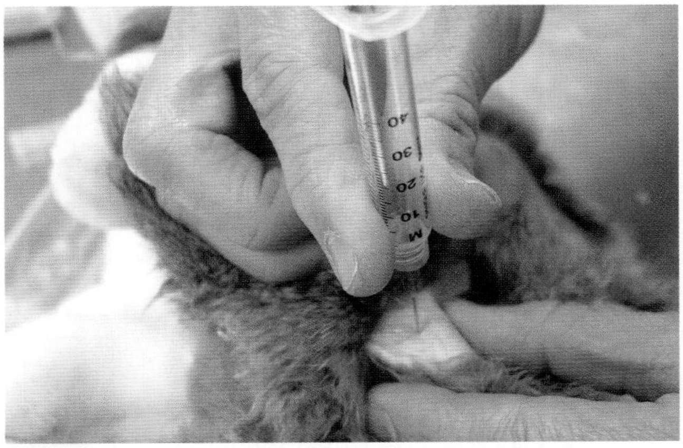

FIGURE 9-13 Collection of sample by the fine needle biopsy non-aspiration technique. Note that the syringe plunger has been removed.

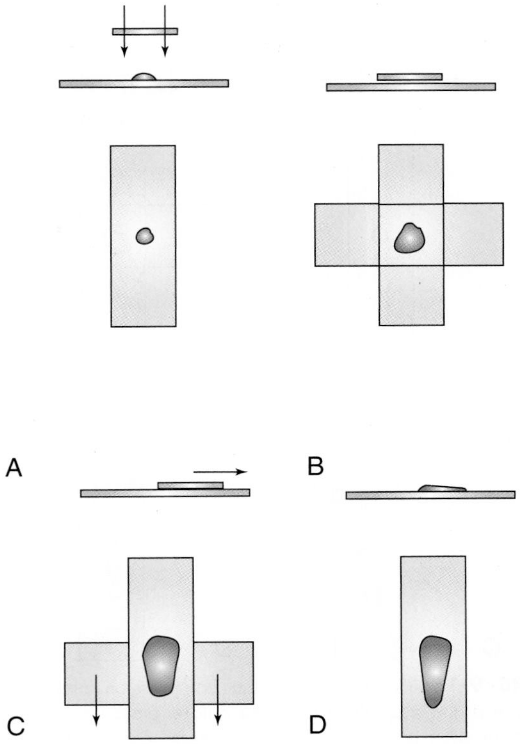

FIGURE 9-14 Compression preparation. **A,** A portion of the aspirate is expelled onto a glass microscope slide. **B,** Another slide is placed over the sample, spreading the sample. If the sample does not spread well, gentle digital pressure can be applied to the top slide. Care must be taken not to place excessive pressure on the slide, which could cause the cells to rupture. **C,** The slides are smoothly slipped apart, which usually produces well-spread smears (**D**) but may result in excessive cell rupture.

PROCEDURE 9-3 Preparing Compression Smears

Materials

- Glass slides

Procedure

1. Place one drop of aspirated material on one end of a slide.
2. Place a second slide gently on top of and parallel or at a right angle to the first.
3. Allow material to spread by capillary action.
4. Pull the second slide across the surface of the first slide using a smooth motion.
5. Allow the slides to air-dry.

the smear must be made quickly to avoid deterioration of the sample. Several smears should be made and rapidly air dried.

Compression Technique

This method has been widely used for many years for preparation of cytology specimens (Procedure 9-3). A small amount of sample is placed on a clean glass slide or cover slip. A second slide or cover slip is placed on top at a 90-degree angle to the first. The second slide is then gently pulled away from the first (Fig. 9-14).

Modified Compression Technique

This technique can be useful for samples that are highly viscous or are likely to contain cells that are very fragile. The technique involves placing a small amount of sample near the middle of a clean glass slide. A second slide is placed on top at a right angle. The top slide is then rotated 45 degrees and then removed (Fig. 9-15).

Combination Method

This technique involves placing a small amount of sample near the middle of a clean glass slide. The edge of a second slide is then placed on top and at a right angle to the first so that it covers about one-third of the specimen. The second slide is then gently slid across the specimen, leaving the middle one-third portion of the specimen untouched. The final one-third portion of the specimen is then smeared in a manner similar to that used for preparation of a routine blood smear, with somewhat less pressure applied to the smear (Fig. 9-16).

COLLECTION AND PREPARATION OF FLUID SAMPLES

Removal of fluid from the abdominal, thoracic, and pericardial cavities can be accomplished in a manner similar to that for fine-needle aspiration of tissue samples (Procedure 9-4). Aspirated fluid samples should be well mixed with an appropriate anticoagulant (e.g., EDTA) and the specimen prepared as quickly as possible to prevent cellular deterioration. Slides can be prepared directly from the nonconcentrated fluid or from concentrated sediment following centrifugation of the sample.

> *TECHNICIAN NOTE* Centesis refers to fluid samples collected from body cavities.

TRANSTRACHEAL AND BRONCHIAL WASHES

Evaluation of mucus secretions from the trachea, bronchi, and bronchioles can aid in differential diagnosis of inflammation, neoplasia, mycosis, and bacterial and protozoal

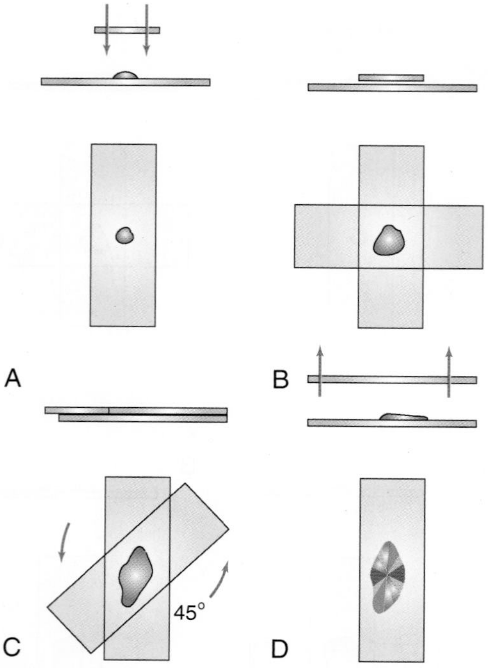

FIGURE 9-15 Modification of the compression preparation. **A,** A portion of the aspirate is expelled onto a glass microscope slide. **B,** Another slide is placed over the sample, causing the sample to spread. If necessary, gentle digital pressure can be applied to the top slide to spread the sample more. Care must be taken not to place excessive pressure on the slide, which could cause the cells to rupture. **C,** The top slide is rotated approximately 45 degrees and lifted directly upward, producing a squash preparation with subtle ridges and valleys of cells (**D**).

diseases. There are various techniques for collecting these samples, such as the percutaneous (jugular catheter) and endotracheal tube methods (Procedure 9-5). Both methods involve infusion of saline into the trachea. Fluid is collected either by aspirating the fluid or waiting for the animal to cough. It is important to collect all fluid coughed up by the animal, even if it requires that the sample be collected in a nonsterile fashion (e.g., from the bottom of the cage floor). Specimens collected in this manner should be noted as such before performing any testing.

Concentration Techniques

Fluid samples may be centrifuged in order to concentrate the solid material before preparing smears. The technique is similar to that used for preparation of urine sediment for microscopic analysis. The anticoagulated fluid is placed in a standard clinical centrifuge and spun for 5 minutes at 1000 to 2000 rpm (165 to 400 G). The supernatant is poured off, leaving a few drops in the tube. The sediment is then gently resuspended in the remaining supernatant. A few drops of this concentrate are then used to prepare several smears. Ideally several preparations should be made using several different techniques.

Slide Preparation

The compression technique described previously may be used for fluid samples, particularly ones that are highly

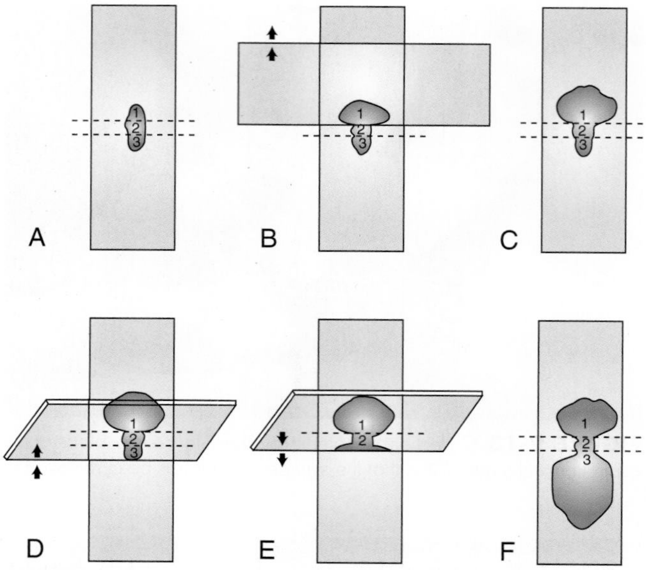

FIGURE 9-16 Combination cytologic preparation. **A,** A portion of the aspirate is expelled onto a glass microscope slide (prep slide). **B,** Another glass microscope slide is placed over approximately one-third of the preparation. If additional spreading of the aspirate is needed, gentle digital pressure can be used. Excessive pressure should be avoided. **C,** The spreader slide is smoothly slid forward. This procedure makes a compression preparation of approximately one-third of the aspirate (area 1). The spreader slide also contains a squash preparation (not depicted). Next, the edge of a tilted glass microscope slide (second spreader slide) is slid backward from the end opposite the compression preparation until it makes contact with approximately one-third of the expelled aspirate (**D** and **E**). **F,** Then the second spreader slide is slid rapidly and smoothly forward. These steps produce an area (3) that is spread with mechanical forces like those of a blood smear preparation. The middle area (2) is left untouched and contains a high concentration of cells.

PROCEDURE 9-4 Abdominocentesis and Thoracentesis

Materials

- Surgical prep materials
- Local anesthetic
- 18- or 20-gauge, over-the-needle catheter or needles (cats, dogs)
- 2- or 3-inch teat cannula, bitch catheter, 18-gauge, 1½-inch needle (cattle, horses)
- 6- to 12-ml syringe
- Red-top and lavender-top tubes
- 3-way stopcock (thoracentesis)
- Sterile IV extension tubing (horses)

Procedure

1. Anesthetize or tranquilize the animal as necessary.
2. Surgically prepare the site (thorax: cranial rib ventral to the fluid line; abdomen: ventral midline). Local anesthetic may be used to infiltrate the site of the catheter, needle, or cannula insertion.
3. Insert the needle or catheter in the appropriate location. If using a needle, use care to avoid lacerating internal organs. Attach the needle or catheter to a three-way stopcock or syringe when entering the thoracic cavity to avoid causing pneumothorax.

PROCEDURE 9-4 Abdominocentesis and Thoracentesis—cont'd

4. Use a three-way stopcock between the catheter and syringe if you are collecting multiple syringefuls from thoracic cavity. IV extension tubing is also helpful, particularly when draining large volumes of thoracic fluid from a horse. Collect samples in a red-top and lavender-top tube if the sample is very bloody.
5. Note the volume of fluid removed.
6. Place a small amount of fluid in a sterile tube.
7. Place a small amount of fluid in EDTA.
8. Note gross appearance of fluid.
9. Prepare slides from the fluid samples. Allow the slides to air-dry.
10. Perform a cell count. Assess protein content using a refractometer.

PROCEDURE 9-5 Tracheal Wash and Bronchoalveolar Lavage

Materials

- Surgical prep materials
- Local anesthetic
- 18-gauge jugular catheter
- Sterile polyethylene tubing and trocar (horses)
- Sterile scalpel blade
- 20- to 30-ml syringe
- Sterile buffered saline
- Endotracheal tube

Procedure

1. A standing animal is preferred; sedation may be necessary. If an endotracheal tube is used, general anesthesia is necessary.
2. The transtracheal approach requires surgical preparation over the cricothyroid area.
3. Infiltrate a local anesthetic agent over the cricothyroid membrane and skin (dogs, cats) or over the tracheal rings (horses, cattle).
4. Make a stab incision with the scalpel blade in the anesthetized area.
5. Insert the catheter (or trocar) into the trachea and direct toward the tracheal bifurcation.
6. Attach a saline-filled syringe (approximately 10 ml for small dogs and cats, 20 ml for large dogs, 30 ml for large animals) and flush into the trachea. An animal that is not anesthetized typically coughs.
7. Bronchoalveolar lavages are done with an endoscope or through an endotracheal tube. Move the catheter or endoscope as far down the trachea as possible (until wedged in a bronchus) before infusing the fluid and aspirating.
8. Aspirate fluid into the syringe by pulling back on the plunger while gently pulling the catheter back and forth within the trachea. Only a portion of the fluid will be recovered.
9. Note volume of fluid recovered. Collect additional fluid if animal coughs after procedure and note this as a nonsterile collection.
10. Place a small amount of fluid in a sterile tube for culture and sensitivity testing.

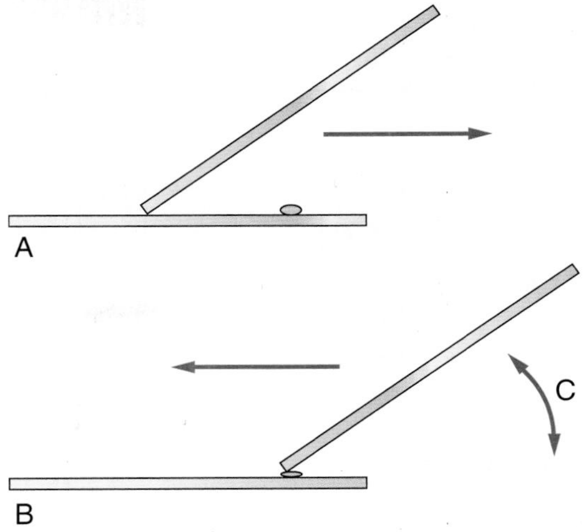

FIGURE 9-17 Wedge smear. **A,** The upper slide is slowly drawn back into the drop of fluid. The fluid is allowed to spread along the edge of the slide until it nearly reaches the edges. **B,** The slide is then pushed along the surface of the first slide to make the smear. **C,** The length of the smear can be varied by altering the pushing speed, changing the amount of fluid on the slide, or changing the angle of the top slide.

viscous or contain a large amount of particulate material. Wedge films (blood smear) are usually suitable for fluid samples (Fig. 9-17). An alternative technique, the line smear, will also provide excellent specimens.

Line Smear

This technique is primarily used when fluid samples cannot be concentrated or when the amount of sediment is very small. A small drop of the sample is placed near the end of a clean glass slide, and a second slide used to spread the specimen in a manner similar to that used for preparation of a peripheral blood film. When the smear covers approximately three-fourths of the slide, the second slide is abruptly lifted off the first. This produces a smear with a thick edge, rather than a feathered edge (Fig. 9-18). The thick edge should contain a line of concentrated sediment from the sample.

Starfish Smear

Although used infrequently, this technique can be used for sample preparation from both solid masses and viscous fluid aspirates. The aspirate is gently spread onto the slide by dragging the point of the needle across the slide in several directions (Fig. 9-19). This technique is probably the least damaging to the cells but often results in cells that are surrounded by large volumes of tissue fluid.

STAINING OF CYTOLOGY SPECIMENS

A variety of stains can be used for cytologic examination. The most commonly used stains in veterinary practice are Romanowsky-type stains. Although there is some variation in staining patterns of cells when using different Romanowsky-type stains, these rarely complicate evaluation once the cytologist becomes familiar with the staining pattern of the particular stain used. In general, stains should be applied according to the recommendations

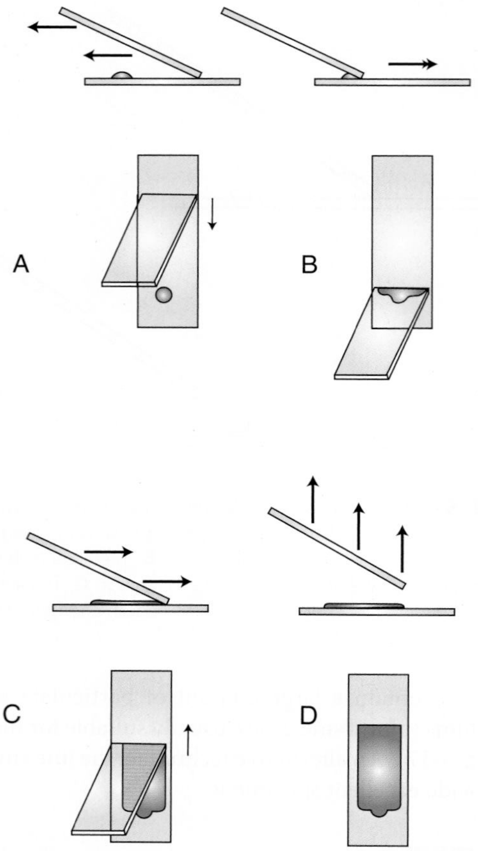

FIGURE 9-18 Line smear concentration technique. **A,** A drop of fluid sample is placed on a glass microscope slide close to one end, then another slide is slid backward to make contact with the front of the drop (**B**). When the drop is contacted, it rapidly spreads along the juncture between the two slides. **C,** The spreader slide is then smoothly and rapidly slid forward. **D,** After the spreader slide has been advanced approximately two-thirds to three-fourths of the distance required to make a smear with a feathered edge, the spreader slide is raised directly upward. This procedure produces a smear with a line of concentrated cells at its end instead of a feathered edge.

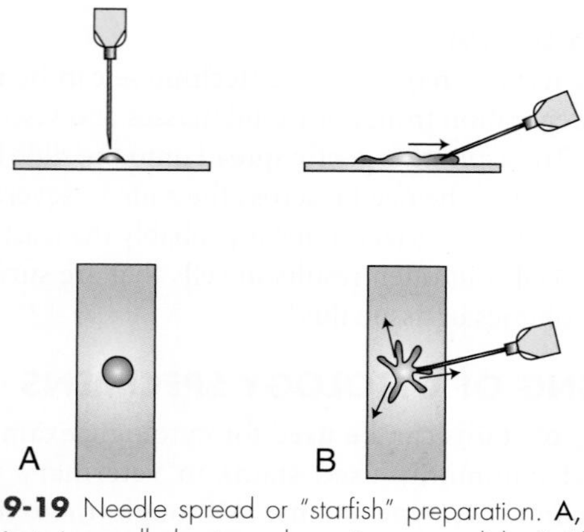

FIGURE 9-19 Needle spread or "starfish" preparation. **A,** A portion of the aspirate is expelled onto a glass microscope slide. **B,** The tip of a needle is placed in the aspirate and moved peripherally, pulling a tail of the sample with it. This procedure is repeated in several directions, resulting in a preparation with multiple projections.

of he manufacturer. In some cases the density or thickness of the tissue may require alteration of that technique. Denser, thicker preparations tend to require longer amounts of time in order to stain structures correctly, usually twice the time required for staining of blood films. Although many stains incorporate a cellular fixative, accomplishing this as a separate step in the procedure is advantageous to ensure the highest quality preparation. The preferred fixative for cytology specimens is 95% methanol. The methanol must be fresh and not contaminated with stain or cellular debris. Methanol containers must be protected from evaporation and dilution resulting from environmental humidity, which will introduce humidity artifacts onto the slide. The prepared cytology slides should remain in the fixative for 2 to 5 minutes. Longer fixative times will improve the quality of the staining procedure and not harm the samples.

> TECHNICIAN NOTE Prepared cytology slides should remain in fixative for a minimum of 2 to 5 minutes before staining.

EXAMINATION OF CYTOLOGY SPECIMENS

The primary goal of the initial cytology evaluation is differentiation of inflammation and neoplasia. In general, samples that are inflammatory are characterized by a predominance of neutrophils and macrophages or eosinophils. Neoplastic processes are characterized by large numbers of tissue cells. There may be a combination of cell types present. This mixed cell population often indicates neoplastic disease with secondary inflammation.

The initial evaluation of the cytology preparation should be performed on low magnification (100×) to determine if all areas are adequately stained and to detect any localized areas of increased cellularity. Large objects such as parasites, crystals, and fungal hyphae will normally also be evident on the low-power examination. This initial evaluation should be used to characterize the cellularity and composition of the sample by recording the types of cells present and relative numbers of each type. A high-power (450× to 1000×) should then be performed to evaluate and compare individual cells and further characterize the types of cells present. A systematic approach is vital to achieving high-quality results. Figure 9-20 contains a sample flowchart for use in evaluating cytology specimens.

Terminology

Consistent terminology must be used when describing cell types. Specific details on the morphology of each cell type will also assist the clinician in making the diagnosis. Neutrophils and macrophages should be evaluated for presence of vacuoles or phagocytized material. Neutrophils should be evaluated for the presence of degenerative changes, such as pyknosis, karyorrhexis, and karyolysis. Squamous epithelial cells should be characterized as cornified or noncornified. Neoplastic cells should be evaluated for malignant changes in the cell, such as mitotic figures, multiple nuclei and nucleoli, and basophilic cytoplasm.

> TECHNICIAN NOTE Fluid samples are classified as transudates, modified transudates, or exudates based on their gross appearance, total protein, and total nucleated cell count.

The gross appearance, total protein, and total nucleated cell count are also recorded for all fluid samples. The total nucleated cell count (TNCC) and total protein values for the sample will allow it to be classified as transudate, modified transudate, or exudate (Procedure 9-6). **Transudate** samples are noninflammatory, appear clear or colorless, and have a TNCC less than 500/microliter and total protein less than 2.5 g/dl. Modified transudates are noninflammatory and represent fluids that are passively

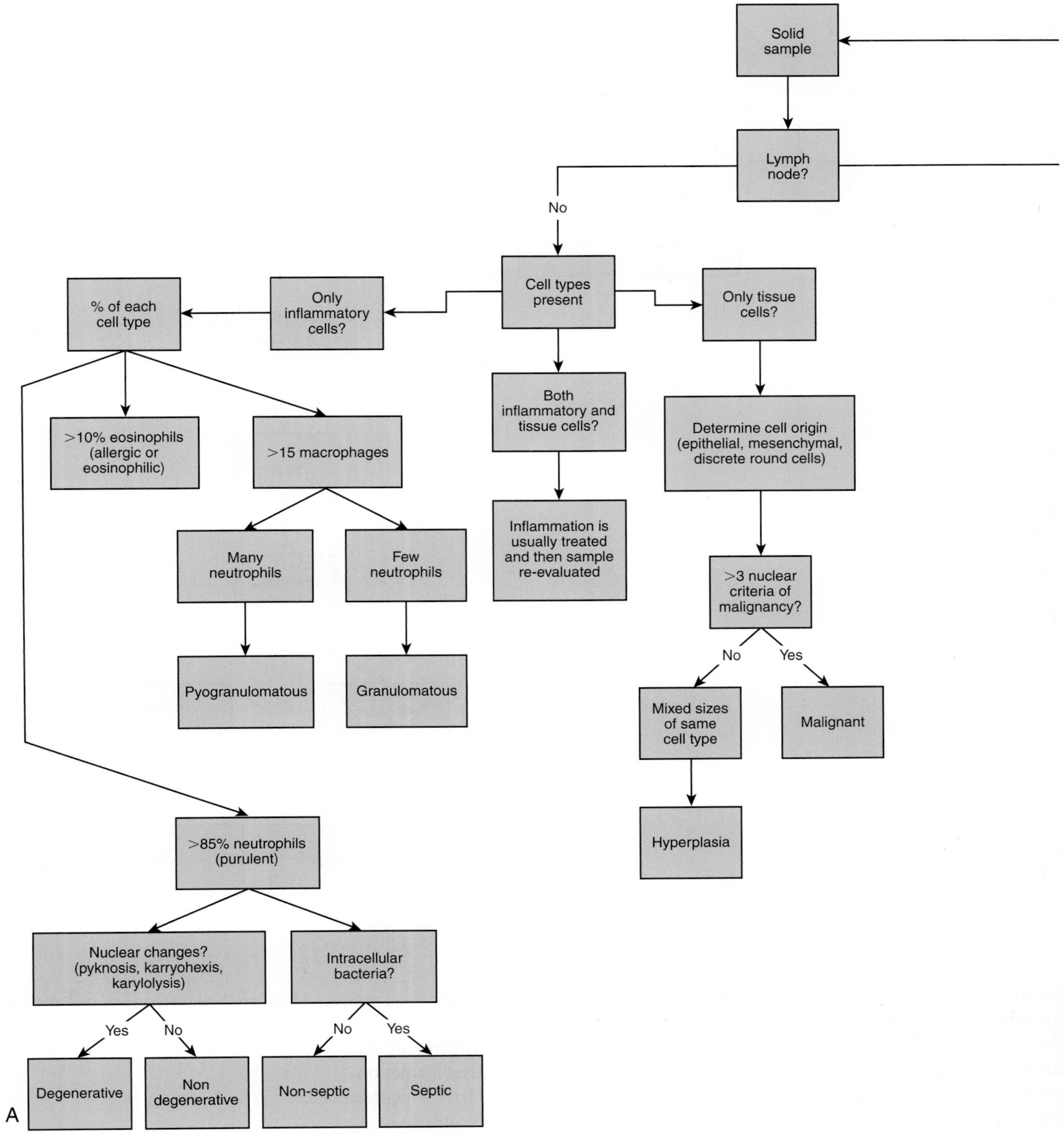

FIGURE 9-20 Flowchart for use in evaluating cytology specimens.

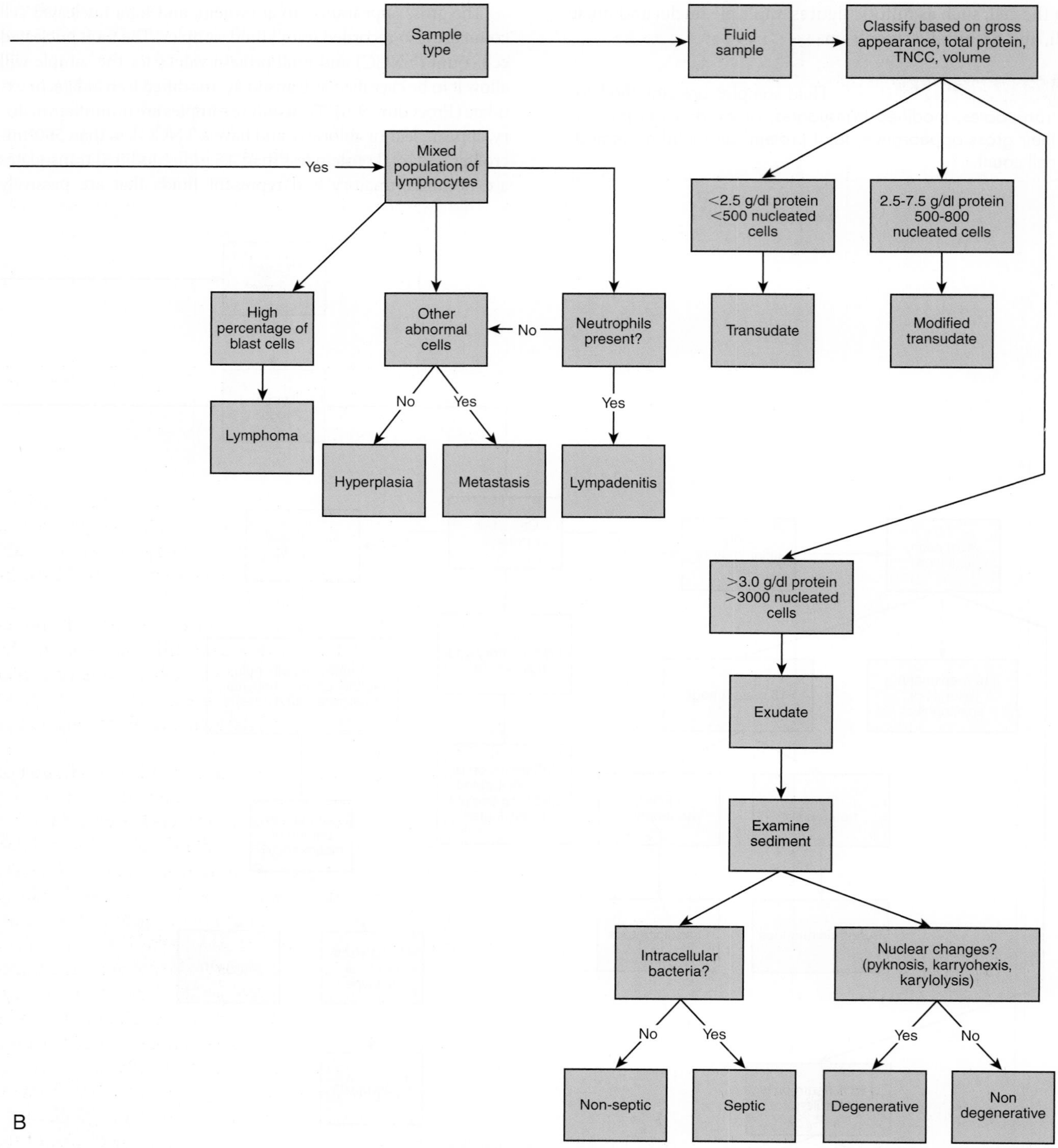

FIGURE 9-20 cont'd

leaked into tissues with a cell count between 500 and 800/microliter and total protein between 2.5 and 5.0 g/dl. **Exudates** are characterized by increased cellularity of greater than 3000/microliter and total protein greater than 3.0 g/dl. This higher cell count and protein value is usually indicative of inflammation. Exudates must be evaluated for the presence of intracellular bacteria and then further classified as septic or nonseptic.

Cytology samples can be classified into one of five general categories:

1. Inflammation
2. Cyst formation
3. Hemorrhagic lesions
4. Neoplasia
5. Mixed cell population

PROCEDURE 9-6 Classifying Fluid Samples

1. Note volume removed from cavity.
2. Save a small amount of fluid in EDTA.
3. Save a small amount of fluid in a sterile tube.
4. Complete gross examination.
5. Perform TNCC and total protein evaluations.
6. Classify fluid as transudate, modified transudate, or exudate.

	Transudate	Modified Transudate	Exudate
Protein	<2.5 g/dl	2.5-5.0 g/dl	>3.0 g/dl
Appearance	Clear, colorlesss	Lightly turbid, white	Turbid, pink
Cellularity	<500/µl	500-800/µl	>3000/µl

It is usually not necessary to collect cytology samples from hemorrhagic lesions or cysts. In most cases, the veterinary technician will be responsible for describing the sample characteristics to allow for an initial determination to classify a lesion as inflammatory, neoplastic, or mixed.

Inflammation

Inflammation is a normal physiologic response to tissue damage or invasion by microorganisms. This damage releases substances that have a chemotactic effect on certain white blood cells. These chemotactic factors, therefore, are involved in attracting white blood cells to the site of inflammation. The first white blood cells to arrive are the neutrophils. Neutrophils phagocytize dead tissue and microorganisms. The process of phagocytosis creates pH changes both within the neutrophils and in the site. As the pH changes, neutrophils become unable to phagocytize any further and the cells quickly die. At this point, macrophages move in to the site and pick up the phagocytic activity. Cytology samples from inflammatory sites are therefore characterized by the presence of white blood cells, particularly neutrophils and/or macrophages. Occasionally eosinophils or lymphocytes also may be present. In fluid samples, total nucleated cell counts of greater than 5000/µl are a common finding with inflammation. The fluid is often turbid and may be white or pale yellow. Total protein is often greater than 3 g/dl.

Once designated as inflammatory, the cells must also be evaluated for evidence of degeneration and presence of microorganisms. Nuclear changes that may be found in inflammatory cells (e.g., neutrophils) include karyolysis, karyorrhexis, and pyknosis. These terms describe a nucleus that is condensed, fragmented, or lysed. Cells should also be evaluated for the presence of bacteria. Inflammatory cells that contain phagocytized bacteria or fungal organisms are referred to as septic. Additional phagocytized material may include erythrocytes or parasites.

Neoplasia

Unlike inflammation, neoplastic specimens normally contain rather homogeneous populations of a single cell type. Although mixed cell populations are sometimes seen, these usually involve a neoplastic area with a concurrent inflammation. Neoplasia is indicated when the cells present are of the same tissue origin. Once identified as neoplastic, the technician should identify the tissue origin and evaluate the cells for presence of malignant characteristics.

Neoplasia must first be differentiated as either **benign** or malignant. Benign neoplasia is represented by hyperplasia with no criteria of malignancy present in the cells. Although there may be some minor morphologic variations, the cells are of the same type and are relatively uniform in appearance. Cells that display at least three abnormal nuclear configurations are identified as malignant. Nuclear criteria of malignancy can include any of the abnormalities listed in Table 9-4.

TECHNICIAN NOTE Samples are generally considered malignant if a significant number of cells display three or more nuclear criteria of malignancy.

In general, if three or more nuclear criteria of malignancy are present in a significant number of cells, the specimen is identified as malignant. Exceptions to this general rule would be indicated if inflammation is also present or only a few cells display malignant characteristics.

Specimens that have been classified as malignant should be further evaluated to determine the cell type involved. The basic tumor categories seen in mammals include epithelial cell tumors, mesenchymal cell tumors, and discrete round cell tumors. Table 9-5 summarizes the overall characteristics of samples from each cell type.

Epithelial cell tumors are also referred to as **carcinoma** or adenocarcinoma. The samples tend to be highly cellular and often exfoliate in clumps or sheets. **Mesenchymal** cell tumors are also referred to as **sarcoma** and are usually less cellular. The cells tend to exfoliate singly or in wispy spindles. Discrete round cell tumors exfoliate very well but are usually not in clumps or clusters. Round cell tumors include histiocytoma, lymphoma, mast cell tumors, plasma cell tumors, transmissible venereal tumors, and melanoma. Histiocytoma and transmissible venereal tumors appear similar except that histiocytoma is not usually highly cellular. Plasma cell tumors can be recognized by the presence of large numbers of cells with a prominent perinuclear clear zone. **Mast cells** can be recognized by their prominent dark purple granules. Melanoma is characterized by cells with prominent dark black granules.

Examination of lymph node tissue is perhaps one of the most complex of cytology evaluations. Normal lymph nodes usually have a mixture of small, intermediate, and large lymphocytes in relatively even percentages (Table 9-6). Lymph nodes may show evidence of inflammation (lymphadenitis), **hyperplasia** (benign neoplasia), mixed (both inflammatory and neoplastic cells present), neoplasia (lymph node cells with abnormal nuclear features), and **metastasis** (neoplastic cells from other body tissues that spread to lymph nodes). Each of these has specific cell types associated with the abnormality.

TABLE 9-4 Nuclear Criteria of Malignancy

CRITERIA	DESCRIPTION	SCHEMATIC REPRESENTATION
Macrokaryosis	Increased nuclear size. Cells with nuclei larger than 10 μ in diameter suggest malignancy.	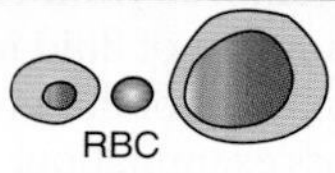 See "Macrokaryosis"
Increased nucleus: cytoplasm ratio (N:C)	Normal nonlymphoid cells usually have an N:C of 1:3 to 1:8; depending on the tissue. Ratios ≥1:2 suggest malignancy.	(see Macrokaryosis)
Anisokaryosis	Variation in nuclear size. This is especially important if the nuclei of multinucleated cells vary in size.	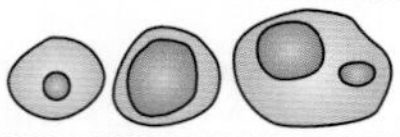
Multinucleation	Multiple nucleation in a cell. This is especially important if the nuclei vary in size.	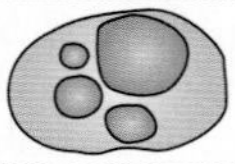
Increased mitotic figures	Mitosis is rare in normal tissue.	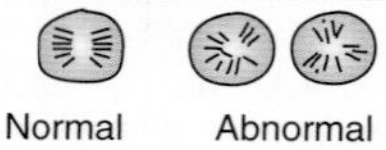
Abnormal mitosis	Chromosomes are improperly aligned.	(see Increased mitotic figures)
Coarse chromatin Pattern	The chromatin pattern is coarser than normal. It may appear ropy or cordlike.	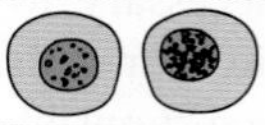
Nuclear molding	Nuclei are deformed by other nuclei within the same cell or adjacent cells.	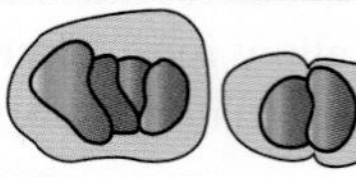
Macronucleoli	Nucleoli are increased in size. Nucleoli greater than or equal to 5 μ strongly suggest malignancy. For reference, RBCs are 5 to 6 μ in cats and 7 to 8 μ in dogs.	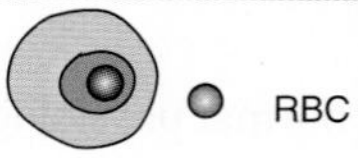
Angular nucleoli	Nucleoli are fusiform or have other angular shapes; instead of their normal, round to slightly oval shape	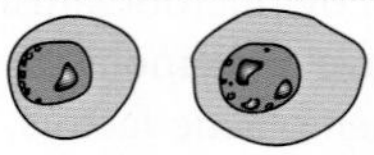 See "Angular nucleoli"
Anisonucleoliosis	Nucleolar shape or size varies. This is especially important if the variation is within the same nucleus.	(see Angular nucleoli)

TABLE 9-5 General Appearance of the Three Basic Tumor Categories

TUMOR TYPE	GENERAL CELL SIZE	GENERAL CELL SHAPE	SCHEMATIC REPRESENTATION	CELLULARITY OF ASPIRATES	CLUMPS OR CLUSTERS COMMON
Epithelial	Large	Round to caudate	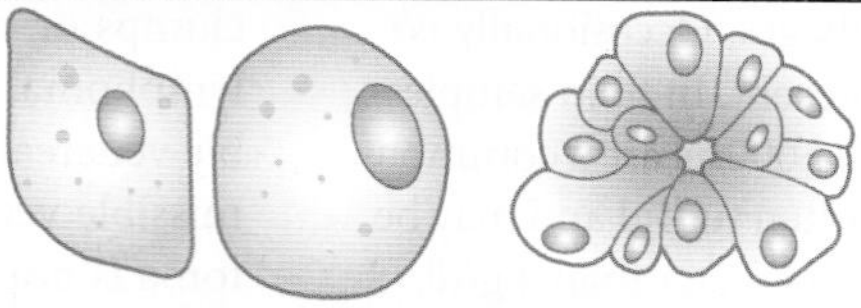	Usually high	Yes
Mesenchymal (spindle cell)	Small to medium	Spindle to stellate	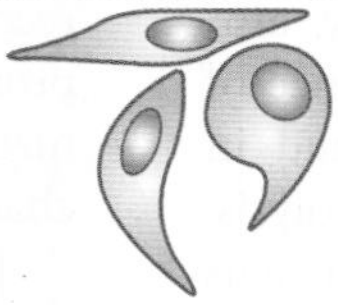 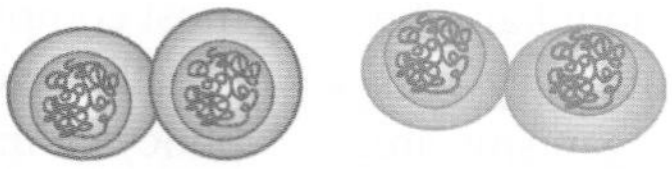 Mast cell Lymphosarcoma	Usually low	No
Discrete round cell	Small to medium	Round	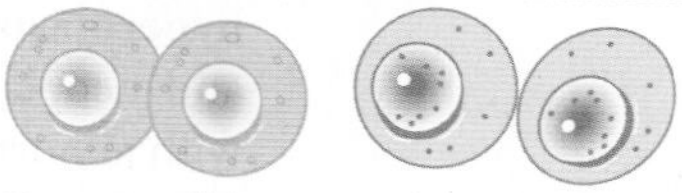 Transmissible veneral tumor Histocytoma	Usually high	No

TABLE 9-6 Cell Types Found in Lymph Node Aspirates

CELL TYPE	CHARACTERISTICS
Lymphocytes, small	Similar in appearance to the small lymphocyte seen on a peripheral blood film. Slightly larger than a Scanty cytoplasm, dense nucleus
Lymphocytes, intermediate	Nucleus approximately twice as large as an RBC. Abundant cytoplasm.
Lymphoblasts	Two to four times as large as an RBC. Usually contain a nucleolus. Diffuse nuclear chromatin
Plasma cells	Eccentrically located nucleus, trailing basophilic cytoplasm, perinuclear clear zone. Vacuoles and/or Russell bodies may be present.
Plasmablasts	Similar to lymphoblasts with more abundant, basophilic cytoplasm. May contain vacuoles.
Neutrophils	May appear similar to neutrophils in peripheral blood or show degenerative changes.
Macrophages	Large phagocytic cell. May contain phagocytized debris, microorganisms, etc. Abundant cytoplasm
Mast cells	Round cells that are usually slightly larger than lymphoblasts. Distinctive purple-staining granules may not stain adequately with Diff-Quik.
Carcinoma cells	Epithelial tissue origin. Usually found in clusters; pleomorphic
Sarcoma cells	Connective tissue origin. Usually occur singly with spindle-shaped cytoplasm
Histiocytes	Large, pleomorphic, single or multinuclear; nuclei are round to oval.

VAGINAL CYTOLOGY

Cytologic evaluation of vaginal tissues is used to determine the stage of estrous in the dog and cat, and as an aid in timing of mating or artificial insemination. Samples are collected with the animal in a standing position with the tail elevated. The external genitalia should be cleaned and rinsed. A lubricated vaginal speculum is inserted into the vagina, followed by a sterile moistened swab. The swab is gently rolled against the vaginal wall and then prepared for evaluation. Two preparations should be made by gently rolling the swab onto two clean glass slides. Approximately ⅔ of each slide should contain material from the vaginal wall. The slides must be air-dried before staining. Any stain appropriate for general staining of blood films is adequate for vaginal cytology preparations. The slide is initially examined on low power, and quality of preparation is determined. High power can then be used to determine the presence of specific cell types. The cells seen in vaginal cytology samples include epithelial cells (intermediate, large, and cornified), blood cells, and bacteria (Table 9-7). Some references may use the terms parabasal (for the youngest epithelial cells), small intermediate, and large intermediate. Cornified cells are also referred to as superficial cells and further characterized as either anuclear or pyknotic. Interpretation of results of vaginal cytology is combined with recent behavioral history and clinical signs in determining estrous stage.

TECHNICIAN NOTE The presence of specific types of epithelial cells, blood cells, and bacteria in a vaginal cytology sample is combined with behavioral history and clinical signs to determine estrous stage.

SEMEN EVALUATION

Evaluation of semen is commonly performed when preparing for artificial insemination to determine quality and quantity of sperm present in a sample. Methods used for collection of semen vary with different species. A "teaser" female may be used, and techniques include massage, electroejaculation, and use of an artificial vagina. Once collected, samples must be protected from rapid changes in temperature and pH and must not contact water, disinfectants, or other chemicals. All equipment and supplies used to collect, store, or process samples must be clean, dry, free of detergent residue, and warmed to 37° C before use. Tests used to evaluate semen include volume, gross appearance, wave motion, motility, concentration of sperm, live-to-dead sperm ratio, morphology, and determination of the presence of foreign cells and other materials.

Semen volume demonstrates significant species variation and is also affected by method of collection. The largest volumes are obtained with electroejaculation combined with the use of a teaser female. Volume is evaluated with the use of a volumetric flask. Gross appearance involves evaluation of degree of opacity. This is considered to be a rough indication of sperm concentration and is usually recorded as creamy, thick, opaque, or milky.

Sperm motility can be assessed with either the wave motion tests or progressive motility tests. Wave motion is a subjective assessment based on the amount of activity seen when observing a drop of semen at 40× magnification. If distinct, vigorous swirling activity is seen, the sample is rated as very good (VG). Moderate, slow swirling is rated as good (G). Barely discernible swirling is rated fair (F). Lack of obvious swirling activity is rated poor (P). Progressive motility testing requires dilution of 1 drop of semen in 1 drop of isotonic saline. The sample is examined at 100× magnification for rate of motility and relative percent of motile sperm.

Concentration of sperm is determined by diluting the sample with saline and formalin. A blood dilution pipette is used to dilute the sample, and a hemacytometer is used to count and calculate the numbers of sperm present. The live-to-dead sperm ratio requires a small drop of warmed eosin/nigrosin stain added to a drop of sperm on a glass slide. The slide is air-dried and examined under high power. Live sperm resist staining and appear pale/clear against a background of stain. Dead sperm stain pink/red. Two hundred sperm are counted and the ratio of live to dead sperm is recorded.

TABLE 9-7 Epithelial Cells Seen in Vaginal Cytology Samples

CELL TYPE/ILLUSTRATION	CELL TYPE/ILLUSTRATION
Parabasal cells	**Superficial epithelial cell**
Parabasal vaginal epithelial cells from a dog.	Superficial epithelial cell with a slightly pyknotic nucleus and folded angular cytoplasm.
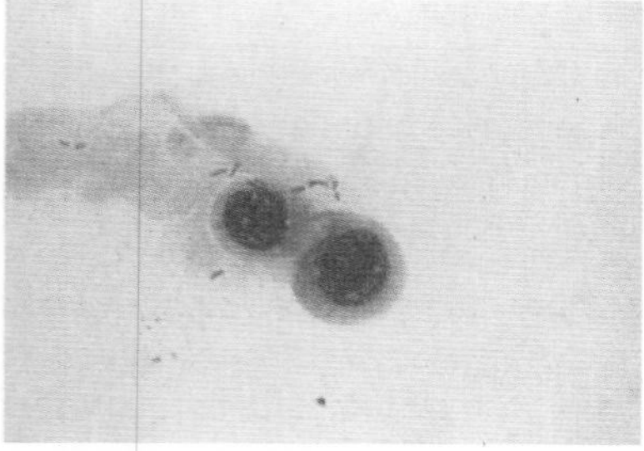	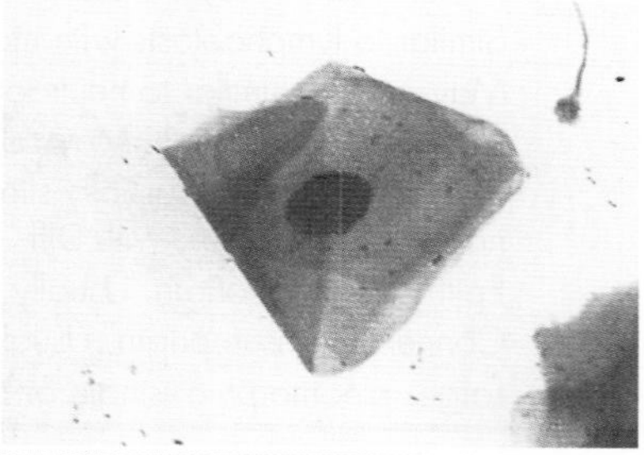
Intermediate vaginal epithelial cells	**Anuclear superficial epithelial cell**
Large intermediate vaginal epithelial cells from a dog.	Anuclear superficial (cornified) vaginal epithelial cells from a dog.
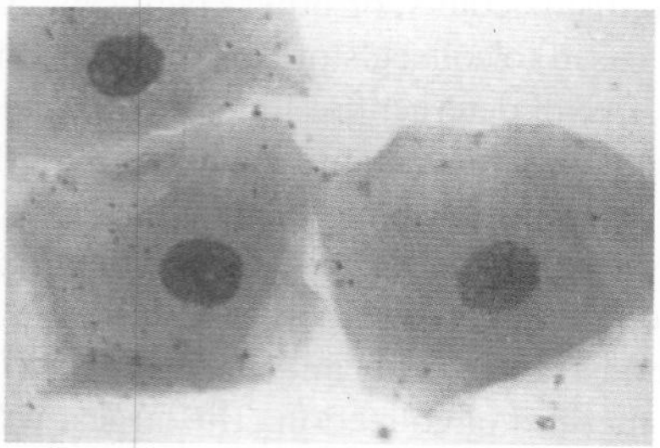	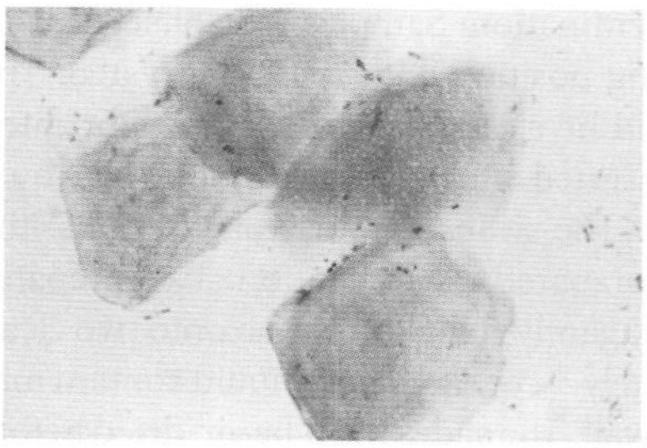

Figures from Cowell RL, Tyler RD, Meinkoth JH: *Diagnostic cytology and hematology of the dog and cat*, ed 2, St Louis, 1999, Mosby.

Morphology of sperm is species variable. Morphologic examination is used to detect the presence of abnormal sperm. Abnormalities may be seen in the head (bicephaly, microcephaly, pyriform, etc.), tail (coiled, double, etc.), or midsection of the sperm. One hundred sperm are counted, and the number of abnormal sperm seen is expressed as a percentage. Other components that may be seen in semen include blood cells, epithelial cells, and other contaminants from the prepuce (Figures 9-21 to 9-24).

HISTOLOGY

Many samples collected for cytology analysis will also require histologic evaluation. Histology samples are usually collected by biopsy and require special preparation in order to preserve the cells for detailed evaluation. The steps required for preparation of permanent histology samples are listed in Box 9-3. Fixation of tissues is a critical first step. The fixative must rapidly denature cellular proteins to avoid autolysis of the sample. Fixatives are chosen based on their speed and penetrating ability. They must not excessively harden or soften tissues and, ideally, be nontoxic to the user and inexpensive. Common fixatives include acetic acid, isopropyl or isobutyl alcohol, chromic acid, and formalin. The size of the tissue sample also affects rate of fixation. Samples must be sectioned so that the fixative can penetrate the entire tissue within 24 to 48 hours. For large tissue samples, several cuts should be made into the tissue to allow the fixative to penetrate rapidly. Most fixatives are capable of penetrating approximately 2 to 4 mm per 24 hours. The amount of solution needed is generally 10 to 20 times the volume of the sample. Once adequately fixed, the sample can be transferred into a smaller container.

TECHNICIAN NOTE Samples to be used for histopathology must be sectioned so that the fixative can penetrate the entire tissue within 24 to 48 hours.

Dehydration and washing of the tissue usually involves transferring the sample into increasingly greater concentrations of alcohols over a 24- to 30-hour time period. The sample is then cleared (alcohol removed) using one of several clearing agents. Xylene, toluene, and/or benzene may all be used as clearing agents. Once cleared of alcohols, the sample is infiltrated with paraffin and then imbedded in a block of paraffin. The paraffin block is sectioned, and the sections are

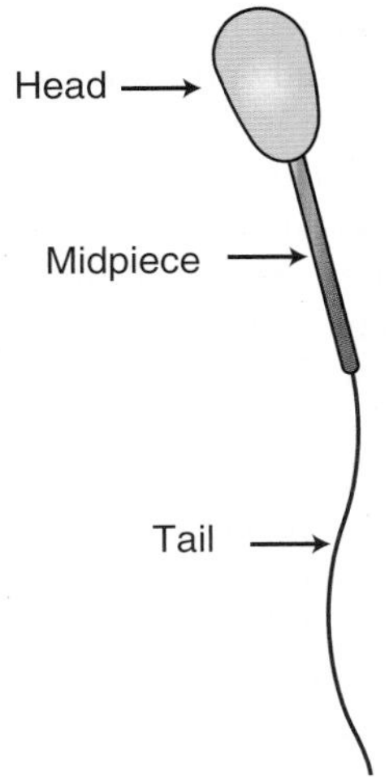

FIGURE 9-21 Diagram of normal spermatozoa. (From Figure 54-28 in Sirois M: *Laboratory procedures for veterinary technicians,* ed 6, St Louis, 2015, Mosby.)

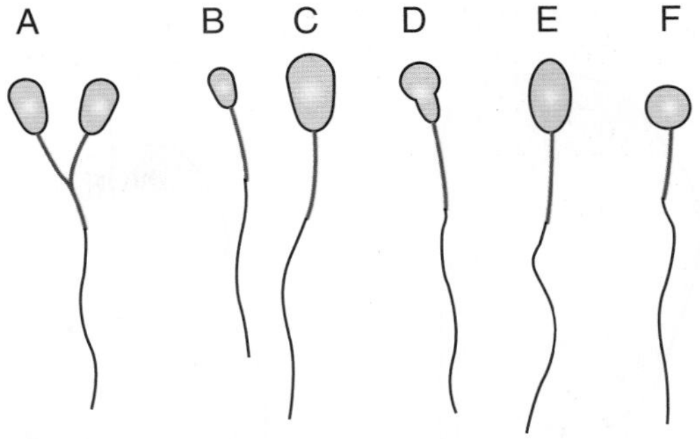

FIGURE 9-22 Diagrammatic representation of primary spermatozoal abnormalities involving the head. Abnormalities depicted are double head (bicephaly) (**A**), small head (microcephaly) (**B**), large head (macrocephaly) (**C**), pear-shaped head (pyriform) (**D**), elongated head (**E**), and round head (**F**). (From Figure 54-29 in Sirois M: *Laboratory procedures for veterinary technicians,* ed 6, St Louis, 2015, Mosby.)

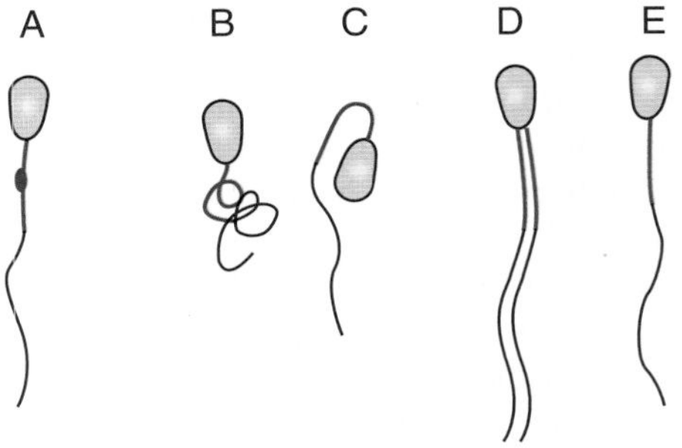

FIGURE 9-23 Diagrammatic representation of primary spermatozoal abnormalities involving the midpiece and tail. Abnormalities depicted are swollen midpiece (**A**), coiled midpiece and coiled tail (**B**), bent midpiece (**C**), double midpiece (**D**), and abaxial midpiece (**E**). (From Figure 54-30 in Sirois M: *Laboratory procedures for veterinary technicians,* ed 6, St Louis, 2015, Mosby.)

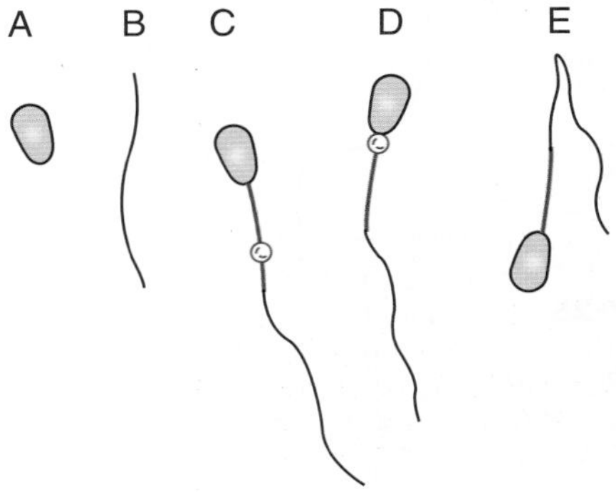

FIGURE 9-24 Diagrammatic representation of secondary spermatozoal abnormalities involving the midpiece and tail. Abnormalities depicted are tailless head (**A**), headless tail (**B**), distal protoplasmic droplets (**C**), proximal protoplasmic droplets (**D**), and bent tail (**E**). (From Figure 54-31 in Sirois M: *Laboratory procedures for veterinary technicians,* ed 6, St Louis, 2015, Mosby.)

mounted on glass slides. Stains are then added and the tissue examined microscopically. Slides can be permanently maintained by adding a cover slip with mounting media.

BOX 9-3 Preparation of Samples for Histopathology

- Tissue fixation
- Dehydration and washing
- Clearing
- Paraffin infiltration
- Sectioning
- Mounting
- Permanent cover slip

URINALYSIS

The urinary system is the primary means by which waste products are removed from the blood and consists of two kidneys, two ureters, the urinary bladder, and the urethra (Fig. 9-25). The left and right kidneys are located in the dorsal part of the abdominal cavity, just ventral to the most cranial lumbar vertebrae. Blood and lymph vessels, nerves, and the ureter enter and leave the kidney through the indented area, the hilus. The area deep to the hilus region is the renal pelvis, the funnel-like beginning of the ureter. The work of the kidneys is done within the nephrons. Depending on the animal's size, each kidney may contain from several hundred thousand to several million nephrons. Each nephron is a tube with several bends. The nephron (tubule) has the following parts: renal corpuscle, proximal convoluted tubule, loop of Henle, distal convoluted tubule, and collecting tubule (Fig. 9-26). Each renal corpuscle is composed of a glomerulus surrounded by a Bowman's capsule. The glomerulus is a tuft of capillaries between the arterioles entering and leaving the renal corpuscle.

FORMATION OF URINE

When blood enters the renal corpuscles, a portion of the plasma, along with its wastes, is filtered out through this filtration membrane into the next portion of the tubule, the

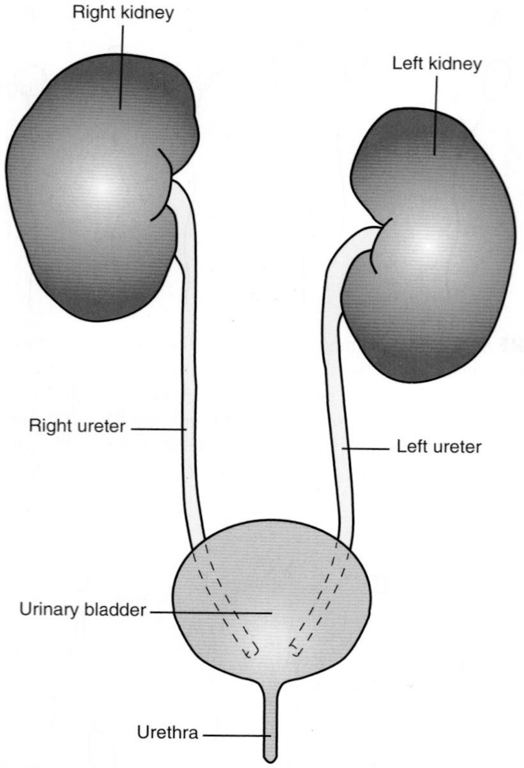

FIGURE 9-25 Parts of urinary system. The urinary system is made up of two kidneys, two ureters, one urinary bladder, and one urethra. (From Colville T, Bassert JM: *Clinical anatomy and physiology for veterinary technicians*, ed 2, St Louis, 2008, Mosby.)

proximal convoluted tubule. The filtered fluid passes slowly through the rest of the nephron and is modified as it moves along. Substances, such as water and glucose, are resorbed back into the blood of the capillary network. The nephron has a specific limit for resorption of specific substances, known as the renal threshold. Should the filtrate contain extremely high concentrations of any of those substances, the excess is not resorbed and is excreted in the urine. By the time the fluid in the nephron reaches the collecting tubules, it has become urine. Collecting tubules of all nephrons drain urine into the renal pelvis to the opening of the ureter.

Complete examination of urine is a relatively simple, rapid, and inexpensive diagnostic procedure that can provide crucial information to the veterinarian. Urinalysis is a valuable diagnostic procedure for evaluating patients. Abnormalities in the urine may reflect a variety of disease processes involving several different organs. The basic equipment needed to perform a urinalysis is minimal and readily available in most veterinary clinics.

SAMPLE COLLECTION

Collect urine samples in clean glass or plastic containers. Sterile containers are not necessary unless you are performing a urine culture. Urine samples are collected using one of the following methods.

- Free-flow or clean catch: collecting a specimen as the animal urinates
- Expressing the bladder: manual compression of the bladder using gentle, steady pressure applied through the abdominal wall
- Catheterization: placing a urinary catheter through the urethra into the bladder
- Cystocentesis: inserting a needle into the bladder through the ventral abdominal wall

Bladder expression and cystocentesis require the bladder to be full enough to palpate and hold in position. Cystocentesis requires sterile collection equipment and aseptic technique. Only specimens collected by cystocentesis are suitable for urine culture. Cystocentesis and catheterization are also performed to relieve bladder distention in animals unable to urinate. Manual compression cannot be performed on an obstructed animal because this could rupture the bladder. Bladder expression, catheterization, and cystocentesis all cause some degree of trauma. It is not unusual to find some red blood cells on microscopic examination of the urine. A first-morning urine sample is the preferred specimen because this sample is the most concentrated. The first few drops should be discarded because there is a high incidence of contamination by the debris normally present at the urethral opening in the first few drops. In females the first drops of urine may also be contaminated with material from the genital tract, such as blood from an intact bitch in proestrus.

Because physical, chemical, and microscopic characteristics of a urine specimen begin to change as soon as urine is voided, urine specimens should be analyzed immediately after collection. Samples left at room temperature for an hour or more will have increases in pH, turbidity, and bacteria and decreases in glucose, bilirubin, and ketones. If specimens are left at room temperature for longer than one hour, cells and casts may also disintegrate, especially in dilute alkaline urine, or urine color may change because of oxidation or reduction of metabolites. If analysis cannot be done immediately, refrigeration will minimize deterioration of the specimen. The specimen should be brought to room temperature before testing. Chemical preservatives can also be added to urine. However, preservatives usually act as antimicrobial agents, so chemically preserved urine cannot be used for culture and may interfere with biochemical testing.

THE COMPLETE URINALYSIS

A complete urinalysis has the following four parts:

1. Gross examination
2. Specific gravity
3. Biochemical analysis
4. Sediment examination

A systematic approach is vital to achieving high-quality, reproducible results. The gross examination includes an evaluation of color, clarity, odor, and volume. Normal canine and feline urine is light amber-colored, clear, and has a characteristic odor. Normal urine output for canine and feline patients is 10 to 20 cc per pound in a 24-hour period. Common changes found during gross examination of the urine sample are summarized in Table 9-8.

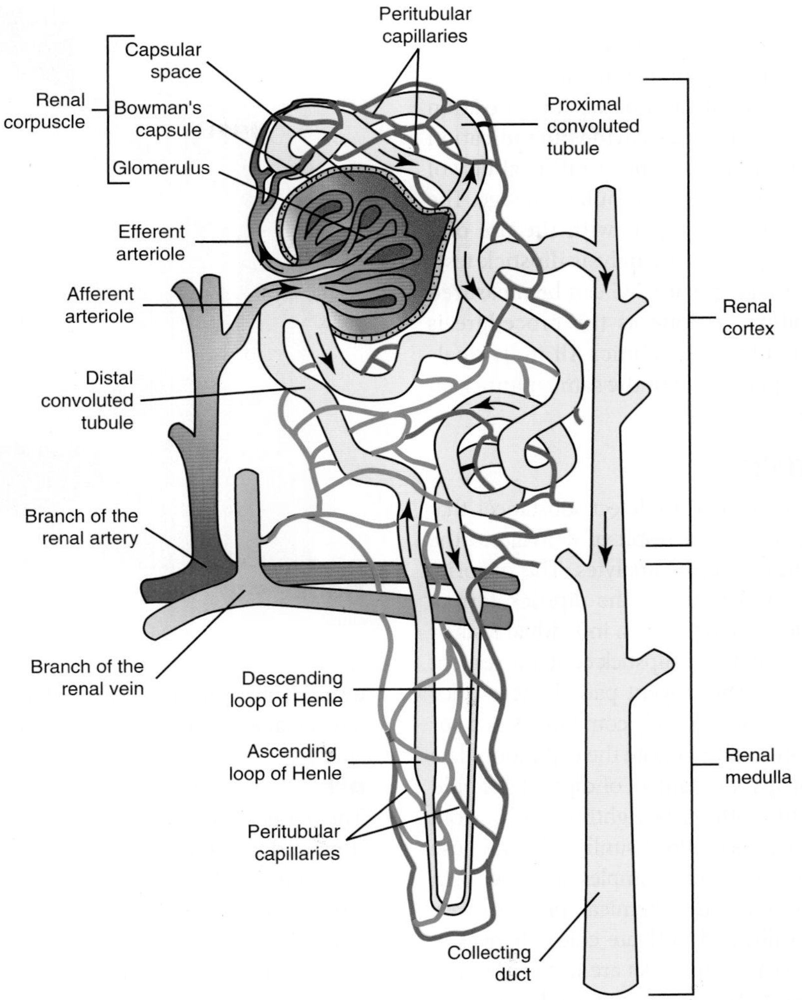

FIGURE 9-26 Microscopic anatomy of nephron. Arrows indicate direction of fluid flow through the nephron. (From Colville T, Bassert JM: *Clinical anatomy and physiology for veterinary technicians*, ed 2, St Louis, 2008, Mosby.)

TABLE 9-8 Gross Examination of Urine

QUALITY	SHOWS EVIDENCE OF
Changes in Color	
Colorless	Dilute urine with low SG; often seen in conjunction with polyuria
Deep amber	Highly concentrated urine (low SG); associated with oliguria
White	Associated with presence of leukocytes
Red to red/brown	Usually indicates presence of RBCs and/or hemoglobin
Changes in Turbidity	
Cloudy	Usually indicates presence of cells (e.g., WBCs, epithelial cells, bacteria)
Milky	Usually indicates presence of fatty material
Changes in Odor	
Sweet	Usually indicates presence of ketones
Pungent	Associated with presence of bacteria
Changes in Volume	
Polyuria	Increase in volume of urine voided in a 24-hour period
Oliguria	Decrease in volume of urine voided in a 24-hour period
Anuria	Absence of urine voiding

SPECIFIC GRAVITY

Specific gravity (SG) is a measure of the ratio of a volume of urine to the weight of the same volume of distilled water at a constant temperature. SG is an indicator of the concentration of dissolved materials in the urine and provides an indication of kidney function. Alteration in the concentrating ability of the kidneys is an early indicator of renal tubular damage. The preferred method for determining SG is with the use of a refractometer. SG indicator pads on urinalysis dipstick tests may be unreliable in veterinary species. SG can be measured before or after centrifugation, as long as the procedure is always performed consistently in the clinic. All individuals performing the test should perform it in the same manner on the same type of sample.

BIOCHEMICAL TESTING

Chemical evaluation of urine is used to detect substances that may have passed into the urine as a result of damage to the nephron or overproduction of specific analytes. The majority of in-house urinalysis chemical tests use the dipstick format (Fig. 9-27). Dipsticks can be used to perform individual tests or multiple tests. Each reagent pad on the dipstick contains reagent for one specific chemical test. The reagent pad changes color during the reaction, and the color is visually compared to a color chart. Before using the dipstick, always note the expiration date and general condition of strips. Containers of dipsticks should be stored at room temperature with the lid tightly capped. Avoid placing containers or color charts in direct sunlight. Always use well-mixed, room temperature urine samples and perform chemical testing before adding any chemical preservatives. Read the instructions carefully, and evaluate color changes at the correct time interval. Because dipsticks are not configured for veterinary species, some tests (i.e., SG, nitrite, leukocytes) may be unreliable with some species.

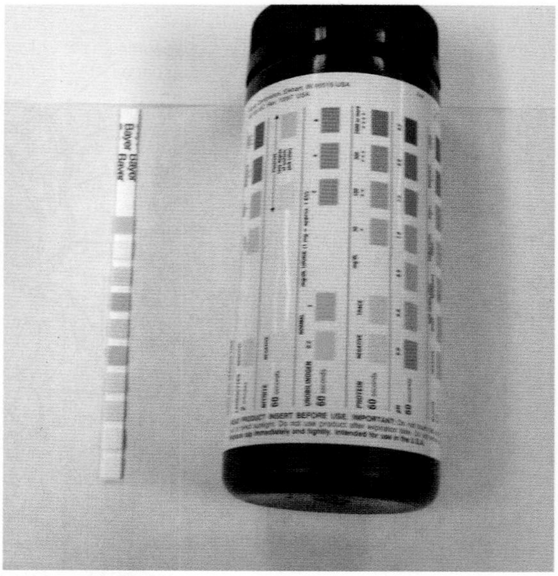

FIGURE 9-27 Reagent strip test container and combination dipstick strip.

Protein

Protein is normally present in very low quantities in the urine (at or below the limit of sensitivity of the urine reagent strips). Physiologic (nonpathologic) proteinuria can occur with fever or strenuous exercise that results in increased permeability of the glomeruli to plasma proteins. Postrenal proteinuria is the result of serum proteins being added from hemorrhage or inflammation in the lower urinary tract (bladder) or genital tract. Renal proteinuria is fairly common and may be caused by glomerular damage.

Glucose

Glucose is normally not present in the urine in quantities detectable on dipsticks. The presence of glucose in the urine is called glucosuria or glycosuria. Glucosuria occurs with any condition that causes the blood glucose level to exceed the renal threshold for resorption. Diabetes mellitus is a common cause of glucosuria resulting from excessive blood glucose concentrations.

Ketones

Ketonuria can occur with diabetes mellitus in small animals, during lactation in cows, and during pregnancy in cows and ewes. It also occurs with high-fat diets, starvation, fasting, anorexia, and impaired liver function.

pH

The pH is an indication of the hydrogen ion (H^+) concentration, and it is a measure of the degree of acidity or alkalinity of urine. A pH greater than 7.0 is alkaline; a pH less than 7.0 is acidic. High-protein diets produce a lower urine pH, whereas vegetable diets result in high urine pH. Carnivores typically have acidic urine, whereas herbivores have alkaline urine. Nursing herbivores have acidic urine from consumption of milk.

Bilirubin

Normal dogs occasionally have small amounts of bilirubin in their urine. Any bilirubinuria is abnormal in other species. Bilirubinuria can be seen with a number of diseases, including hemolytic diseases, hepatic insufficiency, and diseases that cause obstruction of bile flow.

Occult Blood

The occult blood reagent detects both myoglobin and hemoglobin in urine. The hemoglobin may be free hemoglobin (hemoglobinuria) or within intact erythrocytes (hematuria). Hematuria is detected by a positive occult blood test, along with observation of intact red blood cells on urine sediment examination. Cloudy urine that appears red, brown, or wine-colored denotes the presence of moderate to large amounts of blood. Similar colors, but with a transparent appearance, that remain after centrifugation indicate hemoglobinuria. Hemoglobinuria is usually caused by intravascular hemolysis. Myoglobin is a protein found in muscle. Myoglobinuria is usually seen in horses with rhabdomyolysis. A positive occult blood reading is most commonly associated with hematuria, rather than with hemoglobinuria.

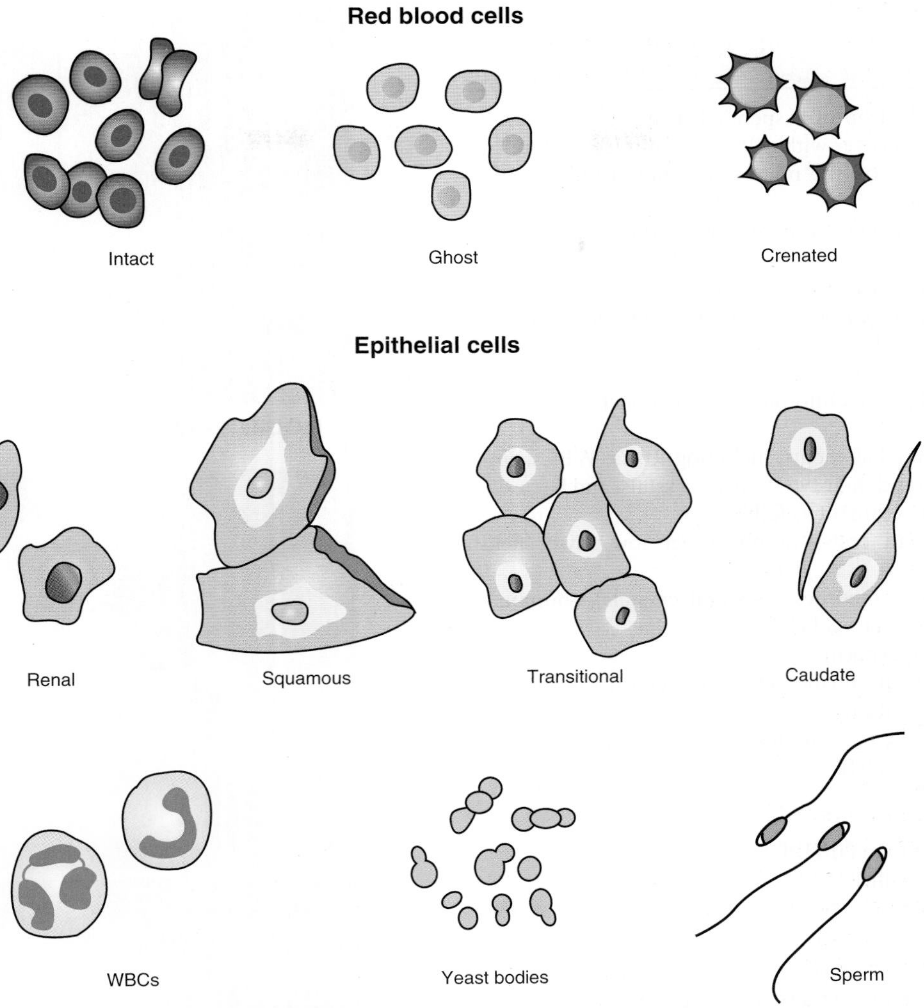

FIGURE 9-28 Cell types that may be found in urine.

MICROSCOPIC EXAMINATION OF URINE SEDIMENT

The primary purpose of microscopic examination of urine is to determine the presence of abnormal formed elements (i.e., cells, casts, crystals) in the sample (Fig. 9-28). The presence of specific formed elements usually provides detailed diagnostic information to the clinician. The examination requires 5 to 10 ml of fresh urine. The sample should be centrifuged at low speed for about 5 minutes and then the supernatant poured off, leaving about 1 ml of supernatant with the sediment. The remaining sediment is resuspended in the supernatant and mixed gently. A drop of this suspension is then placed on a microscope slide, a cover slip is added, and the specimen is examined microscopically. Although stain may be added to the sample, this often creates artifacts and can add bacteria to the sample. When stain is needed to classify cell types, they should be added after the initial evaluation of the specimen.

The specimen should first be scanned with a low-power lens. Large formed elements (e.g., casts) are evident at lower magnifications. A minimum of 10 microscopic fields with a high-power lens should be observed. The results of the microscopic examination are reported as the number of elements seen per low-power field (LPF) or high-power field (HPF). Report cells and bacteria in numbers/HPF and casts in numbers/LPF. Procedure 9-7 contains a summary of the steps required to perform a complete urinalysis.

ELEMENTS IN URINARY SEDIMENT

Cells

Erythrocytes and Leukocytes. The presence of intact erythrocytes (RBCs) in urine may indicate bleeding within the urogenital tract. Up to five RBCs per high-power field is considered normal. RBCs are smaller than leukocytes (WBCs) or epithelial cells; they are round and slightly refractile and lack internal structure (Fig. 9-29). In concentrated urine, the RBCs crenate (shrivel); in dilute urine they swell and lyse, and appear as colorless rings (ghost cells) that vary in size and shape.

Up to five WBCs per high-power field can be found in the urine sediment of normal animals (Fig. 9-30). Greater than 5 WBC/HPF can indicate inflammation. These cells are round

PROCEDURE 9-7 Microscopic Examination of Urine Sediment

1. Place a small drop of suspended urine sediment on a glass slide and cover with a 22- to 22-mm coverslip.
2. Place the slide on the microscope and swing the 10× lens into place.
3. Reduce the light intensity and lower the substage condenser.
4. Focus on the material on the slide.
5. Scan the slide and identify larger elements, such as casts and crystals. Both the center and edges of the slide should be examined.
6. Swing the 40× lens into place and readjust the light, if necessary.
7. Identify formed elements, including RBCs, WBCs, epithelial cells (and their type), casts, crystals, and bacteria.
8. Evaluate the sediment as follows:
   - Crystals and casts—numbers per low-power field (LPF)
   - Cells (and sometimes casts and crystals)—numbers per high-power field (HPF)
   - Bacteria and sperm
9. Semi-qualify any formed elements seen using the following information:
   Rare = Only 2 or 3 seen on scanning several HPF
   1+ = Less than 1/HPF
   2+ = 1-5/HPF
   3+ = 6-20/HPF
   4+ = Greater than 20/HPF
10. Record the results.

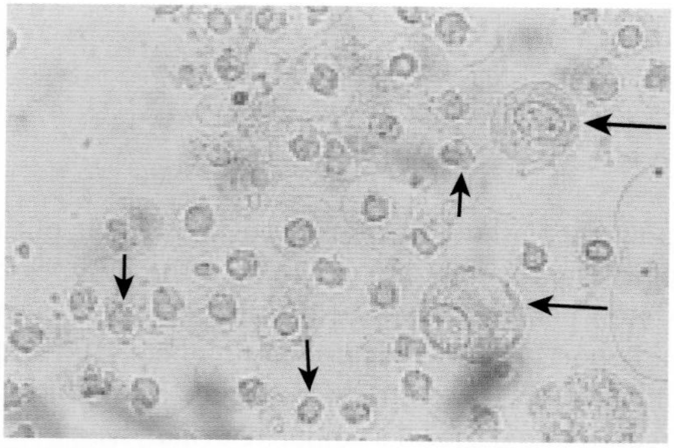

FIGURE 9-29 Unstained urine showing crenated RBCs *(short arrows)* and two epithelial cells *(long arrows)*. (From Raskin RE, Meyer DJ: *Atlas of canine and feline cytology*, St Louis, 2001, Saunders.)

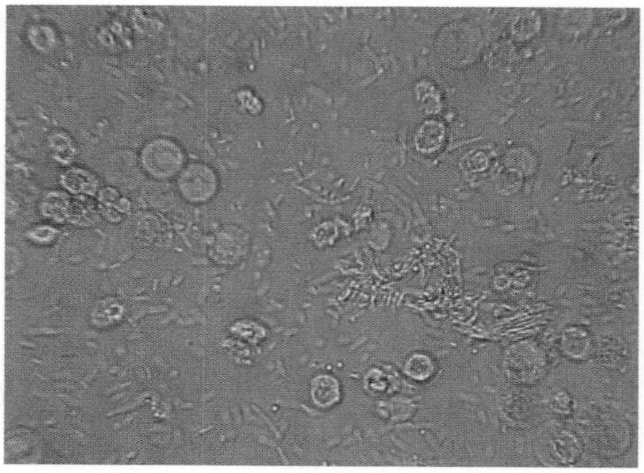

FIGURE 9-30 WBCs and bacteria in canine urine.

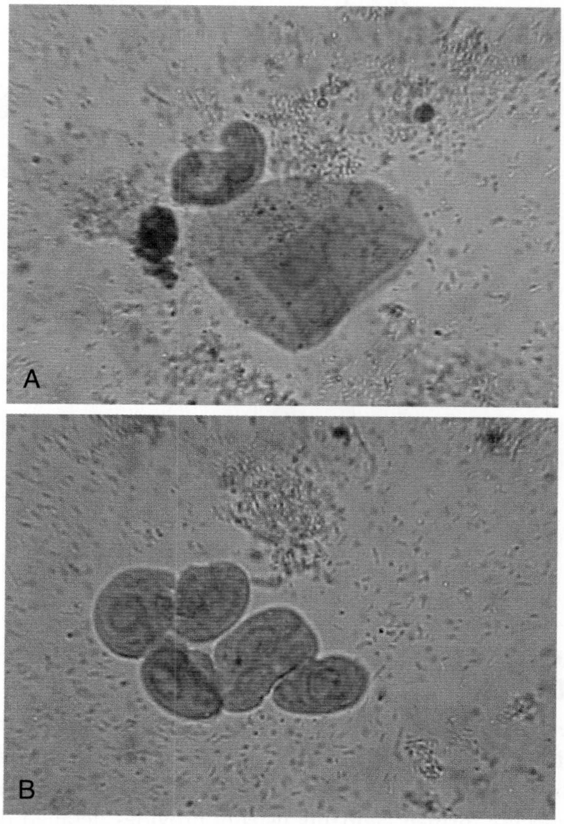

FIGURE 9-31 **A,** Squamous epithelial cells in canine urine. **B,** Transitional epithelial cells in canine urine.

and granular, larger than RBCs, and smaller than epithelial cells. They degenerate in old urine and may lyse in hypotonic or alkaline urine. WBCs should be evaluated for the presence of intracellular bacteria.

Epithelial Cells. Urine samples may contain squamous epithelial cells, transitional epithelial cells, or renal tubule epithelial cells (Fig. 9-31). Unless the sample was collected by cystocentesis, squamous epithelial cells are a common finding in urine samples. They are the largest of the three types of epithelial cells found in urine samples. The cells are thin and flat with angular borders and large nuclei. The cells originate in the distal urethra, vagina, vulva, or prepuce. The presence of squamous cells is usually not significant. Transitional epithelial cells originate in the bladder, ureters, renal pelvis, and proximal urethra. They are usually round, but can be oval or caudate. The nucleus is dense and round.

Transitional epithelial cells may occur in clumps, especially if the urine was collected by catheterization. Sheets of transitional cells in a free-flow sample may reflect transitional cell carcinoma. The morphology of these cells requires close examination for changes suggestive of malignancy. An increase in the number of transitional cells of normal appearance suggests inflammation. Renal epithelial cells are the smallest epithelial cells seen in urine. They originate in the renal tubules, and their presence may represent tubular

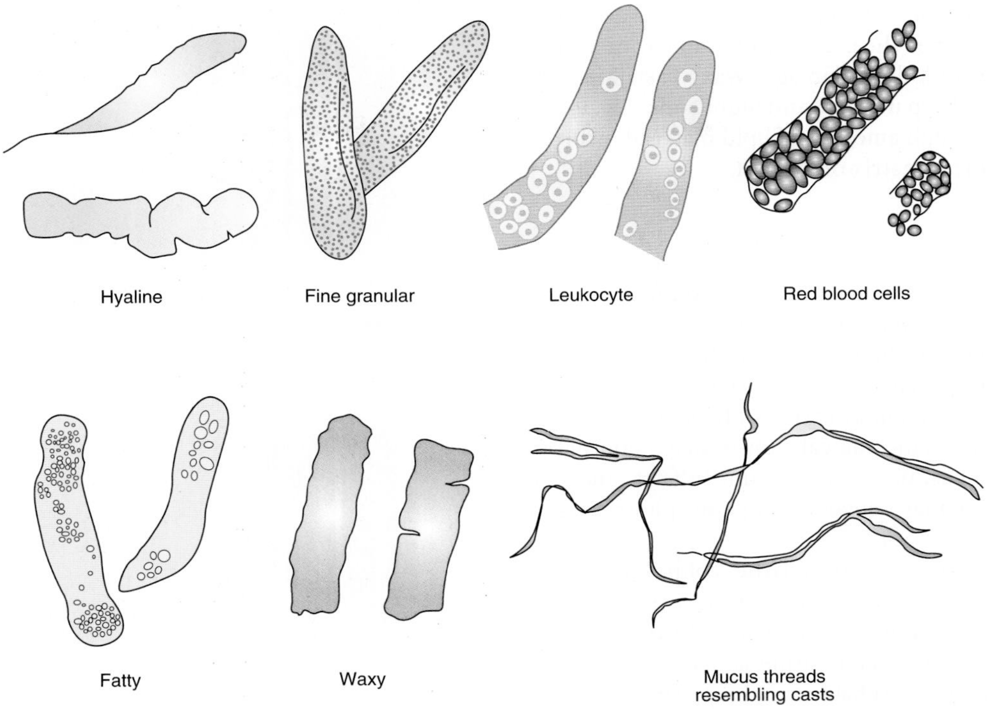

FIGURE 9-32 Various types of casts that may be found in urine sediment.

degeneration. They are small, round, and slightly larger than WBCs.

> **TECHNICIAN NOTE** Types of casts that may be found in urine sediment include hyaline casts, cellular casts, granular casts, and waxy casts.

Casts

Urinary **casts** are cylindrical structures formed from a matrix of protein secreted by the renal tubules. They form in the loop of Henle and distal tubules of the kidney. The cast takes on the shape of the tubule. Any component in the urine can be incorporated into the cast, such as cells or bacteria. Cast types include hyaline casts, cellular casts, granular casts, and waxy casts, depending on the material trapped in the protein matrix at the time of formation and the age of the casts (Fig. 9-32). Therefore, the presence of a specific type may aid in identification of the location of damage within the nephron. Casts dissolve in alkaline urine, so identification and quantification is best done with fresh urine samples. Although a few casts may be seen in normal urine, the presence of casts in urine samples usually indicates tubular damage. The formation of casts requires slow-moving filtrate. Casts are fragile structures that are easily destroyed with improper preparation of sample. Hyaline casts are colorless and translucent (Fig. 9-33). Cellular casts (Fig. 9-34) contain specific recognizable cells (WBCs, RBCs, epithelial cells). Granular casts are formed when cellular casts degenerate or when granular material from damaged renal cells becomes embedded in the protein

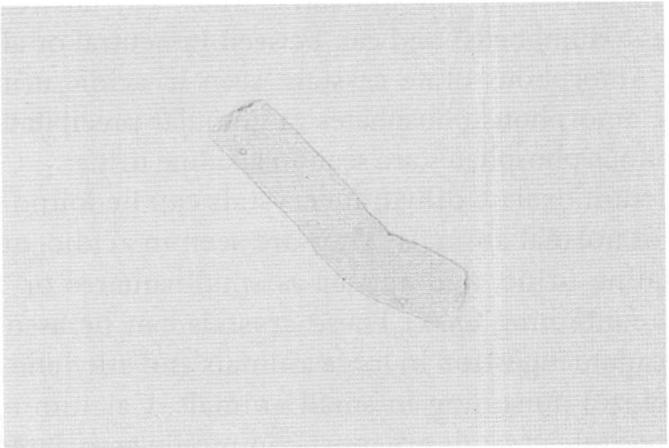

FIGURE 9-33 Hyaline cast. (From Cowell RL et al: *Diagnostic cytology and hematology of the dog and cat*, ed 3, St Louis, 2008, Mosby.)

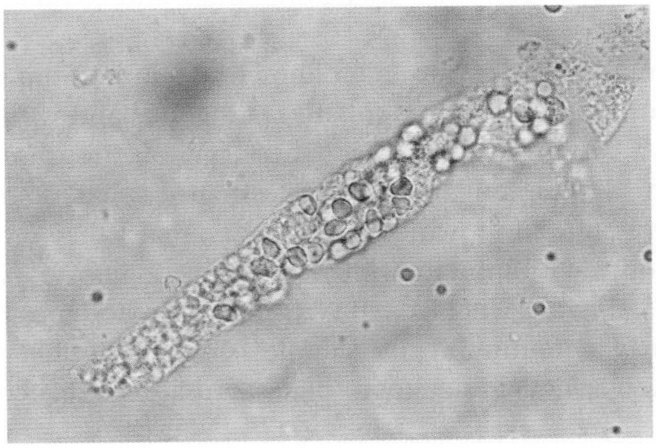

FIGURE 9-34 RBC cast, unstained. (From Raskin RE, Meyer DJ: *Atlas of canine and feline cytology*, St Louis, 2001, Saunders.)

matrix of a hyaline cast. Granular casts should be described as either coarse or fine. The presence of granular casts usually indicates severe kidney damage. Waxy casts are wide and smooth, with sharp margins and blunt ends (Fig. 9-35). Fatty casts contain high amounts of lipid material incorporated into the protein matrix of the cast.

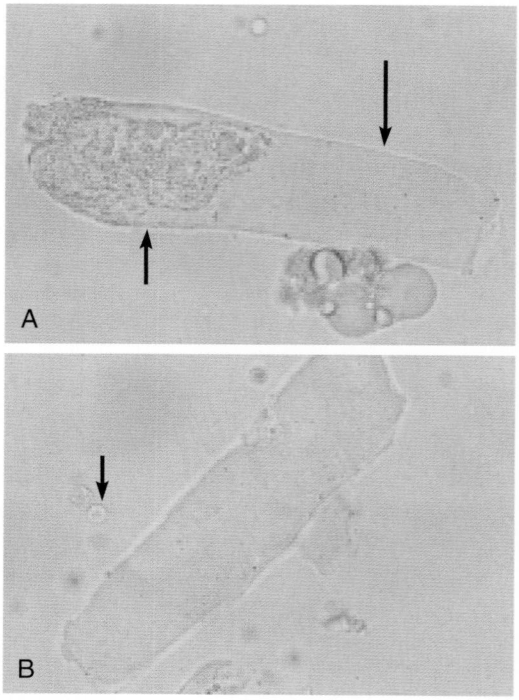

FIGURE 9-35 **A,** Granular casts develop into waxy casts as illustrated by this cast that has characteristics of both a waxy cast *(long arrow)* and a granular cast *(long arrow)*. **B,** Waxy cast, unstained. (From Raskin RE, Meyer DJ: *Atlas of canine and feline cytology*, St Louis, 2001, Saunders.)

Crystals

The presence of crystals in the urine is called crystalluria (Fig. 9-36). Crystals are common in urine sediment, but only a few types are significant. Formation of crystals is dependent on the amount of the substance in the urine and the solubility of the particular crystal type. The pH and SG of the urine affects the formation of crystals (Table 9-9). Crystals found in acidic urine include calcium oxalate, amorphous urates, sodium urates, uric acid, calcium sulfates, and cystine. Alkaline urine may contain amorphous phosphates or **struvite** crystals.

Struvite crystals have a characteristic "coffin lid" appearance (Fig. 9-37). This type of crystal, formerly referred to as triple phosphate, is a common finding in **urolithiasis** in dogs and cats but may also be seen in urine samples from normal patients. Amorphous phosphate crystals appear as a granular precipitate. Calcium oxalate crystals and stones are also found in normal urine and are common in urine from older dogs and cats.

Calcium carbonate crystals are commonly found in the urine of normal horses and cattle. These crystals resemble colorless "dumbbells" and can be seen in neutral or alkaline urine. Amorphous urate crystals, seen in acidic urine, resemble amorphous phosphates (a granular precipitate), but amorphous phosphates are seen in alkaline urine.

Calcium oxalate dihydrate crystals can be found in the urine of normal animals. They are seen in acidic, neutral, or alkaline urine, and appear as small squares or "envelopes" containing an *x*. These crystals can be associated with oxalate ingestion in large animals and ethylene glycol (antifreeze) poisoning in small animals. Calcium oxalate monohydrate crystals are most commonly associated with ethylene glycol poisoning but can also be seen in animals with calcium oxalate urolithiasis. Uric acid crystals can be seen in alkaline urine and are associated with a metabolic defect (most common in Dalmatians) and formation of uroliths.

Ammonium biurate (also known as ammonium urate) crystals are found commonly in Dalmatians and with presence of certain liver diseases. These crystals are round and brownish, with long, thorny, apple-shaped spicules, and are not present in the urine of normal animals; they are seen in the urine of animals with liver disease or portosystemic shunts. Cystine, leucine, and tyrosine are pathologic crystals that may be found in urine samples. Cystine crystals appear as flat, hexagonal (six-sided) plates and are associated with congenital defects in cystine metabolism and are common in certain canine breeds (e.g., Newfoundland). Leucine and tyrosine crystals often occur together and are present in acute liver disease.

Bacteria

Bacteria may be present as the result of infection or contamination. Normal urine is free of bacteria but may be contaminated by bacteria from the distal urethra and genital tract. Urine obtained by cystocentesis is the preferred sample for evaluation of bacteria because contamination is avoided. Bacteria numbers are reported as few, moderate, or many. Evaluate the sample based on the presence or absence of phagocytized bacteria present in the WBCs. Because bacteria often proliferate in urine that has been left standing for some time, it is important to examine a fresh sample.

Miscellaneous

Parasites and/or their ova may be seen in urine sediment. *Capillaria plica, Dichtophyma renale,* and some liver flukes may be present. Additional organisms such as mites are seen as contaminants when samples are collected improperly. Fungal organisms, microfilaria of *D. immitis,* and sperm may also be seen.

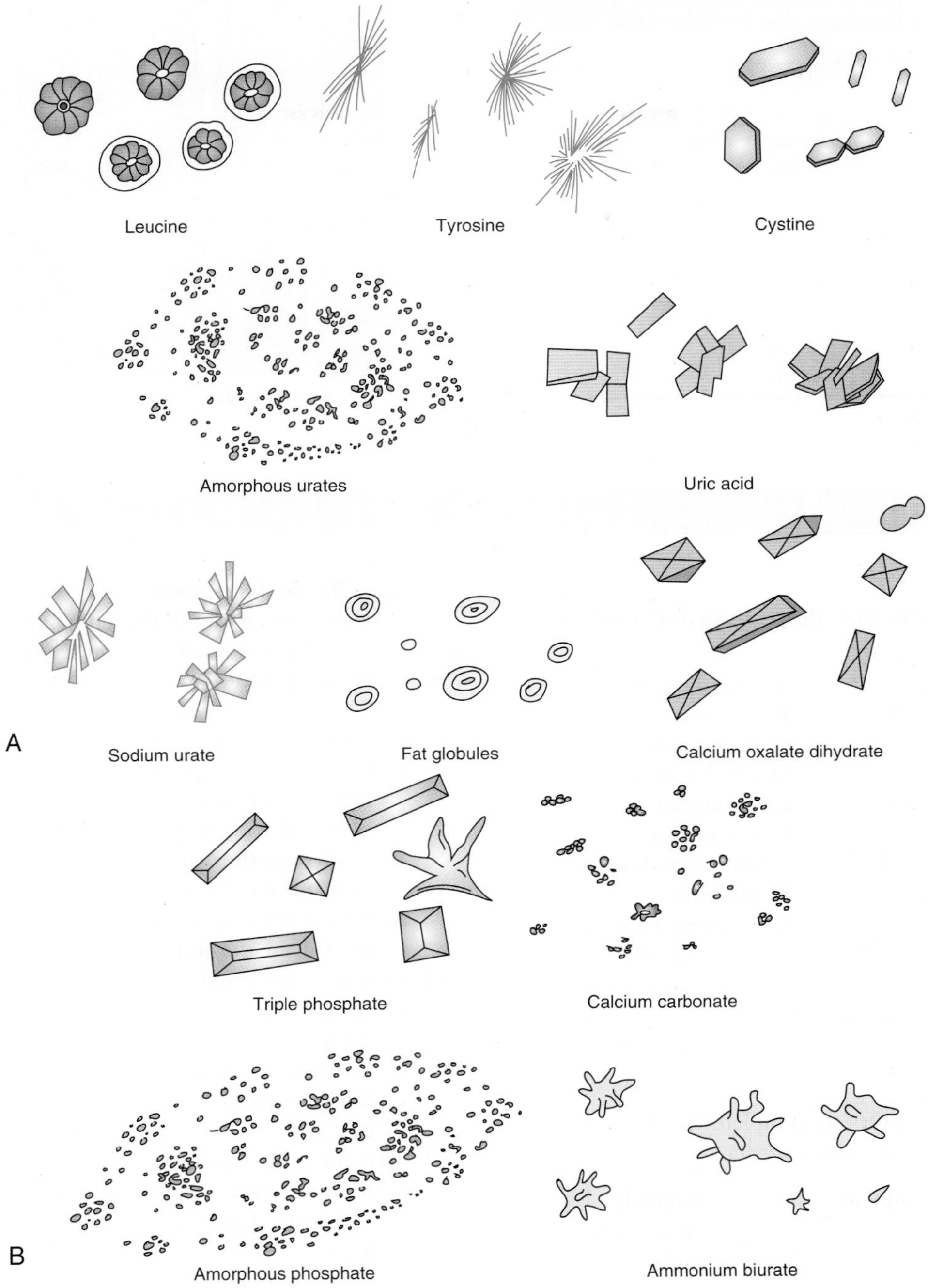

FIGURE 9-36 Crystals that may be found in urine.

TABLE 9-9 pH Chart for Urine Crystals

CRYSTAL	pH
Ammonium biurate	Slightly acidic, neutral, alkaline
Amorphous phosphate	Neutral, alkaline
Amorphous urates	Acidic, neutral
Bilirubin	Acidic
Calcium carbonate	Neutral, alkaline
Calcium oxalate	Acidic, neutral, alkaline
Cystine	Acidic
Leucine	Acidic
Triple phosphate	Slightly acidic, neutral, alkaline
Tyrosine	Acidic
Uric acid	Acidic

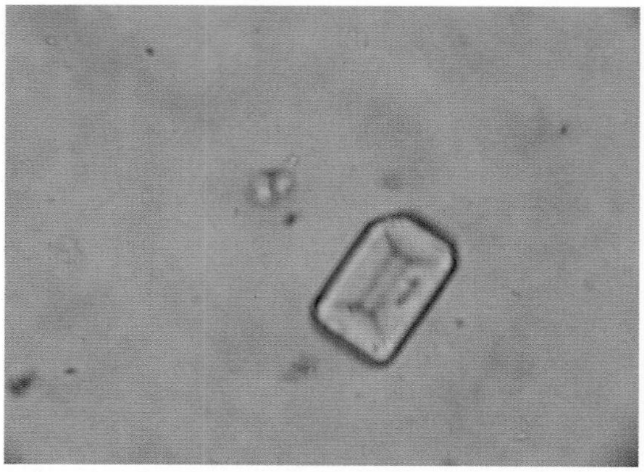

FIGURE 9-37 Struvite crystal in canine urine.

REVIEW QUESTIONS

Matching

Match the terms with their description or definition.

_____1. pyknosis
_____2. epithelial cell tumor
_____3. cocci
_____4. karyorrhexis
_____5. bacillus
_____6. mesenchymal cell tumor
_____7. fungi
_____8. round cell tumor
_____9. bacteria
_____10. karyolysis

A. round bacteria
B. histiocytoma
C. prokaryotic
D. condensed nucleus
E. eukaryotic
F. carcinoma
G. rod-shaped bacteria
H. sarcoma
I. fragmented nucleus
J. lysed nucleus

Fill in the Chart

Provide the best answers to complete the following chart about the three types of culture media.

Culture	Description	Example
Selective	________________ ________________ ________________ ________________	MacConkey EMB
________	Contains specific growth factors for bacteria with strict nutrient requirements	________
Differential	________________ ________________ ________________ ________________	________

Choose the Best Response

Choose the best answer to the following questions.

1. What is the best way to differentiate between hematuria and hemoglobinuria?
   a. Check for occult blood with a dipstick: a positive reading indicates hematuria.
   b. Look for reddish-brown discoloration of the urine (caused by hematuria); hemoglobinuria is detectable only with a reagent strip.
   c. Centrifuge the urine and examine the sediment microscopically for red blood cells.
   d. Spin down a blood sample: if the serum or plasma is red-tinged, the animal will have hemoglobinuria.
2. Which urine crystal is commonly associated with ethylene glycol toxicity in small animals?
   a. triple phosphate
   b. ammonium biurate
   c. calcium oxalate
   d. uric acid
3. To confirm the diagnosis of ringworm (dermatophytosis), which type of specimen should you collect and submit to the diagnostic laboratory?
   a. feces
   b. stomach contents
   c. blood sample
   d. skin scrapings
4. A tumor type in which the cells exfoliate singly is:
   a. mesenchymal
   b. TVT
   c. epithelial
   d. carcinoma
5. A tumor type in which the cells exfoliate in clusters is:
   a. mesenchymal
   b. TVT
   c. sarcoma
   d. carcinoma

6. Samples with very low cellularity are best prepared as:
   a. wedge films
   b. line smears
   c. starfish smear
   d. squash prep
7. Total nucleated cell counts greater than 5000/microliter are characteristic of:
   a. inflammation
   b. neoplasia
   c. hemorrhagic lesions
   d. mixed inflammation
8. A cell with dark purple granules is most likely a:
   a. plasma cell
   b. macrophage
   c. mast cell
   d. eosinophil

RECOMMENDED READING

Baker R, Lumsden J: *Color atlas of cytology of the dog and cat*, St Louis, 2000, Mosby.

Cowell R, Tyler R, Meinkoth J, DeNicola D: *Diagnostic cytology and hematology of the dog and cat*, ed 3, St Louis, 2008, Mosby.

Dow SW, Jones RL, Rosychuk RA: Bacteriologic specimens: selection, collection, and transport for optimum results. In *Veterinary laboratory medicine in practice*, Trenton, NJ, 1997, Veterinary Learning Systems.

Graff L: *A handbook of routine urinalysis*, Philadelphia, 1992, Lippincott Williams & Wilkins.

Meyer DJ: The management of cytology specimens. In *Veterinary laboratory medicine in practice*, Trenton, NJ, 1997, Veterinary Learning Systems.

Raskin R, Meyer DJ: *Canine and feline cytology: a color atlas and interpretation guide*, ed 3, St Louis, 2015, Saunders.

Sirois M: *Laboratory procedures for veterinary technicians*, ed 6, St Louis, 2014, Mosby.

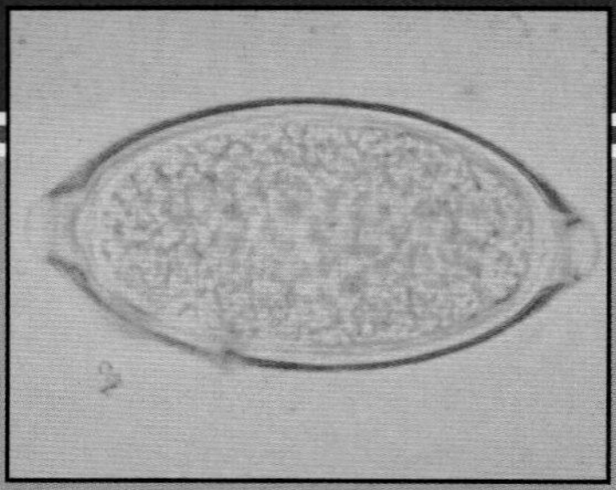

10 Parasitology

OUTLINE

LEARNING OBJECTIVES

After reviewing this chapter, the reader will be able:

1. List common internal parasites of domestic animals.
2. List common external parasites of domestic animals.
3. Discuss life cycles of common parasites of domestic animals.
4. Describe treatment and control strategies for common parasites of domestic animals.
5. Describe procedures used to diagnose parasites.

KEY TERMS

Acariasis
Arthropod
Baermann technique
Bladder worm
Cercaria
Cestode
Cysticercus
Definitive host
Diptera
Ectoparasite
Endoparasite
Hexacanth
Intermediate host
Merozoite
Microfilaria
Miracidium
Myiasis
Nit
Oocyst
Operculum
Pediculosis
Prepatent period
Proglottid
Redia
Scolex
Sporocyst
Sporozoite
Tick paralysis
Trematode
Trophozoite
Vector
Warble
Zoonotic

PARASITOLOGY

Parasitology is the study of organisms that live in (internal parasites, **endoparasites**) or on (external parasites, **ectoparasites**) another organism, the host, from which they derive their nourishment. Parasitism is a type of symbiotic relationship. Symbiosis involves two organisms living together and can be of three types:

- Commensalism: one organism benefits, the other is unaffected
- Mutualism: both organisms benefit
- Parasitism: one organism benefits, the other is harmed

The organism that the parasite lives in or on is called its host. The host may be a **definitive host,** sheltering the sexual, adult stages of the parasite, or an **intermediate host,** harboring asexual (immature) or larval stages of the parasite. There are also paratenic hosts or transport hosts for some parasites, in which the parasite survives without multiplying or developing. Parasite life cycles can be simple with direct transmission, or complex and involve one or more **vectors.** A vector can be mechanical or biological. Mechanical vectors transmit the parasite but the parasite does not develop in the vector. Biological vectors serve as intermediate hosts for the parasite. The term life cycle refers to maturation of a parasite through various developmental stages in one or more hosts. For a parasite to survive, it must have a dependable means of transfer from one host to another and the ability to develop and reproduce in the host, ideally without producing serious harm to the host. This requires the following:

- Mode of entry into a host (infective stage)
- Availability of a susceptible host (definitive host)
- Accommodating location and environment in the host for maturation and reproduction (gastrointestinal, respiratory, circulatory, urinary, or reproductive system)

- Mode of exit from the host (feces, sputum, blood, urine, smegma), with dispersal into an ecologically suitable environment for development and survival.

For parasites that have one or more intermediate hosts, the definitive host is the one in which sexual maturity takes place.

Parasites have a wide distribution within host animals. They can have a negative impact in a number of ways, including the following:

- Injury on entry (e.g., creeping eruption)
- Injury by migration (e.g., sarcoptic mange)
- Injury by residence (e.g., heartworms)
- Chemical and/or physiologic injury (e.g., digestive disturbances)
- Injury caused by host reaction (e.g., hypersensitivity, scar tissue)

CLASSIFICATION OF PARASITES

Parasites of domestic animals are found in the Kingdom Protista and the Kingdom Animalia and in a large number of phyla in those kingdoms. There is some variation in classification schemes in different references and organisms are often re-classified when new information on their biochemistry is obtained. Box 10-1 contains a summary of the taxonomic classifications of common parasites of domestic animals.

BOX 10-1 Taxonomic Classifications of Parasites of Animals

Kingdom: Animalia (animals)
  Phylum: Platyhelminthes (flatworms)
    Class: Trematoda (flukes)
      Subclass: Monogenea (monogenetic flukes)
      Subclass: Digenea (digenetic flukes)
    Class: Cotyloda (pseudotapeworms)
  Phylum: Nematoda (roundworms)
  Phylum: Acanthocephala (thorny-headed worms)
  Phylum: Arthropoda (animals with jointed legs)
   Subphylum: Mandibulata (possess mandibulate mouthparts)
    Class: Crustacea (aquatic crustaceans)
    Class: Insecta
      Order: Dictyoptera (cockroaches)
      Order: Coleoptera (beetles)
      Order: Lepidoptera (butterflies and moths)
      Order: Hymenoptera (ants, bees, and wasps)
      Order: Hemiptera (true bugs)
      Order: Mallophaga (chewing or biting lice)
      Order: Anoplura (sucking lice)
      Order: Diptera (two-winged flies)
      Order: Siphonaptera (fleas)
  Phylum: Sarcomastigophora
   Subphylum: Mastigophora (flagellates)
  Phylum: Sarcomastigophora
   Superclass: Sarcodina (amoebae)
  Phylum: Ciliophora (ciliates)
  Phylum: Apicomplexa (apicomplexans)
  Phylum: Proteobacteria
    Class: Alpha Proteobacteria
      Order: Rickettsiales
        Family: Rickettsiaceae
        Family: Anaplasmataceae

KINGDOM PROTISTA, SUBKINGDOM PROTOZOA

There are about 65,000 known protozoans in a wide variety of habitats. Only a small percentage of protozoans are parasitic. Protozoa are single-celled organisms with one or more membrane-bound nuclei containing DNA and specialized cytoplasmic organelles. Parasitic protozoa can be found in three primary phyla: (1) Sarcomastigophora; (2) Apicomplexa; and (3) Ciliophora. The life cycles of protozoa can be simple or complex. Reproduction may be asexual (binary fission, schizogony, budding) or sexual (syngamy, conjugation). With certain groups of protozoa, reproductive stages are useful in identification. The **trophozoite** (also known as vegetative form) is that stage of the protozoal life cycle that is capable of feeding, movement, and reproduction. Table 10-1 summarizes some common protozoal parasites of veterinary species.

Organelles for locomotion consist of flagella (long whiplike structures), cilia (short flagella usually arranged in rows or tufts), pseudopodia (temporary extensions and retractions of the body wall), and undulatory ridges (small snakelike waves that form in the cell membrane and move posteriorly). Locomotor organelles and modifications of them are frequently used to help identify the type of protozoa recovered from animals. The trophozoite is often too fragile to survive transfer to a new host and generally is not infective. Transmission to a host often occurs when the protozoan is in the cyst stage. Most metabolic functions are suspended when the parasite is encysted. The cyst wall prevents desiccation. The cyst stage occurs under certain conditions that include:

- Lack of nutrients
- Low oxygen tension
- Lack of water
- Low pH
- Accumulation of waste
- Overcrowding

Phylum Sarcomastigophora (Sarcodina)

This phylum includes the amoebas and flagellates. There are about 44,000 known species in this phylum, but only about 2300 are parasitic. Genera of veterinary importance in this phylum include:

- *Trypanosoma* (see Fig. 10-1)
- *Leishmania*
- *Giardia* (see Fig. 10-2)
- *Trichomonas*
- *Histomonas*
- *Entamoeba* (see Fig. 10-3)

TABLE 10-1 Select Protozoal Parasites of Veterinary Species

	INTERMEDIATE HOST(S)	LOCATION IN FINAL HOST
Dogs		
Ciliates		
Balantidium coli		Cecum/colon
Sarcodines (Amoebas)		
Entamoeba histolytica		Large intestine
Flagellates		
Giardia species		Small intestine
Trypanosoma cruzi	Reduviid bugs	Peripheral blood
Leishmania species	Phlebotomine sandfly	Macrophages
Apicomplexans		
Babesia canis	Ticks	Erythrocytes
Cryptosporidium canis		Small intestine
Hepatozoon americanum	Ticks	Leukocytes
Hepatozoon canis	Ticks	Leukocytes
Cystoisospora canis (formerly *Isospora canis*)		Small Intestine/cecum
Cystoisospora felis (formerly *Isospora felis*)		Small Intestine/ileum
Cystoisospora ohioensis (formerly *Isospora ohioensis*)		Small Intestine/cecum/colon
Cystoisospora rivoltas (formerly *Isospora rivolta*)		Small Intestine/cecum/colon
Cystoisospora burrowsi (formerly *Isospora burrowsi*)		Small Intestine/cecum/colon
Sarcocystis species		Small intestine
Cats		
Flagellates		
Giardia species		Small intestine
Apicomplexans		
Cryptosporidium felis		Small intestine
Cytauxzoon felis	Ticks	Erythrocytes
Cystoisospora felis (formerly *Isospora felis*)		Small Intestine/ileum
Cystoisospora rivoltas (formerly *Isospora rivolta*)		Small Intestine/cecum/colon
Sarcocystis species		Small intestine
Toxoplasma gondii		Intestinal mucosal cells
Horses		
Babesia caballi	Ticks	Erythrocytes
Babesia equi	Ticks	Erythrocytes
Eimeria leuckarti		Small intestine
Giardia equi		Small intestine
Sarcocystis neurona		Spinal cord, other CNS tissue
Ruminants		
Babesia bigemina	Ticks	Erythrocytes
Cryptosporidium species		Small intestine
Eimeria bovis		Small intestine
Tritrichomonas foetus		Reproductive system
Swine		
Eimeria species		Small intestine
Cryptosporidium species		Small intestine
Cystoisospora suis (formerly *Isospora suis*)		Small intestine
Rabbits		
Eimeria irresidua		Small intestine
Eimeria magna		Small intestine
Eimeria media		Small/large intestine
Eimeria perforans		Small intestine
Eimeria stiedai		Bile ducts

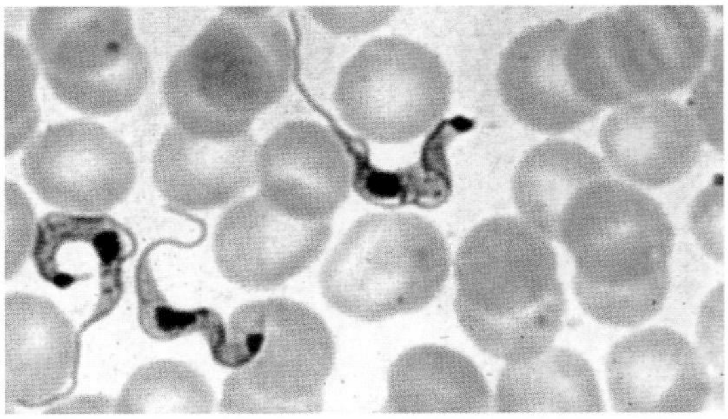

FIGURE 10-1 *Trypanosoma cruzi*. Trypomastigote. (From Bowman DD: *Georgis' parasitology for veterinarians*, ed 9, St Louis, 2009, Saunders.)

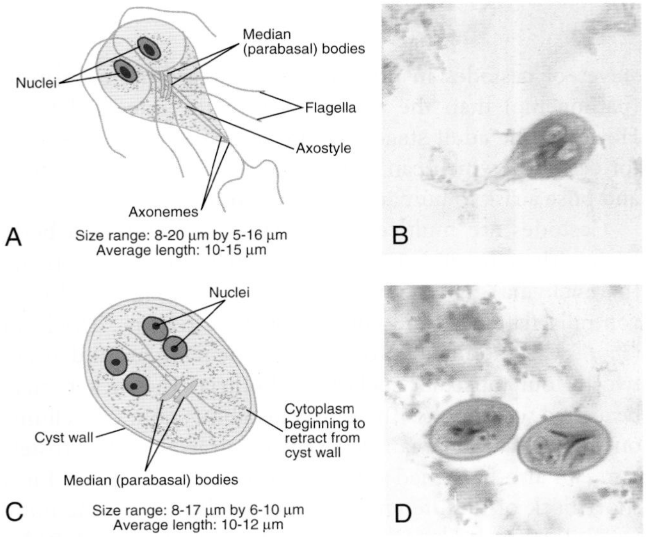

FIGURE 10-2 A, Giardia intestinalis trophozoite. B, Giardia intestinalis trophozoite. C, Giardia intestinalis cyst. D, Giardia intestinalis cyst. (From Forbes BA, Sahm DF, Weissfeld AS: *Bailey & Scott's diagnostic microbiology*, ed 12, St Louis, 2007, Mosby.)

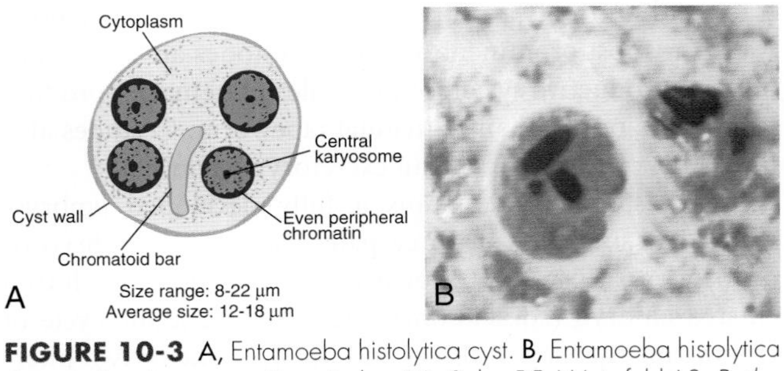

FIGURE 10-3 A, Entamoeba histolytica cyst. B, Entamoeba histolytica -Entamoeba dispar cyst. (From Forbes BA, Sahm DF, Weissfeld AS: *Bailey & Scott's diagnostic microbiology*, ed 12, St Louis, 2007, Mosby.)

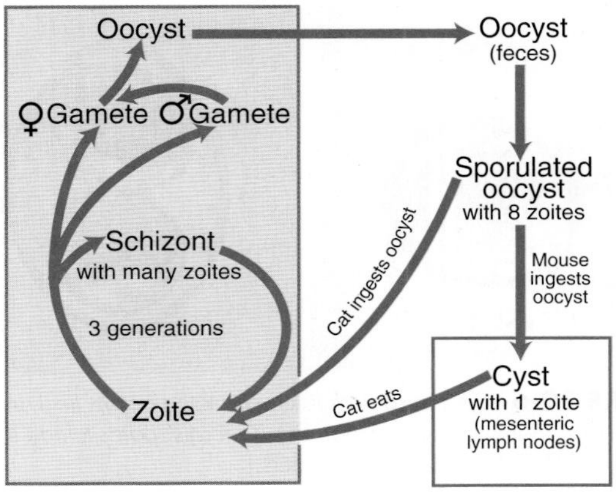

FIGURE 10-4 Life cycle of *Cystoisospora felis*. (From Bowman DD: *Georgis' parasitology for veterinarians*, ed 9, St Louis, 2009, Saunders.)

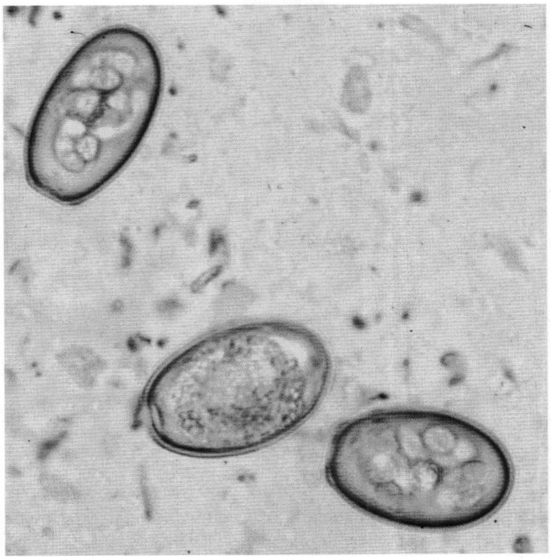

FIGURE 10-5 *Eimeria magna* oocysts, sporulated, from the feces of a domestic rabbit. (From Bowman DD: *Georgis' parasitology for veterinarians*, ed 9, St Louis, 2009, Saunders.)

Phylum Apicomplexa

These are the sporozoans. There are about 4600 species and all are parasitic. Sporozoans are unique in that all their life cycle stages are haploid except for the zygote. Figure 10-4 contains a sample sporozoan life cycle. Sporozoal parasites are found within the host cells and commonly occur in the intestinal tract cells and blood cells. **Oocyst** is the name given to the cyst stage of this group of intestinal protozoa. The genera of veterinary importance include the following intracellular parasites:

- *Eimeria* (Fig. 10-5)
- *Cystoisospora* (formerly *Isospora*) (Fig. 10-6)
- *Cryptosporidium*
- *Klossiella*
- *Toxoplasma* (Fig. 10-7)
- *Sarcocystis*
- *Plasmodium*
- *Babesia* (Fig. 10-8)

Phylum Ciliophora

There are about 7200 species in the phylum Ciliophora, of which about 2200 are parasitic. Only one genus, *Balantidium*, is of veterinary significance.

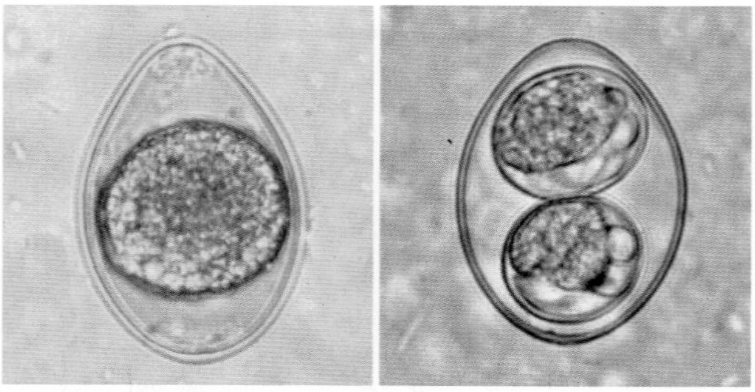

FIGURE 10-6 *Cystoisospora felis* unsporulated oocyst *(left)* and sporulated oocyst *(right)*. (From Bowman DD: *Georgis' parasitology for veterinarians,* ed 9, St Louis, 2009, Saunders.)

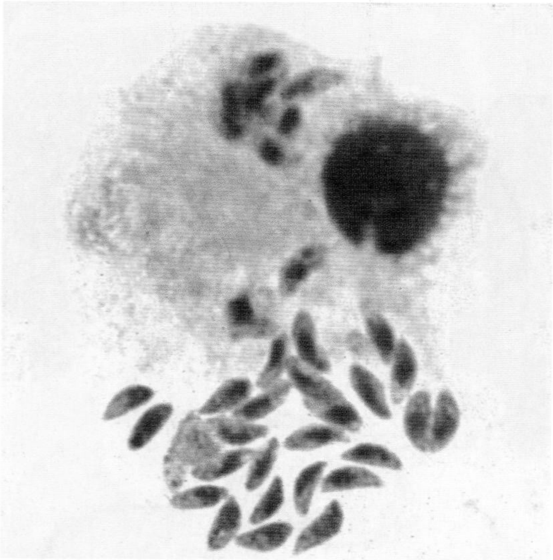

FIGURE 10-7 Tachyzoites of *Toxoplasma gondii* and the pulmonary macrophage of a naturally infected cat (Giemsa stain). (From Bowman DD: *Georgis' parasitology for veterinarians,* ed 9, St Louis, 2009, Saunders.)

KINGDOM ANIMALIA

Three of the phyla in this kingdom contain hundreds of species that are of veterinary significance. These include (1) Platyhelminthes: the flatworms; (2) Nematoda: the roundworms; and (3) Arthropoda: ticks, mites, and lice. The phylum Acanthocephala contains just a few species of veterinary significance.

Phylum Platyhelminthes

Organisms in the phylum Platyhelminthes are commonly called flatworms because of the dorsoventral flattening of their body tissues. The two groups of veterinary importance are the **cestodes** (tapeworms) and **trematodes** (flukes).

Cestodes. Two major groups of tapeworms are important in veterinary medicine. The first group is composed of the cyclophyllidean tapeworms, which typically have one intermediate host (Fig. 10-9). Organisms in this group include *Dipylidium caninum, Taenia* spp., *Echinococcus* spp., and *Moniezia* spp. The second group is composed of the pseudophyllidean tapeworms, which have two intermediate hosts (such as *Diphyllobothrium latum*). Typically the larval

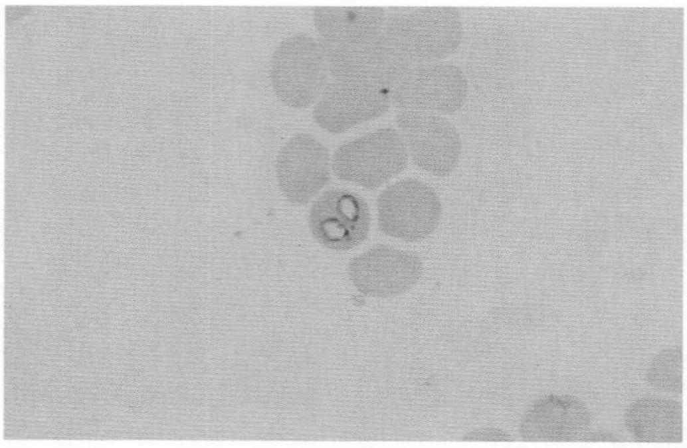

FIGURE 10-8 Peripheral blood from a dog with a Babesia canis infection. Two piroplasms are seen in a single red blood cell in this field. (Wright stain. Original magnification 330x.) (From Valenciano A, Cowell R: *Cowell and Tyler's diagnostic cytology and hematology of the dog and cat,* ed 4, St Louis, 2014, Mosby.)

stages of cestodes in domestic animals are more harmful (pathogenic) than the adult stages in the intestinal tract. However, the adult stages are the source of eggs, especially for cestodes, which can use people as an intermediate host and pose a risk to human health (**zoonotic**).

Cestodes are multicellular organisms that lack a body cavity. Their organs are embedded in loose cellular tissue (parenchyma). The body of tapeworms is long and dorsoventrally flattened, and consists of three regions. The head (**scolex**) is modified into an attachment organ and bears two to four muscular suckers, or bothria. The suckers may be armed with hooks. There may also be a snout (rostellum) on the head, which can be fixed or retractable. The rostellum can also be armed with hooks. Caudal to the head is a short neck of undifferentiated tissue, followed by the body (strobila). The body is composed of segments (**proglottids**) in different stages of maturity. Those near the neck are immature, followed by sexually mature proglottids, and terminating with gravid segments containing eggs. Gravid proglottids break off and pass out of the body of the definitive host in the feces. New proglottids are continually formed from the undifferentiated tissue of the neck. Cestodes lack a digestive tract, and nutrients are absorbed directly through the body wall. The most prominent organs in cestodes are the organs of the reproductive system. Both male and female reproductive organs occur in an individual tapeworm. Cestodes also have a nervous system and an excretory system.

The cestode egg contains a fully developed embryo, which has six hooks in three pairs (**hexacanth** embryo or oncosphere) (Fig. 10-10), or a zygote that develops into a ciliated embryo (coracidium) (Fig. 10-11) The life cycle of tapeworms is always indirect and involves one or two intermediate hosts. The intermediate hosts may be arthropods, fish, or mammals. Domestic animals can be definitive hosts and/or intermediate hosts for tapeworms. The larval stages of some tapeworms found in domestic animals are called **bladder worms** because they resemble fluid-filled sacks with one or multiple scoleces. When ingested by a definitive host, the bladder worms are released from the tissue of the intermediate host and develop into adult tapeworms within the

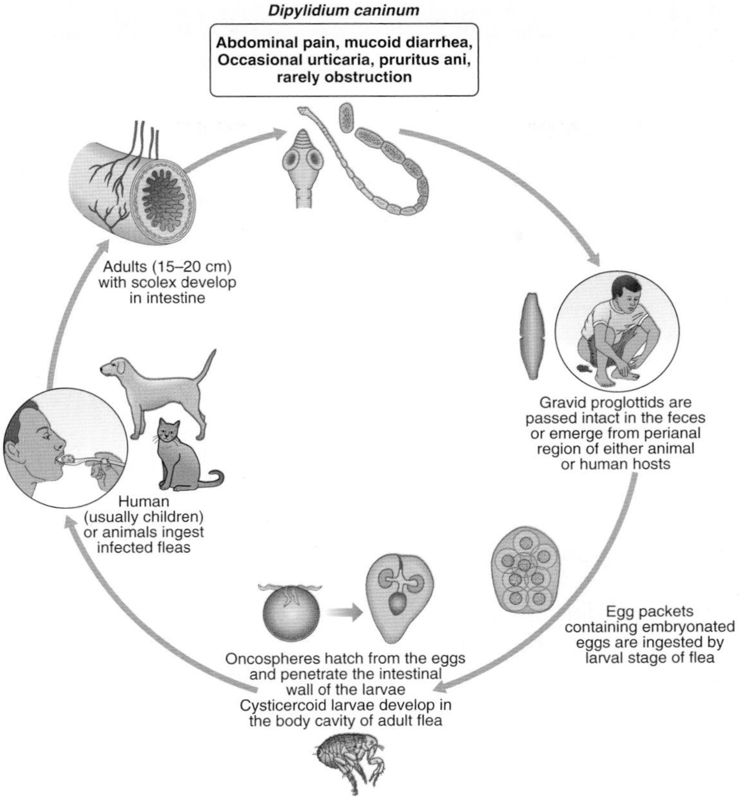

FIGURE 10-9 *Dipylidium caninum* life cycle. (From Guerrant R, Walker D, and Weller P: *Tropical infectious diseases,* ed 3, St Louis, 2011, Saunders.)

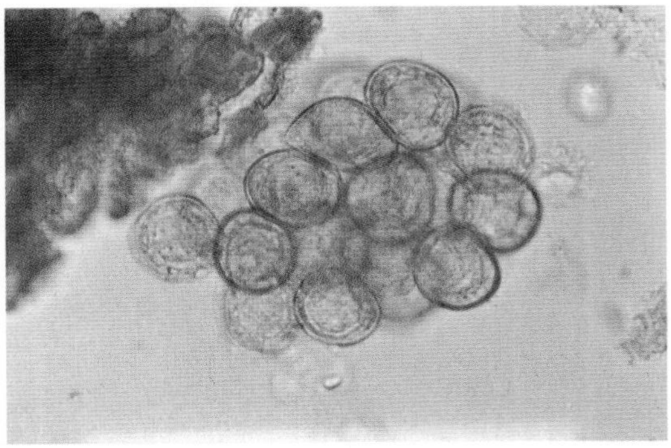

FIGURE 10-10 *Dipylidium caninum* egg packet. (From Mahon C, Lehman D, Manuselis G: *Textbook of diagnostic microbiology,* ed 4, St Louis, 2010, Elsevier.)

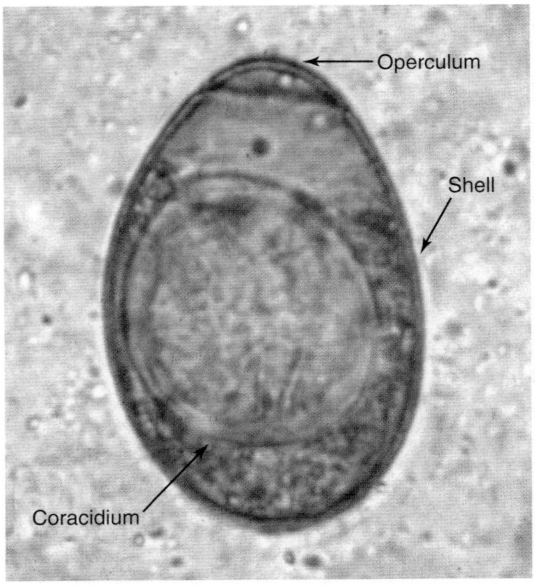

FIGURE 10-11 Egg of *Spirometra mansonoides* (Diphyllobothriidae). The capsule of diphyllobothriid eggs is operculate; this one contains a fully developed coracidium. (From Bowman DD: *Georgis' parasitology for veterinarians,* ed 9, St Louis, 2009, Saunders.)

digestive tract of the definitive host. Some cestodes have larval forms that are solid bodies (procercoid, plerocercoid, and tetrathyridium). Domestic animals become infected with the larval stages of tapeworms by ingestion of the cestode egg or procercoid. Table 10-2 summarizes the cestode parasites of veterinary species.

Trematodes. The trematodes (flukes) are flatworms that, like cestodes, lack a body cavity. They are unsegmented and leaflike. The organs are embedded in loose tissue (parenchyma), and they also possess two muscular attachment organs or suckers. One sucker, the anterior sucker, is located at the mouth. The other sucker, the ventral sucker or acetabulum, is located on the ventral surface of the worm near the middle of the body or at the caudal end. There are three main groups of trematodes, but only the digenetic trematodes are parasites of domestic animals.

TABLE 10-2 Selected Cestode Parasites of Veterinary Species

SCIENTIFIC NAME	COMMON NAME	INTERMEDIATE HOST(S)	PREPATENT PERIOD
Dogs			
Diphyllobothrium species	Broad fish tapeworm	Copepod/fish	40 days
Dipylidium caninum	Cucumber seed tapeworm	Flea	14-21 days
Mesocestoides species		Mites and mouse/reptile	20-30 days
Spirometra species	Zipper tapeworm	Copepod/fish/amphibians	15-30 days
Echinococcus granulosus	Hydatid disease tapeworm	Ruminants	45-60 days
Echinococcus multilocularis		Mice/rats	
Taenia multiceps		Sheep	30 days
Taenia serialis		Rabbit	30-60 days
Taenia hydatigena		Rabbit/sheep	51 days
Taenia ovis		Sheep	42-63 days
Taenia pisiformis		Rabbit/ruminant	56 days
Cats			
Echinococcus multilocularis	Hydatid disease tapeworm	Rodents	28 days
Taenia taeniaeformis or *Hydatigera taeniaeformis*	Feline tapeworm	Mice/rats	40 days
Diphyllobothrium species	Broad fish tapeworm	Copepod/fish	40 days
Dipylidium caninum	Cucumber seed tapeworm	Flea	14-21 days
Mesocestoides species		Mites and mouse/reptile	
Spirometra species	Zipper tapeworm	Copepod/fish/amphibians	15-30 days
Ruminants			
Cysticercus bovis	Larval *T. Saginata*		
Cysticercus cellulosae	Larval *Taenia solium*		
Cysticercus tenuicollis	Larval *Taenia hydatigena*		
Moniezia benedini		Grain mites	40 days
Moniezia expansa		Grain mites	22-45 days
Taenia saginata or Taeniarhynchus saginata	Beef tapeworm of humans	Cattle	70-84 days
Thysanosoma actinoides	Fringed tapeworm	Psocids (lice)	not known
Horses			
Anoplocephala magna		Orabatid mites	4-6 weeks
Anoplocephala perfoliata		Orabatid mites	4-6 weeks
Paranoplocephala mamillana	Dwarf tapeworm	Orabatid mites	4-6 weeks
Pigs			
Taenia solium		Pigs	35-84 days
Rodents			
Hymenolepis diminuta		None	
Hymenolepis nana		Flea, grain beetle, or cockroach	

Digenetic trematodes have an outer body wall or cuticle. They have a simple digestive tract consisting of a mouth, pharynx, esophagus, and an intestine that divides into two blind sacs (ceca). The main organs visible in trematodes are the reproductive organs. Most trematodes have both male and female reproductive organs in the same individual, but a few have separate sexes (e.g., *Schistosoma*). A nervous system and an excretory system are also present.

The life cycle of digenetic trematodes is complicated (Fig. 10-12). They pass through several different larval stages (miracidium, **sporocyst**, **redia**, cercaria, and metacercaria) and typically require one or more intermediate hosts, one of which is nearly always a mollusk (snail, slug). Multiplication takes place in both the definitive (sexual) and intermediate (asexual) hosts. The eggs of digenetic trematodes are capped (operculated), and they contain a ciliated embryo called a **miracidium.** Through penetration or ingestion, the miracidium enters a suitable snail and develops through several stages that eventually give rise to a motile, tailed stage referred to as a **cercaria.** Cercariae are released from the snail and swim actively. Sometimes, depending on the species of fluke, the cercariae encyst on vegetation. This encysted stage, the metacercaria, is infective for the definitive host. In other species, the cercaria may

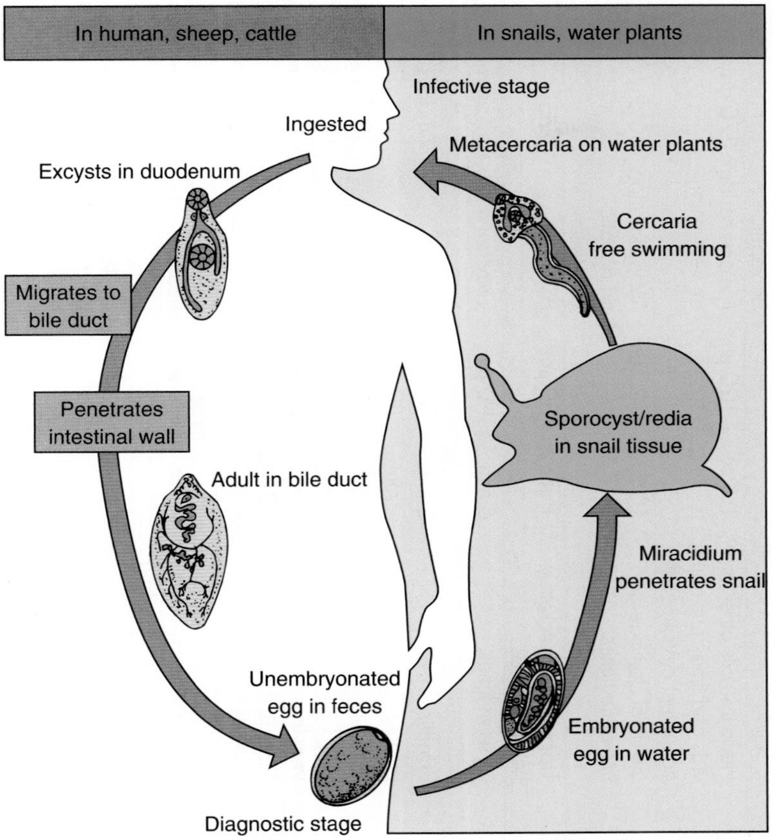

FIGURE 10-12 Life cycle of *Fasciola hepatica*. (From Pfaller M, Rosenthal K, Murray P: *Medical microbiology*, ed 5, St Louis, 2005.)

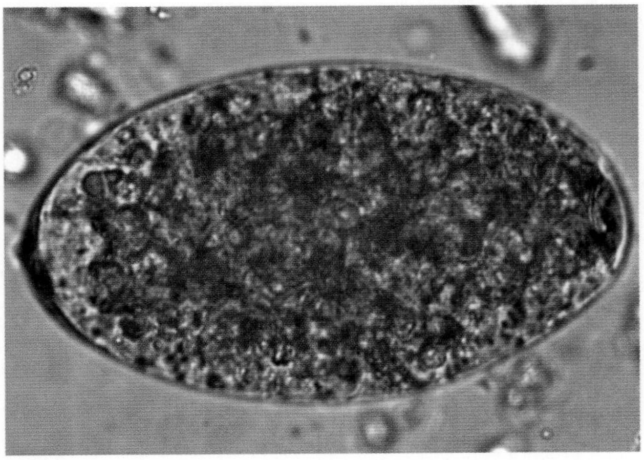

FIGURE 10-13 Egg of *Fasciola hepatica* from feces. (From Bowman DD: *Georgis' parasitology for veterinarians*, ed 9, St Louis, 2009, Saunders.)

penetrate the skin of the definitive host or encyst in another intermediate host. Examples of digenetic trematodes of domestic animals are *Fasciola hepatica* (Fig. 10-13), *Heterobilharzia americana, Paramphistomum cervi, Nanophyetus salmincola,* and *Paragonimus kellicotti.* Table 10-3 summarizes the trematode parasites of veterinary species.

Phylum Nematoda

Organisms in the phylum Nematoda are commonly called roundworms because of their cylindrical body shape.

Nematodes are multicellular, and possess a body wall composed of an external, acellular, protective layer called the cuticle; a cellular layer beneath the cuticle called the hypodermis; and a layer of longitudinal, somatic muscles that function in locomotion. The digestive tract and reproductive organs of roundworms are tubular and are suspended in the body cavity (pseudocoelom). The digestive tract is a straight tube that runs the length of the body from the mouth to the caudal end (anus). The sexes for most nematodes are separate. The reproductive organs are also tubular, but typically are longer than the body and coil around the intestinal tract of the worm. Nematodes have a nervous system and an excretory system, but no respiratory system.

The life cycle of nematodes follows a standard pattern consisting of several developmental stages: the egg, four larval stages that are also wormlike in appearance, and sexually mature adults. The infective stage may be an egg containing a larva, a free-living larva, or a larva within an intermediate host or transport host. A life cycle is considered direct if no intermediate host is necessary for development to the infective stage. If an intermediate host is required for development to the infective stage, the life cycle is considered indirect. Transmission to a new definitive host can occur through ingestion, skin penetration of infective larvae, ingestion of an intermediate host, or deposition of infective larvae into or on the skin by an intermediate host (Fig. 10-14).

TABLE 10-3 Information on Some Trematodes of Veterinary Importance

FAMILY	GENERA AND SPECIES	GEOGRAPHIC DISTRIBUTION	HOSTS	LOCATION IN HOST	DISEASE	LENGTH OF ADULT	LENGTH OF EGG	SECOND INTERMEDIATE HOST	PREPATENT PERIOD
Fasciolidae	*Fasciola hepatica*	Tropics and U.S.	Herbivorous mammals and	Bile ducts	Hepatic fibrosis	3 cm	120 µm	Metacercariae on vegetation	60 days
	Fasciola gigantica	Africa	Humans	Bile ducts	Hepatic fibrosis	5 cm	120 µm	Metacercariae on vegetation	60 days
	Fasciolopsis buskii	Asia	Pigs and humans	Intestine	Intestinal upset	8 cm	120 µm	Metacercariae on vegetation	90 days
	Fascioloides magna	U.S. and Europe	White-tailed deer	Liver (cysts)	Hepatitis, kills other cervids and small ruminants, nonpatent cysts in cattle	10 cm	120 µm	Metacercariae on vegetation	270 days
Paramphistomoidea	*Paramphistomum* and *Cotylophoron*	Worldwide	Ruminants	Rumen	Intestinal damage by immature flukes	10 mm	120 µm	Metacercariae on aquatic vegetation	80 days
Troglotrematidae	*Nanophyetus salmincola*	North Pacific rim	Dogs and cats	Intestine	Transmits Neorickettsia helminthoeca	1 mm	80 µm	Fish	7 days
	Paragonimus kellicotti	Eastern U.S.	Minks, dogs, cats	Lungs	Cysts in lungs	6 mm	90 µm	Crayfish	30 days
Heterophyidae	*Cryptocotyle*	U.S.: East coast	Birds	Intestine	Enteritis	2 mm	30 µm	Fish	14 days
	Heterophyes	Middle East	Dogs and cats	Intestine	Enteritis	2 mm	30 µm	Fish	14 days
Opisthorchidae	*Opisthorchis*	Asia and Europe	Dogs and cats	Bile ducts	Very little	6 mm	30 µm	Fish	30 days
	Metorchis	U.S.	Foxes, pigs	Bile ducts	Very little	6 mm	30 µm	Fish	17 days
	Clonorchis	Asia	Dogs and cat	Bile ducts	Very little	6 mm	30 µm	Fish	60 days
Dicrocoelidae	*Dicrocoelium dendriticum*	New York, Quebec, British Columbia, Europe	Sheep, cattle, pigs, deer, woodchucks	Bile ducts	Fibrosis with chronic disease	10 mm	40 µm	Ants	80 days
	Platynosum fastosum	Caribbean and southern U.S.	Cats	Bile ducts and gall bladder	Hepatitis, fibrosis, vomiting, jaundice, diarrhea	7 mm	45 µm	Lizards	30 days
Diplostomatidae	*Alaria canis*	Northern U.S. and Canada	Dogs and foxes	Intestine	Very little	4 mm	100 µm	Frogs, paratenic hosts	35 days
	Alaria marcianae-Fibricola texensis	Southern U.S.	Raccoons and opossums						

Schistosomatidae	*Schistosoma mansoni*	Worldwide	Humans	Mesenteric veins	Hepatic fibrosis	10-20 mm; sexes separate	55-145 μm; lateral spine	None, penetrate skin	60 days
	Schistosoma haematobium	Africa	Humans	Veins of urinary bladder	Erosion of bladder wall	10 mm; sexes separate	60 × 140 μm; terminal spine	None, penetrate skin	70-84 days
	Schistosoma japonicum	Asia	Humans, cats, mammals	Mesenteric veins	Hepatic fibrosis	10 mm; sexes separate	58 × 85 μm; no spine	None, penetrate skin	35-42 days
	Schistosoma bovis	Africa	Cattle	Mesenteric veins	Hepatic fibrosis	10 mm; sexes separate	62 × 207 μm; terminal spine	None, penetrate skin	42 days
	Schistosoma margrebowiei	Africa	Horses, ruminants	Mesenteric veins	Hepatic fibrosis	10 mm; sexes separate	60 × 80 μm; no spine	None, penetrate skin	38 days
	Bivitellobilhania loxodontae	Africa	Elephants	Mesenteric veins	Hepatic fibrosis	10 mm; sexes separate	71 × 87 μm; no spine	None, penetrate skin	Not known
	Heterobilharzia americana	U.S.	Raccoons, dogs, opossums	Mesenteric veins	Hepatic fibrosis	10 mm; sexes separate	70 × 87 μm; no spine	None, penetrate skin	60 days
	Bird genera	Worldwide		Skin	Dermatitis in mammals	10 mm; sexes separate	Varied	None, penetrate skin	

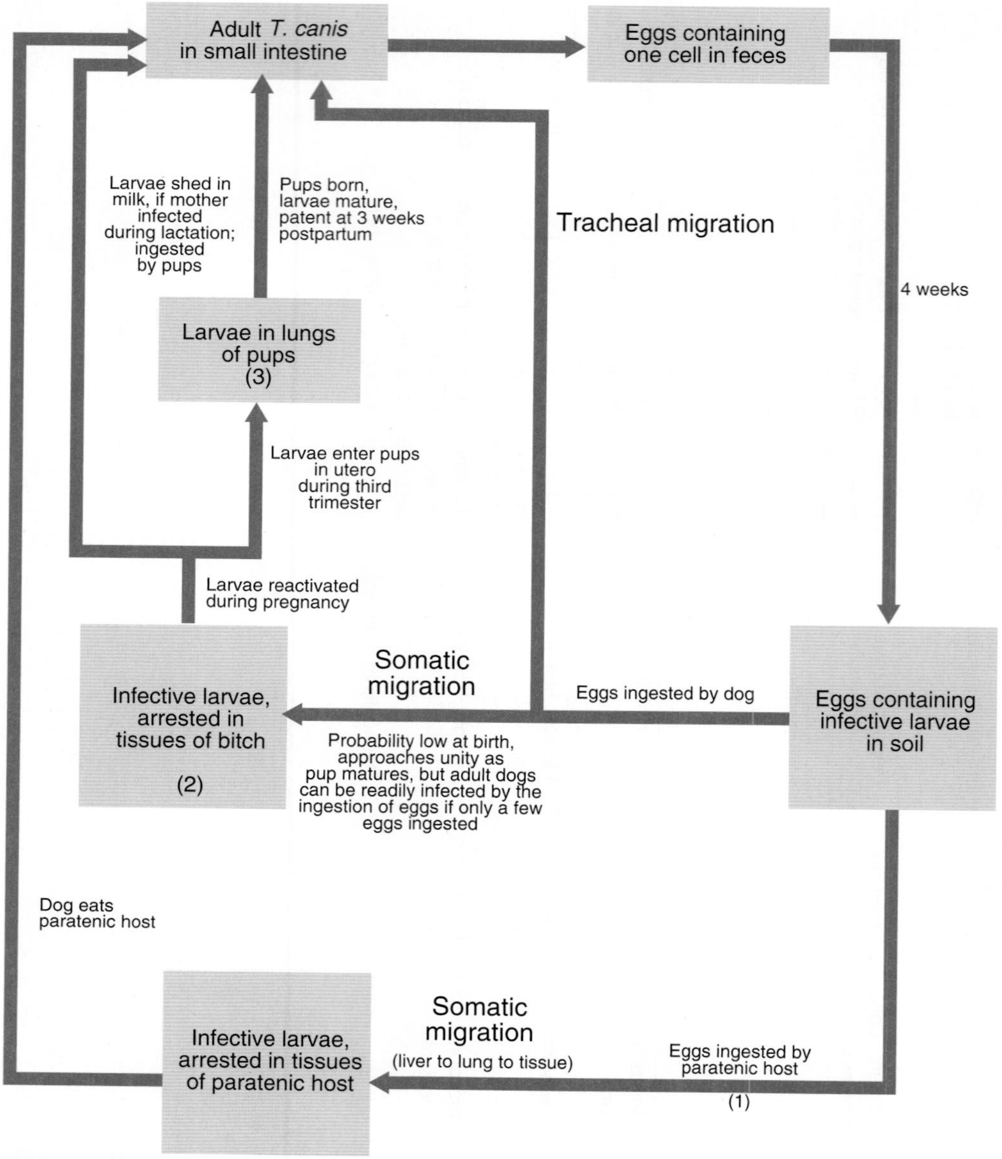

FIGURE 10-14 Alternative life histories of *Toxocara canis.* (From Bowman DD: *Georgis' parasitology for veterinarians*, ed 9, St Louis, 2009, Saunders.)

Once a nematode gains entry into a new host, development to the adult stages may occur in the area of their final location or may occur after extensive migration through the body of the definitive host. The diagnostic stages of parasitic nematodes are typically found in feces, blood, sputum, or urine. Most parasitic nematodes are found in the intestinal tracts of their respective definitive hosts, but some are found in the lungs, kidney, urinary bladder, or heart.

Table 10-4 summarizes the nematode parasites of veterinary species.

The following 11 taxonomic superfamilies of nematodes are significant in veterinary medicine:

1. Ascaroidea (Toxocara spp. (Fig. 10-15), *Toxascaris* spp., *Ascaris* spp., *Parascaris equorum, Toxocara vitulorum*)
2. Strongyloidea (*Strongylus* spp., *Ancylostoma* spp., *Bunostomum* spp., *Uncinaria* spp., *Syngamus* spp., *Oesophagostomum* spp.)
3. Trichostrongylidae (*Haemonchus* spp., *Ostertagia* spp., *Trichostrongylus* spp., *Cooperia* spp., *Nematodirus* spp., *Ollulanus tricuspis, Dictyocaulus* spp.)
4. Metastrongyloidea (*Metastrongylus* spp., *Protostrongylus* spp., *Muellerius capillaris, Filaroides* spp., *Aelurostrongylus abstrusus*)
5. Oxyuroidea (*Oxyuris equi* (Fig. 10-16), *Skrjabinema ovis*)
6. Trichuroidea (*Trichuris* spp. (Fig. 10-17), *Eucoleus* spp., *Trichinella spiralis*)
7. Filaroidea (*Dirofilaria immitis* (Fig. 10-18), *Acanthocheilonema reconditum, Onchocerca* spp., *Setaria* spp.)
8. Rhabditoidea (*Strongyloides* spp.)
9. Spiruroidea (*Habronema* spp., *Thelazia* spp., *Spirocerca lupi, Ascarops strongylina, Physalopetera* spp.)
10. Dracunculoidea (*Dracunculus* spp.)
11. Dioctophymoidea *(Dioctophyma renale)* (Fig. 10-19)

TABLE 10-4 Selected Nematodes of Veterinary Species

SCIENTIFIC NAME	COMMON NAME	PRIMARY LOCATION IN HOST
Dogs		
Acanthocheilonema reconditum (formerly *Dipetalonema reconditum*)	Skin filariid	Small intestine
Ancylostoma braziliense	Hookworm	
Ancylostoma caninum	Hookworm	Stomach
Pearsonema plica (formerly *Capillaria plica*)	Bladder worm	Urinary bladder
Dioctophyma renale	Giant kidney worm	Urinary bladder
Dirofilaria immitis	Canine heartworm	Right kidney
Dracunculus insignis	Guinea worm	Right ventricle of heart/pulmonary arteries
Eucoleus aerophilus (formerly *Capillaria aerophila*)		Bronchioles/alveolar ducts
Eucoleus böehmi		Skin
Filaroides hirthi	Canine lungworm	Trachea/bronchi
Filaroides milksi	Canine lungworm	Nasal cavity/frontal sinus
Filaroides osleri	Canine lungworm	Lung parenchyma
Pelodera strongyloides		Bronchioles
Physaloptera species	Stomach worm	Skin
Spirocerca lupi	Esophageal worm	Small intestine
Strongyloides stercoralis	Threadworms	Trachea
Strongyloides tumiefaciens	Threadworms	Stomach
Thelazia californiensis	Eyeworm	Small intestine
Toxocara canis	Roundworm/ascarid	Skin
Trichuris vulpis	Whipworm	Mucosal surface of stomach
Uncinaria stenocephala	Northern canine hookworm	Esophageal wall
Cats		
Aelurostrongylus abstrusus	Lungworm	
Ancylostoma braziliense	Hookworm	
Ancylostoma tubaeforme	Hookworm	
Aonchotheca putorii (formerly *Capillaria putorii*)	Gastrid capillarid of cats	Conjunctival sac/lacrimal duct
Capillaria feliscati	Bladder worm	Lumen of small intestine
Eucoleus aerophilus (formerly Capillaria aerophila)		Bronchioles/alveolar ducts
Ollulanus tricuspis	Feline trichostrongyle	Lumen of small intestine
Physaloptera species	Stomach worm	Skin
Spirocerca lupi	Esophageal worm	Small intestine
Thelazia californiensis	Eyeworm	Small intestine
Toxascaris leonina	Roundworm/ascarid	Small intestine
Toxocara cati	Roundworm/ascarid	Lumen of small intestine
Trichuris campanula	Whipworm	Cecum and colon
Trichuris serrata	Whipworm	Cecum and colon
Ruminants		
Bunostomum species	Cattle hookworm	Abomasum/intestine
Chabertia species	Trichostrongyle	Abomasum/intestine
Ruminants		
Cooperia species	Trichostrongyle	Abomasum/intestine
Dictyocaulus filaria	Lungworm of sheep/goats	Bronchi
Dictyocaulus viviparus	Lungworm of cattle	Bronchi
Elaeophora schneideri	Arterial worm of sheep	Carotid arteries
Gongylonema pulchrum	Ruminant esophageal worm	Esophagus
Haemonchus species	Bovine trichostrongyle	Abomasum/intestine
Marshallagia species	Bovine trichostrongyle	Abomasum/intestine
Muellerius capillaris	Hair lungworm or sheep/goats	Bronchioles
Nematodirus species	Bovine trichostrongyle	Abomasum/intestine
Oesophagostomum species	Bovine trichostrongyle	Abomasum/intestine

Continued

TABLE 10-4 Selected Nematodes of Veterinary Species—cont'd

SCIENTIFIC NAME	COMMON NAME	PRIMARY LOCATION IN HOST
Ostertagia species	Bovine trichostrongyle	Abomasum/intestine
Protostrongylus species	Sheep and goat lungworm	Bronchioles
Setaria cervi	Abdominal worm	Peritoneal cavity
Stephanofilaria stilesi		Skin
Strongyloides papillosus	Intestinal threadworm	Intestine
Thelazia gulosa	Eyeworms	Conjunctival sac
Thelazia rhodesii	Eyeworms	Conjunctival sac
Trichostrongylus species	Trichostrongyle	Abomasum/intestine
Trichuris ovis	Whipworm	Cecum/colon
Horses		
Dictyocaulus arnfieldi	Lungworm	Bronchi/bronchioles
Draschia megastoma		Stomach mucosa
Habronema microstoma		Stomach mucosa
Habronema muscae		Stomach mucosa (adults); skin (larvae)
Onchocerca cervicalis	Filarial worm	Ligamentum nucha
Oxyuris equi	Pinworm	Cecum/colon, rectum
Parascaris equorum	Roundworm	Small intestine
Setaria equina	Abdominal worm	Peritoneal cavity
Strongyloides westeri	Intestinal threadworm	Large intestine
Strongylus edentatus		Large intestine
Strongylus equinus		Large intestine
Strongylus vulgaris		Large intestine
Thelazia lacrymalis	Eyeworm	Conjunctival sac/lacrimal duct
Trichostrongylus axei		Stomach
Pigs		
Ascaris suum	Swine ascarid	Small Intestine
Ascarops strongylina	Stomach worm	Stomach
Hyostrongylus rubidus	Red stomach worm	Stomach
Metastrongylus elongatus	Lungworm	Bronchi/bronchioles

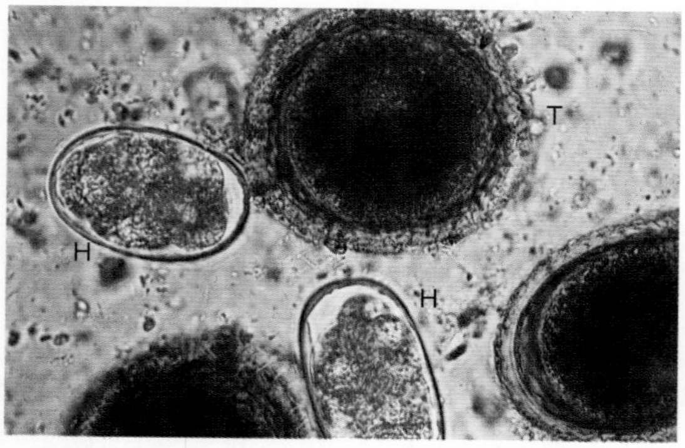

FIGURE 10-15 Photomicrograph of a fecal flotation analysis from a dog demonstrating characteristic ova from hookworms *(H)* and *Toxocara canis (T)*. (Magnification ×400.) (From Nelson R, Couto G: *Small animal internal medicine*, ed 4, St Louis, 2008, Mosby.)

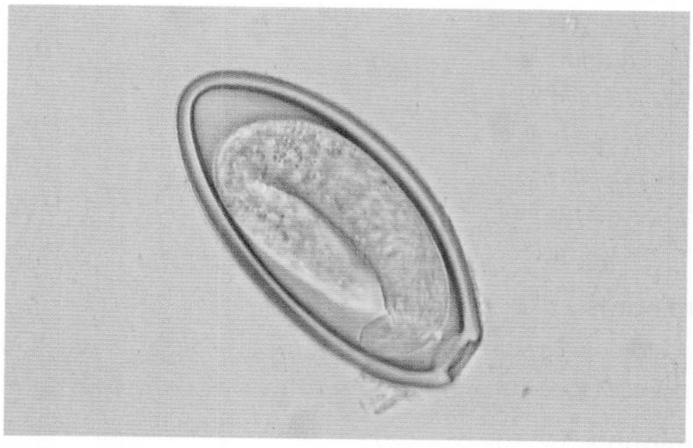

FIGURE 10-16 Egg of *Oxyuris equi*, the equine pinworm. (From Hendrix CM, Robinson E: *Diagnostic parasitology for veterinary technicians*, ed 3, St Louis, 2006, Mosby.)

Phylum Acantocephala

Acanthocephalans are commonly referred to as "thorny-headed worms." This group of intestinal parasites is rarely encountered, but they are occasionally found in pigs and dogs. They are wormlike in appearance after fixation, and have a spiny, protrusible snout (proboscis). They have a body cavity and lack a digestive tract; the sexes are separate. The life cycle of an acanthocephalan is complex and involves an intermediate host, usually a crustacean or an insect. Mature adults produce eggs that are shed through the feces of the definitive host. The eggs contain an embryo, the acanthor, which is surrounded by three to four envelopes. This gives the eggs a layered appearance, which is useful for identification. When an aquatic crustacean or insect ingests the eggs, continuous development through two stages occurs to produce the infective stage (cystacanth). Infection of the definitive host occurs by ingestion of the intermediate host. The main acanthocephalan of concern is *Macracanthorhynchus hirudinaceus,* which is found in the small intestines of pigs. *Oncicola canis* is an acanthocephalan found in dogs. Other hosts for acanthocephalans are aquatic birds, fish, amphibians, and monkeys.

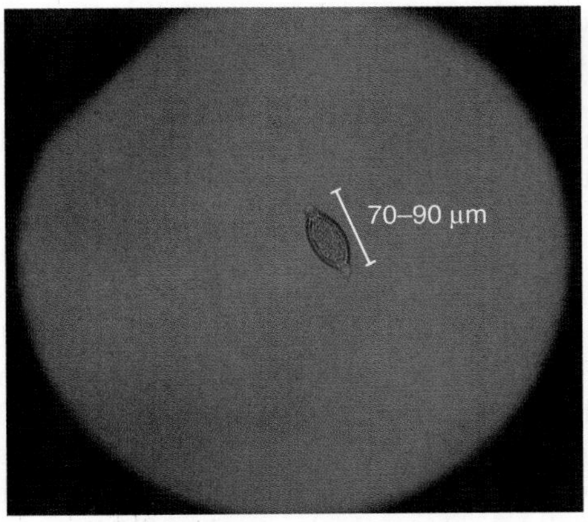

FIGURE 10-17 *Trichuris vulpis* egg. Note the prominent plugs at both ends. (From Aspinall V: *The complete textbook of veterinary nursing,* ed 2, St Louis, 2011, Elsevier.)

Rickettsial Parasites

The rickettsiae are a group of obligate intracellular gram-negative bacteria. The major taxonomic families are the Rickettsiaceae (Table 10-5), which include the genera *Rickettsia, Orientia,* and *Coxiella,* and the Anaplasmataceae (Table 10-6), which include the genera *Anaplasma* (Fig. 10-20), *Ehrlichia* (Fig. 10-21). *Wolbachia,* and *Neorickettsia.* The organisms are transmitted by **arthropod** or helminth vectors.

Phylum Arthropoda

Organisms in the phylum Arthropoda are characterized by the presence of jointed legs. They have a chitinous exoskeleton composed of segments. In the more advanced groups, some segments have fused together to form body parts, such as a head, thorax, and abdomen. Arthropods have a true body cavity (coelom), a circulatory system, a digestive system, a respiratory system, an excretory system, a nervous system, and a reproductive system. The sexes are separate, and reproduction is by means of eggs. Only certain groups of arthropods are parasitic. Members of other groups may act as intermediate host for the other parasites previously discussed. When a parasite resides on the surface of its host, it is called an ectoparasite. Most ectoparasites are either insects (fleas, lice, flies) or arachnids (ticks, mites).

The following general characteristics differentiate the two major classes of arthropods of veterinary importance: Insects

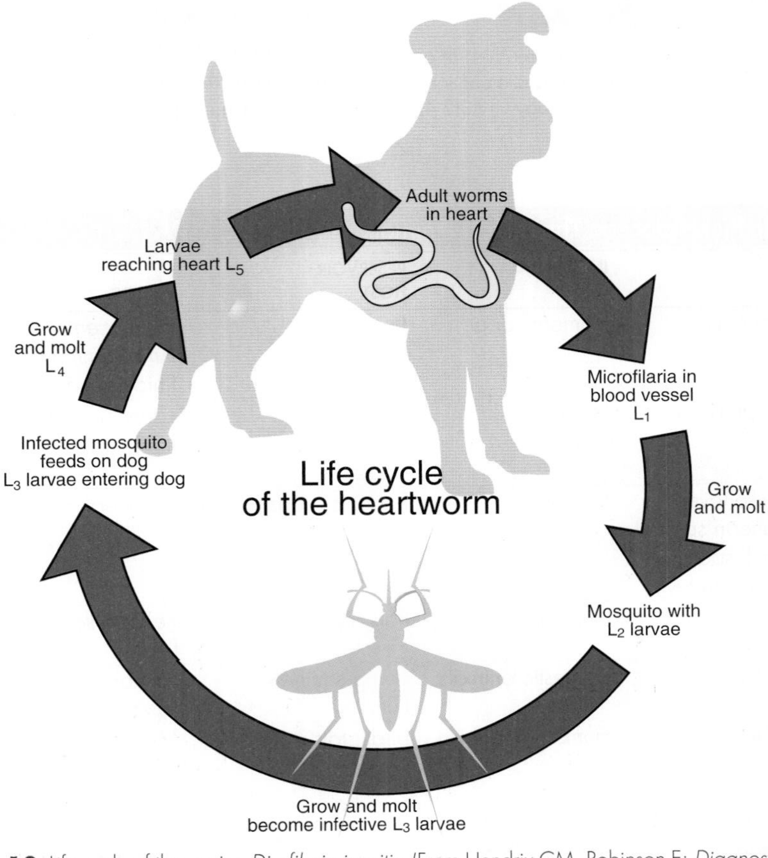

FIGURE 10-18 Life cycle of the canine *Dirofilaria immitis.* (From Hendrix CM, Robinson E: *Diagnostic parasitology for veterinary technicians,* ed 3, St Louis, 2006, Mosby.)

have three pairs of legs, three distinct body regions (head, thorax, and abdomen), and a single pair of antennae. Arachnids (adults) have four pairs of legs, a body divided into two regions (cephalothorax, abdomen), and no antennae. Pentastomids (tongue worms) are another group of parasitic arthropods rarely encountered in the respiratory passages of vertebrates. They resemble worms rather than arthropods in the adult stage. Adults have two pairs of curved, retractile hooklets near the mouth. Immature stages are mitelike, with two or three pairs of legs.

The mouth parts of insects vary in structure, depending on feeding habits, with adaptations for chewing-biting, sponging, or piercing-sucking. The thorax may have one or two pairs of functional wings, in addition to the three pairs of jointed legs. The sexes are separate, and reproduction results in production of eggs or larvae. Development often involves three or more larval stages called instars, followed by formation of a pupa and a change in form or transformation (complete metamorphosis) to the adult stage. In other insects development occurs from the egg through several immature stages (nymphs), which resemble the adult in form but are smaller (incomplete metamorphosis). Fleas and flies demonstrate complete metamorphosis, and lice demonstrate incomplete metamorphosis. Insects may produce harm to their definitive host as adults and/or larvae.

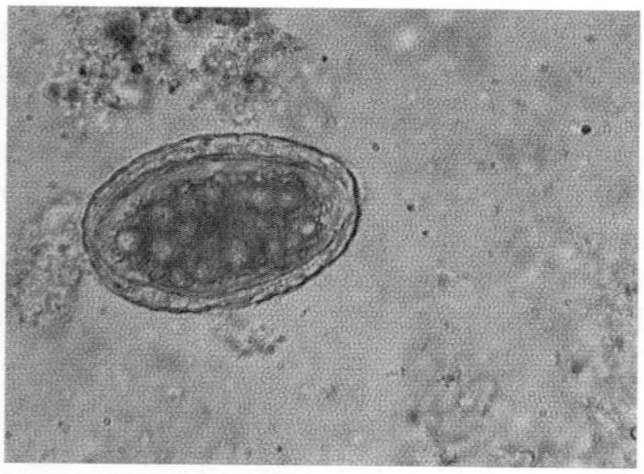

FIGURE 10-19 Egg *Dioctophyma renale*. (From Ishizaki MN, et al: *Dioctophyma renale* (Goeze, 1782) in the abdominal cavity of a capuchin monkey (Cebus apella), Brazil, *Veterinary Parasitology* 173(3-4): 340-3, 2010.)

The arachnids include ticks, mites, spiders, and scorpions. Ticks and mites are the more important groups of arachnids in veterinary medicine, although some spiders and scorpions can harm domestic animals by way of toxic venoms. Arachnids are generally small, often microscopic. Their mouth parts are borne on a structure called the basis capituli and consist of a pair of mobile digits adapted for cutting (chelicerae) and a pair of sensory structures (palps). The hypostome is a structure with recurved teeth that maintains attachment to the host and bears a groove that permits the flow of arthropod saliva and host blood or lymph. Life cycle stages consist of egg, larva, nymph, and adult. There can be more than one nymphal instar. Nymphs resemble the adult in form but are smaller. There is usually only one larval stage, which differs from the nymphs and adults in size and has only three pairs of legs.

Fleas. Fleas are blood-sucking parasites of dogs, cats, rodents, birds, and people. They are vectors of several diseases, such as bubonic plague and tularemia. Cat and dog fleas, *Ctenocephalides felis* and *C. canis,* respectively, can act as intermediate hosts for the common tapeworm, *Dipylidium caninum.* Heavy infestations with fleas, especially in young animals, produce anemia. Flea saliva is antigenic and

TABLE 10-5 Pathogenic Rickettsiaceae That Affect Animals

AGENT	DISEASE	INCIDENTAL HOST	RESERVOIR HOST	VECTOR	GEOGRAPHIC DISTRIBUTION
Rickettsia rickettsii	Rocky Mountain spotted fever	Humans, dogs	Rodents	*Dermacentor* spp. ticks, *Amblyomma cajennense* Rhipicephalus sanguineus	Western Hemisphere
Rickettsia felis	Cat flea typhus	Humans	Norway rat, domestic cat, opossum	*Ctenocephalides felis* (cat flea)	Western Hemisphere, Europe
Rickettsia conorii	Boutonneuse fever Mediterranean spotted fever, Israeli spotted fever, Astrakhan fever	Humans	Rodents, dogs	*Rhipicephalus* spp. ticks	Southern Europe, Africa, Asia
Rickettsia typhi	Murine typhus	Humans	Rats, opossums, cats	*Xenopsylla cheopis* (rat flea)	Worldwide
Rickettsia prowazekii	Epidemic typhus	Domestic animals	Flying squirrels, humans	Human body louse, flying squirrel louse, squirrel flea	Worldwide
Orientia tsutsugamushi	Scrub typhus	Humans, dogs	Birds, rats	Mites	Eastern Asia, northern Australia, western Pacific Islands
Piscirickettsia salmonis	Piscirickettsiosis	Salmonid fish	Unknown	Unknown	Chile, Norway, Ireland, Canada

From Songer JG, Post KW: *Veterinary microbiology: bacterial and fungal agents of animal disease*, St Louis, 2005, Saunders.

TABLE 10-6 Anaplasmataceae of Veterinary Importance

ORGANISM	HOST	DISEASE	VECTOR RESERVOIR	INFECTED CELLS	GEOGRAPHIC DISTRIBUTION
Aegyptianella spp.	Birds, reptiles, amphibians	Anemia, sudden death	*Argus, Amblyomma, Ixodes* spp. Unknown	RBC	Africa, Asia, South America, Southern Europe, South Texas
Anaplasma (Ehrlichia) bovis	Cattle	Bovine ehrlichiosis	*Rhipicephalus appendiculatus, Amblyomma variegatum, A. cajennense, Hyalomma excavatum*Rabbits, ruminants	Mononuclear leukocytes	Africa, Asia, South America
Anaplasma caudatum, centrale, marginale, ovis	Ruminants	Anaplasmosis	*Boophilus, Dermacentor, Ixodes,* or *Rhipicephalus* spp. Ruminants, wild cervids	RBC	Worldwide
Anaplasma phagocytophilum (Ehrlichia equi, HGE agent, *E. phagocytophila)*	Humans, horses, small ruminants	Human and equine granulocytic ehrlichiosis, tick-borne fever	*Ixodes* spp. Deer, sheep, white-footed mice	Granulocytes	Worldwide
Anaplasma (Ehrlichia) platys	Dogs	Infectious cyclic thrombocytopenia	*Rhipicephalus sanguineus* Ruminant	Platelets	United States, Southern Europe, Middle East, Venezuela, Taiwan
Ehrlichia canis	Canidae	Canine monocytic ehrlichiosis	*Rhipicephalus sanguineus, Amblyomma americanum* Canids	Mononuclear leukocytes	Worldwide
Ehrlichia chaffeensis	Humans, dogs, deer	Human monocytic ehrlichiosis	*Amblyomma americanum, Dermacentor variabilis* Domestic dogs, white-tailed deer	Mononuclear leukocytes	United States
Ehrlichia ewingii	Dogs, humans	Canine granulocytic ehrlichiosis	*Amblyomma americanum* Canids	Granulocytes	United States
Ehrlichia muris	Mice	Not named	*Haemaphysalis flava* Not known	Mononuclear leukocytes	Not known
Ehrlichia (Cowdria) ruminantium	Ruminants	Heartwater	*Amblyomma* ticks Ruminants	Granulocytes, endothelium, macrophages	Sub-Saharan Africa, Caribbean
Neorickettsia helminthoeca	Canidae	Salmon poisoning disease	Ingestion of fluke-infested salmonid fish Fluke-infested fish	Mononuclear leukocytes	U.S. Pacific Northwest
Neorickettsia (Ehrlichia) risticii	Horses	Potomac horse fever, equine monocytic ehrlichiosis	Ingestion of fluke-infested insects Flukes	Mononuclear leukocytes, enterocytes	North and South America
Neorickettsia (Ehrlichia) sennetsu	Humans	Sennetsu fever	Ingestion of fluke-infested fish Fluke-infested fish	Mononuclear leukocytes	Japan, Southeast Asia

HGE, Human granulocytic ehrlichiosis; RBC, red blood cell.
From Songer JG, Post KW: *Veterinary microbiology: bacterial and fungal agents of animal disease,* St Louis, 2005, Saunders.

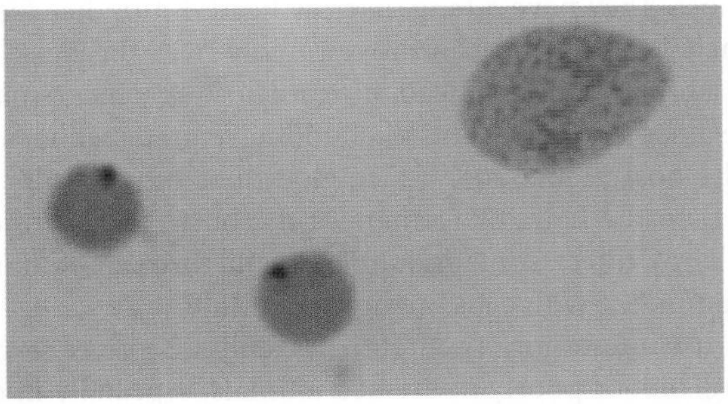

FIGURE 10-20 Blood smear from cow with anaplasmosis, showing two typically parasitized erythrocytes and an immature form. (From Songer, JG: *Veterinary microbiology: bacterial and fungal agents of animal disease,* St Louis, 2007, Saunders.)

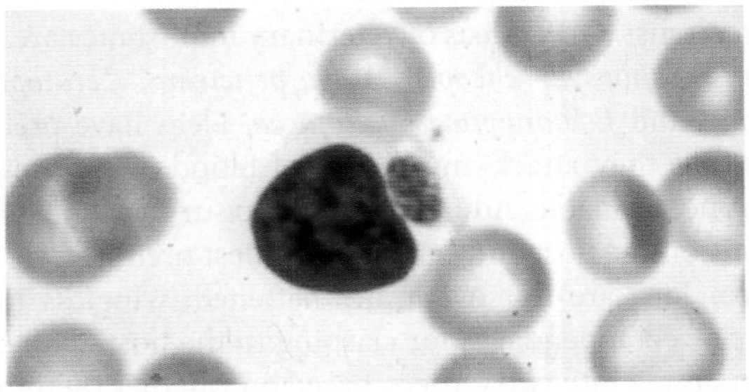

FIGURE 10-21 *Ehrlichia canis*-infected lymphocyte. (From Songer, JG: *Veterinary microbiology: bacterial and fungal agents of animal disease,* St Louis, 2007, Saunders.)

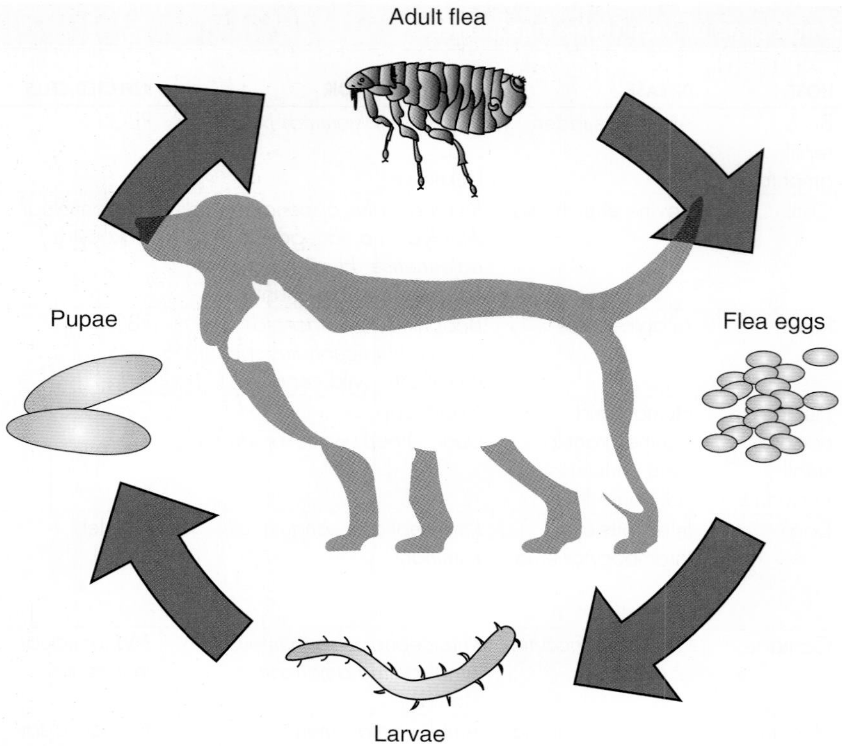

FIGURE 10-22 Life cycle of the flea. (From Bill R: *Clinical pharmacology and therapeutics for the veterinary technician,* ed 3, St Louis, 2006, Mosby.)

irritating, causing intense pruritus (itching) and hypersensitivity, known as flea-bite dermatitis or miliary dermatitis.

Fleas are laterally compressed, wingless insects with legs adapted for jumping. They move rapidly on the host and from host to host. Flea infestations are encountered most frequently on dogs and cats. They can be detected around the tailhead, on the ventral abdomen, and under the chin.

Fleas demonstrate complete metamorphosis (Fig. 10-22). Eggs deposited on the host fall off and develop to larvae in the environment. The larvae can occasionally be found in the animal's bedding, on furniture, or in cracks and crevices of the animal's environment. The larvae are maggotlike, with a head capsule and bristles. Flea larvae feed on organic debris, including the excrement of adult fleas. Flea droppings are reddish brown, comma-shaped casts of dehydrated blood (Fig. 10-23). Flea droppings in the animal's haircoat indicate flea infestation.

Specific identification of fleas requires the expertise of an entomologist. Other fleas of veterinary importance are *Pulex irritans, Xenopsylla cheopis, Tunga penetrans, Ceratophyllus gallinae,* and *Echidnophaga gallinacea.* Fleas have preferred hosts, but they attack any source of blood if the preferred host is not available. Adult fleas can also survive for extended periods off the host and can heavily infest premises.

Lice. Lice are dorsoventrally flattened, wingless insects with clawed appendages for clasping to the host's hairs. Lice are separated into two Orders, based on whether their mouth parts are modified for chewing *(Mallophaga)* or sucking *(Anoplura).* Sucking lice feed on blood and move slowly on the host. They have a long, narrow head. Biting lice feed on epithelial debris and can move rapidly over the host. They have a broad, rounded head. Lice are host-specific, remain in close association with the host, and have preferred locations on the host (Table 10-7). Lice glue their eggs or **nits** (Fig. 10-24) to the hairs or feathers of the host. Transmission is usually by direct contact but can occur through equipment contaminated with eggs, nymphs, or adults.

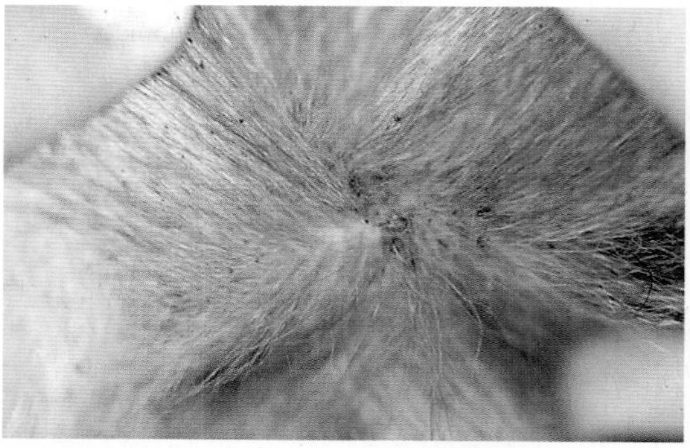

FIGURE 10-23 Black debris in a cat's hair, suggestive of flea feces ("flea dirt"). (From Taylor S: *Small animal clinical techniques,* St Louis, 2009, Saunders.)

Louse infestations (**pediculosis**) tend to be more severe in young, old, or poorly nourished animals, especially in overcrowded conditions and during the colder months. Sucking lice produce anemia, whereas biting lice are irritating

TABLE 10-7 Lice Found on Domestic Animals and Humans

HOST	ANOPLURA	MALLOPHAGA
Dog	*Linognathus setosus*	*Trichodectes canis*
		Heterodoxus spiniger
Cat	None	*Felicola subrostratus*
Cow	*Haematopinus eurysternus*	*Damalinia bovis*
	Haematopinus quadripertusus	
	Haematopinus tuberculatus	
	Linognathus vituli	
	Solenopotes capillatus	
Horse	*Haematopinus asini*	*Damalinia equi*
Pig	*Haematopinus suis*	None
Sheep	*Linognathus ovillus*	*Damalinia ovis*
	Linognathus pedalis	
	Linognathus africanus	
Goat	*Linognathus africanus*	*Damalinia caprae*
	Linognathus stenopsis	*Damalinia crassipes*
		Damalinia limbata
Rat	*Polyplax spinulosa*	None
Mouse	*Polyplax serrata*	None
Guinea pig	None	*Gliricola porcelli*
		Gyropus ovalis
		Trimenopon hispidum
Human	*Pediculus humanus capitus*	None
	Pediculus humanus humanus	
	Pthirus pubis	

From Bowman DD: *Georgis' parasitology for veterinarians*, ed 9, St Louis, 2009, Saunders.

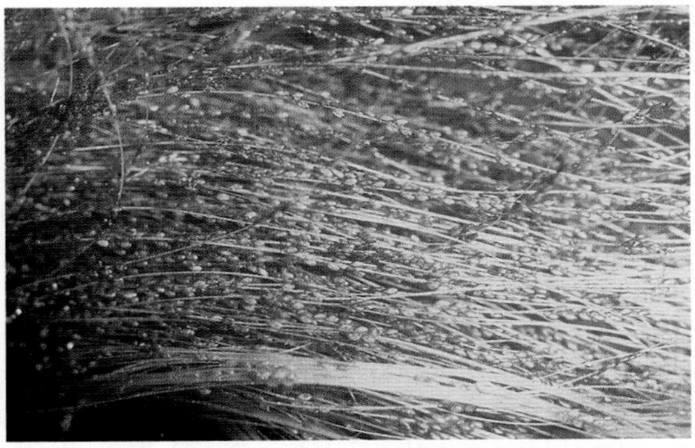

FIGURE 10-24 Thousands of nits can be cemented by female lice to hair coat of domesticated animals. (From Hendrix CM, Robinson E: *Diagnostic parasitology for veterinary technicians*, ed 3, St Louis, 2006, Mosby.)

and disturbing to the animal. Common biting lice of domestic animals include *Trichodectes canis* (dog) (Fig. 10-25), *Damalinia equi* (horse), *D. bovis* (cow), *D. ovis* (sheep), *D. caprae* (goat), and *Felicola subrostratus* (cat). Common sucking lice of domestic animals include *Linognathus setosus* (dog) (Fig. 10-26), *Haematopinus asini* (horse), *Haematopinus vituli, Haematopinus eurysternus, Solenopotes capillatus,*

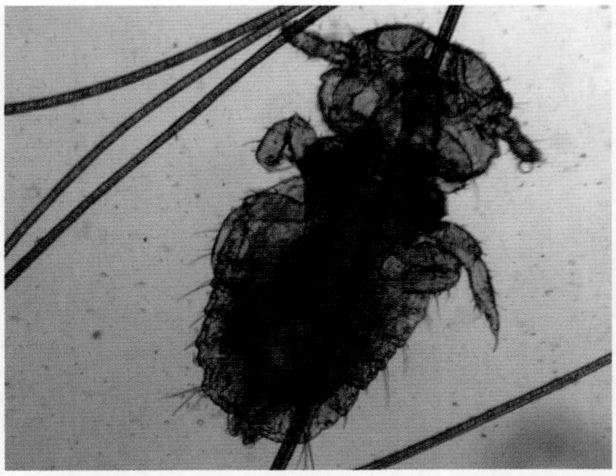

FIGURE 10-25 *Trichodectes canis*, a biting louse of dogs. Adult is 1–2 mm in length. (From Aspinall V: *The complete textbook of veterinary nursing*, ed 2, St Louis, 2011, Elsevier.)

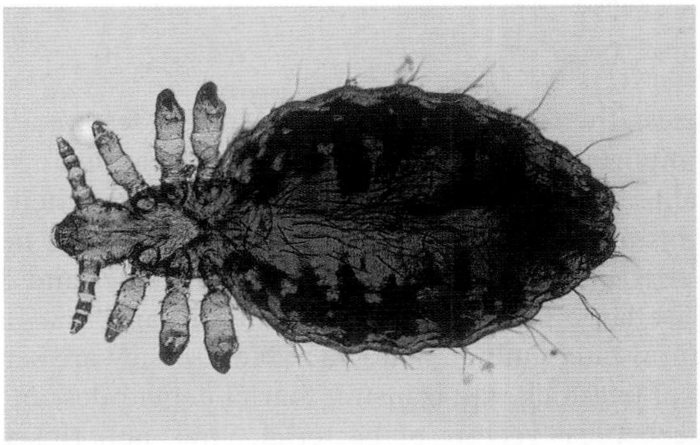

FIGURE 10-26 Sucking louse *Linognathus setosus* of dogs. (From Hendrix CM, Robinson E: *Diagnostic parasitology for veterinary technicians*, ed 3, St Louis, 2006, Mosby.)

Haematopinus quadripertusus (cow), *Linognathus ovillus, Linognathus pedalis* (sheep), and *Haematopinus suis* (pig). Identification of lice beyond their Order is difficult, but not usually necessary.

Flies. Flies are a diverse group of insects that undergo complete metamorphosis. They have one pair of wings, which may be scaled or membranous, and a pair of balancing structures called halters. The mouth parts may be adapted for sponging or piercing-sucking. Flies produce harm by inflicting painful bites, blood sucking, producing hypersensitive reactions, depositing eggs in sores, migration of larval stages through tissues of the host with escape through holes in the skin (**warbles**), causing annoyance, and acting as vectors and intermediate hosts to other pathogenic agents.

Biting midges ("no-see-ums"), *Culicoides* spp., are small flies (Fig. 10-27). The females are blood suckers that inflict a painful bite. Some species cause allergic dermatitis, and others transmit helminths, protozoa, and viruses. Blackflies (buffalo gnats) are small flies with a characteristic humped back. They produce similar harm as no-see-ums and in great numbers can exsanguinate a host. Sandflies (*Phlebotomus* spp.) are mothlike flies, known primarily for their role in the transmission of leishmaniasis and viral

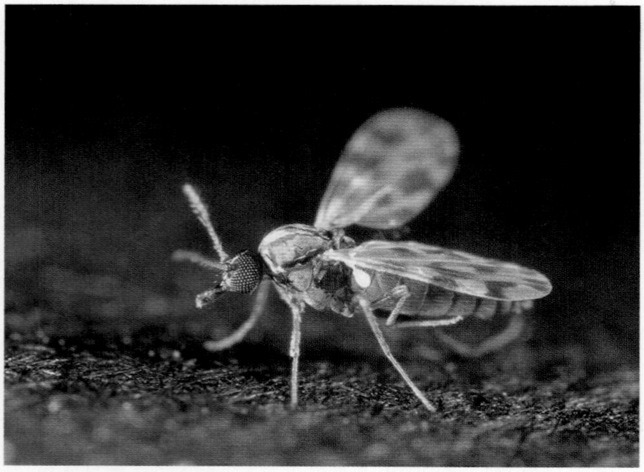

FIGURE 10-27 *Culicoides imicola,* a vector of *Akabane* virus. (From Mahy B, van Regenmortel M: *Encyclopedia of virology*, ed 3, Oxford, 2009, Elsevier.)

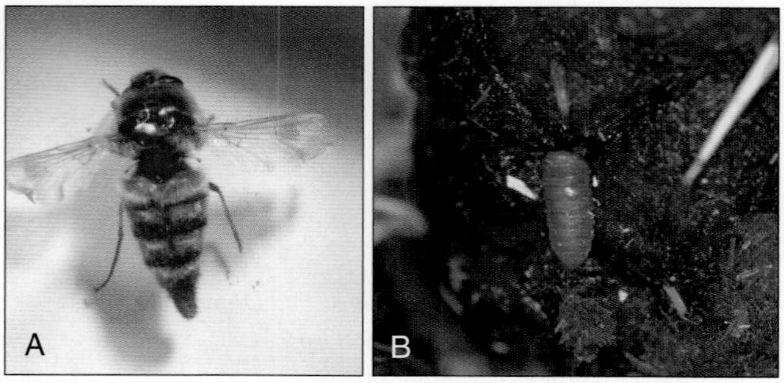

FIGURE 10-28 **A,** Adult *Gasterophilus intestinalis* fly. **B,** Third–stage (mature) larva in faeces. These are the outwardly visible signs of the infestation. (From Knottenbelt D: *Pascoe's principles and practice of equine dermatology*, ed 2, St Louis, 2009, Saunders.)

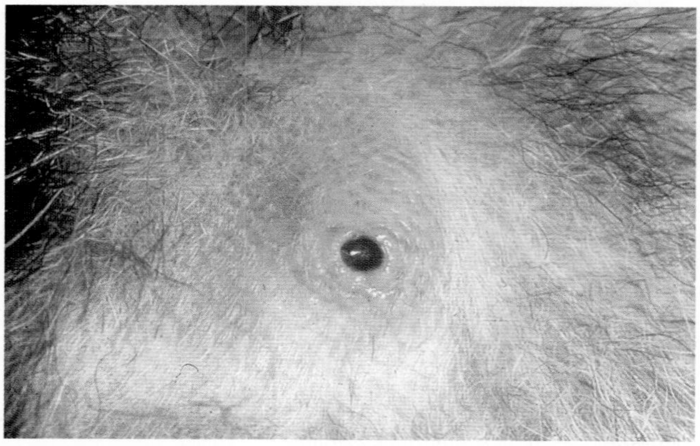

FIGURE 10-29 Larval *Cuterebra* species are usually found in swollen, cystlike subcutaneous sites, with a fistula (pore, or hole) communicating to outside environment. (From Hendrix CM, Robinson E: *Diagnostic parasitology for veterinary technicians*, ed 3, St Louis, 2006, Mosby.)

diseases. The females suck blood. Mosquitoes are a large and important group of flies known for the annoying bites of the females, which suck blood, and also for their role in transmission of numerous protozoal, viral, and nematode diseases to animals and people. Horseflies and deerflies are large flies with serrated mouth parts that inflict a painful bite. Only females suck blood. They are serious pests of livestock, can transmit filarial nematodes, and act as mechanical vectors of bacterial, viral, and rickettsial disease agents.

Muscid flies include the house fly, face fly, horn fly, and stable fly. The house fly and face fly do not suck blood, but are annoyances because they are attracted to excrement and secretions. Both act as intermediate hosts for spirurid parasites (*Habronema* spp., *Thelazia* spp.) and can mechanically transmit bacteria. The horn fly and the stable fly inflict painful bites and suck blood. Horn flies spend most of their life on the host (cattle). Stable flies feed intermittently and rest on fences and in barns. The stable fly can spread bacterial and viral diseases to cattle and horses and is an intermediate host for the stomach worm of horses (*Habronema*).

Blowflies, flesh flies, and screwworm flies are larger flies with bright coloration. The adults do not suck blood but deposit their eggs in decaying organic matter, septic wounds, or living flesh. The larvae of *Callitroga hominovorax* and *Wohlfahrtia opaca* are the only primary invaders of living tissue in North America. Other members are attracted to septic wounds and are known as secondary invaders. *Botflies* (Fig. 10-28) (*Gasterophilus* spp., *Hypoderma* spp., *Cuterebra* spp., *Oestrus ovis*) are beelike flies, the adults of which do not feed. The adult flies glue their eggs to the hairs of the host or deposit them at the entrance of animal burrows. The larvae hatch and penetrate the skin of the host (**myiasis**). Some migrate extensively through the host's body, and others develop locally. They produce large pockets in the subcutaneous tissues of the host with air holes in the skin, and are known as warbles (Fig. 10-29). Hippoboscids or sheep keds (*Melophagus ovinus*) are dorsoventrally flattened, wingless flies that resemble ticks. They suck blood and spend their entire life on the host (sheep). They cause pruritus and damage the wool.

Ticks. Ticks are blood-sucking arachnids. They are dorsoventrally flattened in the unengorged state. There are two types of ticks: hard ticks (Ixodidae) and soft ticks (Argasidae).

Hard ticks are important vectors of protozoal, bacterial, viral, and rickettsial diseases. The saliva of female ticks of some species is toxic and produces flaccid, ascending paralysis in animals and people (**tick paralysis**). The adults, larvae, and nymphs attach to the host and feed on blood. Eggs are deposited in the environment (Fig. 10-30). Hard ticks are dorsoventrally flattened, with well-defined lateral margins in the unengorged state. They have a hard, chitinous covering (scutum) on the dorsal surface of the body. Hard ticks may have grooves, margins, and notches (festoons), which are useful for identification purposes. They may attach to and feed on one to three different hosts during a life cycle and are referred to as one-host, two-host, or three-host ticks.

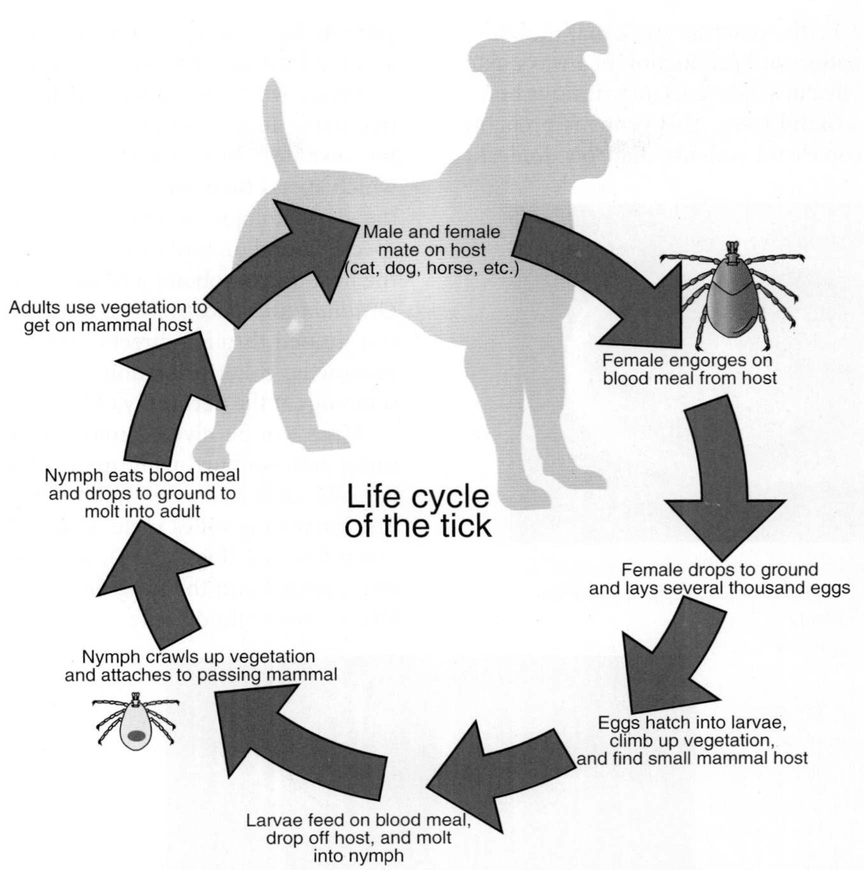

FIGURE 10-30 Life cycle of the tick. (From Hendrix CM, Robinson E: *Diagnostic parasitology for veterinary technicians,* ed 3, St Louis, 2006, Mosby.)

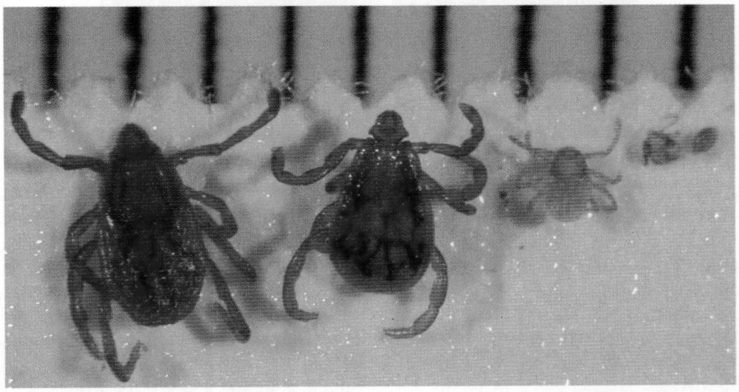

FIGURE 10-31 *Rhipicephalus sanguineus* (the brown dog tick), female *(left)*, male *(2nd of left)*, nymphs, larve, and egg, the main vector of MSF and sometimes vector of RMSF. (From Schaechter M: *Encyclopedia of microbiology,* ed 3, St Louis, 2009, Elsevier.)

Important hard ticks in North America include *Rhipicephalus sanguineus* (Fig. 10-31), *Dermacentor variabilis* (Fig. 10-32), *Dermacentor andersoni, Dermacentor occidentalis, Dermacentor albipictus, Ixodes scapularis, Ixodes cookei, Ixodes pacificus, Amblyomma americanum* (Fig. 10-33), *Amblyomma maculatum, Haemaphysalis leporispalustris,* and *Rhipicephalus annulatus. R. sanguineus* is unusual in that it can become established in indoor dwellings and kennels.

Soft ticks lack a scutum, and their mouth parts are not visible from the dorsal surface. The lateral edges of the body are rounded. The females feed often, and eggs are laid off the host. Soft ticks are more resistant to desiccation than hard ticks, and they can live for several years in arid conditions. There are three genera of veterinary importance: *Argas* spp., *Otobius megnini,* and *Ornithodoros* spp.

Argas spp. are ectoparasites of birds. The larvae, nymphs, and adults live in cracks and crevices of poultry houses and feed at night about once a month. They cause restlessness, loss of productivity, and severe anemia. They also serve as a vector for bacterial and rickettsial diseases of birds. *O. megnini,* the spinose ear tick, occurs on housed stock, dogs, and even people. Only the larval and nymphal stages are parasitic. They live in the external ear canal and suck blood, causing inflammation and production of a waxy exudate. *Ornithodoros* spp. live in sandy soils, in primitive housing, or in shady areas around trees. This genus is probably more important on people and rodents than on domestic animals, but *Ornithodoros coriaceus* is known to transmit the agent of Epizootic bovine abortion in California.

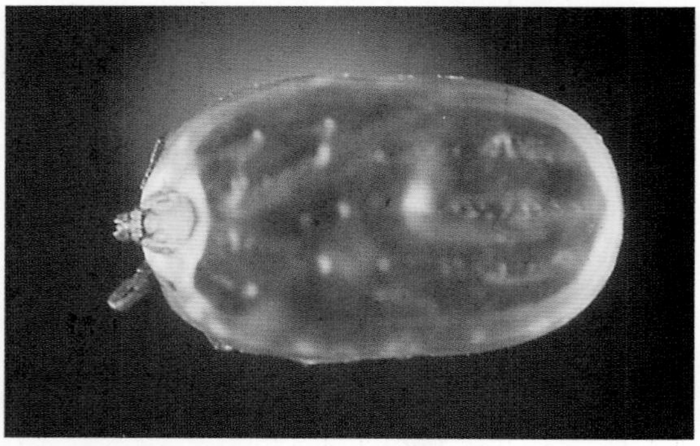

FIGURE 10-32 Engorged, adult female *Dermacentor variabilis*. (From Hendrix CM, Robinson E: *Diagnostic parasitology for veterinary technicians*, ed 3, St Louis, 2006, Mosby.)

Mites. Mites are arachnids that occur as parasitic and free-living forms, some of which act as intermediate hosts for cestodes. Most parasitic mites are obligate parasites, which spend their entire life cycle on the host and produce the dermatologic condition referred to as mange. A few species found on birds and rodents live off the host and visit the host only to obtain a blood meal *(Dermanyssus gallinae, Ornithonyssus bacoti)*. Most mite infestations (**acariasis**) are transmitted through direct contact with an infested animal. Burrowing mite infestations are diagnosed with deep skin scrapings at the periphery of lesions.

Mites can be divided into two main groups: burrowing mites and nonburrowing mites. Another group of mites is parasitic only as larvae, the trombiculid mites or "chiggers." The burrowing mites include *Sarcoptes scabiei* (Fig. 10-34), *Notoedres cati* (Fig. 10-35), and *Knemidokoptes* spp. These mites tunnel into the superficial layers of the epidermis and feed on tissue fluids. Infestations begin as localized areas of

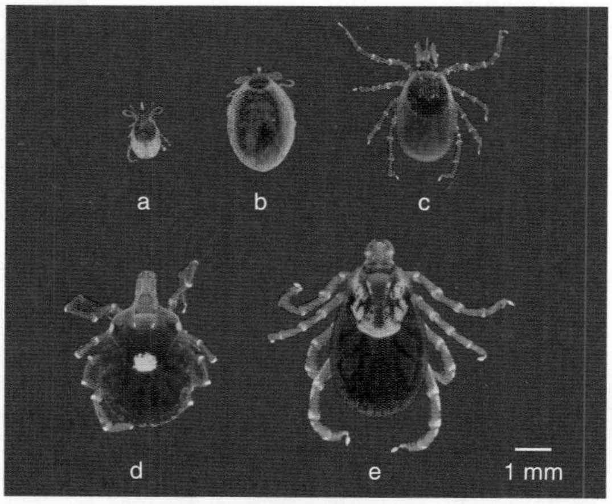

FIGURE 10-33 Tick vectors of agents of human *rickettsial* diseases. An unengaged nymph *(a)*, engorged nymph *(b)*, and adult female *(c)* of *Ixodes scapularis* (deer tick), the vector of *Anaplasma phagocytophilum*, the cause of human granulocytic anaplasmosis. An adult female *(d)* of *Amblyomma americanum* (lone star tick), the vector of *Ehrlichia chaffeensis* and *Ehrlichia ewingii*, the causes of human monocytic ehrlichiosis and ewingii ehrlichiosis, respectively. An adult female *(e)* of *Dermacentor variabilis* (American dog tick), the vector of Rickettsia rickettsii, the cause of Rocky Mountain spotted fever. (From Kliegman R: *Nelson textbook of pediatrics*, ed 19, St Louis, 2011, Saunders.)

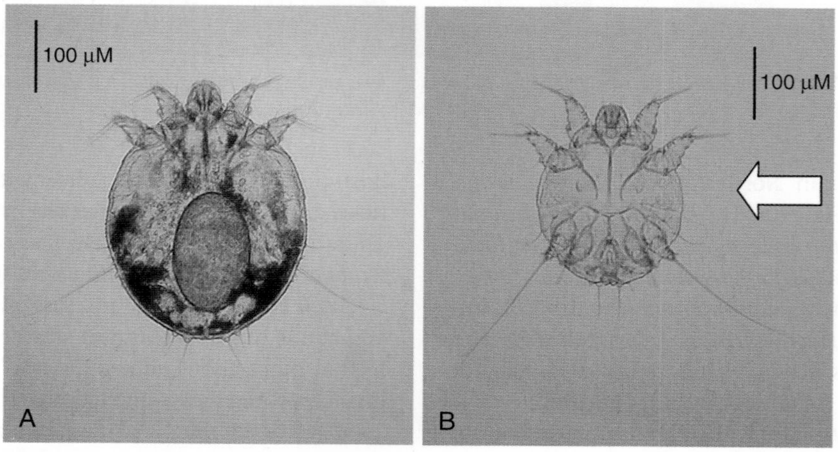

FIGURE 10-34 Photomicrographs of sarcoptic mites from case 1, at higher magnification. **A,** A female mite, containing an egg, is present. **B,** A male is identified by the large arrow. (From Malik R, et al: *Journal of Feline Medicine and Surgery*, Oct 2006, Elsevier.)

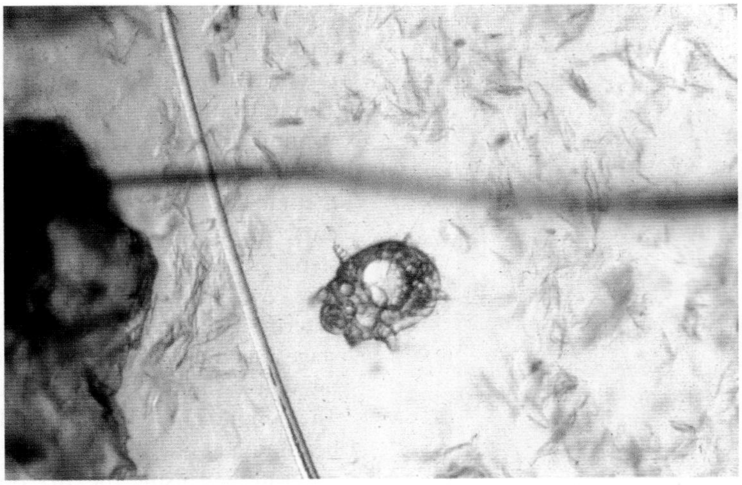

FIGURE 10-35 Feline scabies. Microscopic image of *Notoedres cati* mite from a skin scraping as seen with a 10× objective. (From Hnilica K: *Small animal dermatology,* ed 3, St Louis, 2011, Saunders.)

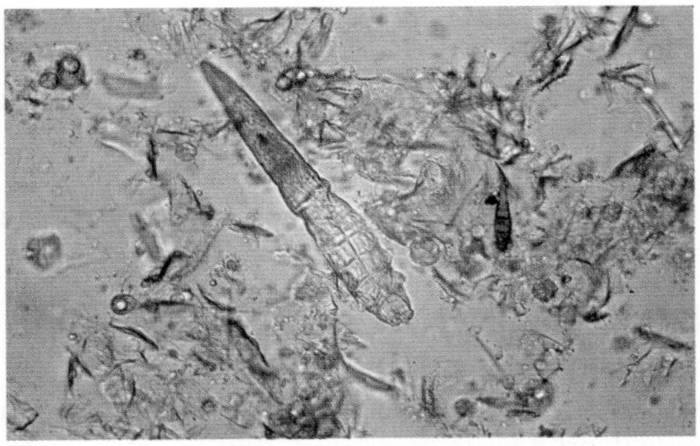

FIGURE 10-36 Adult *Demodex canis.* (From Hendrix CM, Robinson E: *Diagnostic parasitology for veterinary technicians,* ed 3, St Louis, 2006, Mosby.)

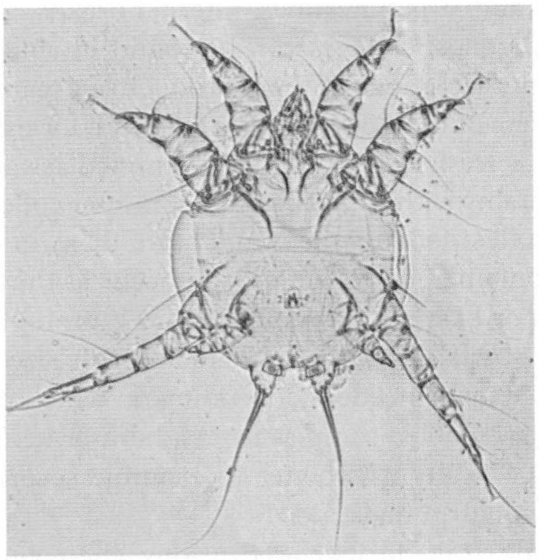

FIGURE 10-37 An adult male *Psoroptes.* (From Bowman DD: *Georgis' parasitology for veterinarians,* ed 9, St Louis, 2009, Saunders.)

inflammation and hair loss, but they spread rapidly to become generalized. Females deposit their eggs in the tunnels. Mating occurs on the surface of the skin. Sarcoptic mange caused by *S. scabiei* can affect most animal species, including people, but it is most commonly seen on dogs and pigs. It is characterized by loss of hair and intense pruritus. Each animal species has its own variety of *S. scabiei,* and cross-transmission does not occur. However, temporary infestation may take place without colonization of the skin. Notodectic mange (caused by *Notoedres*) is more restricted in host range and occurs in cats and occasionally rabbits. Knemidokoptic mange (caused by *Knemidokoptes*) affects birds.

Demodex spp. are also burrowing mites that live in the hair follicles and sebaceous glands of the skin. They are considered part of the normal skin fauna of most mammals. Demodectic mange is most common in dogs and can be localized or generalized. Immunodeficiency, both genetic and induced by the mites, is necessary for an infestation to become clinically apparent. The disease is characterized by loss of hair, thickening of the skin, and pustule formation. Pruritus is not a manifestation of this type of mange. Deep skin scrapings are used to recover the cigar-shaped mites for diagnosis (Fig. 10-36).

Nonburrowing mites live on the surface of the skin and feed on keratinized scale, hair, and tissue fluids. *Psoroptes* spp. (Fig 10-37), *Chorioptes* spp., *Otodectes cynotis, Psorergates ovis,* and *Cheyletiella* spp. are examples of nonburrowing mites. Psoroptic mange is important in sheep. The mites are active in the superficial keratinized layer of the skin but also pierce the skin with their mouth parts. Vesicles develop, with crusting and intense pruritus. Chorioptic mange is less severe and tends to remain localized. *Chorioptes bovis* is the more important species and a common parasite of cattle.

Cheyletiella and *Otodectes* are parasites of dogs and cats. *Cheyletiella* produces a mild condition referred to as "walking dandruff." *Otodectes cynotis* (Fig. 10-38) lives in the external ear canal of dogs and cats. A brownish, waxy exudate accumulates, with crust formation, ulceration, and secondary bacterial infections. Infested animals scratch frequently at the ears and shake their heads. Head shaking can result in rupture of blood vessels and hematomas of the pinna. The mites can be found in the waxy exudate and crust within the ear canal.

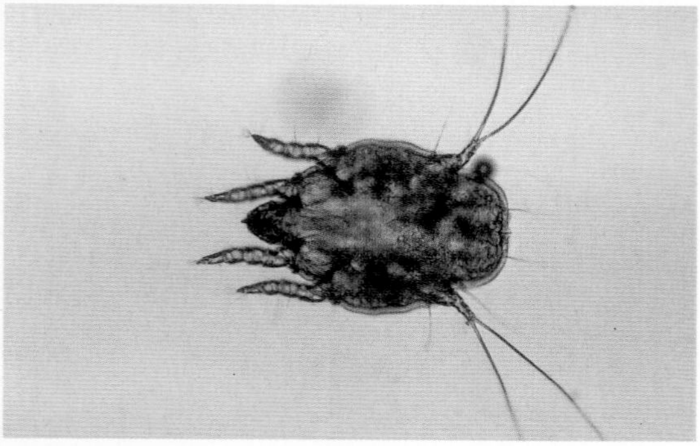

FIGURE 10-38 Adult male ear mite, *Otodectes cynotis*. (From Hendrix CM, Robinson E: *Diagnostic parasitology for veterinary technicians*, ed 3, St Louis, 2006, Mosby.)

DIAGNOSTIC TECHNIQUES IN PARASITOLOGY

Parasites may be located in the oral cavity, esophagus, stomach, small and large intestines, internal organs, and skin of animals. Diagnostic stages can be found in sputum, feces, blood, urine, secretions of the reproductive organs, and epidermal layers of the skin. Samples collected for examination should be as fresh as possible and examined as soon as possible, preferably within the first 24 hours after collection. Clients can collect fecal samples and store them in any clean, sealable container, or collection can occur at the clinic. Refrigeration or fixation may be necessary if prompt examination is not possible. A sample of 5 to 50 g (the size of a pecan or walnut) may be needed, depending on which procedures are necessary. Pooled samples from a herd or kennel can be used, but generally it is better to examine several samples from individual animals.

It is vital to take proper precautions when working with samples to prevent contamination of the work environment and to ensure personal health when handling agents transmissible to people. Wear gloves and/or wash your hands frequently with warm water and soap. Clean and disinfect work areas after examinations. Also, clean equipment frequently.

Maintenance of good records is important. Label samples with the client's name, date of collection, species of host, and identification of the animal. Records should include identification information, procedures performed, and the results. An adequate history, including clinical signs, duration of signs, medications given, environment, vaccinations, stocking density, and number of animals affected, should accompany the sample.

Parasitologic examination of feces begins with gross examination of the sample, noting consistency, color, presence of blood, mucus, odor, adult parasites, or foreign bodies such as string. Normal feces should be formed yet soft. Diarrhea or constipation can occur with parasitic infections. Most secretions are clear and moderately cellular. A yellowish discoloration with excessive mucus could signal infection. Blood in a sample can be fresh and bright red or partially digested (hemolyzed), appearing dark reddish brown to black and tarry. Excessive mucus in a sample generally indicates irritation to a mucosal membrane, with proliferation of mucus-producing cells. This is common in parasitic infections of the respiratory system and lower digestive tract. Adult parasites, such as roundworms and tapeworm proglottids, can be found in vomitus or feces, and can be identified.

Microscopic examination of samples is the most reliable method for detection of parasitic infections. A binocular microscope with 10×, 40×, and 100× objectives is needed. A stereo microscope is also helpful for identifying gross parasites. A calibrated ocular micrometer may be necessary to determine sizes and specific differentiation of some parasitic stages, such as **microfilariae.** Samples are generally mounted on a glass slide in a fluid medium with a cover slip on top. The sample should be thoroughly and systematically viewed, beginning at one corner of the cover slip and ending at the opposite end using the 10× objective. Parasite stages usually are in the same plane of focus as air bubbles or the edge of the cover slip. Any materials or objects observed can be viewed and verified with more powerful objectives. A good working knowledge of the parts of the binocular microscope is essential to produce proper illumination for parasitology examinations.

Parasitology testing is one of the most common activities of the practicing veterinary technician. This section provides an overview of sample collection and handling as well as principles and general procedures for the most common parasitology tests performed.

SAMPLE COLLECTION AND HANDLING

Fecal Samples

For tests to be valid, the fecal sample must be fresh and stored properly if testing is to be delayed. With small animals, it is common to provide the client with a collection container. Instruct the client to witness the animal defecating and collect the sample immediately. Samples can also be collected directly from the rectum using a fecal loop. A sample collected with a fecal loop is the least desirable as only a small quantity of sample is obtained and the quantity may not be sufficient to recover evidence of parasites. The sample should be refrigerated until it is to be examined. Large animal specimens are often collected directly from the rectum. Herd animal samples are normally collected as pooled samples. Several samples are taken from the area where the animals are confined.

Blood Samples

The specific collection procedure varies somewhat depending on the tests to be performed. Whole blood in EDTA or serum may be required. Standard collection methods for these sample types will yield appropriate samples for parasitologic testing.

Miscellaneous Samples

Skin scrapings, cellophane tape collections, transtracheal washes, urine sample collections, and swabbings are all performed in parasitology. Standard protocols for these collections will yield appropriate samples. These methods are described in more detail in Chapter 9.

EVALUATION OF FECAL SPECIMENS

Depending on clinical signs and patient history, it is likely that specific parasite infestations may be suspected. This information helps to guide the choice of test to be performed. All parasitology samples should undergo gross evaluation for the presence of abnormalities such as blood, mucus, and parasites that are large enough to see with the unaided eye (e.g., tapeworm segments). Additional tests can then be performed.

Direct Smear

Fecal direct smears are the simplest of the evaluation procedures. Feces, sputum, urine, smegma, and blood can be observed with the technique described in Procedure 10-1. It requires a minimum amount of equipment and materials and is a rapid scan for parasite stages. The procedure involves placing a small amount of feces on a clean glass slide and examining it microscopically for the presence of eggs and larvae. This method will also allow visualization of the trophozoite stages of protozoal parasites such as *Giardia*.

Unfortunately, a direct smear alone is not an adequate examination for parasites, because only a small quantity of sample is examined and parasitic infections can be missed. However, it should be incorporated as a routine part of any parasitology examination.

PROCEDURE 10-1 Direct Smear of Feces

Materials

- Glass microscope slides (25-mm)
- Glass cover slips (22-mm^2 #1)
- Wooden applicator sticks
- Water or saline

Procedure

1. Dip the applicator stick into the feces (only a small amount should adhere to the stick) (Fig. 1).

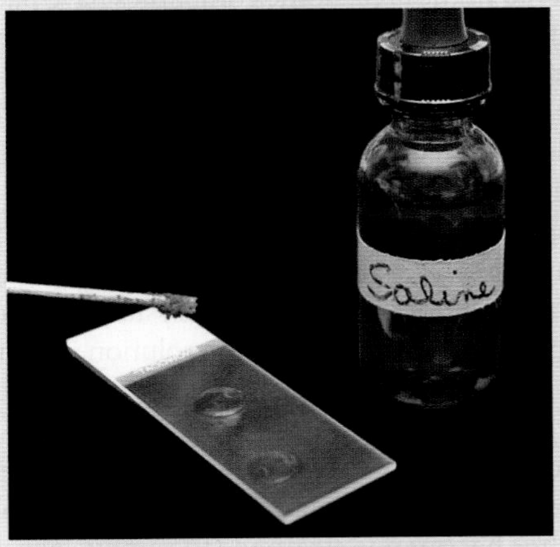

FIGURE 1 (From Greene CE: *Infectious diseases of the dog and cat*, ed 4, Philadelphia, 2012, W.B. Saunders.)

2. Place a drop of saline on a slide (Fig. 2).

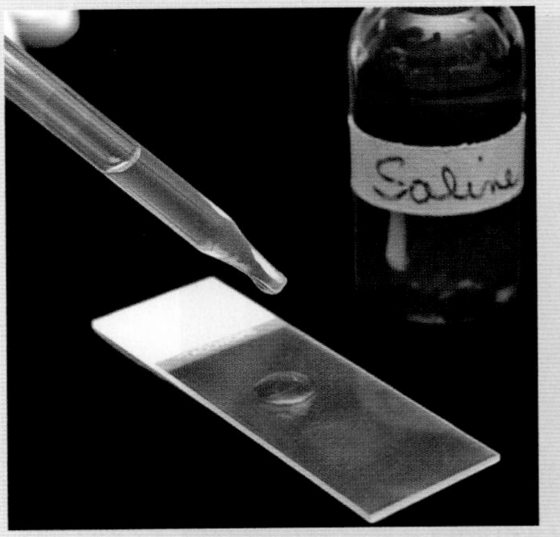

FIGURE 2 (From Greene CE: *Infectious diseases of the dog and cat*, ed 4, Philadelphia, 2012, W.B. Saunders.)

3. Mix the feces with the saline to produce a homogeneous emulsion that is clear enough to read newsprint through it. (A common mistake is to make the smear too thick.) (Fig. 3).

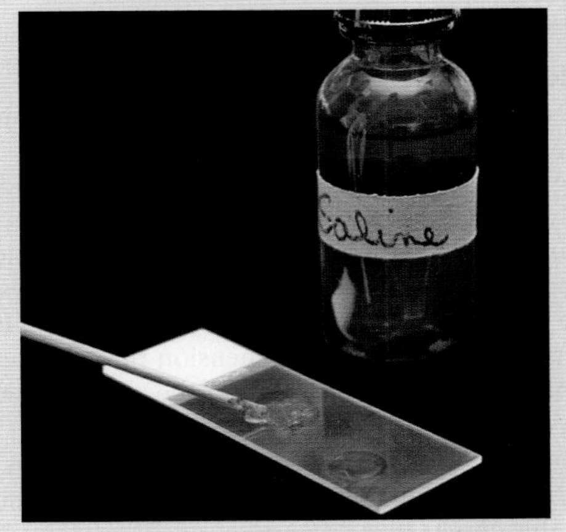

FIGURE 3 (From Greene CE: *Infectious diseases of the dog and cat*, ed 4, Philadelphia, 2012, W.B. Saunders.)

4. Place the cover slip over the emulsion.
5. Examine the slide at 100× and 400× magnification for eggs, cysts, trophozoites, and larvae.
   Optional: To demonstrate diagnostic features of protozoa, add a drop of Lugol's iodine:
   1. To make a 5% Lugol's stock solution, add 5 g iodine crystals to 10 g potassium iodide/100 ml distilled water.
   2. Store solution in an amber bottle away from light.
   3. Dilute 1 part 5% Lugol's stock solution to 5 parts distilled water to make a staining solution.

Fecal Flotation

Flotation methods are based on differences in the specific gravity of life cycle stages of parasites found in feces and fecal debris. Simple fecal flotation is an example of a flotation method (Procedure 10-2). Specific gravity refers to the weight of an object compared with the weight of an equal volume of distilled water, and is a function of the total amount of dissolved material in the solution. Most parasite eggs have a specific gravity between 1.10 and 1.20 g/ml. Flotation solutions are formulated with a specific gravity that is higher than that of common parasite ova. Therefore, the ova float to the surface of the solution. Saturated solutions of sugar and various salts are used as flotation solutions and have a specific gravity ranging between 1.18 and 1.40. Fecal debris and eggs with a specific gravity greater than that of the flotation solution do not float. Fluke eggs are generally heavier than the specific gravity of most routinely used flotation solutions, with a few exceptions (e.g., *Paragonimus, Nanophyetus*), and are not usually recovered using this technique. Nematode larvae can be recovered but frequently are distorted from crenation, making identification difficult. If the specific gravity of the flotation solution is too high, a plug of fecal debris floats and traps parasite stages in it, obscuring them from view.

Commonly used flotation solutions are sugar, sodium chloride, sodium nitrate, magnesium sulfate, and zinc sulfate. Each solution has advantages and disadvantages, including cost, availability, efficiency, shelf life, crystallization, corrosion of equipment, and ease of use. Selection is often determined by the type of practice and common parasites encountered in the area. Some companies have packaged flotation kits using prepared solutions of sodium nitrate or zinc sulfate, disposable plastic vials, and strainers (Fig. 10-39). They are convenient but more expensive. Supplies to conduct simple flotations can be acquired through suppliers of scientific equipment and chemicals.

The specific gravity of flotation solutions can be checked using a hydrometer and adjusted by adding more salts or more water to the solution. Leaving extra crystals of salt on the bottom of the solution ensures that the solution is saturated.

PROCEDURE 10-2 Simple Fecal Flotation

Materials

- 75 glass microscope slides (25-mm)
- Glass cover slips (22-mm^2 #1)
- Wooden tongue depressors
- Waxed paper cups (90-150 ml)
- Cheesecloth or 10 cm gauze squares or metal screen tea strainer
- Shell vial, (1.25-2.0 cm or 5.0-7.5 cm); or 15-ml conical centrifuge tube
- Saturated salt or sugar flotation solution

Procedure

1. Place approximately 2-5 g of feces in the paper cup.
2. Add 30 ml of flotation solution.
3. Using the tongue depressor, mix the feces to produce an evenly suspended emulsion.
4. If using cheesecloth, bend the sides of the cup to form a spout and cover the top with the cheesecloth squares while pouring the suspension into the shell vial. If using a metal strainer, pour the suspension through the metal strainer into another cup and fill the shell vial with the filtered solution.
5. Fill the shell vial to form a convex dome (meniscus) at the rim. *Do not overfill the vial.* Fresh solution can be used to form this dome.
6. Place a cover slip on top of the filled shell vial.
7. Allow the cover slip to remain undisturbed for 10 to 20 minutes.
8. Pick the cover slip straight up and place it on a glass slide, fluid side down.
9. Systematically examine the surface under the cover slip at 100× magnification.

Centrifugal Flotation

This procedure is similar in principle to the flotation procedure except that once the sample and solution are mixed, the specimen is strained (to remove excess debris). Add a coverslip and centrifuge the specimen at 400 to 650 G for 5 minutes. Centrifugal force holds the cover slips in

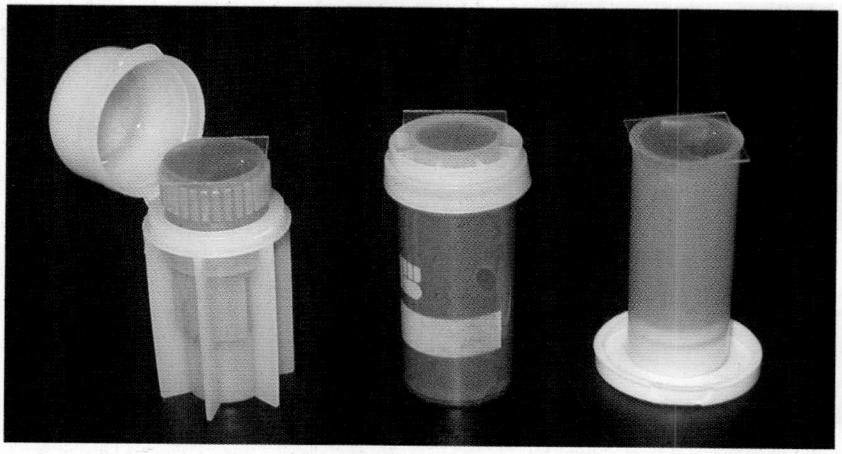

FIGURE 10-39 Three commercially available fecal flotation kits: Fecalyzer *(left)*, Ovassay *(center)*, and Ovatector *(right)*. These kits are based on the principles of the simple flotation procedure. (From Hendrix CM, Robinson E: *Diagnostic parasitology for veterinary technicians*, ed 3, St Louis, 2006, Mosby.)

place during spinning, provided the tubes are balanced. A bacteriology loop is then used to remove a drop of liquid from the surface of the tube, and the drop is examined microscopically. Centrifugal flotation is more sensitive than simple flotation. It recovers more eggs and cysts in a sample in less time (Procedure 10-3). However, it requires access to a tabletop centrifuge with a head for rotation buckets. Fixed-angle heads do not work as well for this procedure as described. They can be adapted for this procedure by not filling the tubes and omitting the coverslip during centrifugation.

Fecal Sedimentation

The sedimentation procedure is used when suspected parasites produce ova too large to be recovered with standard flotation (i.e., fluke ova). The fecal sample is mixed in a small volume of water and strained into a centrifuge tube. The sample can be centrifuged at 400 G for 5 minutes or allowed to remain undisturbed for 20 to 30 minutes. The supernatant is poured off, and a pipette is used to remove a drop of the sediment. A drop from the upper, middle, and lower portions of the sediment is removed. These drops are then examined microscopically. Sedimentation concentrates parasite stages as

PROCEDURE 10-3 Centrifugal Flotation

Materials

- Glass microscope slides (25-mm)
- Glass cover slips (22-mm^2 #1)
- Waxed paper cups
- Cheesecloth or 10 cm gauze squares, or metal screen tea strainer
- Funnel
- Conical centrifuge tubes (15-ml)
- Test tube rack
- Flotation solution
- Centrifuge with rotating buckets
- Wooden tongue depressors
- Balance scale

Procedure

1. Prepare a fecal emulsion using 2-5 g of feces and 30 ml of flotation solution (Fig. 1).

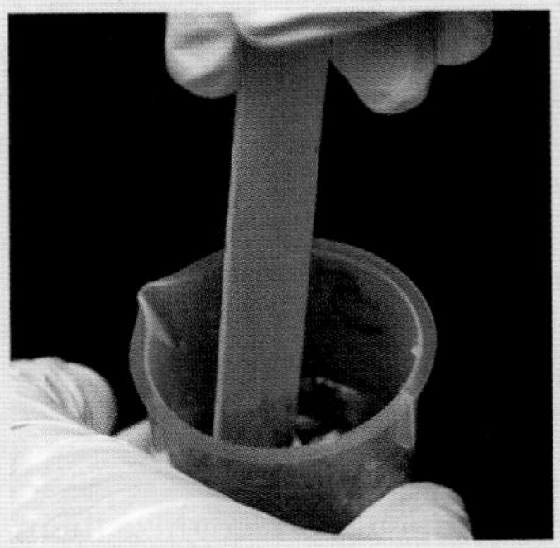

FIGURE 1 (From Greene CE: *Infectious diseases of the dog and cat*, ed 4, Philadelphia, 2012, W.B. Saunders.)

2. Strain the emulsion through the cheesecloth or tea strainer into the centrifuge tube. (Suspending a funnel over the tube facilitates filling the tube.) (Fig. 2).

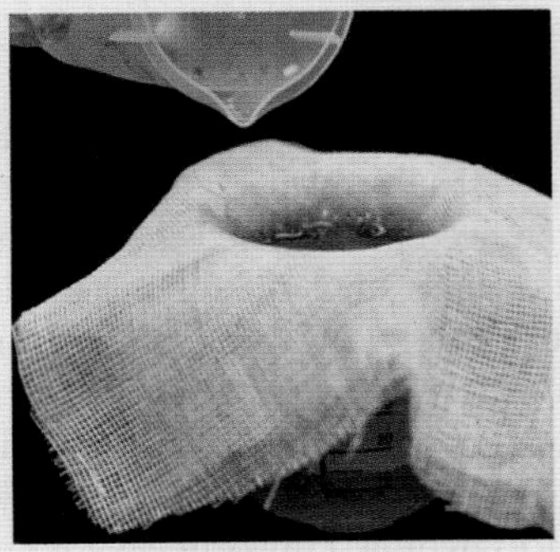

FIGURE 2 (From Greene CE: *Infectious diseases of the dog and cat*, ed 4, Philadelphia, 2012, W.B. Saunders.)

3. Fill the tube to create a positive meniscus with flotation solution (Fig. 3).

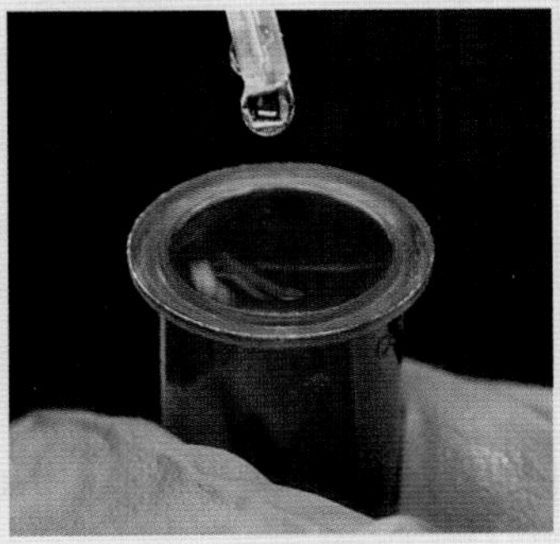

FIGURE 3 (From Greene CE: *Infectious diseases of the dog and cat*, ed 4, Philadelphia, 2012, W.B. Saunders.)

4. Place a cover slip on top of the tube (Fig. 4).

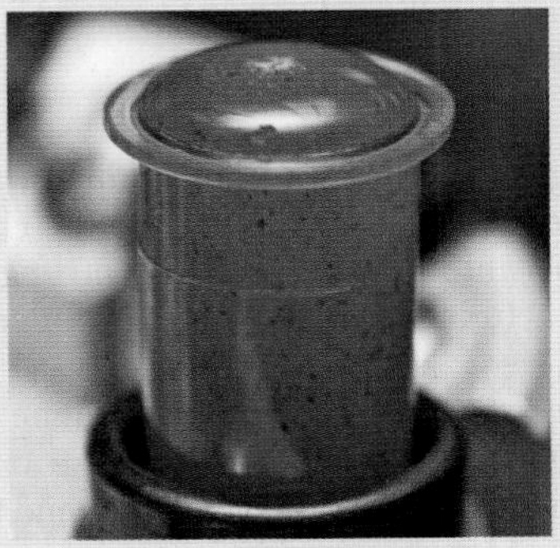

FIGURE 4 (From Greene CE: *Infectious diseases of the dog and cat*, ed 4, Philadelphia, 2012, W.B. Saunders.)

5. Create a balance tube of equal weight, containing another sample or water (Fig. 5).

Continued

PROCEDURE 10-3 Centrifugal Flotation—cont'd

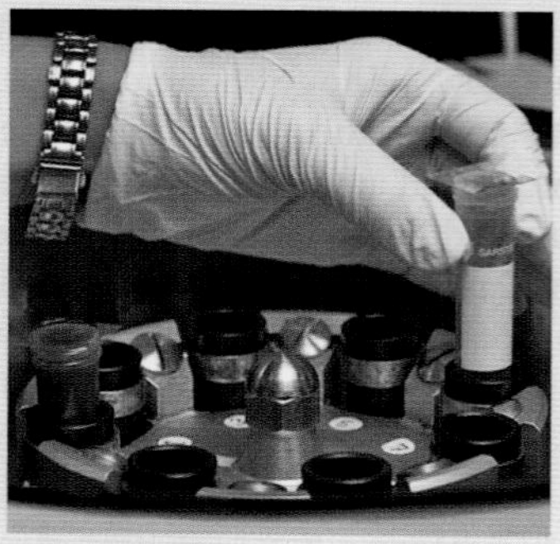

FIGURE 5 (From Greene CE: *Infectious diseases of the dog and cat*, ed 4, Philadelphia, 2012, W.B. Saunders.)

6. Place the tubes in the centrifuge buckets, and weigh them on a balance. You may add water to the buckets to make them equal weights.

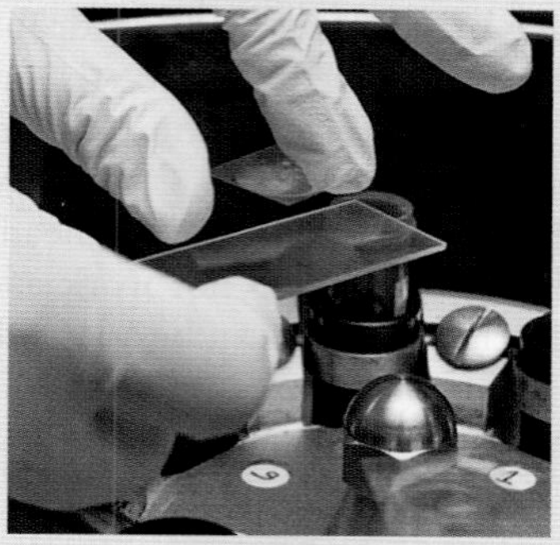

FIGURE 6 (From Greene CE: *Infectious diseases of the dog and cat*, ed 4, Philadelphia, 2012, W.B. Saunders.)

7. Centrifuge the tubes for 5 minutes at 400-650 gravities (approximately 1500 rpm).
8. Remove the cover slips from the tubes by lifting straight up, and place them on a slide (Fig. 6).
9. Systematically examine the slides at 100× magnification.

PROCEDURE 10-4 Fecal Sedimentation

Materials

- Waxed paper cups (90-150 ml)
- Wooden tongue depressors
- Cheesecloth or 10 cm gauze squares, or metal screen tea strainer
- Funnel
- Conical centrifuge tubes (50-ml)
- Disposable pipettes (2-ml)
- Glass microscope slides (25-mm)
- Glass cover slips (22-mm^2 #1)

Procedure

1. Mix 2-5 g of feces in a cup with 30 ml of water.
2. Strain the fecal suspension through the cheesecloth or tea strainer into a 50-ml conical centrifuge tube. (Suspending a funnel over the tube facilitates filling the tube.)
3. Wash the sample with water until the tube is filled.
4. Allow the tube to sit undisturbed for 15 to 30 minutes.
5. Decant the supernatant off, and resuspend the sediment in water.
6. Repeat steps 4 and 5 two more times.
7. Decant the supernatant without disturbing the sediment.
8. Using a pipette, mix the sediment and transfer an aliquot to a slide.
9. Place a cover slip over the sediment, and systematically examine the slide with 100× magnification.
10. Repeat steps 8 and 9 until all sediment has been examined.

PROCEDURE 10-5 Cellophane Tape Preparation

Materials

- Transparent adhesive tape
- Wooden tongue depressors
- Glass microscope slides (25-mm)

Procedure

1. Place adhesive tape in a loop around one end of the tongue depressor, with the adhesive side facing out.
2. Press the tape firmly against the skin around the anus.
3. Place a drop of water on the slide. Undo the loop of tape and stick the tape to the slide, allowing the water to spread out under the tape.
4. Examine the taped area of the slide microscopically for the presence of pinworm eggs.

well as fecal debris (Procedure 10-4). Because of the debris, parasite stages may be obscured from view; this technique is also more laborious. Sedimentation is used primarily when fluke infections are suspected. Most fluke eggs do not float, or they are distorted by flotation solutions with a higher specific gravity, making it difficult to recognize them. A few drops of liquid detergent can be added to the water as a surfactant to help remove excess fats and debris from the sample.

Cellophane Tape Preparation

This method is often used to recover ova of *Oxyuris* (pinworms). It can also aid in identification of tapeworms. A piece of cellophane tape is wrapped around a tongue depressor with the adhesive side out. The animal's tail is raised and the tongue depressor firmly pressed against the anus. The tape is then removed and applied to a glass slide that has a small amount of water on it and then examined microscopically (Procedure 10-5). Pinworms can be found in primates, horses, and ruminants. The adult female worms migrate out of the anus and deposit their eggs on the skin around the anus (perianal region). The activity of the female worms is irritating and produces itching. Pinworm eggs are not consistently found on fecal flotations and are suspected when animals rub

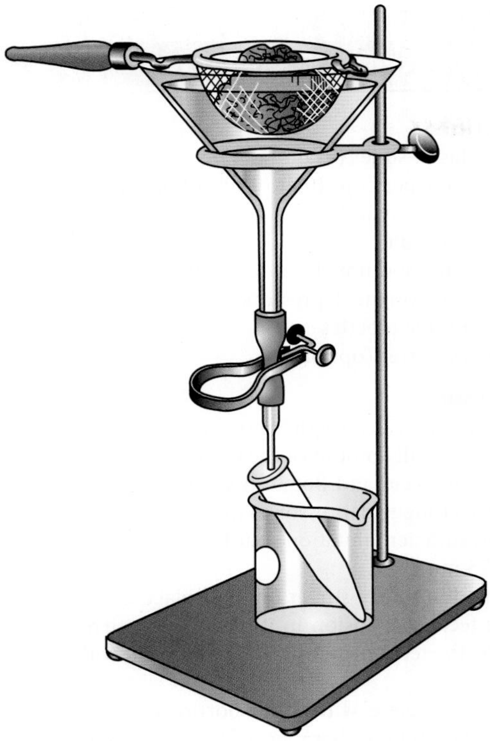

FIGURE 10-40 Baermann apparatus for separating and concentrating nematode larvae from feces, minced tissues, and soil samples. (From Bowman DD: *Georgis' Parasitology for Veterinarians,* ed 9, St Louis, 2009, Saunders.)

their tails on objects, resulting in loss of hair. *Oxyuris equi,* the pinworm of horses, can be a problem. Pinworm species of domestic animals are not transmissible to people. People can be infected with *Enterobius vermicularis* through direct contact with another infected person or premises contaminated with *Enterobius* eggs. Frequently, infected people are misinformed and believe that their infections came directly from their animals.

Baermann Technique

The **Baermann technique** is sometimes used to recover larvae from fecal samples. The procedure requires construction of a Baermann apparatus that consists of a large funnel supported in a ring stand. A piece of rubber tubing is attached to the end of the funnel and placed in a collection tube. The fecal sample is placed in the funnel on top of a piece of metal screen (Fig. 10-40). Warm water or warmed physiologic saline is passed through the sample. The larvae are stimulated to move by the warm water and then sink to the bottom of the apparatus. A drop of the material in the collection container is examined microscopically for presence of larvae. The Baermann technique is used to recover nematode larvae from feces, fecal culture, soil, herbage, and animal tissues (Procedure 10-6). The warm water stimulates larvae to migrate out of the sample and relax. They then sink to the bottom of the apparatus, where they can be collected relatively free of debris. Free-living larvae must be distinguished from parasitic ones, especially if the sample is collected off the ground, from soil, or from herbage. This may require the expertise of an experienced helminthologist. Preserve samples by adding 5% to 10% formalin to the pellet for submission to an expert. Kill free-living larvae by adding 1% hydrochloric acid to the pellet, and examine the preparation without heat fixation. Unfortunately, identification of motile larvae is more difficult.

The Baermann technique is routinely performed on feces of domestic animals when lungworm infections (e.g., *Dictyocaulus, Aelurostrongylus, Filaroides, Crenosoma, Muellerius, Protostrongylus*) are suspected. Ideally, samples should be fresh and collected rectally. In dogs and cats a Baermann technique should be conducted when *Strongyloides* spp. infections are suspected. If the sample is not fresh, a fecal culture may be needed to distinguish first-stage hookworm larvae from first-stage larvae of *Strongyloides.* The third-stage filariform larva of *Strongyloides* is diagnostic and characterized by an esophagus that is half the length of the larva and a forked (bipartite) tail. Care should be taken when handling *Strongyloides* fecal cultures because of the zoonotic potential.

PROCEDURE 10-6 Baermann Technique

Materials

- Baermann apparatus (ring stand, ring, funnel, rubber tubing, clamp, wire screen)
- Cheesecloth or Kimwipes
- Disposable pipettes
- Centrifuge tubes (15-ml) or Petri dishes
- Pinch clamps

Procedure

1. Construct a Baermann apparatus by fastening the ring to the ring stand. Attach 3 to 4 inches of rubber tubing to the narrow portion of the funnel. Ensure that there is a good seal (tubing can be glued on). Place the funnel in the ring. Place the wire screen in the top portion of the funnel to support the feces. Put several layers of cheesecloth or Kimwipes over the wire screen. Place the pinch clamps at the end of the rubber tubing and check, using water, to ensure a tight seal. Put 30 to 50 g of feces on top of the Kimwipes and fill the funnel with warm water (not hot) to a level above the fecal sample. (An alternative method, which is more practical in a practice setting, is to use long-stem, plastic champagne glasses with hollow stems. The feces are wrapped in several layers of Kimwipes, similar to a tea bag. The fecal pouch is then set in the glass. Fill the glass with warm water to a level above the fecal sample.)
2. Allow the apparatus to remain undisturbed for a minimum of 1 hour up to 24 hours.
3. Collect the fluid in the rubber tubing (stem of the glass) and transfer to a petri dish or centrifuge tube.
4. Examine the petri dish for larvae using a stereo microscope, or centrifuge the solution to pellet the larvae. Remove the supernatant from the centrifuge tube and place the pellet on a microscope slide.
5. Examine the slide for larvae and identify them. The slide can be passed over the flame of a Bunsen burner several times to kill the larvae in an extended position before identification.

PROCEDURE 10-7 Fecal Culture

Materials
- Glass jar with tight-fitting lid
- Charcoal or vermiculite
- Wooden tongue depressors

Procedure
1. Moisten 50 g of charcoal or vermiculite with water. The charcoal or vermiculite should be damp but not wet.
2. Using the tongue depressor, mix an equal amount of feces with the moistened substrate.
3. Place the fecal mixture in a glass jar, and seal with the jar lid.
4. Place the jar in indirect light at room temperature for up to 7 days.
5. Check the jar periodically to ensure that the contents remain moist. A spray bottle of water can be used to moisten the fecal mixture if it becomes too dry. Be sure not to saturate the material.
6. Do a Baermann technique on the fecal culture at 48-hour intervals to recover developing stages. Some larvae migrate up the wall of the jar and congregate in condensation droplets. These can be collected by flushing the sides of the jar with water and collecting the excess fluid in a centrifuge tube or petri dish.
7. Identify the larvae recovered.

Miscellaneous Fecal Examinations

Some parasites produce intestinal bleeding. This bleeding may be evident as frank blood in the fecal sample or as darkened feces. Some intestinal bleeding can only be identified with chemical testing. This is referred to as fecal occult blood testing. Several types of kits are available for this procedure. They primarily act to identify the presence of hemoglobin in the sample.

Examination of vomitus may also aid in diagnosis of parasitism. Some parasites (e.g., *Toxacara canis*) are often present in vomitus of infected patients.

Fecal culture is used to differentiate parasites whose eggs or larvae are not easily distinguished by examination of a fresh fecal sample (Procedure 10-7). Trichostrongyle eggs in ruminant feces are indistinguishable from strongyle eggs. Small strongyle eggs in a horse sample cannot be distinguished from large strongyle eggs. First-stage hookworm larvae in a dog or cat sample and some free-living nematode larvae in soil or on grass cannot be easily distinguished from first-stage *Strongyloides* larvae. After fecal culture, the third-stage larvae of many of these parasites can be identified to genus level. Because the life cycles, pathogenicity, and epidemiology of some species may differ, identification may be necessary for proper treatment and control. Identification may require the help of an experienced helminthologist.

An additional type of fecal flotation test is the modified McMaster technique. This technique provides an estimate of the number of eggs or oocysts per gram of feces, primarily with livestock species and horses (Procedure 10-8). Originally it was adapted from a technique used in people infected with hookworms to estimate the worm population in the host. However, it is impossible to calculate the actual worm

PROCEDURE 10-8 Modified McMaster Quantitative Egg Counting Technique

Materials
- McMaster slides (Wallowa, OR)
- Waxed paper cups (90 to 150 ml) or beakers
- Graduated cylinder
- Balance scale
- Saturated sodium chloride solution
- Wooden tongue depressors
- Disposable pipettes
- Rotary stirrer (optional)

Procedure
1. Using the scale, weigh 5 g of feces into a cup.
2. Add a small amount of the flotation solution to the cup.
3. Mix the feces and flotation solution together thoroughly with a tongue depressor to make an even suspension.
4. Add sufficient flotation solution to bring the total volume to 75 ml.
5. Turn the rotary stirrer on, and place the cup containing the fecal suspension in it. If a rotary stirrer is not available, the fecal suspension can be mixed with a tongue depressor.
6. Using a pipette, withdraw a portion of the mixing suspension and fill the chambers of the McMaster slide.
7. Allow the slide to sit undisturbed for 10 minutes.
8. Using the 10× objective, focus on the grid etched in the McMaster slide. Count all eggs or oocysts seen in the six columns of the etched square, keeping a separate count for each species of parasite seen.
9. Multiply the numbers counted by the appropriate dilution factor (dependent on the number of squares counted), and record the results as eggs per gram (epg) of feces The volume under the etched area is 0.15 ml. If 5 g per 75 ml total volume equals 1 g per 15 ml total volume, then 0.01 g is contained in 0.15 ml. Therefore if one chamber is counted, multiply by 100. If two chambers are counted, multiply by 50 to arrive at the total epg.

population in a host, especially in livestock and horses, because many factors influence egg production, and the number of eggs produced varies with the species and number of worms present.

Typically, livestock and horses are infected with several species of worms at one time, and some species are more prolific and pathogenic than others. Also, lesions often result from damage produced by immature stages of the parasites. In ruminants the parasites of interest are coccidia and trichostrongyles. In horses the parasites of interest are large and small strongyles. Both trichostrongyles and strongyles infect ruminants and horses. The eggs of trichostrongyles and strongyles cannot be readily distinguished from one another and are referred to as strongyle eggs. Nevertheless, counts in excess of 1000 are considered indicative of heavy infections, whereas those greater than 500 indicate moderate infections. A low egg count can indicate a low level of infection, or severe infections in which the parasites are just becoming mature. Egg counts must always be interpreted in view of the clinical signs observed, age, sex and nutritional level of the animals, and stocking density of a herd or flock.

More recently, egg counts have been used in epidemiologic investigations and herd health management programs as predictors of peak pasture contamination and transmission potential for different geographic regions and individual farms. This information is applied toward prevention programs involving strategic use of broad-spectrum anthelmintics and pasture rotation schemes aimed at reducing the infective levels of pastures and exposure rates. When herd studies are conducted, individual samples are taken from at least 10% of the herd. Egg counts are also used to monitor development of resistance to anthelmintics. Egg counts are done before treatment and again three weeks following treatment, to determine the effectiveness of the anthelminthic used and development of resistance in a given worm population.

EVALUATION OF BLOOD SAMPLES

Examination of blood samples may reveal adult parasites and/or their various life cycle stages either free in the blood or intracellularly. A variety of methods can be used for this determination. Thin or thick blood smears are prepared in the same way that smears for a WBC differential count are prepared. Preparation of smears for a WBC differential count is described in Chapter 7. Most parasites are carried with the laminar flow to the feathered edge of the slide. Parasites may be located between cells, on the surface of cells, or in the cytoplasm of cells. Thin blood films are most effectively used to study the morphology of protozoan and rickettsial parasites. If parasitemia is low, infections can be missed. A thick blood film or a buffy coat smear is more effective because it concentrates a larger volume of cells (Procedure 10-9).

The buffy coat smear is a concentration technique for detection of protozoa and rickettsiae in white blood cells. A microhematocrit tube is centrifuged as for a PCV determination. Microfilariae and some protozoa may also be found at the top of the plasma column. The technique is quick but cannot be used to differentiate *D. immitis* from *A. reconditum.*

Direct Drop

This is the simplest of the blood evaluations, although it is also the least accurate because of the small sample size. A drop of anticoagulated whole blood is examined microscopically. The movement of parasites that are extracellular can be detected with this method.

Filter Test

The filter technique is a method designed to concentrate microfilariae in blood (Procedure 10-10). The principles applied are similar to those of the modified Knott's test, except that the blood is passed through a Millipore filter, which collects the microfilariae. Commercial kits use a detergent lysing solution and a differential stain (Fig. 10-41). This procedure is quicker and easier than the modified Knott's test, but the differential characteristics of the microfilariae are not as obvious. Identification using the characteristics listed in Table 10-8 is not

PROCEDURE 10-9 Buffy Coat Smear

Materials

- Hematocrit tubes
- Sealant
- Hematocrit centrifuge
- Glass microscope slides (25-mm)
- Glass cover slips (22-mm^2 #1)
- File
- Permount

Procedure

1. Fill the hematocrit tube with the blood sample, and plug one end with sealant.
2. Centrifuge for 5 minutes.
3. The buffy coat is located in the middle of the centrifuged sample, between the red blood cells and the plasma.
4. Use the file to etch the glass below the buffy coat. Snap the tube by applying pressure opposite the etched spot.
5. Take the end of the tube containing the buffy coat and plasma, and tap the buffy coat onto a glass slide with a small amount of plasma. If too much plasma is released, use a clean Kimwipe to wipe away excess.
6. Apply a clean slide over the buffy coat, and rapidly pull the two slides across each other in opposite directions.
7. Allow the slides to air-dry, and stain with Romanowsky stain.
8. After staining, apply mounting medium and a cover slip.
9. Examine the slides microscopically at 400× and 1000× magnification.

PROCEDURE 10-10 Millipore Filtration Procedure

Materials

- 5-μ Millipore filters
- Millipore filter holders
- 2.5% methylene blue stain
- 2% formalin or commercial lysing solution
- Glass microscope slides (25-mm)
- Glass cover slips (22-mm^2 #1)
- 12-ml disposable syringes

Procedure

1. Assemble the filter holder with a Millipore filter.
2. Place 1 ml of blood in the syringe.
3. Add 9 ml of 2% formalin or lysing solution to the blood in the syringe, and insert the plunger.
4. Connect the syringe to the filter apparatus, and slowly apply pressure to the syringe plunger.
5. Remove the syringe and fill it with tap water. Allow a few milliliters of air to remain in the syringe. Flush the water through the filter apparatus.
6. Remove the filter from the filter holder, and place top-side-up on a glass slide.
7. Place a drop of the methylene blue stain on the filter, and add a cover slip.
8. Examine the slide microscopically at 100× magnification for microfilariae.

possible with commercial kits, because the characteristics of the microfilariae are based on fixation with 2% formalin.

Modified Knott's Test

This method is used to concentrate microfilaria and can help in differentiation of *Dirofilaria* from *Acanthocheilonema.* The procedure requires a mixture of blood and formalin in a centrifuge tube. The mixture is incubated at room temperature for 1 to 2 minutes and then centrifuged for 5 minutes. The supernatant is poured off, and a drop of methylene blue is added to the sediment in the tube. A drop of this mixture is transferred to a glass slide for microscopic evaluation. The modified Knott's technique is a rapid method for detection of microfilariae (heartworm larvae) in the blood (Procedure 10-11). It is used primarily for differentiating *Dirofilaria immitis* and *Acanthocheilonema reconditum* infections in dogs. The technique concentrates microfilariae while fixing them and lyses red blood cells. When preparing the 2% formalin solution, it is important to remember that 37% formaldehyde is equivalent to 100% formalin. It is also important to use water, not physiologic saline, to prepare this solution because physiologic saline does not lyse red blood cells. For accurate differentiation of the microfilariae, the microscope must have a calibrated ocular micrometer. The most accurate differentiating characteristics are body width, body length, and shape of the cranial end. The other characteristics are not consistent. The modified Knott's technique cannot detect occult heartworm infections.

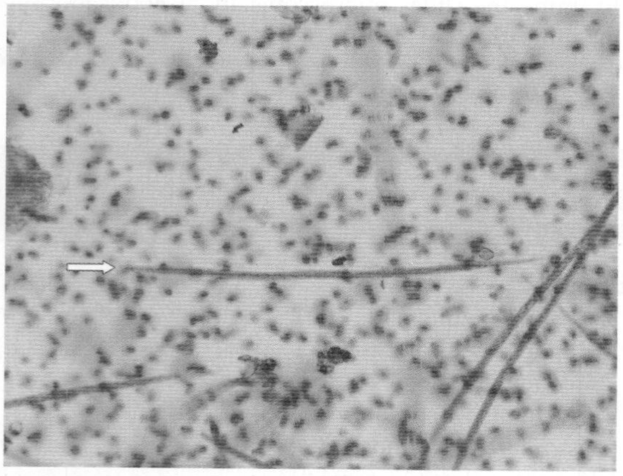

FIGURE 10-41 Microfilariae of *Dirofilaria immitis* on a Millipore filter (stained). (From Hendrix CM, Robinson E: *Diagnostic parasitology for veterinary technicians,* ed 3, St Louis, 2006, Mosby.)

TABLE 10-8 Differential Characteristics of *Dirofilaria immitis* and *Acanthocheilonema reconditum* Microfilariae

CHARACTERISTIC	*DIROFILARIA IMMITIS*	*ACANTHOCHEILONEMA RECONDITUM*
Body shape	Usually straight	Usually curved
Body width	5-7.5 μ	4.5-5.5 μ
Body length	295-325 μ	250-288 μ
Cranial end	Tapered	Blunt
Caudal end	Straight	Curved or hooked
Numbers	Numerous	Sparse
Movement	Undulating	Progressive

Immunologic Tests

A variety of tests are available to identify antigen and/or antibody to specific parasites. The majority of tests are based on the enzyme-linked immunosorbent assay (ELISA) principle. The tests are highly accurate and precise and can detect occult infections. Canine heartworm infections and *Toxoplasma* infections are routinely diagnosed with these methods. In the ELISA method, monoclonal antibodies are used to detect antigens of adult heartworms in the serum or plasma of dogs. These procedures are rapid and easy to perform. They are also more sensitive and specific than microfilariae detection methods. The American Heartworm Society currently recommends using antigen-detection methods for routine screening in addition to microfilaria concentration methods. Antigen-detection methods are preferred to microfilariae concentration methods in cats because such aberrant hosts circulate microfilariae only for a very short time. However, antigen levels in the blood of infected cats may also be too low to detect. Other methods, such as radiography, may be employed to make a diagnosis in cats.

Approximately 25% of heartworm-infected dogs have occult infections. Occult infections are characterized by a lack of circulating microfilaria and occur if the infection is not yet patent, if the population of adult heartworms consists of only one sex, or if immune reactions of the host to microfilariae eliminate this stage from the bloodstream. Occult infections can also occur if animals infected with adult heartworms are given heartworm preventive medications of the ivermectin group. These interfere with oogenesis and sterilize the worms.

PROCEDURE 10-11 Modified Knott's Technique

Materials

- Blood collection materials
- 15-ml conical centrifuge tubes
- 2% formalin (2 ml 37% formaldehyde/98 ml water)
- 2.5% methylene blue (2.5 g methylene blue/100 ml water)
- Tabletop centrifuge
- Glass microscope slides (25-mm)
- Glass cover slips (22-mm^2 #1)
- Pipettes

Procedure

1. Mix 1 ml of blood with 9 ml of 2% formalin in a centrifuge tube. Agitate the tube and mix well.
2. Centrifuge the tube at 1500 rpm for 5 minutes.
3. Pour off the supernatant, and add 1 to 2 drops of methylene blue stain to the pellet at the bottom of the tube.
4. Using a pipette, mix the stain and sediment, and transfer the mixture to a glass slide.
5. Apply a cover slip, and examine the sediment microscopically for microfilariae at 100× and 400× magnification.

Miscellaneous Parasitologic Evaluations

Cellophane tape preparations (described in Chapter 9) can be used to recover external parasites that live primarily on the surface of the skin (i.e., mites, lice, fleas). Parasites that live in hair follicles or burrows are usually diagnosed with skin scraping using standard procedures.

Samples may be collected from the ear or the respiratory or genital tracts with cotton swabs. These can be examined microscopically using standard preparations as for cytology samples. Transtracheal/bronchial washes can also be used to recover parasites of the respiratory system. Parasites of the urinary system are usually recovered using standard urine sediment examination techniques. Impression smears can be used for diagnosis of intracellular parasites. They can be useful for diagnosis of parasitic, neoplastic, and fungal diseases antemortem and postmortem. These procedures are described in more detail in Chapter 9. Frequently, protozoal organisms produce systemic disease and are located in the reticuloendothelial cells of lymph nodes, liver, lung, bone marrow, spleen, brain, kidneys, or muscles. Also, the liver, lung, lymph nodes, bone marrow, and spleen filter out damaged and abnormal cells of the blood, collecting parasitized cells. Toxoplasmosis, leishmaniasis, ehrlichiosis, and babesiosis are examples of parasitic diseases that can be diagnosed using this technique.

Skin scrapings are used as a diagnostic tool for dermatologic conditions, especially mange in domestic animals. Because some mange mites dwell in burrows and hair follicles deep in the epidermis, superficial scrapings are not productive. Other mites live in the more superficial layers of the skin and produce crusty or scaly lesions; deep scrapings are not required to diagnose these infestations. Sometimes the thick crusts interfere with seeing the mites. Soaking the crust in a 10% potassium hydroxide solution helps to dissolve the keratinized skin and releases the mites. Mite infestations usually localize in specific locations (ear margin, tail head) initially, depending on the species of mite involved. Later they may become generalized and more difficult to diagnose. *Sarcoptes* and *Cheyletiella* mites can be transmitted to people and produce pruritic reactions requiring attention. Specific identification of mites can be accomplished with the aid of taxonomic keys.

Cheyletiella infestation can be diagnosed by combing the coat of infested animals over a piece of black paper and observing the paper for "walking dandruff." *Otodectes cynotis* infestations of the external ear canal can be diagnosed by otoscopic examination or by taking a swab of the dark waxy debris found in the ear and microscopically examining it in mineral oil.

Tritrichomonas foetus is a flagellated protozoan parasite of the reproductive tract of cattle that causes early-term abortions and repeat breeding. Bulls remain permanently infected and must be identified and slaughtered to prevent spread of this organism. The organism can be found in fluid from the abomasum of aborted fetuses, uterine discharges, and vaginal and preputial washes. However, the numbers present are usually low and culture of these materials facilitates diagnosis. Occasionally intestinal flagellates can contaminate a sample. These must be differentiated from *T. foetus,* which has three cranial flagella and one caudal flagellum attached to an undulating membrane. Isolates of *T. foetus* can be propagated through several passages of culture medium, whereas intestinal flagellates usually cannot. Materials may also be collected and shipped to diagnostic facilities for culture and identification. InPouch TF (Biomed Diagnostics, San Jose, Calif.) is an excellent transport medium.

Tables 10-9 and 10-10 list diagnostic characteristics of internal parasites of domestic animals. Table 10-11 lists some zoonotic internal parasites.

TABLE 10-9 Diagnostic Characteristics of Internal Parasites of Domestic Animals

PARASITE	PREPATENT PERIOD	DIAGNOSTIC STAGE	DIAGNOSTIC TEST
Aelurostrongylus abstrusus	4-6 weeks	L1 with S-shaped tail and a dorsal spine; 360 μ long; esophagus one-third length of body	Baermann
Ancylostoma braziliense	3 weeks	Hookworm egg; 75-95 × 41-45 μ	Fecal flotation
Ancylostoma caninum	2-3 weeks	Clear, smooth, thin-walled hookworm egg; 8-16-cell morula zygote; 55-65 × 27-43 μ	Fecal flotation
Anoplocephala spp.	1-2 months	Clear, thick-walled, square eggs with a pear-shaped (piriform) apparatus containing a hexacanth embryo	Fecal flotation
Ascaris suum	7-9 weeks	Brownish yellow, thick-walled, mammillated egg; single-celled zygote; 50-80 × 40-60 μ	Fecal flotation
Ascarops strongylina	6 weeks	Oblong, clear, smooth, thick-walled, larvated egg; 34-40 ×18-22 μ	Fecal flotation
Balantidium coli		Thin-walled, greenish cyst with hyaline cytoplasm; 40-60 μ; trophozoite with rows of cilia 30-150 × 25-120 μ	Fecal flotation Direct smear
Bunostomum spp.	2-3 weeks	Strongyle egg	Fecal flotation
Eucoleus aerophilus (formerly *Capillaria aerophila*)	6 weeks	Rough, granular, thick-walled, barrel-shaped, straw-colored egg with asymmetric bipolar plugs; single-celled zygote; 58-79 × 29-40 μ	Fecal flotation
Pearsonema plica	60 days	Rough, striated, thick-walled, barrel-shaped, amber-colored egg with asymmetric bipolar plugs; single-celled zygote; 60-68 × 24-30 μ	Sedimentation of urine
Cryptosporidium muris	4-10 days	Clear, smooth, thin-walled oocyst containing 4 sporozoites; 5 × 7μ	Fecal flotation

Continued

TABLE 10-9 Diagnostic Characteristics of Internal Parasites of Domestic Animals—cont'd			
PARASITE	PREPATENT PERIOD	DIAGNOSTIC STAGE	DIAGNOSTIC TEST
Cryptosporidium spp.	4-10 days	Clear, thin-walled, spherical oocyst containing 4 sporozoites; 5 × 5 μ	Fecal flotation
Cyathostoma (small strongyles)	2-3 months	Smooth, thin-walled, clear strongyle egg zygote 8- to 16-cell morula; size varies with species	Fecal flotation
Dicrocoelium dendriticum	10-12 weeks	Dark brown, operculated egg; 36-45 × 22-30 μ	Sedimentation of feces
Dictyocaulus arnfieldi	2-4 months	L1 with dark, granular intestines; esophagus one-third length of larva; tapered tail	Fecal flotation Baermann
Dictyocaulus spp.	3-4 weeks	L1 with dark granular intestines; esophagus one-third length of larva; straight pointed tail; 550-580 μ long	Baermann
Dioctophyma renale	5 months	Dark brown, thick-walled, barrel-shaped egg with a pitted shell and an operculum at each pole; single-celled zygote; 71-84 × 46-52 μ	Sedimentation of urine
Acanthocheilonema reconditum (formerly *Dipetalonema reconditum*)	9 weeks	Microfilaria	Modified Knott's Millipore filtration
Dipylidium caninum	3 weeks	Proglottid with bilateral genital pores; eggs containing six-hooked hexacanth embryos in packets; 35-60 μ	ID proglottids fecal flotation
Dirofilaria immitis	6-8 months	Microfilaria (L1) lacks an esophagus	Modified Knott's Millipore filtration, ELISA, antigen test
Dracunculus insignis	309-410 days	Comma-shaped larva with an esophagus and a straight tail; 500-750 μ long	Direct smear of fluid in blister
Echinococcus spp.	47 days	Similar to Taenia eggs	Fecal flotation
Eimeria leuckarti	15-33 days	Dark brown, piriform, thick-walled oocyst 70-90 × 49-69 μ	Fecal flotation
Eimeria spp.	4-30 days	Smooth or rough, thin-walled, clear to yellowish brown oocysts; single-celled zygote; size varies with species	Fecal flotation
Elaeophora schneideri	4-5 months	Microfilaria in skin of the poll; 207 ×13 μ	Skin biopsy
Fasciola hepatica	10-12 weeks	Dark amber, oval, operculated egg; 130-150 × 63-90 μ	Sedimentation of feces
Filaroides spp.	5-10 weeks	L1 with S-shaped tail lacking a dorsal spine; esophagus one-third length of body; 230-266 μ long	Fecal flotation, Baermann
Gasterophilus spp.		2.5 cm, robust grub with rows of spines and straight spiracular slits (breathing tubes)	ID 3rd instar at necropsy
Giardia spp.	7-10 days	Smooth, clear, thin-walled cyst with 2-4 nuclei; 4-10 × 8-16 μ	Fecal flotation
Giardia spp.		Piriform, bilaterally symmetric greenish trophozoite with 2 nuclei and 4 pair of flagella; 9-20 × 5-15 μ	Direct smear
Habronema and *Draschia* spp.	2 months	Thin-walled, larvated egg (rarely seen)	ID adults at necropsy
Hyostrongylus rubidus	15-21 days	Strongyle egg	Fecal flotation
Isospora spp.	4-12 days	Clear, spherical to ellipsoid thin-walled oocyst, size varies with species	Fecal flotation
Macracanthorhynchus hirudinaceus	2-3 months	Dark brown, thick-walled egg with 3 membranes; zygote an acanthor with anterior hooks; 67-110 × 40-65 μ	Fecal flotation
Mesocestoides spp.	16-20 days	Smooth, thin egg capsule containing six-hooked hexacanth embryo; 20-25 μ; globular proglottid with parauterine body	Fecal flotation ID proglottid
Metastrongylus spp.	24 days	Rough, clear, thick-walled, larvated egg with a corrugated surface; 45-57 × 38-41 μ	Fecal flotation
Moniezia spp.	6 weeks	Thick-walled, clear, triangular to square egg with a piriform apparatus containing a hexacanth embryo	Fecal flotation
Nanophyetus salmincola	1 week	Rough, brown, operculated egg; 52-82 × 32-56 μ	Sedimentation of feces
Oesophagostomum spp.	32-42 days	Strongyle egg	Fecal flotation
Onchocerca spp.	1 year	Unsheathed microfilaria in the skin of ventral midline; 200-370 μ long	Skin biopsy

TABLE 10-9 Diagnostic Characteristics of Internal Parasites of Domestic Animals—cont'd

PARASITE	PREPATENT PERIOD	DIAGNOSTIC STAGE	DIAGNOSTIC TEST
Oxyuris equi	5 months	Clear, smooth, thin-walled egg with one side flattened; operculated; 90 × 42 μ	Cellophane tape preparation
Paragonimus kellicotti	1 month	Smooth, golden brown, urn-shaped, operculated egg; 75-118 × 42-67 μ	Sedimentation of urine
Paramphistomum spp.	7-10 weeks	Light greenish, oval, operculated egg; 114-176 × 73-100 μ	Sedimentation of feces
Parascaris equorum	10 weeks	Rough, brown, thick-walled, spherical egg single-celled zygote; 90-100 μ	Fecal flotation
Physaloptera spp.	56-83 days	Smooth, clear, thick-walled, larvated egg 45-53 × 29-42 μ	Fecal flotation
Physocephalus sexalatus	6 weeks	Clear, smooth, thick-walled, larvated egg; 31-45 ×12-26 μ	Fecal flotation
Platynosomum fastosum	8-12 weeks	Dark amber, oval, operculated egg containing a miracidium; 34-50 × 20-35 μ	Sedimentation of feces
Protostrongylus rufescens	30-37 days	L1 with a straight, pointed tail 48 × 56 m long without a dorsal spine; 340-400 × 19-20 μ	Baermann
Sarcocystis spp.	7-33 days	Thin-walled oocyst with 2 sporocyst containing 4 sporozoites each or sporocyst; size varies with species	Fecal flotation
Setaria equina	Sheathed microfilaria in the blood; 190-256 μ long	Blood smear ID adults at necropsy	
Spirocerca lupi	5-6 months	Clear, smooth, thick-walled, paper-clip-shaped, larvated egg; 30-37 × 11-15 μ	Flotation
Spirometra mansonoides	10-30 days	Unembryonated, thin-walled, smooth, amber-colored operculated egg; 70 × 45 μ	Fecal flotation
Stephanofilaria stilesi		Microfilaria in the skin along ventral midline; 45-60 μ	Skin biopsy
Stephanurus dentatus	3-4 months	Strongyle egg	Sedimentation of urine
Strongyloides ransomi	3-7 days	Smooth, thin-walled, larvated egg with parallel sides; 45-55 × 26-35 μ	Fecal flotation
Strongyloides stercoralis	8-14 days	L1 with a rhabditiform esophagus and a straight pointed tail; L3 with a filariform esophagus and a bipartite tail	Baermann fecal culture
Strongyloides westeri	8-14 days	Smooth, thin-walled, larvated egg; 40-50 × 32-40 μ	Fecal flotation
Taenia spp.	2 months	Dark brown, thick, radially striated eggshell; six-hooked hexacanth embryo; 32-37 μ; rectangular proglottids with unilateral genital pore	ID proglottid
Thelazia californiensis	3-6 weeks	Adult worm in conjunctival sac	ID adult
Thysanosoma actinoides		Thin-walled egg with hexacanth embryos; 21-45 μ	Fecal flotation
Toxascaris leonina	11 weeks	Clear, smooth, thick-walled eggshell with wavy internal membrane; single-celled zygote; does not completely fill egg; 75 ×85 μ	Fecal flotation
Toxocara canis	3-5 weeks	Dark brown, thick-walled, pitted egg, single-celled zygote 90-75 μ	Fecal flotation
Toxocara cati	8 weeks	Dark brown, thick-walled, pitted egg; single-celled zygote; 65-75 μ	Fecal flotation
Toxoplasma gondii	1-3 weeks	Clear, smooth, thin-walled spherical oocyst; single-celled zygote; 8-10 μ	Fecal flotation
Trichinella spiralis	2-6 days	L3 encysted in striated muscles; esophagus composed of stichocytes (single cells stacked on top of one another); cysts are 400-600 × 250 μ	Compression preparation of muscle
Trichomonads		Spindle-shaped to piriform trophozoite with 3-5 anterior flagella, an undulating membrane and 1 posterior flagellum	Direct smear
Trichostrongyles Haemonchus, Ostertagia, Cooperia, Trichostrongylus	15-28 days	Strongyle egg	Fecal flotation
Trichuris suis	2-3 months	Brownish yellow, smooth, thick-walled egg with symmetric bipolar plugs; single-celled zygote; 50-56 × 21-25 μ	Fecal flotation
Trichuris vulpis	3 months	Smooth, amber, thick-walled, barrel-shaped egg with bipolar plugs; single-celled zygote; 72-90 × 32-40 μ	Fecal flotation
Uncinaria stenocephala	2 weeks	Hookworm egg; 63-93 × 32-55 μ	Fecal flotation

TABLE 10-10 Diagnostic Characteristics of Blood Parasites of Domestic Animals

PARASITE	DEFINITIVE HOST(S)	LOCATION IN HOST	PREPATENT PERIOD	DIAGNOSTIC STAGE	DIAGNOSTIC TEST
Babesia spp.	People, dogs, cattle, horses	Erythrocytes	10-21 days	Paired piriform (tear-shaped) merozoites in erythrocytes	Romanowsky stained blood film, indirect fluorescent antibody test
Trypanosoma spp.	People, dogs, cats, cattle, sheep, horses	Blood and lymph, heart, striated muscle, reticuloendothelial muscle	Acute and chronic disease	Trypanosome form, spindle-shaped flagellate with undulating membrane, central nucleus and kinetoplast, found in blood	Blood smears, xenodiagnosis (clean vector allowed to feed on suspect patient and organism isolated from the vector), biopsy, animal inoculation, serology
				Amastigote form, intracellular spherical bodies with single nucleus and rod-shaped kinetoplast, found in myocardium, striated muscle cells, and macrophages	
Leishmania donovani	People, dogs	Intracellular in cytoplasm of macrophages of reticuloendothelial system	Several months up to a year	Amastigote form, oval, single nucleus, with a rod-shaped kinetoplast, in clusters within the cytoplasm of macrophages	Impression smears and biopsy of skin, lymph nodes, and bone marrow

TABLE 10-11 Zoonotic Internal Parasites

PARASITE	HOST	RESERVOIR	INFECTIVE STAGE	CONDITION
Toxocara spp.	Dogs, cats	Dogs, cats	Egg with L2	Visceral larva migrans
Ancylostoma spp.	Dogs, cats	Dogs, cats	L3	Cutaneous larva migrans
Uncinaria stenocephala	Dogs, cats	Dogs, cats	L3	Cutaneous larva migrans
Toxoplasma gondii	Cats	Cats, raw meat	Sporulated oocyst, bradyzoite, tachyzoite	Toxoplasmosis
Strongyloides stercoralis	Dogs, cats, people	People, dogs, cats	L3	Strongyloidiasis
Dipylidium caninum	Dogs, cats, people	Flea	Cysticercoid	Cestodiasis
Taenia saginata	People	Bovine muscle	Cysticercus	Cestodiasis
Taenia solium	People	Porcine muscle	Cysticercus	Cestodiasis
	People	People	Egg	Cysticercosis
Echinococcus granulosus	Dogs	Dogs	Egg	Hydatidosis
Echinococcus multilocularis	Dogs, cats	Dogs, cats	Egg	Hydatidosis
Spirometra mansonoides	Dogs, cats	Unknown	Procercoid in arthropod	Sparganosis
Sarcocystis spp.	People	Cattle, pigs	Sarcocyst in muscle	Sarcocystiasis
	Dogs, cats	Dogs, cats	Oocyst	Sarcosporidiosis
Cryptosporidium	Mammals	Mammals	Oocyst	Cryptosporidiosis
Balantidium coli	People, pigs	People, pigs	Cyst, trophozoite	Balantidiasis
Ascaris suum	Pigs	Pigs	Egg with L2	Visceral larva migrans
Trichinella spiralis	Mammals	Porcine and bear muscle	Encysted L3	Trichinellosis
Thelazia spp.	Mammals	Flies	L3	Verminous conjunctivitis
Giardia spp.	Mammals	Mammals	Cyst	Giardiasis
Babesia spp.	Rodents, people	Hard ticks	Sporozoite	Babesiosis
Trypanosoma	Mammals	Reduviids	Trypanosomal form in kissing bug	Chagas' disease

REVIEW QUESTIONS

True or False

Indicate whether each of the following statements is True or False.

____ 1. The organism that the parasite lives in or on is call its host.
____ 2. All protozoa are parasitic.
____ 3. Trematodes lack a body cavity.
____ 4. Nematodes are commonly called roundworms because of their cylindrical body shape.
____ 5. The thorax of insects may have one or two pairs of functional wings.
____ 6. Fleas demonstrate incomplete metamorphosis.
____ 7. Some adult flies glue their eggs to the hairs of the host.
____ 8. Ticks are arachnids.
____ 9. Most mite infestations are transmitted by indirect contact with an infested animal.
____10. Mites can be divided into two groups.
____11. Yellowish discoloration of feces can signify infection.
____12. Fecal direct smears are the most complicated of the evaluation process.
____13. Centrifugal flotation is more sensitive than simple flotation.
____14. The modified Knott's technique is a rapid method of microfilariae detection.
____15. Mite infestations are usually initially generalized.

Fill in the Blank

Provide the best answers to complete the following statements.

1. Normal stool should be ________ yet ________.
2. Trematodes pass through several different________ ________.
3. Most parasitic eggs have a specific gravity between ________ g/ml.
4. Some parasites produce ________ ________.
5. When herd studies are conducted individual samples are taken from at least ________.
6. Buffy coat smear is a concentration technique for detection of ________ and ________ in white blood cells.
7. Direct drop is the least accurate due to ________.
8. ELISA tests are highly accurate and precise and can detect ________ ________.
9. *Tritrichomonas foetus* is a ________ protozoan.
10. Fleas are laterally compressed ________ insects.
11. Flea larvae feed on ________ ________.
12. Phylum Arthropoda organisms are characterized by the presence of ________ ________.
13. Parasites residing on the surface of the host are called ________.
14. Trematodes are unsegmented and ________.
15. Cestode eggs contain a fully developed ________.

Matching

Match the terms with their description or definition.

____1. trematodes
____2. flagella
____3. undulatory ridges
____4. ectoparasite
____5. endoparasite
____6. commensalism
____7. mutualism
____8. parasitism
____9. cestodes
____10. scolex
____11. proglottids
____12. strobila
____13. gravid
____14. scutum
____15. *Demodex*
____16. sarcoptic mange
____17. *Cheyletiella*
____18. *Otodectes*
____19. *Oxyuris*
____20. microfilaria

A. segments
B. contains eggs
C. loss of hair and intense pruritus
D. pinworms
E. heartworm larvae
F. body
G. whiplike structure
H. organism that lives on another organism
I. both organisms benefit
J. head of a cestode
K. organism that lives in another organism
L. one organism benefits; the other is harmed
M. small snakelike waves that form in the cell membrane
N. flatworms that lack a body cavity
O. mite living in the external ear canal of dogs and cats
P. walking dandruff
Q. burrowing mite that lives in the hair follicles and sebaceous glands of the skin
R. hard chitinous covering
S. multicellular organisms that lack a body cavity
T. one organism benefits; the other is unaffected

RECOMMENDED READING

Bowman DD: *Georgi's parasitology for veterinarians*, ed 10, St Louis, 2013, Saunders.

Hendrix CM, Robinson E: *Diagnostic parasitology for veterinarians*, ed 4, St Louis, 2011, Mosby.

Sirois M: *Laboratory procedures for veterinary technicians*, ed 6, St Louis, 2014, Mosby.

Sloss MW, Kemp RL, Zajac AM: *Veterinary clinical parasitology*, ed 6, Ames, Iowa, 1994, Iowa State University Press.

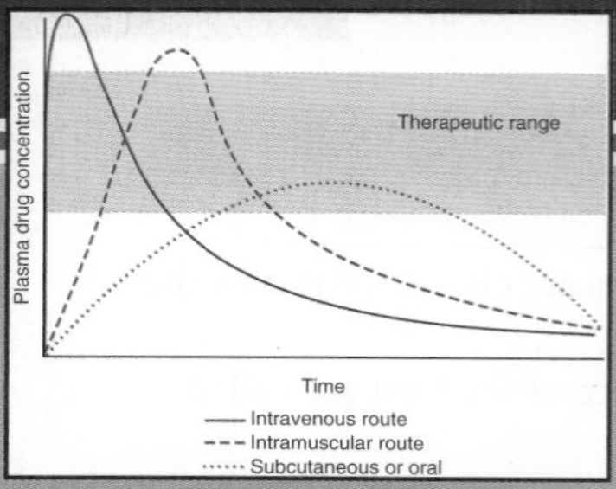

11 Pharmacology and Pharmacy

OUTLINE

LEARNING OBJECTIVES

After viewing this chapter, the reader will be able to:

1. List the various categories of drugs and their clinical uses.
2. Identify dosage forms in which drugs are available.
3. Calculate drug dosages.
4. List and compare routes by which various types of drugs are administered.
5. Describe ways in which drugs exert their effect and affect body tissue.
6. Explain procedures used to safely store and handle drugs.
7. List the primary drugs affecting various body systems.

KEY TERMS

Analgesics
Anthelmintic
Antibiotic
Anticonvulsants
Anti-inflammatory drugs
Antimicrobial
Antiseptics
Bactericidal
Bacteriostatic
Bronchodilator
Continuous rate infusion
Controlled substance
Corticosteroid
Disinfection
Decongestant
Diuretic
Dose
Elixir
Emetics
Enteric-coated tablet
Expectorants
Fungicidal
Neuroleptanalgesia
NSAIDs
Osmotic diuretic
Per os
Pharmacokinetics
Positive inotropic drugs
Prescription
Proprietary name
Residue
Ruminatorics
Sanitizer
Subcutaneous injection
Therapeutic range
Tincture
Vasodilator
Vermicide
Virucidal
Withdrawal time

DRUG NAMES

Drugs are generally referred to by three different names. Their chemical name, such as D-alpha-amino-p-hydroxy-benzyl-penicillin trihydrate, describes the drug's chemical composition. The nonproprietary name (sometimes called the generic name) is a more concise name given to the specific chemical compound. Examples of nonproprietary names are aspirin, acetaminophen, and amoxicillin. The **proprietary** or trade name is a unique drug name given by a manufacturer to its particular brand of drug. Examples of proprietary or trade names include Excedrin, Tylenol, and Amoxitabs. Because the trade name is a proper noun, it is capitalized and the superscript® is added to signify that the trade name is a registered trademark and cannot be legally used by other manufacturers. Because many drug manufacturers produce similar products, a single generic drug can be sold under multiple trade names. For example, the antibiotic amoxicillin is manufactured by several different companies, each of which has its own trade name for amoxicillin (e.g., Amoxi-Tabs, Robamox-V, Amoxil).

> TECHNICIAN NOTE Most drugs are referred to by the generic name in veterinary clinics.

When a drug company develops and patents a new drug (not just a new trade name for an old drug, but a new chemical), and obtains FDA approval to sell the new drug, the company has the exclusive rights to manufacture this drug for a number of years. During that time no other drug manufacturer can produce the same drug. This allows the drug company to recover, at the expense of the consumer, the costs of the research, development, and testing the company has invested to bring the drug to market. After these patent rights expire, other companies can legally produce the drug. These copycat drugs are called generic equivalents, because they have properties equivalent to those of the original compound. Generic equivalents are usually sold at a much lower price than the original manufacturer's product, because the generic manufacturer has not had to underwrite development of the original drug.

DOSAGE FORMS

Drugs are also described by their dosage form. The form of a drug is usually either solid, semisolid, or liquid (Table 11-1). Solid dosage forms include tablets, which are powdered drugs compressed into pills or disks; and capsules, which are powdered drugs enclosed within gelatin capsules. **Enteric-coated tablets** have a special covering that protects the drug from the harsh acidic environment of the stomach

TABLE 11-1 List of Dosage Forms

SOLID FORMS	SEMISOLID FORMS	LIQUID FORMS
Tablet	Suppositories	Syrup
Capsule	Liniment	Elixir
Enteric-coated tablet	Ointment	Tincture
Sustained release	Cream	Lotion
Implant	Paste	Injectable

and prevents dissolving of the tablet until it enters the intestine. Sustained-release forms of oral drugs release small amounts of the drug into the intestinal lumen over an extended time. Suppositories are inserted into the rectum, where they dissolve and release the drug to be absorbed across the membranes of the intestinal wall.

A solution is a drug dissolved in a liquid vehicle that does not settle out if left standing. In contrast, a suspension contains drug particles that are suspended, but not dissolved, in the liquid vehicle. These drug particles usually settle to the bottom of the container when the container is left standing, so one must shake it back into suspension before administration to ensure consistent dosing. Syrups, such as cough syrups, are solutions of drugs with water and sugar (e.g., 85% sucrose).

Elixirs are solutions of drugs dissolved in sweetened alcohol. Elixirs are used for drugs that do not readily dissolve in water. It is therefore important that you do not dilute an elixir with water, because the water will stratify into a layer separate from the elixir solution.

Tinctures are alcohol solutions meant for topical application (applied onto the skin). Topical products are available as liniments, which contain a drug in an oil base that are rubbed into the skin; or lotions, which are drug suspensions or solutions that are dabbed, brushed, or dripped onto the skin without rubbing (e.g., poison ivy medications).

Ointments, creams, and pastes are semisolid dosage forms that are applied to the skin (e.g., ointments, creams) or given orally (e.g., pastes). Ointments and creams are designed to liquefy at body temperatures, whereas pastes tend to keep their semisolid form at body temperature.

Injectable drugs are administered via a needle and syringe. Repository forms of injectable drugs are formulated to prolong absorption of the drug from the site of administration and thus provide a more sustained effective drug concentration in the body. Implants are solid dosage forms that are injected or inserted under the skin and dissolve or release a drug over an extended period.

PRESCRIPTIONS AND DISPENSING MEDICATION

WRITING PRESCRIPTIONS

A **prescription** is an order from a licensed veterinarian directing a pharmacist to prepare a drug for use in a client's animal. Drugs that do not require a prescription are referred to as over-the-counter (OTC). When writing prescriptions, veterinarians must adhere to the following guidelines:

- Veterinary prescription drugs must be used only by or on the order of a licensed veterinarian.
- A valid veterinarian/client/patient relationship must exist.
- Veterinary prescription drugs must meet proper requirements for labeling.
- Veterinary prescription drugs should be dispensed only in quantities necessary for the treatment of the animal(s). Unlimited refills are limited to lifelong treatments to decrease the potential of misuse of the drugs.

HOMETOWN VETERINARY ASSOCIATES
2000 West Chelsea Ave., Momack, PA
(324) 555-4313

Date: November 22, 2011

Patient: Cricket **Species:** Canine

Owner: Lee Ann Wozniak **Phone:** 555-0127

Address: 929 Christopher Robin Lane, Brookside, PA 13235

℞ Amoxicillin tablets 100mg #30 tabs
Sig: 1 tab q8h POPRN until gone

Robert L. Bill **D.V.M.**

FIGURE 11-1 Typical prescription for a veterinary drug.

- Appropriate records of all prescriptions issued must be maintained.
- Veterinary prescription drugs must be appropriately handled and stored for safety and security.

TECHNICIAN NOTE There must be a client/patient/veterinarian relationship for a veterinarian to prescribe medications.

COMPONENTS OF A PRESCRIPTION

A sample prescription is shown in Figure 11-1. Box 11-1 shows common abbreviations used in prescriptions and their meanings. Valid prescriptions must contain the following items:

- Name, address, and telephone number of the person who wrote the prescription
- Date on which the prescription was written
- Owner's name and address, animal's name, and species of animal
- Rx symbol (abbreviation of *recipe,* Latin for "take thou")
- Drug name, concentration, and number of units to be dispensed
- *Sig.* (abbreviation of *signa,* Latin for "write" or "label"), indicating directions for the client in treating the animal
- Signature of the person who wrote the prescription
- Drug Enforcement Administration (DEA) registration number if the drug is a controlled substance.

TECHNICIAN NOTE Always double check a prescription label that has been written or printed to make sure it is accurate.

CONTAINERS FOR DISPENSING MEDICATION

Many veterinary practices dispense tablets and capsules in plastic containers with a childproof lid. If medication is dispensed in a paper envelope and a child becomes poisoned,

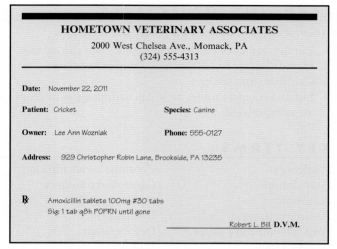

BOX 11-1 Abbreviations Commonly Used in Prescriptions

BID twice a day	**po** by mouth
cc cubic centimeter	**prn** as needed
disp dispense	**q** every
g gram	**q8h** every 8 hours
gm gram	**qd** every day
gr grain	**QID** four times daily
h hour	**QOD** every other day
lb pound	**SID** once a day
mg milligram	**stat** immediately
ml milliliter	**TID** three times daily
od right eye	**tsp** teaspoon
os left eye	

Note: SID is rarely used or recognized by pharmacists outside of the veterinary profession.

the veterinarian could be found negligent in dispensing the medication in a manner that placed the child at risk.

Liquids are dispensed either in individual syringes or a bottle. The bottle usually has a syringe or dropper to draw up the amount needed at each treatment.

CALCULATING DRUG DOSES

Calculating the dose of drug to be administered involves the following steps:

1. Weigh the animal and convert the weight in pounds to kilograms (if necessary).
2. Depending on how the drug is usually dosed (e.g., mg/kg, U/kg), use the animal's weight to calculate the correct dose (e.g., in mg, ml, units, g).
3. Based on the concentration of the drug (e.g., mg of drug/ml of solution or mg of drug/tablet), determine what volume or number of tablets to administer. Simple algebra helps calculate the amount (dose) of drug to be given (e.g., mg or ml), along with the animal's weight and the recommended drug dosage (e.g., mg/kg). You can also calculate the number of units to give (e.g., tablets or ml) if you know the amount of drug in each unit (e.g., mg/ml or mg/tablet) and the duration of treatment (days). Common metric conversion factors used in calculating drug doses are listed in Box 11-2.

Step 1. Set up an equation so that the units (e.g., kg, lb) are the same on the top (numerator) and bottom (denominator) on both sides of the equation. Then solve for *X* (e.g., kg of body weight). This is shown in Step 1 of Box 11-3.

Step 2. Once the animal's weight has been converted to the appropriate units (in this case, kg), determine the amount of drug (dose) to be given. On the left of the equation is the drug dosage (e.g., milligrams of drug/kilogram body weight), and the *X* you are solving for is the total drug dose (in milligrams). This is shown in Step 2 of Box 11-3.

Step 3. After the total dose is determined (in mg or some other measure), calculate the volume (e.g., ml) or number of solid units (tablets, capsules) to be administered using the concentration of drug in the solution (mg of drug/ml of solution) or in each solid unit (mg of drug/tablet), solving for ml of liquid or number of tablets. This is shown in Step 3 of Box 11-3.

When dispensing solid units (tablets, capsules), round to the nearest unit (or half or quarter tablet if the tablet is designed to be broken and greater accuracy is essential). The steps for calculating the total number of solid units required during a course of treatment are detailed in Box 11-4. Always check the rounded dosage with the veterinarian as some drugs have a very narrow margin of safety and may need to be rounded *down* versus up.

BOX 11-2 Metric Conversion Factors

1 kg = 1000 g = 100,000 milligrams (mg)
1 kg = 2.2 lb
1 gram = 1 gm = 1000 mg = 0.001 kg
1 gram = 1 g = 15.43 grains (gr)
1 grain = 64.8 milligrams (usually rounded to 60 or 65 mg)
1 lb = 0.454 kg = 16 ounces (oz)
1 mg = 0.001 g = 1000 micrograms (μg or mcg)
1 liter (L) = 1000 ml = 10 deciliters (dl)
1 ml = 1 cc = 1000 microliters (μl or mcl)
1 tablespoon (tbsp) = 3 teaspoons (tsp)
1 tsp = 5 ml
1 gallon (gal) = 3.786 L
1 gal = 4 quarts (1qt) 8 pints (pt) = 128 fluid ounces (fl oz)
1 pt = 2 cups (c) = 16 fl oz = 473 ml

BOX 11-3 Simple Algebraic Calculation Used to Calculate a Drug Dose

What volume of a drug solution should we give to a 44-lb dog if the recommended dosage is 5 mg/kg and the concentration of the solution is 50 mg/ml?

Step 1: Convert pounds to kilograms.

$$X\text{ kg} = 44\text{ lb} \times \frac{1\text{ kg}}{2.2\text{ lb}} = \frac{44}{2.2} = 20\text{ kg}$$

Step 2: Calculate the total drug dose.

$$X\text{ mg} = \frac{5\text{ mg}}{\text{kg}} \times 20\text{ kg} = 5 \times 20 = 100\text{ mg}$$

Step 3: Calculate the volume of solution needed.

$$\frac{50\text{ mg}}{\text{ml}} = \frac{100\text{ mg}}{X\text{ ml}} = \frac{100\text{ mg}}{50\text{ mg/ml}} = 2\text{ ml}$$

EXAMPLES

1. A 55-lb canine is prescribed amoxicillin twice a day for 7 days. Normal dosing is 10 mg/lb and the tablets come in 50 mg, 100 mg, 250 mg, and 500 mg. What is the prescribed dose, and which concentration of tablet should be prescribed?
   a. 10 mg/lb × 50 lb = 500 mg is the dose and therefore 500 mg tablets should be prescribed. The prescription would then be (1) 500 mg tablet orally every 12 hours for 7 days, a total of 14 tablets.

BOX 11-4 Calculating the Number of Tablets to Dispense

How many 25-mg tablets should we dispense for a 10-lb cat if the recommended dosage is 5 mg/lb twice daily for 7 days?

Step 1: Calculate the number of tablets needed per dose.

$$10 \text{ lb} \times \frac{5 \text{ mg}}{\text{lb}} = 50 \text{ mg per dose}$$

$$50 \text{ mg} \times \frac{1 \text{ tablet}}{25 \text{ mg}} = 2 \text{ tablets per dose}$$

Step 2: Calculate the number of tablets needed daily.
2 tablet per dose × twice daily = 4 tablets daily

Step 3: Calculate the number of tablets needed for 7 days.
4 tablets daily × 7 days = 28 tablets

2. A 14-lb feline is prescribed furosemide at 2 mg/kg. This medication comes in the following tablet forms: 12.5 mg, 50 mg. What is the prescribed dose and which tablet should he get?
   a. 14 lb ÷ 2.2 kg/lb = 6.36 kg
   b. 2 mg/kg × 6.36 kg = 12.7 mg dosage
   c. The 12.5 mg tablets should be prescribed.
3. A 25-lb canine is prescribed doxycycline at 10 mg/kg. The owners have requested liquid, not pill, form. The doxycycline comes in 5 mg/ml liquid dosing.
   a. 25 lb ÷ 2.2 kg/lb = 11.3 kg
   b. 10 mg/kg × 11.3 kg = 113 mg dosage
   c. The liquid is 5 mg/ml so 113 mg ÷ 5 mg/ml = 22.7 ml of liquid at each dosing.
4. The vet asks you to give a 985-lb equine an injection of banamine at 1.1 mg/kg. Banamine comes in 50 mg/ml concentration for injection. How much will you be giving?
   a. 985 lbs ÷ 2.2 kg/lb = 447.7 kg
   b. 1.1 mg/kg × 447.7 kg = 492.5 mg
   c. 492 mg ÷ 50 mg/ml = 9.85 ml of banamine

TECHNICIAN NOTE Become familiar with the medications commonly used in practice so you will have a general idea of the amount that should be given, and you can catch a mistake in figuring out the dosage if you make one.

STORING AND HANDLING DRUGS IN THE PHARMACY

Drugs that are improperly stored (e.g., exposed to extreme temperature or light) can degenerate or become inactivated, providing little or no benefit to the animal in which they are used. Drugs still on the pharmacy shelf after the listed expiration date on the container may be less effective. In some cases, such as with tetracycline, these expired drugs can become hazardous to the animal. Store drugs at their optimum temperature to prevent damage. Temperatures used for drug storage, according to label specifications, are found in Table 11-2.

TABLE 11-2 Drug Storage Temperatures

Cold	not exceeding 8° C (46° F)
Cool	8 to 15° C (46 to 59° F)
Room Temperature	16 to 30° C (60 to 86° F)
Warm	31 to 40° C (87 to 104° F)
Excessive Heat	greater than 40° C (104° F)

Drugs that are sensitive to light are usually kept in a dark amber container. Tablets and powders tend to be sensitive to moisture, and their containers usually contain silica packets to absorb moisture. Some drugs are destroyed by physical stress, such as vibrations. Insulin is one such drug that can be inactivated by violent shaking of the vial.

TECHNICIAN NOTE Make sure drugs are stored properly to ensure their effectiveness.

STORING AND PRESCRIBING CONTROLLED SUBSTANCES

A **controlled substance** is defined by law as a substance with potential for physical addiction, psychological addiction, and/or abuse. Controlled drugs are sometimes called schedule drugs. Controlled substances must be stored securely under lock and key to prevent access by unauthorized personnel. By law, a written record must be kept describing when, for what purpose, and how much of the controlled drug was used. These records must include receipts for purchase or sale of controlled substances and must be maintained for 2 years.

Drug manufacturers and distributors are required to identify a controlled substance on its label with a capital *C*, followed by a Roman numeral, which denotes the drug's theoretical potential for abuse.

C-I denotes extreme potential for abuse with no approved medicinal purpose in the United States. These include such drugs as heroin, LSD, and marijuana (marijuana does have some controversy as being in this classification but as of publication has not been changed to a different class).

C-II denotes a high potential for abuse. Use may lead to severe physical or psychological dependence. These include such drugs as opium, pentobarbital, and morphine.

C-III denotes some potential for abuse but less than for C-II drugs. Use may lead to low to moderate physical dependence or high psychological dependence. These include such drugs as ketamine, buprenorphine, and anabolic steroids.

C-IV denotes low potential for abuse. Use may lead to limited physical psychological dependence, including such drugs as phenobarbital and diazepam (Valium).

C-V also denotes low potential for abuse, but these drugs are subject to state and local regulation (e.g., Robitussin AC, which contains small amounts of codeine).

For veterinarians to legally use, prescribe, or buy a controlled substance from an approved manufacturer or distributor, they must have obtained a certification number from

TABLE 11-3 Commonly Used Controlled Substances in Veterinary Medicine and Their Classifications

CLASSIFICATION OF CONTROLLED SUBSTANCE	EXAMPLES OF COMMONLY USED DRUGS
C- I	None used in veterinary medicine
C- II	Pentobarbital, Morphine, Hydromorphone, Fentanyl, Oxymorphone
C-III	Ketamine, Buprenorphine, Telazol, Hydrocodone, Testosterone
C-IV	Phenobarbital, Diazepam, Butorphanol
C-V	Tussigon, Codeine products

the DEA. This DEA certification number must be included on all prescriptions or any order forms for schedule (controlled) drugs. Even with a valid DEA number, veterinarians cannot prescribe Schedule I (C-I) drugs.

Prescriptions for Schedule II (C-II) drugs, which have the most potential for abuse, must be in written form (many states have special forms for C-II drug prescriptions) and cannot be telephoned to a pharmacist. In the event of an emergency, when the prescription must be ordered by telephone, the verbal prescription must be followed by a written order within 72 hours. Schedule II drug prescriptions may not be refilled; a new prescription must be written for each treatment period. Table 11-3 lists some commonly used controlled substances in veterinary medicine and their classifications.

HANDLING TOXIC DRUGS

Veterinary professionals may be exposed to toxic drugs in various ways, including the following:

- Absorption through the skin via spillage from a syringe or vial, or other contact
- Inhalation of aerosolized drug as a needle is withdrawn from a vial that is pressurized by injection of air to facilitate removal of the drug
- Ingestion of food contaminated with drug via aerosolization or direct contact
- Inhalation resulting from crushing or breaking of tablets and subsequent aerosolization of drug powder
- Absorption or inhalation during opening of glass ampules containing antineoplastic agents

The best way to avoid exposure is to educate all involved personnel about safe handling and storage of these drugs. Training may be in-house or formal. Such safety training should be periodically repeated to emphasize the importance of handling precautions and as a refresher for staff members.

THERAPEUTIC RANGE

The concentration of a drug in the body must be such that the detrimental effects are minimized and benefits are maximized. This ideal range of drug concentration is referred to as the **therapeutic range.** If an excessive dose results in accumulation of too much drug in the body, drug concentrations are said to be toxic, and signs of toxicity develop. If a small drug dose does not produce drug concentrations within the therapeutic range, drug concentrations are said to be at subtherapeutic levels, and the drug's beneficial effect is not achieved.

DOSAGE REGIMEN

There are three components of therapeutic administration of drugs: the dose, the dosage interval, and the route of administration. Altering any of these components can result in drug concentrations that are too high or too low.

A drug's **dose** is the amount of drug administered at one time. For accuracy and clarity in communicating with pharmacists or other veterinary professionals, always state the dose in units of mass (e.g., mg, g, gr). Do not state the dose in number of product units (e.g., tablets or capsules) or volume (ml, L), because manufacturers may produce the same drug in solid dosage forms of various sizes or solutions with various concentrations. For example, writing in an animal's record that the animal received "1 tablet of amoxicillin" is of no value because amoxicillin is available in tablet sizes ranging from 50 mg up to 500 mg. The same is true if you state, "Give 3 ml of xylazine," because 3 ml of a xylazine solution with a concentration of 20 mg/ml contains much less xylazine than 3 ml of a solution with a concentration of 100 mg/ml.

The time between administrations of separate drug doses is referred to as the dosage interval. Dosage intervals are often expressed with the Latin abbreviations shown in Box 11-1.

The dose and the dosage interval together are often referred to as the dosage regimen. The total amount of drug delivered to the animal in 24 hours is determined by multiplying the dose by the frequency of administration (e.g., 100 mg given 4 times daily results in a total daily dose of 400 mg).

> *TECHNICIAN NOTE* Always make sure you record the actual concentration amount of a drug given because most drugs come in multiple concentrations.

ROUTES OF ADMINISTRATION

The amount of a drug that reaches the target tissues in the body can be significantly altered if the proper route of administration is not used. The route of administration is how the drug enters the body. Drugs given by injection are said to be parenterally administered. Drugs given by mouth, or **per os** (PO), are said to be orally administered. If a drug is applied to the surface of the skin, as with lotions and liniments, it is said to be topically administered.

Parenteral administration of drugs is further broken down into specific routes. Intravenous (IV) administration involves injecting the drug directly into a vein. Intravenous injections can be given as a single volume at one time, called a bolus, or they can be slowly injected or dripped into a vein over several seconds, minutes, or even hours as an intravenous infusion. Drugs that are given over long periods of time ranging from hours to days are termed as being given

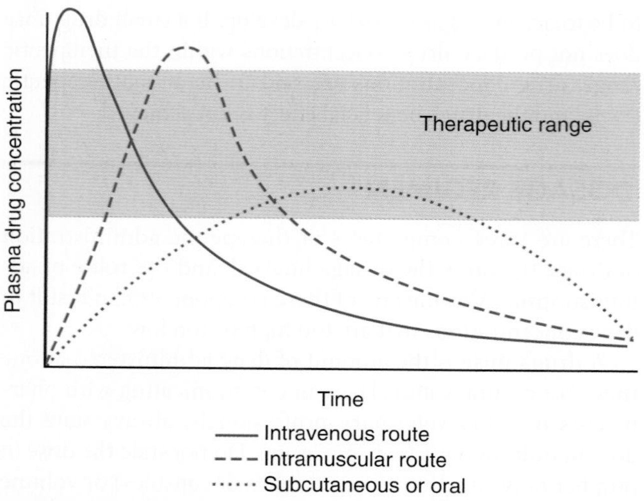

FIGURE 11-2 Plasma drug concentrations attained after intravenous, intramuscular, subcutaneous, and oral administration.

by **continuous rate infusion** (CRI). The differences in drug concentrations achieved by various routes of administration are shown in Figure 11-2.

Note that intravenous injection is not the same as intra-arterial injection. Drugs given by intraarterial injection are injected into an artery (not a vein), quickly producing high concentrations of drug in tissues supplied by that artery. After intravenous injection, blood containing the drug passes to the heart and is mixed and diluted with the remaining blood in circulation before it is delivered to body tissues. Inadvertent injection of drugs intraarterially (e.g., injection into the carotid artery instead of the jugular vein) delivers a bolus of a drug directly to tissues. These accidental intraarterial injections can produce severe effects, such as seizures or respiratory arrest. Injection of a drug outside of the blood vessel (not within the vessel lumen) is an extravascular or perivascular injection.

Some drugs cause extreme local inflammation and tissue death if accidentally injected extravascularly. Intramuscular (IM) administration involves injecting the drug into a muscle mass. **Subcutaneous injections** are administered deep to (beneath) the skin, into the subcutis. Intradermal (ID) injections are administered within (not beneath) the skin with very small needles. The intradermal route is usually reserved for skin-testing procedures, such as testing for tuberculosis or reaction to allergenic substances. Intraperitoneal (IP) injections are administered into the abdominal body cavity and may be used when IV or IM injections are not practical (as in some laboratory animals), or large volumes of solution must be administered for rapid absorption.

MOVEMENT OF DRUG MOLECULES IN THE BODY

Pharmacokinetics describes how drugs move into, through, and out of the body. Knowledge of a drug's pharmacokinetics facilitates understanding of why the drug must be given by different routes or dosage regimens to achieve therapeutic success under different clinical circumstances. Pharmacokinetics involves absorption, distribution, metabolism, and elimination.

Movement of drug molecules from the site of administration into the systemic circulation is called absorption. After a drug has been ingested, injected, inhaled, or applied to the skin, it must be absorbed into the blood and travel to the body areas where it will have its intended effect (target tissues). IV injections almost instantaneously achieve their peak concentration (highest level) in the blood (Fig. 11-2). Drugs given by IM administration take some time to diffuse from the injection site in the muscle, into the systemic circulation. Drugs given by PO administration and SC injection take longer to be absorbed because they must diffuse farther to reach the systemic circulation (SC injection) or they must pass through several barriers to be absorbed (PO administration). Drugs given IM, SC, or PO attain therapeutic concentrations more slowly than drugs given IV.

Distribution describes movement of a drug from the systemic circulation into tissues. Drugs generally are distributed most rapidly and in greater concentrations to well-perfused (rich blood supply) tissues. Examples of well-perfused tissues include active skeletal muscle, the liver, kidney, and brain. In contrast, inactive skeletal muscle and adipose (fat) tissue are relatively poorly perfused, so it takes more time for drugs to be delivered to these tissues. Some drugs bind to proteins in the blood; these protein-bound drug molecules are unable to leave the systemic circulation and so are not distributed to tissues. Thus a significant portion of a highly protein-bound drug remains in systemic circulation, where these protein-bound drug molecules act as a "reservoir" of additional drug.

Many drugs are altered by the body before being eliminated. This process is referred to as biotransformation, or drug metabolism. The altered drug molecule is referred to as a metabolite. The liver is the primary organ involved in drug metabolism, or biotransformation. However, other tissues, such as the lung, skin, and intestinal tract, may also biotransform drug molecules. The product of biotransformation (metabolite) is usually readily eliminated by the kidney or liver. Removal of a drug from the body is called drug elimination or excretion. The two major routes of elimination are via the kidney (into the urine) and via the liver (into the bile and subsequently into the feces). Inhalant anesthetics and other volatile agents are mostly eliminated via the lungs, although some inhalant anesthetics (methoxyflurane and halothane) have some hepatic biotransformation and renal excretion. Drug elimination is greatly affected by dehydration; kidney, liver, or heart disease; age; and a variety of other physiologic and pathologic (disease) conditions.

By law, all drugs approved for use in food animals have mandated withdrawal times. The **withdrawal time** is the period after drug administration during which the animal cannot be sent to market for slaughter, and the eggs or milk must be discarded.

HOW DRUGS EXERT THEIR EFFECT

For cells to respond to a drug molecule, usually the drug must combine with a specific protein molecule on or in the cell, called a receptor. A given receptor combines only with the molecule of certain drugs, based on their shape or molecular makeup.

This concept is illustrated by a key and lock, in which the drug is the key and the receptor is the lock into which only the correct key will fit (produce an effect). The effect of the correct drug molecule-receptor combination is some cellular change, such as causing the cell to secrete substances, muscle cells to contract, or neuronal cells to depolarize (fire). Cells do not have receptors for all drugs; only certain cells respond to certain drugs.

DRUGS AFFECTING THE GASTROINTESTINAL TRACT

Drugs or functions related to the stomach are called gastric, as in gastric ulcers, gastric blood flow, or gastric emptying. Drugs or functions related to the duodenum, jejunum, or ileum are usually referred to as enteric. Drugs and functions related to the colon are termed colonic.

> TECHNICIAN NOTE Gastric, enteric, and colonic all refer to the GI tract.

EMETICS

Emetics are drugs that induce vomiting (Box 11-5). The complex process of emesis is controlled by a group of neurons in the medulla of the brain stem, known as the vomiting center. Emetics are most often used to induce vomiting in animals that have ingested toxic substances. They should not be used in all cases of poisoning, however, because the risk of aspiration (inhalation) of stomach contents into the lungs may outweigh the benefit of induced vomiting. Also, vomiting should not be induced if a corrosive substance or volatile liquid was ingested.

Apomorphine quickly causes emesis in dogs when given by IV or IM injection, or when an apomorphine tablet is placed in the conjunctival sac of the eye. Apomorphine is a less effective emetic in cats. An effective emetic for cats is the sedative xylazine (Rompun, Anased, and others), which produces emesis within minutes of injection.

Hydromorphone is not commonly used to induce vomiting but does have that side effect so it has been used. The main side effect of using this medication is significant sedation and possible bradycardia, which in most cases are not desirable when trying to induce vomiting.

Syrup of ipecac was formerly used as an emetic but had fallen out of favor because of the lag time before vomiting was produced (10 to 30 minutes) and potential for overdosing. The global manufacture of this drug ended in 2010. Other local emetics include hydrogen peroxide; a warm, concentrated solution of salt and water; and a solution of powdered mustard and water. These emetics do not work consistently.

BOX 11-5 Commonly Used Emetics

Apomorphine
Xylazine
Hydrogen peroxide

BOX 11-6 Commonly Used Antiemetics

Chlorpromazine
Maropitant citrate (Cerenia)
Metoclopramide (Reglan)
Cisapride (Propulsid)
Ondansetron (Zofran)

ANTIEMETICS

Antiemetics are drugs that prevent or decrease vomiting (Box 11-6). Antiemetics should only be used when the vomiting reflex is no longer of benefit to the animal. Phenothiazine tranquilizers, such as acepromazine (PromAce), chlorpromazine (Thorazine), and prochlorperazine (Compazine, Darbazine), are commonly used to combat vomiting caused by motion sickness. Maropitant citrate (Cerenia), a neurokinin receptor antagonist, was approved for use in 2008 to help with acute vomiting and vomiting caused by motion sickness. This drug works to block the pharmacological action of substance P in the CNS.

Atropine, aminopentamide (Centrine), and isopropamide (combined with prochlorperazine in Darbazine) are anticholinergic drugs that prevent vomiting by blocking the impulses traveling to the CNS via the vagus nerve and the motor impulses traveling via the vagus nerve to the muscles involved with the vomiting reflex. These drugs are used less commonly because of the availability of other more locally effective drugs.

Metoclopramide (Reglan) is a centrally acting antiemetic that also has local antiemetic activity. Metoclopramide has been useful in helping animals that vomit because of slowed gut motility. Cisapride (Propulsid) has been used to reduce regurgitation in dogs with megaesophagus (dilated esophagus) and in cats with chronic constipation or cats that frequently vomit hairballs.

Ondansetron (Zofran) is a selective serotonin reuptake inhibitor (also known as a 5-HT3 receptor antagonist). It is unclear as to whether it acts centrally, peripherally, or both because the 5-HT3 receptors for serotonin are located peripherally (the vagus nerve) and centrally (the chemoreceptor trigger zone in the brain). Ondansetron is used when other more widely used antiemetics are not effective because of the expense and the limited experience in veterinary medicine. The antihistamines meclizine (Bonine, nondrowsy Dramamine, other), dimenhydrinate (Dramamine) and diphenhydramine (Benadryl)

BOX 11-7 Commonly Used Antidiarrheals

Diphenoxylate (Lomotil)
Loperamide (Imodium)
Bismuth subsalicylate (Pepto-Bismol)

BOX 11-8 Commonly Used GI Adsorbents/Protectants

Activated charcoal (Toxiban)
Kaolin pectate (Kaopectate)

are also used occasionally for prevention of motion sickness, although these are not FDA approved for use in animals.

ANTIDIARRHEALS

Antidiarrheals are drugs used to combat various types of diarrhea (Box 11-7). Narcotics commonly used to combat diarrhea include diphenoxylate (Lomotil), paregoric (tincture of opium), and loperamide (Imodium). A disadvantage of narcotics when used as antidiarrheals is that their analgesic effect can mask pain that otherwise could be used to monitor progression or resolution of disease. Another disadvantage is that narcotics can cause excitement in cats ("morphine mania").

The anticholinergics atropine, propantheline bromide, isopropamide (Darbazine), and aminopentamide (Centrine) are used as antispasmodics because they decrease spastic colonic contractions and combat diarrhea associated with these contractions. These drugs are not particularly effective for most small-bowel diarrhea.

Bismuth subsalicylate, the active ingredient in Pepto-Bismol, breaks down in the gut to bismuth carbonate and salicylate. The bismuth tends to coat the intestinal mucosa, perhaps protecting it from enterotoxins, and seems to have some antibacterial activity. The major antisecretory effect, however, is probably from the salicylate (an aspirin-like compound), which decreases inflammation and blocks formation of prostaglandins that would normally stimulate fluid secretion.

ADSORBENTS AND PROTECTANTS

Locally irritating substances, such as bacterial endotoxins, can produce acute diarrhea. Any drug that prevents these agents from contacting the intestinal mucosa could theoretically reduce the diarrheal response. That is the underlying principle of adsorbents and protectants. An adsorbent causes another substance to adhere to its outer surface, thus reducing contact of that substance with the intestinal tract wall (Box 11-8).

Activated charcoal adsorbs enterotoxins to its surface, preventing them from contacting the bowel wall. The charcoal and the adsorbed enterotoxin then pass out in the feces. Activated charcoal comes with or without a sorbitol additive, which is a cathartic. The cathartic helps to eliminate the charcoal from the body before it releases the toxin it was bound to. Sorbitol additives should not be used in very dehydrated animals or animals with severe diarrhea already. Kaolin and pectin (Kaopectate) are often used together for symptomatic relief of vomiting or diarrhea. The kaolin-pectin combination is thought to adsorb enterotoxins. It is questionable as to whether kaolin-pectin has any significant effect in controlling diarrhea in veterinary patients.

BOX 11-9 Commonly Used Laxatives, Lubricants, and Stool Softeners

Indigestible fiber (bran, Metamucil)
Metamucil
Phosphate salts (Fleet enema)
Psyllium
Mineral oil
Glycerin
Docusate sodium succinate (Colace)
Lactulose

LAXATIVES, LUBRICANTS, AND STOOL SOFTENERS

Laxatives, cathartics, and purgatives facilitate evacuation of the bowels. Laxatives are considered the most gentle of this class of drugs, whereas cathartics are more marked in their evacuating effect, and purgatives are quite potent in their actions. Irritant laxatives, including castor oil and phenolphthalein, work by irritating the bowel, resulting in increased peristaltic motility (Box 11-9).

Bulk laxatives are much gentler than irritant laxatives. These drugs osmotically pull water into the bowel lumen or retain water in the feces. Hydrophilic colloids or indigestible fiber (bran, methylcellulose, Metamucil) are not digested or adsorbed to any degree and therefore create an osmotic force to produce their laxative effect. Psyllium is a hydrophilic compound that has gained popularity for its supposed health benefits. Hypertonic salts, such as magnesium (Milk of Magnesia, Epsom salts) and phosphate salts (Fleet enema), are poorly absorbed and create a strong osmotic force to attract water into the bowel lumen.

Lubricants (mineral oil, cod liver oil, white petrolatum, glycerin) are given to make the stool more "slippery" for easy passage through the bowel. Mineral oil is most commonly used for horses with impactions and is administered by stomach tube. The greatest danger associated with use of this oil is aspiration into the lungs, with subsequent pneumonia. Glycerin is most commonly used as a suppository.

Docusate sodium succinate (Colace) is a stool softener that acts as a "wetting agent" by reducing the surface tension of feces and allowing water to penetrate the dry stool. Docusate sodium succinate and related calcium and phosphate compounds may also stimulate colonic secretions, resulting in increased fluid content of feces.

Lactulose is another laxative that increases osmotic pressure by drawing water into the colon and making fecal material contain more liquid. It has an acidifying aspect as well that is used in treatment of hepatic encephalopathy as it traps

BOX 11-10 Commonly Used Antacids

OTC products (Tums, Rolaids)
Aluminum products (Amphojel)
Magnesium and aluminum (Maalox)
Ranitidine (Zantac)
Famotidine (Pepcid)

ammonia in the form of ammonium. It is used most commonly in small animals with chronic constipation problems. The most common danger with the use of Lactulose is excessive fluid loss leading to dehydration. Fluids may be warranted with initial use.

ANTACIDS

Antacids reduce acidity of the stomach or rumen (Box 11-10). Nonsystemic antacids, in liquid or tablet form, are composed of calcium, magnesium, or aluminum, and they directly neutralize acid molecules in the stomach or rumen. Such over-the-counter (OTC) products as Tums and Rolaids are nonsystemic antacids made primarily of calcium. Other nonsystemic antacids include magnesium products (Riopan, Carmilax), aluminum products (Amphojel), and combinations of magnesium and aluminum products (Maalox).

Systemic antacids decrease acid production in the stomach. Systemic antacids include cimetidine (Tagamet), ranitidine (Zantac), and famotidine (Pepcid).

ANTIULCER DRUGS

Sucralfate (Carafate) is an antiulcer drug used to treat ulcers of the stomach and upper small intestine. The drug has been called a "gastric Band-Aid" because it forms a sticky paste and adheres to the ulcer site, protecting it from the acidic environment of the stomach. Omeprazole (Gastrogard, Prilosec OTC, others) is a gastric acid pump inhibitor that binds irreversibly to the secretory surface of cells in the stomach. It therefore decreases acid secretion (antacid) and helps to support the stomach lining (antiulcer). Misoprostol (Cytotec) is a synthetic prostaglandin that helps decrease acid secretion in the stomach and increases production of the stomach lining (mucosa). Misoprostol is mostly used to combat insults to the stomach caused by nonsteroidal anti-inflammatory agents. It only comes in 100 mcg and 200 mcg tablets, making it difficult to use in very small animals (Box 11-11).

APPETITE STIMULANT DRUGS

Cyproheptadine is a serotonin antagonist antihistamine that is mostly used as an appetite stimulant for cats. Diazepam (Valium), a benzodiazepine, can also be used as an appetite stimulant but again only in cats. Neither drug works in other species (Box 11-12).

RUMINATORICS AND ANTIBLOAT MEDICATIONS

Ruminatorics, such as neostigmine (Stiglyn), are drugs used to stimulate an atonic ("limp") rumen. Antibloat medications

BOX 11-11 Commonly Used Antiulcer Drugs

Sucralfate (Carafate)
Omeprazole (Gastrogard, Prilosec OTC, others)
Misoprostol (Cytotec)

BOX 11-12 Commonly Used Appetite Stimulants

Cyproheptadine
Diazepam (Valium)

BOX 11-13 Commonly Used Ruminatorics and Antibloat Medications

Neostigmine (Stiglyn)
Mineral oil
Dioctyl sodium succinate (DSS)

act by reducing numbers of gas-producing rumen microorganisms or by breaking up the bubbles formed in the rumen with frothy bloat (Box 11-13). Mineral oil or ordinary household detergents mixed with mineral oil are often used to decrease the viscosity of the rumen contents, decrease the stability of the bubbles, and remove the froth. Some commercial antibloat preparations contain poloxalene. Dioctyl sodium succinate (DSS) also reduces the viscosity of rumen contents, allowing the foam to dissipate.

DRUGS AFFECTING THE CARDIOVASCULAR SYSTEM

ANTIARRHYTHMIC DRUGS

An arrhythmia is any abnormal pattern of electrical activity in the heart. Arrhythmias are divided into two general groups: arrhythmias that result in an increased heart rate (tachycardia) and those that cause a decreased heart rate (bradycardia). Once the type of arrhythmia has been determined, an effective antiarrhythmic drug (Box 11-14) is used to re-establish a normal conduction sequence (sinus rhythm).

Lidocaine, mexiletine, quinidine, and procainamide reverse arrhythmias primarily by decreasing the rate of movement of sodium into heart cells. Lidocaine, which is also used as a local anesthetic under the name of Xylocaine, is only available in injectable form. Veterinary technicians must realize that lidocaine is packaged in vials with or without epinephrine. Lidocaine with epinephrine is designed for use as a local anesthetic, not as an antiarrhythmic drug. Accidental IV injection of lidocaine containing epinephrine in an animal with an arrhythmia could cause death. For this reason, it is important to always check the lidocaine bottle before use in treating arrhythmias to be sure it does not contain epinephrine.

BOX 11-14 Commonly Used Antiarrhythmic Drugs

Lidocaine
Quinidine
Propanolol
Atenolol
Verapamil
Diltiazem
Amlodipine (hypertension)

Procainamide and quinidine have been used for supraventricular arrhythmias in horses, but they are not very effective against atrial fibrillation in dogs or cats. Hence they are more commonly used for their ventricular antiarrhythmic effects. Because quinidine and procainamide are available in oral forms, they are used for long-term maintenance of patients with ventricular arrhythmias.

When stimulated by the sympathetic nervous system or by sympathomimetic drugs (drugs that mimic the effects of the sympathetic nervous system), beta-1 receptors in the heart cause the heart to beat more rapidly and with greater strength. Such beta-1 stimulation can produce arrhythmias. Drugs that block beta receptors are known as beta-blockers. Beta-blockers cause the heart to contract with less force. Propranolol (Inderal) blocks stimulation of beta-1 receptors by epinephrine, norepinephrine, and other beta-stimulating drugs. It decreases the heart rate and prevents tachycardia in response to stress, fear, or excitement. Atenolol (Tenormin) and metoprolol (Lopressor) act similarly to propranolol, but at high doses the beta-1 receptor activity may be lost, causing beta-2 blockade. Atenolol and metoprolol are preferred in animals with asthma.

Calcium channel blockers include verapamil and diltiazem. Although calcium channel blockers are not commonly used to treat arrhythmias in veterinary patients, verapamil and diltiazem have been used successfully for treatment of supraventricular tachycardia, atrial fibrillation, and atrial flutter. A more common use of diltiazem is in cats with hypertrophic cardiomyopathy, in which the heart becomes very thickened and enlarged to the point where it cannot contract very efficiently. These drugs combat arrhythmias by blocking calcium channels of cardiac muscle cells, resulting in decreased conduction of depolarization waves and decreased automaticity of parts of the conduction system.

Another calcium channel blocker most commonly used for hypertension in small animals is amlodipine. It acts by dilating the peripheral arteries and thereby reducing afterload. It is eliminated quickly from the system, and hypertension can return rapidly if any doses are missed.

POSITIVE INOTROPIC AGENTS

Drugs that increase the strength of contraction of a weakened heart are referred to as **positive inotropic drugs** (positive inotropes) (Box 11-15). Digoxin is the drug of choice for maintaining long-term positive inotropic effects. Digoxin exerts its positive inotropic effect primarily by making more calcium available for the contractile elements within cardiac muscle cells. Digoxin, available as tablets and an elixir, is often used to control supraventricular tachycardia caused by atrial fibrillation. Digoxin has a small therapeutic index, meaning that therapeutic concentrations are very close to toxic concentrations. Early signs of digoxin toxicity include anorexia, vomiting, and diarrhea. Owners of animals receiving digoxin should be instructed to watch for these early signs of toxicity and to contact the veterinarian immediately if they should occur.

BOX 11-15 Commonly Used Inotropic Agents

Digoxin
Pimobendan

BOX 11-16 Commonly Used Vasodilators

Hydralazine
Nitroglycerin
Pimobendan (see inotropic drugs)
Enalapril (Enacard)
Benazepril

Pimobendan is an inodilator as it has both inotropic and vasodilator effects. This drug is used in conjunction with other medications in dogs to treat congestive heart failure secondary to dilated cardiomyopathy or chronic mitral valve insufficiency.

Dobutamine is also an inotropic agent that is used mostly commonly for short-term management of heart failure and in shock patients when fluid therapy alone is not working. It is used only as a CRI because of its limited availability and quick metabolization by the system. This drug is most commonly used in the ICU setting.

VASODILATORS

Vasoconstriction of peripheral blood vessels is a normal physiologic response to the drop in blood pressure caused by congestive heart failure, hemorrhage, and dehydration. **Vasodilators** open (dilate) constricted vessels, making it easier for the heart to pump blood through these vessels (Box 11-16).

Hydralazine is a vasodilator that causes arteriolar smooth muscle to relax, which benefits animals with a poorly functioning left atrioventricular (mitral) valve (mitral insufficiency). Hydralazine allows more blood to flow into the aorta and less to flow back into the left atrium. Although the valve itself remains poorly functional, blood flow through the left heart is improved.

Nitroglycerin relaxes the blood vessels on the venous side of the circulation; it may also help dilate coronary arterioles. The drug is well absorbed through the skin and mucous membranes. In animals, nitroglycerin cream and nitroglycerin in patch form are applied to the skin to improve cardiac output and reduce pulmonary edema and ascites (abdominal fluid accumulation). Nitroglycerin cream is applied every 4 to 6 hours to the hairless inner aspect of the pinna, thorax, or

BOX 11-17 Commonly Used Diuretics

Furosemide (Lasix)
Spironolactone
Mannitol

groin. A nitroglycerin patch provides drug diffusion for 24 hours and can be cut into small pieces to adjust the dose for smaller patients.

Nitroprusside acts much like nitroglycerin but is usually found only in the ICU setting because of the necessity to constantly monitor blood pressure and the need to give the drug as a CRI.

Other vasodilators are enalapril (Enacard), captopril, and benazepril, which block angiotensin-converting enzyme and prevent formation of angiotensin II (potent vasoconstrictor) and aldosterone. For this reason, they are sometimes referred to as angiotensin-converting enzyme (ACE) inhibitors. Enalapril, captopril, and benazepril are "balanced" vasodilators that relax the smooth muscles of both arterioles and veins, so they are useful in treating animals with cardiac disease that involves the right and the left ventricle (e.g., severe cardiac valvular disease, cardiomyopathy).

DIURETICS

Diuretics are drugs that increase urine formation and promote water loss (diuresis) (Box 11-17). In animals with congestive heart failure, sodium retention from aldosterone secretion and concomitant retention of water in the blood and body tissue lead to pulmonary edema, ascites, and an increased cardiac workload. Removing water from the body with diuretics reduces these deleterious conditions. Diuretics should be used cautiously in animals with hypovolemia (low blood volume) or hypotension (low blood pressure), because they further decrease the fluid component of blood and reduce blood pressure.

Loop diuretics, such as furosemide (Lasix), produce diuresis by inhibiting sodium resorption from the loop of Henle in nephrons. When sodium resorption is inhibited, osmotic forces are exerted that retains additional water in the urine. Retention of sodium in the forming urine osmotically retains water in the urine and prevents its resorption. In the distal convoluted tubule, potassium is exchanged for sodium so that sodium is still resorbed and conserved by the body to some degree. Because loop diuretics cause potassium to be excreted in the urine, prolonged use of loop diuretics may result in hypokalemia (low blood potassium).

Thiazide diuretics, such as chlorothiazide, are not often used in veterinary medicine because of the safety and effectiveness of furosemide. Thiazides are less potent than loop diuretics because of their site of action in the distal convoluted tubule. Thiazide diuretics can cause loss of potassium, with resultant hypokalemia.

Spironolactone is a diuretic that is a competitive antagonist of aldosterone, the hormone that normally causes sodium resorption from the distal renal tubules and collection ducts. When aldosterone is inhibited, more sodium remains in the lumen of the renal tubules, osmotically retaining water and preventing its resorption. Because sodium is excreted and potassium is conserved in the body, drugs like spironolactone are called potassium-sparing diuretics.

Mannitol is a carbohydrate (sugar) used as an **osmotic diuretic.** Mannitol is poorly resorbed from the renal tubule, thus providing a solute that osmotically retains water in the renal tubular lumen. Mannitol is not used in treatment of cardiovascular disease but is used to reduce cerebral edema associated with head trauma and as a diuretic for flushing absorbed toxins from the body.

BOX 11-18 Commonly Used Antitussives

Butorphanol (Torbugesic)
Hydrocodone (Hycodan)
Dextromethorphan (Robitussin, other OTC cough medications)

DRUGS AFFECTING THE RESPIRATORY SYSTEM

ANTITUSSIVES

Antitussives are drugs that block the cough reflex, which is coordinated by the cough center in the brain stem (Box 11-18). A productive cough refers to a cough that produces mucus and other inflammatory products that are coughed up into the oral cavity. A nonproductive cough is "dry" and "hacking," and no mucus is coughed up. Antitussives suppress the coughing that normally removes mucus, cellular debris, exudates, and other products that accumulate within the bronchi as a result of infection or inflammation. For this reason, in animals with a very productive cough (much mucus produced), antitussive drugs should be used cautiously and large doses should be avoided. In such situations, suppression of coughing with cough suppressants can result in accumulation of excessive mucus and debris.

Antitussives should be used in animals with a dry, nonproductive cough producing little or no inspissated mucus. Often these coughs keep the animal (and owner) awake, preventing the animal from getting the rest it needs to recover. Antitussives are commonly used in treating uncomplicated tracheobronchitis ("kennel cough") in dogs. This "retching" type of cough is often punctuated by gagging up small amounts of mucus the owner interprets as vomitus. This type of cough is extremely irritating to the upper airway mucosa; such irritation stimulates more coughing, which further irritates the airway. This pattern can continue for weeks if the cough is not treated.

Butorphanol (Torbutrol) is a centrally acting opioid cough suppressant that, unlike most other opioid cough suppressants, is not classified as a controlled substance in most locations. In antitussive doses, butorphanol causes little sedation, as compared with stronger opioid drugs.

Hydrocodone (Hycodan) is a C-III narcotic available only by prescription from a veterinarian with a DEA clearance for writing C-III prescriptions. Sedation is often noted in treated animals, and long-term administration can result in constipation.

Codeine is a relatively weak opioid/narcotic that is a component of many cough suppressant preparations. Most products containing codeine are prescription preparations with a C-V controlled substance rating. The sedative effect of codeine is similar to that of hydrocodone, and use of the compound can become habit forming.

Dextromethorphan is a common ingredient in OTC non-prescription cough, flu, and cold preparations. Its actions are similar to those of the more potent narcotic antitussives, but it is not a controlled substance. Dextromethorphan is generally not as effective in controlling coughs in veterinary patients as butorphanol or other prescription antitussives; however, owners often initially use human cold products containing dextromethorphan to curtail coughing in their pets. Although dextromethorphan in OTC products is fairly harmless, the other compounds in cold or flu preparations can cause significant harm to animals (e.g., acetaminophen can be very toxic in cats); therefore, it is unwise to recommend that pet owners use OTC products to control coughing in their animals.

MUCOLYTICS, EXPECTORANTS, AND DECONGESTANTS

Mucolytic agents are designed to break up ("lyse") mucus and reduce the viscosity of mucus so that the cilia can move it out of the respiratory tract. Acetylcysteine (Mucomyst) is a mucolytic agent that decreases the viscosity of mucus. Acetylcysteine may be administered by nebulization (inhalation of a fine mist containing the drug) or given PO (although the taste is awful and must be masked with flavoring agents, or it must be administered by feeding tube). Nebulized saline and other fluids are used to increase the fluid content of respiratory mucus in the lower airways. Acetylcysteine is also used as the treatment for acetaminophen toxicity in cats.

Expectorants are compounds that also increase the fluidity of mucus in the respiratory tract by generating liquid secretions by respiratory tract cells. Guaifenesin and saline expectorants (ammonium chloride, potassium iodide, sodium citrate) are given PO. The volatile oils, such as terpin hydrate, eucalyptus oil, and pine oil, directly stimulate respiratory secretions when their vapors are inhaled.

Many OTC human cold preparations that contain expectorants also contain decongestants, such as phenylephrine or phenylpropanolamine, for relief of nasal congestion. **Decongestants** reduce congestion (vascular engorgement) of the mucous membranes (Box 11-19).

BOX 11-19 Commonly Used Mucolytics, Expectorants, and Decongestants

Mucolytic
Acetylcysteine (Mucomyst)

Expectorant
Guaifenesin

Decongestant
Phenylephrine

BRONCHODILATORS

Bronchoconstriction is caused by contraction of smooth muscles surrounding the small terminal bronchioles deep within the respiratory tree. Drugs that inhibit bronchoconstriction are called **bronchodilators** (Box 11-20). Terbutaline, albuterol, and clenbuterol are available in an oral dosage form and as an inhaler. The methylxanthines include such bronchodilators as theophylline and aminophylline. The difference between theophylline and aminophylline is that aminophylline is approximately 80% theophylline and 20% ethylenediamine salt. Because 100 mg of aminophylline contains only 80 mg of active theophylline, the dose of theophylline must be adjusted if the animal is switched to aminophylline or vice versa based on the amount of active ingredient (theophylline) in the compound. Aminophylline is used more commonly in the clinical settings because it is available in injectable form.

BOX 11-20 Commonly Used Bronchodilators

Terbutaline
Albuterol
Clenbuterol
Aminophylline

DRUGS AFFECTING THE ENDOCRINE SYSTEM

DRUGS USED TO TREAT HYPOTHYROIDISM

Drugs used to treat hypothyroidism (insufficiency of thyroid hormone) include levothyroxine (T_4) and synthetic liothyronine (T_3) (Box 11-21). Supplementing a hypothyroid animal with levothyroxine (T_4) provides the various organs and tissues with the appropriate amount of thyroid hormone, as each organ or tissue converts T_4 to T_3. With T_3 supplementation, the local tissue regulation of thyroid hormone conversion is bypassed.

Another advantage of synthetic levothyroxine is its ability to trigger the natural negative-feedback mechanism, thus emulating the normal regulatory mechanism for thyroid hormone production. Levothyroxine (e.g., Synthroid, Soloxine) is usually the drug of choice for treating hypothyroidism. Also, T_3 products (e.g., Cytomel) are generally more expensive than T_4 products and must be administered three times daily, rather than once daily.

DRUGS USED TO TREAT HYPERTHYROIDISM

Hyperthyroidism is an increase in thyroid hormone production. It is most common in cats and is associated with a hormone-secreting thyroid tumor. Hyperthyroidism is treated by surgical removal of the thyroid gland, with drugs that

BOX 11-21 Commonly Used Drugs for Thyroid Disease

Levothyroxine (Soloxine)
Methimazole (Tapazole)
Radioactive iodine (I-131)

decrease thyroid hormone production or drugs that destroy the thyroid tissue (antithyroid drugs).

Methimazole (Tapazole) and propylthiouracil have been used to control hyperthyroidism in cats by blocking the thyroid tumor's ability to produce T_3 and T_4. Of the two drugs, methimazole causes fewer complications and is preferred over propylthiouracil for decreasing thyroid hormone production. Methimazole can be compounded for topical application (onto the ear pinna) as well.

Radioactive iodine (I-131) is an alternative to oral treatment of hyperthyroidism. The radioactive iodine is injected IV. The iodine, a normal component of thyroid hormone, is taken up and concentrated by the active thyroid tumor cells, which are then destroyed by the radioactivity.

ENDOCRINE PANCREATIC DRUGS

Insulin is responsible for movement of glucose from the blood into tissue cells. Lack of insulin results in diabetes mellitus, a condition characterized by high blood glucose levels (hyperglycemia) and passage of glucose in the urine (glucosuria). Blood glucose levels can be controlled by one or two SC insulin injections a day (Box 11-22). The insulins of choice for maintaining diabetic dogs are NPH insulin (Humilin N, Novolin N, PZI), which are of intermediate duration. Diabetic cats sometimes require the longer-acting insulin (Glargine), which is administered once or twice daily. Prozinc is a human-recombinant long-acting PZI insulin also used in cats. Regular insulin is not commonly used to maintain diabetic cats or dogs because its short duration of activity requires multiple doses during a 24-hour period. However, because regular insulin is the only type that can be given IV, it is used initially to stabilize the glucose concentrations of animals with severe, uncontrolled diabetes or diabetic ketoacidosis.

BOX 11-22 Commonly Used Endocrine Pancreatic Drugs

Injectable (Insulin)
Porcine origin lente (Vetsulin)
NPH (Humulin N, Novolin N)
Glargine (Lantus)
Protamine zinc (ProZinc)

Oral Forms
Glipizide (human use)

DRUGS USED TO TREAT HYPOADRENOCORTICISM

Hypoadrenocorticism (Addison's disease) is characterized by a lack of glucocorticoid and/or mineralocorticoid secretion from the adrenal cortex. It can result from the gland itself or from a hormone (ACTH) that aids in telling the gland to secrete the corticoids. Hypoadrenocorticism is treated with corticoids supplementation (Box 11-23). Mineralocorticoid supplementation is achieved with desoxycorticosterone pivalate (DOCP) or fludrocortisone acetate (Florinef). Desoxycorticosterone is a long-acting mineralocorticoid that requires functioning kidneys to work properly. It is used only in dogs as an injection once every 23 to 25 days. Desoxycorticosterone may require the use of concurrent glucocorticoids. Fludrocortisone has both mineral and glucocorticoid activity and is used in both dogs and cats. It is used daily by oral administration. Because fludrocortisone has some glucocorticoid activity, additional supplementation may not be necessary.

BOX 11-23 Commonly Used Drugs for Adrenal Disease

Desoxycorticosterone pivalate (DOCP)
Fludrocortisones acetate (Florinef)
Prednisone/Prednisolone
Mitotane (o,p′DDD, lysodren)
l-Deprenyl (Anipryl)

Glucocorticoid supplementation is achieved using any number of glucocorticoid agents including betamethasone, dexamethasone, fludrocortisone, flumethasone, hydrocortisone, methylprednisolone, prednisolone, prednisone, or triamcinolone. The glucocorticoids vary in duration of effectiveness, which is usually the determining factor for the choice of drug used.

DRUGS USED TO TREAT HYPERADRENOCORTICISM

Hyperadrenocorticism (Cushing's disease) is characterized by excess glucocorticoids in the system. This can be caused by bilateral adrenocortical hyperplasia (caused by a pituitary microadenoma), functional adrenal tumors (benign or cancerous), or by excessive or prolonged administration of oral, parenteral, or topical corticosteroids (termed iatrogenic hyperadrenocorticism).

Treatment of hyperadrenocorticism is based on suppressing the adrenal gland, by discontinuing the corticosteroid use, or by surgically removing the adrenal gland. Mitotane (o,p′-DDD, Lysodren) causes selective necrosis of two sections of the adrenal gland, decreasing the release of corticosteroids. It is administered daily at first and eventually is tapered to twice-weekly dosing. Ketoconazole reversibly inhibits the development of corticosteroids by twice-daily administration but has fallen out of favor because of the lack of response from about 50% of patients it is used on. L-Deprenyl (Anipryl) is a selective monoamine oxidase-B (MAOB) inhibitor. MAOB causes dopamine depletion. In dogs with pituitary-based disease this dopamine depletion causes an increase in

BOX 11-24 Commonly Used Drugs Affecting the Reproductive System

Estradiol
Altrenogest (Regu-Mate)
Dinoprost tromethamine (Lutalyse)
Fluprostenol (Equimate)
Megestrol acetate (Ovaban)
Mibolerone (Cheque drops)
Oxytocin

production of cortisol. In essence, l-deprenyl helps to stop the dopamine depletion and therefore reducing the amount of cortisol produced. All forms of treatment can lead to hypoadrenocorticism.

DRUGS AFFECTING REPRODUCTION

Hormone drugs, either natural or synthetic, are used in food animals and horses to synchronize estrous cycles, terminate pregnancies, and induce ovulation (Box 11-24). In dogs and cats, they are used primarily to prevent pregnancy or alter the state of the uterus.

Gonadotropin-releasing hormone (GnRH) drugs (e.g., Cystorelin) stimulate release of luteinizing hormone (LH) and/or follicle-stimulating hormone (FSH) from the pituitary gland, causing the ovary to develop follicles. The FSH and LH produced by the pituitary gland are also called gonadotropins. In addition to pituitary gonadotropins, some species produce chorionic gonadotropins from the placenta. These can be used as drugs and include human chorionic gonadotropin (HCG), a hormone produced by pregnant women, and equine chorionic gonadotropin (ECG), formerly known as pregnant mare serum gonadotropin (PMSG). These drugs are sometimes used in food animals to induce superovulation (release of ova from multiple follicles) and occasionally in dogs and cats to induce estrus.

Estrogens, such as estradiol cypionate, have been used to induce estrus in anestrual mares. Their most common use in small animals is to prevent pregnancy after "mismating." Progestins are reproductive hormones that are similar to progesterone. Progestins can prevent an animal from coming into full estrus. The progestins used in veterinary medicine include altrenogest (Regu-Mate) and norgestomet.

In livestock breeding systems, the estrous cycles of females can be synchronized so that many animals can be artificially inseminated at the same time. Injecting cows with prostaglandins during diestrus lyses the corpus luteum, causing return to estrus within two to five days. Prostaglandin drugs used include dinoprost tromethamine (Lutalyse), cloprostenol (Estrumate), fluprostenol (Equimate), and fenprostalene (Bovilene).

Because equine breed registries encourage birth of foals as soon as possible after January 1, veterinarians are often asked to help mares conceive during spring. To stimulate more predictable ovulation during this period of transitional estrus, progesterone or a progestin is given for 10 to 14 days to mimic diestrus. Drug use is then halted to mimic lysis of the corpus luteum. Such hormonal therapy is often coupled with exposing the mares to artificial lighting to artificially lengthen the photoperiod. This causes the mare to cycle as though it were summer.

Pregnancy can be prevented (contraception) by suppressing the estrous cycle or by preventing implantation of the fertilized ova in the uterine wall. Megestrol acetate (Ovaban) is an oral progestin used for contraception in female dogs and cats. Megestrol use increases the risk of cystic hyperplasia of the endometrium, endometritis, or pyometra. Prolonged use of megestrol can result in mammary hyperplasia (proliferation of mammary tissue). Mibolerone (Cheque Drops) is another contraceptive used in female dogs. Because mibolerone is a testosterone analog (similar structure), it produces effects similar to those of high levels of testosterone, including increased production of anal sac secretions, masculinization of developing female fetuses, and increased vulvar discharge.

Estradiol cypionate (ECP) is an injectable estrogen used after mismating in dogs. Estrogens prevent pregnancy by increasing the number and thickness of folds within the oviducts, preventing passage of the ova to the uterus. Because there are safer alternatives to estradiol therapy, such as ovariohysterectomy (spaying), many theriogenologists (specialists in animal reproduction) do not recommend use of estradiol in dogs.

Prostaglandin administration causes lysis of the corpus luteum, resulting in a decrease in progesterone levels and subsequent fetal death. Fluprostenol (Equimate) and dinoprost tromethamine (Lutalyse) are both approved for termination of pregnancy in mares. Prostaglandins are only effective in cows if given before the fourth month of pregnancy. Corticosteroids (e.g., dexamethasone) may induce abortion in mares or cows by mimicking the elevated levels of cortisol that occur at the beginning of normal parturition.

Oxytocin is commonly used to increase uterine contractions in animals with dystocia (difficult birth) related to a weakened or fatigued uterus. Anabolic steroids, such as testosterone and progesterone, have been used to increase the weight and conditioning of feedlot cattle. Progestins (e.g., megestrol acetate) have been used to modify behavior in cats.

DRUGS AFFECTING THE NERVOUS SYSTEM

ANESTHETICS

Barbiturates are used to produce short-term anesthesia (infrequently), induce general anesthesia (infrequently), control seizures (frequently), and euthanize animals (frequently). Thiobarbiturates contain a sulfur molecule on the barbituric acid molecule; oxybarbiturates contain an oxygen molecule. Thiamylal and thiopental are thiobarbiturates; methohexital, pentobarbital, and phenobarbital are oxybarbiturates. Thiobarbiturates have a more rapid onset but shorter duration of action than oxybarbiturates.

Propofol is usually injected as an IV bolus and provides rapid injection of anesthesia and a short period of unconsciousness. It is relatively expensive and may cause pain when injected IV.

Ketamine and tiletamine are short-acting injectable anesthetics that produce a rather unique form of anesthesia in which the animal feels dissociated (apart) from its body. Retention of laryngeal, pharyngeal, and corneal reflexes; lack of muscular relaxation (often rigidity); and an increased heart rate characterize this dissociative effect.

The lack of muscular relaxation makes ketamine unsuitable as a sole anesthetic agent for major surgery. Ketamine and tiletamine produce good somatic (peripheral tissue) analgesia (pain relief) and are suitable for superficial surgery; however, they are much less effective in blocking visceral (internal organ) pain and should not be used alone as anesthesia for internal procedures. Tiletamine is included with zolazepam, a benzodiazepine tranquilizer, in a product marketed as Telazol. Zolazepam reduces some of the CNS excitation and side effects produced by tiletamine.

Nitrous oxide, also referred to as "laughing gas," is very safe when used properly and has much weaker analgesic qualities than other inhalant anesthetics. The major role of nitrous oxide is to decrease the amount of the more potent inhalant anesthetics needed to achieve a surgical plane of anesthesia.

Methoxyflurane (Metofane, Penthrane) is an inhalant anesthetic characterized by good muscle relaxation, a relatively slow rate of anesthetic induction (as compared with halothane and isoflurane), and a prolonged recovery period. Unlike halothane and isoflurane, methoxyflurane does not require a precision vaporizer for administration. Methoxyflurane is not readily available in the United States.

Like methoxyflurane, halothane (Fluothane) is a nonflammable, nonirritating inhalant anesthetic that can be used in all species. Anesthesia is induced much more rapidly with halothane than with methoxyflurane. Because of its chemical and physical properties, halothane should be administered with a precision vaporizer. Halothane is not readily available in the United States.

Isoflurane (Forane, AErrane) is an inhalant anesthetic that has gained popularity in veterinary practice because of its rapid, smooth induction of anesthesia and short recovery period. Other inhalant agents with similar properties of isoflurane include enflurane (Ethrane), desflurane (Suprane), and sevoflurane (Ultane). Chapter 14 contains additional information on anesthetic agents (Box 11-25).

TRANQUILIZERS AND SEDATIVES

Acepromazine maleate is a phenothiazine tranquilizer that reduces anxiety and produces a mentally relaxed state. It is often used to calm animals for physical examination or transport. Unlike xylazine or detomidine, phenothiazine tranquilizers have no analgesic effect (do not relieve pain).

Droperidol is a butyrophenone with much more potent sedative effects than most phenothiazine tranquilizers. Droperidol has been combined with fentanyl, a strong narcotic analgesic with emetic activity, and marketed as a neuroleptanalgesic product called Innovar-Vet.

Diazepam (Valium), zolazepam (contained in Telazol), midazolam (Versed), and clonazepam (Klonopin) are benzodiazepine tranquilizers often used with other agents as part of a preanesthetic protocol for their calming and muscle relaxing effects.

BOX 11-25 Commonly Used Anesthetics

Phenobarbital
Propofol
Ketamine/Tiletamine
Isoflurane
Sevoflurane

BOX 11-26 Commonly Used Tranquilizers and Sedatives

Acepromazine
Fentanyl
Diazepam (Valium)
Zolazepam
Xylazine
Dexmedetomidine

Xylazine (Rompun, Anased), dexmedetomidine (Dexdomitor), and detomidine (Dormosedan) produce a calming effect and somewhat decrease an animal's ability to respond to stimuli. These drugs also have some analgesic activity. A disadvantage of xylazine is that sedative doses produce vomiting in about 90% of cats and 50% of dogs (Box 11-26).

ANALGESICS

Analgesics are drugs that reduce the perception of pain without loss of other sensations (Box 11-27). Oxymorphone (Numorphan) and hydromorphone are commonly used for preanesthesia and anesthesia. Butorphanol (Torbutrol, Torbugesic) is used for cough control and GI-related pain in small animals and for reducing colic pain in horses. Tramadol is also used for generalized pain and cough control but has less sedating effects than butorphanol. Fentanyl has an analgesic effect 250 times greater than that of morphine. Meperidine (Demerol) is a fairly weak analgesic/sedative and is often injected SC to restrain cats. Pentazocine (Talwin) is a weak analgesic used in horses with colic and dogs recovering from painful surgery.

Buprenorphine (Buprenex) is commonly combined with sedatives or tranquilizers (acepromazine, xylazine, detomidine). It is also used alone in dogs and cats as an analgesic, both for its potency (30 times the analgesic potency of morphine) and its long duration of analgesia (6 to 8 hours). Etorphine (M-99) is an extremely potent narcotic (1000 times the analgesic potency of morphine) used to sedate and capture wildlife or zoo animals. Butorphanol, pentazocine, and buprenorphine are sometimes used to partially reverse some of the respiratory depression and sedation caused by stronger narcotic agents. Nalorphine is another reversal agent.

Neuroleptanalgesia refers to a state of CNS depression (sedation or tranquilization) and analgesia induced by a combination of a sedative (e.g., xylazine) or tranquilizer (e.g., acepromazine), and an analgesic (oxymorphone).

BOX 11-27 Commonly Used Analgesics

Hydromorphone
Oxymorphone
Butorphanol (Torbugesic, Torbutrol)
Tramadol
Fentanyl
Buprenorphine (Buprenex)

Phenothiazine tranquilizers or butyrophenone tranquilizers (droperidol) calm the animal and also decrease or block the emetic (vomiting) side effect of a narcotic analgesic.

ANTICONVULSANTS

Seizures are periods of altered brain function characterized by loss of consciousness, altered muscle tone or movement, altered sensations, or other neurologic changes. Drugs used to control seizures are called **anticonvulsants** (Box 11-28). Phenobarbital is one of the drugs of choice for long-term control of seizures in dogs and cats. This barbiturate is inexpensive and, because of its long half-life, may be given orally once or twice a day. The main side effect is increased blood levels of liver enzymes and possible liver damage. The dose of phenobarbital is often measured in grains (1 grain = approximately 60 mg). Although primidone has some anticonvulsant activity, most of its efficacy is attributable to phenobarbital, produced by metabolism of primidone.

Phenytoin (Dilantin) is a human anticonvulsant that was once popular for use in treating epilepsy in animals. The major disadvantage of phenytoin is that it is difficult to maintain therapeutic plasma concentrations in dogs. Diazepam (Valium) is the drug of choice for emergency treatment of convulsing animals. Diazepam is very effective when given IV, but it is poorly effective when given PO and is absorbed irregularly if injected SC or IM. Clonazepam (Klonopin) is occasionally used with phenobarbital in animals in which plasma concentrations of barbiturate are in the therapeutic range, but the seizures are not adequately controlled.

Potassium bromide (KBr) has been used for long-term seizure control in dogs. It can be used alone or in conjunction with phenobarbital. The exact mechanism is not fully understood, but it is thought that it has generalized depressant effects on neuronal excitability and activity. The bromide also competes for chloride transport, raising the seizure threshold. The main disadvantage of bromides is the long half-life and consequent necessity to take it for at least one month before seeing therapeutic effects. Bromides are commonly used in dogs but not in cats.

Methocarbamol (Robaxin-V) is not an anti-seizure medication but is a muscle relaxant that is used to help seizure-like tremors in dogs that have metaldehyde poisoning (active ingredient in slug and snail baits). It is also used for acute inflammatory and traumatic conditions of the skeletal muscle and to reduce muscle spasms (such as in a back injury) in dogs and horses. The exact mechanism of how it relaxes the muscles is unknown.

BOX 11-28 Commonly Used Anticonvulsants

Phenobarbital
Diazepam (Valium)

BOX 11-29 Commonly Used Central Nervous System Stimulants

Doxapram (Dopram)
Yohimbine
Atipamezole

CENTRAL NERVOUS SYSTEM STIMULANTS

Central nervous system (CNS) stimulants (Box 11-29) are primarily used to stimulate respiration in anesthetized animals or to reverse CNS depression caused by anesthetic or sedative agents.

Doxapram (Dopram) is a CNS stimulant that increases respiration in animals with apnea (cessation of breathing) or bradypnea (slow breathing). Doxapram is most often used in animals that have received large amounts of respiratory depressant drugs. For example, doxapram is commonly used to stimulate respiration in neonates following cesarean section. It can be administered through the umbilical vein or sublingually. Yohimbine, tolazoline, and atipamezole increase respiration through reversal of CNS depression caused by such drugs as xylazine, detomidine, and dexmedetomidine.

ANTIMICROBIALS

Antimicrobials are drugs that kill or inhibit the growth of microorganisms or "microbes," such as bacteria, protozoa, viruses, or fungi. The term **antibiotic** is often used interchangeably with the term antimicrobial. An antimicrobial can be classified by the type of microorganism against which it is effective and whether the antimicrobial kills the microorganism or prevents the microorganism from replicating and proliferating.

The suffix *-cidal* generally describes drugs that kill the microorganism (e.g., **bactericidal**). The suffix *-static* usually describes drugs that inhibit replication but generally do not kill the microorganism outright (e.g., fungistatic). Examples include the following:

- *Bactericidal:* kills bacteria
- ***Bacteriostatic:*** inhibits bacterial replication
- ***Virucidal:*** kills viruses
- *Protozoastatic:* inhibits protozoal replication
- ***Fungicidal:*** kills fungi

Antimicrobials work by different mechanisms to kill or inhibit bacteria and other microorganisms. Antimicrobials generally exert their effects on the cell wall, cell membrane, ribosomes, critical enzymes or metabolites, or nucleic acids of microorganisms.

BOX 11-30 Summary of Commonly Used Penicillins

Ampicillin
Amoxicillin
Penicillin G
Amoxicillin/Clavulanate (Clavamox)

Some microorganisms have developed the ability to survive in the presence of antimicrobial drugs. This ability to survive is referred to as resistance. Bacteria may become resistant to certain drugs because of genetic changes inherited from previous generations of bacteria, or they may acquire resistance by spontaneous mutations of chromosomes.

A **residue** is an accumulation of a drug or chemical or its metabolites in animal tissues or food products, resulting from drug administration to an animal or contamination of food products. Use of drugs in animals intended for food (meat, egg, milk, etc.) must be stopped a specific number of days (the withdrawal period) before the animal is slaughtered or the food products are to be marketed as food for people. Most antimicrobial residues in food are not degraded by cooking or pasteurization.

PENICILLINS

Penicillins (Box 11-30) are bactericidal and can usually be recognized by their *-cillin* suffix on the drug name. The most frequently used penicillins in veterinary medicine include the following: the natural penicillins, penicillin G and penicillin V; the broad-spectrum aminopenicillins, ampicillin, amoxicillin, and hetacillin; the penicillinase-resistant penicillins, cloxacillin, dicloxacillin, and oxacillin; and the extended-spectrum penicillins, carbenicillin, ticarcillin, piperacillin, and others. Penicillins are generally effective against gram-positive bacteria and varying types of gram-negative bacteria. Penicillins are generally well absorbed from injection sites and the GI tract. A penicillin that should not be given PO is penicillin G. Penicillin G is inactivated by gastric acid and so is used only in injectable form.

Amoxicillin/Clavulanate acid (Clavamox) is another bactericidal aminopenicillin with beta-lactamase inhibitor, which expands its spectrum of coverage. It is most commonly used in dogs and cats for urinary tract, soft tissue, and skin infections by susceptible organisms.

CEPHALOSPORINS

Cephalosporins are bactericidal beta-lactam antimicrobials with a *ceph-* or *cef-* prefix in the drug name (Box 11-31). Cephalosporins are classified by generations, according to when they were first developed. First-generation cephalosporins are primarily effective against gram-positive bacteria (*Streptococcus, Staphylococcus*). They are less effective against gram-negative bacteria than the second- or third-generation cephalosporins. Veterinary products include cefadroxil (first-generation, Cefa-Tabs), cefazolin (first-generation, Kefzol, Ancef, Zolicef, and cefazolin sodium), cephapirin (first-generation, Cefa-Lak and Cefa-Dri intramammary infusions), ceftiofur (third-generation, Naxcel injectable), Cefovecin sodium (Convenia, 2-week injectable), and cefpodoxime proxetil (third-generation, Simplicef). Human products used in veterinary medicine include cefixime (third-generation, Suprax), cefoperazone (third-generation, Cefobid), cefpodoxime proxetil (third-generation, Vantin), cefotetan disodium (second- or third-generation, Cefotan), cephalothin (first-generation, Keflin), ceftriaxone (third-generation, Rocephin), cephalexin (first-generation, Keflex), cefoxitin (second-generation, Mefoxin), and cefotaxime (third-generation, Claforan). First-generation cephalosporins are well absorbed from the GI tract.

BOX 11-31 Commonly Used Cephalosporins

Cefadroxil
Cefazolin
Cephapirin
Ceftiofur
Cefovecin (Convenia)
Cefpodoxime (Simplicef)

BOX 11-32 Summary of Commonly Used Aminoglycosides

Gentamicin
Amikacin
Neomycin
Tobramycin

BACITRACINS

Bacitracins are a group of polypeptide antibiotics, of which bacitracin A is the major component. Bacitracin is a common ingredient in topical antibiotic creams or ointments. It is often combined with polymyxin B and neomycin to provide a broad spectrum of antimicrobial activity.

AMINOGLYCOSIDES

Aminoglycosides (Box 11-32) used in veterinary medicine include gentamicin, amikacin, neomycin, streptomycin, dihydrostreptomycin, apramycin, kanamycin, and tobramycin. With the exception of amikacin, most aminoglycosides can be recognized by the *-micin* or *-mycin* suffix in the nonproprietary name. Aminoglycosides are bactericidal and are quite effective against many aerobic bacteria (bacteria that require oxygen to live) but are not effective against most anaerobic bacteria (those that do not require oxygen). Aminoglycosides are potentially nephrotoxic (toxic to the kidney) and ototoxic (toxic to the inner ear), even at "normal" dosages.

FLUOROQUINOLONES

Fluoroquinolones (quinolones) are bactericidal antimicrobials (Box 11-33) used commonly for their effectiveness against a variety of pathogens. Quinolones are not effective against anaerobes. Enrofloxacin (Baytril) is approved for use in dogs,

BOX 11-33 Commonly Used Fluoroquinolones

Enrofloxacin (Batyril)
Ciprofloxacin (Cipro)
Marbofloxacin (Zeniquin)
Ofloxacin (Ocuflox)

BOX 11-34 Commonly Used Tetracyclines

Tetracycline
Oxytetracycline
Doxycycline

cats, cattle, horses, ferrets, reptiles, birds, and rodents. It has also been used extra-label (in unapproved ways) to treat neonatal diseases in swine. Ciprofloxacin (Cipro) is similar to enrofloxacin and mostly used when larger dosages are necessary. Orbifloxacin (Orbax) is also similar to enrofloxacin and is approved for use in dogs and cats against susceptible infections. Difloxacin (Dicural) and marbofloxacin (Zeniquin) are approved for use against susceptible infections in dogs only. Ofloxacin (Ocuflox) is used as an ophthalmic medication only. The quinolones are effective against common gram-negative and gram-positive bacteria found in skin, respiratory, and urinary infections. Quinolones can cause arthropathies in immature, growing animals and therefore should not be used in these animals.

TETRACYCLINES

Tetracyclines (Box 11-34) are bacteriostatic drugs with a nonproprietary name ending in *-cycline*. They work most effectively against mycoplasma, spirochetes (including *Borrelia*), chlamydia, and rickettsia. The gram-positive organisms they have been effective against in the past are becoming more resistant. Tetracycline and oxytetracycline have similar spectra of antibacterial activity and actions in the body. The newer and more lipophilic doxycycline and minocycline are human drugs that are being used more frequently in animals (unapproved use) because of their longer half-life (increased duration of activity), broader spectrum of antibacterial action, and better penetration of tissues than the older tetracyclines. After oral administration, doxycycline and minocycline are absorbed better than oxytetracycline or tetracycline. Oxytetracycline is the most commonly used injectable tetracycline because of its good absorption from IM injection sites. Chlortetracycline is used as a food or water treatment or as an ophthalmic agent.

SULFONAMIDES AND POTENTIATED SULFONAMIDES

Because sulfonamides ("sulfa drugs") have been in use for many years, many strains of bacteria have become resistant to them. To increase the efficacy of sulfonamides and convert them from bacteriostatic to bactericidal drugs, they are sometimes combined with other compounds, such as trimethoprim and ormetoprim, to potentiate (increase) their antibacterial effects. Some of the more common sulfonamides used in veterinary medicine include sulfadimethoxine (combined with ormetoprim in Primor), sulfadiazine (combined with trimethoprim in Tribrissen), sulfamethoxazole (combined with trimethoprim in Septra), and sulfasalazine (used for its anti-inflammatory effect in inflammatory bowel disease). Potentiated sulfas used in veterinary medicine have a fairly broad spectrum of antibacterial activity, including many gram-positive organisms (e.g., *Streptococcus, Staphylococcus, Nocardia*). Although sulfas and potentiated sulfas are not very effective against gram-negative organisms, they are the drugs of choice for treating some protozoal infections, including *Coccidia* and *Toxoplasma* (Box 11-35).

BOX 11-35 Commonly Used Sulfonamides

Trimethoprim/Sulfas (various types)
Sulfadimethoxine
Sulfasalazine

BOX 11-36 Commonly Used Lincosamides

Lincomycin
Clindamycin (Antirobe)
Pirlimycin

LINCOSAMIDES

Lincosamide antibiotics, including lincomycin and clindamycin (Antirobe), can be bacteriostatic or bactericidal, depending on the concentrations attained at the site of infection (Box 11-36). The lincosamides are generally effective against many gram-positive aerobic cocci. Lincomycin is approved for use in a variety of species (dogs, cats, swine, poultry), but clindamycin is approved only for use in dogs, cats, and ferrets. Pirlimycin is approved for use only in cattle.

MACROLIDES

The macrolide antibiotics erythromycin, azithromycin, and tylosin (Tylan) are approved for use in a variety of companion animals and food animals, including dogs, cats, swine, sheep, cattle, and poultry. Although tylosin is approved for use in dogs and cats, its primary use is in livestock. Both drugs are bacteriostatic and share similar spectra of antibacterial activity and bacterial cross-resistance. Tilmicosin (Micotil) is a macrolide approved for SC administration for treatment of bovine respiratory diseases (Box 11-37).

METRONIDAZOLE

Metronidazole (Flagyl) is a bactericidal antimicrobial that is also effective against protozoa that cause intestinal disease, such as *Giardia* (giardiasis), *Entamoeba histolytica* (amebiasis), *Trichomonas* (trichomoniasis), and *Balantidium coli* (balantidiasis).

BOX 11-37 Commonly Used Macrolides

Erythromycin
Tylosin (Tylan)
Tilmicosin (Micotil)

BOX 11-38 Commonly Used Antifungal Drugs

Amphotericin B
Nystatin
Flucytosine
Fluconazole
Ketoconazole
Griseofulvin

NITROFURANS

The nitrofurans are a large group of antimicrobials, of which nitrofurantoin (Furadantin) is most commonly used in veterinary medicine. Nitrofurantoin is bacteriostatic or bactericidal, depending on concentrations attained at the site of infection. Because about half of the drug administered is secreted into the renal tubule, it is used to treat infections of the lower urinary tract (bladder, urethra) in dogs, cats, and occasionally horses.

CHLORAMPHENICOL AND FLUORFENICOL

Chloramphenicol is an antimicrobial that is bacteriostatic at low concentrations but may become bactericidal when used at higher dosages. Chloramphenicol has produced fatal aplastic anemia in humans. For this reason, chloramphenicol is totally banned from any use in food animals. Fluorfenicol is a new drug similar to chloramphenicol but without the risk of aplastic anemia. It is approved for treatment of respiratory disease in cattle.

RIFAMPIN

Rifampin is a bactericidal or bacteriostatic antimicrobial belonging to the rifamycins. It is primarily used with or without erythromycin for treatment of *Rhodococcus equi* infections in young foals, and sometimes in conjunction with antifungal agents for treatment of aspergillosis or histoplasmosis in dogs and cats.

ANTIFUNGALS

Box 11-38 contains a summary of commonly used antifungal drugs.

AMPHOTERICIN B AND NYSTATIN

Amphotericin B is an antifungal that is administered IV for treatment of deep or systemic mycotic infections. Nystatin, because of its toxicity to tissues, is used only to treat *Candida* infections (candidiasis) on the skin, mucous membranes (e.g., mouth, vagina), and lining of the intestinal tract in dogs, cats, and birds.

BOX 11-39 Commonly Used Antiparasitics

For Treatment of Internal Parasites
Piperazine
Fenbendazole
Ivermectin
Praziquantel (Droncit)
Epsiprantel (Cestex)
Pyrantel (Strongid, Nemex)
Febantel
Melarsomine (Immidicide)
Milbemycin (Interceptor, Sentinel)
Sulfadimethoxine (Albon)

For Treatment of External Parasites
Pyrethrins
Permethrins (Advantix, Vectra)
Amitraz (Mitoban, Preventic)
Imidacloprid (Advantage, Advantix)
Fipronil (Frontline)
Selamectin (Revolution)
Lufenuron (Program, Sentinel)
Spinosad (Comfortis)

FLUCYTOSINE

Flucytosine is an antifungal agent used mostly against *Cryptococcus* and *Candida.* It is often used in conjunction with amphotericin B as resistance is quite common when used alone.

FLUCONAZOLE, KETOCONAZOLE, AND ITRACONAZOLE

Fluconazole, ketoconazole, and itraconazole are imidazole antifungals with fewer side effects than amphotericin B. Of the imidazoles, fluconazole has the least side effects and is apparently safe for use in multiple species.

GRISEOFULVIN

Griseofulvin is a fungistatic drug used primarily to treat infections with *Trichophyton, Microsporum,* and *Epidermophyton* dermatophytes (superficial fungi) in dogs, cats, and horses. These fungi usually infect the skin, hair, nails, and claws, causing the condition known as ringworm. Griseofulvin is available as a veterinary product (Fulvicin) for oral use as a powder (for horses) or tablets.

ANTIPARASITICS

Anthelmintic is a general term used to describe compounds that kill various types of internal parasites (helminths or "worms") (Box 11-39). A **vermicide** is an anthelmintic that kills the worm, as opposed to a vermifuge, which only paralyzes the worm and often results in passage of live worms in the stool. Antinematodal compounds are used to treat infections with nematodes (roundworms). Nematodes include hookworms, ascarids, whipworms, and strongyles. Anticestodal compounds are used to treat infections with cestodes (tapeworms or segmented flatworms). Antitrematodal compounds are used to treat infection with trematodes (flukes or unsegmented flatworms), including *Paragonimus, Fasciola,* and *Dicrocoelium.* Antiprotozoal compounds are used to treat infection with protozoa (single-celled organisms), including *Coccidia, Giardia,* and *Toxoplasma.* Coccidiostats are drugs that inhibit the growth of coccidia specifically.

INTERNAL ANTIPARASITICS

Piperazine, a vermicide and vermifuge, is the active ingredient in most of the "once-a-month" dewormers sold in grocery stores and pet shops. Piperazine is very safe but is only effective against ascarids. The benzimidazoles include fenbendazole (Panacur), mebendazole (Telmin, Telmintic), thiabendazole (Equizole, Tresaderm Otic), oxibendazole (Anthelcide EQ, Filaribits-Plus), albendazole, oxfendazole, and cambendazole.

Organophosphates are used as internal antiparasitics (Task, Combot), as well as external antiparasitics to combat fleas, ticks, and flies. The organophosphates most commonly used internally are dichlorvos and trichlorfon. Ivermectin (Ivomec, Eqvalan, Heartgard-30) is an avermectin widely used in almost every species treated by veterinarians. Ivermectin can produce adverse reactions in Collies and Collie cross-breeds. Anticestodals used in animals include praziquantel (Droncit) and epsiprantel (Cestex).

Anthelmintics containing pyrantel (Strongid, Nemex, Banminth, Imathal) safely remove a variety of nematodes in domestic species. They are marketed as pyrantel pamoate and a more water-soluble salt, pyrantel tartrate. Morantel tartrate (Nematel) is very similar to pyrantel and has similar uses. Febantel is marketed in a palatable paste formulation for horses or in combination with the anticestodal drug praziquantel (Vercom) for dogs and cats or with the organophosphate trichlorfon (Combotel) for horses.

For years, thiacetarsamide sodium (Caparsolate) had been the only drug approved for treatment of adult heartworms; thiacetarsamide is given by IV injection. In 1996, melarsomine dihydrochloride (Immiticide) was approved as an adulticide; it is given by IM injection. After adulticide treatment, a microfilaricide can be administered to eliminate circulating heartworm microfilariae. Ivermectin (e.g., 1% Ivomec injectable, approved for use in livestock) is the microfilaricide of choice. Milbemycin oxime (Interceptor, Sentinel), a drug very similar to ivermectin, is also used as a microfilaricide. After microfilariae have been cleared from the blood, the animal can begin receiving heartworm preventive to prevent reinfection. Diethylcarbamazine (DEC), marketed as Caricide, Nemacide, and Filarbits, is given daily during seasons when an animal could be bitten by a mosquito and for 2 months thereafter. Because they must be given only once a month, ivermectin (Heartgard-30) and milbemycin (Interceptor, Sentinel) have captured a significant percentage of the heartworm preventive market. Ivermectin is also available as a heartworm preventive for cats (Heartgard-30 for Cats).

Antiprotozoals are most commonly used against coccidia, *Giardia,* and other protozoa. They include sulfonamide antimicrobials, such as sulfadimethoxine (Albon, Bactrovet), metronidazole, and amprolium (Corid).

EXTERNAL ANTIPARASITICS

Chlorinated hydrocarbons constitute one of the oldest groups of the synthetic insecticides. The only chlorinated hydrocarbon currently used in veterinary medicine is lindane, which is incorporated in some dog shampoos. Lindane is easily absorbed through the skin and can produce harmful side effects if absorbed in sufficient quantities.

Organophosphates and carbamates are usually grouped together because of their similar mechanism of action, effects on insects, and toxic effects. Unlike the chlorinated hydrocarbons, organophosphates and carbamates decompose readily in the environment and do not pose a significant threat to wildlife. Included in this group are chlorpyrifos, carbaryl (Sevin), and propoxur (Baygon).

Pyrethrins and pyrethroids (synthetic pyrethrins) constitute the largest group of insecticides marketed for use against external parasites and as common household insect sprays. They are generally quite safe. Pyrethrins and pyrethroids produce a quick "knockdown" effect, but the immobilized flies or fleas may recover after several minutes. Pyrethroids include resmethrin, allethrin, permethrin, tetramethrin, bioallethrin, and fenvalerate.

Amitraz is a diamide insecticide that was one of the first effective agents available for treatment of demodectic mange in dogs. Since its introduction, amitraz has been incorporated into other insecticidal products. Amitraz is toxic to cats and rabbits, so it should not be used in those species. The liquid form, available as a dip or sponge-on bath product (Mitaban), is used to treat demodectic mange in dogs. Amitraz is also available as Preventic, a tick collar for dogs, and as Taktic, a liquid topical or a collar for use in cattle.

Imidacloprid (Advantage) is a chloronicotinyl nitroguanidine insecticide used topically to kill adult fleas on dogs and cats. Imidacloprid is applied to the back of the neck in cats or between the shoulder blades in dogs (and over the rump area of large dogs), and kills adult fleas on contact. Fipronil (Frontline and Top Spot) and selamectin (Revolution) are once-a-month flea spray and topical applications that resemble ivermectin in their insecticidal activity.

Rotenone (Derris Powder) is a natural insecticide derived from derris root. It may be included with other insecticides in dips, pour-ons, and powders. D-limonene, derived from citrus peels, purportedly has some slight insecticidal activity. When included in insecticidal products, it imparts a pleasant citrus smell to the haircoat. Sulfur is sometimes included in "tar and sulfur" shampoos to help reduce skin scaling and to treat sarcoptic mange. These products are usually recognized by their strong sulfur odor.

Insect growth regulators are compounds that affect immature stages of insects and prevent maturation to adults. They are insecticidal without toxic effects in mammals.

Methoprene (Siphotrol, Ovitrol) and fenoxycarb (Basus, Ectogard, and others) were some of the first insect growth regulators incorporated into topical products or flea collars. These compounds are distributed over the animal's skin. Female fleas absorb the drug, and it is incorporated into the flea eggs. The drug-impregnated eggs hatch and the larvae do not mature to adult fleas. Lufenuron (Program, Sentinel) is an insect development inhibitor given once a month as a tablet for dogs and cats and as an oral liquid for cats.

Lufenuron interferes with development of the insect's chitin, which is essential for proper egg formation and development of the larval exoskeleton. If flea larvae survive within the egg despite a defective shell, they will be unable to hatch. Because lufenuron is orally ingested and distributed throughout the animal's tissue fluids, a flea must bite the animal to be exposed to the drug. Spinosad (Comfortis) is a neurotoxin that works on fleas only and like lufenuron is orally ingested and distributed throughout the animal's tissue. This should not be given to dogs and cats with epilepsy or those already on ivermectin.

Insect repellents are used to repel insects and keep them off of animals. Butoxypolypropylene glycol (Butox PPG) has been incorporated into flea and tick spray products for use in dogs and cats. It is also used in equine fly repellents.

Diethyltoluamide (DEET) is a common ingredient in repellent products formulated for use in people.

ANTI-INFLAMMATORIES

Drugs that relieve pain or discomfort by blocking or reducing the inflammatory process are called **anti-inflammatory drugs.** There are two general classes of anti-inflammatories: steroidal anti-inflammatory drugs (glucocorticoids) and nonsteroidal anti-inflammatory drugs (**NSAIDs**). Most of these drugs relieve pain indirectly by decreasing inflammation; however, some also have direct analgesic (pain-relieving) activity.

GLUCOCORTICOIDS

When veterinarians use the terms cortisone or **corticosteroid,** they are usually referring to glucocorticoids (Box 11-40). A glucocorticoid, such as hydrocortisone, that exerts an anti-inflammatory effect for less than 12 hours is considered a short-acting glucocorticoid. Many glucocorticoids used in veterinary medicine are classified as intermediate-acting glucocorticoids, with activity for 12 to 36 hours. These include prednisone, prednisolone, triamcinolone (e.g., Vetalog), methylprednisolone, and isoflupredone. Long-acting glucocorticoids, such as dexamethasone, betamethasone, and flumethasone, exert their effects for more than 48 hours.

Glucocorticoids are generally available in three liquid forms: aqueous solutions, alcohol solutions, and suspensions. Glucocorticoids in aqueous (water) solution are usually combined with a salt to make them soluble in water. Dexamethasone sodium phosphate (Azium SP) and prednisolone sodium succinate (Solu-Delta-Cortef) are aqueous solutions of glucocorticoids. The advantage of aqueous forms is that they can be given in large doses IV with less risk than alcohol solutions and suspensions (suspensions should never be given IV). The aqueous forms are often used in emergency situations (shock, CNS trauma) because they can be delivered IV in large amounts and have a fairly rapid onset of activity. If the label of a vial of dexamethasone specifies the active ingredient as dexamethasone, without mention of sodium phosphate, it is likely an alcohol solution. Suspensions of glucocorticoids contain the drug particles suspended in the liquid vehicle. Suspensions are characterized by their opaque appearance (after shaking), the need for shaking the vial before use, and the terms acetate, diacetate, pivalate, acetonide, or valerate appended to the glucocorticoid name. When injected into the body, the drug crystals dissolve over several days, releasing small amounts of glucocorticoid each day and providing prolonged action. Topical preparations of glucocorticoid suspensions using the acetate ester are used in topical ophthalmic medications. Oral tablets are available for prednisone and prednisolone.

Overuse of glucocorticoid drugs can produce Cushing's syndrome. The signs of Cushing's syndrome are related to the effects of glucocorticoids and include alopecia (hair loss), muscle wasting, pot-bellied appearance, slow healing of wounds, polyuria, polydipsia, and polyphagia. Physical changes (alopecia, muscle wasting) do not become apparent until the animal has been treated for weeks.

NONSTEROIDAL ANTI-INFLAMMATORY DRUGS

The advantage of nonsteroidal anti-inflammatory drugs (Box 11-41) over glucocorticoids centers around the many side effects of glucocorticoids as compared with the few adverse effects associated with NSAIDs. NSAIDs decrease protective prostaglandins in the stomach and kidney. In large doses or in sensitive animals, NSAIDs can produce gastric ulcerations or decreased blood flow to the kidneys.

BOX 11-40 Commonly Used Glucocorticoids

Prednisone
Prednisolone
Triamcinolone (Vetalog)
Methylprednisolone
Dexamethasone
Dexamethasone sodium phosphate
Prednisolon sodium succinate (Solu-Delta-Cortef)

BOX 11-41 Commonly Used NSAIDs

Ketoprofen
Flunixin meglumine (Banamine)
Carprofen (Rimadyl)
Deracoxib (Deramaxx)
Meloxicam (Metacam)
Firocoxib (Previcox)
Dimethyl sulfoxide (DMSO)

Aspirin (acetylsalicylic acid) is a fairly safe NSAID in most animal species. Like other NSAIDs, aspirin is metabolized by the liver. Aspirin is metabolized much more slowly in cats than in other species. Aspirin has a half-life of 1.5 hours in people, approximately 8 hours in dogs, and 30 hours in cats. Thus, as with many other drugs, the aspirin dosage for cats is lower than dosages used in other species and usually consists of one "baby aspirin" tablet (81 mg) every two or three days. If used prudently, however, aspirin is one of the safest and most effective NSAIDs for cats.

Ibuprofen, ketoprofen, and naproxen are available as OTC medications (ibuprofen is marketed as Advil, naproxen is marketed as Aleve, ketoprofen is marketed as Orudis). Naproxen is marketed as the veterinary product Naprosyn. A ketoprofen product, Ketofen, is approved for use in horses. Flunixin meglumine (Banamine) is also is a potent analgesic used primarily in equine medicine for treatment of colic; dogs are very sensitive to the GI side effects of flunixin. Both dogs and cats are very sensitive to these OTC medications and can develop liver and kidney failure with overdosing so these are not generally recommended for clients to give to their pets. Carprofen (Rimadyl), deracoxib (Deramaxx), etodolac (Etogesic), meloxicam (Metacam), and firocoxib (Previcox) are all cyclooxygenase-inhibiting (coxib) class, non-narcotic NSAIDs with anti-inflammatory and analgesic properties. There are two main cyclooxygenase enzymes, COX-1 and COX-2, and a newly discovered third enzyme, COX-3, which has yet to be fully characterized. Cyclooxygenase-1 (COX-1) is the enzyme responsible for helping with physiologic processes (e.g., platelet aggregation, gastric mucosal protection, and renal perfusion). Cyclooxygenase-2 (COX-2) is responsible for the synthesis of inflammatory mediators. Cyclooxygenase-3 (COX-3) is still undetermined as to its effects. These coxib class NSAIDs therefore decrease prostaglandins associated with inflammation but do not significantly reduce the protective prostaglandins of the stomach and kidneys. Tepoxalin (Zubrin) is a coxib class NSAID but also has 5-lipoxygenase (LOX) inhibition that may be useful in allergic conditions.

Meclofenamic acid (Arquel) was commonly administered to horses as granules mixed in the feed but no longer is marketed in the U.S. Dimethyl sulfoxide (DMSO) is used topically and parenterally, primarily in horses. DMSO is also a component of some otic (ear) preparations used in dogs and cats. Orgotein (superoxide dismutase) is most commonly used to treat horses with joint and vertebral disease.

OTHER ANTI-INFLAMMATORIES

Although acetaminophen is not an anti-inflammatory drug, it is included here because its analgesic and antipyretic (fever-reducing) properties often cause it to be grouped with NSAIDs. Acetaminophen (e.g., Tylenol) does not cause the GI upset, ulcers, or interference with platelet clumping associated with NSAIDs. Unfortunately, the metabolites of acetaminophen can have other severe side effects, especially in cats. A single "extra-strength" acetaminophen tablet (500 mg) can kill an average-sized cat. In dogs a higher dosage (above 150 mg/kg) is required before signs of hepatic necrosis, weight loss, and icterus (jaundice) become evident.

Phenacetin is a compound found in many "cold preparations." This drug is metabolized to acetaminophen and thus can produce acetaminophen toxicity in susceptible species and individual animals. Gold salts, such as aurothioglucose, have been used to treat severe immune-mediated skin problems, such as the various forms of pemphigus. The anti-inflammatory activity of dipyrone is weak compared with its analgesic properties and its ability to decrease fever.

DISINFECTANTS AND ANTISEPTICS

Disinfection is the destruction of pathogenic microorganisms or their toxins. **Antiseptics** are chemical agents that kill or prevent the growth of microorganisms on living tissues. Disinfectants are chemical agents that kill or prevent growth of microorganisms on inanimate objects (surgical equipment, floors, tabletops). Antiseptics and disinfectants may also be described as sanitizers or sterilizers. **Sanitizers** are chemical agents that reduce the number of microorganisms to a "safe" level, without completely eliminating all microorganisms. Sterilizers are chemicals or other agents that completely destroy all microorganisms. As with antimicrobials, it is important to know against what organisms the antiseptic or disinfectant is effective (Table 11-4).

TABLE 11-4 Relative Efficacy of Disinfectants and Antiseptics*

	CHLORHEXIDINE	QUATERNARY AMMONIUM COMPOUNDS	ALCOHOL	IODOPHOR	CHLORINE	PHENOLS
Bactericidal	3+†	2+	2+	3+	2+	2+
Lipid-enveloped virucidal	3+	2+	2+	2+	3+	1+
Nonenveloped virucidal	2+	1+	(—)‡	2+	3+	(—)
Sporicidal	(—)	(—)	(—)	1+	1+	(—)
Effective in presence of soap	1+	(—)	2+	2+	2+	2+
Effective in hard water	1+	1+	1+	2+	2+	1+
Effective in organic material	3+	1+	1+	(—)	(—)	(—)

*Ratings are relative indicators, and the effectiveness is dependent upon concentration of compound used.
†The higher the positive number, the greater the efficacy.
‡Hyphens (—) indicate lack of efficacy.

PHENOLS

Phenols are used as scrub soaps and surface disinfectants. Phenols are also the main disinfecting agents found in many household disinfectants (Lysol, pine oil, and similar cleansers). They are very effective against gram-positive bacteria but generally not effective against gram-negative bacteria, viruses, fungi, or spores. Hexachlorophene is a phenolic surgical scrub that has decreased in popularity because of its suspected neurotoxicity (damage to the nervous system) and teratogenic effects (birth defects) in pregnant nurses who performed hexachlorophene scrubs on a regular basis.

ALCOHOLS

Alcohols, such as ethyl alcohol or isopropyl alcohol, are among the most common antiseptics applied to skin. Solutions of 70% alcohol are used to disinfect surgical sites, injection sites, and rectal thermometers. Nonenveloped viruses are not susceptible to the virucidal effects of alcohol. Alcohol is also ineffective against bacterial spores and must remain in contact with the site for several seconds to be effective against bacteria (several minutes for fungi). Therefore a cursory swipe with an alcohol-soaked swab on an animal's skin, especially if the skin is encrusted with dirt or feces, does little to disinfect an injection site.

QUATERNARY AMMONIUM COMPOUNDS

Quaternary ammonium compounds are used to disinfect the surface of inanimate objects. One of the most commonly used quaternary ammonium compounds in veterinary medicine is benzalkonium chloride. Quaternary ammonium compounds are effective against a wide variety of gram-negative and gram-positive bacteria, but they are ineffective against bacterial spores and have poor efficacy against fungi. Although quaternary ammonium compounds can destroy enveloped viruses, they are ineffective against nonenveloped viruses, such as parvovirus. They act rapidly at a site of application and are not normally irritating to the skin or corrosive to metals.

CHLORINE COMPOUNDS

Chlorine compounds, such as sodium hypochlorite (Clorox, household bleach), can kill enveloped and nonenveloped viruses and are the disinfectant of choice against parvovirus. Chlorines are also effective against fungi, algae, and vegetative forms of bacteria. Like many other disinfectants, chlorine is not effective against bacterial spores.

IODOPHORS

Iodophors are used as topical antiseptics before surgical procedures or for disinfection of tissue. An iodophor is a combination of iodine and a carrier molecule that releases the iodine over time, prolonging the antimicrobial activity. The most common iodophor is iodine combined with polyvinylpyrrolidone, more commonly known as povidone-iodine. Iodophors are bactericidal, virucidal, protozoacidal, and fungicidal.

BIGUANIDES

Chlorhexidine, a biguanide antiseptic, is commonly used to clean cages and to treat various superficial infections in animals. Its wide variety of uses is likely related to its low tissue irritation and its virucidal, bactericidal (both gram-positive and gram-negative), and fungicidal activity. Because chlorhexidine binds to the outer surface of the skin, it is thought to have some residual activity for up to 24 hours if left in contact with the site.

REVIEW QUESTIONS

Dosage Calculations

Calculate the amount of medication required in each of the following scenarios.

1. A 6-lb feline is prescribed amoxicillin at 5 mg/kg twice a day for 7 days. The oral medication has a concentration of 50 mg/ml. How many ml will the cat need per day?
2. A 30-lb Cocker Spaniel is to get a ketamine and diazepam induction IV and the dose is 0.025 ml/lb for each drug. How much ketamine and diazepam will you draw up?
3. A 1200-lb Holstein cow requires a ketoprofen injection and the vet prescribes 1 mg/lb and the concentration is 100 mg/ml. How much ketoprofen will you give?

Matching—Drug Formulations

Match the terms with their description or definition.

_____1. Solid dosage forms injected or inserted under the skin
_____2. Tablets and capsules
_____3. Drugs dissolve, release, and are absorbed by intestinal wall
_____4. Drug particles not dissolved in a liquid vehicle
_____5. Solutions of drugs with water and sugar
_____6. Administered via a needle and syringe
_____7. Alcohol solutions meant for topical application
_____8. Semisolid dosage forms that are applied to the skin
_____9. Drugs dissolved in sweetened alcohol
_____10. Drug dissolved in a liquid vehicle
_____11. Semisolid dosage forms given orally

A. ointments
B. elixirs
C. suspension
D. implants
E. tinctures
F. solution
G. injectables
I. pastes
H. solid
J. syrups
K. suppositories

Matching—Anesthetic Drugs With Their Actions

Match the anesthetic drug action or use with the drug name.

____**1.** Cough control, GI-related and colic pain
____**2.** Long-term control of seizures and for euthanasia
____**3.** Reversal of CNS depression from xylazine and dexmedetomidine
____**4.** Inhalant anesthetic
____**5.** Commonly used dissociative anesthetic
____**6.** A strong narcotic analgesic often on a patch
____**7.** CNS stimulant that increases respiration
____**8.** Calming effect, decreased stimulus response, light analgesic
____**9.** Benzodiazepine tranquilizer with good muscle relaxation
____**10.** Laughing gas—weak analgesic
____**11.** Phenothiazine tranquilizer—reduces anxiety
____**12.** Potent, with long duration of analgesia

A. ketamine
B. barbiturates
C. nitrous oxide
D. isoflurane
E. acepromazine
F. fentanyl
G. diazepam
H. xylazine
I. butorphanol
J. buprenorphine
K. doxapram
L. yohimbine

RECOMMENDED READING

Bill RL: *Pharmacology for veterinary technicians*, ed 3, St Louis, 2006, Mosby.

Papich MG: *Saunders handbook of veterinary drugs*, ed 3, St Louis, 2011, Saunders.

Plumb DC: *Plumb's veterinary drug handbook*, ed 6, Ames, IA, 2008, Wiley Blackwell.

Riviere JE, Papich MG: *Veterinary pharmacology and therapeutics*, ed 9, Ames, IA, 1995, Wiley Blackwell.

Veterinary pharmaceuticals and biologicals 1997/1998, ed 10, Lenexa, KS, 1997, Veterinary Medicine Publishing.

Wanamaker BP, Massey KL: *Applied pharmacology for the veterinary technician*, ed 4, St Louis, 2009, Saunders.

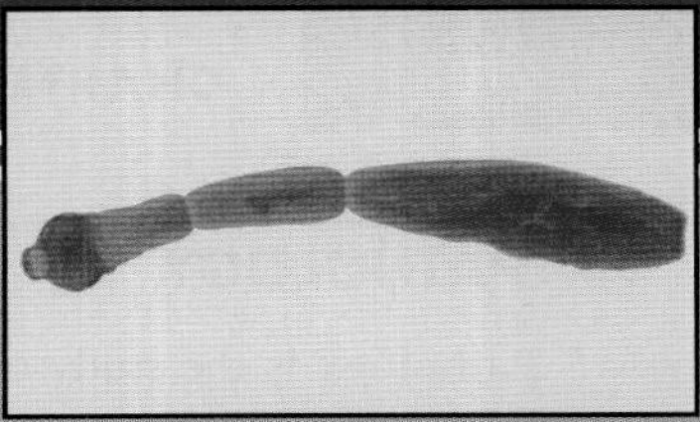

12 Pathology, Response to Disease, and Preventive Medicine

OUTLINE

LEARNING OBJECTIVES

After reviewing this chapter, the reader will be able to:

1. Describe ways in which tissues respond to injury.
2. List the phases of inflammation and the cells involved.
3. Describe ways in which injured tissues heal.
4. List and describe ways in which pathogens affect tissues.
5. Discuss types of immune responses.
6. Discuss the physiologic basis for vaccination.
7. Describe hypersensitivity reactions.
8. List and describe common zoonotic diseases and ways in which they can affect people.
9. Discuss methods used to control spread of zoonotic diseases.
10. Explain the general principles of epidemiology and their applications to public health.
11. Explain the general principles of food hygiene and their applications to public health.
12. Explain the general principles underlying disease prevention.
13. Discuss features of appropriate housing and nutrition for animals.
14. List and discuss types of vaccinations and schedules of vaccinations for domestic animal species.
15. Explain the principles of sanitation that relate to disease prevention.
16. Describe factors that predispose to disease.
17. Discuss general principles of incorporating a wellness program into a veterinary facility.

KEY TERMS

Anaphylaxis
Autoimmune disease
Blood group antigens
Capsid
Caseous exudate
Concussion
Contusion
Cyclozoonosis
Endemic
Endotoxin
Enzootic
Epidemic
Epidemiology
Epizootic
Etiology
Exotoxin
Exudate
Fibrosis
Granulation tissue
Interstitium
Isotype
Laceration
Lymphocytes
Lymphokine
Macrophage
Monokine
Necropsy
Negri bodies
Neurotropic
Opsonization
Pathology
Phagocytosis
Plasmacyte (plasma cell)
Public health
Pyogenic
Pyrexia
Pyrogen
Recombinant vaccine
Reservoir
Toxoid
Urticaria
Vaccine
Virus
Wound

PATHOLOGY

Pathology is the study of disease. Disease is any alteration from the normal state of health. Disease may range from a superficial skin laceration to widely disseminated metastatic neoplasia (malignant tumors spread to many different organs). A pathologist is one who studies diseases and often is responsible for accurate diagnosis, as well as determining the cause, or etiology, of those diseases. Pathologists are trained in different areas of expertise, including either anatomic pathology or clinical pathology. A veterinary pathologist is a specialist who, after receiving an advanced degree in veterinary pathology, is employed by veterinary schools, state diagnostic laboratories, or pharmaceutical companies.

The primary responsibility of a veterinary anatomic pathologist is the prosection (dissection) of cadavers (carcasses) presented for **necropsy**, which is analogous to an autopsy in humans. During necropsy the pathologist collects tissue sections from lesions, which are grossly observable diseased tissues, and examines them with a microscope. Evaluating tissues with a microscope is called histopathology. The study of causes of disease, or sometimes the causes themselves, are referred to as the **etiology**. Histopathology may allow the pathologist an insight into the etiology and prognosis of the disease. The prognosis is the expected outcome of the patient affected by the disease, and is usually stated as good, guarded, or poor. Veterinary anatomic pathologists also evaluate tissues that have been surgically removed by the veterinarian. Thus, these tissues are often referred to as surgical biopsies.

Veterinary clinical pathologists evaluate components of the blood as well as types of bodily fluids such as transudates and exudates. These provide valuable information regarding the causes and prognoses of diseases.

TERMINOLOGY

Pathologists use specific terms to describe the lesions observed at necropsy and with the microscope. Gross lesions are described by stating the location, color, size, texture, and appearance of the altered tissue (Box 12-1). The diagnosis may be a morphologic (anatomic) diagnosis or an etiologic (cause) diagnosis. The morphologic diagnosis is usually limited to describing the lesion within that organ system. An example of a morphologic diagnosis is "acute necrotizing enteritis," which states that the intestine is inflamed and necrotic and that it occurred very suddenly. The corresponding etiologic diagnosis may be "enteric salmonellosis," which means that the animal had the intestinal form of infection with *Salmonella* bacteria. Other bacterial and viral agents may also cause the lesions described in the morphologic diagnosis, so acute necrotizing enteritis does not always indicate a specific diagnosis of enteric salmonellosis.

Fever, Inflammation, and Response to Injury

Fever and inflammation are protective responses of the animal's body to fight infection resulting from pathogens (disease-causing agents). Pathogens include viruses, bacteria, parasites, fungi, and molds. Pathogens are described in more detail later in the chapter.

Fever, Inflammation, and Response to Injury

Fever, also called **pyrexia,** is an abnormal increase in body temperature caused by the release of agents, called **pyrogens,** within the body. Pyrogens can be thought of as substances that cause the body to adjust its biological "thermostat" to a higher setting. This differs from hyperthermia, in which the body temperature increases above the body's "thermostat setting" because of such things as drugs, toxins, or external temperatures, as in heatstroke. Many pyrogens are released by the body's own immune cells when they encounter pathogens; however, some pathogens also produce substances that act as pyrogens. Fever serves important functions in the body: It activates phagocytes, including neutrophils, and causes iron to be sequestered out of the blood, thereby depriving many pathogens of a mineral they need for survival.

> **TECHNICIAN NOTE** Pyrogens are agents that cause an abnormal increase in body temperature.

Signs of Inflammation

The five cardinal signs of inflammation are heat, redness, swelling, pain, and loss of function (Box 12-2). These signs result from complex interactions between the cells and fluids in the involved area. Initial vasodilation (dilation of blood vessels) increases the flow of blood to the site of inflammation, resulting in an increase in temperature and redness. The dilation causes the blood vessels to leak, thereby allowing more blood, including phagocytes, other white blood cells, clotting factors, and fluid to enter an area. The swelling is caused by decreased flow of blood away from the site of inflammation, as well as possible edema, or increased fluid in the tissues. The pain and loss of function (if the inflammation is severe) are the result of pressure on the peripheral nerves at the site of inflammation. Additionally, the immune system and hemostatic (blood clotting) factors may be involved in

BOX 12-1 Description of Gross Lesions

Location
Color
Size
Texture
Appearance of altered tissue

BOX 12-2 Signs of Inflammation

Heat
Swelling
Pain
Redness
Loss of function

the inflammatory process, making it a very integrated and complex series of biochemical events.

Cells of the Inflammatory Process

The cells involved in the inflammatory process are the leukocytes (white blood cells). Leukocytes include neutrophils, eosinophils, lymphocytes, and monocytes. Other cells throughout the body (but not within the bloodstream), such as mast cells, and **macrophages** also play a key role in the inflammatory process.

Neutrophils are the first leukocytes participating in the chain of events that occurs during an inflammatory reaction. The cells exit the blood vessels at the site by "squeezing" through the microscopic space between the endothelial cells lining the blood vessels. This process is called diapedesis. The primary function of neutrophils in the inflammatory process is **phagocytosis,** or ingestion of pathogens, as well as release of lysosomal enzymes, which destroy the pathogens. Neutrophils are very short lived; they survive for only 24 to 48 hours once they leave the blood vessels and enter the host tissues.

Eosinophils, so named because they have eosinophilic (pink to reddish-orange) granules, also participate in inflammatory reactions. However, they are more specific than neutrophils and usually are prominent only in inflammation associated with parasitic infestations and allergic reactions. Like neutrophils, eosinophils have two major roles: (1) phagocytosis and (2) lysosomal enzyme release.

Lymphocytes are another type of important leukocytes in the inflammatory process. Like neutrophils, lymphocytes migrate to the tissue site of inflammation, but they have a very different role in the inflammatory process. They are responsible for humoral antibody production and cellular immunity. Lymphocytes can be divided into B-lymphocytes and T-lymphocytes; however, these two groups cannot be distinguished microscopically. B-lymphocytes can be transformed into **plasma cells** (also known as plasmacytes), which produce antibodies. T-lymphocytes are capable of directly killing cells. They also secrete **lymphokines,** chemical substances that influence and help to activate many other cells of the immune system.

Monocytes are a stage in the development of tissue macrophages. Once monocytes leave the bloodstream and enter the tissue at the site of the inflammatory process, they become activated macrophages. Macrophages are the workhorses of the inflammatory process; they contain a large number of lysosomal enzymes that kill pathogens. They are capable of phagocytosis, in which they extend their cell membranes around a pathogen, engulfing it, and thereby incorporating it into the macrophage where lysosomal enzymes will destroy it. Other macrophages are present in fixed locations in the body and have different names depending on their location. In the liver, they are referred to as Kupfer cells. They are called microglial cells in the brain and histiocytes in loose connective tissue.

Inflammatory Exudates

An **exudate** is the visible product of the inflammatory process. It is usually composed of cellular debris, fluids, and cells that are deposited in tissues as well as on tissue surfaces, such as the serosal, mucosal, and skin surfaces. Exudates may be classified based on their primary constituent, such as serous, fibrinous, purulent (or suppurative), or others.

> *TECHNICIAN NOTE* Exudate classifications include serous, fibrinous, purulent (or suppurative), hemorrhagic, mucopurulent (or catarrhal), eosinophilic, and nonsuppurative.

Serous exudates consist primarily of fluid with low protein content. Cutaneous blisters are examples of lesions that contain a serous exudate. Fibrinous exudates are composed chiefly of fibrin, which is derived from a plasma protein, fibrinogen. Fibrinous exudate is observed in traumatic reticulopericarditis ("hardware disease"). This disease can occur when a cow ingests a metallic foreign body (nail or wire) that penetrates the forestomach (reticulum) and subsequently penetrates the diaphragm and pericardium, the membranous sac surrounding the heart. As a result, a large amount of fibrin collects in the pericardial sac. The proper morphologic diagnosis for this lesion is fibrinous pericarditis.

Purulent or suppurative exudates are composed primarily of large numbers of neutrophils and cellular debris (Fig. 12-1). Abscesses contain a purulent or suppurative exudate (pus).

Hemorrhagic exudates consist primarily of erythrocytes that have collected in a tissue after disruption of the vascular system. Other less common types of exudate include mucopurulent (or catarrhal), eosinophilic, and nonsuppurative.

Mucopurulent exudates consist of a mixture of purulent and mucous exudates. They are commonly found in tissues that secrete mucus (i.e., have a mucous membrane), such as the intestinal and respiratory tracts.

Eosinophilic exudates are composed primarily of eosinophils and are associated with such diseases as eosinophilic granuloma complex of cats, eosinophilic myositis of dogs, and salt poisoning of pigs (Fig. 12-2).

Nonsuppurative exudates are composed primarily of monocytes or histiocytes along with lymphocytes. The term

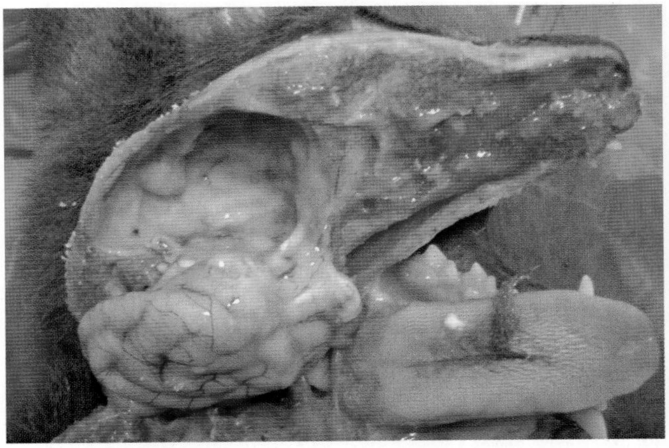

FIGURE 12-1 Purulent exudates in braincase of a cat.

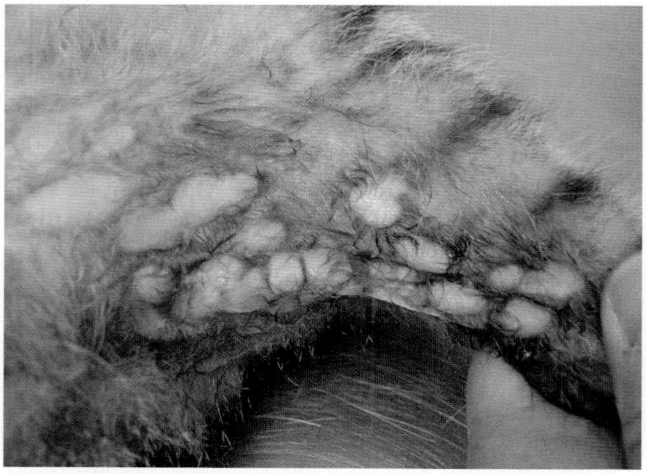

FIGURE 12-2 Eosinophilic granuloma complex in a cat.

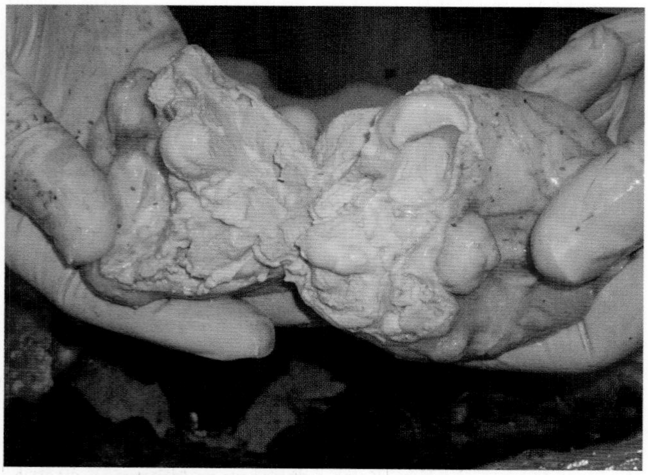

FIGURE 12-3 Caseopurulent abdominal abscess in a rabbit.

nonsuppurative is usually restricted to exudates in only two anatomic sites: (1) the central nervous system and (2) the integumentary system (skin). Occasionally, purulent material tissue can change into a thick, pasty material, which resembles cheese. This is called a **caseous exudate.** Finally, exudates may consist of intermediate stages or combinations of the previously mentioned types, such as fibrinopurulent, necrohemorrhagic, or caseopurulent exudates (Fig. 12-3).

Vascular Changes Associated With Inflammation

The cellular response associated with inflammation is only a part of the inflammatory process; the blood vessels or vascular system are also involved. Blood vessels are highly dynamic structures that respond rapidly during inflammation. The first response of the blood vessel to vascular injury is dilation, which means the diameter of the blood vessel increases, allowing more blood to flow into the affected area. This is caused by local release of histamine from mast cells. Next there is increased vascular permeability, which means the blood vessels become slightly "leaky." This is the result

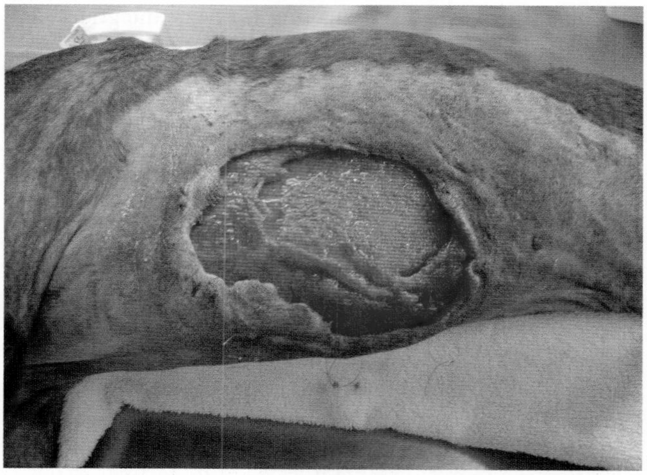

FIGURE 12-4 Granulation tissue forming under an area of sloughed skin on a dog's abdomen.

of contraction of endothelial cells lining the inside of blood vessels. Increased vascular permeability allows a wide array of proteins to pass through the vessel walls to the site of inflammation. Immediately after vascular permeability increases, the process of exudation allows an influx of leukocytes and red blood cells to the inflammatory site. Congestion of the blood vessels occurs in the next step, which means stasis or "sludging" of blood flow in the vessels from fluid loss through exudation.

All of these events work in concert with the cells associated with inflammation such that the host is able to repair the injured site and defend itself against infection. The entire process occurs rapidly, beginning with vascular dilation, which occurs within minutes of the initial insult, and ending with initiation of congestion within 8 hours of the initial vascular dilation.

Healing and Repair of Damaged Tissues

The repair process really starts as soon as injury occurs, but healing is the last event to be completed in the inflammatory process. In almost every organ system, the end result of tissue repair is **fibrosis,** or scarring. The exception to this is in the central nervous system, which includes the brain and the spinal cord. Fibrosis does not occur in the central nervous system because it would be detrimental to the functioning of these vital tissues. A **wound** is an injury caused by physical means, with disruption of normal structures.

> TECHNICIAN NOTE The end result of tissue repair is usually fibrosis or scarring.

Granulation tissue is a highly vascularized connective tissue that is only produced after extensive tissue damage (Fig. 12-4). Re-epithelialization eventually occurs unless excessive granulation tissue forms, a condition commonly referred to by lay people as "proud flesh." It is a difficult and lengthy process for re-epithelialization to occur over

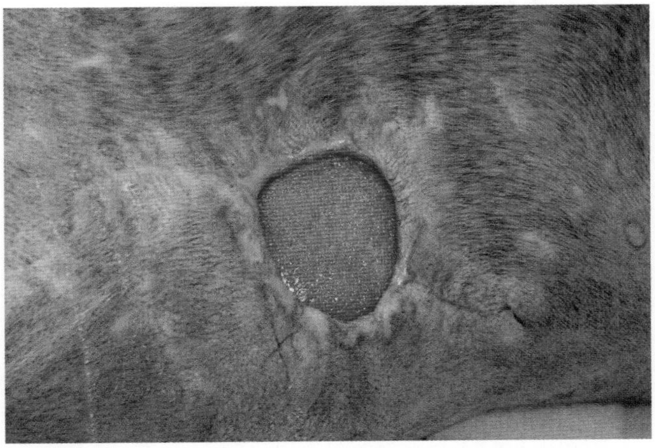

FIGURE 12-5 Same wound from Fig. 12-4, 1 month later.

large amounts of granulation tissue. Therefore, it is optimal for wound edges to be brought together whenever possible in wound closure. Otherwise, the excessive granulation tissue must be removed before the wound surface can be re-epithelialized.

Fibrosis or scar tissue primarily comprises dense fibrous connective tissue and collagen and contracts when mature. In parenchymatous organ systems, such as the lungs, kidneys, liver, and spleen, scar tissue is usually characterized as a small, irregular focus that has shrunken beneath the capsule of the organ. On the skin, a scar or cicatrix is the contracted area of fibrous tissue that remains under the re-epithelialized dermis after the healing of wound (Fig. 12-5).

PATHOGENS

Pathogens are infectious organisms that can cause disease in a host. Pathogenic agents include multicelled and single-celled parasites, protozoans, bacteria, fungi, rickettsiae, mycoplasmas, chlamydiae, and viruses. Many of these organisms are very specific in their ability to cause disease in only certain animal species. In some cases, they affect very specific organs or organ systems of the body.

Parasites

Parasites are organisms that have adapted to live on or within a host organism, deriving all of their nutrients from that host, ideally without killing the host. Nomenclature can be confusing because all the pathogens described in the preceding may live on or in a host organism from which they derive a benefit while the host may experience disease. However, we generally use the word parasite only in conjunction with multicelled organisms such as worms, flukes, and arthropods, or single-celled protozoans; whereas we tend to classify bacteria, fungi, rickettsiae, mycoplasmas, chlamydiae, and viruses separately. Chapter 10 contains an extensive discussion of internal and external parasites.

Bacteria

Bacteria make up another group of pathogens that cause disease in animals. Bacteria are single-celled organisms referred to as prokaryotes, because they lack a nucleus and organelles, and their DNA consists of one double-stranded chromosome. These are some of the things that differentiate them from all other types of cells, the eukaryotes. Most bacteria have a cell wall outside their cell membrane, as do plant and fungal eukaryotic cells, although composed of different materials. It is the staining characteristics of this cell wall that form two major classifications of bacteria. Bacteria are classified as either gram-positive or gram-negative, depending on the staining characteristics of their cell walls with Gram stain. Gram-positive organisms stain purple, and gram-negative organisms stain red. As a general rule, gram-negative bacteria contain **endotoxins** (substances that cause disease) in their cell walls, while gram-positive bacteria contain preformed **exotoxins,** which they secrete into the surrounding medium. Some bacteria are **pyogenic** and cause the host to produce a purulent exudate. Within the infected host, bacteria may be found in the **interstitium** (between cell layers), within inflammatory cells, or on epithelial surfaces. See Chapter 9 for more information on identification of bacteria.

Animals with bacterial infections are often febrile, lethargic, and anorexic. In part this is caused by the associated endotoxins, which stimulate release of an endogenous pyrogen from the host's neutrophils. Endogenous pyrogen is a protein that causes fever and associated lethargy and inappetence. However, this protein aids the animal by increasing its body temperature and allowing neutrophils to be more effective in killing bacteria. Bacterial virulence factors determine the pathogenicity of bacteria. In addition to the cell wall, the surface of bacteria may contain such structures as pili and capsules. These virulence factors allow the bacteria to more easily attach to and colonize tissues and minimize the host immune response. Additionally, bacteria may possess a wide variety of enzymes or proteins, known as soluble factors, which inhibit host functions and provide the bacteria a "foothold" within the host.

Viruses

Viruses are extremely small infectious agents, ranging from 30 to 450 nm in diameter, which can cause disease in a wide variety of animals. To put their size in perspective, assume that an average mammalian red blood cell was the size of a large house. Using this scale, an average bacterium would be about the size of a car and viruses would range from the size of a penny to the size of a small child. For viruses to cause disease, they must enter the animal's body, bind to the surface of a host cell, enter the cell, and destroy it. Viruses are technically nonliving agents, which consist of genetic material in the form of either DNA or RNA surrounded by a protein coat, called a **capsid.** Some viruses may have an envelope, derived in part from the host cell membrane, which surrounds the protein coat. After the virus enters a host cell, it uses the host cell's machinery to transcribe, translate, and replicate the viral genetic material, thereby creating new viral proteins and new viruses. Viruses can destroy the cells by suppressing the cells' metabolic activity or causing the cells to lyse, releasing the newly formed viruses. In some instances, viruses may cause no immediate damage and may remain latent in cells for years.

Certain viruses are specific for the type of cells they attack. For example, epitheliotropic viruses attack epithelial cells, such as respiratory, intestinal, or urinary epithelium. The clinical signs of these viral diseases are often associated with death of the infected cells. For example, canine distemper virus, a morbillivirus, attaches to and destroys the epithelium of the dog's lungs. Dogs with distemper may develop coughing and respiratory distress because of the effect of viral infection of the lung. The result is interstitial pneumonia caused by the inflammatory infiltrates within the interstitium of the lung. Transmissible gastroenteritis virus of pigs, caused by a coronavirus, destroys the gastric and intestinal epithelium of preweanling pigs. A lesion of transmissible gastroenteritis virus is villous atrophy; affected intestinal villi become shortened and blunted and have an atrophic appearance. Clinical signs include vomiting, diarrhea, dehydration, and death.

Viruses classified as **neurotropic** invade and destroy cells of the central nervous system. Examples of disease caused by these viruses include rabies and equine encephalitis. Rabies is caused by a rhabdovirus and has a worldwide distribution. Most cases of rabies are spread by animal bites; the virus is present in the saliva of infected animals. After the virus enters the body, it travels to the central nervous system by way of peripheral nerves. Once it enters the central nervous system, it infects and destroys neurons. Animals infected with this virus develop behavioral changes and sometimes become aggressive, which may result in biting other animals or humans. The lesions of rabies are those of nonsuppurative encephalitis. Diagnosis is dependent on demonstration of characteristic **Negri bodies** (eosinophilic inclusion bodies) within affected neurons (Fig. 12-6).

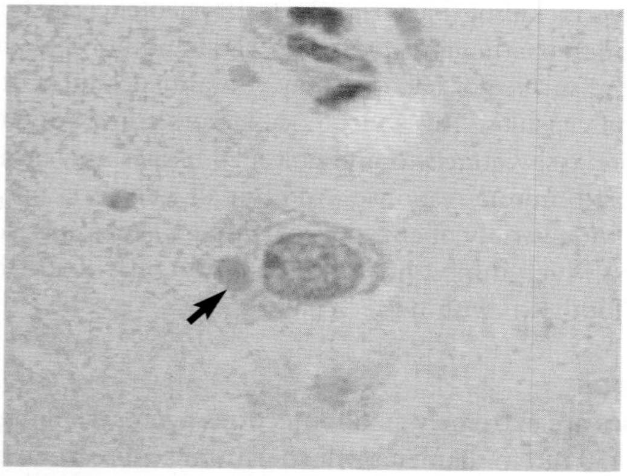

FIGURE 12-6 Negri body in rabies-infected neuron.

As is the case of parasites and bacteria, a large number of viruses can infect animals. A list of some common viruses that cause disease in animals is presented in Table 12-1.

NONPATHOGENS

Disease can also be produced in animals by nonpathogens. Nonpathogenic causes of disease include trauma associated with mechanical, sonic, thermal, and electrical injuries, temperature extremes, and irradiation.

The primary effects of trauma, regardless of the initiating cause, are tissue necrosis and hemorrhage. Trauma is a physical wound or injury. Internal, localized mechanical injury can be associated with such things as intestinal foreign bodies, which can cause necrosis by strangulating blood supply to the intestines (Fig. 12-7). An abrasion is an injury whereby the epithelium is removed from the tissue surface. A **contusion** is a bruise or injury with no break in the surface of the tissue. A **laceration** is a tear or jagged wound. A **concussion** is a violent shock or jarring of the tissue, a common injury to the brain after blunt trauma to the head. In all of these instances, the inflammatory process occurs as described previously in this chapter, with the exception of destruction and removal of the pathogen.

IMMUNE RESPONSE

The immune system is another inherent protective mechanism of the body. This highly complex and complicated system has many components that, along with the inflammatory process, prevent pathogens from causing disease or aid in recovery from disease. The immune system consists of nonspecific defenses and specific defenses.

Nonspecific defenses include the body's defenses against pathogens in general, regardless of pathogen type. These include mechanical barriers to infection, such as skin and

TABLE 12-1 Some Viruses That Cause Disease in Animals

VIRUS CLASSIFICATION	DISEASE	HOST	LESIONS
Morbillivirus	Canine distemper	Canidae, mink, raccoon, ferret	Pneumonia, encephalitis
Herpes virus	Pseudorabies	Pig	Abortion, encephalitis
Herpes virus	Infectious laryngotracheitis	Avian	Laryngotracheitis
Adenovirus	Infectious canine hepatitis	Canidae	Acute necrotizing hepatitis
Papillomavirus	Sarcoid	Horse	Sarcoids (neoplasm)
Rhabdovirus	Rabies	Mammals	Fatal encephalomyelitis
Coronavirus	Transmissible gastroenteritis (TGE)	Pig	Enteritis, villous atrophy
Coronavirus	Feline infectious peritonitis (FIP)	Cat	Peritonitis, pleuritis
Alphavirus *(Arbovirus)*	Eastern, western, Venezuelan equine encephalitis	Horse	Encephalitis

mucous membranes, chemical barriers such as lysozymes in tears, salt in sweat, antiviral substances such as interferon in blood, and acid in the stomach. Fever and inflammation, discussed earlier, are also part of the nonspecific defenses.

Specific defenses comprise what is normally thought of as immunity: the body's protection against very specific pathogens. Specific defenses include antibodies, complement, lymphocytes, and macrophages and are divided into humoral immune responses and cell-mediated immune responses. The primary components of the humoral response are antibodies produced by plasma cells, which are transformed B-lymphocytes. B-lymphocytes are one of two major subsets of lymphocytes. The other major subset, referred to as T-lymphocytes, plays a major role in the cell-mediated response. B-lymphocytes are distributed throughout the body within the lymph nodes, spleen, Peyer's patches, and other organs. B-lymphocytes are so named because they were first discovered in the bursa of Fabricius, a lymphoid organ of birds. T-lymphocytes are so designated because they arise from the thymus, a lymphoid organ of birds and mammals. All mammals, as well as birds, possess both B-lymphocytes and T-lymphocytes. These lymphocytes cannot be distinguished by their morphology because they look identical under the microscope; however, they can be differentiated by their function. They may also be differentiated by their cell surface markers, which are molecules attached to their surface, necessary for binding with substances such as antigens, antibodies, and other immune cells.

Humoral Immunity

Humoral immunity implies that antibodies are produced against a particular pathogen. When the pathogen enters the host's body, it becomes coated with antibodies, allowing it to be more easily destroyed by cells of the inflammatory process. Antibodies are protein molecules that can attach to the surface of cells and coat pathogens. Antibodies bind to portions of certain molecules, usually proteins or polysaccharides, on the surface of the cell or pathogen. The molecule to which an antibody attaches is called an antigen, and the particular part of the antigen that binds the antibody is more specifically known as the antigenic determinant, or epitope. Antigens can be any substances that elicit a response upon exposure to the immune system, and can range from molecules in a pathogenic bacterium's cell wall to usually harmless substances such as pollen. Pollen antigens do not normally elicit abnormal immune reactions unless the body is allergic to pollen. Even normal body cells contain antigen; unfortunately, sometimes those antigens also elicit an abnormal immune response. This is known as an **autoimmune disease,** and examples include such diseases as systemic lupus erythematosus and rheumatoid arthritis.

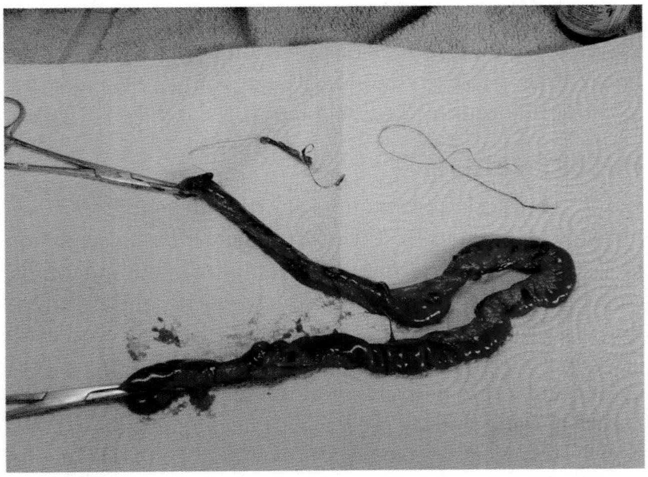

FIGURE 12-7 Necrotic jejunum in cat that had a linear foreign body. Note the piece of string.

Antibodies can be detected in the serum of animals; the study and application of this science is known as serology. The principles of serology and immunology are discussed in more detail in Chapter 8. The level of antibodies present in the serum (blood) is reported as an antibody titer. Antibody titers provide a measure of the highest dilution of the serum containing antibody that still gives a positive reaction to the serologic test being performed. Although a very high antibody titer to certain pathogens may indicate protection against or immunity to a specific pathogen, it may be very difficult to differentiate between vaccine-induced immunity, natural immunity, or current infection. For example, with feline immunodeficiency virus (FIV), a cat that is infected with the virus will have a positive antibody titer; however, a cat that is vaccinated against the virus will also have a positive titer. It is not possible to distinguish an infected cat from a vaccinated cat. With other diseases, special tests may be performed to make the distinction. This used to be the case with Lyme disease, when a test called Western blot needed to be done to differentiate between vaccine-induced immunity and natural immunity from exposure; however, recent advances have resulted in tests that measure antibodies induced by infection, as opposed to antibodies induced by vaccination.

Natural immunity implies that the animal has been exposed to the pathogen by natural means rather than through vaccination. With natural immunity, the animal may have previously become ill from infection with a specific pathogen and may have produced antibodies against the pathogen during the disease.

Antibodies, or immunoglobulins, can be separated by their molecular weight into different classes or **isotypes,** including IgG, IgM, IgA, and IgE. The antibody isotype IgG is the most common antibody and is found in the highest concentration in the blood. It helps defend tissues by coating the outer surface of pathogens, a process called **opsonization,** which allows them to be more easily phagocytized by macrophages. The isotype IgM is the second most common antibody in the blood. It is the major immunoglobulin isotype produced in a primary immune response. It is more efficient than IgG in opsonization and neutralization of viruses. The isotype IgA is of primary importance for mucosal immunity. This antibody is secreted onto the mucosal surface of such organs as the lungs and gastrointestinal tract. It binds to pathogens to prevent them from adhering to mucosal surfaces, preventing them from gaining a foothold in the body. The isotype IgE is the primary immunoglobulin associated with Type-1 hypersensitivity reactions, which are discussed later in the chapter. It also plays a role in helminth infestations, along with certain cells from the inflammatory process, including eosinophils.

> **TECHNICIAN NOTE** Humoral immunity involves production of antibody, whereas cell-mediated immunity primarily involves actions of T-lymphocytes.

Cell-Mediated Immunity

The cell-mediated immune response primarily involves T-lymphocytes and macrophages. Cell-mediated immunity may begin in several ways. A macrophage may phagocytize a pathogen, then present an antigen from the pathogen on its surface. When a type of T-lymphocyte known as a helper T-cell binds to the antigen on the macrophage surface, both cells secrete specific cytokines; **monokines** are produced by the macrophage and lymphokines are produced by the T-lymphocyte. These cytokines stimulate macrophages to become more efficient in phagocytosis and pathogen destruction, and recruit more T-lymphocytes to the area, including a type of T-lymphocyte called a cytotoxic T-cell. Cytotoxic T-cells will then search for the pathogen in infected body cells and destroy them.

Hypersensitivity Reactions

Abnormally severe inflammatory responses mediated by the immune system are called hypersensitivity reactions. These allergic reactions have been classified into four types: Type I (immediate), Type II (cytotoxic), Type III (immune complex), and Type IV (delayed).

Type-I hypersensitivity reactions occur within minutes after exposure to an antigen. Animals may be exposed to antigens by direct contact, inhalation, ingestion, insect bites or stings, or injection. Examples of antigens include pollen, proteins (e.g., in food, milk, or bacterial cell walls), and plant resins (e.g., in poison ivy or poison oak). Antigens are often referred to as allergens when they evoke an allergic reaction.

Type-I reactions are mediated by IgE antibodies on the surface of mast cells located on mucosal surfaces (airways, intestines) and in connective tissues. Upon exposure, the antigen is bound by IgE, causing the mast cells to release granules containing various factors, such as histamine, serotonin, and leukotrienes. These factors cause vasodilation, increased vascular permeability, smooth muscle contraction, and other inflammatory changes.

The severity and manifestation of a Type-I hypersensitivity reaction depend on the location and number of mast cells stimulated as well as the route of exposure and amount of antigen involved. Reactions may be relatively mild, such as **urticaria** (hives) after a bee sting or diarrhea after eating a particular food ingredient. However, Type-I reactions can also be very severe, such as acute **anaphylaxis,** which is characterized by profound hypotension (low blood pressure), pulmonary edema, and collapse, caused by massive exposure to an antigen.

Type-II hypersensitivity reactions involve destruction of certain cells by neutrophils and macrophages or activation of complement. Complement is a group of enzymes that act in sequential fashion, leading to disruption of tissue or bacterial cell membranes and resulting in the cell's destruction. An adverse reaction to blood transfusion is an example of a Type-II reaction.

On their surface, red blood cells contain antigens called **blood group antigens.** In some species, animals of the same species may develop antibodies against blood groups other than their own. The red cells function normally, and no immune response results if blood from one animal is transfused to a recipient with the same blood group. However, if blood is transfused into a recipient with a different blood group, the donor's red cells are destroyed by hemolysis (rupture) because of complement, phagocytosis because of macrophages, or become agglutinated (clumped) because of massive antibody binding with numerous red blood cells. Depending on the species, the first of such incompatible transfusions may be tolerated. However, the transfusion stimulates production of antibodies, and these antibodies immediately modulate destruction of the red cells in a second transfusion.

In Type-III hypersensitivity reactions, antigens and antibodies interact to form immune complexes that become lodged in various tissues, such as the skin, joints, eyes, lungs, or blood vessel walls. Macrophages gather in these areas to destroy the immune complexes, resulting in inflammation. Examples of Type-III reactions include rheumatoid arthritis and equine viral arteritis.

Type-IV hypersensitivity reactions occur hours after sensitized animals are again exposed to a particular antigen. These delayed hypersensitivity reactions reach their peak at about 24 hours after exposure and are mediated by sensitized T-cells. The tuberculin test used in cattle is a classic example of Type-IV hypersensitivity. A small volume of extract of *Mycobacterium tuberculosis* is injected into the skin of the animal. Normal cattle show no significant response to the injection. Cattle previously exposed to *Mycobacterium tuberculosis,* however, develop a large, warm swelling at the injection site within 12 to 24 hours.

PUBLIC HEALTH

Public health is a community's effort to prevent disease and promote life and health. The effort usually includes sanitation of the environment, control of communicable infections, education of individuals in personal hygiene, and organization of medical and nursing services to ensure proper health care. Veterinary public health plays an important role in protecting and improving human well-being by using veterinary knowledge and skills to preserve the healthy relationship between humans and animals. The veterinary profession's major roles in preventing disease in people are in epidemiology, food hygiene, and zoonotic disease.

EPIDEMIOLOGY

Epidemiology is the study of the occurrences of disease and the risk factors that cause disease in a population. Some texts refer to the study of disease in an animal population as epizootiology, but the term epidemiology is appropriate for both human and animal populations and is a more widely recognized term. Descriptive epidemiology studies the frequency of disease in a population and describes the type of animals affected and how and when they are affected. In other words, it describes the disease in terms of the animal or people affected and the time and geographic region in which they are affected. This information gives epidemiologists clues about the cause of disease, allows them to form hypotheses about the cause, and helps them determine the risk that animals or people will become ill. Epidemiologists can then design more elaborate analytic epidemiologic studies to test these hypotheses. Once the cause of the disease and the risk factors that influence the disease are identified, programs for control or prevention of the disease can be implemented. Epidemiologists are essential professionals in veterinary and human public health efforts to study the cause and initiate the control of disease.

FOOD HYGIENE

The field of food hygiene involves making sure that food is safe and wholesome for human consumption. Proper food hygiene is important in preventing food-borne diseases. An estimated 10 million people in the United States become ill with food-borne diseases. Primarily, veterinarians are involved in the food-hygiene process through inspection and processing of animals for food. Proper inspection and processing are essential in prevention of food-borne diseases that originate from contamination with bacteria at the slaughterhouse. These organisms are the cause of significant disease in people. Some of the most common organisms involved are *Salmonella* spp., *Campylobacter* spp., and *E. coli* 0157:H7. Outbreaks of *E. coli* have occurred periodically over the past few years in a number of people, especially children, who ate undercooked foods that were contaminated with the pathogen. *E. coli* 0157:H7 infection causes hemolytic uremia and may result in death. The most common source of *Salmonella* in the United States is poultry or poultry products, such as eggs. In fact, *Salmonella enteritidis* infection has become a highly reported food-borne disease in the United States and has generated new recommendations for the public in handling raw egg products. Proper cooking and handling of meat can help prevent serious disease. Other food-borne diseases can be caused by contamination of food and improper handling, such as *Staphylococcus* infection, *Clostridium* infection (botulism), and hepatitis.

An important step in food hygiene before an animal reaches the slaughterhouse is prevention of adulterating residues. Residues are hormonal compounds, antibacterials, antimycotics, anthelmintics, antiprotozoals, or pesticides in meat or milk that have accumulated to levels that are above the established safe tolerance levels. The U.S. Department of Agriculture (USDA) monitors foodstuffs for the presence of residues and is responsible for inspection of food. The U.S. Environmental Protection Agency (EPA) sets the residue limits for pesticides. The U.S. Food and Drug Administration (FDA) sets the limits for drug residues.

How do drugs become residues? Most drug residues are caused by misuse of drugs. Misuse of drugs includes not following label directions, using drugs in unapproved species, and not adhering to withdrawal times. Residues can occur in meat or milk through misuse of drugs in mastitis treatments or with injectable antibiotics. In addition, feed or drinking water can be contaminated with drugs or pesticides.

Residues are important to public health because they can cause toxic or allergic reactions in people. For example, penicillin residues in milk can cause a severe, life-threatening reaction in a person who is allergic to penicillin. Veterinarians and veterinary technicians are responsible for using drugs in food animals according to standard veterinary practice.

ZOONOTIC DISEASES

Zoonoses are the major area of involvement for veterinarians in public health. Zoonoses are diseases that are transmitted between animals and people; however, this definition is not always very clear-cut. Some diseases are indirect zoonoses and can be transmitted to animals and humans, and between species, by arthropods such as ticks or mosquitoes. Still other infectious diseases are common to but not transmitted between animals and people; these can be caused by similar exposures to the same infectious organism. More than 150 zoonoses have been reported, and diseases not previously thought to be zoonotic are frequently added to the list. For example, *Bordetella bronchiseptica,* one of the pathogens associated with the canine infectious respiratory disease (CIRD) complex, was previously not believed to be zoonotic; however, recently it has been discovered to be transmissible to humans. Zoonoses are a significant cause of human disability, hospitalization, death, and high economic cost in the United States and underdeveloped countries. Table 12-2 lists the causative organism, hosts, and mode of transmission for some common zoonoses.

Veterinarians are concerned with monitoring and surveillance of zoonoses, evaluating risks to people, and planning and coordinating prevention and control programs with appropriate agencies and individuals. Part of that surveillance is looking for an outbreak or epizootic of the disease. An **epizootic** is an increase over the normal expected number of disease cases in a geographic area or a certain period. In human medicine, the term **epidemic** is used; however, this term has become accepted in veterinary medicine as well and has largely replaced the term epizootic. An **enzootic** disease is one that has maintained a certain level of disease over time in a given geographic area. In human medicine, the term **endemic** is used, and once again, this has become the term of choice in veterinary medicine as well. For example, rabies is endemic or always present at a certain level in raccoons in the eastern United States. However, in the late 1970s and early 1980s, when rabies began appearing more frequently in the mid-Atlantic area, it was considered

TABLE 12-2 The Causative Organisms, Animal Hosts, and Modes of Transmission for Selected Common Zoonoses

	CAUSATIVE ORGANISMS	SMALL ANIMAL HOSTS	LIVESTOCK HOSTS	WILDLIFE HOSTS	MODES OF TRANSMISSION
Viral Diseases					
Rabies	Rhabdovirus	Most	Most	Most	Animal bite
Encephalitis (EEE, WEE)	Togavirus	Horses, poultry	Birds, rodents	Mosquito bite	
Lymphocytic choriomeningitis	Arenavirus	Mice	Varied		
Contagious ecthyma (orf)	Pox virus	Sometimes dogs	Sheep, goats	Contact	
Simian herpes (B virus)	Herpesvirus simiae	Primates	Animal bite, direct contact		
Newcastle disease	Paramyxovirus	Domestic birds	Poultry	Wild fowl	Contact, inhalation
Yellow fever	Togavirus	Primates	Mosquito bite		
Hantavirus infection	Hantavirus	Rodents	Contact		
Rickettsial Diseases					
Q fever	*Coxiella burnetii*	Cattle, sheep, goats	Birds, rabbits, rodents	Inhalation, milk ingestion, contact	
Rocky Mountain spotted fever	*Rickettsia rickettsii*	Dogs	Rodents, rabbits	Tick bite	
Psittacosis	*Chlamydia psittaci*	Psittacine birds	Turkeys, ducks	Birds	Inhalation
Mycoses					
Ringworm	*Trichophyton* spp., *Microsporum* spp.	Cats, dogs	Cattle, horses, pigs, sheep	Rodents	Contact
Parasitic Diseases					
Trichinosis	*Trichinella spiralis*	Pigs	Rats, bears, carnivores	Ingestion	
Scabies	*Sarcoptes scabiei*	Dogs, rodents, cats	Horses	Primates	Contact
Taeniasis, Cysticercosis	*Taenia* spp., *Cysticercus*	Pigs, cattle	Boars	Ingestion	
Hydatid disease	*Echinococcus* spp.	Dogs	Herbivores	Wolves	Ingestion
Schistosomiasis	*Schistosoma* spp.	Dogs, cats	Pigs, cattle, horses	Rodents	Contact
Larva migrans	*Toxocara, Ancylostoma, Strongyloides*	Dogs, cats	Pigs, cattle	Raccoons	Ingestion
Bacterial Diseases					
Anthrax	*Bacillus anthracis*	Dogs	Most	Most except primates	Contact
Brucellosis	*Brucella* spp.	Dogs	Cattle, pigs, sheep, goats	All except primates	Contact, inhalation, ingestion
Plague	*Yersinia pestis*	Cats	Rodents, rabbits	Flea bite	
Campylobacteriosis	*Campylobacter fetus fetus*	Dogs, cats	Cattle, poultry, sheep, pigs	Rodents, birds	Ingestion, contact
Cat-scratch disease	*Bartonella henselae*	Cats	Cats	Cat bite, scratch	
Leptospirosis	*Leptospira* spp.	All, especially dogs	All, especially cattle, pigs	Rats, raccoons	Contact with urine
Salmonellosis	*Salmonella* spp.	All, especially dogs, cats	All, especially pigs, poultry, cattle	Rodents, reptiles	Ingestion
Tuberculosis	*Mycobacteria* spp.	Dogs, cats	Cattle, pigs, goats, sheep, poultry	All except rodents, monkeys	Ingestion, inhalation
Tularemia	*Francisella tularensis*	All	All except horses	Rodents, rabbits	Tick bites, contact with tissue
Erysipelas	*Erysipelothrix rhusiopathiae*	Pigs, sheep, cattle, horses, poultry	Rodents	Contact	
Tetanus	*Clostridium tetani*	Horses	Reptiles	Wound	

Continued

TABLE 12-2 The Causative Organisms, Animal Hosts, and Modes of Transmission for Selected Common Zoonoses—cont'd

	CAUSATIVE ORGANISMS	SMALL ANIMAL HOSTS	LIVESTOCK HOSTS	WILDLIFE HOSTS	MODES OF TRANSMISSION
Lyme disease	*Borrelia burgdorferi*	Dogs, cats	Cattle, horses	Deer, birds, rodents	Tick bite
Protozoal Diseases					
Cryptosporidiosis	*Cryptosporidium* spp.	Most	Calves, sheep	Birds	Ingestion
Toxoplasmosis	*Toxoplasma gondii*	Cats, rabbits, guinea pigs	Pigs, sheep, cattle, horses	Cats	Ingestion
Balantidiasis	*Balantidium coli*	Pigs	Rats, primates	Ingestion	
Sarcocystosis	*Sarcocystis* spp.	Dogs, cats	Pigs, cattle	Ingestion	
Giardiasis	*Giardia lamblia*	Dogs, cats	Pigs, cattle	Beavers, zoo monkeys	Ingestion

epidemic. Surveillance of zoonoses or any other disease depends on knowledge about the cause of the disease, transmission of the disease, and how the disease is maintained in the population.

Disease Transmission

For an infectious disease to survive in a population, the agent causing the disease must be transmitted. The mode of transmission is an important epidemiologic clue in understanding the disease. It is important for the veterinary profession to be aware of how specific diseases are transmitted so that preventive measures can be taken and the public educated. Reservoirs and hosts of a specific disease are important to identify because these are essential in transmission of a disease and its maintenance in the population. Control programs for a disease are often aimed at the **reservoirs**, or hosts of the disease. For example, spraying programs aimed at controlling mosquito populations are initiated when there is an outbreak of encephalitis.

> TECHNICIAN NOTE Diseases can be transmitted via the direct route or indirect routes.

Reservoirs can be inanimate (e.g., soil) or animate (e.g., mammals, people, birds). Reservoirs are essential and necessary for the survival and reproduction of the organism. Hosts are living beings that offer an environment for maintenance of the organism, but they are not necessary for the organism's survival. Depending on the disease, the infectious organism may be transmitted through several hosts of different species. This is particularly true of helminth and protozoal diseases. Several hosts or reservoirs are required for the egg to develop to a larva and then to an adult. An infectious disease can be transmitted from the reservoir to a host or from one host to another host.

Direct transmission of disease requires close association or contact between a reservoir of the disease and a susceptible host. Contact with infected skin, mucous membranes, or droplets from an infected human or animal can cause disease. Examples of disease that are transmitted directly are rabies transmitted by a bite, leptospirosis by contact with contaminated urine, and brucellosis by contact with infected tissues. Another example of direct transmission is through contact with the wool, hair, or hide of an infected animal. Anthrax, although not very common in the United States, is transmitted to people through skin contact with contaminated bone meal from infected cattle or direct contact with infected wool or hair.

Animal bites can be a source of infections, trauma, and even zoonotic disease. *Pasteurella* is responsible for 50% of dog bite infections and 90% of cat bite infections. Cat bites are 10 times more likely to become infected than dog bites. Mixed infections include *Staphylococcus aureus, Staphylococcus epidermidis, Streptococcus* spp., *Bacteroides* spp., *Fusobacterium* spp., and other gram-negative bacteria that can cause fever, septicemia, meningitis, endocarditis, and septic arthritis.

Soil or vegetation contaminated with parasites, bacteria, or spores may be another source of direct transmission. Visceral larva migrans is transmitted when children eat soil or vegetables that have been contaminated with feces that contain *Toxocara* (roundworm) eggs. The eggs hatch in the individual's gastrointestinal system and the larvae migrate through the organs. The disease is usually mild and chronic, with eosinophilia, fever, hepatomegaly, and pulmonary signs. If the larvae migrate to the eye, there may be loss of vision or the eye. A similar disease occurs with ancylostoma (hookworm). The signs of cutaneous larva migrans are those of dermatitis, which is caused by the hookworm larvae migrating in the skin.

Droplet spread is differentiated from air-borne transmission by the fact that the droplets travel only a short distance (i.e., a few feet) and involve larger particles that often are removed by mechanisms in the upper respiratory passages. Psittacosis is an occupational risk at poultry processing plants. People are infected by inhalation of *Chlamydia psittaci* from the droppings or secretions of infected birds. Cage and aviary birds, especially infected large birds that are shipped into pet stores from foreign countries and not properly treated with antibiotics, can also infect people.

Indirect transmission of disease is more complicated and involves intermediaries that carry the agent of disease from one source to another. The intermediary may be air-borne, vector-borne (an arthropod), or vehicle-borne through water, food, blood, or an inanimate object. A vector is a living organism that transports the infectious agent. A vehicle is simply the mode of transmission of an infectious agent from the reservoir to the host. Indirect airborne transmission involves spread of the agent through tiny dust or droplet particles over long distances. Particles smaller than 5 microns in diameter can be inhaled into the alveoli deep within the lungs. Q fever is most commonly transmitted by air-borne transmission. It is transmitted by inhalation of the rickettsia, *Coxiella burnetii,* in dust from areas that are contaminated by tissue or excreta from infected animals. Airborne particles with the infective organism can travel a long distance, which makes it difficult to locate the source of the infection. Q fever can also be transmitted by direct contact with contaminated wool, other materials, and milk. Infected individuals may have an inapparent infection or they may have chills, headache, weakness, and sweats.

Various types of arthropods may serve as vectors. These may include mosquitoes, ticks, and fleas. Each type of arthropod has its own life cycle that is often reflected by seasonal and geographic patterns in transmission of disease. For example, ticks may have two- or three-host maturation cycles and may take 2 years to complete a life cycle. Arthropods may carry the agent mechanically to a susceptible host, or they may be involved biologically in multiplication of the organism or a stage of development.

Plague is the best-known vector-borne disease and involves the flea as a vector. Plague still occurs in the western United States. The natural reservoir for plague is wild rodents, such as ground squirrels and prairie dogs. Infected fleas that spend time on rabbits and especially on domestic cats are a source of infection for people. The most common source of transmission is through the bite of an infected flea. In addition, people can be infected by handling infected tissues during hunting of small ground animals or even by airborne transmission. The mortality (death rate) from untreated plague can be 50%.

Several diseases are transmitted by ticks. Lyme disease (borreliosis) is a commonly reported tick-borne disease, but Rocky Mountain spotted fever is the deadlier disease. Other tick-borne diseases include anaplasmosis, ehrlichiosis, and babesiosis. Rocky Mountain spotted fever causes high fever, headache, chills, severe muscle pain, and malaise. In about 50% of patients, a rash occurs on the palms and soles and then spreads to the rest of the body. Mortality is about 15% to 20% if the disease is not treated. Rocky Mountain spotted fever is maintained in nature by ticks, primarily either the dog tick *Dermacentor* or the Lone Star tick *Amblyomma.* People are infected by the tick bite during outdoor activities in tick-infested areas or from contact with ticks on pets. Wearing tick repellents in areas infested with ticks and keeping pets free of ticks prevents tick-borne transmitted diseases.

Food and water are also vehicles of indirect transmission of disease. Both are sources of bacterial, viral, and parasitic diseases. Food-borne diseases are acquired by consumption of contaminated food or water and include food-borne intoxications and food-borne infections. Food-borne intoxications are caused by toxins produced by certain bacteria that may contaminate food, such as *Staphylococcus aureus, Clostridium* spp., and *Vibrio* spp. The toxins may be present in the food or may be formed in the intestinal tract after the contaminated food is eaten. Food-borne infections are caused by bacterial or viral organisms that cause infection. These include *Salmonella* spp., *Campylobacter* spp., hepatitis virus, and *Vibrio* spp. The type of organism involved determines the incubation period and how quickly the clinical signs appear. Each organism also causes certain clinical signs, such as diarrhea, vomiting, or nausea. These specific incubation periods and particular clinical signs help epidemiologists determine the organism's identity and source.

Parasitic diseases are also transmitted through food and water. Nematode and trematode infections are most often transmitted either through ingestion of eggs or undercooked meat that contains cysts. *Giardia* is a protozoan that causes gastrointestinal disease in people; giardiasis can be quite serious in immunosuppressed individuals. Although *Giardia* is most often transmitted from person to person, it is also a source of water-borne outbreaks when people use mountain streams as community water sources without proper filtration techniques or drink the water during outdoor activities. Beavers and other domestic animals are reservoirs.

Cryptosporidiosis is another disease that can be transmitted by contaminated water and is a serious disease in immunosuppressed individuals. Cattle and other domestic animals are reservoirs. Proper water filtration and treatment are essential in preventing water-borne diseases.

Pasteurization of milk is important to prevent diseases that can be transmitted through milk. Milk can transmit disease directly from animal to animal or from animals to people through ingestion of contaminated milk. Diseases directly transmitted through milk include brucellosis, Q fever, tuberculosis, toxoplasmosis, and listeriosis. Milk can be contaminated with disease-causing bacteria, such as *Campylobacter* spp., *Salmonella* spp., and *E. coli,* either from the animal or the environment.

Maintenance of Disease

Included in the transmission cycle of disease is maintenance of disease in the human or animal population. There are several ways in which zoonotic diseases are maintained in a population. A direct zoonosis is transmitted by a single vertebrate species. For example, the organism that causes cat-scratch fever is maintained in the feline population. In the eastern United States, rabies virus is maintained in the raccoon and bat population.

A **cyclozoonosis** requires several cycles of disease, usually a parasitic disease, to occur in several different vertebrate species. An example of this is hydatid disease caused by the

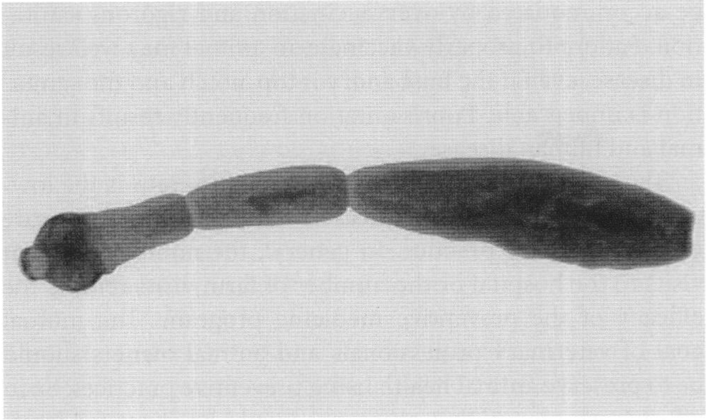

FIGURE 12-8 Adult *Echinococcus* tapeworm. (Photo from CDC website.)

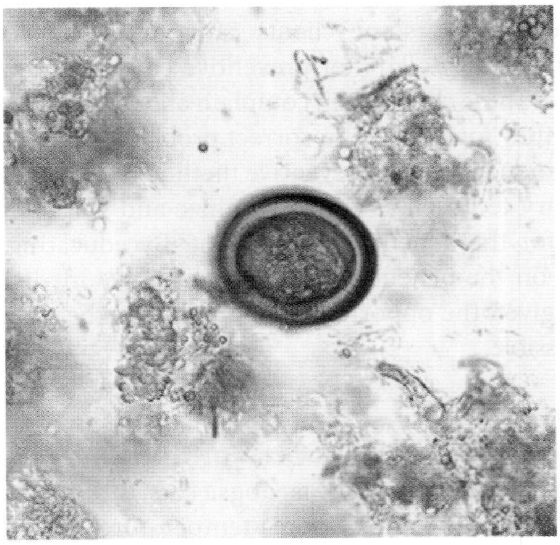

FIGURE 12-9 *Echinococcus* tapeworm egg in a dog's feces (400×). (Photo from CDC website.)

tapeworm *Echinococcus* (Fig. 12-8). The primary reservoir of the adult tapeworm is the dog; eggs are produced and are shed in dog feces (Fig. 12-9). The intermediate hosts are cattle, sheep, pigs, and goats. These species eat grasses and plants that are contaminated with feces. The eggs hatch and become larvae in the intermediate hosts; the larvae migrate throughout the intermediate host and form hydatids or cysts in various organs. Within each hydatid, numerous protoscoleces develop, each with the capability of becoming an adult tapeworm. Dogs are reinfected by eating the organs and tissues of dead cattle, sheep, and other infected livestock, thereby ingesting the hydatids and releasing the protoscoleces into the dog's intestines. There they mature into adults and the cycle begins again. People are infected by ingesting the eggs while handling contaminated materials or soil, or infected dogs. People are then treated as the intermediate host by the larvae, which migrate through the body and become encysted hydatids in human organs (Fig. 12-10). The signs of echinococcosis in infected people depend on the number, size, and location of the cysts of *Echinococcus*.

A metazoonosis is maintained by both invertebrate (tick or mosquito) and vertebrate species. An example is encephalitis. This viral disease is maintained in the vertebrate population

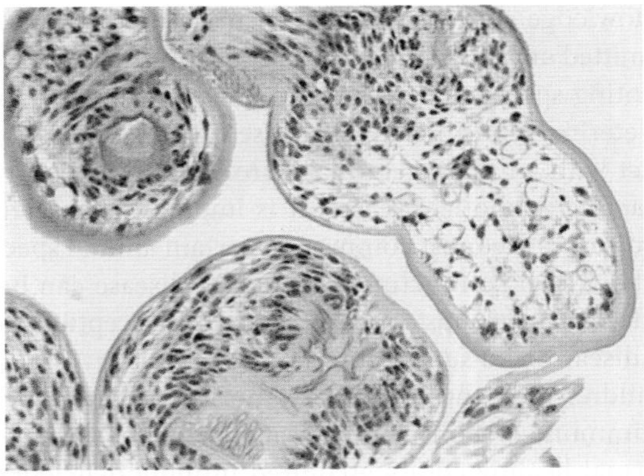

FIGURE 12-10 Numerous *Echinococcus* protoscoleces in a hydatid cyst removed from human lung tissue (600×). (Photo from CDC website.)

of wild or domestic birds and horses through transmission by a mosquito. People are often infected accidentally.

A saprozoonosis depends on an inanimate reservoir to maintain the cycle of infection. Visceral larva migrans, caused by *Toxocara* spp., is considered a saprozoonosis, although the disease also involves vertebrate reservoirs. Soil is essential for transmission of the disease to people and for reinfection of dogs and cats. Infected dogs and cats shed *Toxocara* eggs in their feces. Humid soil is most favorable for survival of the eggs.

Control of Zoonotic Diseases

Because of their regular contact with animals, animal tissues, animal environments, and pet owners, veterinarians and veterinary technicians are often the first to notice a zoonotic disease or the potential for one. In fact, animals can act as sentinels for a potential epidemic or outbreak of infection in people. Good examples are the arboviral diseases, such as eastern equine encephalitis, western equine encephalitis, California and St. Louis encephalitis, and Japanese encephalitis. Fever and headache characterize mild forms of these diseases; the most serious forms can cause death in people. Mortality depends on the specific type of virus involved. The diseases are transmitted by the bite of an infected mosquito. Mosquitoes acquire the infection from birds, horses, and even pigs (Japanese encephalitis). Eastern equine encephalitis is transmitted among birds; horses and people are uncommon hosts. Both eastern equine encephalitis and western equine encephalitis viruses can cause encephalitis in horses. Venezuelan equine encephalomyelitis rarely causes encephalitis in humans, but rather causes a flulike viral infection in people. Horses are the reservoir for infection in people. Cases of encephalitis in birds or horses can signal a potential problem for humans; consequently, preventive programs can be implemented before a large outbreak of disease occurs in the human population.

TECHNICIAN NOTE Veterinary professionals are at risk of contracting zoonotic diseases and must have knowledge of the ways diseases are transmitted to aid in their prevention and control.

Knowledge of the ways in which zoonotic diseases are transmitted and maintained in a population is important for preventing spread of diseases and infection in veterinarians and veterinary technicians. Because of their close working contact with animals, veterinary professionals are at risk of contracting zoonotic diseases. It is important to determine what diseases are most common in certain animal species so that the risk of contracting a particular disease can be estimated. Certain groups of people are more susceptible to zoonotic diseases and suffer more serious effects.

Children and the elderly are more susceptible because their immune systems function at a lower level than those of normal healthy adults. Acquired immunodeficiency disease (AIDS), lupus, and chemotherapeutic medications suppress function of the immune system, making an individual more susceptible to disease. Children are also more likely to put contaminated soil or materials in their mouth. Pregnant women are also highly susceptible. Some diseases, such as toxoplasmosis, may represent a serious disease threat to the fetus.

Control of zoonotic diseases is aimed at the reservoir of disease or the intermediaries that transmit the disease. Control measures include spraying for mosquitoes, use of tick repellent, pasteurization of milk, adequate water filtration, and proper cooking and handling of food. Control programs also include treatment of infected animals in the reservoir population and decrease of contact with infected animals in the reservoir to prevent further transmission. Prevention programs require a thorough knowledge of the disease and how it is maintained and transmitted so as to break the cycle of disease in the population or prevent disease transmission. Prevention programs include vaccination of animals in the reservoir population, potential hosts, and people, if vaccines against that disease are available. Prevention of human infection is possible by treatment of infected animals that may transmit the disease to people. For example, treating puppies and kittens for roundworms and hookworms can prevent contamination of soil by feces containing infective eggs. Veterinarians and veterinary technicians can also test animals for infection, such as for tuberculosis and brucellosis.

PREVENTIVE MEDICINE

Veterinary preventive medicine is the science of preventing disease in animals. The three major components of a preventive medicine program include husbandry, vaccination or prevention through medication, and sanitation. Husbandry involves the housing, diet, and environment of animals. Vaccination involves the use of vaccines or bacterins to prevent such diseases as rabies or equine encephalomyelitis. Medication can be given regularly to prevent certain diseases such as heartworms or infestations with fleas. Sanitation focuses on cleanliness and the use of disinfectants to prevent infection or disease transmission. All three components are interrelated; disease is prevented only by attention to all components. For example, poor husbandry practices cannot be accommodated by overvaccination and rigorous sanitation. Failure to properly vaccinate an animal may well result in disease, even if the husbandry is top-notch and the sanitation is impeccable. Poor sanitation frequently results in animal and human disease.

The goal of any preventive medicine program is the lowest possible incidence of disease in animals under the care of the veterinary practice. In general, the number of client visits to the hospital or the number of farm visits reflects the efficacy of the preventive medicine program. The mutual goal of veterinary professionals and animal owners should be to preserve animal health using preventive practices. Such efforts save money that otherwise would be spent for treatment of disease. Preventive medicine also prolongs the life span, improves the well-being of animals, and fosters a good client-veterinarian relationship.

Unfortunately, some clients cannot see the benefit of spending a few dollars for preventive care, such as for vaccination. These clients then complain about the large sums of money they must spend to correct problems that could have been avoided through preventive methods. The challenge for veterinary technicians is to empathize and work with these clients for the benefit of the patient. By educating animal owners on the benefits of proper preventive medicine, you will be given the opportunity to provide the best veterinary care possible.

HUSBANDRY

Temperature, Light, and Ventilation

For small animals, such as dogs, cats, birds, and small mammals, the ambient (room) temperature should ideally be 65° to 84° F (18° to 29° C). Birds, very young pets, old pets, and those with a sparse haircoat should be maintained at the higher end of this temperature range. Those that are well-furred or overweight should be kept at the lower end of this range. Livestock can survive extremes in outdoor temperatures if sheltered from precipitation and wind. In a barn or stable, good ventilation is more important than ambient temperature. Smaller animals of any species generally require warmer temperatures, whereas larger animals, with their greater body mass, generally require cooler temperatures.

Light sufficient for a human is adequate for most animals. Excessive light can cause eye problems in albino rats. Too little light makes sanitation difficult. Rodents do well in low-light environments. Breeding stock may require adjustment of the photoperiod (periods of daylight and darkness) to maximize breeding potential. Most rodents are best housed with 14 hours of light and 10 hours of darkness. Stallions have improved breeding behavior with long light cycles. All species do better when there is a definite difference between day and night. Animals should never be kept in direct sunlight without access to shade, as they may become sunburned and overheated. Such environmental stress can also predispose to disease.

Ventilation is extremely important in maintaining good health. Inadequate air exchange in an enclosure increases urine odors, ammonia levels, and numbers of airborne bacteria and viruses. Such conditions irritate the respiratory tract and predispose to respiratory disease. Drafty conditions or excessive ventilation can be dangerous. Excessive cool airflow can cause chilling. In a low-humidity environment, as with air conditioning, high airflow can dehydrate an animal. Small pets caged indoors must be kept away from air conditioning drafts or heater vents. It is usually best to place a cage along an interior wall away from ventilation or heating ducts.

Housing

An important aspect of husbandry is housing, such as in cages, pens, or stalls. It is important to keep in mind the following considerations. Housing should:

- Prevent contamination of the animal with feces or urine
- Provide for the psychosocial comfort of companion animals
- Be appropriate for the species
- Be structurally sound
- Be free of dangerous surfaces
- Be constructed so that the animal cannot escape and vermin are not allowed access
- Be easy for the owner to clean

Housed animals should be dry, clean, and protected from environmental extremes. Walls and roofing should be sufficient to protect animals from the sun, wind, rain, and snow. Rabbits held in outdoor hutches can become sunburned. Horses can develop conjunctivitis from wind-driven dust. Pens and corrals must be free of exposed nails, sharp metal edges, or other dangerous features. Attention should be paid to escape-proofing cages. Rodents can squeeze through 1-inch openings; many other small pets learn to flip the latch on their cage door.

Accommodation must also be made for species-specific behavior. For example, pigs should have access to dirt lots for rooting and mud wallowing. Rodents need sufficient bedding for burrowing. Cats need scratching posts. Chinchillas require dust baths.

A major failure of many animal enclosures is that they do not allow sufficient room for normal movement or even postural changes. Cages, pens, and stalls that are too small increase the risk of disease and may predispose to abnormal behavior, such as pacing or excessive barking. Pets may be kept in close confinement for short periods, such as a dog kept for a few hours in a portable kennel or carrier. However, such enclosures should have sufficient room for normal postural movements and stretching. A useful general rule for holding enclosures is that the enclosure be a minimum of 10 times the body size of the animal. This recommendation assumes the animal will be given opportunity to exercise routinely outside of the primary enclosure. Also, housing too many animals in a single primary enclosure of insufficient size can create problems. A high concentration of animals in a primary enclosure, whether hamsters or ponies, dramatically increases the risk of stress, aggression, and disease transmission.

Animals of different species should be housed separately, or in some cases, at least in separate rooms. Do not house natural predators and prey animals in the same room, such as cats with mice or birds, as this leads to stress and possible attack. Also, there are medical reasons for housing different species separately. A disease considered inconsequential in one species can be deadly in another species. For example, healthy rabbits may carry *Bordetella* and *Pasteurella* bacteria, but these agents can quickly kill guinea pigs.

Enclosures should be cleaned and sanitized frequently, from once per day to once per week. Few pet owners clean their pets' cages or pens too often. For large animals, stalls or stanchion areas should be "mucked" daily and new straw or other bedding should be spread. Barn gutters and pens should be shoveled or cleared of manure with a tractor as needed and periodically hosed down. Small cages can be sanitized by hand or even in a dishwasher. Generally speaking, any good dishwashing detergent will effectively clean holding areas. Additional sanitation can be obtained with a dilute solution of laundry bleach, using 1 part bleach to 19 parts of water. All surfaces should be rinsed thoroughly after cleaning and disinfecting. Wet items should be left to dry completely before returning the animal to the cage.

Nutrition

Animals must have free access to fresh potable water. Water in containers should be changed sufficiently to prevent accumulation of slime, algae, or dirt. Bowls should be kept clean and sanitized in a dishwasher (180° F) at least once per month. Water troughs for livestock should be periodically emptied and sanitized. Automatic watering devices must be kept clean and free of ice. Water containers should be sufficient for the number of animals in an enclosure.

Animals should be fed a wholesome, palatable diet on a regular schedule and in sufficient quantity. Feeding devices must be designed to prevent contamination by wastes. Usually this is accomplished with an appropriately sized feeder, positioned off of the floor, in close proximity to the water source. As with water containers, feeding devices should be sanitized routinely, at least monthly or more often as needed.

Clients should be encouraged to purchase good-quality feedstuffs and refrain from feeding outdated or off-brand diets. In general, commercial diets more than 3 months old should not be fed as a sole food source, because certain nutrients deteriorate with long storage. Clients should be cautioned not to buy feeds that show large amounts of oil uptake by the bag or box. Such products have likely been held for considerable time in a warehouse that was warm enough to cause oil to bleed out of the feed.

The diet fed should be formulated for that species. Cats should not be fed food formulated for dogs. Rat rations are of little value for rabbits, dogs, or cats. Guinea pigs require vitamin C in their diet. Rat or mouse diets can produce disease in guinea pigs. Pig rations, with their high carbohydrate component, can cause bloat in horses. Rabbit rations can cause metabolic disease in sheep. Feeding an improperly formulated diet produces nutritional deficiencies, excesses, or imbalances that can predispose to bacterial infections or metabolic disease. Chapter 23 contains detailed information on nutrition.

Animal Identification

An often overlooked aspect of preventive medicine is animal identification. The method of identification depends on the species. For pets allowed outdoors, an implanted microchip or a tattoo is preferred to a collar with a name tag. Collars may be removed or fall off, and tags may be lost. Permanent identification ensures that a lost pet can be identified for return to its owner.

VACCINATION AND PREVENTIVE MEDICATION

There are two basic ways that an animal can acquire the immunity that it needs: passively and actively. Passive immunity occurs when the animal acquires preformed antibodies to various pathogens. This can take place naturally, such as when maternal antibodies cross the placenta into the fetus or neonates ingest the dam's colostrum. It can also occur artificially, such as when antibodies are administered exogenously. An example of artificially acquired passive immunity is through administration of rattlesnake antivenin. Antivenin contains antibodies harvested from serum of horses that have developed immunity to the rattlesnake venom. Active immunity is when an animal develops its own antibodies to pathogens. This can also occur naturally, through infection or exposure to the pathogen, or artificially through vaccination. Both artificially acquired passive and artificially acquired active immunity can exist for the same disease. For example, the tetanus antitoxin is an example of artificially acquired passive immunity. It consists of preformed antibodies to the toxin produced by the bacterium *Clostridium tetani,* the causative agent of tetanus. There is also a tetanus **toxoid,** which consists of inactivated antigenic toxin molecules that stimulate development of the animal's own antibodies. Because the preformed antibodies only persist for a few weeks, the antitoxin is usually given in a situation when the animal may have been exposed to the toxin or has developed tetanus. The tetanus toxoid is administered as a preventive because it provides long-lasting immunity.

Animals can be vaccinated against a wide variety of diseases, ranging from blackleg in cattle to distemper in dogs. These vaccines are commonly administered by injection and are critical in disease prevention. After injection, the vaccine does not cause disease but stimulates the cells of the immune system to develop antibodies against the portion of the pathogen that is antigenic. Upon the next exposure to the pathogen, a vaccinated animal will not become infected because it has been immunized.

The vaccine consists of a particular antigen unique to a pathogen, such as the cell wall of the causative bacterium or a small unit of the virus. The pathogen can be in several forms, including modified-live, inactivated, or recombinant. A modified-live vaccine consists of a weakened version of the pathogen, which will induce an immune response but is attenuated enough so that it will not cause disease. An inactivated or noninfectious vaccine consists of whole killed pathogens or selected antigenic subunits—enough to induce immunity. A **recombinant vaccine** consists of a live, nonpathogenic virus into which the gene for a pathogen-related antigen has been inserted. When the virus is injected into the animal, viral genes, including the inserted gene for the antigen of interest, will be expressed. This will cause the animal to produce antibodies to the antigen without ever having been exposed to the pathogen.

Certain diseases are readily prevented by vaccination. Domestic animals should be routinely vaccinated against prevalent diseases. Such serious diseases as parvovirus infection and distemper in dogs, panleukopenia and feline leukemia virus infection in cats, and equine encephalomyelitis and tetanus in horses can be prevented by vaccination. In some cases, vaccination is beneficial to humans as well as animals. For example, animals at risk of developing rabies from the bite of rabid animals should receive regular rabies prophylaxis.

Most small mammals kept as pets (rodents and rabbits) are not routinely vaccinated because of the relatively small risk of contracting certain diseases for which vaccines are available for the species. Mice can contract rabies, but pet mice housed in a cage in a home are unlikely to encounter a rabid animal. Vaccination recommendations for some species are changing. In years past, rabies vaccination was not considered necessary for pet ferrets; with the improved rabies vaccines now available, ferret vaccination is considered appropriate.

The decision whether or not to vaccinate an animal is influenced by the risk of contracting the disease, the effects of the disease, and the benefits and cost of vaccination. Vaccination may not be warranted if the disease is unlikely to develop or causes only mild illness. For example, veterinarians do not routinely vaccinate dogs or cats against tetanus because they are unlikely to contract the disease; however, horses are vaccinated against tetanus because they are more likely to develop it. Vaccination against a very rare disease may not be necessary. However, vaccination is worthwhile if the disease poses a substantial threat to human and animal health, such as with rabies. Vaccination also benefits the offspring of vaccinated females; for instance, a vaccinated female will develop antibodies to the disease and then transfer maternal immunity through her colostrum.

The attitude toward vaccination also varies with circumstances. Kennel and cattery owners, breeding farm managers, and ranchers are very concerned with diseases that could sweep through the animal population, with devastating economic effects. The canine infectious respiratory disease (CIRD) complex, traditionally referred to as "kennel cough," and historically attributed to *Bordetella bronchiseptica,* can range from a fairly mild upper respiratory infection to tracheobronchitis to pneumonia. This could cause great harm in the form of bad public relations if it infected dogs in a boarding facility; however, an individual owner is often not overly concerned with "kennel cough" in his or her pet. Fortunately, good client education is beginning to change owner attitudes. The disease complex may consist of several respiratory pathogens, including canine distemper virus (CDV), canine respiratory coronavirus (CRCV), canine influenza virus (CIV), canine adenovirus Type-1 (CAV-1), canine parainfluenza virus (CPIV), canine herpesvirus (CHV), and *Bordetella bronchiseptica.* Signs of these diseases may be similar, yet some of the pathogens cause fatal disease. *Bordetella bronchiseptica* often plays only a minor contributory role or is absent altogether, and currently there are vaccines for all of the pathogens except CRCV. Respiratory coronavirus is a different pathogen from the canine coronavirus that causes enteric disease in dogs (CCV) for which there is a vaccine.

A growing number of practitioners are concerned about the apparent association between vaccines and a particular type of cancer (sarcoma) at the injection site in cats. The American Association of Feline Practitioners (AAFP) currently recommends using different vaccines at different locations on the body. It is recommended that feline leukemia virus (FeLV) vaccine be given below the left stifle and rabies vaccine be given below the right stifle. FPV, FHV-1, and FVC vaccines should be administered below the right elbow. All feline vaccines should be administered as distally as possible at each location.

Animal vaccines are available in many combinations. For example, Duramune PC (Boehringer Ingelheim, St. Joseph, MO) is a canine vaccine against two viruses: CPV and CCV. Duramune Max 5 protects against five viruses: CDV, CAV-1, CAV-2, CPV, and CPIV, but not CCV. Canine adenovirus Type-1 is the causative agent of infectious canine hepatitis. The vaccine for CAV-2 is protective against CAV-2 but is cross-protective against CAV-1; therefore, it is given instead of the vaccine for CAV-1. The CAV-1 vaccine is not used because it may cause adverse effects, including kidney infections and ocular problems such as uveitis and corneal opacity ("blue eye"). Duramune Max 5-CvK/4L and Vanguard Plus 5/CV-L (Zoetis, Florham Park, NJ) protect against six viruses and *Leptospira* spp. There are many such products available with multiple combinations of pathogens to accommodate different animal needs based on their lifestyles. It is also because some vaccines are considered core vaccines and others are noncore. Core vaccines are recommended for all dogs, whereas noncore vaccines are recommended based on a dog's lifestyle. For instance, the vaccine against *Borrelia burgdorferi,* the causative agent of Lyme disease, is a noncore vaccine; it is recommended for dogs that have a likelihood of contact with ticks that transmit *B. burgdorferi.* A similarly wide variety of vaccine products is also available for cats, horses, cattle, pigs, and other species.

Vaccination of Dogs

The following vaccines are available for dogs:

- Rabies
- Distemper
- Parvovirus
- Coronavirus
- Canine adenovirus (CAV-1 or CAV-2)
- *Bordetella bronchiseptica*
- Parainfluenza
- Leptospirosis
- *Borrelia burgdorferi*

Puppies are usually immunized with one to three doses in the first few months of life and then annually as adults (Table 12-3).

The American Animal Hospital Association (AAHA) vaccination guidelines for dogs offer specific recommendations as to which vaccines are core and noncore, and when vaccinations should be administered.

Newer or less common vaccines available for dogs include *Crotalus atrox* toxoid, which protects against rattlesnake venom, and canine influenza vaccine. There is limited information available regarding their efficacy. There is also a vaccine against *Giardia,* but this is not recommended.

Vaccination of Cats

The following vaccines are available for cats:

- Rabies
- Panleukopenia (feline distemper)
- Feline herpesvirus-1
- Calicivirus
- *Chlamydophila felis*
- Feline leukemia virus
- Feline immunodeficiency virus
- *Bordetella bronchiseptica*

Most cats begin receiving vaccines as kittens, usually around 6 weeks of age. Kittens require boosters after an original series of vaccines. Adult cats may require annual boosters against each of these diseases (Table 12-4).

The AAFP vaccination guidelines for cats offer specific recommendations as to which vaccines are core and noncore, and when vaccinations should be administered.

Other vaccines available for cats include vaccines against feline infectious peritonitis and *Microsporum* spp. ("ringworm"), but these are not recommended.

Vaccination of Horses

The following vaccines are available for horses:

- Rabies
- Encephalomyelitis (eastern and western)
- Tetanus
- Influenza
- Equine herpesvirus 1 and 4
- Potomac horse fever
- Strangles
- Rotavirus
- Botulism
- Anthrax

Most horses begin receiving vaccines as foals. Horses of unknown vaccination status should receive an initial series of vaccines, which is repeated in 4 weeks for maximal antibody production. Adult horses generally require annual boosters against each of these diseases (Table 12-5).

TABLE 12-3 2011 AAHA Canine Vaccination Guidelines

VACCINE	INITIAL VACCINATION (<16WK OF AGE)	INITIAL VACCINATION (>16 WK OF AGE)	REVACCINATION RECOMMENDATION (BOOSTER)	COMMENTS
Core Vaccines				
CDV (MLV) or rCDV	Every 3–4 wk between the ages of 6 and 16 wk. Final dose of the initial series should be administered between 14 and 16 wk of age.	One dose is considered protective and acceptable. Revaccination is recommended every ≥3 yr after completion of the initial vaccination.	Dogs completing the initial vaccination series by 16 wk of age or younger should receive a single booster vaccination no later than 1 yr after completion of the initial series and be revaccinated every ≥3 yr thereafter.	• Among healthy dogs, all commercially available distemper vaccines are expected to induce a sustained protective immune response lasting at least ≥5 yr. • Among healthy dogs, the rCDV vaccine has been shown to induce a protective immune response lasting at least 5 yr. • Although rare, some dogs are genetically predisposed "nonresponders" and are incapable of developing protective immunity subsequent to CDV vaccination. • The rCDV vaccine can be used interchangeably with MLV-CDV vaccine. • It is recommended that all CDV vaccines be administered within 1 hr after reconstitution; vaccine held more than 1 hr should be discarded. • MLV-CDV vaccine is particularly vulnerable to inactivation after reconstitution.
CPV-2 (MLV)	Puppies should be vaccinated every 3–4 wk between the ages of 6 and 16 wk. To minimize the risk of maternal antibody interference with vaccination, the final dose of the initial series should be administered between 14 and 16 wk of age.	One dose is considered protective and acceptable. Revaccination is recommended every ≥3 yr after completion of the initial vaccination.	Dogs completing the initial vaccination series by ≤16 wk of age should receive a single booster vaccination not later than 1 yr after completion of the initial series and be revaccinated every ≥3 yr thereafter.	• All MLV-CPV-2 vaccines available today are expected to provide immunity from disease caused by any field variant recognized today (CPV-2a, -2b, and -2c). • As new variants of CPV-2 occur, those variants will need to be evaluated, as the previous ones have, to ensure vaccines in use at the time are protective. • Among healthy dogs, all commercially available MLV-CPV-2 vaccines are expected to induce a sustained protective immune response lasting at least 5 yr. • Although rare, some dogs are genetic nonresponders and are incapable of developing protective immunity subsequent to CPV-2 vaccination no matter how often vaccine is administered. • Specific breed-susceptibility to CPV-2 nonresponsiveness is not recognized. • There is no value in extending initial CPV-2 vaccination series beyond 16 wk of age. • It is recommended that CPV-2 vaccine, especially when administered in combination with CDV vaccine, be administered within 1 hr after reconstitution; vaccine held more than 1 hr should be discarded.

CAV-2 (MLV parenteral)	Puppies should be vaccinated every 3–4 wk between the ages of 6 and 16 wk. To minimize the risk of maternal antibody interference with vaccination, the final dose of the initial series should be administered between 14 and 16 wk of age.	One dose is considered protective and acceptable. Revaccination is recommended every ≥3 yr after completion of the initial vaccination.	Dogs completing the initial vaccination series by ≤16 wk of age should receive a single booster vaccination not later than 1 yr after completion of the initial series and be revaccinated every ≥3 yr thereafter.	• CAV-2 induces protection against CAV-1 (canine hepatitis virus) as well as CAV-2. • Among healthy dogs, all commercially available MLV-CAV-2 vaccines are expected to induce a sustained protective immune response lasting at least 7 yr. • It is recommended that CAV-2 vaccine, especially when administered in combination with CDV vaccine, be administered within 1 hr after reconstitution; vaccine held more than 1 hr should be discarded.
Rabies 1 yr (killed)	Administer a single dose not earlier than 12 wk of age or as required by state, provincial, and/or local requirements.	Administer a single dose of a "1-yr" rabies vaccine.	Administer a single dose of a "1-yr" rabies vaccine annually. State, provincial, and/or local laws apply.	• State, provincial, and local statutes govern the frequency of administration for products labeled as "1-yr" rabies vaccine. • Route of administration may not be optional; see product literature for details.
Rabies 3 yr (killed)	Administer a single dose of a "3-yr" rabies vaccine not earlier than 12 wk of age or as required by state, provincial, and/or local requirements.	Administer a single dose of a "3-yr" rabies vaccine or as required by state, provincial, and/or local requirements.	Administer a single dose of a "3-yr" rabies vaccine within 1 yr after administration of the initial dose, regardless of the animal's age at the time the initial dose was administered. Revaccination with a "3-yr rabies" vaccine should be administered every 3 yr thereafter, unless state, provincial, and/or local requirements stipulate otherwise.	• State, provincial, and local statutes govern the frequency of administration for products labeled as "3-yr rabies" vaccines. • Use of rabies vaccine multidose vials in companion animals is not recommended. • Route of administration may not be optional; see product literature for details.
Non-Core Vaccines				
MV (MLV)	A single dose is recommended for administration to healthy dogs between the ages of 6 and 12 wk.	Not recommended.	Not recommended.	• Measles vaccine is only intended to provide temporary immunization of young puppies against CDV. • MV has been shown to cross-protect puppies against CDV in presence of MDA to CDV. • These vaccines should not be administered to dogs less than 6 wk or female dogs more than 12 wk of age that will be used for breeding, • After administration of a single dose of measles virus-containing vaccine, subsequent vaccination with a CDV vaccine that does not contain MV is recommended at 2–4 wk intervals until the patient is 14–16 wk of age. • Vaccine that contains MV must be administered by the IM route. • It is recommended that MV-containing vaccine be administered within 1 hr after reconstitution; vaccine held more than 1 hr should be discarded.

Continued

TABLE 12-3 2011 AAHA Canine Vaccination Guidelines

VACCINE	INITIAL VACCINATION (<16WK OF AGE)	INITIAL VACCINATION (>16 WK OF AGE)	REVACCINATION RECOMMENDATION (BOOSTER)	COMMENTS
CPiV (MLV) For parenteral administration only. (Available only as a combined product for parenteral administration)	Parenteral CPiV vaccine is only available in combination with core vaccines (CDV-CPV-2 and CAV-2). Veterinarians who elect to administer parenteral CPiV vaccine should follow the same administration recommendations as outlined above for the core vaccines.	Veterinarians who elect to administer parenteral CPiV vaccine should follow the same administration recommendations as outlined above for the core vaccines.	Veterinarians who elect to administer parenteral CPiV vaccine should follow the same administration recommendations as outlined above for the core vaccines.	• Parenterally administered CPiV vaccine does prevent clinical signs but has not been shown to prevent infection and shedding • Use of the parenteral vaccine is recommended for use in those patients that aggressively resist IN vaccination.
Bb (inactivated-cellular antigen extract) For parenteral administration only.	Administer first dose at 8 wk of age and second dose at 12 wk of age (see comments).	Two doses, 2–4 wk apart are required.	Annually.	• There is no known advantage to administering parenteral and IN Bb vaccines simultaneously. • On initial vaccination, administration should be scheduled such that the second dose can be administered at least 1 wk before exposure (kennel, dog show, daycare, etc.). • The parenteral vaccine is not immunogenic if administered by the IN route.
Bb (live avirulent bacteria) For IN administration only.	A single dose should be administered in conjunction with 1 of the core vaccine doses. Note: The initial IN dose may be administered to dogs as young as 3–4 wk of age (depending on manufacturer) when exposure risk is considered to be high (see comments).	A single dose is recommended.	Annually or more often in high-risk animals.	• Transient (3–10 days) coughing, sneezing, or nasal discharge may occur in a small percentage of vaccinates. • IN Bb vaccine must not be administered parenterally.
CPiV (MLV) For IN administration only. (IN CPiV vaccine is only available in combination with IN Bb vaccine or Bb 1 CAV-2)	A single dose should be administered in conjunction with 1 of the core vaccine doses. Note: The initial IN dose may be administered to dogs as young as 3–4 wk of age (depending on manufacturer) when exposure risk is considered to be high (see comments).	A single dose is recommended.	Annually or more often in high-risk animals.	• When feasible, IN vaccination is recommended over parenteral vaccination. • Parenterally administered CPiV vaccine does prevent clinical signs, but has not been shown to prevent infection and shedding. • IN CPiV vaccine prevents not only clinical disease but also infection and viral replication (shedding).
CAV-2 (MLV) (for IN administration only) (Available only in combination with IN Bb and CPiV vaccine)	A single dose should be administered in conjunction with 1 of the core vaccine doses. Note: The initial IN dose may be administered to dogs as young as 3–4 wk of age (depending on manufacturer) when exposure risk is considered to be high (see comments).	A single dose is recommended.	Annually or more often in high-risk animals.	• Administration of IN CAV-2 vaccine is recommended for use in dogs considered at risk for respiratory infection caused by the CAV-2 virus. • IN CAV-2 vaccine may not provide protective immunity against CAV-1 (canine hepatitis virus) infection and should not be considered a replacement for parenteral MLV-CAV-2 vaccination.

Canine influenza vaccine (killed virus)	Administer 1 dose not earlier than 6 wk of age and a second dose 2–4 wk later.	Two doses, 2–4 wk apart are required. A single initial dose will not immunize a seronegative dog.	Annually.	
Borrelia burgdorferi (Lyme disease) (killed whole cell bacterin) or *Borrelia burgdorferi* (rLyme: rOspA)	Administer 1 dose not earlier than 12 wk of age and a second dose 2–4 wk later. For optimal response, do not administer to dogs <12 wk of age.	Two doses, 2–4 wk apart. A single initial dose will not immunize a seronegative dog.	Annually. Alternatively, it has been recommended that initial vaccination or revaccination (booster) be administered before the beginning of tick season, as determined regionally.	• Generally recommended only for use in dogs with a known risk of exposure, living in or visiting regions where the risk of vector tick exposure is considered to be high, or where disease is known to be endemic. • In addition to vaccination, prevention of canine Lyme borreliosis includes regular utilization of tick-control products.
Leptospira interrogans (4-way killed whole cell or subunit bacterin) Contains serovars canicola + icterohemorrhagiae + grippotyphosa + pomona	Administer 1 dose not earlier than 12 wk of age and a second dose 2–4 wk later. For optimal response, do not administer to dogs <12 wk of age.	Two doses, 2–4 wk apart. A single initial dose will not immunize a seronegative dog.	Annually. Administration of booster vaccines should be restricted to dogs with a reasonable risk of exposure.	• Specific vaccination recommendations vary on the basis: (1) known geographic occurrence/prevalence, and (2) exposure risk in the individual patient. • It is recommended that the first dose of leptospira vaccine be delayed until 12 wk of age. • DOI based on challenge studies has been shown to be approximately 1 yr.
Leptospira interrogans (2-way killed bacterin) Contains serovars canicola + icterohemorrhagiae only	Not recommended.	Not recommended.	Not recommended.	Not recommended.
Canine oral melanoma (plasmid DNA vaccine-expresses human tyrosinase). Availability is currently limited to practicing oncologists and selected specialists.	Not applicable. See manufacturer's indications for use.	See manufacturer's indications for use.	See manufacturer's indications for use.	• Use of this vaccine is limited to the treatment of dogs with malignant melanoma. • This vaccine aids in extending survival times of dogs with Stage II or III oral melanoma and for which local disease control has been achieved (negative local lymph nodes or positive lymph nodes that were surgically removed or irradiated). • The human tyrosinase protein will stimulate an immune response that is effective against canine melanoma cells that over express tyrosinase. • Vaccination is not indicated for the prevention of canine melanoma.

Continued

TABLE 12-3 2011 AAHA Canine Vaccination Guidelines

VACCINE	INITIAL VACCINATION (<16WK OF AGE)	INITIAL VACCINATION (>16 WK OF AGE)	REVACCINATION RECOMMENDATION (BOOSTER)	COMMENTS
Crotalus atrox (Western Diamondback rattlesnake vaccine) (toxoid)	Initial vaccination recommendation may depend on size of the individual dog. Refer to manufacturer's label. Current recommendations are to administer 2 doses, 1 mo apart, to dogs as young as 4 mo.	Initial vaccination recommendation may depend on size of the individual dog. Refer to manufacturer's label. Current recommendations are to administer 2 doses 1 mo apart.	Refer to manufacturer's label. Annual revaccination requirements vary depending on prior exposure, size of dog, and risk of exposure. Refer to manufacturer's label.	• Field efficacy and experimental challenge data in dogs are not available at this time. • Intended to protect dogs against the venom associated with the bite of the Western Diamondback rattlesnake. • Some cross-protection may exist against the venom of the Eastern Diamondback rattlesnake. • There is currently no evidence of cross-protection against the venom (neurotoxin) of the Mojave rattlesnake. • Vaccine efficacy and dose recommendations are based on toxin neutralization studies conducted in mice. • Conventional challenge studies in dogs have not been conducted. Neither experimental nor field data are currently available on this product. • Note: Veterinarians should advise clientele of vaccinated dogs that vaccination does not eliminate the need to treat individual dogs subsequent to envenomation
Canine coronavirus (CCoV) (killed and MLV)	Not recommended.	Not recommended.	Not recommended.	• Not recommended. • Neither the MLV vaccine nor the killed CCoV vaccines have been shown to significantly reduce disease caused by a combination of CCoV and CPV-2. • Only CPV-2 vaccines have been shown to protect dogs against a dual-virus challenge. • DOI has never been established. In controlled challenge studies, neither vaccinates nor control dogs developed clinical evidence of disease after experimental virus challenge.

Bb, *Bordetella bronchiseptica;* CAV-1, canine adenovirus, type 1 (cause of canine viral hepatitis); protection from CAV-1 infection is provided by parenterally administered CAV-2 vaccine; CAV-2, canine adenovirus, type 2; CCoV, canine coronavirus cause of enteric coronavirus infection (antigenically distinct from the canine respiratory coronavirus [CRCoV]); CDV, canine distemper virus; CIV, canine influenza virus—H3N8; CPiV, canine parainfluenza virus; CPV-2, canine parvovirus, type 2; DOI, duration of immunity; IN, intranasal; MLV, modified live virus, attenuated virus vaccine; MV, measles virus; OspA outer surface protein A (antigen) of *Borrelia burgdorferi;* RV, rabies virus.

TABLE 12-4 American Association of Feline Practitioners Feline Vaccination Guidelines for Pet Cats

VACCINE	KITTENS (<16 WEEKS OLD)	ADULTS (16+ WEEKS OLD)	REVACCINATION (BOOSTERS)	COMMENTS
Panleukopenia + herpesvirus-1 + calicivirus (FPV, FHV-1, FCV)	Administer the first dose as early as 6 weeks of age, then every 3–4 weeks until 16–20 weeks of age 7–11	Administer two doses, 3–4 weeks apart	Revaccinate 1 year after primary series; thereafter, boost every 3 years, lifelong	Modified-live and inactivated vaccines are available for parenteral administration; Recommended for all cats For cats going into boarding or another high exposure, stressful situation, a booster 7–10 days prior to boarding may be warranted.
Feline leukemia (FeLV)	Administer two doses, 3–4 weeks apart, beginning as early as 8 weeks of age	Administer two doses, 3–4 weeks apart	Administer a single dose 1 year following administration of the initial two-dose series. Thereafter, revaccination every 2 years for cats at low risk of infection and annually for cats at higher risk.	Inactivated and recombinant Test first to verify FeLV antigen-negative status. Recommended for all kittens up to and including 1 year of age. At-risk adult cats should continue to be vaccinated against FeLV
Rabies	Administer a single dose at not less than 12 weeks/ 3 months of age	Administer a single dose	Administer a single dose 1 year following the initial dose; then repeat annually (or every 3 years if using a vaccine licensed for this interval)	Inactivated and recombinant. Necessary for all cats where legally mandated or in an endemic region Where rabies vaccination is required, the frequency of vaccination is based on local statutes or requirements.

TABLE 12-5 Preventive Medicine Programs Generally Recommended for Horses

FOALS AND WEANLINGS	YEARLINGS AND ADULTS
Physical examination at time of vaccination	Physical examination at time of vaccination
Deworm every 2 months (rotate products)	Deworm at least every 2 months (rotate products)
	Check teeth and float as needed
Trim feet as needed	Trim feet as needed
Vaccinate for tetanus, EEE, WEE, VEE, equine influenza, rhinopneumonitis	Vaccinate for tetanus, EEE, WEE, VEE, equine influenza, rhinopneumonitis
	Review stall cleaning schedule
Discuss feeding regimen	Discuss feeding regimen
Discuss exercise program	Discuss exercise program
Monitor body condition	Monitor body condition

Vaccination of Cattle

The following vaccines are available for cattle:

- Rabies
- Trichomoniasis
- Brucellosis
- IBR
- BVD
- Parainfluenza-3
- Campylobacteriosis
- Leptospirosis
- Rotavirus
- Coronavirus

- *E. coli*
- Clostridial diseases
- Anthrax
- Anaplasmosis

Most cattle begin receiving vaccines as calves, with booster doses after 6 months of age. Cattle of unknown vaccination status should receive an initial series of vaccines, which is repeated in 4 weeks for maximal antibody production. Adult cattle generally require annual boosters against each of these diseases (Table 12-6).

Vaccination of Pigs

The following vaccines are available for pigs:

- Rabies
- Leptospirosis
- Parvovirus
- TGE
- Rotavirus
- Clostridial diseases
- *E. coli*
- *Bordetella*
- *Pasteurella*
- *Actinobacillus*
- *Mycoplasma*
- PRRS
- Erysipelas
- Pseudorabies
- *Streptococcus*
- Encephalomyocarditis

Most swine begin receiving vaccines as piglets. Pigs of unknown vaccination status should receive an initial series of vaccines, which is repeated in 4 weeks for maximal antibody production. Adult pigs generally require annual boosters against each of these diseases (Table 12-7).

Vaccination of Goats

The following vaccines are available for goats:

- Rabies
- Clostridial diseases
- Tetanus
- Contagious ecthyma
- Anthrax
- Leptospirosis
- Caseous lymphadenitis
- *E. coli*

Most goats begin receiving vaccines as kids, usually around 4 to 6 weeks of age. Kids require boosters after an original series of vaccines. Adult goats require annual boosters against each of these diseases (Table 12-8).

Vaccination of Sheep

The following vaccines are available for sheep:

- Clostridial diseases
- Tetanus
- Vibriosis
- Foot rot
- Bluetongue
- Contagious ecthyma

TABLE 12-6 Preventive Medicine Programs Generally Recommended for Cattle

NEONATAL PERIOD	1 TO 3 MONTHS	5 TO 6 MONTHS	ANNUALLY
Physical examination	Physical examination	Physical examination	Physical examination
Deworm (rotate products)	Deworm (rotate products)	Deworm (rotate products)	
Vaccinate for bovine rotavirus and coronavirus infection (if necessary)	Vaccinate for clostridial diseases	Vaccination for clostridial diseases, infectious bovine rhinotracheitis, parainfluenza-3, bovine virus diarrhea	Vaccinate for infectious bovine rhinotracheitis, parainfluenza-3, bovine virus diarrhea
Review stall-cleaning schedule	Review stall-cleaning schedule	Review stall-cleaning schedule	Review stall-cleaning schedule
Monitor body condition	Monitor body condition	Monitor body condition	Monitor body condition
	Discuss feeding regimen	Discuss feeding regimen	Discuss feeding regimen

TABLE 12-7 Preventive Medicine Programs Generally Recommended for Pigs

NEONATAL PERIOD	1 TO 3 WEEKS	4 TO 5 WEEKS	8 TO 10 WEEKS	ANNUALLY
Physical examination	Physical examination	Physical examination	Physical Examination	Physical examination
Dock tails	Vaccinate for transmissible gastroenteritis, atrophic rhinitis, porcine parvovirus infection	Vaccinate for atrophic rhinitis, erysipelas, *Haemophilus* infection, swine dysentery		Vaccinate as necessary
Castrate (if necessary)	Monitor body condition	Monitor body condition	Monitor body condition	Monitor body condition
Clip needle teeth	Review stall-cleaning schedule	Review stall-cleaning schedule		Review stall-cleaning schedule
Iron dextran injection			Treat for ectoparasites	Check for ectoparasites
Identify with ear notching			Deworm	Deworm (rotate products)
			Discuss feeding regimen	Discuss feeding regimen

- *E. coli*
- Caseous lymphadenitis

Most lambs begin receiving vaccines at 4 to 6 weeks of age. Lambs require boosters after an original series of vaccines. Adult sheep need annual boosters against each of these diseases (see Table 12-8).

Vaccination of Llamas

The following vaccines are available for llamas:

- Rabies
- Clostridial diseases
- Anthrax
- Brucellosis
- Leptospirosis

Most crias (immature llamas) begin receiving vaccines before 4 weeks of age. Crias require boosters after an original series of vaccines. Adult llamas require annual boosters against each of these diseases (see Table 12-8).

ANTIBODY TITERS IN LIEU OF VACCINATION

Although mostly safe, annual vaccinations are a source of controversy because of risks that may be associated with vaccine use. Reactions to vaccine administration ranging from localized swelling to anaphylaxis and sarcoma formation (e.g., in cats) have been reported. Also, although there are recommendations for appropriate vaccination protocols, optimal intervals have not been established for most vaccines. It is likely that the vaccinations currently in use provide long-term immunity; however, some patients that are at risk for contracting common diseases may still need vaccination. In particular, pets that are exposed to other dogs or cats on a routine basis or are ill with some other disease (e.g., FIV or FeLV) may still need routine vaccinations.

Many veterinarians are now recommending the measurement of antibody titers to diseases normally vaccinated against as an alternative to routine annual vaccination. An antibody titer may help determine whether or not a patient is likely to need booster vaccinations. Although this is a promising alternative to vaccination, there is still much uncertainty surrounding titer use. Different outside laboratories have different measurement standards. Also, there is disagreement and inconsistency as to the level of antibodies that constitutes protection against a disease if the animal were infected or challenged with the pathogen. Titers also measure humoral immunity and do not address the issue of cell-mediated immunity. Finally, antibody titers are often more costly than vaccines.

Use of Preventive Medication

Certain diseases can be prevented by regular administration of preventive medication. This is best exemplified by use of anthelmintics and other parasiticides to prevent heartworm infection and control internal and external parasites in dogs and cats.

SANITATION

The third aspect of the preventive medicine triad is sanitation. A good preventive medicine program involves the judicious use of selected sanitizing agents. Asepsis is a condition of free from infection. It involves disinfection, sterilization, and antisepsis. Disinfection is the destruction of vegetative forms of bacteria on inanimate or nonliving objects; however, this may not necessarily include spores or spore-forming bacteria. Sterilization is the destruction of all organisms, including bacteria and spores. Antisepsis is the prevention of infectious agent growth on animate (living) objects. Sterilization generally involves heat and pressure or gas agents that can only be used in objects that can fit in a sterilizer, such as an autoclave. Therefore, for most purposes, sanitation involves asepsis of inanimate objects by disinfectants, which is discussed in this section. Gross accumulations of dirt and organic matter must be removed by cleaning before application of disinfectants. The ideal sanitizing agent has the following characteristics: broad spectrum of antimicrobial activity, no odor, rapid microbicidal effect, no tissue toxicity, no corrosive action, no inactivation by urine or other organic matter, ability to be used at normal environmental temperatures; reasonably priced, readily obtainable, and easily applied. Because no single disinfectant meets all of these criteria, selection is based on the specific needs of the client's preventive medicine program.

A practical way to assess sanitation is to avoid use of highly scented products, such as cedar shavings, pine-scented cleaners, or perfumes, on animals or in their surroundings. Although deodorants make the animal or its enclosure smell good, they also mask odors that can be associated with poor sanitation. Chapters 11 and 15 contain additional information on disinfectants as well as sterilization and antiseptics.

TABLE 12-8 Preventive Medicine Programs Generally Recommended for Goats, Sheep, and Llamas

NEONATAL PERIOD	1 TO 3 MONTHS	5 TO 6 MONTHS	ANNUALLY
Physical examination	Physical examination	Physical examination	Physical examination
Vaccinate for clostridial diseases, tetanus	Vaccinate for clostridial diseases		Vaccinate as needed
	Deworm (rotate products)	Deworm (rotate products)	Deworm (rotate products)
Review stall-cleaning schedule	Review stall-cleaning schedule	Review stall-cleaning schedule	Review stall-cleaning schedule
Monitor body condition	Monitor body condition	Monitor body condition	Monitor body condition
	Discuss feeding regimen	Discuss feeding regimen	Discuss feeding regimen

FACTORS PREDISPOSING TO DISEASE

Some factors that predispose to disease can be controlled, but others cannot. Although some factors are beyond our control, we can often establish conditions so that even uncontrollable factors have only minimal impact on our animals. Animals are predisposed to disease by genetic, dietary, environmental, and metabolic factors.

Genetic Factors

Genetic factors are largely beyond our control, although they can be reduced to some extent by selective breeding. These include such things as gender predispositions, inherited mutations, immunodeficiencies, and the effect of inbreeding. Most male tricolored cats are sterile, whereas tricolored female cats are usually fertile. Inherited malocclusions can interfere with chewing. Immunodeficiencies may be noted by an increased incidence of infections. Inbreeding can lead to physical abnormalities or diminished mental (intellectual) capacities.

Dietary Factors

Dietary factors are generally controllable. Animal owners determine most aspects of an animal's diet, such as feed type, quality, amount, and regimen. A high-quality balanced ration is of little value if the feeder is inaccessible. This is occasionally seen with young bunnies, which are too short to reach the feeder. Limited feeding can prevent obesity but can lead to malnutrition if not applied properly. A diet formulated for one type or age of animal may not be healthful for another group of the same species. For example, hard pellets may not be chewable by aged animals, kitten diets may have some nutrients in excess of that required by an adult cat, etc. The diet must change as the needs of the animal change.

> *TECHNICIAN NOTE* Genetic, dietary, environmental, and metabolic factors may predispose an animal to specific diseases.

Environmental Factors

Environmental factors also require consideration in the preventive health plan. Climatic extremes or sudden climatic changes can clearly cause distress or even death. Although we cannot change the weather, we can adjust the animal's housing to reduce environmental stress. Additional bedding improves the insulation around animals housed in extremely cold conditions. Overhead cover is needed to prevent sunburn and heat prostration and shield animals from precipitation.

Inadequate ventilation increases the incidence of respiratory diseases through increased ammonia levels and large numbers of microorganisms in the air. Inadequate ventilation also impairs cooling in animals that use respiration to regulate body temperature (e.g., dogs) and prevents radiation of body heat (e.g., heat loss from the ears of rabbits). Inadequate ventilation inhibits the drying of bedding, favoring proliferation of bacteria or parasites. At the other end of the spectrum, excessive ventilation is also stressful. Drafts or excessive ventilation can cause chilling, dehydration, or inflamed ocular tissues.

The level of ventilation should be appropriate for the animal, rather than for the animal owner. We must take the time to experience the same conditions that the animal is experiencing. We must evaluate airflow not at the 5-foot level, but at the 5-inch level. A draft along the floor could lead to respiratory disease in a small mammal but may not be evident to the animal owner. A 2-hour period of sunshine directly on a hamster each day could dehydrate the pet, while the owner remains unaware of it. Inadvertent spraying of perfume or other aerosols near a fish tank could kill the fish. If the air in a poorly ventilated barn or stable causes discomfort in farm personnel, such as burning eyes or a sore throat, it is also causing discomfort in the animals.

Metabolic Factors

Metabolic factors also must be considered in preventive health programs. Factors beyond our control include the age of the animal and reproductive status; concurrent disease; and nonspecific stressors. Young, old, pregnant, and lactating animals have different physiologic needs than other animals. These needs may require alteration of the animal's diet and housing.

A common metabolic problem that influences the health of many companion animals, and that can be effectively managed by the animal owner, is obesity from overfeeding and lack of exercise. We often focus on the animal's age group and manage health problems as they relate to age; however, a more effective preventive approach is to address factors under the client's control. Veterinary professionals should discuss proper nutrition and exercise programs with clients so that their animals can benefit from that knowledge.

WELLNESS PROGRAMS

There is no doubt that preventive medicine and specifically the use of vaccines has been responsible for saving the lives of countless animals over the past few decades. For years the veterinary community has relied on the annual booster vaccination as a means of encouraging yearly visits to the veterinarian. Because of recent controversies surrounding the use of vaccines, and client knowledge of these issues, the veterinary community is trying to shift emphasis from yearly booster vaccines to health and wellness examinations.

Because companion animals mature at approximately seven times the rate of humans, annual wellness examinations are essential to ensure their health and identify developing diseases in their early stages.

Implementing a Wellness Program

Creating a wellness program for patients should begin with client education. Veterinary technicians should look for ways to maximize opportunities to educate clients on wellness. Written materials with specific wellness goals can be reviewed with each client. Use an age equivalence chart to help clients see that a year in the life of a dog or cat can be as much as 20% of its life expectancy (Tables 12-9 and 12-10).

TABLE 12-9 Age Equivalents for Dogs
Comparative Age in Human Years

DOG'S AGE	0-20 LB	21-50 LB	51-90 LB	>90 LB
5 years	36	37	40	42
6 years	40	42	45	49
7 years	44	47	50	56
10 years	56	60	66	78
12 years	64	69	77	93
15 years	76	83	93	115
20 years	96	105	120	

Adapted from senior@seven wellness exam brochures. Antech Diagnostics.

TABLE 12-10 Age Equivalents for Cats

CAT'S AGE	COMPARATIVE AGE IN HUMAN YEARS
1	15
2	24
5	36
7	45
12	64
15	76
18	88
21	100

Adapted from senior@seven wellness exam brochures. Antech Diagnostics.

BOX 12-3 In-House Laboratory Supplies*

General Supplies
- Binocular microscopes
- Glass slides and coverslips
- Lens tissue
- Immersion oil
- Lab timer and stopwatch
- Disposable pipettes
- Test tube rack
- Refractometer
- OSHA supplies: labels, manuals, personal protective equipment
- Blood collection supplies

Hematology Supplies
- Microhematocrit centrifuge
- Microhematocrit tubes and sealant
- Microhematocrit card reader
- Differential stain
- New Methylene Blue stain
- Multi-place tally counter
- Staining jars
- Hematology analyzer supplies: sample cups/dilution vials, dilution fluids, quality control material, hemoglobin lysing reagent

Clinical Chemistry Supplies
- Chemistry analyzer and supplies
- Clinical centrifuge and centrifuge tubes
- Sample/dilution cups
- Quality control material

Urinalysis Supplies
- Urine collection containers
- Conical centrifuge tubes
- Variable speed clinical centrifuge
- E.R.D. screen test kit
- Quality control material

Coagulation Testing Supplies
- Hemacytometer and coverglass
- Hand tally counter
- Bleeding time lancets
- Blotting paper
- Automated coagulation analyzer and supplies or ACT tubes and heat block

Parasitology and Immunodiagnostic Supplies
- Fecal sample collection supplies
- Fecal flotation solution
- Heartworm antigen test kits
- Antibody test kits

*This list is not meant to be an all-inclusive presentation of supplies needed. The most commonly used equipment and supplies needed for an in-house laboratory performing wellness exams are included.

Many clinics have special testing programs for senior pets. However, even healthy young adult pets should be evaluated for early detection and prevention of disease. Once the client agrees to the wellness examination, be sure to provide a written "report card" of the exam and take time to explain recommendations to the client.

What to Include

Wellness programs vary at different veterinary facilities and different ages and life stages of pets. In general, a complete physical examination should be performed annually. Blood test results, antibody titers, parasite testing, urinalysis, nutritional assessment, behavioral evaluations, and assessment of the pet's home environment may be included. Patients that are considered geriatric (usually over the age of 7) may also need electrocardiography, radiography, and other tests for common problems of senior pets.

The In-House Laboratory

Although the wellness test profiles can be sent to outside labs, providing these services in-house improves service by sparing the client the several hours-to-overnight wait for test results. In addition, the treatment benefit of rapid test turnaround time is one of the goals of a successful wellness program. In-house laboratory testing is also a source of additional revenue for the clinic. Many of the basic supplies needed for in-house testing are already present in most veterinary clinics. Clinics that do not currently perform in-house laboratory services may have additional equipment and supply needs. Box 12-3 lists some commonly used supplies for in-house laboratory testing.

TABLE 12-11 In-House Analyzers

	CHARACTERISTICS	MANUFACTURER
In-House Chemistry Analyzers		
Analyst	Rotor technology Profiles or miniprofiles Semiautomated dilution	Hemagen Diagnostics www.hemagen.com
Irma	Cartridge technology Portable Miniprofiles Limited chemistry menu Includes electrolytes	Diametrics Medical, Inc. www.diametrics.com
Phoenix	On-board sealed reagents Ideal for small samples Multiple simultaneous sample processing	Oxford Science http://www.oxfordscienceinc.com
VetStat	Cassette technology Single tests or profiles	Idexx Laboratories www.idexx.com
Hematology Analyzers		
COULTER A^c T	Impedance counter Includes WBC histogram Automated quality control	Beckman Coulter www.beckmancoulter.com
Genesis	Combines impedance and laser flow cytometry methods	Oxford Science http://www.oxfordscienceinc.com
LaserCyte	Laser flow cytometry Differential WBC count	Idexx Laboratories www.idexx.com
Miscellaneous Analyzers		
CoagDx	aPTT and PT tests Automated Portable	Idexx Laboratories www.idexx.com
Element POC	Multi-parameter blood gas/electrolyte analyzer Portable	Heska www.heska.com

During the past two decades, in-house laboratory equipment has become increasingly user-friendly and cost-effective. Laboratory equipment for in-house wellness testing requires a blood chemistry analyzer, hematology analyzer, and supplies for urinalysis and coagulation profiles. Table 12-11 provides an overview of some of the common in-house analyzers marketed to veterinary facilities. Some of these analyzers are also capable of performing electrolyte testing, although most patients will not require those tests. Most of these analyzers are similar in their degree of accuracy. The veterinary staff should determine cost per test based on anticipated test volume. Additional costs include supplies and technician time to prepare and run samples, as well as time required for routine maintenance, calibration, and quality control.

Physical Examination

A complete systems examination should be performed on all pets. The pet's weight and overall nutritional status should be evaluated. A complete behavioral history and assessment of the environment in which the pet lives should also be performed. These data will help to determine whether the patient is at any risk of exposure to specific diseases. There are several approaches to performing the physical examination. Box 12-4 provides a systematic method of physical examination. Additional information on physical examination techniques is located in Chapter 22. Remember that "normal" can vary among species and even among individuals at different times. Appropriate words to use for finding no abnormalities are "characteristic" or "adequate." Each of the systems has a minimum number of parameters that you can and should be evaluating.

Every attempt should be made to show the client the thoroughness and importance of the physical examination. The client should see the veterinarian and/or veterinary technician using the tools that they would expect to see in their own physician's office (stethoscope, otoscope, ophthalmoscope, etc.). This adds value to the client's perception of the physical examination.

Blood Tests

Depending on the age and life stage of the patient, a complete blood count (CBC) and chemistry panel should be performed. These tests can detect hundreds of internal diseases, such as diabetes, liver diseases, and kidney diseases. The complete blood count includes tests that can identify the presence of anemia and can aid in evaluating the pet's nutritional status. The CBC includes red and white blood cell counts,

BOX 12-4 Systematic Method of Physical Examination

- Record TPR.
- Evaluate and record animal's general condition (i.e., disposition, activity level, overall body condition, etc.).
- Evaluate and record condition of each body system:
  - ✓ *Integument:* Note overall condition of hair coat, presence or absence of alopecia, parasites, lumps, wounds, rashes, etc., note hydration status with skin turgor test.
  - ✓ *Respiratory:* Evaluate respiratory rate and rhythm; record presence or absence of rales, rhonchi, crepitus, dyspnea, nasal discharge, etc.
  - ✓ *Cardiovascular:* Evaluate cardiac rate and rhythm; CRT, presence or absence of pulse; deficit, etc.
  - ✓ *Gastrointestinal:* Record presence or absence of diarrhea, vomiting (note character, if present). Palpate abdomen and record presence or absence of tenderness, impaction, etc.
  - ✓ *Genitourinary:* Palpate kidneys, bladder. Note presence of characteristic urine volume; note any blood, etc., in urine. [In male, check for presence/absence of testicles in scrotum; penile discharge. In female, record evidence of pregnancy, lactation, vaginal discharge (note character, if present)].
  - ✓ *Musculoskeletal:* Evaluate presence or absence of swelling (particularly in joints); manipulate limbs; record any abnormal gait, limping, guarding, tenderness; note overall musculature.
  - ✓ *Nervous:* Record presence or absence of head tilt, tremors, etc. Evaluate pupillary light reflexes. Evaluate and record triceps, patellar, and gastrocnemius reflexes.
  - ✓ *Eyes:* Evaluate and record, presence or absence of abrasions, ulcers, discharge (note character, if present).
  - ✓ *Ears:* Evaluate and record presence or absence of tenderness, parasites, odor, ulcers, discharge (note character, if present).
  - ✓ *Mucosa:* Note color of mucous membranes, evaluate odor of mouth, evaluate periodontal tissues.
  - ✓ *Lymphatic:* Palpate peripheral lymph nodes, evaluate characteristic size and location of lymph nodes.

hemoglobin concentration, packed cell volume, and differential blood film. All adult patients under the age of 7 years should have at least one baseline CBC and chemistry panel.

It is common for patients to have one or more laboratory values that are outside of accepted "normal" or "reference" ranges. Normal values are a guideline only. It may be that a particular patient normally has a value that is somewhat beyond the normal range. This may be perfectly acceptable for that patient. If a patient becomes ill and the veterinarian has no baseline data, it is difficult to determine if an abnormal result is to the result of the illness or is an idiosyncrasy of the patient.

Other tests may be included because of the pet's potential risk. For example, patients that are obese may need thyroid evaluations. As discussed earlier in this chapter, antibody titers for common diseases may also be performed. Pets that are older than 7 years and those with chronic illnesses such as Cushing's disease, diabetes, etc. should have more detailed wellness examinations.

Coagulation Profile

Veterinary patients can be affected by a number of genetic and acquired diseases of the coagulation mechanisms. There are several simple and inexpensive evaluations that can identify these defects. All patients should have a coagulation profile before any surgery to identify potential bleeding problems in these patients. Patients with chronic disease, especially those with poor nutrition, should also be evaluated. Some coagulation abnormalities may be subclinical; that is, the patient does not always have visible signs or symptoms of disease. When these patients have surgery or are involved in traumatic events, bleeding problems become evident and are much more difficult to manage. A platelet count, bleeding time, and activated clotting time test should be performed at least once on all adult patients. Other coagulation tests that may be included in wellness exams include prothrombin time and activated partial thromboplastin time. Both of these tests require special instrumentation but can be performed easily in-house.

Parasite Exams

Wellness exams should include a fecal direct smear, fecal flotation, and serum tests for heartworm antigen. The blood smear can be used to detect other parasites such as *Ehrlichia, Mycoplasma,* and *Babesia.* The fecal direct smear is useful for detecting protozoal parasites such as *Giardia* and *Coccidia.* Fecal flotation can detect the presence of common parasites such as *Toxocara canis, Trichuris vulpis,* and *Ancylostoma caninum.*

Urinalysis

Evaluation of the overall health and function of the urinary system is arguably one of the most valuable sets of tests that can be performed. The kidneys perform many functions in maintaining the health of the patient. Changes in urine chemistry and the presence of certain types of cells and crystals in the urine can provide a great deal of information on the patient's overall health status. Renal disease is a leading cause of mortality in small animals. Early detection can halt or slow progression of a disease. In addition to the CBC and chemistry panel, senior pets should also be tested for microalbuminuria to detect early changes in kidney function. The presence of any protein in urine indicates alteration in glomerular filtration. The microalbuminuria test acts to detect the protein, albumin in the urine and can be performed with in-clinic test kits (E.R.D.-HealthScreen, Heska, Fribourg, Switzerland). Because the test is more sensitive to urine protein, it provides for detection of changes in the glomerulus before a reduction in kidney function occurs.

Radiography and Electrocardiography

Although not required for every pet, chest radiographs and an electrocardiograph should be performed on all senior pets. Patients that have had prior treatment for heartworm infection and those with chronic illnesses or chronic coughing should also be screened for cardiac health. Chest radiographs should be performed routinely in cats, especially those that are not on heartworm prophylaxis because heartworm disease is more difficult to detect in cats than in dogs. Also, cats tend to clear immature heartworms, which can lead to a pulmonary condition known as heartworm associated respiratory disease (HARD). Many cardiac and respiratory diseases in dogs and cats can be successfully treated in their early stages. Early detection of these diseases can greatly improve prognosis; however, in late-stage disease, tissue damage is often too great for treatment to be effective.

Miscellaneous Tests

Keratoconjunctivitis sicca is one of the most common ocular diseases in dogs and a common cause of blindness. The Shirmer tear test can identify this condition. Certain dog breeds such as Cocker Spaniels, Lhasa Apsos, and Shih Tzus are especially prone to this condition. Glaucoma is also a common cause of blindness in dogs and cats. Glaucoma screening can be accomplished with a tonometer or by ocular ultrasound.

REVIEW QUESTIONS

Matching

1. Match the following cells to their function:

_____**A.** neutrophils
_____**B.** eosinophils
_____**C.** lymphocytes
_____**D.** monocytes

a. responsible for humoral antibody production
b. primary function is phagocytosis
c. a more specific phagocytosis and lysosomal enzyme release
d. become macrophages when they enter tissue at the site of inflammation

2. Match the following terms:

_____**A.** wound
_____**B.** parasites
_____**C.** fibrosis tissue
_____**D.** granulation tissue
_____**E.** disease
_____**F.** virus

a. are organisms that have adapted to live on or within a host organism
b. is any alteration from the normal state of health
c. is an injury caused by physical means, with disruption of normal structures
d. are extremely small infectious agents which can cause disease in a wide variety of animals
e. is a highly vascularized connective tissue that is only produced after extensive tissue damage
f. primarily comprises dense fibrous connective tissue and collagen and contracts when mature

3. Match the cell type to its function

_____**A.** B-lymphocyte
_____**B.** T-lymphocyte

a. antibodies that are produced by plasma cells
b. play a role in cell-mediated responses

Fill in the Blank

Provide answers to complete the following statements.

1. Vaccines that are recommended for all patients of a particular species are considered a _____________ vaccine.
2. Vaccines that are recommended based on a patient's lifestyle are considered a _____________ vaccine.
3. A vaccine that consists of a weaker version of a pathogen is _____________.
4. A vaccine that consists of whole killed or selected antigenic subunits is _____________.
5. A vaccine that consists of a live, nonpathogenic virus into which the gene for a pathogen-related antigen has been inserted is _____________.

RECOMMENDED READING

August JR: Dog and cat bites, *J Am Vet Med Assoc* 193:1394–1398, 1988.

Birchard SJ, Sherding RG: *Saunders manual of small animal practice*, ed 3, St Louis, 2006, Saunders.

Bonagura JD: *Kirk's current veterinary therapy XV, small animal practice*, St Louis, 2014, Saunders.

Breitschwerdt EB: Tick-borne zoonoses, *Vet Tech* 11(5):249–251, 1990.

Colville JL, Berryhill DL: *2013 Handbook of zoonoses: identification and prevention*, St Louis, 2013, Mosby.

Gershwin LJ, et al.: *Immunology and immunopathology of domestic animals*, ed 2, St Louis, 1995, Mosby.

McCapes RH, Osburn BI, Riemann H: Safety of foods of animal origin: responsibilities of veterinary medicine, *J Am Vet Med Assoc* 199:870–874, 1991.

National Association of State Public Health Veterinarians: Inc: Compendium of animal rabies control, *J Am Vet Med Assoc* 208:214–218, 1996.

Smith B: *Large animal internal medicine*, ed 5, St Louis, 2014, Mosby.

Summers A: *Common diseases of companion animals*, ed 3, St Louis, 2013, Mosby.

Tizard IR: *Veterinary immunology: an introduction*, ed 9, St Louis, 2013, Saunders.

Zachary JF: *Pathologic basis of veterinary disease*, ed 4, St Louis, 2013, Mosby.

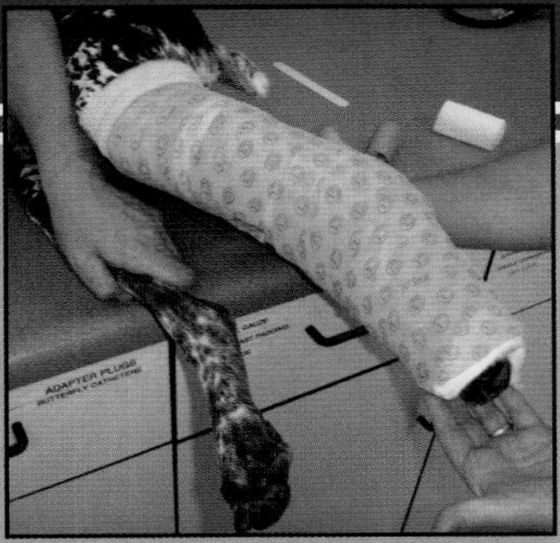

13 Management of Wounds, Fractures, and Other Injuries

OUTLINE

LEARNING OBJECTIVES

After reviewing this chapter, the reader will be able to:

1. Describe the phases of wound healing.
2. Identify the categories of wounds.
3. Explain the principles of first-aid treatment of wounds.
4. Explain the principles of wound closure.
5. Give examples of the types and application of bandages.
6. Give examples of the types and application of splints and casts.
7. Distinguish ways in which specific types of wounds are managed.

KEY TERMS

Closed-suction drains
Debridement phase
Eschar
First-intention healing
Inflammatory phase
Maturation phase
Penrose drain
Porous adhesive tape
Proud flesh
Repair phase
Second-intention healing
Third-intention healing

A wound is a disruption of cellular and anatomic functional continuity. Wound healing is the restoration of this continuity. Acute wounds are those induced by surgery or trauma that heal normally, with healing time determined by the depth and size of the lesion. Examples of acute wounds include surgical incisions, blunt trauma, bite wounds, burns, gunshots, and avulsion injuries. Chronic wounds have various causes and, as determined by their underlying pathology, may take months or years to heal completely. Decubital ulcers (pressure sores), diabetic ulcers, and vascular ulcers are examples of chronic wounds.

WOUND HEALING

PHASES OF WOUND HEALING

Most healing of soft tissue occurs as a result of epithelial regeneration and fibroplasia, both of which occur simultaneously. The epidermis serves as a barrier from the environment and is necessary for optimal appearance, function, and protection. A bed of granulation tissue is required for migration of epithelium across the defect. The four phases of soft tissue wound healing are the **inflammatory phase,** the **debridement phase,** the **repair phase,** and the **maturation phase.** The phases of wound healing are overlapping events; a wound may have more than one phase occurring at the same time. Most of the time the inflammatory and debridement phases can be considered one phase because these two occur simultaneously. Box 13-1 summarizes the phases of wound healing. Details on tissue response to injury were presented in Chapter 12.

TYPES OF WOUND HEALING

Relatively clean, minor wounds, such as small lacerations, heal by primary or **first-intention healing.** The tissues can be pulled together with sutures, and healing progresses without complication. Wounds that are larger, more complicated, or infected may need to heal by second-intention. In this case, the wound is left open and allowed to heal from the inner areas to the outer surface. Although sometimes necessary, **second-intention healing** is a less desirable method of healing.

Some large or grossly contaminated wounds are allowed to heal initially by second intention and then are closed with sutures. After a healthy granulation bed is formed and infection is no longer present, the granulation bed is closed with sutures. This is described as **third-intention healing.** Very large wounds treated with third-intention methods may heal more rapidly than if allowed to heal by second-intention.

First-intention healing of fractures is primary bone healing, with rigid internal fixation (e.g., pins, plates). Second-intention ("normal") healing of fractures is by callus formation, using no internal fixation.

Wound healing is impaired by numerous factors, including infection, debris and necrotic tissue, old age, malnutrition, poor perfusion, drugs (e.g., corticosteroids), and hypothermia.

BOX 13-1 Events in the Three Phases of Wound Healing

Exudative-Inflammatory-Debridement Phase

Inflammation starts immediately and predominates for up to 6 hours
This phase can last for several weeks
Acute vasoconstriction followed by vasodilation
Plasma proteins leak from vessels into interstitial space
Leukocytes (neutrophils, monocytes, macrophages) exit blood vessels
Fibroblasts differentiate
Endothelial cells begin to proliferate

Proliferation-Collagen Phase

Starts at 12 to 36 hours after injury
Fibroblasts and endothelial cells proliferate
Neutrophils decrease while macrophages increase
Collagen synthesis starts after 4 to 6 days
Components of granulation tissue become engaged in healing; endothelial buds grow into damaged or intact blood vessels; mesenchymal cells follow the budding endothelium, secreting ground substance

Remodeling-Maturation Phase

Starts after about 2 weeks
Lasts 2 to 3 weeks in rapidly healing tissues (viscera)
Can last for years in slowly healing tissues (bone, tendon, ligament)
Slow increase in tensile strength
Equilibrium of collagen synthesis and breakdown
Collagen cross-linking slowly increases tissue strength

WOUND CONTAMINATION AND INFECTION

Wound contamination is not the same as wound infection. Microorganisms in the environment contaminate all wounds, even those created during surgery using strict aseptic technique. Initially, these organisms are loosely attached to tissues and do not invade adjacent tissue; there is no host immune response to these organisms. With time, the microorganisms multiply. Infection is the process by which organisms bind to tissue, multiply, and then invade viable tissue, eliciting an immune response. Tissue infection depends on the number and pathogenicity (or virulence) of the microorganisms. In general, a wound is infected when the number of microorganisms reaches 100,000 per gram of tissue or milliliter of fluid. At these numbers, the microorganisms have exceeded the host's defense mechanisms to control them. If the patient is presented for treatment more than 12 hours after injury, any wounds should be considered infected. Infection is characterized by erythema, edema, pus, fever, elevated neutrophil count, pain, change in color of exudate, or uncharacteristic odor. Contaminated wounds may become infected under the following circumstances:

- Foreign bodies are present (e.g., organic material, bone fragments, suture material, glove powder, bone plates, and screws).
- Excessive necrotic tissue is left in the wound.
- Excessive bleeding results in higher levels of ferric ion (necessary for bacterial replication).
- Local tissue defenses are impeded (e.g., excessive hemoglobin in burn patients or patients receiving immunosuppressive drugs).
- The vascular supply is altered.
- Dirt and debris are present.

Appropriate treatment soon after injury is important to avoid infection.

WOUND CATEGORIES

Open traumatic wounds can be categorized according to the degree of contamination present (Box 13-2). Management of these wounds varies according to the severity of the injury and the patient's condition. In general, wounds that are grossly contaminated and/or dirty may not be good candidates for primary closure. Until contamination and infection can be eliminated, open wound management is necessary. Dead and dying tissues must be excised (debrided) to minimize the potential for bacterial infection and create a viable wound bed.

USE OF ANTIBACTERIALS

The decision to use antibacterials systemically or topically in a surgical wound depends on several preoperative factors, including the patient's condition and immune status, the nature of the surgery (emergency versus elective), location of the wound (orthopedic versus abdominal), predicted duration of the surgical procedure, the surgeon's experience, and the environment in which the procedure is performed.

It is generally thought that antibacterials are not needed for patients in good health with an adequate immune status undergoing a relatively short (less than 90 minutes) elective orthopedic or soft tissue surgical procedure (not abdominal) performed by an experienced surgeon using aseptic technique in a clean surgical facility.

In clean surgical wounds, preoperative antibacterials should be considered in cases of shock, severe systemic trauma, long procedures, traumatic procedures, poor blood supply, foreign bodies, dead space (seromas, hematomas), malnutrition, obesity, or other factors altering host defense mechanisms. When systemic (injected) antibacterials are used, they are most effective if administered just before surgery is begun and continued every 90 to 120 minutes thereafter during the surgical procedure.

Traumatic wounds, as opposed to "clean" surgical wounds, may contain devitalized tissue and/or foreign material and are contaminated by microorganisms. Traumatized tissue provides a suitable environment for bacterial multiplication and provides a route of entry for penetration of pathogens into adjacent viable tissue. Chronic (long-standing) wounds offer an ideal environment for bacterial proliferation, with copious wound fluid, necrotic tissue, and deep cracks and crevices on the wound surface. In such cases, antibacterials with a broad spectrum of antimicrobial activity are given systemically.

It is likely that we often do more harm than good by applying topical medications to wounds. The adverse effect of these products on wound healing is independent of their antimicrobial action. Generally, water-soluble antibacterial products tend to impede wound healing more than do ointments or creams. Solutions tend to evaporate, contributing to drying of the wound surface. Ointments and creams remain in contact with the wound longer than solutions, preventing drying of the wound surface but also trapping bacteria in the wound and allowing for infection. A clean wound in a healthy patient can heal optimally without application of ointments, salves, etc. Certain topical products may be beneficial at times; however, a focus on aseptic technique and appropriate "clean" management of wounds is more appropriate.

BOX 13-2 Categories of Wounds

Clean
Surgical wounds
Elective incisions
Highly vascular tissues not predisposed to infection

Clean-Contaminated
Minor contamination evident
Surgical wounds with minor break in aseptic technique
Elective surgery in tissues with normal resident bacterial flora (e.g., gastrointestinal tract, respiratory tract, or genitourinary tract)
No spillage of organ contents

Contaminated
Moderate contamination evident
Fresh traumatic injuries, open fractures, penetrating wounds
Surgery with gross spillage of organ contents
Presence of bile or infected urine
Surgical wounds with major break in aseptic technique

Dirty
Grossly contaminated or infected
Contaminated traumatic wounds more than 4 hours old
Perforated viscera, abscess, necrotic tissue, foreign material

WOUND MANAGEMENT

FIRST AID

In the field and/or before transport to a treatment facility, the wound should be protected with a bandage. An occlusive bandage is preferred. This type of bandage controls hemorrhage, prevents additional contamination, and provides immobilization of the extremity. Open fractures should be splinted. In open or compound fractures, exposed bone should not be forced into position below the skin. This avoids additional soft tissue trauma and reduces chances of deep tissue contamination. The wound should be evaluated for antimicrobial therapy at the treatment facility. The wound should be protected during preparation of the surrounding area (e.g., clipping and scrubbing).

TECHNICIAN NOTE Wound management revolves around three considerations: cleansing, closing, and covering.

WOUND ASSESSMENT

Wound assessment includes evaluation of the wound's location, size, and depth; exudate (drainage); tissue in the wound bed; and any signs of infection. Wound management revolves around three considerations: cleansing, closing, and covering. Control of hemorrhage is usually the first step in wound management. After initial hemostasis, it is important to evaluate the wound for bacterial contamination and the potential for bacterial growth. To avoid introduction of microorganisms, the wound should be cleaned under aseptic or at least sanitary conditions.

CLIPPING

In initial wound treatment, the wound must be protected while areas around the wound are clipped and cleaned.

Before the area around the wound is clipped and cleaned, cover the wound with a water-soluble sterile ointment (e.g., K-Y Lubricating Jelly, Johnson & Johnson, New Brunswick, NJ) or moistened sterile gauze sponges. This helps to prevent loose hairs from further contaminating the wound. The wound can also be temporarily closed with towel clamps or a continuous suture. This may require analgesia. Before clipping and shaving areas around head or face wounds, an ophthalmic ointment should be instilled in the conjunctival sac to protect the cornea and conjunctiva.

If the patient is covered with dirt and debris (and is not in critical condition), it should be bathed before clipping. This reduces further contamination. Clipper blades also stay sharper longer when cutting clean hair. Clipping removes sources of contamination (e.g., hair, dirt, and debris) and allows better visualization of the wound. Two pairs of clipper blades are advantageous; the second set of blades is disinfected for use in areas of elective surgical sites. Hair at wound edges may be trimmed with scissors or a handheld No. 10 scalpel blade dipped in mineral oil, K-Y Jelly, or water so that the hair sticks to the blade and does not enter the wound.

> TECHNICIAN NOTE Cover a wound with K-Y jelly or gauze sponges when clipping and cleaning around it to help reduce potential contamination.

SCRUBBING

After the area around the wound has been clipped, replace the gauze sponges or gel over the wound. Gently scrub the surrounding intact skin, not the wound itself. The most commonly used surgical scrubs for skin preparation contain an antimicrobial agent plus a detergent/surfactant, such as chlorhexidine or povidine-iodine. Rinsing with saline or 70% isopropyl alcohol does not seem to influence the antimicrobial effect.

WOUND LAVAGE

Cleansing and debridement of a wound begins after the surrounding area has been cleaned. Obvious foreign bodies and gross contamination must be removed. Usually, a noncaustic solution is used to clean the wound without creating further irritation. Lavaging with a sterile solution and gentle scrubbing are the primary methods used for cleaning the wound. Take care not to use forceful lavage or scrub too vigorously; this may force bacteria into the wound and spread contamination. Often more than one session of lavage and additional debridement may be necessary to remove debris and necrotic tissue. Bandaging with wet wound dressing can facilitate this process. As a general rule, wound lavage should be discontinued before the tissues take on a "water-logged" appearance.

Lavage solutions are most effective when delivered with a fluid jet impacting the wound with a pressure of at least 7 pounds per square inch (psi) (Figs. 13-1 and 13-2). This can be achieved by forcefully expelling solution from a 35- to 60-ml syringe through an 18-gauge needle. Lavage solutions can also be delivered using a fluid bag (with administration set, three-way stopcock, and 35- to 60-ml syringe on one side and 18-gauge needle on the other) or Water Pik. The Water Pik should be used with care, because it can deliver fluids at up to 70 psi. Adequate fluid pressure cannot be achieved with gravity flow, a bulb syringe, or a turkey baster.

Isotonic ("normal") saline, lactated Ringer's solution, or plain Ringer's solution may be used for lavage. These physiologic (isotonic, isosmotic, and sterile) solutions do not damage tissue but have no antibacterial properties.

Povidone-iodine solution is commonly used to lavage wounds because of its broad antimicrobial spectrum. Dilutions of povidone-iodine in the range of 1% to 2% are more potent and more rapidly bactericidal than commercial 10% povidone-iodine solution, because dilution makes more "free iodine" available. A 1% solution can be prepared by diluting 1 part commercial 10% povidone-iodine with 9 parts sterile water or electrolyte solution. The bactericidal effect of povidone-iodine lasts only 4 to 6 hours. It is inactivated by blood, exudate, and organic soil, reducing the period

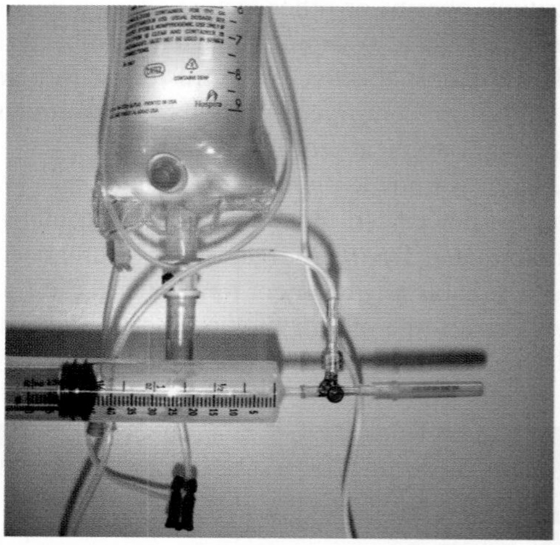

FIGURE 13-1 Lavage system. This shows a setup using fluid bag, syringe, and stopcock.

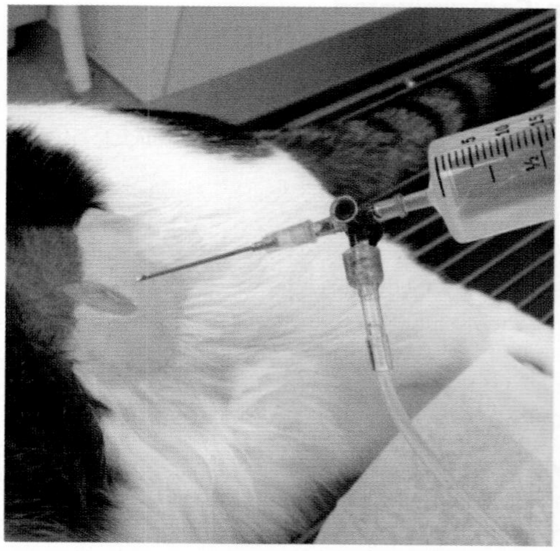

FIGURE 13-2 Demonstration of the lavage system. Lavaging an open wound.

of residual action. The detergent form of povidone-iodine (scrub) is deleterious to wound tissues, causing irritation and potentiation of wound infection.

Chlorhexidine diacetate solution has a broad antimicrobial spectrum and is commonly used on small animals. In dogs, it is more effective against *Staphylococcus aureus* than is povidone-iodine. When chlorhexidine is applied to intact skin, the antimicrobial effect is immediate, with a lasting residual effect. Prolonged tissue contact with solutions concentrated at 0.5% or greater may be harmful. Currently, 0.05% chlorhexidine solutions are recommended for use in wound lavage. A 0.05% solution can be prepared by diluting 1 part 2% stock solution with 40 parts water. Chlorhexidine has sustained residual activity. Systemic absorption, toxicosis, and inactivation by organic material do not seem to be problematic.

Hydrogen peroxide is commonly used as a foaming wound irrigant. It has little antimicrobial effect, except on some anaerobes. It is more effective as a sporicide. In concentrations of 3% and greater, hydrogen peroxide is damaging to tissues. It also causes thrombosis in the microvasculature adjacent to the wound margins, impairing proliferation of blood vessels. Hydrogen peroxide should be reserved for one-time initial irrigation of dirty wounds. It should not be delivered to wounds under pressure, because its foaming action forces debris between tissue planes, enlarging the wound and allowing accumulation of air in tissues.

TECHNICIAN NOTE Hydrogen peroxide can be used only for initial wound cleaning.

ANESTHESIA AND ANALGESIA

After preparation of the surrounding area, the wound is prepared for analgesia and debridement. Local, regional, or general anesthesia may be used for wound management. General anesthesia is preferred if the patient can tolerate it. Tranquilizers or sedatives (e.g., xylazine, acepromazine, diazepam) are often used in conjunction with local and regional anesthesia.

Local anesthetics, such as lidocaine and bupivacaine, are used for pain control if the patient is not a candidate for general anesthesia. It may be beneficial to lavage a wound initially with 2% lidocaine for 1 or 2 minutes before irrigating to make removal of foreign bodies less painful. Local anesthetics do not usually offer sufficient analgesia for surgical debridement.

Epinephrine is included in some local anesthetic products. It causes vasoconstriction and helps reduce hemorrhage and prolong the anesthetic effect. Epinephrine may cause tissue necrosis along the wound edge, adversely affect tissue defenses, and potentiate infection. In general, local anesthetics containing epinephrine should not be used in wound care.

DEBRIDEMENT

Debridement is the removal of devitalized or necrotic tissue. Necrotic tissue must be removed, as epithelium will not migrate over nonviable tissue, a wound will not contract without debridement, and necrotic tissue may act as a growth medium for bacteria. Debridement also removes sources of contamination, infection, and mechanical obstructions to healing.

Debridement is complete when the wound bed consists of only healthy tissue, commonly referred to as a "clean wound." However, this does not mean the wound is free of bacteria. Acute traumatic wounds are usually debrided to facilitate surgical closure, whereas chronic wounds are usually debrided to reduce the risk of infection and facilitate second-intention healing.

Wounds are usually debrided by mechanical means, such as with surgical instruments, irrigation, and dry-to-dry or wet-to-dry dressings (Procedure 13-1). Nonmechanical debridement techniques include application of enzymatic agents or chemicals. In many cases, a combination of techniques is used.

Debridement should be performed as an aseptic procedure. To protect the wound from further contamination, sterile surgical gloves and mask should be worn and the area draped. Ideally, several sets of sterile instruments should be used to prevent reintroducing contaminated instruments into the wound (Fig. 13-3).

After a wound is cleansed and free of devitalized tissue, the surgeon explores the wound using sterile techniques. Other diagnostic procedures, such as radiographic studies

PROCEDURE 13-1 Applying a Wet-to-Dry Dressing

1. This is performed using antiseptic technique and after initial cleaning and debridement of the wound has taken place.
2. Open the sterile dressings (usually gauze pads), the irrigation and cleaning solution (this varies but sterile saline works well), and the instrument set to provide a sterile field.
3. Gently remove and discard the old tape and soiled dressing. If the dressing sticks to the wound, then moisten with sterile saline before removing.
4. Cleanse the wound. Clean from the least to the most contaminated area.
5. Apply saline to sterile gauze and place the wet material directly on the wound.
6. Apply dry gauze on top of the wet gauze.
7. Use cling gauze to hold the material in place followed by vet wrap.

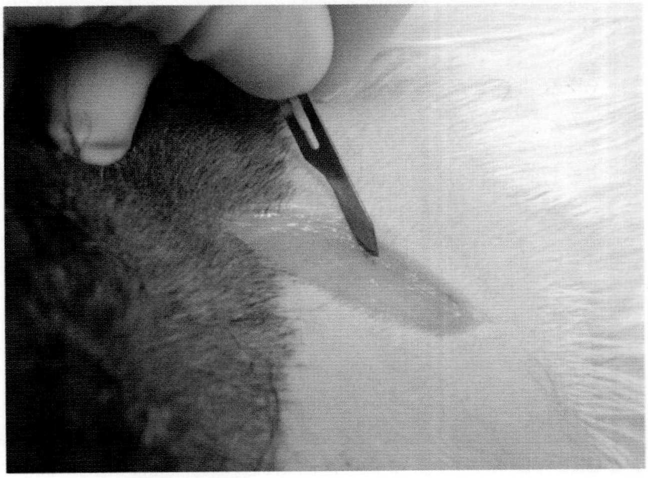

FIGURE 13-3 Debridement of a wound.

using contrast materials, collection and assessment of fluid samples, and cytologic examination, may be performed to assist in the overall evaluation. Once this process is completed, a decision is made regarding how the wound will be managed, including if drainage is required. If primary closure is elected, decisions are made concerning anesthesia, antibacterials, nonsteroidal anti-inflammatory drugs, tetanus status (if the injured animal is a horse), and bandaging (if required). The wound is then prepared for suturing.

DRAINAGE

Drains implanted in a wound provide an escape path for unwanted air and/or wound fluids, thus preventing or reducing seroma or hematoma formation in tissue pockets or dead space.

Accumulation of exudate in a wound favors infection. Excessive fluid prevents phagocytic cells from reaching bacteria within a wound and provides a medium for bacterial growth. Drains are needed when wounds produce fluids and exudates for several days after initial treatment. They are indicated as follows:

- For treatment of an abscess cavity
- When foreign material and nonviable tissue are present and cannot be excised
- When contamination is inevitable (e.g., wounds near anal area)
- To obliterate dead space
- As a prophylaxis against anticipated fluid or air collection after a surgical procedure

Penrose drains are made of soft latex rubber. Their sizes range from ¼ to 1 inch in diameter and 12 to 18 inches long (Fig. 13-4). They provide a simple conduit for gravity flow (Fig. 13-5). If a bandage covers the drain, there may be some capillary action. Fluid flows through the drain's lumen and around the tube and is related to the surface area of the tubing. The fenestrations (holes) in the drain decrease the surface area and reduce its effectiveness. Cutting the Penrose drain in half lengthwise increases the surface area by 100%. Penrose drains should not be left in place for more than 3 to 5 days, because most gravitational drainage has subsided by that time.

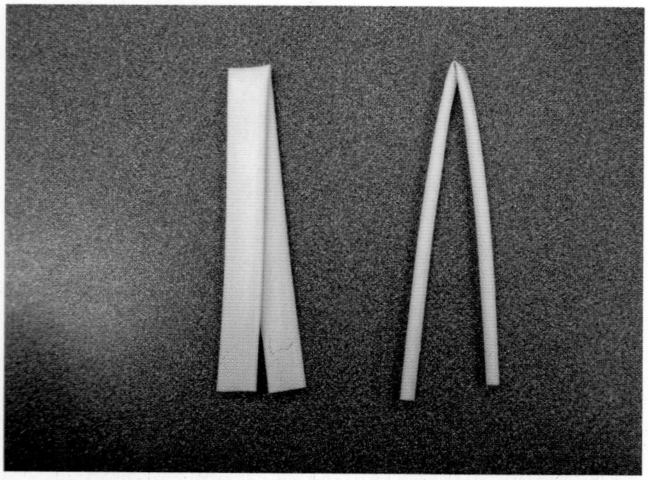

FIGURE 13-4 Penrose drains. A collection of different sized Penrose drains.

Closed-suction drains provide drainage with a vacuum applied to the drain lumen with no air vent. Closed-suction drains allow wounds and dressings to stay dry, prevent bacterial movement through and around the drain, afford continuous drainage, and eliminate the need for irrigation.

These drains help hold the skin grafts in contact with the granulating wound bed to enhance revascularization. Excessively high negative pressure in the drain system can injure tissue. The vacuum for these drain systems can be generated by glass vacuum bottles, a compressible plastic canister (Hemovac), a compressible plastic canister with two one-way valves (Drevac), or a simple syringe (usually a modified 60-ml syringe) (Fig. 13-6).

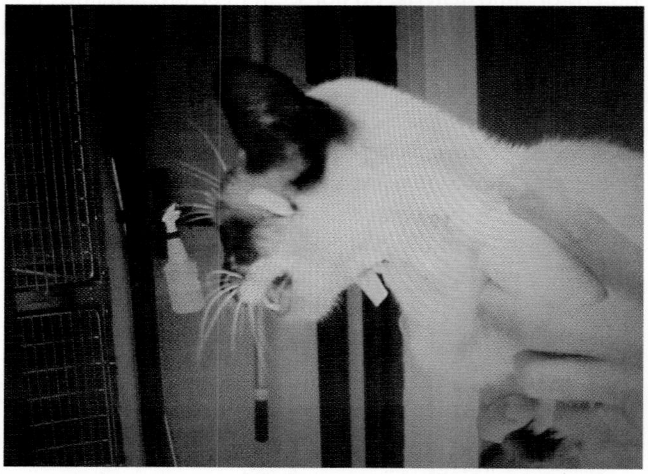

FIGURE 13-5 A Penrose drain placed in an abscess on a cat's face.

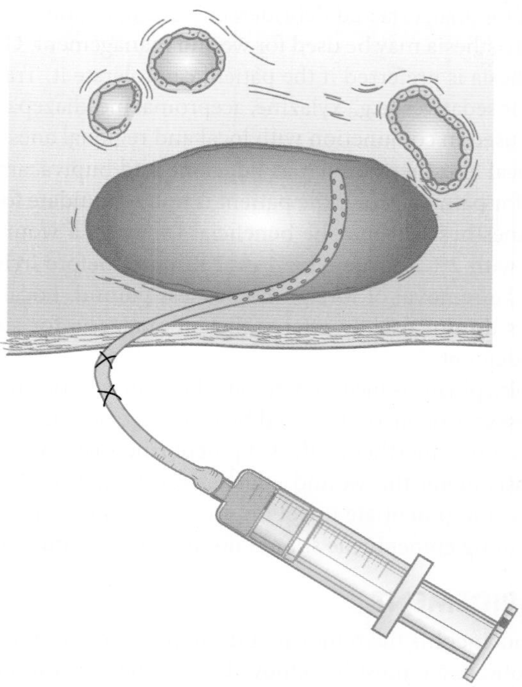

FIGURE 13-6 Fluids can be drained by periodic aspiration with a syringe attached to the drain.

Gauze or umbilical tape "setons" may be passed into a wound opening to keep the wound from closing before all exudates have drained. They are unsatisfactory for drainage purposes because they do not promote drainage once the gauze is saturated. They act as wicks, retaining bacterial contaminants, and can be mechanically irritating.

Box 13-3 presents guidelines for and complications of drain use.

WOUND CLOSURE

The patient's ability to tolerate anesthesia influences initial wound management. It is usually best to close fresh wounds as quickly as possible, when the risk of infection and complication is very low. Wounds with minor contamination may be cleaned, debrided, and closed. Sometimes a drain is installed to facilitate removal of tissue fluids associated with significant soft tissue trauma. Wounds that require optimal wound drainage because of gross contamination, tissue necrosis, and/or infection are managed as open wounds until they can be closed at a later time. Table 13-1 summarizes the types of closure used with different types of wounds.

A wound should be closed only when the veterinarian is certain that all devitalized and contaminated tissue has been removed and there is adequate skin to appose the wound edges. Veterinarians should consider covering the wound and allowing it to heal by second intention or delayed closure. Unfortunately, wounds are sometimes closed

BOX 13-3 Guidelines for Drain Use

Technique

- Provide adequate drainage, using the fewest possible drains with the least number of drain holes.
- Clip a generous area of skin around the drain to prevent contamination of the drain end by hair.
- Do not tunnel the drain too far subcutaneously before entering the wound pocket; this may collapse the drain and prevent proper drainage.
- To minimize the chance of misplaced drains, record the number and size of drains used in the patient, and count them again when the drains are removed.
- Make the stab incision for the drain exit large enough to allow adequate drainage.
- Make the drain exit through a separate stab incision; drains that exit the primary wound/incision may cause dehiscence.
- Place the drain dorsoventrally to allow drainage through the dependent opening.
- Bandage the drain, if possible, to increase drainage by capillary action and prevent ascending infection, self-mutilation, and premature drain removal.
- Use radiopaque drains (evident on radiographs).
- Suture the drain to the skin at the point of exit.

Complications

- Infection from bacteria ascending the drain
- Drain obstruction
- Retention of the drain if the exposed portion of the drain retracts under the skin, requiring surgical removal
- Foreign-body reaction
- Damage to surrounding tissues
- Pain
- Premature loss and/or removal by the patient
- Delayed healing, with increased possibility of wound dehiscence or formation of a fistulous tract

TABLE 13-1 Types of Wound Closures

TYPE OF CLOSURE	TYPE OF WOUND HEALING	CONDITIONS OF USE
Primary closure	First-intention healing	Wound closed with sutures or staples Full-thickness apposition of wound edges Tissues in direct apposition Minimal edema No local infection No serous discharge Minimal scar formation Rapid healing
Nonclosure	Second-intention healing	Wound left open because of infection, extensive trauma, tissue loss, or incorrect apposition of tissues Healing by contraction and epithelialization, from inner layers to outer surface Contraction starts after around 72 hours and stops when wound edges meet or tension exceeds strength of contraction Epithelialization starts within 24 hours after injury and requires a moist, oxygen-rich environment Delayed by healing
Delayed primary closure	Form of third-intention healing	Closure 3 to 5 days after cleaning and debridement, but before granulation tissue forms Wound strength and rate of healing not affected by delaying primary closure
Secondary closure	Form of third-intention healing	Closure after more than 3 to 5 days after granulation tissue has formed in the wound bed
	Third-intention healing	Safe method for repair of dirty, contaminated, or infected wounds with extensive tissue damage Allows for management of infection or necrosis before closure Surgeon debrides damaged tissue and wound is closed, with accurate apposition of tissues
Adnexal re-epithelialization	Second-intention healing	Partial-thickness skin loss with epithelialization primarily from compound hair follicles ("road burns")

prematurely, resulting in dehiscence (opening) and infection a few days later. If there is any doubt about the advisability of a surgical closure, the clinician may cover the wound with a proper dressing and manage the wound with frequent dressing changes (at least daily), lavage, debridement, and reassessment as required.

CLOSURE WITH SUTURES

When wound closures require suturing, certain fundamental considerations apply:

- Potential tissue reaction to the suture material must be acceptable.
- The suture material need not be stronger than the tissue in which it is placed.
- The sutures should retain their strength until healing keeps the wound edges together.
- Suture patterns should not impair blood supply to the wound.
- Knots should be tied securely with sufficient but not excessive "throws."

In selecting suture material, considerations include suture construction (monofilament, braided), suture material (absorbable, nonabsorbable), suture size (diameter), suture pattern, knot type, and needle type. Chapter 15 presents detailed information on suture materials.

There are many different suture patterns used depending on the anatomic area in which it is being used; the need for apposition, inversion, or eversion of tissues; and the amount of tension being placed on the closure site. The three most commonly used suture patterns include simple continuous, simple interrupted, and cruciate. Methods for performing each of these patterns are described in Procedure 13-2. Illustrations of the different sutures are shown in Figure 13-7. The similarities in all three listed procedures are the knot tying and needle placement.

TECHNICIAN NOTE There are many different suture patterns, and the decision on which pattern to use is based on the type of suture, the area being sutured, the amount of tension, and whether the tissue should be everted or inverted.

There are two different types of knots that can be used—regular knot and surgeon's throw. A surgeon's throw occurs when two throws are made on the first portion of the knot followed by a single throw (see Fig. 13-7). All knots should consist of at least four throws (two knots), but the total number of knots is determined primarily by the suture size and type.

Needle placement in general is determined by skin thickness. The needle is placed the same distance from the skin edge as the thickness of the skin. However, that said, sutures should penetrate the skin a minimum of 5 mm from the wound edge. The goal of skin closure is to square the skin edges without overlapping them and placing the sutures close enough together to not allow gaps in the skin closure (Procedure 13-2).

PROCEDURE 13-2 Suturing

1. Positioning the needle: Using needle drivers, gently grasp the needle at the midpoint for general sutures, near the eye for delicate tissue and near the tip for dense tissue.
2. Placing the needle into the tissue: Start at the far side of the incision because this is easiest and place the needle into the tissue at least as far as the tissue is thick.
3. Driving the needle: Because single rotating motion is most efficient, have the needle go from the outside of the tissue, into the tissue, and back out the middle of the tissue.
   a. For the simple interrupted and simple continuous suture patterns, the needle may be inserted into the opposing tissue before being completely pulled through the first tissue.
   b. For the cruciate suture, the needle is usually pulled completely through the first piece of tissue before being inserted into the next piece of tissue.
4. Releasing the needle: Tissue forceps are used to help stabilize the tissue layer during release of the needle and keep it from becoming dislodged.
5. Steps 1 to 4 are then repeated for the opposing piece of tissue, but the needle is inserted in the middle of the tissue and pulled through to the outer portion (again at least the same distance as the tissue is thick).
6. Depending on the suture pattern used, when a piece of tissue is apposed a knot is tied (interrupted and cruciates) or the process is continued until the length of the tissue is apposed (continuous).

NONCLOSURE

In second-intention healing (nonclosure), the wound is not sutured but heals by contraction and epithelialization. Second-intention healing is selected for wounds involving significant tissue loss. In horses, it is especially useful for wounds of the neck, body, and proximal limbs. Although these wounds are prepared with the same care as for primary closure and delayed primary closure, wounds of the extremities in horses are often left uncovered or managed with a pressure bandage or a cast. If left open to heal by second intention, the wound should be cleaned daily at first to remove accumulated exudate. Skin distal to the wound is also cleaned and protected with petroleum jelly or a similar product to prevent skin maceration ("serum burns").

Second-Intention Healing in Horses

Wounds of the distal limbs of horses (carpus and distally) with large tissue deficits present a special problem, mainly the formation of excessive granulation tissue called **proud flesh** (Fig. 13-8). With newly formed moist granulation tissue protruding slightly above the skin edges, application of a corticosteroid-antibacterial combination ointment with an overlying pressure bandage can control granulation tissue growth. The topical corticosteroids seem to have little effect on wound healing and epithelialization at this early stage. If the granulation tissue is mature and protrudes well above the

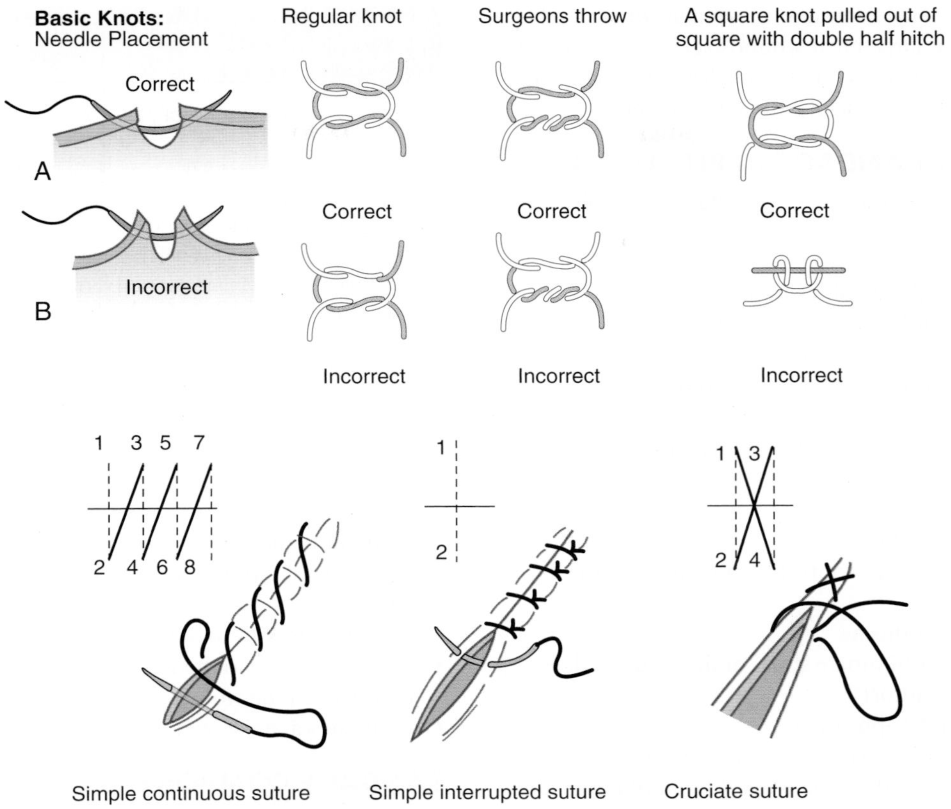

FIGURE 13-7 Suture patterns and knot tying.

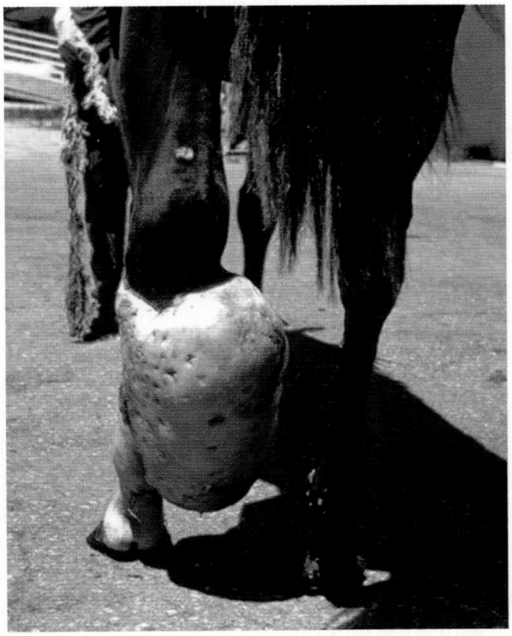

FIGURE 13-8 Exuberant granulation tissue (proud flesh), chronic ulcer, skin, distal hindlimb, horse. Note the large proliferating mass of fibrous tissue on the lower portion of the left hindlimb. It often lacks superficial epithelium. (Courtesy Dr. M.D. McGavin, College of Veterinary Medicine, University of Tennessee.)

skin surface to form a fibrogranuloma, sharp excision is preferred. If excessive granulation tissue must be excised with a scalpel, a pressure bandage is applied immediately after excision to control the considerable hemorrhage. Several hours after surgery, this bandage must be changed.

Topical application of caustics (e.g., silver nitrate or triple dye) and astringents can remove and prevent formation of granulation tissue by chemically destroying it. This destructive chemical action is indiscriminate, however, and also harms migrating epithelial cells. Often this prolongs healing and produces more scarring than sharp resection, bandaging, and casting. Large wounds of the distal extremities with skin deficits tend to heal very slowly because of reduced blood supply, increased movement, and excessive contamination. They heal by formation of scar tissue covered with a thin layer of easily damaged epithelial cells. Skin grafting is often recommended in these cases.

COVERING WOUNDS

Nature provides "natural bandages" as a part of normal healing. A partial-thickness wound that forms a blister rarely becomes infected and heals more rapidly if the blister is not broken. The scab of a full-thickness wound and the eschar (necrotic layer that sloughs off) of a burn also serve as natural bandages. The scab protects from external contamination, maintains internal homeostasis, and provides a surface beneath which cell migration and movement of skin edges occur. The eschar of large burn wounds serves as a biologic dressing that is protective and is considered by many surgeons to be superior to artificial bandaging materials.

PRINCIPLES OF BANDAGE APPLICATION

In veterinary application, bandages have the following functions:

- Protect wounds
- Hold clean or sterile dressings in place
- Absorb exudate and debride a wound
- Serve as a vehicle for therapeutic agents
- Serve as an indicator of wound secretions
- Pack the wound
- Provide support for bony anatomic structures
- Support and stabilize soft tissue
- Secure splints
- Prevent weight-bearing
- Provide compression to control hemorrhage, dead space, and tissue edema
- Discourage self-grooming
- Restrict motion to eliminate stress of the wound edges
- Provide patient comfort
- Provide an aesthetic appearance

The basic principles of bandage application are as follows:

- *Properly prepare the area before application of a bandage.* This may require clipping of the hair, wound debridement, and/or cleaning of surrounding skin.
- *Use porous materials when possible.* This allows circulation of air and escape of excessive moisture.
- *Use absorbent materials when exudates may be a problem.* Change absorbent dressings when they become saturated and before saturation is evident externally.
- *Use appropriate materials of adequate width* to avoid producing a tourniquet effect.
- *Apply bandage materials as smoothly as possible.* Ridges and lumps lead to skin irritation and necrosis.
- *Secure protective wound pads to the skin* so that they do not shift from the site.
- *Check bandages frequently* to determine if there is persistent swelling, skin discoloration, or coolness. A bandage applied too tightly can impair circulation, resulting in serious damage to soft tissues.
- *Instruct clients on basic care of bandages and signs of bandage failure.* This includes the physical appearance of the bandage, as well as behavior of the patient. Box 13-4 lists key points in discharge instructions.

Ideally, materials used for bandaging should have the following properties:

- Permeable to oxygen and other gases
- Conform to body contours
- Acceptable appearance
- Inert
- Long storage life
- Inexpensive
- Easily sterilized
- Unaffected by disinfecting and cleaning solutions
- Nonflammable
- Will not shred (so particles do not contaminate the wound)
- Compatible with topical therapeutic agents
- Will not adhere to the wound but can remove exudate and debris from the wound
- Maintains a moist wound surface that is free from exudate

BOX 13-4 Key Points in Discharge Instructions for Bandages

1. Strict confinement initially and then restricted activity during healing.
2. Keep the pet from licking or chewing the bandage. Many pets require an Elizabethan collar.
3. Monitor the pet for any sign of excessive discomfort. If the pet is trying to remove the bandage, it could mean there is a problem beneath the support. Pay particular attention to the toes and area at the top of the bandage. Look for swelling of the toes or any sores and pay attention to bad odors from the bandage.
4. If the bandage appears loose, soiled, or wet it should be checked.
5. Schedule rechecks as prescribed by the veterinarian.

BANDAGE COMPONENTS

In most situations, bandages are generally composed of three layers, each with its own properties and function. The primary layer rests on the wound and may or may not be adherent. The secondary layer provides absorbency and padding. The tertiary layer is the outer layer that holds the underlying layers in place. This is usually the only layer the client sees. Clients often judge the quality of treatment solely on the appearance of this outer bandage layer.

TECHNICIAN NOTE It is best to have all necessary materials laid out and ready for use (i.e., out of packaging) before starting a bandage.

Primary Layer

The primary layer is in contact with the wound itself (Fig. 13-9). When debridement is the goal, an adherent layer is used for the primary bandage. Once the wound is in the proliferation phase and granulation tissue has formed, use a nonadherent dressing to avoid disruption of the new tissue. The primary layer should be sterile and comfortable, allow fluids to pass to the secondary layer, protect the wound from exogenous contamination, and be nontoxic and nonirritating to tissue.

Adherent bandaging material, such as sterile gauze sponges with wide mesh openings and noncotton filler, can be used to provide debridement during the early stage of wound healing. This layer removes devitalized tissue and wound exudate when it is taken off during a bandage change. Adherent dressings may be wet or dry, depending on the nature of the wound. Some bandages are applied wet and then

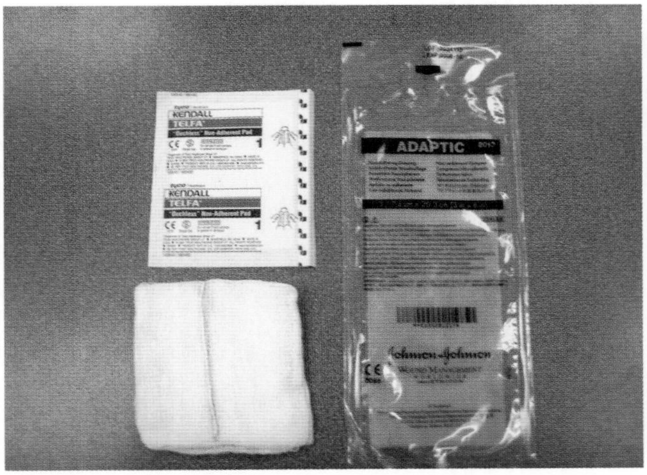

FIGURE 13-9 Examples of primary bandage materials.

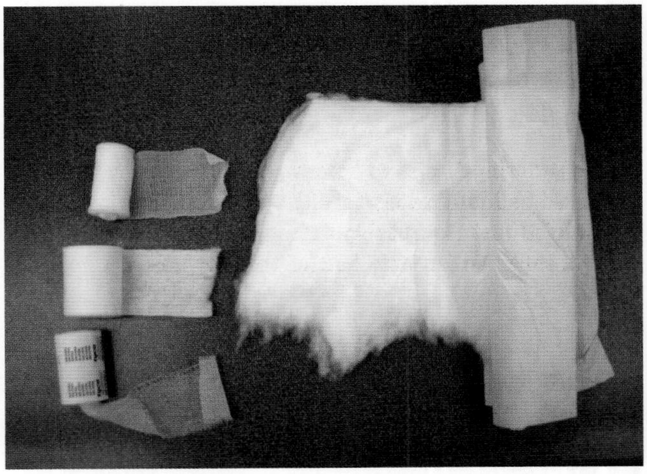

FIGURE 13-10 Examples of secondary layer bandage materials.

allowed to dry. Use of an adherent primary layer should be discontinued after the wound has been cleared of necrotic debris and heavy exudate.

If loose necrotic tissue or foreign material is present on the surface of the wound, a dry-to-dry dressing may be the best type to use. Dry gauze with a large mesh is placed directly on the wound. An absorbent layer is placed over this primary layer, and fluid is absorbed from the wound and allowed to dry. Necrotic material adheres to the gauze and is removed with the bandage. Although this type of bandage removes tissue debris, bandage removal is very painful and may also remove viable tissue. For this reason, dry-to-dry dressings should be used only when necessary.

If the exudate is especially viscous or dried foreign matter must be removed, a wet-to-dry dressing may be appropriate. The bandage is applied wet, which dilutes the exudate for absorption. As the bandage dries, the foreign material adheres to the bandage and is later removed with the bandage. Solutions used to wet the primary layer include physiologic (0.9%) saline or a water-soluble bacteriostatic or bactericidal compound, such as 0.05% chlorhexidine diacetate solution.

For wounds with copious exudate or transudate, a wet-to-wet dressing may be best. Wet dressings absorb fluid more rapidly than dry dressings. They may be used to transport heat to a wound and/or enhance capillary action to promote wound drainage. A water-soluble bacteriostatic or bactericidal solution can be used to wet the dressing to help control microorganisms. The primary layer is applied wet and kept wet after the secondary and tertiary layers have been applied. This bandage is also removed wet. Wet-to-wet dressings cause less pain than dry dressings when removed; by using a warm solution, patient comfort is increased. A disadvantage is that these bandages tend to cause tissue maceration and have little debriding capacity.

A nonadherent primary layer is indicated during the reparative stage of wound healing, with formation of granulation tissue and production of a more serosanguineous exudate. In the early repair stage, petrolatum-impregnated products can be used in the presence of exudate and when little or no epithelialization has taken place. Later, when there is little fluid and during epithelialization, nonadherent dressings are indicated. Nonadherent dressings are used to cover lacerations, skin graft donor sites, minor burns, abrasions, and surgical incisions. The main goal is to minimize tissue injury upon removal. They do not absorb much fluid; draining wounds usually require a secondary dressing. Examples of nonadherent dressing materials include Adaptic (Johnson & Johnson, Langhorne, PA), Release (Johnson & Johnson), and Telfa adhesive pads (Kendall/Curity, Mansfield, MA). These semiocclusive, nonadherent materials leave the granulation bed undisturbed yet still move fluid away from the wound.

Secondary Layer

The secondary (intermediate) layer provides support and moves exudate or transudate away from the wound (Fig. 13-10). Materials used in this layer include gauze bandaging material (e.g., Sof-Band, Kling, Sof-Kling, Johnson & Johnson), cast padding, and bandaging cotton.

The secondary layer should be thick enough to absorb moisture, pad the wound from trauma, and inhibit wound movement. If the bandage allows evaporation of fluid from absorbed exudate, this partially dry environment retards bacterial growth. With wounds producing copious fluids, evaporation does not keep the bandage dry. If such a moist bandage is not changed frequently, the wound fluids serve as a growth medium for bacteria.

Tertiary Layer

The tertiary (outer) layer holds the underlying bandage layers in place (Fig. 13-11). Materials used in this layer include adhesive tapes (e.g., Zonasdont, Johnson & Johnson), elastic bandages (Elastikon, Johnson & Johnson; Vetrap 3M; Conform, Kendall; Medi-Rip, Conco Medical), and conforming stretch gauze. This layer should be applied carefully to provide support without constricting.

TECHNICIAN NOTE If using Vetrap, it is best to unroll the wrap and then loosely re-roll before placing.

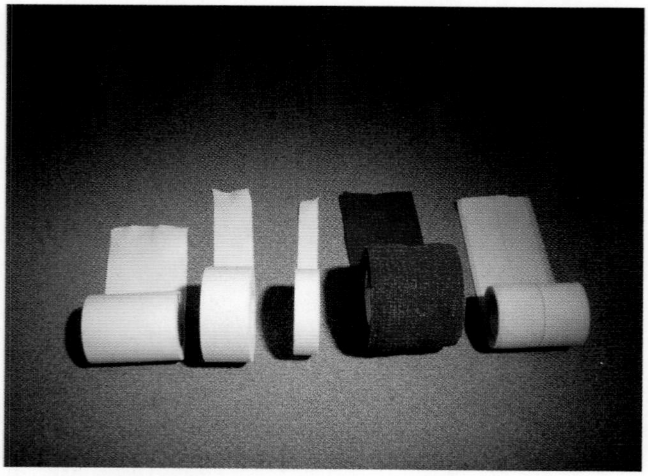

FIGURE 13-11 Examples of tertiary layer bandage materials.

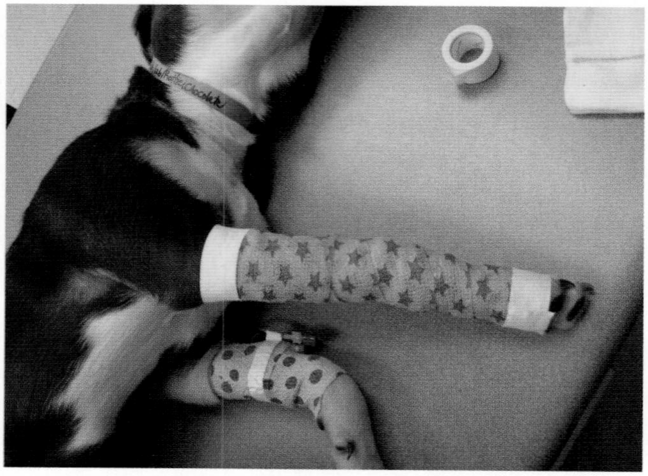

FIGURE 13-12 Example of a leg bandage.

Porous adhesive tape allows evaporation of fluid from the bandage. It can also allow movement of fluid (e.g., saliva, rainwater) into the wound, which may be undesirable. Waterproof adhesive tape repels water but also prevents evaporation. If the wound is producing considerable exudate, the tissues may become macerated from retained fluids. The resultant damp environment favors bacterial growth.

Elastic adhesive tape is compliant and applies continuous, dynamic pressure to the wound as the patient moves. Elastic tape products should be wrapped over the underlying bandage materials carefully to apply even but not excessive pressure. Elastic adhesive tapes tend to adhere to themselves, so minimal external taping is needed. Self-adherent products (e.g., Vetrap, 3M; Medi-Rip, Conco) have no adhesive undercoat. Although these products tend to adhere to themselves, in veterinary practice, some external tape is usually required at the ends to keep the bandage from coming apart during movement.

> TECHNICIAN NOTE Always make sure the bandaging is smooth—if there are any wrinkles in the material, this can cause pressure points or sores to develop.

ORTHOPEDIC BANDAGES AND SPLINTS

ROBERT JONES COMPRESSION BANDAGE

The Robert Jones compression bandage is illustrated in Figure 13-12, and the technique is described in Procedure 13-3.

Indications

The Robert Jones bandage is generally used in large and small animals to temporarily immobilize fractures distal to the elbow or tarsus, support injured soft and bony tissues, and prevent excessive swelling. It may be modified to incorporate the thorax or pelvis to provide additional stabilization of more proximal limb fractures. It absorbs exudates, decreases, or prevents edema and swelling through compression, and reduces (but does not totally inhibit) movement of fracture fragments. It is an excellent emergency treatment for distal limb injuries, reduces or prevents limb swelling postoperatively, and absorbs drainage before or after surgery. In horses, the Robert Jones bandage is used as an emergency method for treating fractures and tendon and ligament disruptions until repair can be made. It is used to immobilize a limb to protect from further damage through weight-bearing or motion.

Precautions

The Robert Jones bandage may act as a heavy pendulum if used for injuries proximal to the elbow or stifle unless modified. It should never be used as a definitive fracture treatment for any type of fracture.

SOFT PADDED AND COAPTATION BANDAGES

Indications

These bandages include the Schanz soft padded bandage, the Mesa-Meta Splint, the coaptation bandage made with a thermoplastic splint (Orthoplast, Johnson & Johnson), fiberglass strips (C-Splint, Johnson & Johnson), or other casting materials. The Schanz soft-padded bandage is the most commonly used limb bandage. It is designed to cover abrasions and lacerations, and provide light support after long bone or joint surgery. For the application technique, see Procedure 13-4.

Modifications

The soft-padded bandage may be modified to provide additional support of a limb by incorporating splint materials. The resultant bandages can support the limb distally to the elbow or hock. They are generally used to provide additional support for fractures or other orthopedic injuries after surgical intervention. For some types of fractures, they may be used as the primary means of stabilization.

Precautions

Bandages in this category should not be used for fractures near the elbow or tibiotarsal joint, severely comminuted or

PROCEDURE 13-3 Applying a Robert Jones Bandage

Materials

- 1-inch adhesive tape
- Dressing for primary layer if needed
- "Pound cotton" rolls (1 lb cotton/10 kg body weight in small animals)
- 4- to 8-inch Kling or roll gauze
- 4- to 8-inch elastic or Ace-type bandage

In Small Animals

1. Suspend the limb vertically, if possible; this allows gravity to work.
2. Dress any wounds; Telfa type of material is preferred.
3. Apply porous tape stirrups, extending to the elbow or knee and considerably past the toes (Fig. 1).

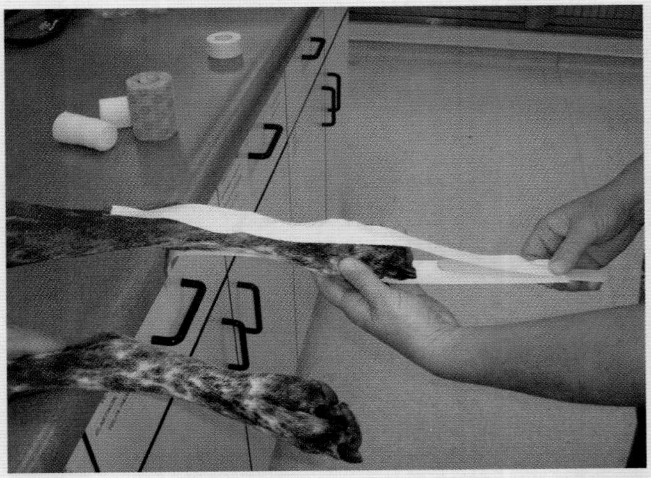

FIGURE 1 Placement of stirrups.

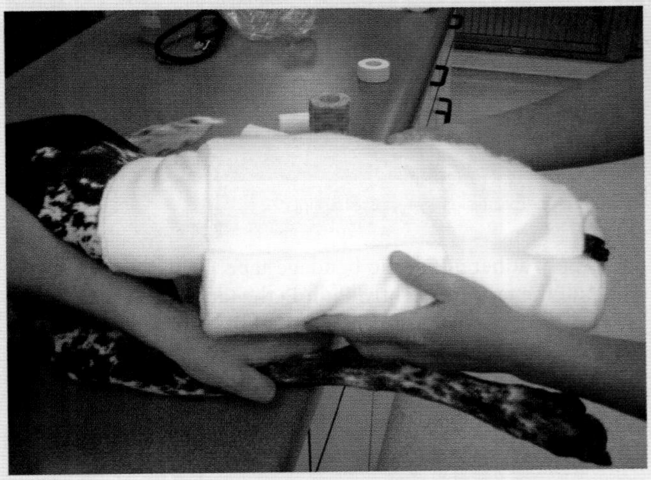

FIGURE 2 Wrapping the leg with large amounts of sheet cotton.

4. Apply a snug layer of Sof-Kling to prevent slippage.
5. Unroll cotton to remove the separation paper, and then re-roll before application. Apply cotton to the limb, starting at the foot and extending to the groin or axilla, overlapping one-fourth to one-half the width of the roll. An assistant should hold the limb in extreme abduction to facilitate this process. Wrap the cotton as tightly as possible, with no wrinkles or twists. The object is to make the limb into a straight cylinder (Fig. 2).
6. Wrap the cotton with Kling or Sof-Kling gauze as tightly as possible, again overlapping half the width of the roll (Figs. 3 and 4).

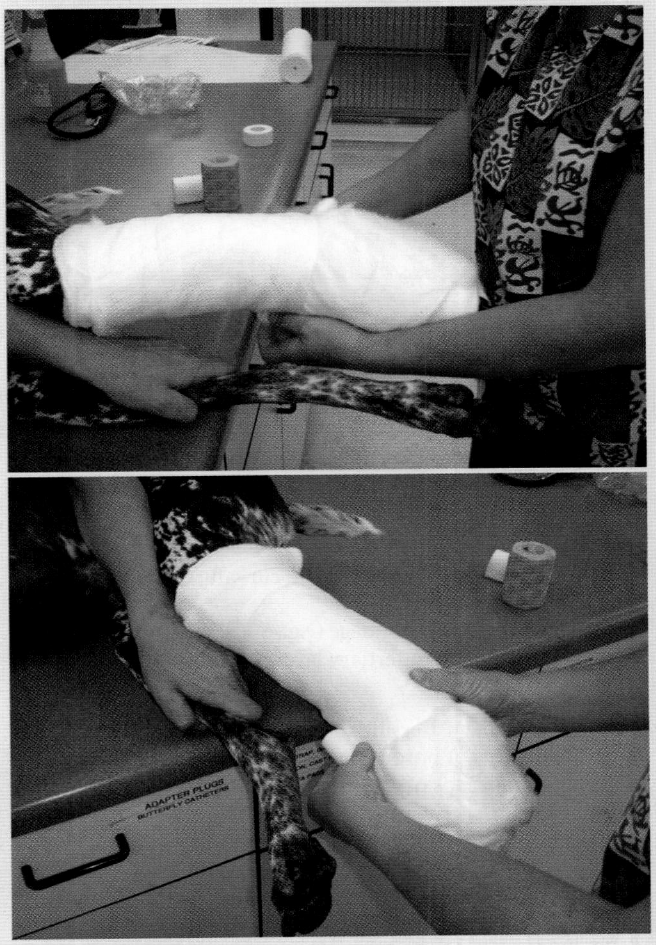

FIGURES 3 AND 4 Wrapping the cotton with roll gauze to compress the cotton.

7. Separate the tape stirrups to the sides of the bulky bandage. This provides a small opening to assess blood flow to the toes.
8. Apply self-adherent elastic adhesive tape, an Ace-type bandage, or Vetrap-type material, starting at the toes and working proximally, overlapping by about half the width (Fig. 5).
9. The completed bandage should be very firm and should produce a sound similar to a ripe watermelon when thumped.

In Horses

1. Stirrups are not used in horses.
2. Apply rolls of cotton to the limb, from the distal limb proximally, in gradual spirals to the proximal forearm. The proximal edge of the bandage should extend as far proximally as possible. It is most important to start the bandage on the inside of the leg. If started on the back, it may damage the tendon.

Continued

PROCEDURE 13-4 Applying Soft Padded Bandages—cont'd

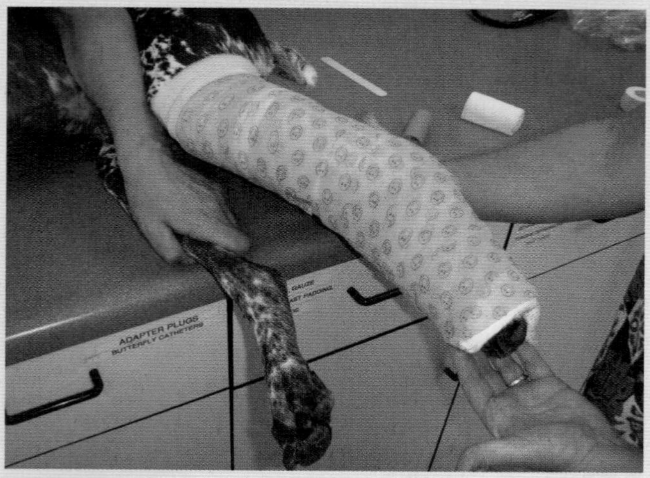

FIGURE 5 Placement of Vetrap and Elastikon.

3. Apply five to eight consecutive rolls of cotton with firm pressure. When the final layer has been applied, the bandage should be of even thickness throughout its length.
4. Secure the bandage in place with one or two layers of 6-inch gauze.
5. The tertiary layer consists of an elastic bandage covered with a 4-inch elastic adhesive tape and or vet-wrap material as the final wrap. Apply the elastic adhesive tape, overlapping by about half, in several layers, depending on the strength and durability of the bandage desired. Then apply the adhesive bandage layer. This bandage requires six to eight rolls of Ace elastic bandage, six or seven rolls of Elastikon, four to six rolls of Sof-Kling, Kling, or other conforming bandage, and a roll of porous tape to secure the ends of each roll of Ace elastic bandage used.

PROCEDURE 13-4 Applying Soft Padded Bandages

Materials

- Wound dressing for the primary layer
- 2-inch porous adhesive tape
- Kling
- Splint of appropriate size (width, curvature, length) (Fig. 1)
- Cast padding or soft bandage (e.g., Sof-Band bulky bandage)
- Elastic self-adherent tertiary layer (e.g., Elastikon, Vetrap)

Procedure

1. Apply a primary dressing to the wound area.
2. Form stirrups of porous tape to prevent bandage slippage. Apply the stirrups on the medial and lateral surfaces of the limb, leaving a tab on the distal end, if possible, to be pulled apart later.
3. Apply cast padding snugly to the limb, starting at the foot and moving proximally, overlapping one-fourth to one-half the roll width, to a point proximal to the elbow joint.
4. Apply a layer of Sof-Kling or other conforming bandage in the same manner.
5. Place the splint (if needed) and then continue to wrap with Sof-Kling gauze.
6. Separate the tape stirrups and attach them to their respective sides.

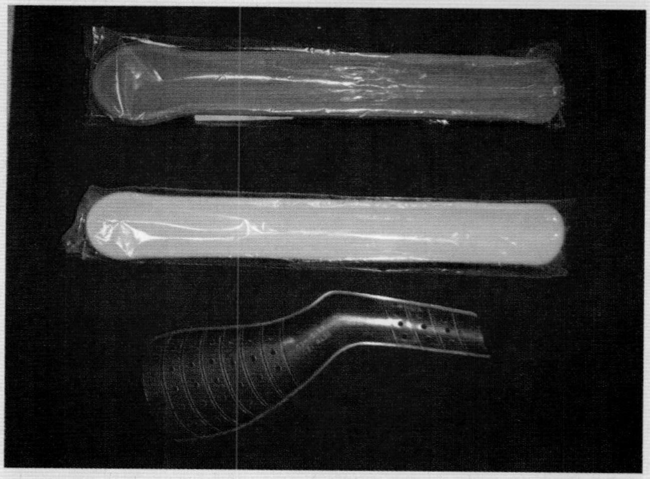
FIGURE 1 Examples of types of splints.

7. Apply adherent elastic bandage tape, being careful not to pull the tape too tightly. Pulling the tape to its elastic limits can compromise the circulation of the limb.
8. Leave the toes exposed to allow assessment of circulation.

collapsing fractures, or as definitive treatment for ligament or tendon ruptures.

SPICA SPLINT

The spica splint is a semirigid splint bandage. It is usually brought over the trunk to immobilize the elbow or shoulder. It is made from casting material or a thermoplastic splint fitted to the lateral portion of the limb, incorporated into a padded bandage, and fixed to the limb with conforming gauze and surgical porous or elastic adherent tape.

SCHROEDER-THOMAS SPLINT

The Schroeder-Thomas splint is an external weight-bearing device. It is best used for closed fractures of the radius/ulna or tibia/fibula in young dogs. These fractures heal rapidly with moderate stabilization. It is also of value in elbow dislocations, because the elbow can be held in position following reduction. Fractures proximal to the elbow or stifle are better repaired by internal fixation than with the Schroeder-Thomas splint. After surgical bone or joint repair, this device can provide additional stabilization and restrict movement of the limb. It is best if the aluminum splint rod is custom made for each individual patient.

EHMER SLING

Indications

An Ehmer sling is applied after reduction of hip luxation. It maintains the hip joint in flexion, abduction, and internal rotation; the sling provides limited abduction. The Ehmer sling helps keep the femoral head deeply seated within the acetabulum by internally rotating and abducting the hip. The technique for applying the Ehmer sling is described in Procedure 13-5.

MODIFIED EHMER SLING

Indications

The modified version maintains hip flexion and abduction but no internal rotation. The modified Ehmer sling can be adjusted to ensure abduction and relieve swelling by simply cutting the tape, repositioning it, and retaping. These adjustments cannot be made easily with the traditional Ehmer sling. The technique for applying the modified Ehmer sling is described in Procedure 13-6.

VELPEAU SLING

Indications

The Velpeau sling prevents weight-bearing on the forelimb by cradling the forelimb against the shoulder and chest wall. It is indicated for scapular fractures not requiring open reduction and internal fixation, postoperative splintage of scapular fractures and shoulder dislocations, and ligament and joint capsule injuries of the shoulder joint. Procedure 13-7 describes the application procedure.

Precautions

The Velpeau sling should not be used in patients with internal or external thoracic trauma or disease; respiratory compromise; limbs with swelling, edema, or cellulitis; lateral luxation of the scapulohumeral joint; scapular neck fractures; or fractures involving the scapulohumeral joint.

CASTS

INDICATIONS

Casts are simple and effective devices for providing support for some fractures in companion animals. Indications include external fixation of noncollapsing fractures of the radius, ulna, tibia, metacarpals, and digits; as an adjunct to internal fixation, including arthrodesis; immobilization of a limb after tendon repair or surgery; protection from self-mutilation; and restriction of motion after plastic or reconstructive surgery.

Bending forces, primarily transmitted perpendicularly to the long axis of a bone, are well neutralized by a cast. Rotational, compressive, shearing, and tensile forces transmitted parallel to the long axis of a bone are poorly neutralized by a cast. Incomplete or minimally displaced, transverse, or short oblique diaphyseal fractures of the radius/ulna and tibia/fibula, especially in younger animals, are ideally suited for cast fixation.

MATERIALS

For many years, plaster was the only cast material available. Disadvantages of plaster casts included heavy weight, permeability to water, and susceptibility to breakage and mutilation.

Fiberglass casting material is now widely used because of its light weight, rigidity, ventilation, and waterproof characteristics. In small animals, fiberglass casts are highly effective for external fracture fixation and as an adjunct to internal fixation techniques (e.g., pinning, plating). Equine practitioners use fiberglass casts to protect heel bulb and flexor tendon lacerations, protect granulation tissue beds in wounds, and treat laminitis. Casts are also used after surgical fracture repair and in management of midbody sesamoid fractures following a bone graft, by keeping the leg in a flexed position. In neonatal calves, fiberglass casts have proven to be of value for external fixation of forelimb fractures caused by assisted deliveries in dystocia.

TECHNIQUE

Proper application of a fiberglass cast requires practice and experience (Procedure 13-8). Patient movement during application can create pressure points. General anesthesia is required for cast application. The skin of the affected area should be clean and dry before casting. If a hoof is to be covered with fiberglass casting material, it should be cleaned and disinfected to prevent foot rot and thrush. Surgical incisions, lacerations, or wounds should be debrided and, if indicated, sutured and covered with a sterile nonadherent primary dressing. Cast padding should be kept to a minimum and applied only at pressure points. Cast padding is used infrequently in equine and bovine patients.

The cast should be of sufficient length to immobilize the joints proximal and distal to the lesion. Assistants should be advised to use the flat portion of the hand to support the limb during cast application to prevent indentations that may cause pressure sores. Any sharp edges at proximal and distal ends of the cast should be well padded. For horses and cattle, tape should be placed around the proximal rim of the cast to prevent foreign material from entering between cast and skin. If horses or cattle are to be kept outside after casting, the hoof should be covered with a rubber boot to prevent excessive moisture from entering the cast. Clients must be instructed about observing the cast, cast care, adverse clinical signs, and limiting the patient's activity.

MAINTAINING BANDAGES, SPLINTS, AND CASTS

A trained staff member should examine every bandage, splint, cast, or orthopedic appliance every 6 to 8 hours during the first day after application. The device should be removed immediately if evidence of constriction is detected.

PROCEDURE 13-5 Applying an Ehmer Sling

Materials

- Cast padding or soft bandage (e.g., Sof-Band bulky bandage)
- 4-inch Elastikon
- 2-inch nonporous adhesive tape

Procedure

The traditional Ehmer sling is based on a modified figure-8 bandage:

1. Wrap cast padding around the metatarsal area.
2. Cover the cast padding with elastic adherent tape (Elastikon) (Fig. 1).
3. Manually flex the stifle, trying to keep the femur rotated slightly inward.
4. Continue the Elastikon from the metatarsal region passing it medial to the stifle.
5. Pass the tape over the stifle and medially, to the hock, creating a figure-8 pattern (Fig. 2).
6. Repeat several times.
7. Cover the limb completely with several more wraps of tape.
8. Abduct the limb by then passing the Elastikon dorsally over the back and fully around the body, incorporating the knee into the wrap (Fig. 3).
9. Continue wrapping several more layers of elastic tape (Fig. 4).
10. (optional) A towel may be used just above the leg on the abdomen to decrease the chances of swelling and rubbing of the bandage.
11. Cover the whole bandage with nonporous tape.
12. Monitor for swelling resulting from impaired circulation.

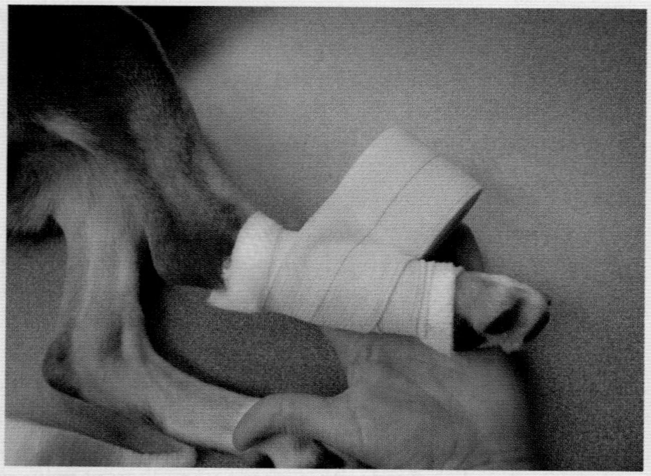

FIGURE 1 Cast padding is first wrapped around the metatarsal region and then covered with Elastikon tape.

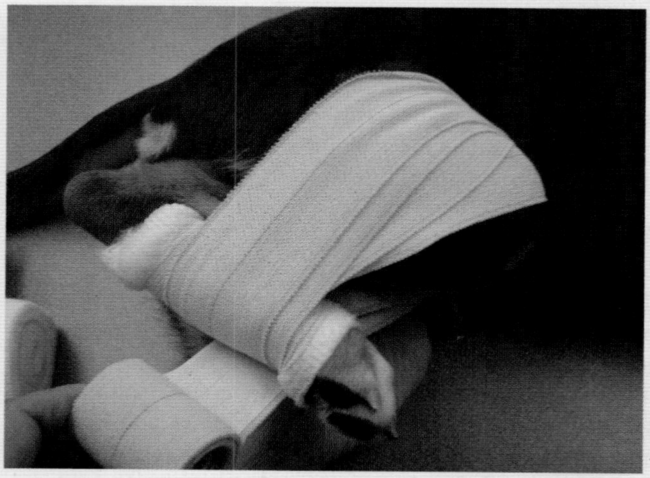

FIGURE 2 The leg is fixed and the Elastikon is then continued around the whole leg in a figure-8 pattern.

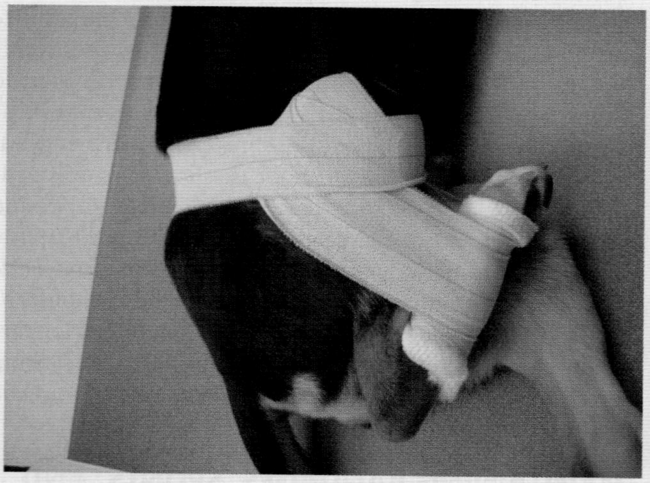

FIGURE 3 The wrap is extended around the abdomen and then covered with white (nonelastic) tape.

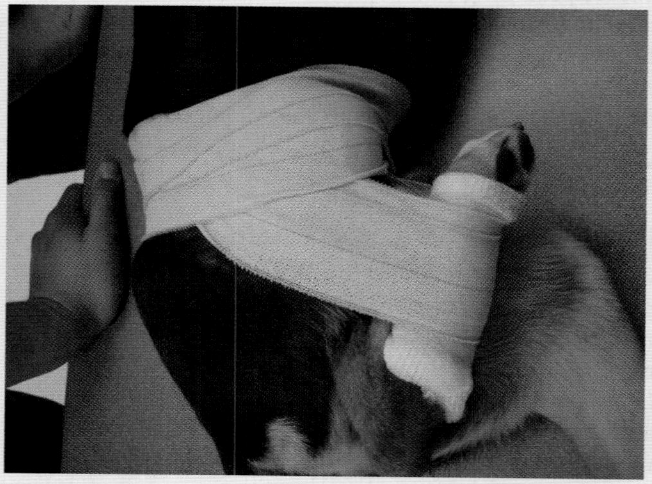

FIGURE 4 Several layers of elastic tape are added. The finished product should then be covered with nonporous tape.

PROCEDURE 13-6 Modified Ehmer Sling

Materials

- 4-inch Elastikon
- 2-inch nonporous adhesive tape

Technique

1. Place elastic wrap around the metatarsals, from medial to lateral, without encircling the limb, and adhere the tape to itself.
2. Carry the tape dorsally and cranially to encircle the trunk at the level of the caudal thorax, and anchor it to the body around the caudal ribs. This location avoids compression of the abdomen and avoids the prepuce in male dogs.
3. Applying tension to the wrap before encircling the trunk provides both hip joint flexion and abduction.
4. Before encircling the trunk, pull the skin from the dorsal back toward the affected limb to prevent the limb from dropping into an abducted position.
5. Once the elastic wrap is secured, apply 2-inch waterproof tape, covering the elastic wrap and eliminating any stretch of the elastic material.
6. Apply the waterproof tape, fanning outward from the metatarsal area to the trunk. This ensures that the stifle joint remains covered and medial to the bandage.

HOME CARE OF BANDAGES

It is important to involve clients in wound management, especially for outpatients. Clients play a significant role in detection of adverse conditions affecting the bandage. Many problems can be avoided by taking the time to instruct clients on care of the bandage, splint, or cast placed on their animals (see Box 13-4). An information sheet with home care instructions is often helpful. However, an instruction sheet cannot replace face-to-face communication between the client and veterinary staff. Before leaving the clinic, the client must be shown how to check the bandage or orthopedic appliance. It is often a good idea to telephone the client the next day to inquire about any problems.

TECHNICIAN NOTE Be specific about what to look for when talking with owners about monitoring bandages and casts. Having a checklist and handout to go over with the owner can be helpful.

BANDAGE, CAST, AND SPLINT REMOVAL

To remove the bandages, it is often easiest and safest to carefully cut the outer layer with scissors or a scalpel blade and then tear the cotton material from distal to proximal along the lateral aspect of the extremity, rather than trying to cut the cotton with bandage scissors. Casts are typically removed with an oscillating saw (e.g., Stryker). Splints can be removed with bandage scissors. With bandages or casts around any body part, be sure to determine the exact location of underlying structures before cutting the bandage. It is very easy to cut off the tip of an ear, toe, foot pad, or the tail if the area is not identified before cutting.

MANAGEMENT OF SPECIFIC WOUND TYPES

PENETRATING WOUNDS

Gunshot Wounds

High-velocity rifles and the more powerful handguns generate tremendous explosive kinetic energy that can shatter bone, cause massive tissue destruction, and propel fragments of metal and bone into surrounding soft tissue. High-velocity projectiles also destroy tissue by shock waves or cavitation. Large exit wounds are common. Treatment of high-velocity missile wounds generally requires extensive debridement that creates a considerable tissue defect. This prolongs the healing time and usually requires more elaborate reconstructive procedures than low-velocity wounds.

Bullets from most handguns are considered low-velocity projectiles; however, they can inflict serious injuries at close range. Handgun bullets produce an entry wound, with or without an exit wound. As these missiles travel through tissues, they create a tract via crushing and laceration, damaging only tissues contacted by the projectile. When these wounds are confined to soft tissues, they may require little or no exploration or debridement unless vital or important structures are involved. The tract is considered contaminated by bacteria. Clipping of hairs around the wound, local wound cleaning, lavage, and application of topical dressings may suffice. Easily accessible projectiles may be removed. Retention of projectiles in the hypodermis, fascia, or muscle poses little health threat to the patient. If perforation or penetration involves the abdomen, surgical exploration is required. Missile fragments in joints should be removed.

Shotguns fire multiple small pellets or a single large slug. At close range, shotguns are among the most lethal and traumatic of weapons, causing massive tissue destruction. At extremely close range, the wadding of the explosive charge may be driven into the tissues.

Arrow Wounds

Broad-head arrows, used for hunting, have razor-sharp blades to lacerate vessels and vascular visceral tissues. Field-point arrows, usually used for target practice, have a rounded point about the size of the arrow shaft. They can penetrate deeply but do not lacerate tissues like broad-head hunting arrows.

Deeply embedded arrows, especially broad-heads, are best removed surgically by the veterinarian, not the client. Clients may cut short arrow shafts with a bolt cutter to transport the patient to the veterinary facility. The client should be discouraged from pulling the arrow out before transport to the clinic. The shaft end of some arrows is threaded for changing heads. If the arrow's head is accessible to the clinician, it can be grasped with a forceps and unthreaded from the shaft to facilitate removal.

Thorough examination is essential to identification and management of injuries caused by projectiles. This includes radiographs of the involved body region. Abdominal cavity wounds require surgical exploration to prevent bacterial

PROCEDURE 13-7 Applying a Velpeau Sling

Materials

- 6-inch Kling gauze, Elastikon, Ace bandage, or Vetrap

Technique

1. Apply tape stirrups. Slightly flex the carpus and metacarpus to a comfortable position and wrap them (Figs. 1 and 2).
2. Comfortably flex the antebrachium across the cranial chest wall (with paw pointing toward the opposite scapulohumeral joint) (Fig. 3).
3. Apply additional wraps around the chest and flexed limb (Fig. 4).

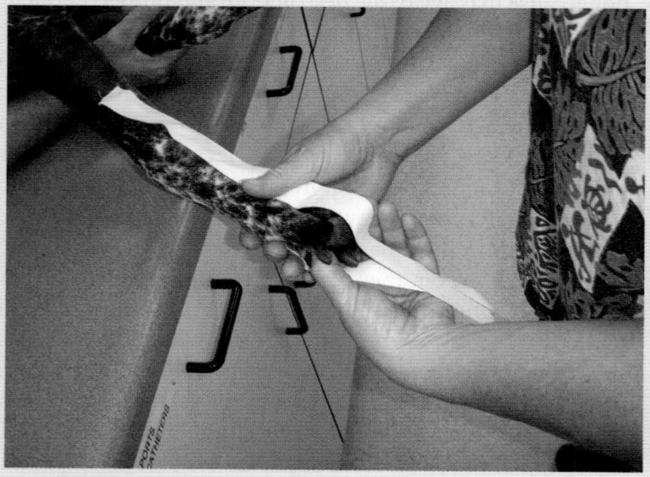

FIGURE 1 Placement of stirrups.

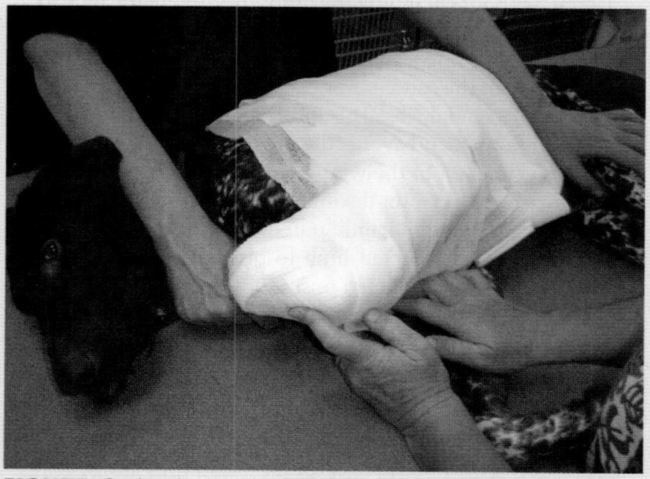

FIGURE 3 Flex the antebrachium across chest wall and wrap with cotton gauze.

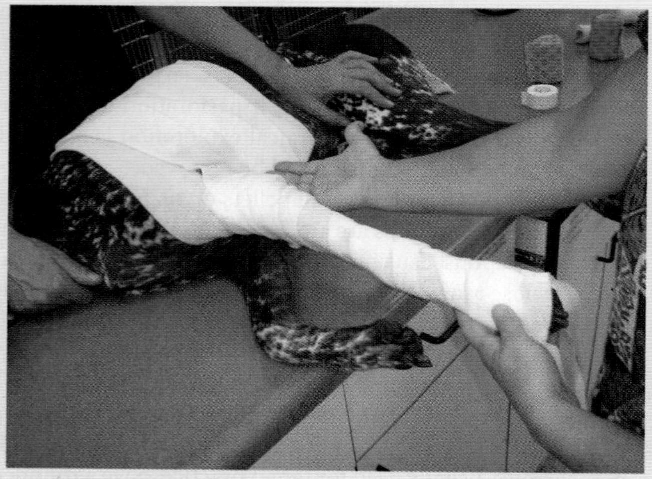

FIGURE 2 Flex the carpus and metacarpus and wrap with cotton gauze.

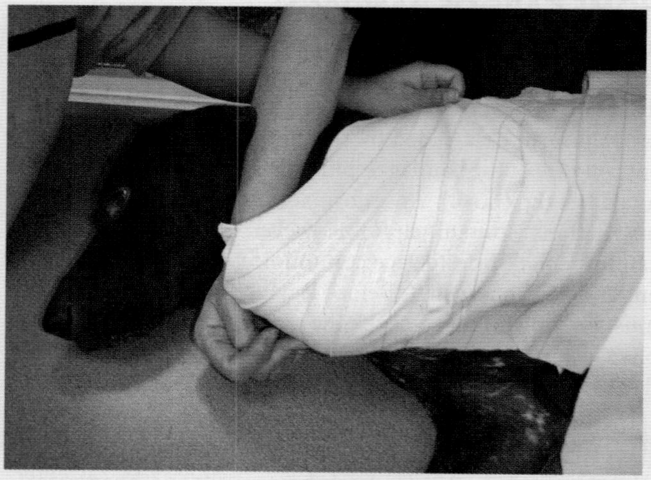

FIGURE 4 Apply additional wraps around the chest and flexed limb.

peritonitis resulting from perforation of the bowel. Penetrating thoracic wounds generally do not require exploration unless there is significant hemorrhage, pneumothorax, or esophageal involvement.

SNAKEBITES

Treatment of snakebites is directed toward preventing and controlling shock, neutralizing venom, minimizing necrosis, and preventing secondary infection. Fatal snake bites are more common in dogs than in any other domestic animal. Dogs are typically bitten in the head region. Because of their size, horses and cattle rarely die from snakebites; however, swelling on the muzzle, head, or neck can produce dyspnea and then death. Domestic animals vary in their sensitivity to the venom of pit vipers.

In North America, venomous snakes of the Crotalidae group, sometimes listed as a subfamily of Viperidae, are most commonly encountered in bite cases. These include the copperhead, cottonmouth, and rattlesnake. Clients should be instructed to bring the dead snake along with the bitten animal when possible, without mutilating the snake's head, because it may be needed for identification.

PROCEDURE 13-8 Cast Application

1. Stirrups of porous tape are applied to the dorsal and palmar aspects of the limb. Make sure to extend well beyond the toes.
2. A stockinette is applied over the limb with excess material at the proximal and distal ends.
3. Padding material is applied to cover bony protuberances.
4. The fiberglass casting material is soaked in warm water and then the excess water is squeezed out.
5. The fiberglass casting material is rolled onto the limb, beginning at the toes and working proximally, overlapping each pass (Fig. 1).
6. The stockinette ends and the tape stirrups are reflected onto the limb and incorporated into the cast by two or three more overlying layers of the fiberglass material (Fig. 2).
7. The completed cast is then molded (if needed) before setting.

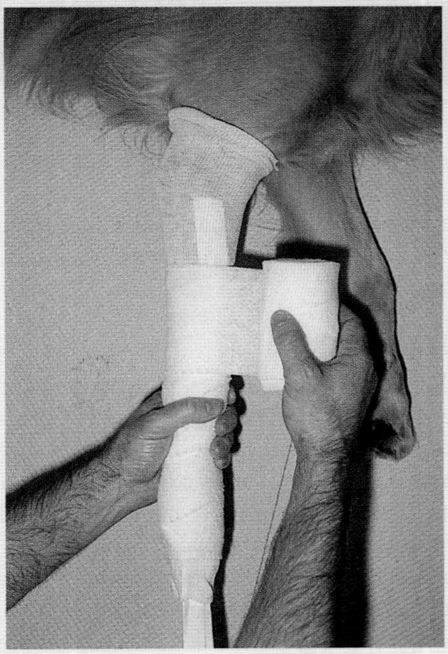

FIGURE 1 When applying a fiberglass cast, place adhesive stirrups on the limb and cover them with a stockinette. Apply cast padding firmly over the stockinette using an overlapping pattern.

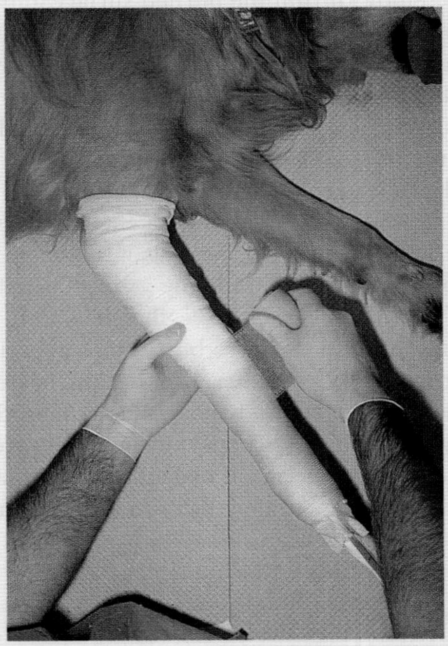

FIGURE 2 Then place four to six layers of casting material on the limb, overlapping each layer 50%. (From Fossum TW: *Small animal surgery*, ed 3, St Louis, 2007, Mosby.)

Systemic effects of envenomation include hypotension, shock, lethargy, salivation, lymph node pain, weakness, muscle fasciculations, and possible respiratory depression. Venomous snakebites often produce tissue necrosis and require reconstructive surgery. Tissue damage varies with the depth of bite and amount of venom injected. Local signs include fang puncture wounds (one or two), bleeding, swelling, tissue discoloration, and pain. The severity of envenomation cannot be judged by local signs alone.

Diphenhydramine hydrochloride (Benadryl, McNeil-PPC) is often given as a pretreatment (10 mg for small dogs and cats, 25 mg for large dogs). After an intravenous catheter has been placed and fluid administration (lactated Ringer's solution, physiologic saline, colloids) has commenced, give half the dose subcutaneously and the remainder intravenously.

Antivenin (polyvalent for Crotalidae, Pfizer Laboratories) should be given, as soon as possible, according to package insert recommendations. Antivenin can prevent systemic reactions and limit tissue necrosis. Although antivenin is expensive, it helps prevent large necrotic sloughs and may reduce costs associated with reconstructive surgery.

Necrotic snakebite wounds should be managed as an open infected wound during sloughing. Broad-spectrum antibacterial therapy is warranted to help prevent wound infection; tetanus antitoxin should be given. When sloughing is complete and healthy granulation tissue has formed, the wound should be assessed for possible reconstruction, grafting, or management as an open wound.

BURNS

Thermal Burns

Thermal burns caused by exposure to excessive heat are classified according to their depth. First-degree burns are superficial and involve only the epidermis. Except in pigs, first-degree burns in animals do not form vesicles or blisters, as commonly seen in humans. Third-degree burns destroy the full thickness of the skin. They form a dark brown, insensitive, leathery covering called an eschar. Second-degree burns fall between these two classifications.

Burn patients may be sedated to relieve pain and provide restraint if cardiovascular function is stable. Fluid therapy with a balanced electrolyte solution or lactated Ringer's solution should be used to treat shock associated with burns.

If started soon after injury, application of ice/cold water compresses or submersion in ice water may relieve pain and arrest progression of the burn. Hair should be clipped or removed from the burned surface and the area washed gently with a detergent antiseptic. The antiprostaglandin effects of topical aloe vera products may reduce the severity of burns.

Burns should be carefully debrided. In first- and second-degree burns, cleaning the burn may constitute debridement. A third-degree eschar may retain infection under it and prevent wound contraction. As the eschar separates from underlying tissue during healing, it should be removed with scissors. This is painful, and the patient's pain tolerance should be considered. After the eschar has been removed from second- and third-degree burns, topical antibacterial medication (e.g., silver sulfadiazine or bacitracin cream) and light bandages are applied. Bandages are changed at least twice daily. Occlusive dressings and ointments are usually contraindicated. The prognosis depends on the total area of the burn, depth of penetration, location, and age and condition of the patient.

Electrical Burns

Electrical burns occur most often when animals chew on electrical cords. The most common signs are tissue damage with necrosis, cardiac dysrhythmias, and acute pulmonary edema. Often, there is charring of tissue at the point of contact (e.g., lips or mouth). Because the electrical current may flow along blood vessels to tissues, ischemic demarcation and sloughing often occur 2 or 3 weeks later. Managing lip and mouth injuries associated with electrical burns requires debridement and possibly reconstructive surgery.

Chemical Burns

Chemical burns cause denaturation and coagulation of tissue protein. They often produce hard and soft eschars, with underlying ulcers. They may also be deeper and more extensive than they initially appear. Chemical burns are managed in much the same manner as thermal burns, with reconstruction or open wound healing.

BITE WOUNDS

Bite wounds usually appear as punctures, lacerations, or avulsions of skin flaps. Massive subcutaneous and muscle contamination, maceration, dead space, serum accumulation, and infection leading to abscess formation (especially in cats) may develop in underlying tissues. Bite wounds in cats commonly form abscesses and draining sinuses. These should be surgically explored, lavaged, and initially managed as a dirty wound. Systemic antibacterials should be used in bite wound patients.

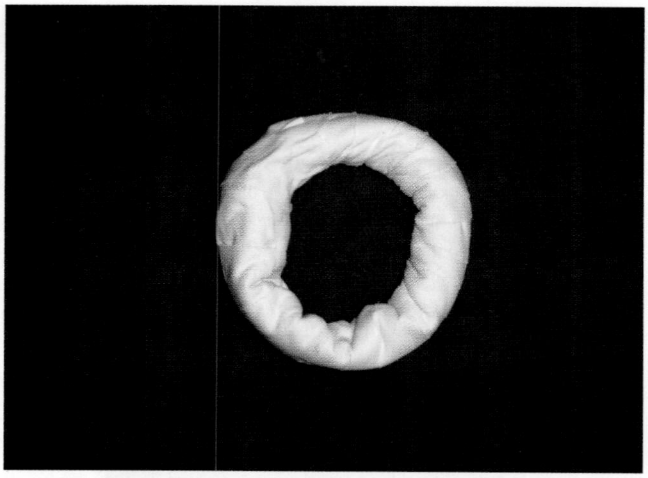

FIGURE 13-13 A donut-shaped pad used to help treat decubital ulcers.

DECUBITAL ULCERS

Decubital ulcers ("pressure sores") are open wounds that develop over bony prominences as a result of pressure in patients recumbent for long periods. Pressure sores can also develop over bony prominences covered by a cast or bandage as a result of insufficient or loose padding or overly tight application of the cast or bandage.

Decubital ulcers should be cleaned thoroughly with a surgical scrub and debrided when necessary.

Following cleaning, the area should be completely dried. Astringents (e.g., Burrow's solution) can be used to help dry the lesion. The decubital ulcer should be padded to prevent further pressure injury by use of a soft padded bandage held in the shape of a donut, with the ulcer in the center (Fig. 13-13). These protective bandages leave the ulcer open to the air and relieve pressure. Use of antibacterial agents may be considered; however, decubital ulcers heal best if kept clean and dry.

In recumbent patients, decubital ulcers can be prevented using the following measures:

- Provide sufficient soft padding or bedding material. This can include water pads, air mattresses, artificial fleece, rubber grids, straw, and towels. The material should be disposable or washable.
- Change the patient's position frequently. Turn the patient from side to side. Intermittent use of slings or carts may be considered.
- Periodically check the skin over bony prominences for signs of ulcer formation. These include hyperemia, moisture, and easily epilated hair.
- Keep the skin clean and dry. Bathe the patient frequently.
- Provide a well-balanced, high-protein diet.
- Apply casts and bandages correctly. Safeguard bony prominences with adequate padding.

REVIEW QUESTIONS

Matching

Match the terms with their description or definition.

_____1. carpal flexion sling
_____2. Ehmer sling
_____3. external coaptation
_____4. nonadherent dressing
_____5. occlusive dressing
_____6. Robert-Jones bandage
_____7. semi-permeable dressing
_____8. Velpeau sling

A. Configures to hold the carpus in flexion, thus reducing tension on the flexor surface.
B. Placed to keep weight-bearing off the coxofemoral joint.
C. Placed to hold the forelimb against the chest and prevent weight-bearing of the limb.
D. When used on a wound this allows for air transfer but not fluid transfer.
E. After orthopedic surgery on a rear limb, this is placed to help protect the limb initially.
F. A granulating wound needs this placed to keep it from sticking to the wound.
G. Using this requires less changing and accelerates epithelialization compared to an exposed wound.
H. This is used on the outside of a limb to join or maintain two ends together, such as a broken bone or cut tendon.

Exercise 2: True or False

Indicate whether each of the following statements is True or False.

______1. Pressure sores and vascular ulcers are types of chronic wounds.
______2. The phases of wound healing occur in this order: debridement, inflammation, repair, maturation.
______3. Infection and corticosteroids delay or stop wound repair.
______4. Contaminated tissue becomes infected if the bacteria multiply to a critical number of organisms per gram of tissue and then invade the tissue.
______5. Third-intention healing is where large or grossly contaminated wounds are allowed to heal completely without any surgery.
______6. Application of topical medications to aid in wound healing is recommended.
______7. Occlusive bandages are preferred when bandaging an injury in the field or before transport.
______8. Drains are used in wounds to help decrease the formation of tissue pockets and dead space.
______9. Formation of excess granulation tissue during wound healing is common in dogs.
______10. Closure of decubital ulcers is usually very successful.
______11. Puncture wounds usually are small holes with extensive deep tissue damage and contain foreign material and bacteria deep in the wound.
______12. Arrows can be removed by the client to help with transport to the hospital.
______13. Burn wounds normally can be managed by primary closure.
______14. Splints and casts should be checked daily in hospital and weekly once an animal has been sent home.
______15. In a modified Schroeder-Thomas splint, the traction should be significant within the splint, so as not to create excessive pressure.

Matching—Bandage Materials

Match the bandage layer with the type of material that may be used (some materials can be used in more than one layer of the bandage).

______1. primary layer
______2. secondary layer
______3. tertiary layer

A. stirrups
B. cast padding
C. cling gauze
D. Vetrap
E. Elasticon

RECOMMENDED READING

Bojrab MJ: *A handbook on veterinary wound management*, Ashland, OH, 1994, KenVet.

Fossum TW: *Small animal surgery*, ed 4, St Louis, 2013, Mosby.

Gfeller RW, Crowe DT: Emergency care of traumatic wounds, *Vet Clin North Am Small Anim Prac* 24:1249–1274, 1994.

Knottenbelt D: *Handbook of equine wound management*, Oxford, UK, 2002, Saunders. Saunders.

Pavletic MM: The clinician's guide to basic wound management, *Proc North Am Vet Conf* 512–513, 1996.

Stashak TS, Theoret CK: *Equine wound management*, ed 2, Ames, IA, 2009, Wiley-Blackwell.

Swaim SF, Henderson RA: *Small animal wound management*, ed 2, Philadelphia, 1997, Lippincott Williams & Wilkins.

Swaim SF, Krahwinkel DJ: Wound management, *Vet Clin Small Anim Pract*, July 15, 2006.

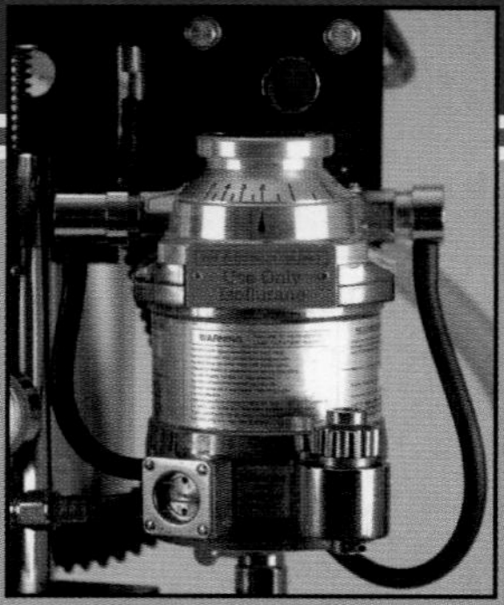

14 Veterinary Anesthesia, Analgesia, and Anesthetic Nursing

OUTLINE

LEARNING OBJECTIVES

After reviewing this chapter, the reader will be able to:

1. Define the role of veterinary technicians in anesthesia and perioperative pain management.
2. State the significance of and methods for managing perioperative pain.
3. Identify the goals and fundamentals of anesthesia.
4. Compare and contrast the types of anesthetic agents, their effects, and their advantages and disadvantages, used in the anesthetic induction and maintenance of small animals.
5. Outline the equipment used for anesthetizing animals, be able to identify the function and use of each component of the anesthetic machine, and differentiate between rebreathing and non-rebreathing circuits, a precision and nonprecision vaporizer, and a VOC and VIC.
6. Describe the rationale for each of the anesthetic machine components and its use.
7. Prepare and maintain anesthetic machines and the associated equipment.
8. List and describe the steps involved in anesthetizing animals for induction.
9. Explain the procedures used in medicating and monitoring animals before, during, and after anesthesia.
10. Prepare a small animal patient, anesthetic equipment, anesthetic agents, and accessories for general anesthesia.
11. Discuss endotracheal intubation, including its advantages and potential complications.
12. State the standards for providing for patient positioning, comfort, and safety during anesthetic maintenance.
13. List factors that affect patient recovery from anesthesia, the signs of recovery, and appropriate monitoring during recovery.

KEY TERMS

Analgesia
Anamnesis
Anesthesia
Bain coaxial circuit
Balanced anesthesia
Barotrauma
Breathing circuit
Central venous pressure
End tidal
Esophageal stethoscope
Flow meter
General anesthesia
Hypercarbemia
Hypercarbia
Hypoxemia
Laryngoscope
Multimodal therapy
Narcosis
Nociception
Non-rebreathing system
Norman mask elbow
Pain
Preemptive analgesia
Pressure manometer
Pulse deficit
Pulse oximeter
Pulse pressure
Pulse quality
Rebreathing system
Reservoir bag
Respiration
Scavenging system
Sedation
Tachycardia
Tidal volume
Transduction
Transmission
Vaporizer
Vasoconstriction
Ventilation

INTRODUCTION

ROLE OF VETERINARY TECHNICIANS

In many settings, technicians assume considerable responsibility for routine **anesthesia** administration and monitoring. Anesthesia or **sedation** is indicated for a wide variety of situations in veterinary medicine including restraint of patients, management of acute or chronic pain, and surgical anesthesia. The necessity for chemical restraint of an animal varies tremendously with the species and procedure. Calm, friendly, domestic animals tolerate more handling than agitated or wild animals. A variety of techniques may be used to produce anesthesia or sedation (Fig. 14-1). Judgment is required to determine the degree of sedation or anesthesia necessary and the delivery technique for patient and personnel comfort and safety (Table 14-1).

The involvement of veterinary technicians in managing perioperative pain before, during, and after a procedure is growing profoundly. Whether resulting from inflammation from tissue injury (trauma, disease) or the controlled trauma of surgery, pain is debilitating and undesirable. Surgical anesthesia continues to be the central focus of providing intraoperative pain relief. Postoperative **analgesia** has received increased attention recently and is expected whenever appropriate. Management of chronic pain is an issue of growing concern to owners of geriatric pets. Recent pharmacologic innovations have enhanced our ability to provide such relief with increased safety and efficacy. Technicians are assuming greater responsibilities for the assessment of patients and alleviation of their discomfort, distress, and pain.

The alert technician is invaluable in bringing patient distress to the attention of the veterinarian. Given the wide variety of species and situations encountered, this chapter can only provide a foundation on which to build and focuses on surgical anesthesia and perioperative analgesia. It is highly recommended that veterinary technicians involved with these procedures expand their knowledge via the recommended reading and continuing education. The opportunity for specialty certification of technicians in anesthesia exists and may be pursued where appropriate.

PAIN MANAGEMENT

Pain is defined as an unpleasant sensory or emotional experience associated with actual or potential tissue damage. Physiologic pain results from the stimulation of nerve endings called nociceptors, which are found throughout the tissues (Fig. 14-2). Pain may be classified as peripheral, neuropathic, clinical, or idiopathic. Pain causes many deleterious effects on the body possibly affecting each of the systems (Box 14-1). **Nociception** is different from pain. General anesthesia controls the perception of intraoperative pain. Anesthetics vary in analgesic efficiency and may not completely disrupt the nociceptive mechanisms of the nervous system.

> *TECHNICIAN NOTE* Unconsciousness or unresponsiveness is not lack of pain—nociception still occurs. This is why it is important to check the depth of anesthesia and monitor the patient closely, using the response to painful stimuli.

Pain recognition is difficult, as responses to pain vary among species and individuals. Some individuals tolerate considerable discomfort without any reaction. Other individuals vocalize loudly when given a minor injection. Anticipation of possible pain enters into the animal's response as well. It is very helpful to know the normal behavior of the individual when assessing them for pain (Box 14-2). Obvious inflammation (redness, swelling, and heat) is generally accompanied by pain. Animals recovering from anesthesia are not able to exhibit a normal range of behavioral signs and may be experiencing pain long before it becomes apparent to the observer. Research guidelines indicate that any condition that would cause pain in humans should be assumed to cause pain in animals. Accordingly, we assume that a dog

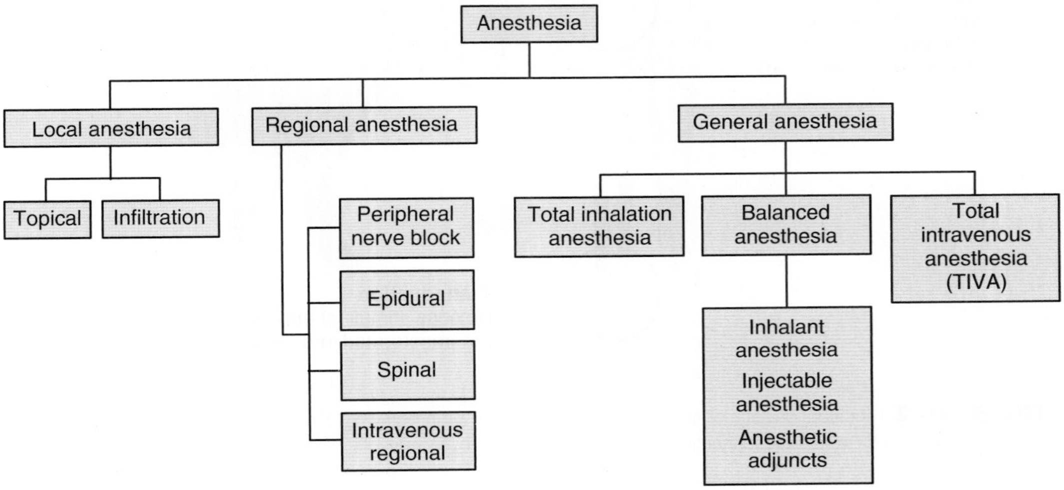

FIGURE 14-1 Types of anesthetic procedures. (From Muir WW, Hubbell JAE: *Equine anesthesia: monitoring and emergency therapy*, ed 2, St Louis, 2009, Mosby.)

TABLE 14-1 Types of Anesthesia

TYPE	COMMENTS
Local anesthesia	May result in less intraoperative pain from the incision site if injected before surgery or in site before suturing
Regional or segmental anesthesia—blocking the nerve or nerves that supply a region or segment of the body	An injection of a local anesthetic agent is made near the nerve at a point proximal to the region being anesthetized. Effective in dental extractions. A paravertebral nerve block is often used to produce regional flank anesthesia in cattle undergoing standing abdominal surgery. Nerve blocks are also commonly used to help diagnose lameness in horses.
Spinal or epidural anesthesia (or analgesia)—injecting a local anesthetic or analgesic agent into the subarachnoid or epidural space of the spinal cord	This is typically done at the lumbosacral junction to provide profound analgesia or anesthesia to the pelvis and rear limbs during fracture repair. *Note:* Animals may perceive numbed body parts with anxiety, and self-mutilation may result. Prevention of these reactions may require tranquilization or sedation.
General anesthesia—purposeful derangement of a patient's normal physiologic processes to produce a state of unconsciousness, relaxation, analgesia, and/or amnesia	Induced by administering an anesthetic agent systemically either by injection (IM or IV) or by inhalation, depending on the agent, that will be distributed to the brain.
Sedation and tranquilization—often used interchangeably but actually have different meanings. *Sedation* is a mild to profound degree of CNS depression in which the patient is drowsy but may be aroused by painful stimuli. *Tranquilization* is a state of relaxation and calmness characterized by a lack of anxiety or concern without significant drowsiness.	Generally drugs that produce tranquilization at low doses may produce sedation at higher doses. Some sedatives also produce significant analgesia. Hence, it is difficult to refer to a drug strictly as a tranquilizer, sedative, or analgesic agent, as any or all of these effects may occur in a dose-dependent fashion.

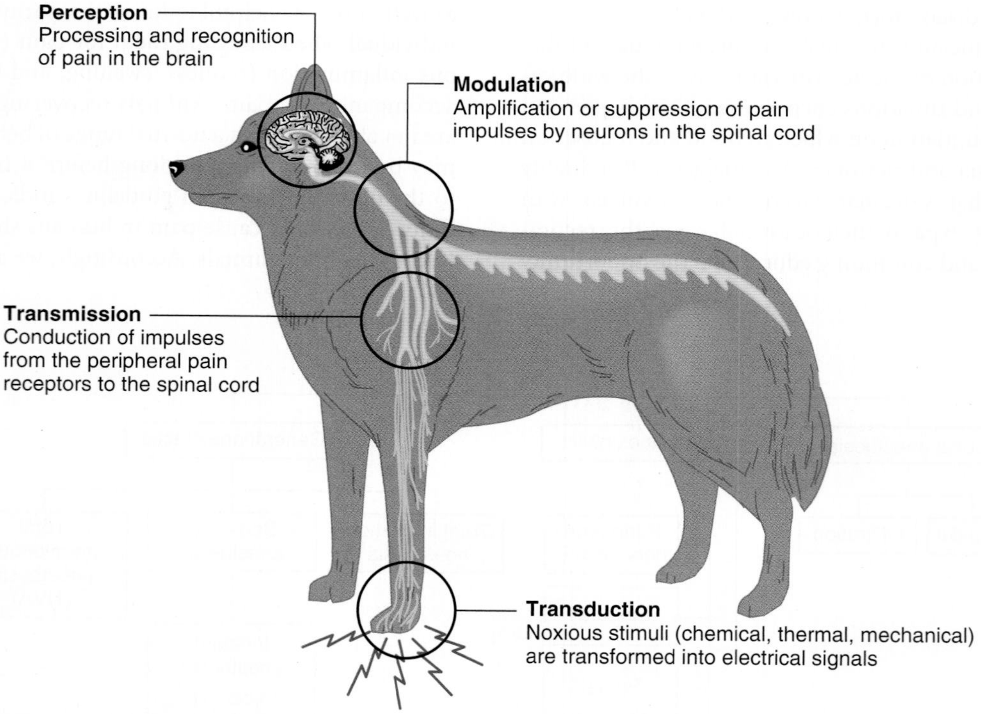
Perception
Processing and recognition of pain in the brain
Modulation
Amplification or suppression of pain impulses by neurons in the spinal cord
Transmission
Conduction of impulses from the peripheral pain receptors to the spinal cord
Transduction
Noxious stimuli (chemical, thermal, mechanical) are transformed into electrical signals

FIGURE 14-2 Nociception. Site of analgesic action along the pain pathway. (From Thomas JA, Lerche P: *Anesthesia and analgesia for veterinary technicians,* ed 4, St Louis, 2011, Mosby.)

BOX 14-1 Effects of Clinical Pain

1. Immunosuppression
2. Increased tissue catabolism
3. Reduced healing
4. Increased autonomic activity, primarily sympathetic
5. Emotional stress/distress

BOX 14-2 Signs of Pain

1. Changes in behavior and temperament (shunning or seeking attention, postural changes, inappetence, changes in voiding behavior, reluctance to move, unusual gait)
2. Protection of the affected area (avoids touching; threatens if approached)
3. Vocalization (especially on movement or palpation of affected area)
4. Licking or biting affected area
5. Scratching or shaking affected area
6. Restlessness, pacing
7. Sweating
8. Tachycardia, hyperpnea, peripheral vasoconstriction, muscle tension, hypertension

undergoing abdominal surgery would experience as much pain as a person would experience from a comparable procedure, even if the dog does not exhibit signs of pain. It has been demonstrated that pain is more easily managed if analgesics are given preemptively (**preemptive analgesia**), before a patient experiences pain. To properly assess the patient, it is essential that a comprehensive and thorough history and physical assessment be completed.

Pain-Relief Modalities

Pain-relief modalities take advantage of one or more means of preventing or interfering with the development or perception of pain (Box 14-3). Refinement of surgical technique to produce less tissue damage will prevent a great deal of postoperative pain. Proponents of laser surgery report that postoperative pain is greatly reduced, for example. To the extent that some tissue trauma is inevitable in any surgical procedure, one or more of the following modalities may be used before, during, and after the procedure to manage the type and level of pain experienced at that time.

ANALGESIA

Most of the drugs used for analgesia cause various other dose-dependent effects. The opioid analgesic agents produce a dose-dependent sedation (called **narcosis**) that may be quite profound. The nonsteroidal anti-inflammatory drugs (NSAIDs) (especially the older ones) have a tendency to cause gastrointestinal irritation, ulceration, and bleeding. Newer analgesic agents are designed to have fewer adverse side effects (Table 14-2). Preemptive analgesia implies the prevention of the "wind-up" phenomenon. "Wind-up" refers to an increased central pain sensitization in which repeated painful stimulation of peripheral nerves increases the strength of pain signal reaching the brain. The process leads to increased pain (hyperalgesia) in which less stimulation is needed to increase pain response to otherwise nonpainful stimuli (allodynia) and spontaneous pain. Use of multiple drugs with different mechanisms of action, which may act at different levels of the nociceptive pathways, produce enhanced (additive, superadditive) analgesic effects. Using several analgesic drugs, each with a different mechanism of action, is called **multimodal** therapy. This results in lower dosages, which increases safety.

BOX 14-3 Concepts of Physiology of Pain: Nociception and the Pain Pathway

1. Nociception: refers to the process by which pain information is carried from the periphery sense receptors in the skin and in the viscera to the cerebral cortex through network of neuronal relays. Has three phases:
   a. Transduction: begins with tissue trauma in which the nociceptors are stimulated, and converted into electrical impulses once the threshold is exceeded.
   b. Transmission: if noxious stimuli exceed the nociceptor's threshold, they travel along peripheral nerves to the spinal cord (dorsal horn) and the brain (thalamus).
   c. Modulation: the descending pathway that allows the brain to modify pain sensory. It does this by sending chemical messages from the brain to close the gates in the spinal cord to ascending messages.
2. Perception: fourth phase of pain pathway that occurs in conscious brain where impulses are processed and recognized as actual pain.
3. Pain wind-up or central stimulation: a phenomenon of increased central pain sensitization in which repeated painful stimulation of peripheral nerves increases the strength of pain signal reaching the brain. The process leads to increased pain (hyperalgesia) in which less stimulation is needed to increase pain response to otherwise nonpainful stimuli (allodynia) and spontaneous pain.

> **TECHNICIAN NOTE** Pain modalities may be used before, during, and after the procedure to manage the type and level of pain experienced at that time.

Tranquilizers and sedatives are typically used as preanesthetic medications to calm the patient and reduce the amount of anesthetic needed (Table 14-3). When inhalation anesthesia is performed, the animal is usually first induced into **general anesthesia** with a short-acting injectable agent to facilitate tracheal intubation and induction with the inhalation agent (Table 14-4).

Analgesic agents are needed to suppress the physiologic pain mechanisms that remain active during anesthesia. These will also allow a reduction in the dose of general anesthetic needed to maintain anesthesia. In human anesthesiology, there have been recent reports of awareness of sound and

TABLE 14-2 Classes of Analgesic Agents

DRUG CLASS	EXAMPLE	ADVERSE EFFECTS
Opioids	Oxymorphone,* morphine, fentanyl, butorphanol, buprenorphine	Sedation, respiratory depression, hypotension
Alpha-2 adrenergic agonists	Xylazine, detomidine, medetomidine, romifidine	Bradycardia, hypertension, cardiac arrhythmia, peripheral vasoconstriction
Nonsteroidal anti-inflammatory drugs (NSAIDs)	Carprofen, aspirin, meloxicam, phenylbutazone, flunixin, ketoprofen	GI bleeding and disturbances, renal disturbances
Local anesthetics	Lidocaine, bupivacaine mepivacaine	If given through CRI, may see nausea, vomiting, seizures, neurologic signs
Adjunctive agents	Ketamine, acepromazine, benzodiazepine, prednisolone, etomidate, alfaxan	Varied depending on the agent

CRI, constant rate infusion.
*Not licensed in Canada.

TABLE 14-3 Tranquilizers and Sedatives for Patients with P1 and P2 ASA Physical Status Classification

DRUG CLASS AND EXAMPLES	TRADE NAMES	COMMENTS
Phenothiazines		
Acepromazine	ProMACE (dogs, cats, horses)	Concentration: 10 mg/ml; dilute to 1 mg/ml for small-animal use
		Dosage 0.01 to 0.1 mg/kg IV, IM or SC (3 mg maximum total dose)
		Major tranquilizer, alpha-adrenergic blocker
		Antiemetic, lowers seizure threshold, no significant analgesia but potentiates or prolongs analgesic effect of analgesic agents, variable sedation
		Potential hypotension/tachycardia due to vasodilation
		Avoid in cardiovascular compromise
Acepromazine + opioid		Consider combination of glycopyrrolate IM at 0.01 mg/kg, acepromazine IM at 0.1 mg/kg (3 mg maximum total dose) and butorphanol IM at 0.1-0.4 mg/kg
		If available oxymorphone IM at 0.05-0.2 mg/kg (3 mg maximum total dose) can be substituted for butorphanol
		Reduce opioid dosage for IV use; administer to effect
		Used as preanesthetic and for chemical restraint
Alpha-2 Agonists		Sedation, analgesia, anxiolysis, sympatholysis, vasoconstriction, arrhythmogenesis
1. Xylazine	Rompun, GeminiAna-Sed Sedazine (different concentrations approved for dogs, cats, horses, deer, elk)	May induce vomiting during induction (especially if given SC or IM) Premedication with anticholinergic prevents bradycardia May be used as epidural for analgesia, especially in large animals. Alpha-2 to Alpha-1 selectivity: 160:1 Concentration: Small-animal: 20 mg/ml; Large animal: 100 mg/ml
2. Detomidine	Dormosedan (horses)	*Dosage:* dogs: 0.25-0.5 mg/kg IM; cats: 0.5-1 mg/kg IM (max 5 mg dose)—when used *Onset/duration:* 10-15 minutes after IM; up to 1 hour of sedation
3. Medetomidine	Domitor (dogs)	Arrhythmogenic effects include bradycardia, AV block, SA block Rompun-ketamine was a classic combination in dogs and cats for many years but has been supplanted by newer agents
4. Romifidine antagonists		The bradycardia and decreased cardiac output are offset by ketamine's sympathomimetic effects, whereas the xylazine offsets the muscle rigidity of ketamine; ruminants are extremely sensitive to alpha-2 agonists, extralabel usage must be cautious

TABLE 14-3 Tranquilizers and Sedatives for Patients with P1 and P2 ASA Physical Status Classification—cont'd

DRUG CLASS AND EXAMPLES	TRADE NAMES	COMMENTS
Xylazine + butorphanol		*Dosage:* glycopyrrolate IM at 0.01 mg/kg with xylazine IM at 0.2 mg/kg (5 mg maximum total dose). Wait 10 minutes, then give butorphanol IM at 0.1-0.4 mg/kg
		Reduce dosage for IV use; administer to effect
		Used as preanesthetic and for chemical restraint. Concentration: 1 mg/ml
		Dosage for sedation (per label): 750-1000 μg/m^2 with butorphone
		Alpha-2 to Alpha-1 selectivity: 260:1 Alpha-2 to Alpha-1 selectivity: 1620:1 Increased selectivity results in more predictable and effective sedation and analgesia with fewer side effects.
		Preanesthetic dosage: 5-10 μg/kg IM; >10 μg/kg produces sedation and bradycardia
		Sedation and analgesia are enhanced by opioids and benzodiazepines and best used as such
		Newest Alpha-2 agonist under investigation Alpha-2 to Alpha-1 selectivity: 340:1 Alpha-2 agonist antagonized by yohimbine (Yobine), Antagonil, tolazoline (Tolazine), atipamezole (Antisedan)
Benzodiazepines		Minor tranquilizers, muscle relaxation, anticonvulsant, appetite stimulant, little or no sedation, no significant analgesia but potentiates or prolongs effect of analgesic agents, antagonized by flumazenil
1. Diazepam Schedule IV	Valium (human)	Concentration: 5 mg/ml Dosage: 0.2-0.4 mg/kg IV
		Lipid based so administer IV only
		Avoid rapid IV injection; may produce pain and hypotension
		Anxiolytic, amnesic, muscle relaxant, anticonvulsant Useful in central nervous system and cardiac patients Little sedative effect in healthy animals; may cause profound depression in compromised patients
		Do not mix with other agents in same syringe (except ketamine)
		Administer cautiously in aggressive patients
		Effects may be prolonged effects in hepatic dysfunction
		Propylene glycol base may cause arrhythmias
		Flumazenil (Romazicon: Roche) is an effective antagonist (0.1 mg/kg IV)
2. Midazolam Schedule IV	Versed (human)	Concentration: 1 mg/ml Dosage: 0.2-0.4 mg/kg IV or IM—lower dosage for IV
		Midazolam 0.2 mg/kg and Butorphanol 0.2 mg/kg IM can be combined
		Effects similar to those of diazepam
		Water-soluble so can be given IM
		More potent, more rapid onset of action, shorter duration of action than diazepam
		Excellent choice in critically ill patients
		May cause excitement and pain if rapidly administered
		Flumazenil is an effective antagonist (0.1 mg/kg IV)
3. Zolazepam Schedule III		Available only in drug combination Telazol (+tiletamine) Approved for use in dogs and cats. (See dissociative agents for information.)

TABLE 14-4 Injectable General Anesthetics

DRUG CLASS AND EXAMPLE	TRADE NAMES	COMMENTS
Barbiturates		
Thiopental sodium	Thiopental Human products: Pentothal	Ultrashort-acting thiobarbiturate Extralabel use: Dogs, cats
		Concentration: 2%-5%; store reconstituted product under refrigeration
		Dosage (if premedicated with tranquilizer/opioid): 5-10 mg/kg slowly IV to effect
		Duration of effects is 5-10 minutes but only provides 2- to 3-minute intubation window at minimal doses
		Used as induction agent for inhalation anesthesia
		Short action because of redistribution from the CNS to the muscle tissue and then the adipose tissue
		Accumulates in tissue: Do not use for anesthetic maintenance
		Provides minimal analgesia
		Use small dose, and dilute concentrations in small or debilitated patients with cardiopulmonary, hepatic, or renal compromise
		May produce arrhythmias and apnea
		Monitor closely and support ventilation
		Administer fluids and oxygen to improve outcome
		Provides smooth transition to unconsciousness
		Premedication with tranquilizer and opioid reduces dose required
		Use with caution in sighthounds
		The ultrashort barbiturates are Class III controlled substances in the US and Schedule G in Canada and must be kept secure.
		Similar but less cumulative than thiopental
		Dosage 6-10 mg/kg for small animals with a duration of 5-10 minutes
Methohexital	Brevane Brevital	Solutions are stable at room temperature
		Metabolized more rapidly than thiopental
Nonbarbiturates		
Propofol	Veterinary products (canine): Rapinovet Propofol Human products: Diprivan	Ultrashort-acting alkyl phenol, Concentration: 10 mg/ml
		Used as induction agent for inhalation anesthesia, maintenance for brief procedures
		Dosage: 2-6 mg/kg IV for induction over 60-90 seconds to effect (if premedicated) Sedation: 0.5-2 mg/kg
		Rapid injection causes apnea
		Duration of effects is 5-10 minutes, but only provides a 2- to 3-minute intubation window at minimal doses
		Maintenance: 0.2-0.8 mg/kg/min IV infusion in conjunction with benzodiazepine and opioid
		Highly lipid-soluble
		Can produce the "five hypos"
		Short action because of redistribution and rapid metabolism by somatic cells
		Tissue accumulation minimal because of rapid metabolism
		Provides minimal analgesia
		Not recommended for pregnant or nursing females
		Considered safer for use in sighthounds and patients with compromised liver and kidney function
		Provide cardiovascular and pulmonary support
		Not a controlled substance
		Aseptic technique is critical: Must be used within 6 hours of opening vial
		Short-acting imidazole-derivative used as a sedative-hypnotic
		Not a controlled substance

TABLE 14-4 Injectable General Anesthetics—cont'd

DRUG CLASS AND EXAMPLE	TRADE NAMES	COMMENTS
		Causes minimal changes in CV and respiratory function
Etomidate	Amidate	Rapid onset and recovery, noncumulative
		Wider therapeutic index than propofol or barbiturates
		Choice of drug for patients with severe heart disease or shock
		Does not provide analgesia but does give good muscle relaxation
		Cannot be given IM
		Can be given as CRI and suggested to give with fluids to reduce adverse effects that can include vomiting, muscle movements, sneezing, and excitement during induction and recovery—an antiglucocorticoid and mineralocorticoid effect—no histamine release
		Can cause phlebitis, and in cats with repeated doses can cause hemolysis
		Is costly
		Give rapidly to effect following premedication with a tranquilizer, or concurrently with IV diazepam or midazolam (use a separate syringe if diazepam is chosen)
		Not usually used to maintain anesthesia
		Narcotic + tranquilizer; e.g., hydromorphone and diazepam. Give an IV bolus of diazepam, followed by a bolus of hydromorphone
		Produces CNS depression and analgesia
		May need additional bolus for intubation—useful for short or minor procedures
		May or may not remain conscious and respond to stimuli
		Side effects are respiratory depression and bradycardia
		The severe respiratory depression can usually be reversed by an opioid antagonist
		Not available in North America at time of writing
		Is an injectable anesthetic agent for induction and maintenance of general anesthesia in dogs and cats
		Clear, colorless, aqueous solution of alfaxalone, which is a neuroactive steroid molecule with properties of a general anesthetic
		Does not contain the combination of alphaxolone/alphadalone of the original Saffan, nor does it contain cremesol, a preservative that caused the histamine release frequently noticed as swollen face and paws
		Should be given slowly over 60 seconds for smoother induction
		Will not cause irritation if perivascular
		Can be used to maintain anesthesia by topping up or as CRI
		Wide safety margin
Alfaxalone	Alfaxan	Metabolized in the liver with a very short plasma elimination half-life in dogs and cats
		Neuroleptanalgesia
Dissociative Agents		
Ketamine	Veterinary Products (cats, primates): Ketaset, Vetalar, Vetaket, extralabel uses; horses, dogs	Concentration: 100 mg/ml
		Dosage: 5-20 mg/kg IM or 1-6 mg/kg IV (slowly)
		Duration: 5-10 minutes IV; 20-40 minutes IM
		Causes catatonia, muscle rigidity, possible convulsions if used alone; do not use alone without a tranquilizer
		The effects of dissociative combinations last longer than the effects of thiobarbiturates or propofol, affecting the patient well beyond the initial induction period, even into the postoperative recovery period
		Rapid onset of profound anesthesia with some somatic but poor visceral analgesia
		Causes apnea, enhancing hypoxemia and hypercarbemia

Continued

TABLE 14-4 Injectable General Anesthetics—cont'd

DRUG CLASS AND EXAMPLE	TRADE NAMES	COMMENTS
		Increases heart rate and blood pressure, increasing myocardial oxygen demand
		Usually maintains cardiac output and blood pressure better than barbiturates
		May increase intracranial and ocular pressure
		Avoid in patients with renal, hepatic, or cardiac disease, ocular surgery, and epileptics
		Transition to inhalation anesthesia may be rougher than with barbiturates
		Apnea reduces uptake of inhalation agent
		Animal awakens abruptly when ketamine wears off
		Oropharyngeal reflexes not completely abolished
		Excessive salivation and respiratory secretions may occur
		Irregular respirations, rapid heart rate, emergence delirium, and the eyes to remain wide open and prone to drying. Ophthalmic ointment must be used to prevent corneal ulceration.
		Dissociative agents have been reclassified as Class III controlled drug in the US and Schedule 1 in Canada
		Dissociative agents are rarely used alone. They are typically combined with other agents that offset the undesirable properties to induce anesthesia in a wide variety of species. Examples include: Ketamine + benzodiazepine:
		• Useful combination for canine induction • Dosage: ketamine at 5 mg/kg and benzodiazepine at 0.25 mg/kg, slowly IV Others (see recommended reading for details of usage): • Ketamine + acepromazine + butorphanol • Ketamine + alpha-2 agonist • Ketamine + butorphanol Ketamine + butorphanol + dexmedetomidine—IV "Kitty Magic"
Tiletamine	Telazol dogs and cats Extralabel use: Exotics	The only commercially available dissociative-tranquilizer combination.
		Concentration: zolazepam 50 mg/ml and tiletamine 50 mg/ml
		Dosage: 2-6 mg/kg IV or IM
		Rapidly induces surgical plane of anesthesia for 10-20 minutes
		Recovery period varies
		Tiletamine has longer duration and greater analgesia than ketamine
		Large doses can produce apnea, leading to hypoxia and hypercarbia
		Excitement may occur during recovery if zolazepam is eliminated from tissues before tiletamine
		Administer an additional sedative IV
		Recovery may be prolonged with use of large doses if zolazepam is not completely metabolized
		Reverse with flumazenil
		In cats, tiletamine is often metabolized first; in dogs, zolazepam is usually metabolized first
		Very effective in exotic and aggressive patients
		In healthy patients, premedication with acepromazine (0.05-0.1 mg/kg IM or SC) 15 minutes before Telazol administration may provide 20-40 minutes of surgical anesthesia
		Recovery varies

pain by apparently anesthetized patients. Postoperatively, they are able to repeat conversations overheard during their procedure and describe the experience of searing pain. It is not fully understood if this situation occurs in anesthetized animals or how to recognize it if it does.

> *TECHNICIAN NOTE* Multimodal therapy involves the use of several analgesic drugs, each with a different mechanism of action.

Goals of an Anesthetic-Analgesic Plan

The goals of every anesthetic-analgesic plan are to predict, prevent, recognize, and correct complications. Complications can be prevented by using the correct equipment and methods, ensuring equipment is in good working order, avoiding drugs that enhance a preexisting condition, and supporting the specific needs of the patient. Supporting respiration with oxygen enrichment and supporting perfusion with appropriate fluids may be adequate to prevent common arrhythmias or hypotension. Appropriate and timely use of analgesic agents prevents complications associated with pain. Knowledge of preexisting conditions is essential (see Patient Evaluation section). Promptly recognizing anesthetic complications requires close, continuous monitoring. Specific attention should be paid to the "five hypos" (Table 14-5) and other predicted complications (anesthetic monitoring). Western medicine has depended almost exclusively on pharmacologic agents for pain management. However, alternative modalities such as acupuncture, electrical nerve stimulation, magnetic field induction, and neurolysis have gained increasing acceptance. Refer to the recommended reading for information on these pain relief modalities.

FUNDAMENTALS OF ANESTHESIA

The fundamentals of anesthesia can be summarized as follows:

- Carefully evaluate the medical history, physical examination findings, and laboratory data.
- Prepare for the expected and unexpected. Work with adequately trained personnel.
- Minimize anesthesia time by planning ahead (e.g., prepare the surgical site before anesthesia).
- Carefully select and use the correct dose of anesthetic drugs based on the patient's health status, species, and breed. Avoid drugs that can enhance preexisting health problems.
- Avoid administration of induction agents until calming agents have taken effect.
- Reevaluate and stabilize (if necessary) vital signs before induction.
- Maintain a patent airway and monitor ventilation; support with supplemental oxygen and assisted ventilation.
- Monitor cardiovascular function; support with fluids and oxygen.
- Monitor body temperature; support by preventing heat loss and providing external sources of heat.

TABLE 14-5 The Five "Hypos"

CONDITION	DESCRIPTION
Hypoxemia	Insufficient oxygenation of the blood (PaO_2 less than 60 mm Hg). A common sign of pulmonary compromise during anesthesia and the reason for oxygen enrichment of inspired air.
Hypoventilation	Reduced rate and depth of ventilation as determined by increased arterial carbon dioxide levels (hypercarbia or hypercapnia) ($PaCO_2$ above 45 mm Hg). Hypercarbia is an early sign of pulmonary compromise.
Hypotension	Inadequate arterial blood pressure. The most common sign of cardiovascular depression. Diastolic/systolic pressures are normally 80/120 mm Hg.
Hypovolemia	Insufficient circulating blood volume. A common cause of hypotension. For this reason, fluid administration is one of the most valuable supportive measures one can provide during anesthesia.
Hypothermia	Abnormally low body temperature (2-3° C below normal). A sign of central nervous system and cardiovascular depression.

- Continually monitor and support all body systems from premedication through recovery.
- Use analgesics to minimize pain and discomfort. Use calming agents to reduce excitement.
- Keep an accurate record of the anesthetic procedure, monitoring efforts, and all major anesthetic events.

STEPS OF ANESTHESIA

STEP 1: PATIENT EVALUATION

Patient evaluation means carefully judging a patient's medical history and physical condition to determine health status and predict potential complications. This is the most important step, because all anesthetic decisions are based on health status. The medical history and physical examination are absolutely critical before anesthesia. All abnormalities discovered should be pursued to determine their potential effect on anesthetic outcome. Patient evaluation includes consideration of patient characteristics, medical history, physical examination, and laboratory data.

See Table 14-6 for physical status classification as suggested by the American Society of Anesthesiologists (ASA), keeping in mind that the classification can be subjective and may change over time.

Patient Characteristics

Patient characteristics such as species, breed, age, and gender may prompt special considerations. Sighthounds (e.g., Greyhounds, Salukis, Borzois) are known to be very excitable during induction and have a prolonged recovery period. Brachycephalic breeds (e.g., Pug, Bulldog, Boston terrier) are known

TABLE 14-6 ASA Physical Status Classifications

CLASSIFICATION	RISK	CRITERIA	REPRESENTATIVE CONDITIONS
P1	Minimal	Normal, healthy patient	Patients undergoing elective procedures (OHE, castration, or declaw)
P2	Low	Patient with mild systemic disease	Neonatal, geriatric, or obese patients Mild dehydration Skin tumor removal
P3	Moderate	Patient with severe systemic disease	Anemia Moderate dehydration Compensated major organ disease
P4	High	Patient with severe systemic disease that is a constant threat to life	Ruptured bladder Internal hemorrhage Pneumothorax Pyometra
P5	Extreme	Moribund patient that is not expected to survive without the operation	Severe head trauma Pulmonary embolus Gastric dilation-volvulus End-stage major organ failure

From Bassert JM, McCurnin DM: *McCurnin's clinical textbook for veterinary technicians*, ed 7, St Louis, 2010, Saunders.

to have problems with airway obstruction during recovery. Pediatric patients are prone to hypothermia and hypoglycemia. Geriatric patients may have difficulty metabolizing drugs and typically require more supportive care.

Medical History

Patient medical history should include signalment, and anamnesis including the vaccine status, medical and surgical history, injuries, diseases, past anesthetic complications, changes in the patient's condition since last observed, purpose of the appointment including specific location, observance of fasting recommendations, and concurrent medication. As much information should be obtained as possible using questions that elicit facts and details. Ask open-ended questions and avoid ones that yield yes-or-no answers. For most of the signs that are noted, it is helpful to question the client so that the four main factors of almost any condition—the duration, volume or severity, character or appearance, and frequency—are covered.

Physical Examination

The physical examination includes general body condition scoring (Fig. 14-3) and evaluation of the cardiovascular, respiratory, hepatic, renal, and central nervous systems (Table 14-7). It is important to examine the animal entirely and systematically and to know the normal physiologic values of the patient (Table 14-8).

> TECHNICIAN NOTE Pale mucous membranes or prolonged capillary refill time indicate decreased perfusion from shock, vasoconstriction, hypotension, or a variety of other issues. Anemia can be association with pale mucous membranes. Cyanotic mucous membranes point to reduced oxygen saturation, which is a medical emergency.

Diagnostic Testing

It is important to stress the value of preanesthetic screening when counseling a client before a procedure. Most clinics use a minimum set of laboratory data for younger, healthier patients and add others when specific concerns arise based on signalment and assessment. A client consent form should be signed. Preanesthetic laboratory tests may include hematocrit (PCV), total plasma protein level, blood smear, liver enzymes (ALT), bile acids, blood urea nitrogen (BUN), blood glucose, heartworm status, fecals, acid-base balance, urinalysis, electrolyte levels, blood gas values, and blood coagulation screens, depending on the condition and age of the animal. Thoracic radiographs and electrocardiography also may be useful in evaluating a patient.

STEP 2: PATIENT PREPARATION

Patient preparation requirements vary depending on the anticipated procedure. It is also important to prepare for the possibility of unanticipated situations. Standard practice is to withhold food for 8 to 12 hours and water for 2 to 4 hours before anesthetic induction. However, special preparation may be required in complex procedures. Pediatric or smaller patients should be fasted for shorter time periods. Chronically compromised patients should have their condition stabilized, when possible, before anesthesia. For example, anemic patients (PCV less than 20%) should have a transfusion to ensure adequate oxygen-carrying capacity. Dehydrated patients should receive sufficient intravenous fluids to restore hydration status. Patients with low total plasma protein levels (less than 3 g/dl) may benefit from administration of plasma.

> TECHNICIAN NOTE An accurate weight should be obtained just before any anesthetic procedure. Use a pediatric scale for animals less than 5 kg and a gram scale for those less than 1 kg.

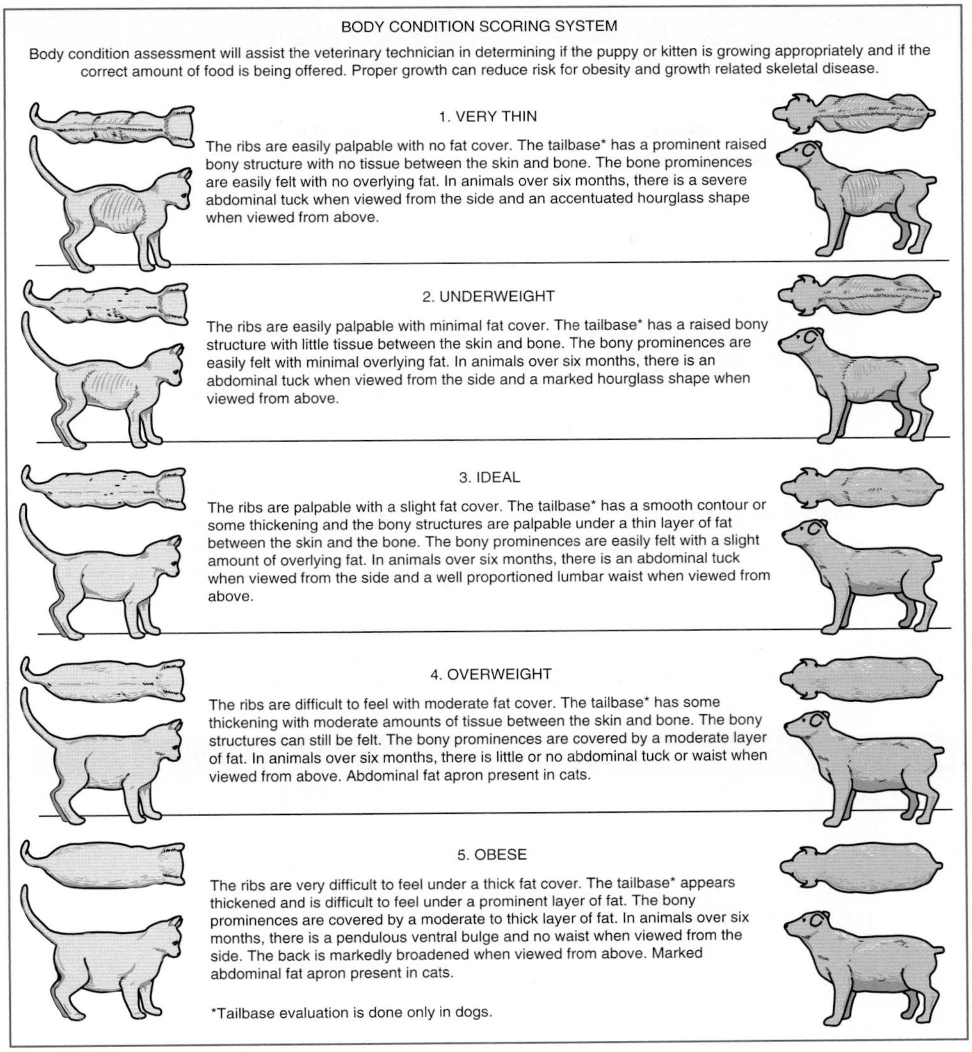

BODY CONDITION SCORING SYSTEM
Body condition assessment will assist the veterinary technician in determining if the puppy or kitten is growing appropriately and if the correct amount of food is being offered. Proper growth can reduce risk for obesity and growth related skeletal disease.
1. VERY THIN
The ribs are easily palpable with no fat cover. The tailbase* has a prominent raised bony structure with no tissue between the skin and bone. The bone prominences are easily felt with no overlying fat. In animals over six months, there is a severe abdominal tuck when viewed from the side and an accentuated hourglass shape when viewed from above.
2. UNDERWEIGHT
The ribs are easily palpable with minimal fat cover. The tailbase* has a raised bony structure with little tissue between the skin and bone. The bony prominences are easily felt with minimal overlying fat. In animals over six months, there is an abdominal tuck when viewed from the side and a marked hourglass shape when viewed from above.
3. IDEAL
The ribs are palpable with a slight fat cover. The tailbase* has a smooth contour or some thickening and the bony structures are palpable under a thin layer of fat between the skin and the bone. The bony prominences are easily felt with a slight amount of overlying fat. In animals over six months, there is an abdominal tuck when viewed from the side and a well proportioned lumbar waist when viewed from above.
4. OVERWEIGHT
The ribs are difficult to feel with moderate fat cover. The tailbase* has some thickening with moderate amounts of tissue between the skin and bone. The bony structures can still be felt. The bony prominences are covered by a moderate layer of fat. In animals over six months, there is little or no abdominal tuck or waist when viewed from above. Abdominal fat apron present in cats.
5. OBESE
The ribs are very difficult to feel under a thick fat cover. The tailbase* appears thickened and is difficult to feel under a prominent layer of fat. The bony prominences are covered by a moderate to thick layer of fat. In animals over six months, there is a pendulous ventral bulge and no waist when viewed from the side. The back is markedly broadened when viewed from above. Marked abdominal fat apron present in cats.
*Tailbase evaluation is done only in dogs.

FIGURE 14-3 Body score chart.

It is important to obtain a current and accurate weight for the patient. Clipping the surgical site and placing an intravenous catheter before induction minimizes anesthesia time. Maintaining patient calmness reduces stress and may lower anesthetic induction requirements. Avoid unnecessary handling and noisy personnel or equipment. Provide an environment free of excitement or anxiety. Oxygenation before and during induction may improve PaO_2 in patients with cardiopulmonary compromise, especially during mask or chamber induction.

Preanesthetic checklists should be completed before all procedures to ensure that appropriate items are readily available, important health issues have been addressed, and all involved persons have communicated. This is especially important in high-volume clinics, when several people are involved in patient evaluation and preparation. Anesthetic induction must not be initiated until the checklist is completed (Box 14-4).

> TECHNICIAN NOTE If food is not withheld, pulmonary aspiration leading to pneumonia, permanent disability, or immediate respiratory arrest and death of the patient may occur. Adhere to veterinary instructions.

STEP 3: EQUIPMENT AND SUPPLIES

More anesthetic mishaps are attributed to poor planning and preparation than to improper use of drugs. Correct selection, preparation, and use of anesthetic equipment are essential to patient safety. All equipment should be prepared and checked to be in good working order before administration of anesthetic compounds; the need for intubation and oxygenation may occur unexpectedly. The use of a preanesthetic checklist ensures that all items are completed before induction (Box 14-5).

Supplies for Intravenous Fluid Administration

Placement of an intravenous catheter is essential for patient safety during anesthesia. Intravenous (IV) catheters provide immediate access for intravenous injection and administration of fluids. Catheters should be placed before induction of anesthesia when possible, as most anesthetic agents produce hypotension or vasoconstriction and may complicate catheter placement. Appropriately sized catheters, infusion sets, needles, syringes, and other supplies

TABLE 14-7 Preanesthetic Physical Examination Checklist

SYSTEM	CHECK	NOTE SIGNS
General body condition	Temperature, weight, body score (Figure 14-3), skin turgor, temperament	Obesity, dehydration, cachexia, hypothermia, hyperthermia, pregnancy, any recent changes in weight, aggressiveness
Central nervous systems	Level of consciousness	Bright, alert, responsive (BAR), quiet (QAR), obtunded, depressed, lethargic, stuporous, comatose, seizures, syncope
Cardiovascular	Heart rate and rhythm, arterial blood pressure quality and regularity, concurrent pulse and auscultation, capillary refill time	Cyanosis or icterus, pale mucous membranes, prolonged CRT, heart murmurs, weak or irregular pulse, arrhythmias
Respiratory	Respiratory rate, depth and effort, character, mucous membrane color	Pallor, cyanosis, increased effort or rate, abnormal lung sounds (wheezing, crackles), dyspnea, nasal discharge
Hepatic	Color	Jaundice, failure of blood to clot, coma, seizures
Renal	Volume and discharges	Vomiting, polyuria/polydipsia, oliguria/anuria, hematuria
Gastrointestinal	Abnormalities	Diarrhea, vomiting, distention
Musculoskeletal	Stance, activity	Weakness, abnormal gait, recumbency
Exterior surfaces	Integument, coat condition, lymph nodes, mammary glands, body openings	Wounds, parasites, tumors, lesions, exudates, hair loss, roughness, redness, inflammation, enlarged lymph nodes, discharges, odors, vaginal discharge
EENT	Ears, eyes, nose, and throat	Discharges, inflammation, swelling, abnormal pupil size and response, redness, odor, stridor, dental tartar
Abdominal palpation	Abnormalities	Hardness, pain, distention

TABLE 14-8 Normal Physiologic Values in Dogs, Cats, Horses, and Cattle

	DOGS	CATS	HORSES	CATTLE
Heart rate (HR)	60-160/min	80-200/min	24-50/min	60-120/min
Respiratory rate (RR)	20-40/min	20-40/min	8-20/min	20-40/min
Tidal volume (V_T)	10-20 ml/kg	10-20 ml/kg	10-20 ml/kg	10-20 ml/kg
Body temperature (° F/° C)	100-102.5° F (37.8-39.2° C)	100-102.5° F (37.8-39.2° C)	99-100.5° F (37.2-38° C)	100 -102.5° F (37.8-39.2° C)
Minute volume (resp. rate × tidal vol)	200-800 ml/kg/min	200-800 ml/kg/min	200-800 ml/kg/min	200-800 ml/kg/min
Blood pH	7.35-7.45	7.35-7.45	7.35-7.45	7.35-7.45
PaO_2	80-110 mm Hg	80-110 mm Hg	80-110 mm Hg	80-110 mm Hg
$PaCO_2$	35-45 mm Hg	35-45 mm Hg	35-45 mm Hg	35-45 mm Hg
HCO_3	22-27 mm Hg	22-27 mm Hg	22-27 mm Hg	22-27 mm Hg
Total CO_2	38-54 mm Hg	38-54 mm Hg	54-72 mm Hg	47-72 mm Hg
Base excess	−4 to +14	−4 to +14 (correct if −5 to −10)	−4 to +14	−4 to +14
Central venous pressure (standing awake)	0-4 cm H_2O	0-4 cm H_2O	5-10 cm H_2O	2-4 cm H_2O
Central venous pressure (anesthetized)		2-7 cm H_2O	2-7 cm H_2O	15-25 cm H_2O
Systolic blood pressure		100-160 mm Hg	120-150 mm Hg	100-120 mm Hg
Diastolic blood pressure		80-120 mm Hg	70-130 mm Hg	60-80 mm Hg
Mean blood pressure		90-120 mm Hg	100-150 mm Hg	80-100 mm Hg

necessary for aseptic catheterization should be arranged for easy access. The correct catheter size is one large enough to deliver large volumes of IV fluids (90 ml/kg/hr)—18- to 24-gauge, depending on the size of the dog or cat. For cats, avoid using the cephalic vein if a front declaw is planned and the femoral vein if a rear declaw is planned. Large animals (horses, cattle) should have a 14- to 16-gauge catheter placed in the jugular vein.

Infusion sets are available as vented or nonvented sets. Vented administration sets are required when using nonvented bottles. Nonvented administration sets can be used with plastic fluid bags or vented bottles. Delivery rates of 10 drops/ml, 12 drops/ml, 15 drops/ml, and 60 drops/ml are commonly used in veterinary medicine. Smaller drop sizes improve the accuracy of delivery in smaller patients. Generally, patients weighing less than 10 kg should receive fluids

BOX 14-4 Preanesthesia Checklist

Personnel
1. Select personnel and identify roles.
2. Review procedure.
3. Review emergency procedures.

Patient
1. Identify patient properly.
2. Verify patient was fasted (as appropriate).
3. Weigh patient.
4. Perform special prep (as needed, e.g., bowel prep).
5. Perform preanesthetic examination (signalment, anamnesis).

Drugs
1. Select drugs; confirm they are available.
2. Review routes of drug administration.
3. Check crash cart inventory.

Fluid Administration
1. Select IV fluids; maintain at proper temperature.
2. Confirm sufficient fluids available for adverse events.
3. Gather necessary equipment.
   - IV catheters (18- to 24-gauge 1- to 2-inch)
   - Injection caps
   - Materials for securing IV catheter (tape, adhesive)
   - Saline flush or heparinized saline (2 to 4 IU/ml), in syringe with needle
   - Fluid delivery sets (60 drops/ml for <10 kg, 15 drops/ml for 11 to 40 kg, 10 drops/ml for >40 kg)

Endotracheal Intubation
1. Select and inspect three sizes of endotracheal tube.
2. Gather necessary equipment.
   - Lubricating gel
   - Rolled gauze for securing
   - Laryngoscope and appropriate blades
   - Stylets
   - Lidocaine spray or swab if needed

Equipment
1. Review anesthetic machine checklist (see Box 14-5).
2. Select and inspect monitoring equipment.

Miscellaneous Supplies
- Ophthalmic ointment
- Circulating warm water blanket, table insulation, or heated table
- Face mask

BOX 14-5 Checklist for Daily Inspection of Anesthetic Equipment

- Sufficient oxygen available—check cylinder pressure
- Flow meter bobbin or float moves freely through length of tube
- Unidirectional valves properly functioning
- Vaporizer filled and filler caps tightened
- All gas lines correctly connected
- Sufficient and fresh CO_2 absorbent time available
- Scavenger system properly connected and operational
- Cuff syringe available
- Attach breathing circuit, tubes, and reservoir bag
- Check for leaks:
  1. Close pop-off valve.
  2. Occlude patient end of breathing circuit (where endotracheal tube attaches).
  3. Fill circuit with oxygen to a pressure of 20 cm H_2O.
  4. Turn on oxygen flow to 100 ml/min (0.1 L/min).
  5. If pressure increases, leaks are within acceptable limits.
  6. If pressure drops, increase the flow rate until pressure remains stable.
  7. Leaks exceeding 200 ml/min (0.2 L/min) must be corrected via machine maintenance.
  8. Open the pop-off valve while occluding Y-piece; pressure should drop to 0 cm H_2O.

through a "microdrip" (60 drops/ml) infusion set to increase accuracy of fluid delivery. Patients requiring large fluid volumes (e.g., horses) need 10 drops/ml sets. Routine fluid delivery rates during anesthesia should be 5 to 10 ml/kg/hour for larger animals and 10 to 20 ml/kg/hr for smaller animals.

Endotracheal Tubes

Endotracheal intubation ensures a patent airway, facilitates patient ventilation, and provides easy delivery of volatile anesthetics. Endotracheal tube diameter and length are important. The diameter should be the largest size that will fit into the trachea with ease. If too large, the larynx and trachea may be traumatized. If too small, the patient will have difficulty breathing through the tube. To illustrate this, try breathing through a soda straw for a couple of minutes. Generally the internal diameter (ID) is used. Cats usually require 3 to 4.5 mm, whereas dogs necessitate 6 to 14 mm (Fig. 14-4).

A fairly accurate assessment for the tube size can be based on the weight of the dog, keeping in mind that body condition, confirmation, brachycephalic breeds, obesity, and small size may alter the final size chosen. Use a 9- to 9.5-mm tube for a 40-pound (18.2-kg) dog. As the weight changes by 5 lb (2.3 kg) change the size of the ETT by 0.5 mm. Thus a 50-lb dog (22.7 kg) would require approximately a 10- to 10.5-mm tube of ID. The trachea also can be palpated to feel the approximate size, or an approximation can be made by measuring the nasal septal width with the outer diameter of an endotracheal tube.

Proper length of endotracheal tube is also important. The inserted tip of the tube should not extend beyond (caudal to) the thoracic inlet to prevent bronchial intubation. The adapter end of the tube should not extend more than 1 or 2 inches beyond (rostral to) the mouth to limit mechanical dead space (Fig. 14-5) and prevent the rebreathing of exhaled gas.

Endotracheal tubes should be clean and free of defects or obstructions. If it has an inflatable cuff, it should be checked for leaks. The connector must be securely attached.

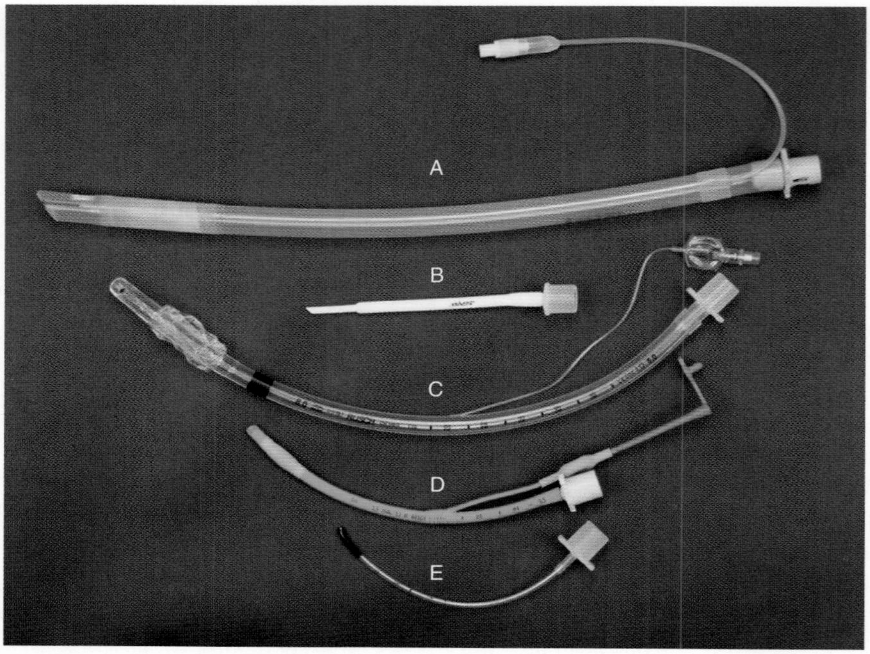

FIGURE 14-4 Endotracheal tube type, material and size comparison. **A,** Cuffed 11-mm silicone rubber tube. **B,** 2.5-mm Cole tube. **C,** Cuffed 8-mm PCV tube. **D,** Cuffed 4-mm red rubber tube. **E,** Uncuffed 2-mm PVC Murphy tube. (From Thomas JA, Lerche P: *Anesthesia and analgesia for veterinary technicians,* ed 4, St Louis, 2011, Mosby.)

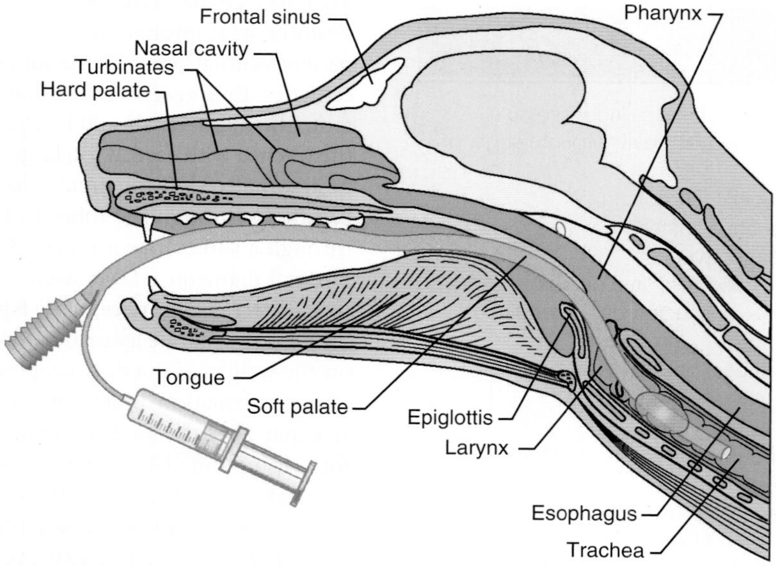

FIGURE 14-5 Correct placement of an endotracheal tube. The connector is located near the incisor teeth, minimizing mechanical dead space. The cuffed end is in the cervical trachea, near the thoracic inlet.

Stylets may be used to facilitate intubation with small-diameter or very flexible tubes. When using a stylet, the tip should not extend beyond (caudal to) the tip of the endotracheal tube; this prevents damage to or penetration of the trachea. The stylet is removed immediately on achieving intubation.

Laryngoscope

The **laryngoscope** facilitates visualization of the glottis as the endotracheal tube passes through into the trachea. Laryngoscopes consist of a handle and detachable blades in a variety of sizes and shapes (Fig. 14-6). The blade is curved to match the curvature of the tongue and allow even pressure along its length.

Medical Gas Supply

Medical gases may be delivered from compressed gas cylinders by central pipeline or direct attachment to the anesthetic machine. Medical-grade oxygen and nitrous oxide are the commonly used gases in veterinary medicine, although the benefits of nitrous oxide in veterinary practice are limited. The nitrous oxide source must be independent of the oxygen

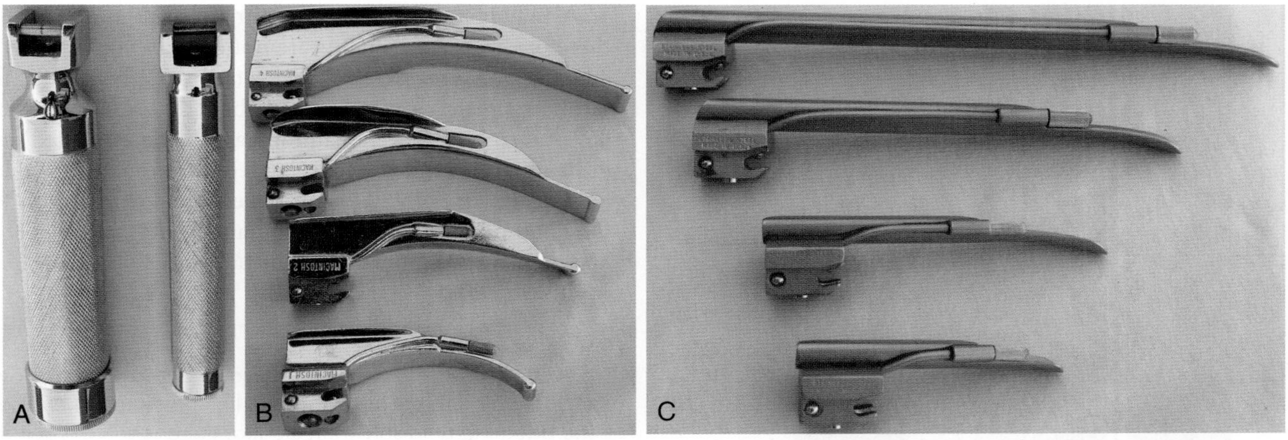

FIGURE 14-6 Laryngoscopes. **A,** Laryngoscope handle. **B,** MacIntosh laryngeal specula. **C,** Miller laryngeal specula. (From Sonsthagen TF: *Veterinary instruments and equipment: a pocket guide,* ed 2, St Louis, 2011, Mosby.)

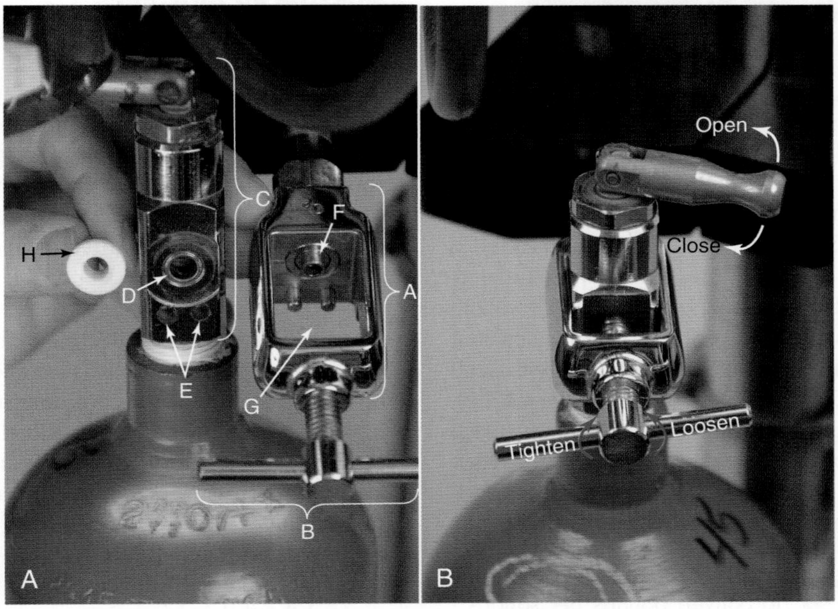

FIGURE 14-7 **A,** Parts of compressed gas cylinder and yoke. *A,* Yoke. *B,* Wing nut. *C,* Outlet valve. *D,* Valve port. *E,* Pin holes. *F,* Nipple of yoke. *G,* Index pins. *H,* Nylon washer. **B,** Opening-closing the outlet valve; loosening-tightening the wing nut. (From Thomas JA, Lerche P: *Anesthesia and analgesia for veterinary technicians,* ed 4, St Louis, 2011, Mosby.)

source; nitrous oxide is mixed with oxygen just before passing through the vaporizer.

The most commonly used sizes of compressed medical gas cylinders are the *E cylinder* (4.25 × 26 in.) and the *H cylinder* (9.25 × 51 in.). All medical gas cylinders are color-coded; oxygen cylinders are green (white in Canada), and nitrous oxide cylinders are blue. E cylinders attached directly to the anesthetic machine for backup should be kept in the *off* position until in use to ensure that they remain full until needed.

Pressure regulators attached to the cylinder valve on H cylinders and near the hanger yokes for E cylinders (Fig. 14-7) passively reduce oxygen pressure to the normal working pressure of the anesthetic machine to 50 pounds per square inch (psi) gauge. If there is a line pressure gauge it should be checked before every procedure to verify correct pressure in the intermediate pressure gas lines (between 40 and 50 psi) (Fig. 14-8). Pressure reduction is necessary to prevent damage to the anesthetic machine and allow a constant rate of oxygen delivery to the flow meter. Cylinder pressure gauges are associated with the pressure regulator and may be used to estimate the relative volume of gas remaining in a cylinder. Oxygen cylinders contain only compressed oxygen vapors, and the pressure is proportional to the content. The pressure in a fully charged oxygen cylinder, regardless of size, is near 2200 psi.

TECHNICIAN NOTE Handle compressed gas cylinders with care. Only turn a tank on when it is attached to a yoke or pressure regulator. Avoid contact with flames, store tanks properly, and make sure the tanks fit properly to the yoke.

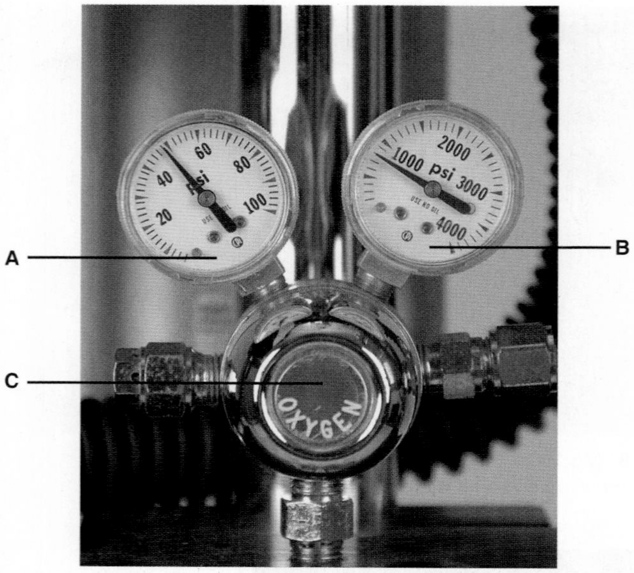

FIGURE 14-8 *A,* Line pressure gauge (registering 48 psi). *B,* Tank pressure gauge (registering 800 psi). *C,* Pressure reducing valve. *(From Thomas JA, Lerche P: Anesthesia and analgesia for veterinary technicians, ed 4, St Louis, 2011, Mosby.)*

To calculate the volume in liters (L) of oxygen in an E-tank, multiply the pressure (in psi) by a factor of 0.3. Thus a full E cylinder of oxygen that contains a pressure of approximately 2200 psi will have about 660 liters of oxygen gas (0.3 × 2200 psi). The volume in liters for the larger H cylinder is calculated by multiplying the pressure (psi) by 3.0. A full tank with 2200 psi contains approximately 6600 liters of oxygen (3 × 2200). One can now calculate the length of time a tank can be used. To do so consider the oxygen flow rate as well. If the oxygen flow rate is 1 L/minute, a full E tank of oxygen containing 660 L of oxygen will last 660 minutes or about 11 hours.

> **TECHNICIAN NOTE** To convert pounds per square inch (psi) to kilopascals (kPa), multiply the PSI value by 6.89. To convert kilopascals to pounds per square inch, multiply the kPa value by 0.145.

Mark tanks as "full," "in use," or "empty" to indicate their status, and be sure that a full backup tank is always kept on the machine as a spare in case the primary tank runs out. Change the tanks at no less than 100 psi of oxygen for an E tank and 680 psi for an H tank.

To determine how long an oxygen tank will last:

1. Calculate the volume in liters (L) of oxygen present in a compressed gas cylinder, keeping in mind that regardless of the size a full tank will contain 2200 psi.
   a. Multiply the pressure (in psi) in an E-tank by a factor of 0.3 or in an H-tank by 3.0. (e.g., if an E-tank is half full it will contain 1100 psi or 330 L of oxygen [0.3 × 1100]).
2. Divide the L of oxygen in the tank by the flow rate (e.g., 2 L/minute flow rate means that you will have 330/2, which is 150 minutes or 2½ hours of oxygen).

A fully charged cylinder of nitrous oxide is 95% liquid; therefore, cylinder contents are not directly proportional to cylinder pressure. Pressure begins to drop only after the liquid is completely vaporized and about 75% of the contents have been used. The remaining gas can be estimated after pressure begins to fall. Fully charged nitrous oxide cylinders have a pressure of 750 psi and need to be changed no less than 500 psi. An H cylinder contains about 16,000 L N_2O, and an E cylinder contains about 1600 L N_2O.

> **TECHNICIAN NOTE** Once the oxygen valve is closed, depress the oxygen flush valve or increase the flow meter to a high rate to remove the line pressure; otherwise, the gauge may falsely indicate that there is still oxygen in the line.

Anesthesia Machines

Several companies manufacture anesthesia machines for small and large animal use. Anesthetic machines deliver a mixture of oxygen and inhalation anesthetic to the **breathing circuit.** The components of an anesthetic machine include the oxygen source, pressure regulator, oxygen pressure valve, flow meter, vaporizer, breathing circuit, reservoir bag, circuit manometer, positive pressure relief valve, carbon dioxide absorbent, and unidirectional dome valves (Fig. 14-9).

Flow Meters

Flow meters receive medical gases from the pressure regulator. Their purpose is to measure and deliver a constant gas flow to the vaporizer, the common gas outlet, and the breathing circuit. The flow meter also further reduces the pressure of the gas in the intermediate-pressure line from about 50 to 15 psi. This pressure is only slightly above atmospheric pressure (about 14.7 psi), making it ideal for the breathing circuit and the patient's lungs

Oxygen enters the flow meter near the bottom and travels upward through a tapered, transparent flow tube. A floating indicator, either a ball or plumb bob, inside the flow tube indicates the amount of gas passing through the control valve. The flow rate is indicated on a scale associated with the flow tube. When the control valve is open, oxygen enters the tube, pushing the floating indicator upward. Where the indicator hovers in equilibrium, the rate of flow is determined by reading the calibrated scale from the center of the ball or the top of the plumb bob (Fig. 14-10).

Flow meters are gas-specific and must not be interchanged; an oxygen flow meter cannot safely be replaced with a nitrous oxide flow meter. Control knobs to regulate flow of medical gases must be distinguishable from each other.

> **TECHNICIAN NOTE** The oxygen control knob must be green, permanently marked with the word or symbol for oxygen, and the valve should be fluted, project beyond other knobs, and be larger in diameter than other knobs.

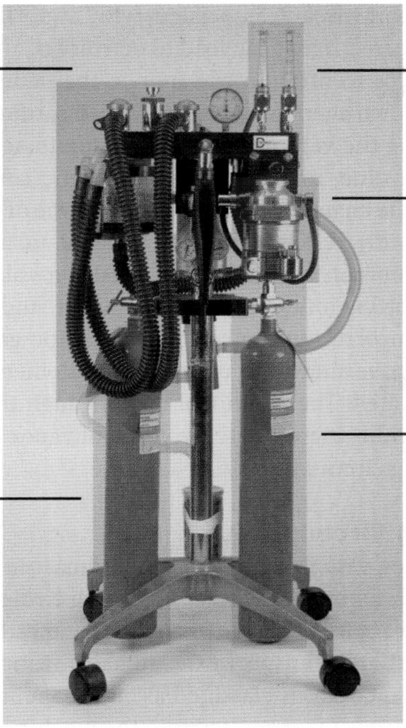

FIGURE 14-9 Small-animal anesthesia machine. Anesthetic machine systems. *A,* Carrier gas supply. Note the two size-E compressed gas oxygen cylinders. *B,* Anesthetic vaporizer. *C,* Breathing circuit. Note that the scavenging system is not visible in this view. (From Thomas JA, Lerche P: *Anesthesia and analgesia for veterinary technicians,* ed 4, St Louis, 2011, Mosby.)

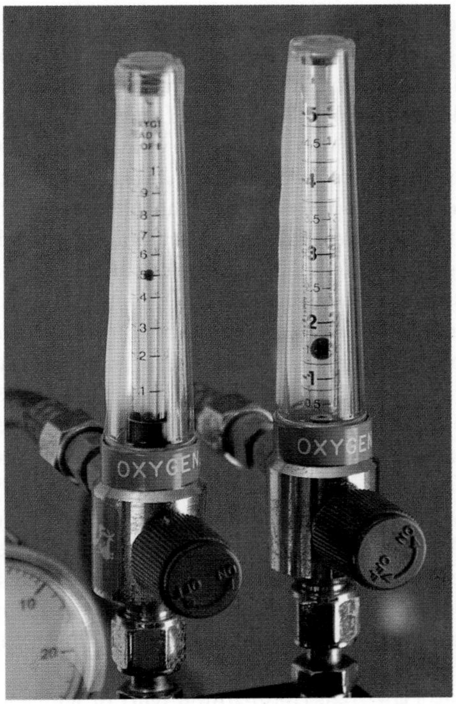

FIGURE 14-10 Oxygen flow meters with ball indicators. The flow meter on the left is adjusted to 0.5 L/min, and the flow meter on the right is adjusted to 1.5 L/min for a total oxygen flow of 2 L/min. (From Thomas JA, Lerche P: *Anesthesia and analgesia for veterinary technicians,* ed 4, St Louis, 2011, Mosby.)

BOX 14-6 Factors Affecting Anesthetic Output of Vaporizers

Nonprecision In-Circle Vaporizers
- Vaporizer setting: Does not equate to a known concentration.
- Fresh gas flow: High flows dilute circuit concentration; low flows increase circuit concentration.
- Patient minute ventilation: Increased ventilation increases vaporizer output.
- Temperature of anesthetic agent: Increased temperature increases vaporizer output.

Precision Out-of-Circle Vaporizers
- Vaporizing setting: Generates a known anesthetic concentration; increased setting increases vaporizer output.
- Fresh gas flow: No effect on vaporizer output.
- Patient minute ventilation: No effect on vaporizer output.
- Temperature of anesthetic agent: No effect on vaporizer output.

Flow meters are common sources of leaks and should be checked at regular intervals for cracks in the flow tube. Dirt or static electricity may cause a float to stick, causing flows to be higher or lower than indicated. Excessive tightening easily damages control knobs, leading to expensive repair. Overtightening may prevent the flow meter from closing completely, causing significant leaking in the off position. Leaking may lead to unexpected shortage of medical gases and exhaustion (saturation) of carbon dioxide absorbent from constant flow of gas through the absorbent.

Vaporizers

Inhalation anesthetic agents are volatile liquids that vaporize at room temperature. The primary function of a **vaporizer** is controlled enhancement of anesthetic vaporization. Vaporizers in common use are of two general types: precision vaporizers (for use with isoflurane, sevoflurane) and nonprecision vaporizers (formerly used for methoxyflurane). Each precision vaporizer is designed to be used with a specific inhalant anesthetic and is color coded—isoflurane is purple, sevoflurane is yellow, halothane is red, and desflurane is blue. Their functional differences apply to the administration of volatile anesthetics (Box 14-6).

Precision vaporizers, designed for a specific anesthetic agent, deliver a constant concentration (%) that is automatically maintained with changing oxygen flow rates and temperature (Fig. 14-11). The percent setting on the control dial approximates delivery to the breathing circuit. Precision vaporizers are designed to function out of the breathing circuit (VOC, vaporizer-out-of-circuit); that is, between the flow meter and the breathing circuit, so that oxygen from the flow meter flows into the vaporizer before entering the breathing circuit. The inherent safety attributed to precision vaporizers is that the anesthetic concentration delivered to the breathing circuit and patient cannot increase above the vaporizer setting. Precision vaporizers

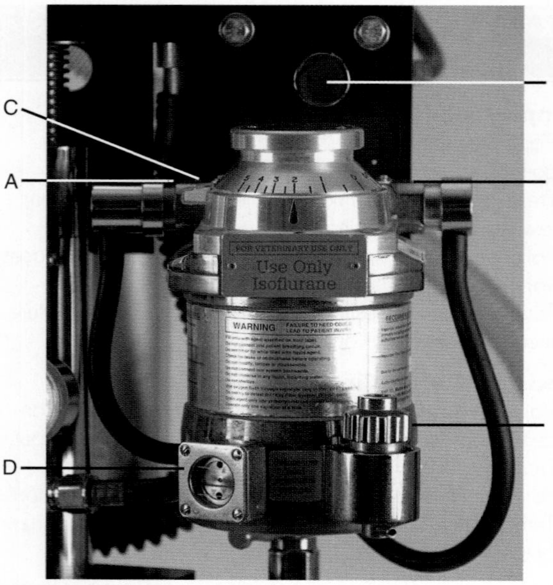

FIGURE 14-11 Precision anesthetic vaporizer for isoflurane set on 2%. *A,* Inlet port with keyed fitting leading from the flow meters. *B,* Outlet port with keyed fitting leading to the fresh gas inlet. *C,* Safety lock. *D,* Indicator window. *E,* Fill port. *F,* Oxygen flush valve (part of the compressed gas supply). (From Thomas JA, Lerche P: *Anesthesia and analgesia for veterinary technicians,* ed 4, St Louis, 2011, Mosby.)

may deliver less than dial settings when flows are very low (250 ml/min or lower) or very high (15 L/min or higher). Sevoflurane requires a precision vaporizer calibrated for this agent. One cannot safely use sevoflurane in a vaporizer calibrated for isoflurane. Precision vaporizers are more expensive than nonprecision vaporizers.

Nonprecision vaporizers are rudimentary, allowing some control of vaporization, but delivering an unknown concentration of the inhalant. The dial scale is not a percent concentration, but rather a relative number based on the agent's vapor pressure and temperature, and the patient's minute **ventilation,** indicating the amount of fresh gas diverted through the chamber. A lever setting of 0 on the Ohio No. 8 vaporizer indicates that no gas flows through the chamber, with no anesthetic delivered to the patient. When the lever is set on 10, all of the circuit gases are diverted through the chamber, increasing the anesthetic concentration delivered to the patient.

Nonprecision vaporizers are designed to function in the breathing circuit (VIC, vaporizer-in-circuit, or "draw over vaporizer"), between the expiratory breathing tube and the expiratory unidirectional valve. Resistance to gas flow is low. Location of the vaporizer in the circle has disadvantages. The anesthetic concentration may increase over time without change in setting because of positive-pressure ventilation, increased minute ventilation, increased room temperature, and/or low fresh gas flow. High fresh gas flow decreases the anesthetic concentration by dilution of anesthetic in the breathing circuit. They were used in the past to deliver low vapor pressure anesthetics such as methoxyflurane, which is no longer available. The Ohio No. 8 or Stephens vaporizer are examples of nonprecision vaporizers.

Several hazards are associated with vaporizers. Filling with the incorrect agent can lead to delivery of an excessively high or low concentration of vapor to the patient. Delivering an unknown agent may present varied cardiovascular effects. Tipping the vaporizer may allow liquid agent to enter the fresh gas line, increasing the anesthetic concentration. Overfilling the chamber decreases the volume of vapor available to mix with fresh gas and may allow liquid anesthetic to reach the common gas outlet line. Leaks are also common at the inlet fitting, outlet fitting, filling port, and drain port. Vaporizers incorrectly located in the common gas outlet can deliver excessive anesthetic concentrations when the oxygen flush is activated. The additional flow through the vaporizer (35 to 75 L/min) increases the volume of vapor delivered to the breathing circuit.

Breathing Circuits

Medical gases pass from the anesthetic machine to the patient through tubing known as a breathing circuit. Breathing circuits deliver "fresh gases" (oxygen and anesthetic vapor) to the patient and transport exhaled gases from the patient. The breathing circuit is classified as either a rebreathing circuit, whereby it is incorporated into the machine and carbon dioxide is eliminated from the circuit by soda lime absorption, or a **non-rebreathing system,** in which the carbon dioxide is eliminated using high gas flow rates and not a carbon dioxide absorber.

Rebreathing Circuits

The term rebreathing means "to breathe again" and refers to exhaled gases (carbon dioxide, oxygen, anesthetic). Rebreathing circuits (circle system) are most commonly used in veterinary practice. The amount of carbon dioxide rebreathed depends on the degree of carbon dioxide absorption and the fresh gas flow rate. The components of the circle system include a reservoir bag, manometer, positive-pressure-relief valve (pop-off valve), carbon dioxide absorbent, unidirectional valves, fresh gas inlet, and a removable set of breathing tubes (Fig. 14-12). Some circuits also have a negative-pressure-relief valve.

Advantages of the rebreathing circuit include conservation of body heat and fluids, reuse of exhaled oxygen and anesthetic gases, and cost-efficient lower flow rates. Disadvantages of the rebreathing circuit include danger of hypercarbia resulting from malfunction of the carbon dioxide absorbent or unidirectional valves, particularly at flow rates low enough to produce a closed system. There exists a potential for the patient to need to work harder because of added resistance from faulty unidirectional valves, carbon dioxide absorbent, or faulty pop-off valves. Additionally, there is a slow change in the inspired anesthetic concentration at lower flows.

The **reservoir bag** (rebreathing bag) provides a gas volume sufficient for the patient to inhale maximally without creating negative pressure in the circuit. It is also used for positive-pressure ventilation or to inflate the lungs when needed. Reservoir bag sizes of 0.5 to 5 L are used for small

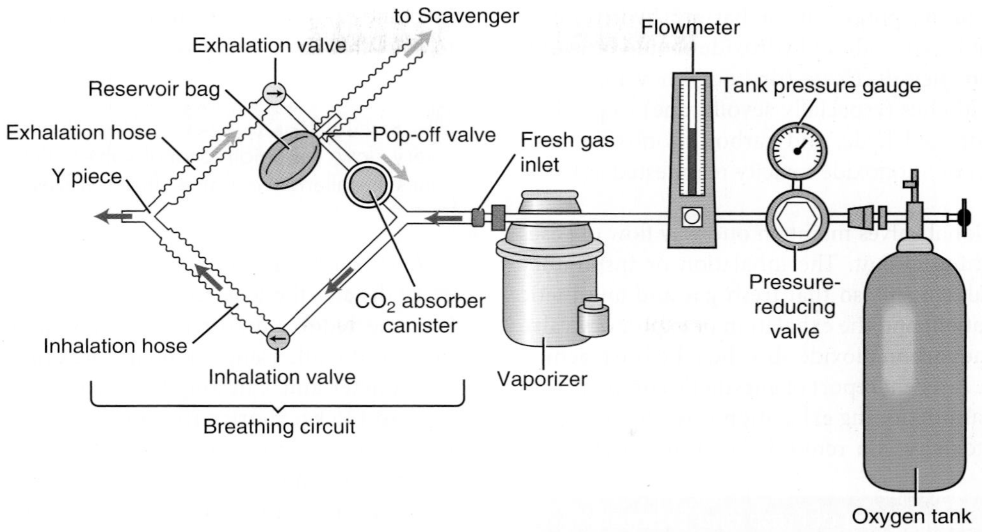

FIGURE 14-12 Diagram of an anesthetic machine with a rebreathing circuit and vaporizer outside of the breathing circuit. (From Bassert JM, McCurnin DM: *McCurnin's clinical textbook for veterinary technicians*, ed 7, St Louis, 2010, Saunders.)

animals and 15 to 30 L for large animals. The ideal reservoir bag is five to six times the patient's normal **tidal volume** of 10 ml/kg.

> *TECHNICIAN NOTE* At peak expiration the reservoir bag should be approximately three fourths full.

The circuit manometer is useful to monitor circuit pressure. Excessive circuit pressure (greater than 4 cm H_2O) may prevent normal respiration and increase intrathoracic pressure, resulting in decreased venous return and a subsequent drop in cardiac output. During positive-pressure ventilation ("bagging"), the manometer allows delivery of the correct circuit pressure. **Barotrauma** (respiratory tract injury from excessive circuit pressure) decreases oxygenation of blood and can rupture lung tissue. Typically, healthy dogs and cats are ventilated to pressures of 15 to 20 cm H_2O to ensure adequate tidal volume. Horses may require positive-pressure ventilation pressures of 30 to 40 cm H_2O to achieve adequate tidal volume. When breathing spontaneously the manometer should not read more than 0 to 2 cm H_2O. It is vital to note that positive pressure ventilation is not the same as normal physiologic inhalation (which is accomplished via negative intrathoracic pressure). The vena cava collapses and venous return stops when intrathoracic pressure exceeds **central venous pressure** (approximately 4 cm H_2O). This, in turn, reduces cardiac output. Ventilation rates should not exceed one third of the heart rate to avoid significant cardiac output decrease.

The positive-pressure-relief (pop-off) valve prevents excessive pressure in the rebreathing circuit and allows removal of excess waste gases. A common cause of anesthetic mishap is leaving the pop-off valve closed after performing positive-pressure ventilation. The pop-off valve is equipped with a scavenger interface, permitting connection to a waste gas removal system to prevent waste gas discharge into the operating room air.

Never allow the reservoir bag to get too empty or too full. If the bag assumes the appearance of an inflated beach ball, it is too full. Pressure in the breathing circuit will exceed safe limits, making it difficult for the patient to exhale, which may lead to ruptured alveoli or pneumothorax. Keep the pop-off valve open unless using a closed system and watch for obstructions in the scavenger system. If the bag is too empty, the animal will have difficulty fully inhaling the anesthetic gases.

> *TECHNICIAN NOTE* Make sure there is adequate fresh gas flow, the bag is the right size, the pop-off valve is not excessively open, and the scavenging system is properly set up.

The carbon dioxide absorbent canister removes carbon dioxide from the exhaled gases before the gases are returned to the patient. The gases are directed to the canister by the expiratory unidirectional valve of the breathing circuit. The canister contains absorbent granules such as calcium hydroxide, which removes CO_2 from the expired air. This causes a chemical reaction with a decrease in pH and by-products that are mainly calcium carbonate ($CaCO_3$), water, and heat. Exhaustion of the granules depends on gas flow rates and patient size. The absorbent should be changed either monthly or after 6 to 8 hours of use, whichever is first. Look for signs if the granules need to be changed earlier (Table 14-9). Precautionary measures to ensure that the absorbent is reasonably fresh include logging of date changed and amount of time used for anesthesia. Inadequate absorbent function may lead to **hypercarbia** (excessive carbon dioxide in the blood), with resultant increased respiratory rate. Initially there may be an increased heart rate followed by cardiovascular depression.

Absorbents containing potassium or barium hydroxide or higher concentrations of sodium hydroxide should be avoided, because when they desiccate (dry out) they may react with volatile anesthetics (especially sevoflurane) to produce excessive heat, formaldehyde, and carbon monoxide sufficient to cause carbon monoxide toxicity manifested as tissue hypoxia.

The unidirectional valves maintain one-way flow of gases within the breathing circuit. The inhalation or inspiratory unidirectional valve opens so that fresh gas and anesthetic can flow to the patient and the exhalation or expiratory valve passes through the carbon dioxide absorbent before reaching the patient again. A recent report of anesthetic complications arising from a malfunctioning exhalation valve and resultant carbon dioxide toxicity is a reminder that any part of the machine can fail unexpectedly. Vigilance and rapid response to complications are always needed.

TABLE 14-9 Comparison of Fresh and Exhausted CO_2 Granules

	FRESH CO_2 GRANULES	EXHAUSTED CO_2 GRANULES
Consistency	$Ca(OH)_2$—chip or crumble with finger pressure	$CaCO_3$—hard and brittle
Color	White	Slightly off-white
pH indicator	Pink or white depending on brand	When ⅓ to ½ of granules change: White (instead of original pink) Violet (instead of original white) Note: May not occur in small patients and returns to original color in a few hours
Capnograph monitor	$[CO_2]$—peak inspiration—near 0 mm Hg	$[CO_2]$—>0 (could also result from other causes, e.g., dysfunctional expiratory unidirectional valve)

TECHNICIAN NOTE When the velocity of the gas is very slow, the unidirectional valves "flutter" in response—thus the alternative name "flutter valves."

Corrugated inspiratory and expiratory breathing tubes carry the anesthetic gases to and from the patient. Each tube is connected to a unidirectional valve at one end, and the Y-piece at the other end. Standard breathing tubes are 22 mm in diameter and 1 m long for small-animal patients weighing 7 to 135 kg. Shorter 15-mm-diameter tubes are preferred for patients weighing less than 7 kg. Large-animal tubes are 500 mm in diameter and 1.7 m long. The classic setup uses separate inhalation and exhalation tubes connected via a Y-piece to the endotracheal tube adapter. The Universal F-circuit was developed to place the inhalation tube inside the exhalation tube. The advantages of this arrangement include warming of inhaled gases by exhaled gases.

The air intake valve admits room air to the circuit in the event that negative pressure (a partial vacuum) is detected in the breathing circuit, a situation indicated by a collapsed reservoir bag. An air intake valve can be present on some machines either separately, or integrated into the inspiratory unidirectional valve or the pop-off valve.

Non-rebreathing Circuits

Non-rebreathing circuits do not have a carbon dioxide absorber. The exhaled gases are immediately vented from the system through another hose and usually into a reservoir bag, where the gases are released into the **scavenging system** through an overflow valve. If properly used, non-rebreathing circuits allow no significant rebreathing of exhaled gases (Fig. 14-13). Because the non-rebreathing system does not resist air, they are recommended for patients less than 7 kg in body weight so that

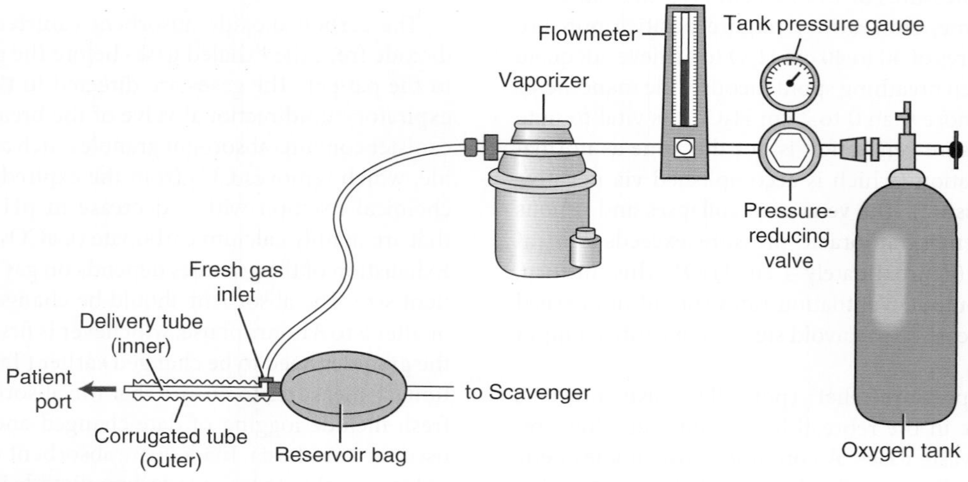

FIGURE 14-13 Diagram of an anesthetic machine with a non-rebreathing system attached to the vaporizer outlet port. (From Bassert JM, McCurnin DM: *McCurnin's clinical textbook for veterinary technicians*, ed 7, St Louis, 2010, Saunders.)

work required to breathe is minimized. As with the rebreathing system, the oxygen or nitrous oxide enters the circuit from the tank, through the flow meter and into the vaporizer, but instead of the fresh gas passing into the circle, as with a rebreathing system, the fresh gas goes directly to the patient. Thus the carbon dioxide absorber canister, pressure manometer, and the unidirectional valves are not present in a non-breathing circuit. The point of entry into the circuit, the flow rate, and the expiratory port location determine the amount of carbon dioxide rebreathed. Ultimately, the composition of the inspired gas mixture depends on the fresh gas flow rate. Flow rates near two to three times the patient's minute ventilation are required to prevent rebreathing. Flow rates below two times minute ventilation allow some rebreathing and warrant monitoring for signs of hypoxemia and hypercarbemia.

Non-rebreathing circuits used in veterinary medicine include the Mapleson A (Magill and Lack circuits), modified Mapleson D (Bain coaxial circuit), Mapleson E (Ayre's T piece and Bain) or Mapleson F circuits (Jackson-Rees' modification of Ayre's T-piece and Norman mask elbow), and the Humphrey ADE, which can switch among Mapleson A, D, and E (Fig. 14-14). Advantages of non-rebreathing circuits include

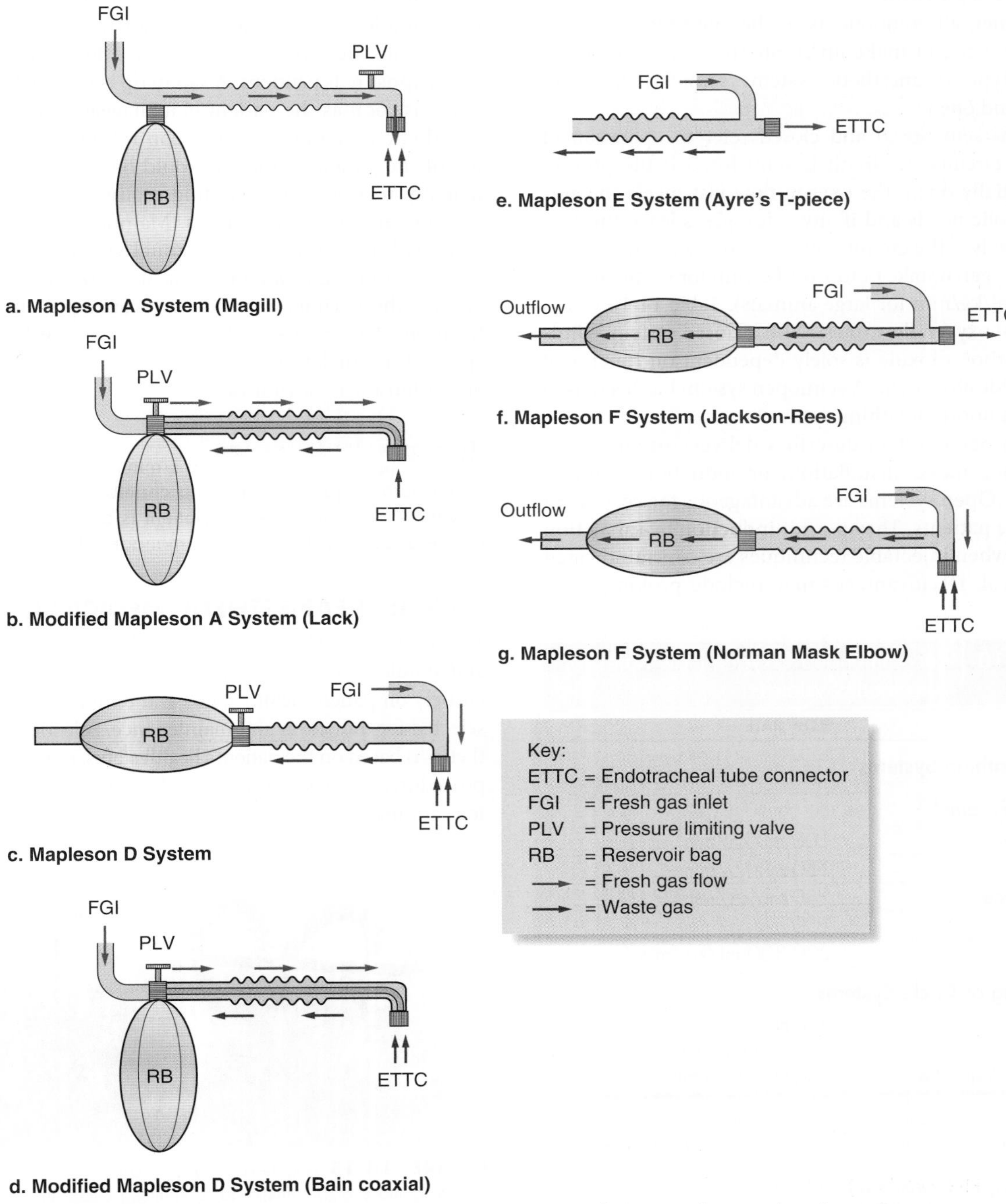

FIGURE 14-14 Non-rebreathing circuits. (From Thomas JA, Lerche P: *Anesthesia and analgesia for veterinary technicians,* ed 4, St Louis, 2011, Mosby.)

decreased resistance to breathing, rapid change of inspired anesthetic concentration, light weight, and ease of cleaning and use. Disadvantages are primarily associated with the required high fresh gas flow rates and include increased use of oxygen and anesthetic, more atmospheric pollution with anesthetic agents, enhanced risk of hypothermia, and dehydration.

> TECHNICIAN NOTE The best way to understand how your anesthetic machine functions is to follow the flow of oxygen right from the source to the patient.

Anesthetic Systems

Taken together, all components of the anesthetic machine and breathing circuit make up an anesthetic system. There are several types of anesthetic systems: semiclosed, closed, semiopen, and open.

The terms semiclosed and closed refer to operation of rebreathing circuits. A circuit is semiclosed if the pop-off valve is partially open, the oxygen flow just meets the animal's metabolic needs and if any waste gases leave through the pop-off valve. The circuit is closed if oxygen flow is equal to patient oxygen uptake (4 to 7 ml/kg/min for small animals and 2 to 3 ml/kg/min for large animals). Table 14-10 shows small-animal oxygen flow rates. With a closed system, elimination of carbon dioxide is solely dependent on functional carbon dioxide absorbent. A semiopen system has been used to describe a non-rebreathing system.

The term open system describes delivery of anesthetic gases via face mask, insufflation, or induction chamber (Fig. 14-15). Open systems are advantageous for very small or aggressive patients. They permit induction by inhalation anesthetics when injectable techniques are contraindicated or impractical. Disadvantages may include prolonged induction time, passage through a stressful excitement phase, inability to monitor the patient, air pollution from waste anesthetics, and increased expense because of high flow. Excitement during inhalation induction by mask or chamber increases the anesthetic risk in compromised patients. If no gases are returned to the patient, the system is also described as open; if some gases return, the system is described as semiopen.

Chambers used for induction should be large enough to permit recumbency without compromising respiration. With mask or chamber induction, patients should breathe oxygen-enriched air for several minutes before induction to optimize alveolar oxygen concentration. Chamber induction allows large amounts of waste anesthetic gases to escape into the surgery area. Serious effort to minimize human exposure is prudent. A safety tip is to switch to the face mask as soon as the patient is manageable. This conserves anesthetic and allows greater control and better monitoring of the patient. Patients should be intubated when sufficiently relaxed, thus avoiding maintenance by mask except in very short procedures. Maintaining anesthesia via face mask does not permit manual ventilation, may allow aspiration of regurgitated stomach contents, permits leaks around the perimeter, which can cause pollution and inhalation of room air, and also increases mechanical dead space. The inhalation agents of choice for open induction are isoflurane or sevoflurane.

TABLE 14-10 Recommended Oxygen Flow Rates for Anesthetic Systems

SYSTEM	FLOW RATE
Non-rebreathing Systems	
*Mapleson Systems**	
Magill system	100 ml/kg/min
Lack system	150 ml/kg/min
Ayre's T piece	150 ml/kg/min
Bain circuit	150 ml/kg/min
Insufflation	200-300 ml/kg/min
Rebreathing or Circle Systems	
Closed	3-5 ml/kg/min†
Semi-closed low flow	5-10 ml/kg/min‡
Semi-closed high flow	20-30 ml/kg/min‡

*Do not use during controlled or assisted ventilation.
†Do not use nitrous oxide in a closed circle unless in-circuit oxygen analyzer is used.
‡If using nitrous oxide, add to the O_2 flow.
From Muir WW et al.: *Handbook of veterinary anesthesia*, ed 4, St Louis, 2007, Mosby.

> TECHNICIAN NOTE To minimize environmental exposure to gases when using chamber induction, switch to the face mask once the patient is down and then intubate as soon as the patient is manageable.

STEP 4: PREANESTHETIC MEDICATION

Preanesthetic medication is usually beneficial to the patient and should be considered for all patients. The need is based entirely on patient health status and temperament and drugs selected for induction and maintenance. Selection of preanesthetics is based on the patient's health status, not on the surgical procedure. Various drugs are used for premedication, including calming agents, analgesics, and anticholinergics.

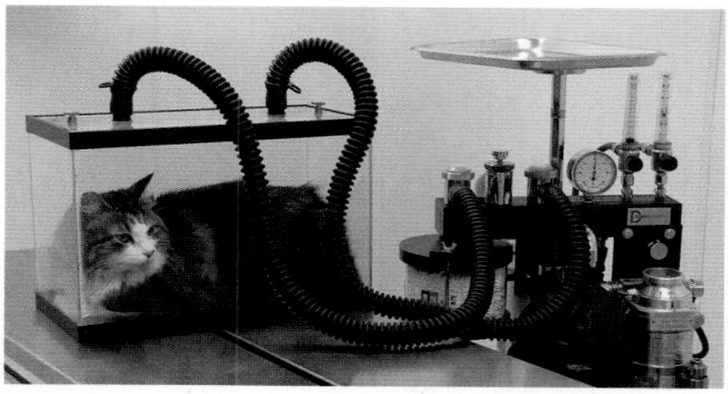

FIGURE 14-15 Anesthetic chamber attached to the corrugated breathing tubes of a semiclosed rebreathing circuit in place of the Y-piece. (From Thomas JA, Lerche P: *Anesthesia and analgesia for veterinary technicians*, ed 4, St Louis, 2011, Mosby.)

Anticholinergics

Anticholinergics (Table 14-11) are sometimes given to decrease excessive salivation. Anticholinergics should be avoided in hypothermic patients because of the increased risk of cardiac arrhythmia.

Calming and Analgesic Agents

Tranquilizers, sedatives, and analgesics (pain relievers) are useful adjuncts to general anesthesia, if given before (preanesthetic), during (maintenance), or after (postanesthetic) anesthesia. Patients that are calm, sedated, and free of pain generally require less anesthetic for induction and maintenance (Box 14-7). Excited patients or those in pain have higher levels of circulating catecholamines, which may increase the likelihood of adverse cardiovascular effects, such as cardiac arrhythmias. Sedation or analgesia may improve recovery from anesthesia. Each of these agents has beneficial as well as adverse effects on physiology.

Drug combinations may have additive, synergistic, complementary, or antagonistic interactions. If the effects are additive or synergistic, less of each drug is needed to produce the desired effect. Complementary effects are useful when a drug lacks a particular effect (e.g., xylazine complements the poor muscle relaxation of ketamine). Drugs commonly used for this purpose fall into several drug categories: phenothiazine derivatives, benzodiazepines, thiazine derivatives, barbiturates, and opioids (Table 14-12).

STEP 5: INDUCTION

A primary goal of proper anesthetic technique is to provide maximum safety for the patient and personnel (Box 14-8). Recognize that induction is short-term general anesthesia and induction agents are frequently used alone to perform short surgical or diagnostic procedures. **Balanced anesthesia** should be used for procedures lasting longer than the duration of the induction agent or performed in patients with

TABLE 14-11 Anticholinergic Agents

TRAIT	DESCRIPTION
Purpose	Block the action of the neurotransmitter acetylcholine at cholinergic receptors in the heart, salivary glands, and smooth muscle fibers throughout the body.
Effects	Effects may include increased heart rate (with concomitant increase in myocardial oxygen demand), decreased salivation and bronchial secretions, mydriasis (dilated pupils), bronchodilation, decreased gastric and intestinal motility, reduced tear formation, and blocking of vagus-mediated reflexes. Central effects (e.g., sedation or excitement) may occur with anticholinergics that cross the blood-brain barrier.
Indications	Anticholinergics are indicated when vagus-mediated reflexes, bradycardia, second-degree AV block, or excessive salivation exist or are anticipated. Because of the expected cardiovascular effects of opioid or alpha-2 agonists (e.g., xylazine) or before reversing the effects of muscle relaxants, an anticholinergic may be indicated. Anticholinergics are used during cardiopulmonary resuscitation (CPR) to alleviate bradyarrhythmias.
Contraindications	They are contraindicated in the presence of tachycardia (>160 beats/min in dogs; >200 beats/min in cats) or ventricular fibrillation. The introduction of isoflurane and sevoflurane has reduced the incidence of bradyarrhythmias and hence the need to routinely premedicate with anticholinergics. Routine preanesthetic use of anticholinergics was common when halothane was the principal inhalation anesthetic, but it is now considered inappropriate by many anesthesiologists.

ANTICHOLINERGIC DRUGS COMMONLY USED	TRADE NAME	COMMENTS
Atropine	Atropine sulfate (dogs, cats, horses, cattle, sheep, swine) Atropine sulfate (human) Also available in tablets and ophthalmic ointment	Concentration: 0.54 mg/ml Dosage: 0.02-0.04 mg/kg IV, IM, or SC Duration of action: 60-90 minutes Anticholinergic; use only when indicated Prevents vagal effects, bradycardia, heart block, excessive salivation Avoid if tachycardia present (dogs, 140/min; cats, 200/min) May increase myocardial oxygen consumption Indications: before use of narcotics and alpha-2 agonists, muscle relaxant reversal, combat bradycardia or bradyarrhythmias
Glycopyrrolate	Robinul-V (dogs, cats) Robinul (human)	Concentration: 0.2 mg/ml Dosage: 0.005-0.01 mg/kg IV, IM, or SC Duration of action: 2-4 hours Anticholinergic; use only when indicated Prevents vagal effects, bradycardia, AV block, excessive salivation Does not cross blood-brain barrier; may be less effective in CPR Longer duration of action and fewer side effects than atropine Indications: before use of narcotics and alpha-2 agonists, muscle relaxant reversal, combat bradycardia or bradyarrhythmia

BOX 14-7 Benefits of Preanesthetic Medication

The benefits of preanesthetic medication include the following:
- Reduces patient stress and minimizes sympathetic effects, which improves handling during preparation for procedures
- Usually decreases the required dose of induction and maintenance agents
- Minimizes adverse or potentially toxic effects of concomitantly administered drugs
- Minimizes sympathetic or parasympathetic autonomic reflex activity
- Facilitates anesthetic induction and maintenance, dampening the sudden changes in anesthetic depth associated with surgical stimulation
- Allows a smoother recovery and reduces pain
- Produces muscle relaxation

organ dysfunction. When gas anesthesia is to be performed, anesthetic induction is the transition from the conscious, preanesthetic state to the level of anesthesia at which the patient may be intubated. The ideal induction agent provides a smooth and calm transition from consciousness to unconsciousness, abolishes oropharyngeal and tracheal reflexes, has a brief duration of effect, produces minimal or no toxicity, and requires minimal metabolism for recovery.

It is important to minimize or avoid personnel exposure to anesthetic waste gases (Box 14-9). Anesthetic techniques have evolved to avoid specific problems previously encountered. Although the consequences of error or mishap in any one step of a procedure may seem negligible, the cumulative effects of marginal technique may produce serious consequences.

Drugs for Anesthetic Induction

Several methods are used for induction before inhalation anesthesia, each having advantages and disadvantages. IV administration of the induction agent is preferred in most

TABLE 14-12 Opiates and Opioids

EXAMPLE	PRODUCT	COMMENTS
Opiates, opioids	General comments	Refers to as opioid agonists, partial agonists, agonist-antagonists, and antagonists Acts by reversible combination with one or more specific receptors in the brain and spinal cord Opioid portion may be reversed, see naloxone (below) Generally sparing to cardiovascular system Depress respiration; assisted ventilation may be necessary May cause excitement and panting Classified according to analgesic activity or addiction potential Repeated or large doses may produce bradycardia Indicated for relief of postoperative pain; more effective if administered before pain develops
Oxymorphone Schedule II—USA	Numorphan (human)	Concentration: 1.5 mg/ml 10 to 15 times more potent than morphine Dosage: 0.05-0.2 mg/kg IV, IM, or SC (3 mg maximum total dose) Reliable pain relief for 2-4 hours Not available in Canada—hydromorphone used in lieu
Hydromorphone Schedule IV—USA Schedule I—Canada	Hymorphan	Pure opioid agonist Similar properties to morphine but fewer side effects—less likely to induce emesis and hypotension Elevated body temperature noted in cats
Butorphanol Schedule IV—USA Schedule I—Canada	Torbugesic, Dolorex (10 mg/ml, horses) Torbutrol inj (0.5 mg/ml) and tablets (dogs)	Agonist—antagonist—causes less pronounced effects than pure agonist Equine product is typically used extralabel for dogs and cats, diluted appropriately for accurate measurement 2-5 times more potent than morphine Dosage: 0.2-0.5 mg/kg IV, IM, or SC Decreases cough reflex (antitussive) Somewhat reliable for pain relief; combine with a sedative for best results Provides 2-4 hours of analgesia
Buprenorphine	ButorPhanol Buprenex (human)	Partial agonist binds to more than one type of receptor 3-5 times more potent than morphine Dosage: 0.005-0.01 mg/kg IV or IM Somewhat reliable for relief of pain Provides 4-12 hours of analgesia May cause excitement; combine with a sedative for best results

TABLE 14-12 Opiates and Opioids—cont'd

EXAMPLE	PRODUCT	COMMENTS
Morphine Schedule II—USA Schedule I—Canada	Infumorph, Astramorph (human)	Pure agonist Dosage: dogs 0.1-0.2 mg/kg IV, IM, or SC; cats 0.05-0.1 mg/kg IV, IM, or SC though higher uses may be used Duration of action: reliable pain relief for up to 4 hours May cause histamine release or panting; combine with a sedative for best results Epidural administration: 0.1 mg/kg; onset of action within 30 minutes; duration 10-24 hours
Naloxone Schedule II—USA Schedule I—Canada	P/M Naloxone HCl inj (dogs) Narcan (human)	Pure narcotic antagonist Dosage: 0.002-0.02 mg/kg IM or slowly IV to effect Concentration of 0.4 mg/ml, dilute to 4 μg/ml if needed with sterile distilled water Observe for return of narcotic effects; redose as needed
Fentanyl Schedule II—USA Schedule I—Canada	Fentanyl	Pure opioid agonist Rapid onset with short duration of action if given IM or IV, can be given as CRI Best used as a transdermal patch for long term analgesia—3 days Onset of action from 12-24 hours, but is continuous if skin shaved and cleaned
Synthetic opioid	Tramadol	Synthetic drug with opioid-like analgesia affect with fewer side effects Most effective with NSAID to control moderate pain Unscheduled Available as oral form and useful for long-term, at-home management

cases. Anesthetic induction may proceed after a vein is catheterized, the equipment is readied, and the surgeon is available. Administration of the induction or maintenance agent should provide a smooth and safe transition to unconsciousness (Box 14-10). When jaw muscle tone and orolaryngeal reflexes are lost, intubate the patient.

Endotracheal Intubation in Dogs and Cats

Dogs and cats are placed in sternal position, with the head and neck extended in a straight line to aid visualization of the larynx. If an assistant is available, have him or her position the head by grasping the maxilla behind the canine teeth while the anesthetist places the endotracheal tube. Lubrication of the cuff with sterile water-soluble lubricant facilitates intubation and protects the tracheal mucosa from drying where the inflated cuff contacts the mucosa. If the mouth is opened fully, the tongue is firmly pulled forward, and a good light source from the laryngoscope is used, the epiglottis can be gently displaced ventrally—either by the tube itself or by the laryngoscope—to visualize the glottis and vocal folds. Avoid the tendency of using only the tip of the laryngoscope blade to depress the tongue, as this puts too much pressure in one place and may cause bruising. Also, the blade should not be used to press down on the epiglottis, as this may damage it and the glottis. If the epiglottis is flipped upward or is trapped behind the soft palate, simply lift the soft palate and gently push the epiglottis down with the tip of the endotracheal tube. Pulling the tongue forward also helps to improve visualization of the glottis.

Using a gently rotating motion, insert the tube past the vocal folds. Place the largest tube that will enter the airway without causing trauma or undue stimulation of vagal reflexes, otherwise cardiac arrhythmias may be induced. Applying lidocaine to the larynx by spray or with a cotton-tipped swab, especially in cats and swine, facilitates intubation. Cetacaine (benzocaine) spray should not be used because it can cause methemoglobinemia. Proper positioning of the endotracheal tube may be confirmed by condensation of respiratory gases on the inside of the tube with expiration, ability to palpate only one tubular structure in the neck (trachea), auscultation of lung sounds when bagging the patient, or the carbon dioxide reading on the capnometer. Secure the endotracheal tube to the maxilla, mandible, or head with gauze or tape to prevent dislodgement or excessive movement during the procedure.

Attach the breathing circuit to the endotracheal tube adapter before inflating the cuff (Box 14-11). The endotracheal tube cuff is inflated to allow positive-pressure ventilation and prevent aspiration in the event of regurgitation. A pressure of 20 to 25 cm H_2O is sufficient for both purposes.

Open the oxygen flow meter to deliver 1 to 3 L/min, and set the vaporizer to the appropriate delivery concentration (1% to 3%). Secure the tube with gauze or tape to the mandible or maxilla, place the animal in lateral recumbency, and begin cardiopulmonary observations. Once the tube is in place and secured and the system is free of leaks, apply ophthalmic ointment to protect the cornea (if not previously done) and proceed with preparation for the procedure. When moving the patient is required, it is prudent to disconnect the breathing circuit from the endotracheal tube to avoid trauma or dislodgement.

TECHNICIAN NOTE Do not inflate the cuff until the need has been determined.

BOX 14-8 Patient Positioning, Comfort, and Safety

Keep the following in mind throughout both the anesthetic induction and maintenance:

- Support patient's body as it is losing consciousness.
- If using an IV agent for induction and if not using an indwelling catheter, remove the needle and syringe once the animal is induced.
- Lay the animal in lateral recumbency after intubation.
- Secure the endotracheal tube before inflating the cuff.
- Constantly check for endotracheal tube patency.
- When turning the patient, temporarily disconnect the endotracheal tube to prevent trauma to the trachea.
- Ensure the anesthetic tubing does not apply force on the endotracheal tube.
- Minimize hyperflexion and hyperextension of the neck or limbs during the procedure.
- Keep the patient warm by placing on a heat-retaining surface.
- Do not apply pressure to the chest with either instruments or restraint devices.
- Ensure that the leg restraint devices are not overly tightened.
- Put sterile lubricant in the eye initially and every 90 minutes.
- To prevent pressure on the diaphragm, do not elevate the caudal aspect of the body more than 15 degrees.
- Record vital signs every 5 minutes throughout the anesthetic as well as postoperatively.
- Constantly note reflexes and other indicators of anesthetic depth.
- Periodically, manually ventilate the lungs to help expand collapsed alveoli, keeping the reading on the pressure manometer reading below 20 cm H_2O.
- Know normal values and when to inform the veterinarian.
- If properly monitoring, you are noting circulation, oxygenation, and ventilation.
- Keep administering O_2 for 5 minutes after anesthetic is turned off—use mask if too light.
- Postoperatively keep the patient warm and turn every 10 to 15 minutes.

BOX 14-9 Techniques for Minimizing Exposure to Waste Anesthetic Gases

1. Check for and correct leaks in anesthesia machine and breathing circuit.
2. Use a cuffed endotracheal tube of the proper size; inflate the cuff if needed.
3. Do not disconnect the patient from the breathing circuit immediately after anesthesia; if possible, wait several minutes for gases to dissipate.
4. Connect pop-off valve to a scavenger system, preferably one that discharges outdoors.
5. Connect non-rebreathing systems to a scavenger system.
6. Avoid use of chamber or mask-induction techniques.
7. Avoid spilling liquid anesthetic while filling the vaporizer; recap bottle and vaporizer immediately.
8. Maintain adequate ventilation of the area.

BOX 14-10 Progression of Anesthetic Depth

1. Analgesia and amnesia
2. Loss of consciousness and motor coordination
3. Reduced protective reflexes
4. Blockade of afferent stimuli
5. Muscle relaxation
6. Respiratory and cardiovascular depression
7. Depression of cardiovascular and respiratory reflexes
8. Apnea
9. Cardiac arrest

BOX 14-11 Endotracheal Cuff Inflation

To determine the need for cuff inflation, perform the following steps:

1. Close the pressure-relief valve and squeeze the reservoir bag while observing the manometer and listening for leakage of gas around the endotracheal tube. Signs of leakage include: a hissing sound as gas escapes around the cuff, inability to hold the pressure at 20 to 25 cm H_2O, the smell of anesthetic agent emanating from the mouth, and/or stertorous breathing from the tube pushing on the side of the larynx.
2. If circuit pressure reaches 25 cm H_2O without leaking around the tube, do not inflate the cuff.
3. If leakage occurs below 25 cm H_2O, inflate the cuff just enough to prevent the leakage. Should the cuff be inflated beyond 25 cm H_2O, the excessive pressure may damage the tracheal mucosa.
4. Changes in the patient's position or a slow leak in the cuff may result in leakage occurring later in the procedure. It is prudent to observe for signs of leakage during routine manual ventilation (bagging).
5. Tissue damage from traumatic intubation or an overinflated cuff is often manifested as coughing a few days after anesthesia.

STEP 6: MAINTENANCE OF ANESTHESIA

Generally, the anesthetic effects of an ultrashort-acting induction agent will dissipate within a few minutes. Once the patient is fully anesthetized by the inhalation anesthetic, the induction period is over and the stage of maintenance anesthesia begins. Surgical or diagnostic procedures that exceed the duration of the induction agent are best maintained with inhalation anesthesia (Box 14-12). Injectable anesthetics are not recommended for long-term maintenance of anesthesia. Repeated injections of the induction agent to maintain anesthesia cause tissue accumulation, with increased risk of adverse events and greater dependence on metabolism for recovery. Steady states of anesthesia and a consistent depth of anesthesia are easier to maintain with inhalants. Once an injection is given it cannot be recovered, while inhalation agents are easily "blown off" via ventilation.

BOX 14-12 Characteristics of Inhalation General Anesthetics

General Induction With Inhalants—Halogenated Hydrocarbon Anesthetic Agents

- Advantages of inhalation induction include avoidance of multiple drugs in the blood and tissues (important for some research protocols), rapid recovery, and ease of induction of very small animals that are difficult to handle (e.g., rats, mice, cats)
- Disadvantages include slower induction with passage through an excitement phase that may be quite stressful to the patient (and the anesthetist), difficulty restraining and monitoring the patient, high potential for pollution of room air with inhalation anesthetics, and the expense of the high flow rates and anesthetic levels needed
- The excitement of inhalation induction increases the risk of anesthetic complications in compromised patients predisposed to cardiac or respiratory insufficiency
- In healthy patients, stress-induced catecholamine release may produce cardiopulmonary compromise
- Mask or chamber induction requires several minutes of preoxygenation to increase the margin of safety
- With chamber induction, large amounts of anesthetic vapor escape into the room air when the chamber is opened, so the procedure should ideally be performed under a hood that removes effluent gases
- The tank size should be just large enough to accommodate the animal comfortably
- Once anesthesia is induced, the patient should be masked or intubated and maintained on the inhalant anesthetic
- When direct inhalant induction is indicated, the agents of choice are isoflurane or sevoflurane. Sevoflurane will induce anesthesia approximately twice as fast as isoflurane
- The high 30% vapor pressure of isoflurane, and sevoflurane concentrations may rise to lethal levels if the amount of vapor being delivered to the breathing circuit is not controlled via a precision vaporizer out of the breathing circuit (VOC)

Isoflurane (Veterinary Products: Aerrane, IsoVet, IsoFlo; Human Products: Isoflurane Forane)

- MAC: dog, 1.3%; cat, 1.63%; horse, 1.31%
- Blood-gas partition coefficient: 1.46
- Elimination: 0.17% by liver metabolism
- Induction is 3 to 5 minutes and recovery is less than 5 minutes
- Currently most popular in small-animal practice
- Provides greatest margin of safety of all currently used gas anesthetics
- Excellent anesthetic for high-risk patients
- Indications: liver disease, renal failure, trauma, arrhythmias, cesarean section, old animals, obese animals, hypersensitivity to other anesthetics
- Stable in contact with soda lime

Sevoflurane (Veterinary Products: SevoFlo, Sevorane, Ultane)

- MAC: dog, 2.34%; cat, 2.58%; horse, 2.34%
- Blood-gas partition coefficient: 0.68
- Elimination: 3% by liver metabolism
- Introduced into veterinary market in 1999
- Induction is 1½ to 3 minutes and recovery within 2½ to 3 minutes
- Induction up to 8%
- Still very expensive compared with isoflurane
- Requires a precision vaporizer calibrated for this agent
- Induction and recovery more rapid than isoflurane because of lower blood solubility
- Cardiovascular effects similar to isoflurane, with less myocardial sensitization to catecholamines
- Marked respiratory depression occurs—more than with halothane
- Potential for production of nephrotoxic olefin because of degradation by desiccated CO_2 absorbents

Desflurane (Veterinary Product: Suprane)

- MAC: averages 7.2%, less potent than other halogenated agents
- Low blood gas partition coefficient of 0.42 for rapid induction and recovery—twice as fast as isoflurane
- Effects similar to isoflurane as structure is identical but fluorine is substituted for chlorine
- Good muscle relaxant and analgesia
- Vaporizer must be electrically heated
- Pungent odor so masking difficult—induce at 10% to 15% concentration
- Anesthetic maintenance 6% to 9%

Nitrous Oxide

- Nitrous oxide is occasionally used in veterinary anesthesia as an adjunct to other agents
- Its very low blood solubility allows very rapid uptake, distribution, and elimination
- Cannot be used alone because of very high MAC (255 in cat)
- Speeds uptake of the anesthetic gas (a second gas) into the blood, decreasing the time required for induction by inhalant anesthetics called the *second gas effect*
- Nitrous oxide is not potent enough to produce general anesthesia alone
- Used to improve analgesia
- Use with caution as it can diffuse into gas-filled body spaces, causing them to expand
- Must use a minimum of 30% O_2 to prevent hypoxia
- Must monitor ratio of N_2O to O_2 constantly with a maximum of 70% N_2O
- Concentrations are usually N_2O:O_2 = 1:1 or 2:1
- Contraindicated in patients with pneumothorax or a diaphragmatic hernia with bowel in the thorax
- Diffusion hypoxia may occur during recovery
- Rapid movement of nitrous oxide from the blood to alveoli may cause hypoxia by displacing oxygen or diluting alveolar carbon dioxide, which may decrease respiratory stimulation and ventilation
- Adequate ventilation should be maintained and a high flow rate of 100% oxygen used for the first 5 to 10 minutes of recovery after nitrous oxide use

> **TECHNICIAN NOTE** All volatile (inhalation) anesthetics decrease cardiac output, and some decrease peripheral vascular resistance in a dose-related fashion. This results in decreased blood pressure.

The amount of anesthetic needed to maintain an appropriate level of anesthesia is not a constant. Anesthetic depth is a product of the amount of drug reaching the brain, degree of painful stimulus applied, and the patient health status (Table 14-13). In a typical abdominal surgical procedure, minimal anesthesia is needed during the surgical preparation, moderate anesthesia during the skin incision, maximal anesthesia during the intraabdominal phase, and moderate anesthesia during skin suturing. Hypothermia and hypotension reduce anesthetic requirements. If anesthetic administration is not reduced in the presence of hypothermia or hypotension, patients may become too deeply anesthetized, with further compromise of tissue perfusion.

Inhalant Anesthetics

Among the inhalant anesthetics commonly used in veterinary medicine are isoflurane and sevoflurane. Desflurane is relatively new in the veterinary field. Nitrous oxide is rarely used, and halothane and methoxyflurane are no longer available in North America. When mixed with oxygen and inhaled by the patient, the gases diffuse rapidly into the bloodstream and are then distributed to all body tissues. As the concentration of drug in the brain rises, the CNS becomes progressively depressed. With the loss of consciousness and response to painful stimuli, the patient enters the plane of surgical anesthesia. Further rise of anesthetic concentrations in the brain continues to depress the CNS until vital functions cease and death ensues. The degree of anesthetic depth required by a patient during a particular procedure and the amount of inhalation anesthetic required to achieve and maintain that depth are unpredictable and variable.

TABLE 14-13 Signs of Anesthetic Depth

	ANESTHETIC DEPTH		
	LIGHT	SURGICAL	DEEP
Spontaneous movement	Possible	None	None
Reflex movement	Possible	None	None
Anesthetic concentration	1 MAC	1.1-1.5 MAC	1.5-2 MAC
Jaw muscle tone	Tense	Moderate	Relaxed
Palpebral reflex	Present	None or slight	None
Nystagmus	Present	Absent	Absent
Globe position	Central	Ventromedial	Central
Corneal reflex	Present	Present	Absent
Corneal moisture	Moist	Moist	Dry
Pupil size	Partially constricted	Moderate	Dilated
Pupillary light response	Present	Gradually non-responsive	Poor to absent
Nystagmus	Present	Absent	Absent
Palpebral reflex	Present	Sluggish to absent	Absent
Response to painful stimuli	Present	Absent to mild—increased HR, BP, or RR	Absent
Respiration (RR) and depth	Increased	Shallow, decreased RR	Depressed
Heart rate (HR)	Increased	Mildly decreased	Depressed
Blood pressure (BP)	Normal	Mildly decreased	Depressed

Advantages of using inhalant agents include the ease and speed of controlling anesthetic depth, good muscle relaxation, and rapid recovery with minimal dependence on metabolism of the agent, and delivery of high levels of oxygen with the agent through an endotracheal tube. Placement of an endotracheal tube provides a patent airway and the ability to support ventilation as needed.

Disadvantages of inhalant agents include the relatively expensive equipment and the knowledge and skill required for their use. Also, halothane sensitizes the myocardium to epinephrine-induced arrhythmias and produces liver damage in some patients. Isoflurane and sevoflurane are the least toxic of the inhalant agents, partially because of their small degree of biotransformation in the body.

A drug's potency is a measure of how much of the drug is needed to produce a standard effect, as compared with similar agents. For inhalant agents, potency is determined largely by the lipid solubility of the agent and is reflected by the minimum alveolar concentration (MAC). The MAC is defined as the lowest alveolar concentration of anesthetic required to prevent gross, purposeful movement in response to a painful stimulus. The MAC varies with species and individuals. The higher the MAC is, the less potent the agent is. Ironically, the inhalants with the most rapid induction time (lowest blood-gas solubility) are also the least potent (highest MAC).

Ideally, the transition from anesthesia by the induction agent to the inhalation agent will be smooth and uneventful. It must be recognized that the uptake of inhalation anesthetics is dependent on adequate ventilation. If the patient is hypoventilating when first placed on the gas machine, inadequate anesthetic will be taken up to maintain anesthesia once the induction agent dissipates.

Once anesthesia with the inhalant agent is accomplished, the vaporizer setting and oxygen flow should be reduced to maintenance levels. The anesthetist's attention now focuses on monitoring and support of vital organ function. Connect all monitoring instruments and begin recording all pertinent information on the patient's anesthetic record. Monitoring should be continuous, and data should be recorded every 5 to 10 minutes or when significant changes occur.

The oxygen flow rate used for maintenance depends on the type of breathing circuit used. Non-rebreathing circuits require high flows throughout maintenance, whereas rebreathing circuits may use reduced flows for semiclosed or closed operation.

Flow Rates for Non-rebreathing Systems

Flow rates for non-rebreathing systems must remain high because this is the means by which exhaled CO_2 is flushed away from the patient. Depending on the system used, flow rates of 100 to 300 ml/kg/min or two to three times the minute ventilation are recommended. Ideally, $ETCO_2$ (end tidal carbon dioxide) should be monitored with a capnometer to ensure adequate removal of CO_2 flow rates for rebreathing systems.

Closed Systems. Maintenance flow rate for a rebreathing circuit operated as a closed system, is equal to the patient's calculated oxygen consumption rate [10 × (kg × 0.75)/kg]. At 4 kg, this will be a total flow of 28 ml/min (7 ml/kg/min), whereas at 38 kg it will be 153 ml/min (4 ml/kg/min). The larger the animal is, the lower its per-kilogram oxygen requirement is. Oxygen consumption is also affected by body temperature and anesthesia. The advantages of closed-system operation include minimal pollution, economy, and minimal loss of moisture and heat. Disadvantages include slow changes in anesthetic concentration, increased use of the CO_2 absorber, necessity to monitor the system volume closely, inability to use N_2O, dilution resulting from patient nitrogen output, and necessity of high flow rates during induction.

Semiclosed Systems. Maintenance flow rate for a rebreathing circuit operated as a semiclosed system exceeds oxygen requirements. These have traditionally been called low flow (up to 22 ml/kg/min) and high flow (up to 44 ml/kg/min) rates. Depending on the size of the animal, low flow is up to 3 to 5 times oxygen needs and high flow is up to 6 to 10 times oxygen needs.

The standard practice of using 1 L/min for the maintenance flow rate exceeds the high flow range (22 to 44 ml/kg/min) for animals less than 23 kg and is in the high flow range for animals 23 to 45 kg. Therefore, 1 L/min is excessively expensive financially and physically for the majority of patients less than 45 kg.

The advantages of maintenance flow rates greater than oxygen needs include less oxygen dilution resulting from patient nitrogen output, less worry about meeting oxygen needs, less dependence on CO_2 absorber, ability to use N_2O safely, and faster changes in anesthetic concentration. Disadvantages include greater loss of heat and moisture and greater expense.

It should be recognized that lower flow rates increase the time it takes to change the anesthetic concentration of the breathing circuit. Any time rapid changes must be made in anesthetic concentration (such as the patient awakening during surgery); a very high flow rate (3 to 4 L/min) must be used in conjunction with an increased vaporizer setting.

> **TECHNICIAN NOTE** The vaporizer setting controls where anesthetic concentration in the circuit is going, and the oxygen flow rate controls how fast it will get there.

One must also remember that the larger the circuit volume, the more time it takes to alter the anesthetic concentration in the circuit. The use of an excessively large reservoir bag adds unnecessary volume to the circuit that slows changes in anesthetic concentration.

Adjust the vaporizer to provide the desired depth. The correct setting provides just enough anesthetic depth to perform the procedure. Excessive concentrations should be avoided. Begin administration of intravenous fluids as soon as possible (10 to 20 ml/kg/hour).

Throughout maintenance, the patient should be ventilated twice per minute or as needed to maintain a $PaCO_2$ of 40 to 45 mm Hg. This is accomplished by closing the pop-off valve and squeezing the reservoir bag to inflate the lungs to a pressure of 15 to 20 cm H_2O. This artificial "breath" should mimic a normal breath in terms of inspiratory time. (Do not hold pressure; just inflate and release.)

Anesthetic Delivery, Uptake, Distribution, and Elimination

The relationship between the vaporizer setting and the time required to achieve effective brain levels of anesthetic is fundamental to inhalation anesthesia. Anesthetic delivery, uptake, and distribution are the processes by which the anesthetic reaches its intended site of action, the brain.

The process of getting anesthetic to the pulmonary alveoli is known as anesthetic delivery. Anesthetic uptake is the movement of anesthetic molecules from the pulmonary alveoli into the bloodstream. It is analogous to the absorption phase of injectable agents. Anesthetic distribution is the movement of anesthetic molecules throughout the body via the bloodstream and diffusion into the tissues. Movement of gas molecules from the blood into the tissues is also called tissue uptake. Gas molecules must pass sequentially through these phases to reach the brain and produce anesthesia. If any one phase is altered, the chain of events leading to anesthesia is altered.

Anesthetic delivery to the alveoli is determined by the inspired concentration and alveolar minute ventilation. Increased anesthetic concentration in the breathing circuit increases the inspired concentration. The primary means of accomplishing this is by increasing the vaporizer setting. Anesthetic uptake (removal of anesthetic from the alveoli by the blood) is determined by solubility of the agent in blood, cardiac output, and the difference between alveolar and venous partial pressure of anesthetic. Uptake by the blood continually removes anesthetic from the alveoli. The more soluble the agent is in blood, the greater this effect is and the longer it takes to produce anesthesia. This is why less soluble agents like isoflurane and sevoflurane induce anesthesia rapidly.

Vessel-rich tissues include the brain, heart, liver, kidney, lungs, and gastrointestinal tract. These organs make up less than 10% of the body weight but receive 75% of cardiac output. Because of this large volume of blood flow, anesthetic is rapidly distributed to these vessel-rich tissues. Muscle makes up about 50% of body mass and receives nearly 20%

of cardiac output. This large tissue group is significant in that, during induction, most of the anesthetic delivered to muscle is removed from the blood. Fat makes up nearly 20% of total body mass but only receives about 4% of cardiac output. Although anesthetics are highly lipid soluble, low blood flow to this group limits anesthetic uptake, with little effect on induction rate. However, fat continually takes up anesthetic over time, and this must be released upon recovery. Prolonged procedures allow fat to accumulate enough anesthetic to significantly delay recovery. Vessel-poor tissues, such as fascia and ligaments, make up 20% of body mass and receive approximately 1% of the cardiac output. This tissue group has an insignificant effect on anesthetic induction or recovery despite the fact that it is significant in proportion.

In summary, anesthesia does not occur until the brain concentration of anesthetic is sufficient to induce loss of consciousness. The more soluble the anesthetic in the blood is, the slower the induction time is. Increasing the inspired anesthetic concentration and patient minute ventilation shortens the induction time.

Anesthetic elimination is the reverse of uptake and distribution, wherein anesthetic molecules move from the tissues into the blood, and then into the pulmonary alveoli to be exhaled.

The speed of uptake and elimination is important in inhalation anesthesia, because this determines how rapidly one may alter anesthetic depth. Major factors that determine the speed of uptake are the inhaled concentration of anesthetic, minute ventilation, alveolar diffusion area, the agent's solubility coefficient and molecular weight, pulmonary blood flow, and the anesthetic partial pressure gradient between alveolar gas and plasma.

> **TECHNICIAN NOTE** Special precautions are needed when using nitrous oxide to avoid diffusion hypoxia. Administer O_2 5 minutes after terminating N_2O and never use more than 70% N_2O. Avoid use during low-flow or closed-system anesthesia. Watch diffusion into closed air cavities.

Following induction, the patient must be maintained in the anesthetized state until the procedure is completed. A common misconception is that maintenance involves only keeping the patient from moving during the procedure, regardless of the patient's needs. Maintenance is the management period of the anesthetic procedure. Monitoring and support of organ function are essential during anesthetic maintenance. An anesthetic record provides important documentation of your vigilance, and it notes adverse trends and important events occurring in the perioperative period (Fig. 14-16). A well-organized anesthetic record serves as legal documentation of anesthetic events, drug dosages used, and patient values during anesthesia, and it guides the actions of the anesthetist by tracking trends in cardiopulmonary function.

> **TECHNICIAN NOTE** To decrease inhalant anesthetic concentrations:
> - Turn up O_2 flow rate or activate O_2 valve
> - Turn vaporizer down or off
>
> To increase inhalant anesthetic concentrations:
> - Turn up O_2 flow
> - Turn up vaporizer
> - Do not activate O_2 flush valve

ANESTHETIC MONITORING

Comprehensive monitoring of the anesthetized patient involves observing anesthetic equipment and evaluating the central nervous system, pulmonary function, and cardiovascular function. Early detection of equipment failure and/or depression of vital organ function allows execution of corrective measures, which are more effective than treating complications (Box 14-13). Corrective actions to maintain or restore tissue perfusion are determined by integrating information from all body systems. Monitoring anesthesia covers a wide range of parameters and situations. It is important to "expect the unexpected."

> **TECHNICIAN NOTE** Common anesthetic complications are hypoxemia and inadequate depth; thus proper equipment maintenance and monitoring are essential. Be skeptical of monitoring devices that suddenly change.

Monitoring Anesthetic Depth

Anesthetic depth refers to the degree of CNS depression, with observable signs grouped into stages and planes of anesthesia (Fig. 14-17). Anesthetic depth is commonly referred to as light if the degree of CNS depression is minimal and deep if it is profound.

Monitoring is actually subjective and requires integration of numerous factors, such as muscle tone, ocular reflexes, heart rate, respiratory rate and depth, and blood pressure. The progressive signs of anesthetic depth vary with the anesthetic drugs used, the species, and the individual patient. One cannot rely on a single sign, but must use all available information to evaluate anesthetic depth.

Anesthetic depth is not a steady state, but rather a product of the anesthetic drugs on board, the patient's physiologic state, and the degree of surgical stimulation applied to the patient at a particular time. Anesthetic depth is dose dependent. More drug produces more CNS depression, but it varies with the general anesthetic used.

Estimating Anesthetic Depth. Jaw muscle tone and eye reflexes are useful signs of anesthetic depth; they diminish with progression toward deeper planes of anesthesia. When noting signs of deep anesthesia, monitor the patient closely for adequate cardiopulmonary function and lighten the anesthetic level if possible.

Direct response to surgical stimulation is the most reliable sign of light anesthesia. In many patients, other signs, such as increased rate and depth of respiration, often precede movement.

MONITORING "EARLY WARNING"					RECOVERY PERIOD
Time:	10 20 30 40 50	10 20 30 40 50	10 20 30 40 50	10 20 30 40 50	
AGENTS:	ml/hr	ml/hr	ml/hr	ml/hr	TOTALS
Fluids:					Fluids:
Blood:					Blood:
Plasma:					Plasma:
Meds:					Meds:
Oxygen Flow:					Vaporizer Off:
Vaporizer Setting:					ETT Removed:
End Tidal Conc:					Sternal:
Light					Standing
					SUPPORT
PLANE:					1. None
Deep					2. Heating
Anesthesia A 250					3. Fluids
240					4. Oxygen
Operation ⊙ 230					5. ICU
220					6. Other
End ⊙⊗ 210					
200					
End A A 190					COMPLICATIONS
180					1. None
Systolic P V 170					2. Arrhythmias
160					3. Aspiration
Diastolic P Λ 150					4. Cardiac Arrest
140					5. Convulsions
Mean P X 130					6. Cyanosis
120					7. Death
Heart Rate • 110					8. Excitement
100					9. Hypothermia
Resp. Rate o 90					10. Injury
80					11. Laryngospasm
Spont. S 70					12. Panting
60					13. Regurgitation
Assist. A 50					14. Resp. Arrest
40					15. Resp. Depression
Ventil. V 30					16. Resp. Obstruction
20					17. Salivation
10					18. Other
0					
Temperature (°F)					
E.C.G.					
pH					
Pco_2					
Po_2					
HCO_3					
Base Balance					
Event					

Complications:

1. None	5. Cardiac Arrest	9. Hyperthermia	13. Panting	17. Resp. Obstruct.
2. Apnea	6. Cyanosis	10. Hypotension	14. Regurgitation	18. Salivation
3. Arrythmias	7. Death	11. Hypothermia	15. Resp. Arrest	19. Tympany
4. Aspiration	8. Hemorrhage	12. Inadequate Relaxation	16. Resp. Depression	20. Variable Depth

Assigned to Student Clinician at:___________

Student Anesthetist:

Student Clinician:

FIGURE 14-16 Anesthetic monitoring record. Typical anesthetic record for recording information related to an anesthetic procedure.

> **TECHNICIAN NOTE** The most essential monitor is a well-prepared, highly skilled individual performing continuous monitoring.

Monitoring Physiologic Conditions

The patient's physiologic conditions are monitored to ensure that excessive derangement of vital functions is not developing. A variety of equipment is available for this purpose (Table 14-14). This process is focused on the respiratory and cardiovascular systems, and the goal is to maintain adequate delivery of oxygenated blood to the tissues or tissue perfusion. Poor perfusion may imply poor blood flow and/or poor blood oxygenation. Shock is defined as inadequate tissue perfusion. Death is a late sign of poor perfusion; patients are not normally well perfused one minute and dead the next.

BOX 14-13 Monitoring of Anesthetic Equipment

1. All anesthetic equipment should be clean, calibrated, and maintained in good working order, and be functionally checked before and continuously throughout the procedure. Observe the oxygen source, anesthetic machine, and breathing circuit for leaks, and check that carbon dioxide absorbent is not exhausted.
2. During anesthesia, frequently check connections to the patient or anesthetic circuit. Power sources to monitoring equipment and heat sources should be verified throughout the procedure.
3. Verify monitoring device readings with quick, simple observations, such as mucous membrane color, capillary refill time, pulse rate, and pulse quality. If the blood pressure reads zero but the mucous membranes are pink and well perfused, common sense dictates that the blood pressure reading is probably incorrect.

Monitoring Respiratory Function

Equipment useful for monitoring respiratory function includes a blood gas machine, pulse oximeter (Fig. 14-18), end-tidal carbon dioxide analyzer (capnometer), rate monitor, and ventilometer. Respiratory function is monitored to ensure adequate oxygenation and removal of carbon dioxide from the blood. Respiratory function may be evaluated by respiratory rate, tidal volume, breathing patterns, hemoglobin saturation, end-tidal carbon dioxide, and arterial blood gases. Arterial blood gas analysis is the most reliable method to assess respiratory function, but it requires an arterial blood sample and special equipment.

Hearing, vision, and touch can be used to monitor the respiratory system and airway. Good indicators that air is moving in and out of the lungs are auscultation of breathing and lung sounds with a standard or esophageal stethoscope (Fig. 14-19), observation of the chest wall and the reservoir bag for movement, and feeling the reservoir bag for resistance. Air movement does not ensure adequate exchange of oxygen and carbon dioxide between the alveoli and blood. Bright red arterial blood at the surgical site as well as observing mucous membranes for pinkness is

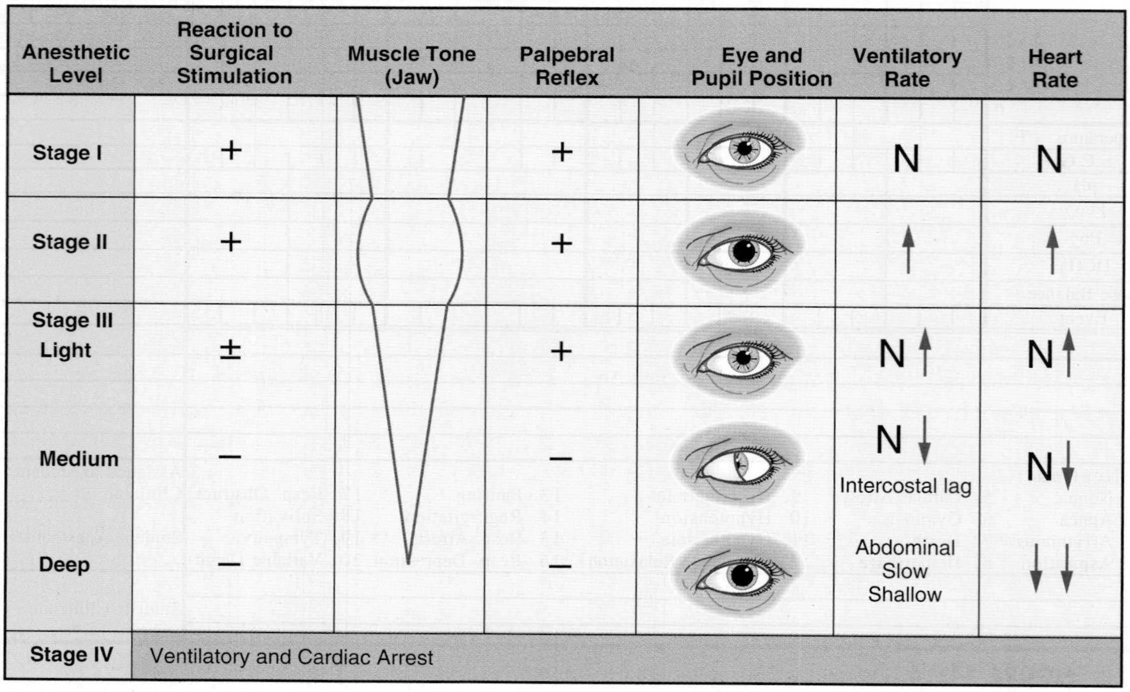

Anesthetic Level
Reaction to Surgical Stimulation
Muscle Tone (Jaw)
Palpebral Reflex
Eye and Pupil Position
Ventilatory Rate
Heart Rate
Stage I
+
+
N
N
Stage II
+
+
Stage III Light
±
+
N
N
Medium
–
–
N
Intercostal lag
N
Deep
–
–
Abdominal Slow Shallow
Stage IV
Ventilatory and Cardiac Arrest

FIGURE 14-17 Increasing depth of anesthesia produces characteristic changes in ocular, motor reflex, respiratory, and cardiovascular responses. Medium levels of stage III anesthesia are ideal for most invasive surgical procedures. Light levels of stage III anesthesia can be used if analgesia is supplemented by local anesthetic or opioids. (From Muir WW, Hubbell JAE, Skard R, et al.: *Handbook of veterinary anesthesia*, ed 4, St Louis, 2007, Mosby.)

desired. Color changes are not evident until severe hypoxemia exists, however.

> TECHNICIAN NOTE An SpO_2 reading of 66% (⅓ of hemoglobin not carrying oxygen) is needed before visible cyanosis (blue mucous membranes) occurs in a patient with normal hemoglobin levels (15 g/dl).

Monitoring Cardiovascular Function

Cardiovascular function is monitored to ensure that cardiac output and forward movement of blood are contributing to tissue perfusion. Vigilance is essential to warn of impending crisis with adequate time to prevent or correct actions. The degree to which different agents produce each of these effects varies. Cardiovascular function is evaluated by the heart rate, heart sounds, pulse quality and rate, mucous membrane color, and capillary refill time. Electrocardiography is recommended for

TABLE 14-14 Monitoring Equipment Used in Veterinary Medicine

MONITORING DEVICE	OVERVIEW	CONCERNS
Stethoscope	Always accessible. Evaluates heart rate (HR), rhythm, and sounds.	More difficult to hear beat in anesthetized patient
Esophageal stethoscope	Amplifies heart beat audible from a distance, can alert to possible arrhythmia, inexpensive	Does not give quantitative information. If sounds are muffled, difficult to hear. Complicated if mouth or throat surgery.
Electrocardiograph	Monitor HR and rhythm	Heart can stop beating even though electrical activity continues.
Pulse oximeter	Detects changes in oxygen saturation of hemoglobin by calculating the difference between levels of oxygenated and deoxygenated blood. Also determines heart rate. During oxygenation saturation level should be >95%. Probe either transmissive—place over nonpigmented skin that allows light transmission (e.g. tongue, lip)—or reflective (in hollow organ; e.g., rectum or esophagus).	To help minimize signal loss the light source must be oriented toward the tissue. Decreased signal strength in hypotension, hypothermia, and altered vascular resistance. Inaccurate if carboxyhemoglobin or methemoglobin is present.
Apnea monitor	Sensor placed between ETT connector and breathing circuit. Audible beep is heard when the patient breathes the difference in temperature between warm expired and cold inspired air is monitored. Will hear an alarm if no breath for a preset time period.	Increased mechanical dead space can be a problem in smaller animals if not using a special ETT connector. Does not warn of inadequate respiratory depth. Alarm may sound with decreased tidal volume (V_T) or hypothermic patient.
Ultrasonic Doppler	Monitors HR and rhythm by detecting flow of blood through small arteries. Converts into an audible beep. When combined with cuff and sphygmomanometer can indirectly determine systolic blood pressure. Fairly accurate in dogs.	Must clip hair, cover skin with ultrasonic gel, be parallel to and directly over artery, and use firm contact. If using cuff must be 30%-50% of circumference of the extremity. Manually performed so is labor intensive. Probe is expensive and easily damaged. Underestimates systolic BP in cats by 15 mm Hg. Prone to artifacts and technical problems such as movement, shivering, contact pressure.
Oscillometric BP monitor	Monitors HR and indirect BP. Cuff with an internal pressure-sensing bladder is placed around tail or leg and then connected to a computerized base that automatically inflates and deflates the cuff and interprets the signals sent by machine. More expensive but measures BP automatically and in addition to the systolic pressure, notes the diastolic and MAP.	Expensive and not as accurate in animals under 7 kg. Also prone to artifacts and technical problems as well as hypotension, tachycardia, and arrhythmias. Best to keep the cuff at the same horizontal plane as the heart. Inaccurate at low BPs.
Capnometer	Determines respiratory rate and the end tidal CO_2 by estimating partial CO_2 in bloodstream at the end of expiration, when CO_2 levels of the expired gas are approximately equal to alveolar and arterial CO_2 ($PaCO_2$). The fitting is placed between ETT and breathing circuit. The monitor measures CO_2 in inspired and expired air. One of best indicators of adequate respiration. Levels for anesthetized patients should be 40-45 mm Hg.	Abnormal readings if lung, CV or tissue disease, hypoventilation, abnormal breathing problems or malfunctioning equipment. Interpretation of capnogram is complex. Levels higher than normal indicate hypoventilation. Lower levels indication hyperventilation.
Central venous pressure	Monitors hydration and efficacy of fluid therapy by inserting catheter into anterior vena cava. Catheter is connected to a water manometer for measurement of mean right arterial pressure.	Invasive. Best used in conjunction with other parameters and to monitor trends. Zero mark of manometer must be at level of distal catheter tip. See Chapter 16 for more details.

Note: If alarm signals occur when using monitoring equipment, it is important to confirm by physically examining the patient.

evaluation of rhythm and conduction disturbances. Ordinarily, smaller patients have faster heart rates than larger patients of the same species. Blood pressure, urine output, and body temperature are also indicators of cardiovascular function.

All anesthetic drugs used today have dose-dependent cardiovascular depressant effects, such as arrhythmias, decreased contractility, vasodilation, or vasoconstriction. Monitoring the cardiovascular system does not require a grand display of electronic instrumentation. Although mechanical devices are appealing, the senses of touch, hearing, and vision are extremely useful for evaluation of cardiovascular function. Pulse palpation, capillary refill time, mucous membrane color, and heart sounds may be determined with simple instrumentation. Monitoring equipment can be used to enhance evaluation of cardiovascular function but can never replace what you observe, feel, or hear. Heart rates are easily determined with a simple stethoscope, esophageal stethoscope, or ECG.

Cardiac output (stroke volume × heart rate) is critical in maintaining adequate perfusion. The heart rate alone is of limited value in judging the adequacy of cardiac output.

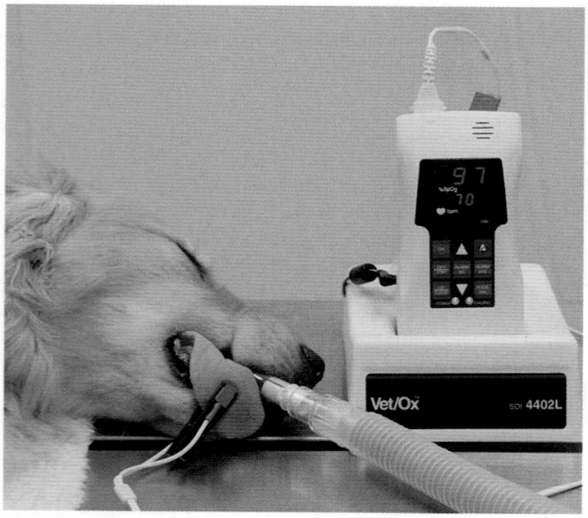

FIGURE 14-18 Pulse oximeter with transmission lingual probe. The upper number (97) represents the percent oxygen saturation (% SpO_2). The lower number (70) represents the HR in beats per minute. (From Thomas JA, Lerche P: *Anesthesia and analgesia for veterinary technicians*, ed 4, St Louis, 2011, Mosby.)

Other factors such as capillary refill time and pulse quality should be considered as well. Changes in heart rate may indicate adverse anesthetic effects, pain, compensation for decreased blood pressure, or vagal reflex stimulation.

Auscultation. Auscultation of the heart with a standard or esophageal stethoscope can provide valuable information, in addition to the heart rate. See Box 14-14 for informative auscultatory sounds. The rhythm and loudness of the heartbeat reflect overall cardiovascular function. Heart sounds are easily amplified by inexpensive monitoring devices. These small amplifiers provide the convenience of easily audible heart sounds while freeing the surgeon or technician to move around within the surgical area.

> TECHNICIAN NOTE Sinus arrhythmia, which is normal in dogs but not cats, results from the vagus nerve slowing the heart as the dog breathes.

Auscultation of the heart while simultaneously palpating the peripheral pulse is an excellent method of recognizing pulse deficits that may result from cardiac arrhythmias. Abnormal heart rates, irregular rhythm, and weak or muffled heart sounds may indicate diminished cardiac function. Altered heart rate and irregular rhythm suggest arrhythmias, whereas diminished heart sounds may indicate low cardiac output from myocardial hypoxemia or hypotension. Integrating this information with mucous membrane color, pulse quality, and capillary refill time provides usable information. However, it is a mistake to simply assume that because there is an audible beep or heart sound, everything is fine.

Electrocardiogram. The electrocardiogram (ECG) provides reliable information concerning heart rate and rhythm, including specific cardiac arrhythmias. When adverse anesthetic events occur, the sequence of adverse events is abnormal ECG, abnormal or skipped beats, decreased blood flow, weak or absent pulse, and finally cardiac arrest.

> TECHNICIAN NOTE Remember that the ECG is only an indicator of the electrical activity of the heart muscle and alone is a poor indicator of normal contraction or blood flow.

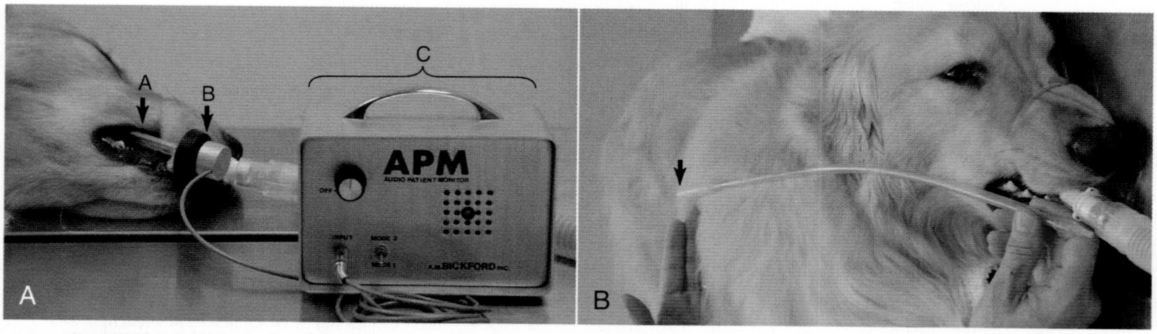

FIGURE 14-19 **A,** Esophageal stethoscope. *A,* Catheter. *B,* Sensor. *C,* Base unit. **B,** Measurement of the catheter to the level of the fifth rib or the caudal border of the scapula *(arrow)*. (From Thomas JA, Lerche P: *Anesthesia and analgesia for veterinary technicians*, ed 4, St Louis, 2011, Mosby.)

BOX 14-14 Informative Auscultatory Sounds

Respiratory Sounds
- Partial airway obstruction: increased or decreased sound volume, harshness
- Severe narrowing of airways: stridor, snoring, squeaking, whistling
- Fluid: crepitation
- Excessive fluid: bubbling
- Profoundly decreased or totally inaudible breath sounds

Cardiac Sounds
- Loudness indicates contractile strength and cardiac output
- Murmurs may mean decreased forward movement of blood
- Simultaneous pulse palpation can reveal arrhythmias
- Diminished heart sounds may indicate myocardial hypoxemia or hypotension

Pulse. The arterial pulse is the result of a pressure wave generated by cardiac contraction and ejection of blood into the aorta. This pressure wave travels down the arterial blood faster than the blood actually flows. Even though the pulse is not a result of blood flow, normal pulse rate and adequate pulse quality are indicators of adequate blood flow. Pulse rate is easily determined by palpation or pulse oximetry. The peripheral pulse rate may be less than the heart rate; a situation called **pulse deficit.** Comparison of heart rate and pulse rate enables detection of pulse deficits. The presence of a heart sound with an absent or extremely weak pulse indicates a pulse deficit and should be investigated before anesthesia proceeds. Significant arrhythmias produce ineffective heartbeats that are audible but do not produce a palpable arterial pulse. Pulse deficits occurring at a rate of 1 per 10 heartbeats (10%) or more may significantly diminish coronary and peripheral perfusion and require immediate attention. Anesthetics produce dose-related decreases in pulse quality. **Pulse quality** describes how the pulse feels when palpated with light digital pressure. Terms that describe pulse quality are strong, moderate, weak, and thread. **Pulse pressure** is the difference between systolic and diastolic arterial pressures. The pulse pressure curve shows changes in the pulse pressure during the cardiac cycle (Fig. 14-20) and can be obtained from direct arterial pressure monitors. Some pulse oximeters display a pulse curve that looks similar to the pulse pressure curve, but is derived from detection of pulsations, not direct pressure.

Pulse quality is affected by several factors, including vascular tone, vascular fluid volume, systolic/diastolic pressure differences, cardiac stroke volume, cardiac ejection rate, and peripheral location. In general, it is a useful indicator of stroke volume. Frequent causes of decreased pulse quality during anesthesia include hypovolemia, hypotension, and anything that causes decreased cardiac stroke volume. If the pulse weakens, decrease the anesthetic concentration, increase the infusion rate of fluids, determine the underlying cause, and make appropriate corrections.

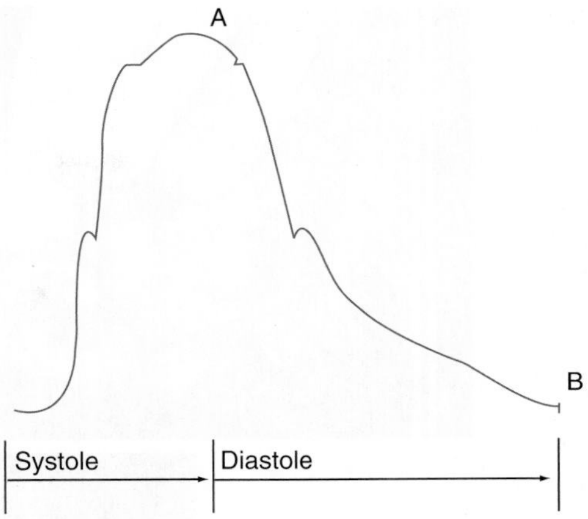

FIGURE 14-20 Pulse pressure curve. Diagram of pulse pressure curve shown in relationship to ECG.

Mucous Membrane Color. Mucous membrane color can be used to estimate tissue perfusion and oxygenation (Fig. 14-21). Mucous membranes are normally pink, indicating adequate respiratory and cardiovascular function. Cherry red mucous membranes may be seen with carbon monoxide poisoning. However, in severe carbon monoxide poisoning, cyanosis may mask the cherry red color. Hemoglobin has 200 times the affinity for carbon monoxide than oxygen, and its presence reduces the oxygen-transporting capability of hemoglobin, resulting in hypoxemia. Carbon monoxide poisoning has occurred during anesthesia of people using halogenated hydrocarbons. It is important to change soda lime frequently, as desiccated soda lime and Baralyme react with halogenated inhalation anesthetics to produce toxic concentrations of carbon monoxide. Pale mucous membranes indicate **vasoconstriction,** or a decrease in circulating red blood cells. Pale mucous membranes are not always a sign of poor hemodynamic status or shock. Cyanosis is a sign of respiratory insufficiency and an indication of hypoxemia.

TECHNICIAN NOTE Absence of cyanosis does not ensure adequate blood oxygenation. Anemic patients may not have sufficient hemoglobin to produce blueness, even when hypoxia is severe.

Capillary Refill Time. Capillary refill time (CRT) provides another indication of cardiovascular tone and a way to estimate tissue perfusion and oxygenation. CRT of less than 2 seconds in small animals and less than 3 seconds in large animals is considered normal. However, in a head-down position or the presence of vasodilation, patients may have normal or reduced CRT in the presence of severely compromised blood flow. This is especially true in horses, cattle, and other very large patients. Vasoconstriction prolongs the CRT. In summary, the presence of shortened or normal CRT may not be a reliable sign of adequate perfusion, but a prolonged CRT is significant.

Arterial Blood Pressure. Arterial blood pressure is an indicator of perfusion and cardiac output but not a true measure of blood flow. Anesthetics produce dose-dependent

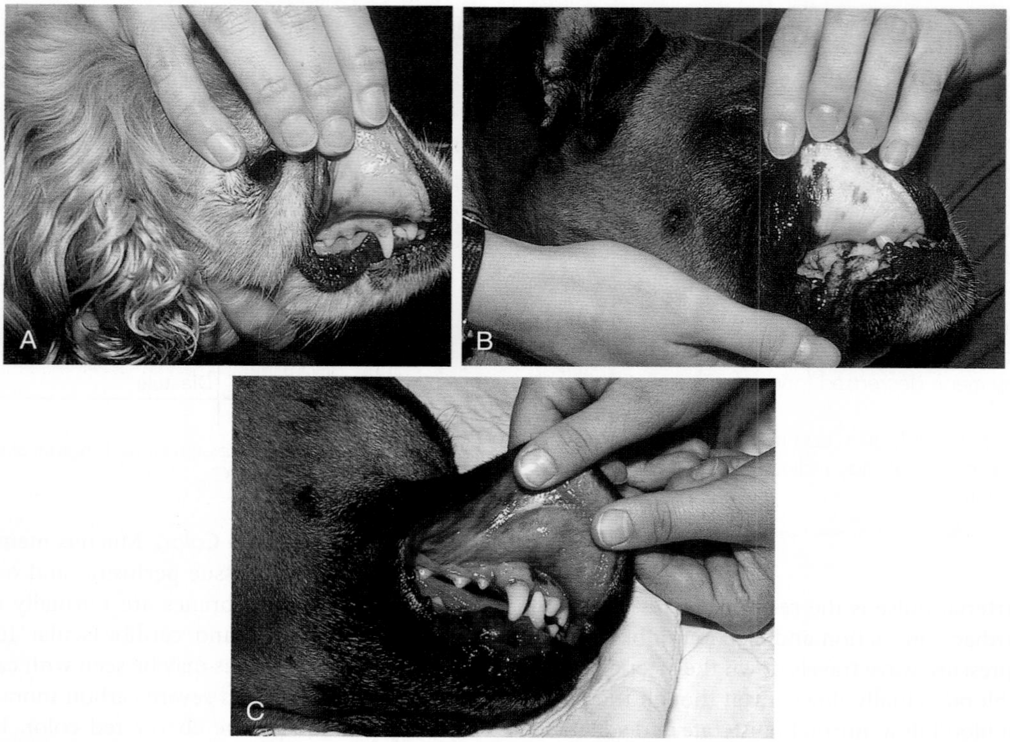

FIGURE 14-21 Mucous membrane color. **A,** Icterus mucous membrane color in a Cocker Spaniel with liver disease. **B,** Pale mucous membrane in a Boxer with a packed cell volume of 13%. **C,** Brick-red mucous membrane in a mongrel with septic shock. (From Battaglia A: *Small animal emergency and critical care,* ed 2, St Louis, 2007, Saunders.)

decreases in blood pressure; therefore, monitoring blood pressure during anesthesia is useful for depth determination and evaluation of patient health status. Blood pressure may be determined by direct or indirect methods.

Direct or invasive monitoring requires special equipment and placement of an arterial catheter. Indirect or noninvasive methods require special equipment but do not require an invasive arterial catheter to measure blood pressure. Doppler (Fig. 14-22) and oscillometric methods are indirect and noninvasive and are frequently used to determine blood pressure in clinical settings. Low arterial blood pressure may be caused by hypovolemia, cardiac depression, or vasodilation. The awake or lightly anesthetized, healthy patient rapidly compensates for hypotension by increasing cardiac output or increasing vascular tone. However, patients anesthetized to surgical planes of anesthesia may be unable to compensate or maintain acceptable blood pressure because of dose-dependent autonomic nervous system depression produced by anesthetic drugs. In most anesthetized patients, hypotension can be prevented by IV administration of crystalloid fluids at 10 to 20 ml/kg/hr, along with careful monitoring of tissue perfusion and anesthetic depth.

Monitoring Body Temperature

Monitoring body temperature during anesthesia provides an indication of CNS and cardiovascular function. Depression of thermoregulatory centers in the brain and decreased blood flow produced by anesthetic agents leads to hypothermia. It may also be produced in response to various drug combinations, specifically halothane, isoflurane, sevoflurane, succinylcholine, and ketamine. Continuous measurement of core temperature with a rectal or esophageal thermometer warns of significant temperature change.

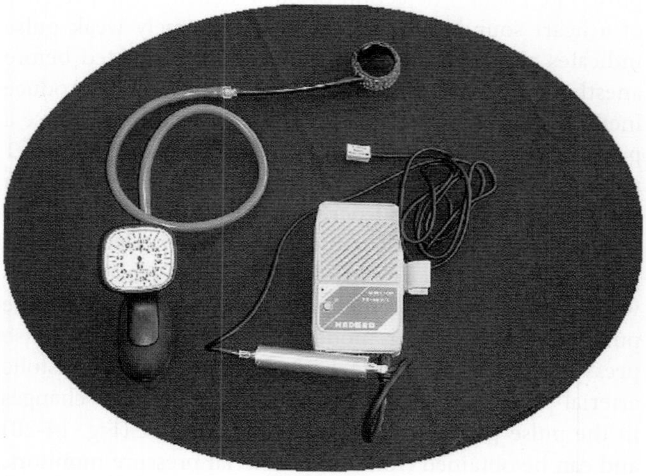

FIGURE 14-22 Doppler ultrasonic blood pressure monitor. (From Sonsthagen TF: *Veterinary instruments and equipment: a pocket guide,* ed 2, St Louis, 2011, Mosby.)

TECHNICIAN NOTE It is much easier to prevent heat loss than to restore heat.

Responding to Adverse Events

All adverse events should be brought to the veterinarian's attention immediately. The role of the technician in responding to adverse events is generally that of being prepared to execute the veterinarian's directives quickly and accurately (Table 14-15). The administration of drugs to counteract specific conditions should be under the veterinarian's direction. However, some situations simply require a common-sense approach.

> **TECHNICIAN NOTE** Hypoxia differs from hypoxemia. Hypoxia literally means decreased oxygen, either generally or locally as in low tissue pO_2. In hypoxemia, it is the oxygen concentration within the arterial blood that is abnormally low, specifically less than 60 mm Hg (8.0 kPa), or causing hemoglobin oxygen saturation of less than 90%. Incorrect use of these terms can lead to confusion, especially as hypoxemia is among the causes of hypoxia (in hypoxemic hypoxia).

TABLE 14-15 Preventing Adverse Effects During Anesthesia

PROBLEM AND SIGNS	TO PREVENT
Hypothermia Body temperature drops <35° C	Decrease the anesthetic concentration, ensure adequate circulation, insulate from cold surfaces, dry the body surface, apply warm blankets and/or hot packs, warm inspired air, and decrease fresh gas flow to minimum requirements.
Tachycardia Heart rate exceeds 160-180 in dogs (depending on breed) or 200 in cats.	If the patient is not moving (anesthetic depth is adequate), decrease the anesthetic concentration, increase oxygen flow, increase the rate of IV fluid delivery, and support ventilation. If tachycardia persists, prepare for cardiac arrest.
Bradycardia Heart rate drops <60.	Bradycardia caused by alpha agonists: may be treated with anticholinergics or a specific alpha antagonist. Opioid-induced bradycardia: can be managed with anticholinergics. Bradycardia resulting from excessive anesthetic depth: usually responds to a decreased anesthetic concentration and support with oxygen and fluids. Vagus-mediated bradycardia is usually transient: discontinue vagal stimulation. If bradycardia worsens or persists, administration of an anticholinergic may be required, along with fluid administration. Hypothermic patients exhibiting bradycardia must be warmed and may require IV fluid administration to correct bradycardia.
Pain If signs are evident as indicated above	Treat with an analgesic that produces less cardiovascular depressant effect than additional general anesthetic.
Hypotension Decreased blood pressure <60 mm Hg	Usually controlled by appropriate fluid administration and lowering the anesthetic concentration.
Hypercapnia Associated with decreased CO_2 elimination during anesthesia, not increased CO_2 production	Monitor perianesthetic drugs as they depress the respiratory center. Prevent respiratory obstruction. Increase ventilation ("bagging") to remove carbon dioxide from the patient. Avoid expired soda lime or faulty unidirectional valves in rebreathing circuits. In non-rebreathing circuits, ensure adequate flow rate. Have correct ET length and proper fitting face mask to prevent excessive mechanical dead space.
Hypoxemia Present if the SpO_2 reading on the pulse oximeter is 90% and below.	Initially treat by increasing inspired oxygen concentration and ensuring adequate ventilation. Ensure clear and nonkinked ET. Proper O_2 tank level.

Continued

TABLE 14-15 Preventing Adverse Effects During Anesthesia—cont'd

PROBLEM AND SIGNS	TO PREVENT
Excessive Depth	
Note signs described in Table 14-14.	Reverse by decreasing the vaporizer setting, increasing the oxygen flow rate, and ensuring adequate ventilation and circulatory support.
Inadequate Depth	
Ensure secure fitting endotracheal tube or face mask.	Keep vaporizer at proper level and ensure it is functioning. Use adequate flow rate and proper vaporizer settings.
Endobronchial Intubation	
Endotracheal tube not properly inserted into the trachea so that there is difficulty maintaining adequate ventilation and anesthetic depth.	Easily corrected by withdrawing the endotracheal tube sufficiently to remove it from the bronchus.
Excessive Circuit Pressure	
The pressure in the breathing circuit exceeds the central venous pressure (approximately 4 cm H_2O) with collapse of the thoracic vena cava and reduction of venous return to the heart. Cardiac output cannot exceed venous return, so it decreases as well, leading to hypotension.	Monitor pop-off valve carefully. Have the correct oxygen flow rate for the animal and system. Scavenger system is not occluded.

STEP 7: RECOVERY

Recovery means "to restore to a normal state" and begins when administration of anesthetic is discontinued. This is a reminder that, during anesthesia, patients are in an abnormal state. Vigilance and support of organ function should continue until the patient is satisfactorily recovered from anesthesia. Pain relief and maintenance of a patent airway are important during recovery. The critical period has passed when the body temperature is normal, sternal recumbency is achieved, and oropharyngeal reflexes are restored. However, observation should continue until the patient can stand and is free of all drug effects.

When recovering, the patient should be maintained on 100% oxygen to ensure oxygenation and allow exhaled anesthetic gases to enter the scavenger system, rather than the room air. As the patient begins to awaken, the endotracheal tube cuff should be deflated and the tie undone. When the patient exhibits swallowing reflexes, the tube should be gently removed. Close observation is essential immediately after extubation, as the patient may regurgitate or have difficulty breathing. Brachycephalic dogs are especially notorious for developing breathing difficulties after extubation.

Fluid administration should continue until recovery is adequate. Premature removal of the IV catheter may result in the inability to quickly administer IV medications in the event of an emergency. Recovery is considered adequate (but not complete) when the body temperature is normal, the patient's vital signs are stable, and sternal recumbency is maintained. Observation should continue until the patient can stand and walk without assistance.

LARGE ANIMAL ANESTHESIA

The basic principles of anesthesia discussed in this chapter apply to large animals as well. Some specialized equipment may be needed to move and position large animals. Many of the same medications are also used in large animals. Box 14-15 contains a summary of equine anesthesia protocols.

TECHNICIAN NOTE Always ensure the horse is sedated before anesthetic induction. To minimize anesthetic complications, keep the horse calm before induction of anesthesia.

BOX 14-15 Quick Reference Guide for Equine Anesthesia

Preparation

1. Withhold food for 24 hours and water for 6 to 12 hours, when possible. Telephone the client to remind about food and water restriction.
2. Obtain the horse's body weight by weighing or chest girth tape measurement for estimation.
3. Avoid or delay elective procedures in horses that are not healthy. Perform a physical examination before administration of any drug. Minimum data should include heart rate, respiratory rate, mucous membrane color, pulse quality, ocular or nasal discharge, lymph nodes, PCV, and total plasma protein assay.
4. Prepare drugs and equipment
   a. Equipment includes clippers, local anesthetic, antiseptic scrub, catheters, tape, heparinized saline, suture material, catheter cap, administration extension set with drip chamber (do not use a simplex), three-way stopcock, syringe pump
      i. Administer fluids to debilitated horses or horses to be anesthetized for long procedures.
   b. Prepare and calculate the volume of the drugs and agents required—preanesthetic agents, fluids, induction agents, maintenance, analgesic agents including local anesthetics if required, and reversal agents.
   c. If using, assemble and check the anesthetic machine for leaks.
   d. Accessories required include scales, syringes, needles, emergency cart, controlled substance log, anesthesia record, monitoring equipment, endotracheal tubes, and adjuncts.
5. Clean hooves and wrap or remove shoes if needed.
6. Place an IV catheter—some horses may need IM sedation.
7. Avoid stress, such as from extreme heat or long trailer rides, before induction of anesthesia, and keep the horse calm before induction of anesthesia.
8. If the horse is to be in lateral recumbency, prevent myopathy and neuropathy by:
   a. Removing the halter upon induction
   b. Ensuring the face and lower limbs are padded
   c. Maintaining an open airway
   d. Ensuring unrestricted blood flow
   e. Applying no pressure to the chest
9. Constantly check and monitor the vital signs and anesthetic depth
10. Standing chemical restraint with the addition of local anesthetic nerve blocks or opioid epidurals are often used for many procedures, such as castration, dental, sinus, or eye surgery, or rectovaginal fistula repair.

Intubation

1. Similar to small animals, but placed in lateral recumbency.
2. Thoroughly flush the oral cavity with water to remove food and debris.
3. Place an oral speculum between the incisor teeth to prevent biting the tube.
4. Select a tube of the largest diameter that will pass without excessive force. A 22- to 30-mm tube is generally used for adults and a 9- to 6-mm tube for foals.
5. Lubricate with copious amounts of water-soluble sterile lubricant
6. Grasp the tongue, pulling it forward between the lips and speculum, and extend the head and neck.
7. Pass the endotracheal tube through the preinserted speculum, avoiding the sharp edges of the check teeth.
8. Rotate the tube about 90 degrees while applying slight pressure; this usually facilitates tube passage if there is difficulty.
9. Check for correct placement by feeling the exhaled gases.

Sedation and Analgesia for Standing Chemical Restraint in Horses

1. Sedation may be maintained either with bolus or CRI (constant rate infusion).
2. Bolus is the most common, but keep in mind that effects occur rapidly post-IV administration.
3. Use lower doses initially and assess until the desired effect is noted.
4. Vigilant monitoring of anesthetic depth and vital signs is essential.

α_2 Agonist IV Doses in Combination with Opioids

1. Give the α_2 agonist first and wait 10 minutes.
   a. Xylazine 0.3 to 1.0 mg/kg
   b. Detomidine: 0.005 to 0.02 mg/kg
   c. Medetomidine 0.0035 to 0.007 mg/kg
   d. Romifidine: 0.03 to 0.1 mg/kg
2. Give the opioid—butorphanol at 0.02 to 0.2 mg/kg or morphine at 0.15 mg/kg
3. Provide neuroleptanalgesia
4. In combination with xylazine, butorphanol provides 20 to 30 minutes of chemical restraint.
5. The sedation for xylazine and butorphanol can be extended if necessary with one-half dosage of each as needed.
6. Detomidine and morphine provide about 60 minutes of sedation. Morphine has a longer duration of action than detomidine.

α_2 Agonist in Combination with Phenothiazines

1. Because of slow onset of effect, the phenothiazine should be administered 15 to 30 minutes before the α_2 agonist.
2. Acepromazine at 0.02 to 0.05 mg/kg followed by xylazine at 0.5 to 1 mg/kg or detomidine at 0.005 to 0.01 mg/kg.

Anesthetic Induction and Maintenance

1. Induction agents should be given to effect monitoring carefully.
2. Induction should include a sedative.
   a. Sedatives used are usually an α_2 agonist alone or with opioids or phenothiazines.
   b. Phenothiazines alone or with opioids or α_2 agonists.

Note: Unless otherwise indicated for the protocols listed below, use the following dosages of α_2 agonist IV as the sedative, administering it before the induction agent:

1. α_2 agonist: a. Xylazine at 1.0 to 1.5 mg/kg
   b. Detomidine at 0.01 to 0.02 mg/kg
   c. Romifidine at 0.05 to 0.12 mg/kg
   d. Medetomidine at 0.005 to 0.075 mg/kg

Continued

BOX 14-15 Quick Reference Guide for Equine Anesthesia—cont'd

2. Proceed once maximum effect is achieved—usually in 3 to 5 minutes if given IV.
3. If given IM, usually three times the IV dose is given with profound sedation usually taking 10 to 15 minutes.
4. Not all horses will respond the same, with higher doses often being required in fractious horses, ponies, donkeys, and mules. Detomidine tends to be more effective than xylazine.
5. Do not disturb the animal during sedation and induction; otherwise, poor induction may result.
6. If the horse is not sedated by the α_2 agonist, administer 10 to 20 mg (total dose) of diazepam or butorphanol IV rather than an additional α_2 agonist.
7. For short procedures under field conditions, such as castration, the most commonly used drugs are α_2 agonist and ketamine.

α_2 Agonist and Ketamine

1. Following the α_2 agonist regime, give ketamine as an IV bolus at 2.0 to 2.5 mg/kg.
   a. In combination with xylazine, the ketamine will give 5 to 10 minutes of surgical anesthesia.
   b. With detomidine and romifidine, ketamine has a longer duration than xylazine.
2. Best to use the high end of the sedative dose.
3. Anesthesia may be prolonged with Triple Drip (see below) or up to two additional doses of α_2 agonist and ketamine, using half the original dosage. Do not give more than two additional doses.

α_2 Agonist and Telazol

1. Following the α_2 agonist regime, Telazol, which is a 1:1 mixture of tiletamine and zolazepam, is given at 1.0 to 1.5 mg/kg, IV.
2. Tiletamine is similar to ketamine in its mode of action and zolazepam is a long-acting benzodiazepine.
3. Telazol is not recommended as an induction agent in the unsedated horse.
4. Inductions are excellent, and the duration of surgical anesthesia is roughly twice as long as with ketamine.
5. Recoveries are not quite as smooth as with ketamine.

Benzodiazepine with α_2 Agonist and Ketamine

1. Following the α_2 agonist regime, combine diazepam or midazolam (0.05 to 0.1 mg/kg) with ketamine (2.0 to 2.5 mg/kg).
2. Not used for standing sedation as both diazepam and midazolam cause ataxia.
3. The sedative, muscle relaxing and anticonvulsant effects of the diazepam improve the quality of anesthesia, but the duration of surgical anesthesia is not extended.

Butorphanol with Xylazine and Ketamine

1. Give butorphanol IM or slowly IV at 0.05 mg/kg.
2. Wait 20 minutes.
3. Give α_2 agonist IV with doses as listed above. The dose may be reduced.
4. When the horse is sedated, give ketamine as an IV bolus at 2.0 to 2.5 mg/kg.
5. Anticipate 12 to 20 minutes of anesthesia and analgesia.
6. Anesthesia may be prolonged with Triple Drip or guaifenesin.

Ketamine and Guaifenesin Following α_2 Agonist

1. Follow the α_2 agonist regime listed above. The dose may be reduced.
2. Administer ketamine 2.0 to 2.5 mg/kg IV combined with guaifenesin at 50 to 100 mg/kg.
3. Improves relaxation.

Thiopental and α_2 Agonist

1. Follow the α_2 agonist regime listed above.
2. Administer Thiopental at 3 to 5 mg/kg IV.
3. Good relaxation, but analgesia only from the α_2 agonist.

Thiopental and Guaifenesin Following α_2 Agonist

1. Follow the α_2 agonist regime listed above. The dose may be reduced if desired.
2. Can mix thiopental at 3 to 5 mg/kg IV and guaifenesin at 50 to 100 mg/kg.
3. Good relaxation.

Propofol Following α_2 Agonist

1. Follow the α_2 agonist regime listed above using the full dose.
2. Administer propofol at 2 mg/kg.
3. Myoclonus and paddling may occur and some horses become excited.

For Anesthetic Maintenance

1. Isoflurane 1.5% to 2.5% or sevoflurane 2.5% to 4%
   a. Feasible in foals
   b. If used as the sole induction and maintenance agent inhalation anesthetics in horses have been associated with higher mortality rates than injectable drugs.
   c. Has a narrow therapeutic index.
2. Short-term prolongation using intermittent bolus injection
   a. Use of α_2 agonist with ketamine—½ to ¼ of induction dose of each.
      i. Extends anesthesia by 5 to 10 minutes.
   b. Thiopental at 1 to 2 mg/kg, and give ¼ to ½ of induction dose.
      i. Extends anesthesia by 5 to 10 minutes.
      ii. Not good choice if thiopental is the sole induction drug.
3. CRI
   a. Triple drip
      i. Add 10 ml of ketamine (100 mg/ml) and 5 mg of xylazine (100 mg/ml) to 1 L of 5% guaifenesin (50 mg/ml).
      ii. Each ml of triple drip will contain 1.0 mg of ketamine, 0.50 mg of xylazine, and 50 mg of guaifenesin.
      iii. Infuse IV at a constant drip rate of approximately 1 to 2 ml/kg/hr.
      iv. Anesthesia is extended by 30 to 40 minutes.
      v. For procedures longer than an hour, double the dosage of ketamine and xylazine.
      vi. Other α_2 agonists may be substituted for xylazine.

BOX 14-15 Quick Reference Guide for Equine Anesthesia—cont'd

vii. Triple Drip is useful for maintenance following induction with xylazine and dissociative anesthetics. Ketamine and α_2 agonist alone provides poor relaxation.

b. An example of TIVA (total intravenous anesthesia)
   i. To achieve balanced anesthesia using two or more drugs in combination.
c. Ketamine in combination with benzodiazepines can also be used, as can propofol either alone or in combination with Ketamine or with an α_2 agonist.
d. If using TIVA it is important to premedicate to help decrease the final dosage.

4. Can also use PIVA (partial intravenous anesthesia) combining intravenous and inhalation anesthesia to achieve balanced anesthesia.
   a. Various injectables can be used.
   b. Injectable drugs do accumulate in the body over time, so best to decrease the doses over prolonged procedures.
   c. The negative cardiorespiratory effects of the inhalants can be reduced as long as they are replaced by intravenous drugs with less depressant effects.
5. Local and regional anesthesia will prolong the effect of the general anesthesia by preventing painful stimuli from reaching the CNS.
   a. For castration, the local anesthetic can be injected directly into the spermatic cord or testicle.
   b. Regional anesthesia can be used for nerve blocks of the head or distal limb.

REVIEW QUESTIONS

Short Answer

List some special anesthesia considerations for each of the four groups listed below.

a. Sighthounds
b. Brachycephalic breeds
c. Pediatric patients
d. Geriatric patients

Fill-In the Blank

Provide answers to complete the following statements.

1. A growing concern in veterinary medicine is ________________ control, pre-, peri-, and post-operative.
2. It is very helpful to know the normal behavior of the __________________ when assessing them for pain.
3. It has been demonstrated that pain is more easily managed if analgesics are given _________________before a patient experiences pain.
4. Using several analgesic drugs, each with a different mechanism of action, is called ____________________ therapy.
5. Tranquilizers and sedatives are typically used as ______________medications to calm the patient and reduce the amount of anesthetic needed.
6. Analgesic agents are needed to suppress the ___________________ pain mechanisms that remain active during anesthesia.
7. The process by which pain information is carried from the periphery sense receptors in the skin and the viscera to the cerebral cortex through a network of neuronal relays is called _________________.
8. The most important step in an anesthetic procedure is the ____________________ ____________________, because all anesthetic decisions are based on health status.
9. Standard practice is to withhold food for ______ to ______ hours and water for ____ to ____ hours before anesthetic induction.
10. In high-volume clinics, when several people are involved in patient evaluation and preparation, ________________ _______________ should be completed before any anesthetic procedure is done to ensure that appropriate items are available, important health issues have been addressed, and all involved persons have been informed.
11. Administration of the induction agent transitions the patient to unconsciousness, when jaw muscle tone and ________________reflexes are lost, the patient can be intubated.
12. Applying ______________________ to the larynx by spray or with a cotton-tipped swab, especially in cats and swine, facilitates intubation.
13. For most procedures and patients the flow meter is set to deliver ________L/min of oxygen, and the vaporizer is set to deliver a concentration of ______to ______ percent.
14. If anesthetic administration is not reduced in the presence of ______________________ or _______________, patients may become too deeply anesthetized, with further compromise of tissue perfusion.
15. For inhalant agents, potency is determined largely by the lipid solubility of the agent and is reflected by the ______________ __________________ __________________.
16. Monitoring should be ________________, and data should be recorded every ____ to ____ minutes or when significant changes occur.
17. Flow rates for non-rebreathing systems are high because it is the only way CO_2 is flushed away from the patient; flow rates of _______ to _______ ml/kg/min or 2 to 3 times the minute ventilation are recommended.
18. Maintenance flow rate for a rebreathing circuit operated as a closed system is equal to the patient's calculated oxygen consumption rate _____________________________.

19. The primary means of increasing ______________________ uptake is to increase the vaporizer setting.
20. Monitoring a patient under anesthesia primarily focuses on the ______________________ and ____________________ systems.
21. A SpO_2 reading of __________ % is needed before visible cyanosis occurs in a patient.
22. The peripheral pulse rate may be less than the heart rate and is called ______________ ______________.
23. Pulse deficits occurring at a rate of ______/________ heartbeats (10%) or more may significantly diminish coronary and peripheral perfusion and require immediate attention.
24. Hemoglobin has ________ times the affinity for carbon monoxide than oxygen, and its presence reduces the oxygen-transporting capability of hemoglobin, resulting in hypoxemia.
25. Capillary refill time (CRT) of less than ________ seconds in small animals and less than ________ seconds in large animals is considered normal.

RECOMMENDED READING

Anon: Commentary and recommendations on control of waste anesthetic gases in the workplace, *J Am Vet Med Assoc* 209:75–77, 1996.

Bassert JM, Thomas J: *McCurnin's clinical textbook for veterinary technicians*, ed 8, St Louis, 2014, Saunders.

Clarke K, Trim C, Hall L: *Veterinary anaesthesia*, ed 11, St Louis, 2014, Saunders.

Gaynor J, Muir W: *Handbook of veterinary pain management*, ed 3, St Louis, 2015, Elsevier.

Mathews KA: Management of pain. *Vet Clin North Am Small Animal Practice*, July 2000 Saunders.

Muir WW, Hubbell JAE: *Equine anesthesia: monitoring and emergency therapy*, ed 2, St Louis, 2008, Mosby.

Muir WW, Hubbell JAE, Skard R, et al.: *Handbook of veterinary anesthesia*, ed 5, St Louis, 2012, Mosby.

Riebold TW: *Large animal anesthesia: principles and techniques*, ed 2, Ames, IA, 1995, Iowa State University Press.

Thomas JA, Lerche P: *Anesthesia and analgesia for veterinary technicians*, ed 4, St Louis, 2011, Mosby.

Thurmon JC, Tranquilli WJ: *Lamb and Jones' veterinary anesthesia*, ed 3, Baltimore, 1996, Williams & Wilkins.

Thurmon JC, Tranquilli WJ, Benson GJ: *Essentials of small animal anesthesia and analgesia*, Philadelphia, 1999, Lippincott.

15 Principles of Surgical Nursing

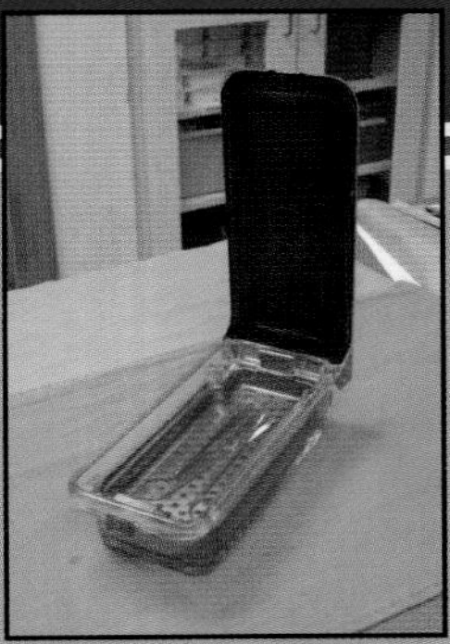

OUTLINE

LEARNING OBJECTIVES

After reviewing this chapter, the reader will be able to:

1. Describe and explain surgical terminology.
2. Discuss principles of aseptic technique.
3. Give examples of methods used to disinfect or sterilize surgical instruments and supplies.
4. Describe procedures for preparing the surgical site and surgical team.
5. Identify surgical instruments and explain their uses and maintenance.
6. Compare and contrast types of suture needles and suture materials.

KEY TERMS

Angiotribes
Aseptic technique
Autoclave
Brown-Adson tissue forceps
Celiotomy
Crile forceps
Curettes
Electrocautery
Electrocoagulation
Enterotomy
Eviscerate
Flank incision
Gastropexy
Gastrotomy
Herniorrhaphy
Intestinal anastomosis
Intramedullary bone pinning
Iris scissors
Kelly forceps
Laparotomy
Mayo scissors
Mayo stand
Mayo-Hegar needle holders
Metzenbaum scissors
Nosocomial infection
Orchiectomy
Osteotome
Ovariohysterectomy
Paracostal incision
Paramedian incision
Peritonitis
Rongeurs
Rumenotomy
Sterilization indicators
Suture
Thoracotomy
Urethrotomy
Ventral midline incision
Weitlaner retractor

GENERAL SURGICAL PRINCIPLES

The role of the veterinary technician in surgical procedures is quite diverse. During the presurgical period, the veterinary technician is responsible for preparation of the patient, the surgical instruments and equipment, and the surgical environment. During surgery, the veterinary technician is usually responsible for anesthesia of the patient. The veterinary technician often assists the surgeon, either directly, by actually scrubbing in, or indirectly, by opening surgical packs, suture materials, and other supplies. It is vital that the veterinary technician know how to function in a sterile surgical environment without causing contamination. In the postsurgical period, the veterinary technician is frequently responsible for postoperative patient care and monitoring, instructing clients on patient care during the recovery period, and removing sutures.

BASIC SURGICAL TERMINOLOGY

Surgical procedures are described using anatomic terms combined with word roots (suffixes) (see Chapter 5). The most common suffixes used for describing surgical procedures are presented in Box 15-1.

BOX 15-1 Common Suffixes Used to Describe Surgical Procedures

- *-ectomy* = to remove (excise). For example, a splenectomy is a surgical procedure to remove the spleen.
- *-otomy* = to cut into. For example, a cystotomy (incision into the urinary bladder) is often performed to remove urinary calculi (bladder stones).
- *-ostomy* = surgical creation of an artificial opening. For example, a perineal urethrostomy is a surgical procedure often performed on male cats for relief of urethral obstruction. It involves excision of the penis (penectomy) and creation of a widened new urethral opening.
- *-rrhaphy* = surgical repair by suturing. For example, abdominal herniorrhaphy is the surgical repair of an abdominal hernia by suturing the defect in the abdominal musculature.
- *-pexy* = surgical fixation. For example, gastropexy (suturing of the stomach to the abdominal wall to fix it in place) is often performed in cases of gastric torsion.
- *-plasty* = surgical alteration of shape or form. For example, pyloroplasty enlarges the pyloric orifice of the stomach to facilitate gastric emptying.

ABDOMINAL INCISIONS

Abdominal surgery is commonly performed in animal species. Entry into the abdomen is usually gained by any of four common abdominal incisions. Named according to its location, each incision offers different advantages and a different exposure of the abdomen (Fig. 15-1).

A **ventral midline incision** is located on the ventral midline of the animal. It offers excellent exposure of the entire abdominal cavity. Because the abdominal cavity is entered through the linea alba, where the abdominal muscles on each side are joined, the abdominal wall can be closed with a single layer of sutures in the linea alba. Closure of a ventral midline incision must be very secure, because the weight of the abdominal organs exerts tension on the incision when the animal stands. Also, any exertion by the animal can create tension on the suture line.

A **paramedian incision** is located lateral and parallel to the ventral midline of the animal. It is usually used when exposure of only one side of the abdomen is needed, such as for removal of a cryptorchid (retained) testis. The muscles of the abdominal wall are individually incised, so closure of the abdominal wall usually requires multiple layers of sutures.

A **flank incision** is generally performed on either a standing animal or one in lateral recumbency. It is oriented perpendicular to the long axis of the body, caudal to the last rib. A flank incision provides good exposure of the organ(s) immediately deep to (beneath) the incision but does not allow exploration of much of the remainder of the abdomen. It is, therefore, useful for such procedures as rumenotomy and nephrectomy, in which the organ in question lies directly beneath the incision. The muscles of the abdominal wall usually require a multiple-layer closure. In contrast to tension exerted on a ventral midline incision, the weight of the abdominal organs generally tends to keep a flank incision closed rather than pulling it apart.

A **paracostal incision** is oriented parallel to the last rib and offers good exposure of the stomach and spleen in monogastric animals. The muscles of the abdominal wall are usually closed in multiple layers.

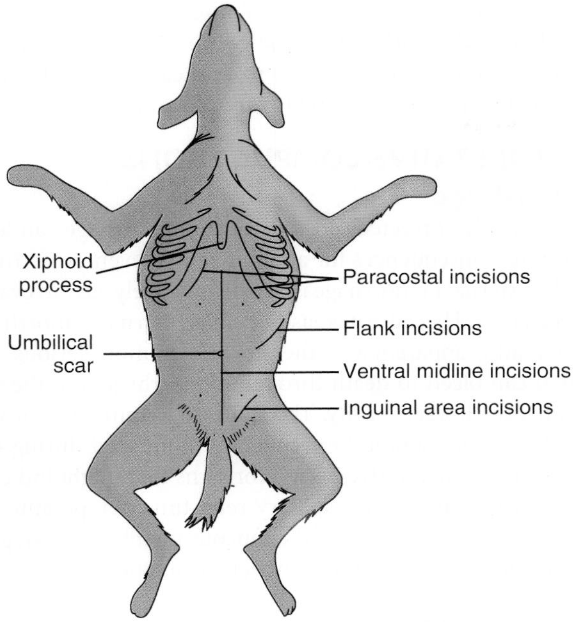

FIGURE 15-1 Surgical incisions for abdominal procedures.

THORACIC INCISIONS

Thoracic surgery may be indicated because of pathology in the chest or traumatic injuries. Two common incisions are used in veterinary medicine.

A median sternotomy is used for many cardiac procedures or when all lung fields need to be visualized or approached. This incision is along the patient's midline, on the ventral thorax, moving cranially from the xiphoid process or caudally from the first sternebrae, always leaving two to three sternebrae intact.

A lateral intercostal thoracotomy may be used if only one side of the chest needs to be approached, such as cases of lung lobe torsion or mass. This is done on the side of the patient's thorax, perpendicular to the spine and between ribs.

COMMON SURGICAL PROCEDURES

Soft Tissue Procedures

- An **ovariohysterectomy,** commonly referred to as a "spay," involves removal of the ovaries and uterus.
- A cesarean section is a method of delivering newborn animals in cases of dystocia (difficult labor). It consists of an abdominal incision (flank or ventral midline) and then an incision into the uterus through which the newborn(s) is (are) delivered.
- An **orchiectomy** (castration) is the surgical removal of the testes.
- A lateral ear resection is often performed in animals with chronic external ear infection. It involves removal of the lateral wall of the vertical portion of the external ear canal to allow improved ventilation and establish drainage for exudates.
- A **laparotomy** is an incision into the abdominal cavity, often through the flank.
- A **celiotomy** is another term for laparotomy.
- A cystotomy is an incision into the urinary bladder, frequently for removal of urinary calculi (bladder stones).
- A **gastrotomy** is an incision into a simple stomach, whereas a **rumenotomy** is an incision into a rumen.
- **Gastropexy** involves suturing of the stomach to the abdominal wall to fix it in place. This procedure is frequently done in cases of gastric torsion.
- A splenectomy is the removal of the spleen.
- A **thoracotomy** is an incision into the thoracic cavity (chest).
- A **herniorrhaphy** is the surgical repair of a hernia by suturing the abnormal opening(s) closed.
- An **enterotomy** is an incision into the intestine, often for removal of a foreign body.
- An **intestinal anastomosis** involves removal of a portion of the intestine (resection) and suturing the cut ends together to restore the continuity of the intestinal tube (anastomosis).
- A perineal urethrostomy involves incision into the urethra and suturing of the splayed urethral edges to the skin to create a larger urethral orifice. This procedure is frequently performed on male cats with recurrent urethral obstruction.
- A **urethrotomy** is an incision into the urethra, most commonly to retrieve stones that have traveled out of the bladder and become lodged in the urethra.
- A mastectomy involves removal of part or all of one or more mammary glands.

Orthopedic (Bone) Procedures

- An onychectomy is the surgical removal of a claw, commonly called declawing.
- An intervertebral disk fenestration is done to remove prolapsed intervertebral disk material causing pressure on the spinal cord.
- An **intramedullary bone pinning** involves insertion of a metal rod (bone pin) into the medullary cavity of a long bone to fix fracture fragments in place.
- Joint stabilization via lateral suture technique or tibial tuberosity advancement is performed when the cranial cruciate ligament in the stifle joint has ruptured. Lack of an intact cranial cruciate ligament creates instability in the stifle, causing abnormal movement. This can damage the joint surfaces of the distal femur and proximal tibia.
- A femoral head ostectomy involves amputation of the head of the femur. It is usually performed in animals with severe damage to the femoral head or neck, or with a damaged acetabulum.

PREOPERATIVE AND POSTOPERATIVE CONSIDERATIONS

PREOPERATIVE EVALUATION

Anesthesia and surgery are stressful events that put an animal's life at risk. The role of a proper preoperative evaluation is to gather enough pertinent information to minimize that risk. That information can be gathered through a patient history, a physical examination, and appropriate laboratory tests. Chapter 14 contains a more detailed review of preoperative evaluation.

POSTOPERATIVE EVALUATION

The postoperative period should be considered critical for all patients. Because of the possibility of unforeseen complications, it is essential that patients be continually monitored after any type of surgery.

Body Temperature

After surgery, every patient should have its rectal temperature measured hourly until it reaches 100° F, and then every 4 to 12 hours based on orders prepared by the doctor. A 1- or 2-degree increase in rectal temperature for the first few postoperative days is a normal physiologic response to the trauma of major surgery. A higher or more prolonged temperature increase may indicate infection.

Body Weight

Daily monitoring of a surgical patient's body weight gives a measure of the animal's nutritional status and general body condition. One of the most frequently neglected aspects of postoperative patient care is provision of adequate nutrition. The healing process after surgery increases an animal's nutritional needs, particularly for protein. Those needs must be met so that healing can proceed without delay.

Attitude/Mentation

An animal's behavior during the immediate postoperative period can give important information about the amount of pain it is enduring and possible complications that might be developing. If a patient is very depressed, the reasons for that state must be determined and appropriate treatment instituted quickly.

Appetite and Thirst

Surgical patients must receive adequate nutrition and fluid intake. Animals should begin eating and drinking as soon as possible after surgery. Opioid medications used for pain control may reduce appetite, so encouragement or temptation to eat is sometimes needed by postoperative patients. A genuine lack of interest in food or obvious nausea may indicate problems that should be investigated without delay.

Urination and Defecation

Elimination patterns give important information about kidney and GI tract function in patients recovering from surgery. GI motility and defecation may be reduced if opioids are used for pain management, but this should resolve within a day or two of discontinuing the medications. Assuming adequate fluid intake, urination should proceed normally.

Appearance of the Surgical Wound

The surgical incision should be examined at least daily during the immediate postoperative period. It should be evaluated by visual inspection as well as gentle palpation. Such abnormalities as excessive or prolonged bleeding, fluid accumulation, dramatic inflammation, and impending dehiscence (opening) of the surgical wound can be detected and corrected early if the incision is carefully evaluated.

POSTOPERATIVE COMPLICATIONS

Hemorrhage

If not quickly corrected, postoperative hemorrhage can lead to serious consequences for an animal, and even death from shock. External hemorrhage is usually relatively easy to evaluate and control because it is easily visible. Internal hemorrhage is not readily apparent and, therefore, often more serious. An animal can bleed to death through hemorrhage into the abdominal or thoracic cavity. The status of an animal's cardiovascular system should be frequently monitored during the immediate postoperative period for signs that might indicate hemorrhage. Pulse rate, capillary refill time, temperature of the extremities, and color of the mucous membranes can give valuable information on cardiovascular function.

Seroma and Hematoma

Seromas (accumulations of serum) and hematomas (accumulations of blood) beneath the surgical incision are usually caused by "dead space" left in the incision that the body naturally fills with fluid. Small seromas and hematomas are usually of cosmetic importance only, unless the skin sutures tear out. Treatment may not be indicated in cases of small seroma or hematoma but will be observed to gauge resolution. Larger seromas or hematomas may be treated with warm compresses, drainage of the fluid via needle and syringe, and possibly application of a pressure bandage.

Infection

A persistently or drastically elevated rectal temperature, depressed attitude, poor appetite, or swollen, inflamed incision are all signs of possible postoperative infection.

Postoperative infections can be superficial, subcutaneous, within a body cavity, or spread throughout the body. Superficial infection often results in a draining wound that does not heal well. Subcutaneous infections frequently progress to abscess formation. Infection in the abdominal cavity (**peritonitis**) or thoracic cavity (pleuritis) often results from a penetrating injury or damage to organs in that body cavity. Septicemia is a generalized infection that spreads via the bloodstream. Fortunately, septicemia is not common after surgery.

When the danger of postoperative infection is high, as with long or potentially contaminated procedures, the patient may be given an antibiotic during and/or following surgery.

Wound Dehiscence

Wound dehiscence (disruption of the surgical wound) is one of the most common and serious postoperative complications that can occur. Possible causes of wound dehiscence include the following:

- Suture failure (loosening, untying, breakage)
- Infection

- Tissue weakness (old or debilitated animals, hyperadrenocorticism, prolonged corticosteroid use)
- Mechanical stress (stormy anesthetic recovery, chronic vomiting, chronic cough, excessive activity)
- Poor nutrition

Early signs of surgical wound dehiscence are frequently seen within the first 3 or 4 days after surgery. They may include a serosanguineous discharge (one containing both serous fluid and blood cells) from the incision, firm or fluctuant swelling deep to (under) the suture line, and palpation of a hernial ring or loop of bowel beneath the skin.

If only the muscle layer of an abdominal incision breaks down and the skin sutures remain intact, a doughy swelling can be palpated under the skin. This is a serious situation but is not an acute emergency. A bandage should be applied for support, and the suture line should be repaired as soon as possible.

If both the muscle layer and the skin sutures of an abdominal incision break down, the animal can **eviscerate** (abdominal organs protrude through suture line). If evisceration occurs, the involved organs can become bruised and grossly contaminated, and may even be mutilated by the animal itself. This is an acute emergency that must be attended to immediately. Carefully gather the exteriorized viscera in a towel moistened with physiologic saline and hold them in place near the incision while others are preparing the animal and operating room for the repair.

PRINCIPLES OF ASEPSIS

Aseptic technique is the term used to describe all of the precautions taken to prevent contamination, and ultimately infection, of a surgical wound. Its purpose is to minimize contamination so that postoperative healing is not delayed.

CONTAMINATION AND INFECTION

Contamination of an object or a wound implies the presence of microorganisms within or on it. Contamination of a wound can, but does not necessarily, lead to infection. With infection, microorganisms in the body or a wound multiply and cause harmful effects. Fungal, protozoal, viral, and bacterial organisms can all cause contamination of the surgical area and harmful effects to the patient. Four main factors determine if infection occurs:

- *Number of microorganisms:* There must be sufficient microorganisms to overcome the defenses of the animal.
- *Virulence of the microorganisms:* This is their ability to cause disease.
- *Susceptibility of the animal:* Some individuals have a greater natural resistance to infection than others.
- *Route of exposure to the microorganisms:* Some routes of exposure are more likely to result in infection than others.

The route of exposure to microorganisms during surgery is determined by the surgical procedure. The factor that can be most significantly influenced is the number of microorganisms that enter the surgical wound, by application of strict aseptic technique before and during surgery. Improper application of methods of sanitation, sterilization, and disinfection can lead to microbial resistance and increase the risk of **nosocomial** (hospital-acquired) **infection.**

> **TECHNICIAN NOTE** Antibiotics should only be used perioperatively and postoperatively when indicated by patient status, surgery performed, or duration of surgery to reduce risk of developing antibiotic resistant microbes.

RULES OF ASEPTIC TECHNIQUE

During surgery, aseptic technique protects the exposed tissues of the patient from four main sources of potential contamination: the operative personnel, the surgical instruments and equipment, the patient itself, and the surgical environment. Proper operating room conduct and adherence to a few general rules will help minimize the possibility of contamination. All personnel must be aware of which items are sterile and which nonsterile. Sterile items should be grouped together in the operating room and kept separate from nonsterile items. Body movements should be restricted to reduce air currents. Only sterile items should touch patient tissues. When the sterility of an item is in question, always consider it contaminated.

STERILIZATION AND DISINFECTION

Sterilization refers to the destruction of all microorganisms (bacteria, viruses, spores) on a surface or object. It usually refers to objects that come in contact with sterile tissue or enter the vascular system (e.g., instruments, drapes, catheters, needles).

Disinfection is the destruction of most pathogenic microorganisms on inanimate (nonliving) objects; antisepsis is the destruction of most pathogenic microorganisms on animate (living) objects. Antiseptics are used to kill microorganisms during patient skin preparation and surgical scrubbing; however, the skin cannot be sterilized. Most disinfectants are microbicidal; that is, they kill microbes. Some disinfectants are bacteriostatic; they inhibit the growth of microbes. Common antimicrobial agents are listed in Table 15-1.

Disinfectants can be classified according to their spectrum of activity as:

- Bacteriocidal (kills bacteria)
- Bacteriostatic (inhibits growth of bacteria)
- Sporicidal (kills spores)
- Virucidal (kills viruses)
- Fungicidal (kills fungi)

Mode of Action

Different physical and chemical methods destroy or inhibit microorganisms in several ways:

Some act by damaging microbial cell walls or membranes. Others act by interfering with microbial cell enzyme activity or metabolism or by destroying microbial cell contents by oxidation, hydrolysis, reduction, coagulation, protein denaturation, or the formation of salt. The effectiveness of all microbial control methods depends on the following factors:

TABLE 15-1 Common Antimicrobial Chemical Agents

AGENTS	MAJOR MODE OF ACTION	APPLICATIONS
Soaps	Disrupt cell membranes and increases permeability	Cleansing, mechanical removal of microorganisms
Detergents	Disrupt cell membranes by combining with lipids and proteins; leak N and P compounds out of cells	Cleansing, bactericidal action
Quaternary ammonium compounds	Cause changes in cell permeability, neutralized phospholipids	Disinfection of surfaces
Bisdiguanide compounds (chlorhexidine)	Alter cell-wall permeability, protein precipitation; rapid action broad spectrum	Routine skin preparation
Povidone-iodophor compounds	Damage cell wall, forms reactive ions and protein complexes; rapid action	Routine skin preparation
Phenol, cresols, Lysol, hexylresorcinol	Bactericidal; denaturation and precipitation of proteins	Disinfection of laboratory equipment, instruments, bench tops, garbage pails, toilets
Bis-phenols (hexachlorophene)	Bacteriostatic	Deodorants in soaps, inhibition of gram-positive bacteria; require repeated use
Cl_2 and sodium hypochlorite (bleach)	Bactericidal, oxidation of SH and NH_2 groups	Purification of water, kennel sanitation
Iodine	Bactericidal, oxidation of indole nucleus of enzymes or coenzymes	Skin disinfection, especially as tincture
H_2O_2 (hydrogen peroxide)	Bacteriostatic; mildly bactericidal	Antisepsis of cuts, minor wounds
$HgCl_2$ (zinc)	Highly bacteriostatic; precipitation of proteins	Antisepsis of cuts, minor wounds
$AgNO_3$, silver nitrate	Chemical cauterizing agent	Stops minor bleeding

1. *Time:* Most methods have minimum effective exposure times.
2. *Temperature:* Most methods are more effective as temperature increases.
3. *Concentration and preparation:* Chemical methods require appropriate concentrations of agent; disinfectants may be adversely affected by mixing with other chemicals.
4. *Organisms:* These are the type, number, and stage of growth of target organisms.
5. *Surface:* The physical and chemical properties of the surface to be treated may interfere with the method's activity; some surfaces are damaged by certain methods.
6. *Organic debris or other soils:* If present, these will dilute, render ineffective, or interfere with many control methods.
7. *Method of application:* Items may be sprayed, swabbed, or immersed in disinfectants; cotton and some synthetic materials used to apply or store chemicals may reduce their activity.

Methods used for control of microorganisms consist of chemical and physical methods. Physical methods include dry heat, moist heat, radiation, filtration, and ultrasonic vibration. Of these methods, only moist heat, in the form of steam under pressure, is routinely used for sterilization in the veterinary clinic. Chemical control methods include application of soaps, detergents, disinfectants, and gases.

Quality Control for Sterilization and Disinfection

The effectiveness of any method of microbial control must be monitored regularly. Verification of the effectiveness of microbial control should be performed at least monthly. Simply placing an item in a sterilizer and initiating the sterilization process does not ensure sterility. Failure to achieve sterility may be caused by improper cleaning (if an item cannot be disassembled and all surfaces cleaned, it cannot be sterilized), mechanical failure of the sterilizing system, improper use of sterilizing equipment, improper wrapping, poor loading technique, and/or failure to understand the underlying concepts of sterilization processes.

Indicators. Chemical indicators, or **sterilization indicators,** are generally paper strips or tape impregnated with a material that changes color when a certain temperature or chemical exposure is achieved (Fig. 15-2). Most also indicate that a specific duration of exposure has been achieved, which is critical to the sterilization process. Therefore, it is important to remember that chemical indicators do not indicate sterility. Their response indicates only that certain conditions for sterility have been met. Chemical indicators can be used with autoclaves and ethylene oxide systems and must be placed deep inside packs before sterilization. Indicator tape (Fig. 15-3) is often used to secure surgical packs and mark smaller packages of sterilized items. The tape incorporates an indicator that changes color when sterilization temperatures or chemical exposure have been reached. The color change in tape does not allow for any evaluation of duration of exposure to sterilization conditions.

Biological Testing. Because the purpose of the sterilization procedures is to eliminate the most hardy microorganisms, the presence or absence of bacterial spores can help

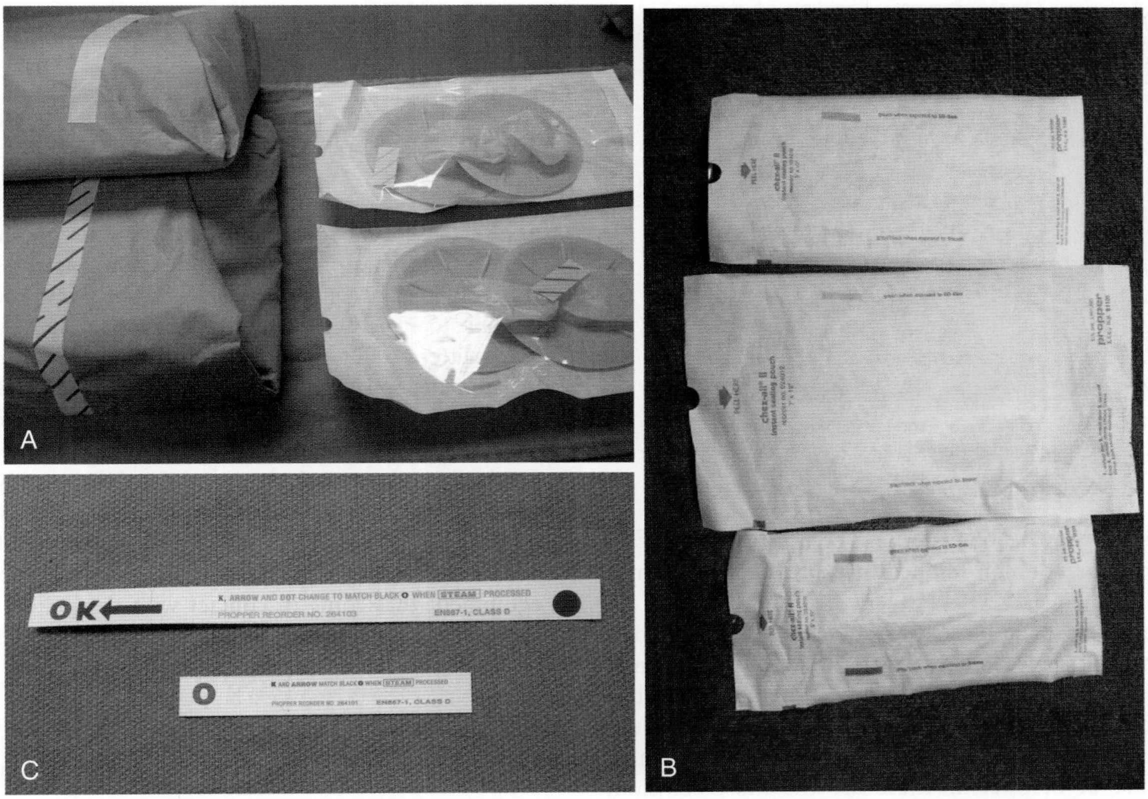

FIGURE 15-2 A, Surgical packs *(left)* and sterilization pouches *(right)*, showing sterilization indicator tape before *(top)* and after *(bottom)* sterilization; pack was autoclaved, pouch was gas sterilized. B, Sterilization pouches, paper side indicators before processing *(top)*, after ethylene oxide (EO) gas sterilization *(middle)*, and after autoclave sterilization *(bottom)*. C, Sterilization indicators typically packed inside surgical instrument packs; after autoclave sterilization *(top)*, and before autoclave sterilization *(bottom)*.

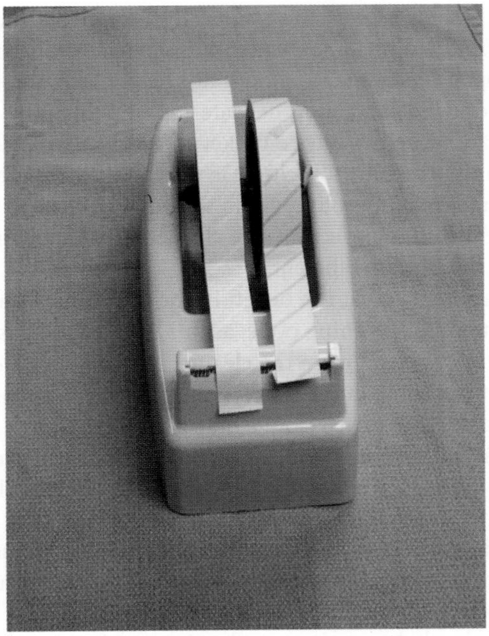

FIGURE 15-3 Sterilization indicator tape may be used on all types of pack wrapping: paper, cloth, or plastic. Autoclave indicator tape *(left)*, ethylene oxide indicator tape *(right)*.

verify proper sterilization conditions. To perform a biological test of sterility conditions, commercially available bacterial spores are exposed to autoclave or ethylene oxide sterilization conditions and then cultured. Bacterial spores should be killed by sterilization so no bacterial colonies should be present after culturing. This is the recommended method for verification of proper autoclave operation in veterinary clinics.

Another test used to verify sterility is the surface sampling technique. The procedure involves swabbing the test surface (i.e., surgical equipment) with a sterile swab. The swab is then transferred to a suitable media plate for growth. This method is recommended for ensuring proper disinfection of surgical suites in veterinary clinics.

Steam Sterilization

Pressurized steam is the most efficient and common method of sterilization used in veterinary clinics. Steam destroys microbes via cellular protein denaturation. To destroy all living microorganisms, the correct relationship among temperature, pressure, and exposure time is critical. If steam is contained in a closed compartment under increased pressure, the temperature increases as long as the volume of the compartment remains the same. If items are exposed long enough to steam at a specified temperature

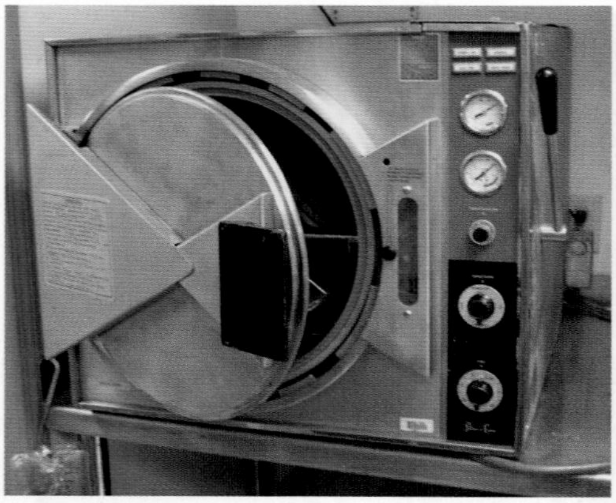

FIGURE 15-4 Large autoclave found in veterinary hospitals. This model is installed on a custom metal shelf. It will process four large surgical packs and numerous individually wrapped items in each load.

and pressure, they become sterile. The unit used to create this environment of high-temperature, pressurized steam is called an **autoclave.**

Several types of autoclaves are available. Gravity displacement autoclaves involve water that is heated in a chamber. The continued application of heat by an electric element creates pressure within the chamber; this pressure raises the boiling point of the water and thus the ultimate temperature of the steam. These are the most common type of autoclave in veterinary clinics and are known as gravity displacement autoclaves because the steam gradually displaces the air contained within the chamber—the air is forced out through a vent (Fig. 15-4). A prevacuum autoclave is a much larger and more costly machine that is equipped with a boiler to generate steam and a vacuum system. Air is forced out of the loaded chamber by means of the vacuum pump. Steam at 121° C (250° F) or more is introduced into the chamber; the steam immediately fills the chamber to eliminate the vacuum.

Autoclaves consistently achieve complete sterility, are inexpensive, and are easy to operate. They are safe for most surgical instruments and equipment, drapes and gowns, suture materials, sponges, and some plastic and rubber items. Achieving complete sterility depends on saturated steam of the appropriate temperature having contact with all objects within the autoclave for a sufficient length of time. Heat is the killing agent in the autoclave, and steam is the vector that supplies the heat and promotes penetration of the heat. Pressure is the means to create adequately heated steam. Complete sterilization of most items is achieved after 9 to 15 minutes of exposure to 121° C (250° F). The temperature of steam at sea level is 100° C (212° F); an increase in pressure results in an increase in the temperature of the steam. The minimum effective pressure of the autoclave is 15 psi, which provides steam at 121° C (250° F). Because the autoclave produces intense heat and pressure, the steam must be vented prior to opening the door once the sterilization cycle is complete. Always keep your face and hands away from the vent when allowing the steam to dissipate and stand back from the autoclave door when opening it to avoid exposure to any residual heat or steam that may be present.

CARE AND MAINTENANCE OF SURGICAL INSTRUMENTS AND SUPPLIES

Good surgical instruments are a valuable investment and must be used and maintained properly to prevent corrosion, pitting, and/or discoloration. Instruments should be rinsed in cool water as soon after the surgical procedure as possible to avoid drying of blood, tissue, saline, or other foreign matter on them. Many manufacturers recommend that instruments be rinsed, cleaned, and sterilized in distilled or deionized water, because tap water contains minerals that may cause discoloration and staining. If tap water is used for rinsing, instruments should be dried thoroughly to avoid staining. Instruments with multiple components should be disassembled before cleaning. Delicate instruments should be cleaned and sterilized separately. All surgical supplies and equipment that come in contact with the patient or other surgical equipment, such as Mayo instrument stands, must be cleaned and disinfected before use.

TECHNICIAN NOTE Daily and weekly cleaning schedules should be maintained for the operating room.

INSTRUMENT CLEANING

Ultrasonic and enzymatic methods of cleaning are effective and efficient (Fig. 15-5). Ultrasonic cleaners work by producing sinusoidal energy waves at a high frequency. Before putting soiled instruments in an ultrasonic cleaner, they should be washed in cleaning solution to remove all visible debris. Dissimilar metals (e.g., chrome and stainless steel) should not be mixed in the same cycle. All instruments should be placed in the ultrasonic cleaner with their ratchets and boxlocks open. Instruments should not be piled on top of each other to avoid damaging delicate instruments. The instruments are placed in a wire basket to be placed in the ultrasonic unit. The ultrasonic unit is then filled with water and ultrasonic cleaning solution and the basket placed in the solution. The lid is closed and the cleaner is switched on. Usually, 15 minutes is sufficient.

Instruments must not be left in the ultrasonic cleaner for longer than the cleaning cycle, as this may lead to rust. They should be removed from the cleaner, rinsed, lubricated, and dried at the completion of the cycle. Dry carefully, as water trapped in areas such as joints may lead to corrosion.

If an ultrasonic cleaner is not available, instruments should be manually cleaned as thoroughly as possible, paying particular attention to boxlocks, serrations, and hinges. Nylon brushes and cool cleaning solution may be used for most instruments. Rasps and serrated parts of instruments may require a wire brush. A cleaning solution with a neutral pH should be used to avoid staining. Cleaning solutions should be prepared as instructed by the manufacturer and changed frequently. Enzymatic solutions may be used to

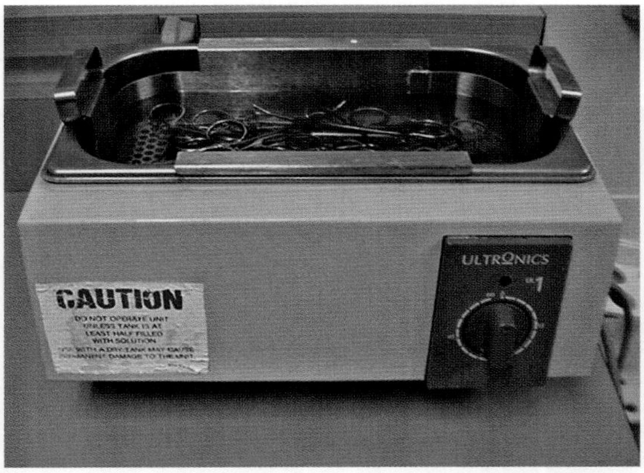

FIGURE 15-5 Ultrasonic cleaning unit. (From Tear M: *Small animal surgical nursing,* ed 2, St Louis, 2012, Mosby.)

remove proteinaceous materials from general surgical instruments and endoscopic equipment.

INSTRUMENT LUBRICATING AND AUTOCLAVING

Autoclaving is not a substitute for proper instrument cleaning. Before they are autoclaved, instruments with boxlocks and hinges and power equipment should be lubricated with instrument milk or surgical lubricants. Do not use industrial oils to lubricate instruments because they interfere with steam sterilization. All instruments should be allowed to thoroughly air dry before packing them into a surgical pack. The procedure for wrapping items is based on enhancing the ease of sterilization and preserving sterility of the item, not for convenience or personal preference. Before they are packed, instruments are separated and placed in order of their intended use. If steam or gas sterilization is used, the selected wrap should be penetrable by steam/gas, impermeable to microbes, durable, and flexible.

Specific guidelines should be followed when preparing packs for steam and gas sterilization to allow maximal penetration. Small items may be wrapped, sterilized, and stored in self-sealing (peel and seal) or heat-sealable paper/plastic peel pouches (Fig. 15-6), or regular cloth/muslin/drape wrapping material.

Packed instruments can be placed in a tray or wrapped individually. The pack is wrapped using at least two layers of material. A presterilization wrap for steam sterilization consists of two thicknesses of two-layer muslin or non-woven (paper) barrier materials. The poststerilization wrap (after sterilization and proper cool down period) consists of a waterproof, heat-sealable plastic dust cover; this wrap is not necessary if the item is used within 24 hours of sterilization. Always take care to wrap packs tightly so that the drape material does not contact the inner wall of the autoclave. The instrument pack is sealed with autoclave tape and labeled with date, contents, and operator. Autoclave tape provides verification that the outside of the pack was exposed to appropriate sterilization temperatures. Surgical packs should not exceed 30 × 30 × 50 cm (12 × 12 × 20 inches) in size and 5.5 kg (12 lb) in weight.

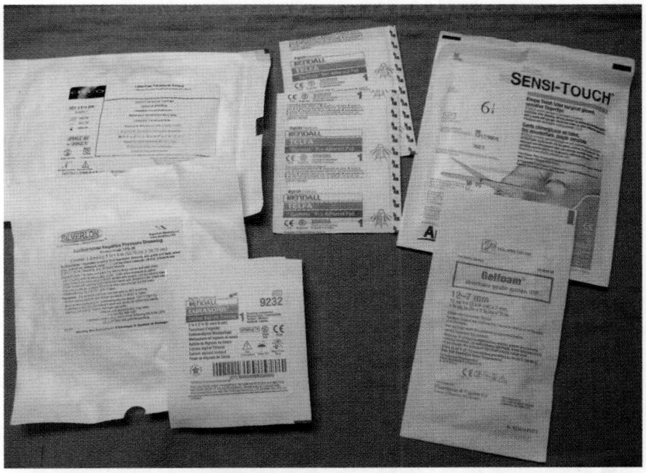

FIGURE 15-6 Presterilized items packaged in paper. Paper is generally suitable for steam or gas sterilization.

Individual instruments can also be placed into sterilization pouches (see Fig. 15-2, *B*). These pouches usually incorporate a chemical sterilization indicator. Many sterilization pouches are transparent, allowing easy visualization of contents. The pouches are often self-sealing or you may use autoclave tape to close the pouch. Double wrapping in pouches can be used for particularly delicate or sharp instruments. Always mark items with the date that the item was autoclaved.

For steam and gas sterilization, instruments should be organized on a lint-free towel placed on the bottom of a perforated metal instrument tray. A chemical sterilization indicator is included in every pack. This provides verification that the inside of the pack was exposed to appropriate sterilization temperatures for the correct amount of time.

Instruments with boxlocks should be autoclaved opened. A 3- to 5-mm space between instruments is recommended for proper steam/gas circulation. Complex instruments should be disassembled when possible and power equipment should be lubricated before sterilization. Items with a lumen should have a small amount of water flushed through them immediately before steam sterilization, because water vaporizes and forces air out of the lumen. Conversely, moisture left in tubing placed in a gas sterilizer may decrease the sterilization efficacy below the lethal point. Containers (e.g., saline bowl) should be placed with the open end facing up or horizontally; containers with lids should have the lid slightly ajar. Multiple basins should be stacked with a towel between each. A standard count of radiopaque surgical sponges should be included in each pack. A sterilization indicator is placed in the center of each pack before wrapping. Solutions should be steam sterilized separately from instruments using the slow exhaust phase. Linens may be steam sterilized.

WRAPPING INSTRUMENT PACKS

Packs may not be completely sterilized if they are wrapped too tightly or improperly loaded in the autoclave or gas sterilizer container (Procedure 15-1). Instrument packs should be positioned vertically (on edge) and longitudinally in an

PROCEDURE 15-1 Wrapping a Pack

1. Place a large unfolded wrap diagonally in front of you.
2. Place the instrument tray in the center of the wrap so that an imaginary line drawn from one corner of the wrap to the opposite corner is perpendicular to the two sides of the instrument tray (Fig. 1).

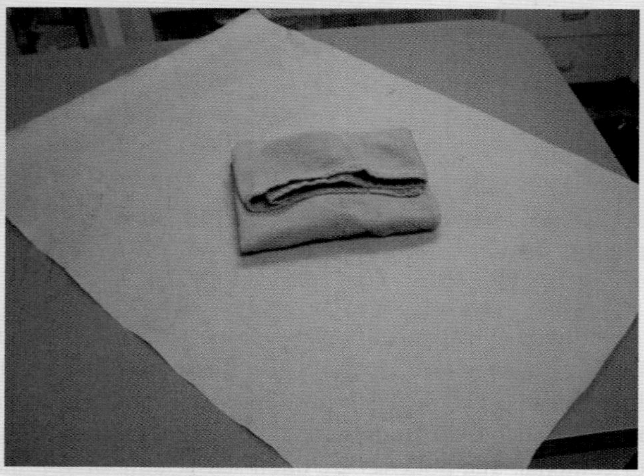

FIGURE 1 Position pack contents on wrapping cloth or paper.

3. Fold the corner of the wrap that is closest to you over the instrument tray and to its far side, tucking it underneath the tray (Fig. 2).

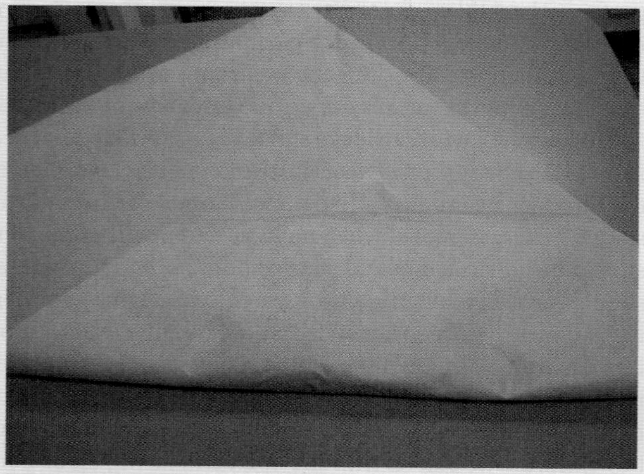

FIGURE 2 Fold first flap away from you, tucking it under pack, with a tab out.

4. Fold the right corner over the pack as shown in Fig. 3.
5. Fold the left corner over the pack similarly (Fig. 4).
6. Fold the final corner over the wrap over the tray, tucking it in tightly under the previous two folds. Fold the tip of the final fold so that it is exposed for easy unwrapping (Fig. 5).
7. Wrap the pack in a second layer of cloth or paper, securing the final tab with autoclave or gas sterilization indicator tape for ease of grasping and opening.

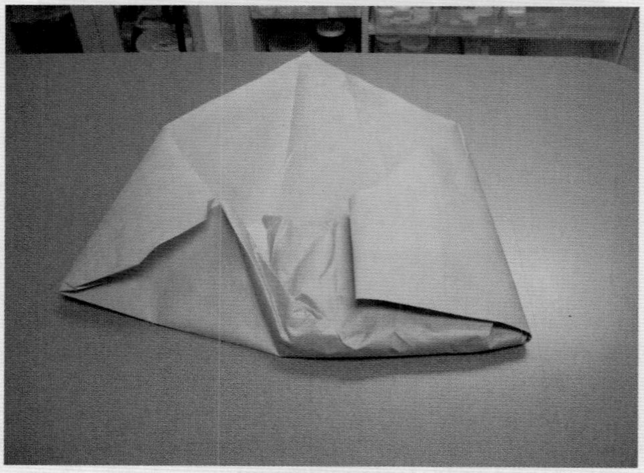

FIGURE 3 Fold right side flap.

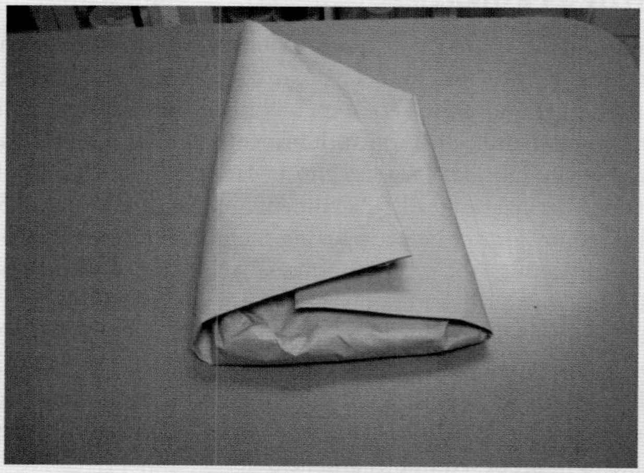

FIGURE 4 Fold left side flap.

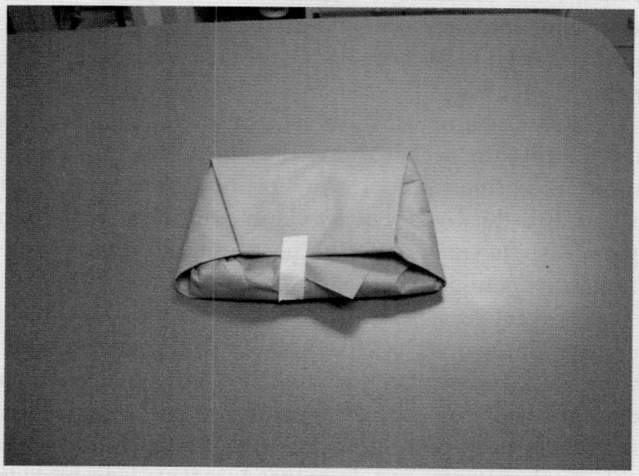

FIGURE 5 Fold final flap under the two side flaps, and seal with indicator tape.

autoclave. Heavy packs should be placed at the periphery, where steam enters the chamber. Allow a small amount of air space between each pack to facilitate steam flow (1 to 2 inches between each pack and surrounding walls). Load linen packs so that the fabric layers are oriented vertically (on edge). Do not stack linen packs on top of one another, because the increased thickness decreases steam penetration. Careful attention to exact standards for preparing, packaging, and loading of supplies is necessary for effective steam and gas sterilization.

GAS STERILIZATION

Ethylene oxide is the most common form of gas sterilization used in the veterinary hospital. It is a flammable, explosive liquid that becomes an effective sterilizing agent when mixed with carbon dioxide or Freon. Equipment that cannot withstand the extreme temperature and pressures of steam sterilization (e.g., endoscopes, cameras, plastics, power cables) can be safely sterilized with ethylene oxide. Environmental and safety hazards associated with ethylene oxide are numerous and severe. It is critical to the safety of the patient and hospital personnel that all materials sterilized with ethylene oxide be aerated according to instructions provided by the manufacturer of an ethylene oxide gas sterilization unit. Porous materials or those that will be used as implants in patients should generally be aerated for 24 hours following gas sterilization.

Items should be clean and dry before ethylene oxide sterilization; moisture and organic material bond with ethylene oxide and leave a toxic residue. If an item cannot be disassembled and all surfaces cleaned, it cannot be sterilized. Items are packed and loaded loosely to allow gas circulation. Complex items (e.g., power equipment) are disassembled before processing. Items that cannot be sterilized with ethylene oxide include acrylics, some pharmaceutical items, and solutions.

COLD CHEMICAL STERILIZATION

Liquid chemicals used for sterilization must be noncorrosive to the items being sterilized. These items are usually placed in a special tray kept in the surgery area (Fig. 15-7). Glutaraldehyde solution is noncorrosive and provides a safe means of sterilizing delicate, lensed instruments (endoscopes, cystoscopes, bronchoscopes). Most equipment that can be safely immersed in water can be safely immersed in 3% glutaraldehyde. Table 15-2 lists some commonly used cold sterilization agents. Items for sterilization should be clean and dry. Organic matter (e.g., blood, pus, saliva) may prevent the chemical sterilization agent from penetrating the instrument crevices or joints. Residual water causes chemical dilution. Complex instruments should be disassembled before immersion. Immersion times suggested by the manufacturer should be followed (e.g., for sterilization in 3% glutaraldehyde, 10 hours at 20° to 25° C; for disinfection, 10 minutes at 20° to 25° C). After the appropriate immersion time, instruments should be rinsed thoroughly with sterile water and dried with sterile towels to avoid damaging the patients' tissues.

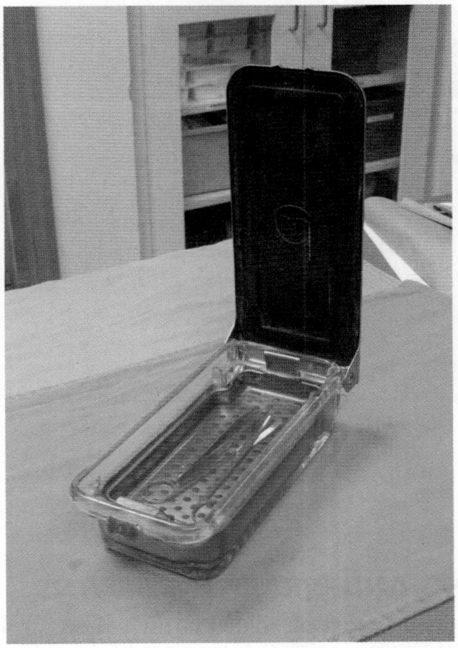

FIGURE 15-7 Cold sterilization tray. Gasket on inner surface of lid will form a seal when lid is closed, preventing airborne microbes from contaminating contents and preventing evaporation of chemical disinfectant.

TABLE 15-2 Antimicrobial Activity of Commonly Used Cold Sterilants

	DESTRUCTIVE ACTION AGAINST				
AGENT	BACTERIA	TUBERCLE BACILLI	SPORES	FUNGI	VIRUSES
Alcohol-ethyl (70% to 90%)	+	+	0	+	±
Alcohol-isopropyl (70% to 90%)	++	+	0	+	±
Alcohol-iodine (2%)	++	+	±	+	+
Formalin (37%)	+	+	+	+	+
Glutaraldehyde (buffered, 2%) (Cidex)	++	+	++	+	+
Iodine (2% to 5% aqueous)	++	+	±	+	+
Iodophors (1%) (povidone-iodine complex)	+	+	±	±	+
Mercurials (Merthiolate)	±	0	0	+	±
Phenolic derivatives (0.5% to 3%)	+	+	0	+	±
Quats (benzalkonium chloride, 1:750 to 1:1000)	++	0	0	+	0

++, Very good; +, good; ±, fair (greater concentration or more time needed); 0, no activity.

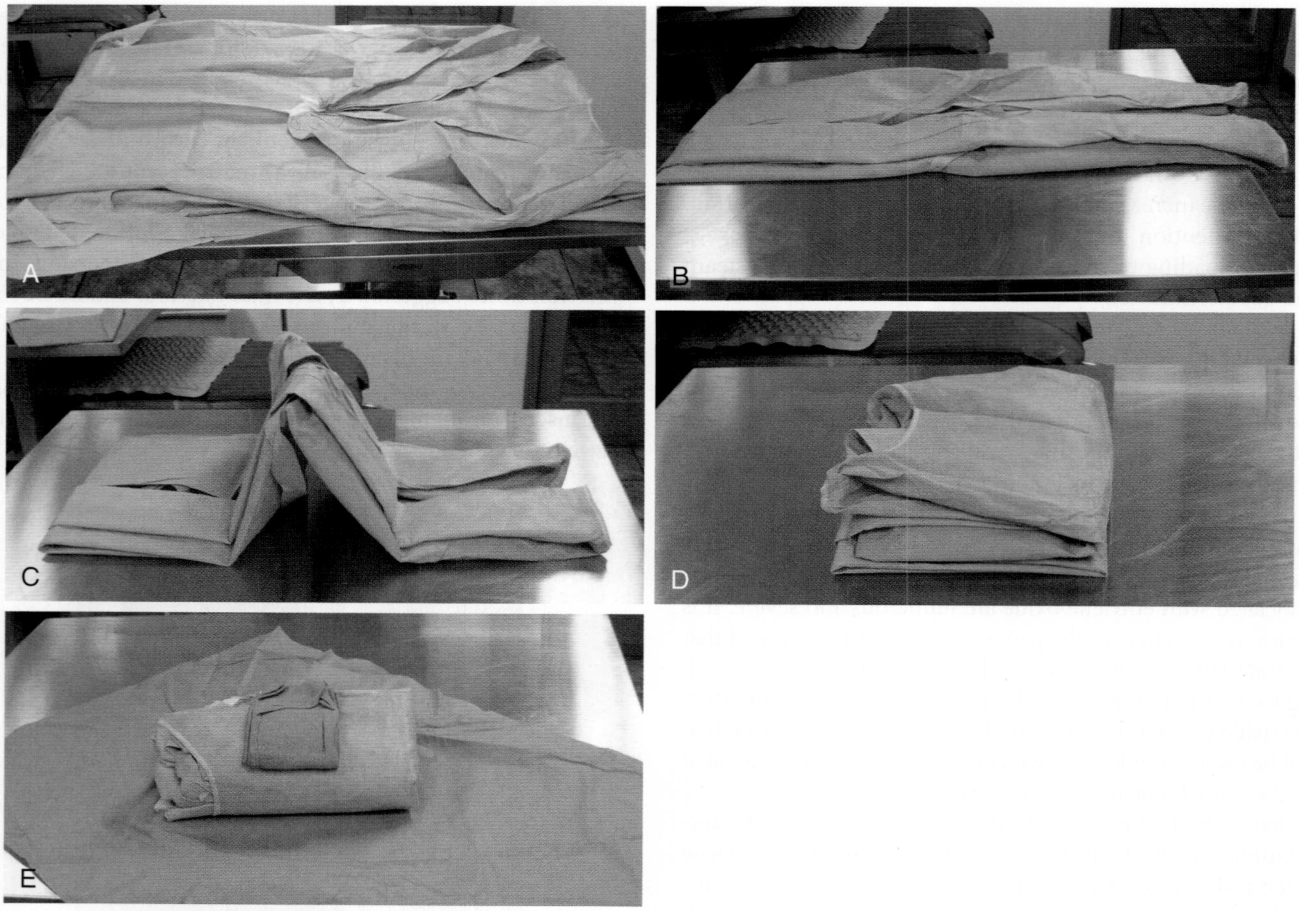

FIGURE 15-8 Wrapping a gown. **A,** Lay gown on flat surface, with front of gown up and sleeves toward center. **B,** Fold sides to the center, and then fold gown in half longitudinally. **C,** Fanfold the gown from the bottom to the neck. **D,** The gown should finish with the interior neck and shoulders on top. **E,** Place a fanfolded hand towel with the gown, and set is ready for wrapping.

FOLDING AND WRAPPING GOWNS

Surgical gowns must be folded so that they can be easily donned without breaking sterile technique (Fig. 15-8). Place the gown on a clean, flat surface with the front of the gown facing up. Fold the sleeves neatly toward the center of the gown with the cuffs of the sleeves facing the bottom hem. Fold the sides to the center so that the side seams are aligned with the sleeve seams. Then, fold the gown in half longitudinally (sleeves inside the gown). Ties should be placed so that they can be touched without contaminating the gown. Starting with the bottom hem of the gown, fanfold it toward the neck. Fanfolding allows compact storage and simple unfolding. Fold a hand towel in half horizontally and fanfold it into about four folds. Place it on top of the folded gown, leaving one corner turned back to allow it to be easily grasped. Wrap the gown and towel in two layers of paper or cloth wrap as described.

FOLDING AND WRAPPING DRAPES

Drapes should be folded so that the fenestration (or the center of an unfenestrated drape) can be properly positioned over the surgical site without contaminating the drape (Fig. 15-9). Lay the drape out flat with the ends of the fenestration perpendicular and the sides of the fenestration parallel to you. Grasp the end of the drape closest to you and fanfold one half of the drape toward the center. Make sure the edge of the drape is on top to allow it to be easily grasped during unfolding. Then, turn the drape around and fanfold the other half toward the center, similarly. Next, fanfold one end of the drape to the center; repeat with the other end. Note that when the drape is properly folded, the fenestration is on the ventral outermost aspect of the drape. Fold the drape in half and wrap it in two layers of paper or cloth wrap as described previously for packs.

TECHNICIAN NOTE Drapes are folded accordion fashion to allow easy unfolding and placement, without the possibility of contamination.

STORING STERILIZED ITEMS

Packs are allowed to cool and dry individually on racks when removed from the autoclave; placing instrument packs on top of each other during cooling may promote

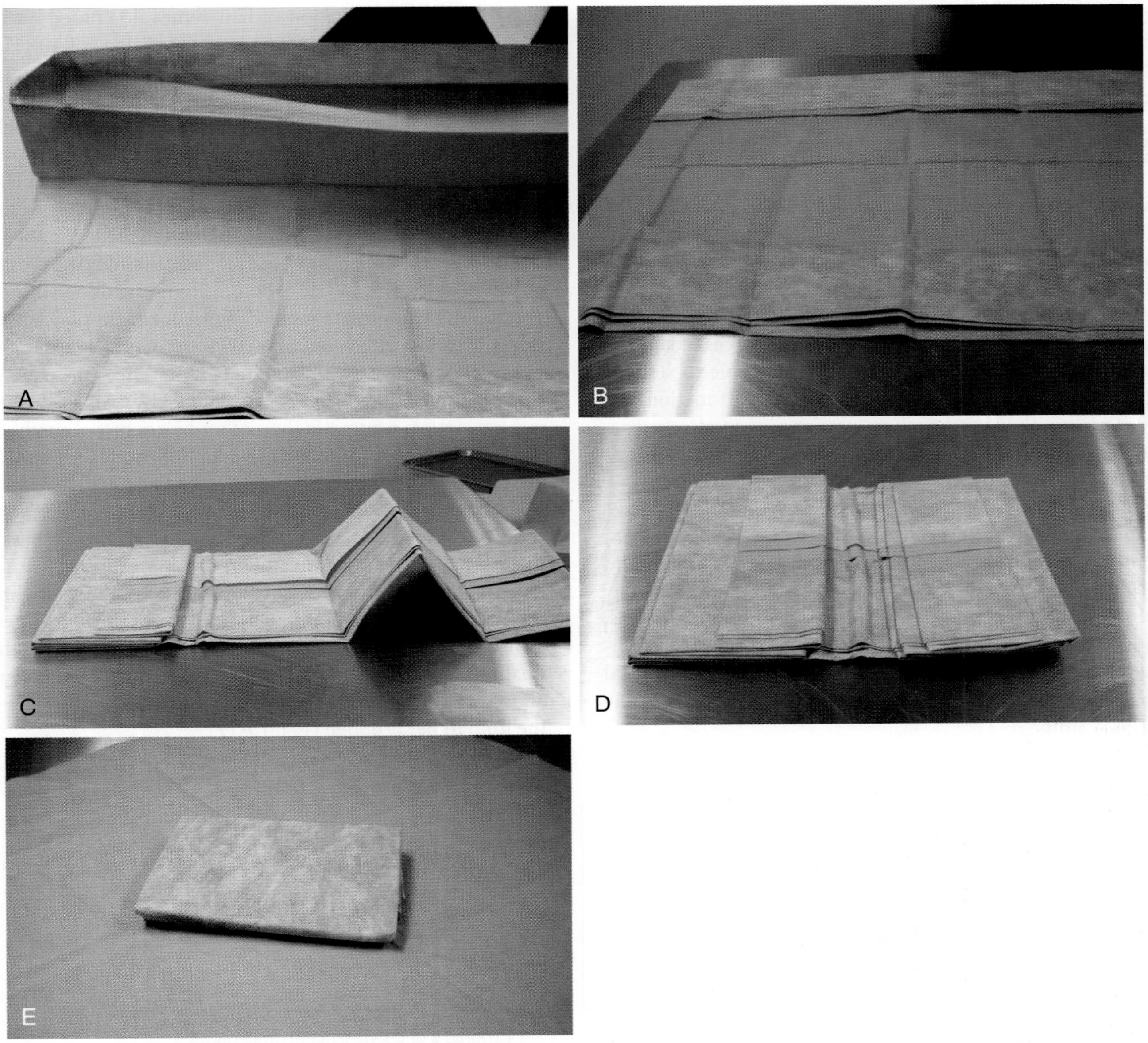

FIGURE 15-9 Accordion pleat folding technique. **A** and **B**, Fold item (drape) lengthwise as shown. **C** and **D**, Fold item accordion style again, widthwise. **E**, Position item as shown to wrap.

condensation of moisture, resulting in contamination via strike-through (wick action). After sterile packs are completely dry, they should be stored in waterproof dust covers in closed cabinets (rather than uncovered on open shelves) to protect them from moisture or exposure to particulate matter, such as dust-borne bacteria. Sterile packs are labeled with the date on which the item was sterilized and a control lot number to trace an unsterile item. Heat-sealed waterproof dust covers are placed on items not routinely used. The shelf life of a sterilized pack varies with the type of outer wrap (Table 15-3). However, in human medicine, current practice is to consider sterile items to be sterile for an indefinite period unless some event occurs that could compromise stability. Examples of events include the pack being opened, becoming wet, or being

TABLE 15-3 Recommended Storage Times for Sterilized Packs*

WRAPPER	SHELF-LIFE
Double-wrapped, two-layer muslin	4 weeks
Double-wrapped, two-layer muslin, heat-sealed in dust covers after sterilization	6 months
Double-wrapped, two-layer muslin, tape-sealed in dust covers after sterilization	2 months
Double-wrapped nonwoven barrier materials (paper)	6 months
Paper/plastic-peel pouches, heat-sealed	1 year
Plastic peel pouches, heat-sealed	1 year

*Note that sterilized items from hospitals adopting event-related sterility assurance have an indefinite shelf-life.

dropped. Best practices in sterilization also include sterilizing only those items that will be used within a few days or a week. Keeping all items sterile at all times wastes storage space and time.

PREPARATION OF THE OPERATIVE SITE

Surgery puts a patient at risk for nosocomial infections. Because most surgical infections develop from bacteria that enter the incision during surgery, proper preparation of the surgical site is crucial to reduce the likelihood of infection. Resident skin flora (particularly *Staphylococcus aureus* and *Streptococcus* spp.) are the most common sources of surgical wound contaminants. Although it is impossible to sterilize skin without impairing its natural protective function and interfering with wound healing, proper preoperative preparation reduces the likelihood of infection.

HAIR REMOVAL AND SKIN SCRUBBING

Before preparing the patient for surgery, verify the patient's identity, surgical procedure being performed, and surgical site. It may be useful to bathe the animal the day before the surgical procedure to remove loose hair, debris, and external parasites. Preparing patients for surgery includes clipping hair and scrubbing the skin at the surgical site. These procedures should be performed outside of the surgical suite.

The extent and location of hair removal is based on the type of surgical procedure to be performed (Fig. 15-10). Hair should be liberally clipped around the proposed incision site so that the incision can be extended if needed, while still remaining within a sterile field. A general guideline is to clip 20 cm on each side of the incision. The hair can be removed most effectively with an Oster-type clipper and a #40 clipper blade. Patients with a dense haircoat may be clipped first with a medium blade (#10). The higher the blade number is, the shorter the remaining hair. Clippers should be held using a "pencil grip" and initial clipping should be done with the grain of the hair growth pattern. Subsequent clipping should be against the pattern of hair growth to obtain a closer clip. This will minimize the likelihood of irritation to the patient's skin (commonly referred to as "clipper burn"). Depilatory creams are less traumatic than other hair removal methods, but they induce a mild dermal lymphocytic reaction. They are most useful in irregular areas where adequate hair clipping is difficult. Razors are occasionally used for hair removal (e.g., around the eye), but they cause microlacerations in skin that may increase irritation and promote infection. After hair has been clipped from the site, loose hair is removed with a vacuum. To enhance manipulation of limbs during surgery, a "hanging-leg" preparation may be done. This requires that the limb be circumferentially clipped; the limb is hung from an intravenous pole during preparation to allow the sides of the limb to be scrubbed (Fig. 15-11).

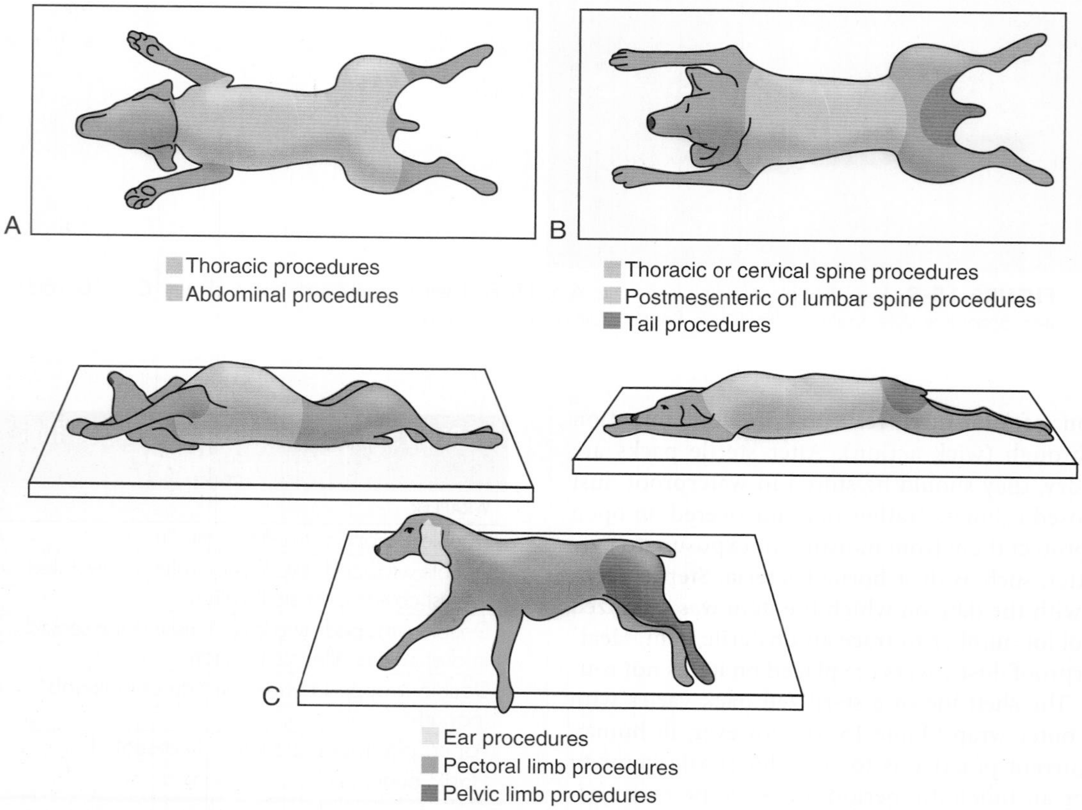

FIGURE 15-10 Hair-removal patterns for selected surgical procedures. A, Dorsal recumbency. B, Sternal recumbency. C, Lateral recumbency.

> TECHNICIAN NOTE Sterile patient preparation generally consists of three rounds of alternating antiseptic solution with saline rinse, and every pass with gauze moves in a circular motion from the anticipated incision site radiating outward.

Before transporting the animal to the surgical site, the incision is given a general cleansing scrub. Some medications may reduce tear production and minimize blink reflex and some clinicians will request that the ophthalmic antibiotic ointment or lubricant be placed on the cornea and conjunctiva preoperatively. In male dogs undergoing abdominal procedures, the prepuce may be flushed with an antiseptic solution. The skin is scrubbed with germicidal soap to remove debris and reduce bacterial populations in preparation for surgery. The area is lathered well until all dirt and oils are removed. This is a generous scrub that often encompasses the hair surrounding the operation site to remove unattached hair and dander that may be disturbed during draping. This "dirty prep" (done outside the OR) will often consist of chlorhexidine and saline, and the lather step may be left in place for 60 to 120 seconds to ensure adequate contact time. Other options for scrubbing solutions include iodophors, alcohols, hexachlorophene, and quaternary ammonium salts. Alcohol is not effective against spores, but it rapidly kills bacteria and acts as a defatting agent. However, it must not be used on critical patients where the possibility of defibrillator use exists. Using alcohol by itself is not recommended, but it is sometimes used in conjunction with povidone-iodine. Hexachlorophene and quaternary ammonium salts are less effective than other available agents.

> TECHNICIAN NOTE Chlorhexidine and povidone-iodine are the most commonly used antiseptic scrub/prep agents.

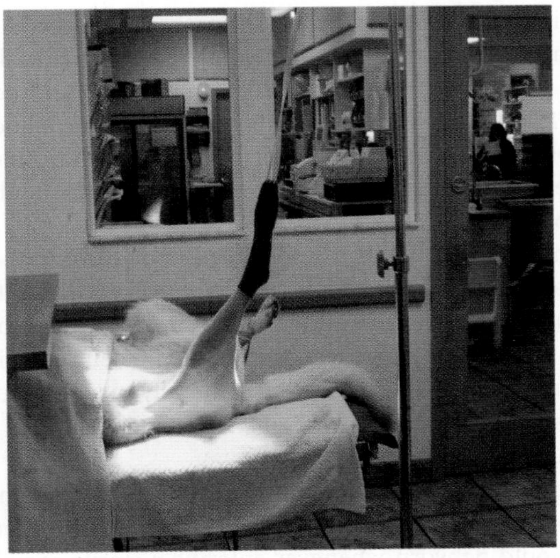

FIGURE 15-11 Manipulation of the limb during orthopedic procedures may be facilitated with a "hanging-leg" preparation. The limb is clipped circumferentially and carefully suspended from an intravenous pole with tape. The patient is positioned for medial rear limb surgery.

POSITIONING

Before sterile application of the epidermal germicide, the animal is moved to the operating room and positioned so that the operative site is accessible to the surgeon and secured with ropes, sandbags, troughs, or tape. The animal is generally placed on a water circulating heating pad and provided with a warm air circulating blanket (Fig. 15-12); if **electrocautery** is being used, a ground plate should be positioned under the patient. Anesthetic monitoring equipment is then attached and baseline vital signs evaluated before proceeding with sterile prep.

STERILE SKIN PREPARATION

Sterile preparation of the surgical site begins after transporting and positioning the animal on the operating table. Scrubbing the skin for surgery is a multistep process (Procedure 15-2). An appropriate antiseptic solution should be applied using sterile gauze.

Frequently, when using povidone-iodine and alcohol, the site is scrubbed alternatively with each solution three times to allow for 5 minutes of contact time. However, using alcohol between the povidone-iodine scrubs decreases contact time of povidone-iodine with skin and may decrease its efficacy. Excess solution on the table or accumulated in body "pockets" should be blotted with a sterile towel or sponges. When the final povidone-iodine scrub is completed, a 10% povidone-iodine solution should be sprayed or painted on the site. If chlorhexidine is the preparation solution, it may be rinsed with saline. Because chlorhexidine binds to keratin, contact time is less critical than with povidone-iodine. Two 30-second applications are considered adequate for antimicrobial activity.

PREPARATION OF THE SURGICAL TEAM

SURGICAL ATTIRE

All persons entering the operating room suite, regardless of whether a surgery is in progress or not, should be dressed in appropriate surgical attire. To minimize microbial

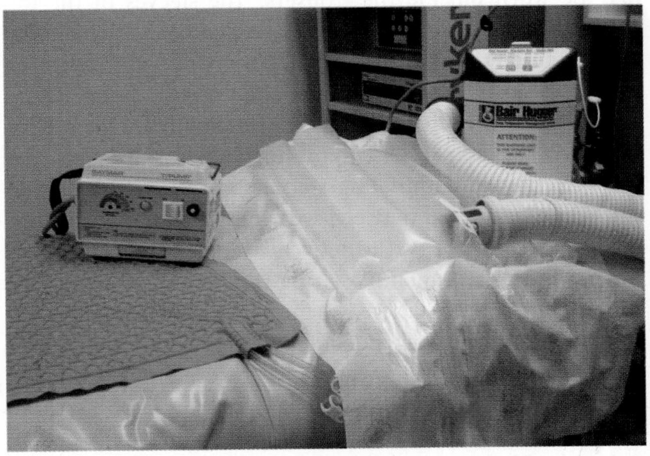

FIGURE 15-12 Patient warming systems used in the operating room: warm water circulating blanket *(left)*, warm air circulating system *(right)*.

PROCEDURE 15-2 Patient Skin Scrub (sterile prep)

1. Gauze sponges for use in the surgical site preparation are sterilized in a pack, along with bowls into which the germicides and rinse can be poured.
2. Sponges are handled with sterile sponge forceps or the gloved hand, using aseptic technique.
3. The scrub should begin at the intended incision (Fig. 1) and continue out in concentric circles to an area at least 2 inches larger than the expected size of the sterile field needed (Fig. 2).
4. The scrub should be completed three times, and may incorporate a rinse with saline or sterile water between each scrub.
5. Sponges are discarded after reaching the periphery (Fig. 3).

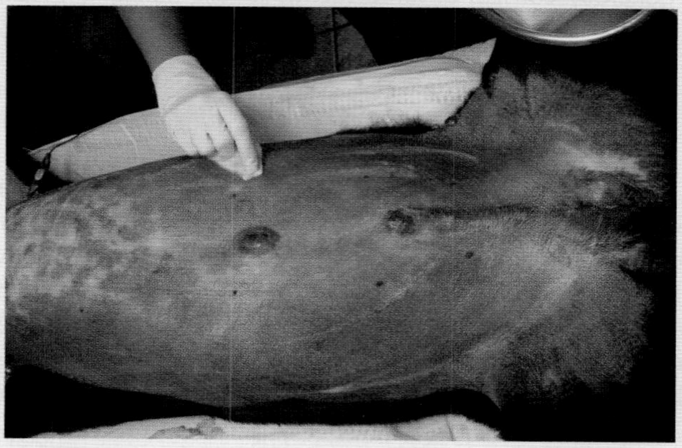

FIGURE 2 The scrub should continue out in concentric circles from the site.

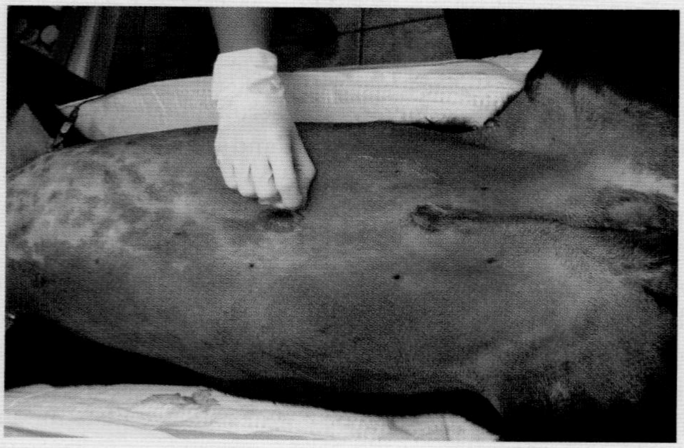

FIGURE 1 The scrub should begin at the intended incision.

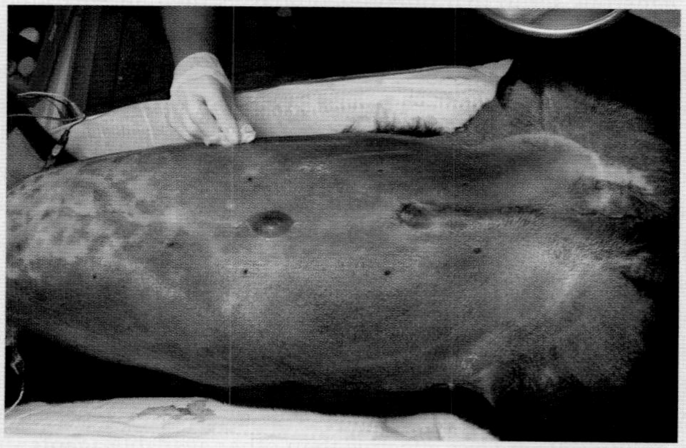

FIGURE 3 When the edge of the shaved area is reached, the gauze is discarded.

contamination from operating room personnel, wear dedicated surgical scrub clothes rather than street clothes in the operating suite. With two-piece pant suits, tuck loose-fitting tops into the trousers. Tunic tops that fit close to the body may be worn outside the trousers. The sleeves of the top should be short enough to allow the hands and arms to be scrubbed. Pants should have an elastic waist or drawstring closure. Nonscrubbed personnel should wear long-sleeved jackets over their scrub clothes. Jackets should be buttoned or snapped closed during use to minimize the risk of the edges' inadvertently contaminating sterile surfaces. Scrub clothes should be laundered between wearings and changed if they are visibly soiled or wet to prevent transfer of microorganisms to the environment. Wearing scrub clothes outside the surgical environment increases microbial contamination. If a scrub suit must be worn outside the surgery room, a laboratory coat or single-use gowns should be used to cover it.

Other surgical attire includes hair coverings, masks, shoecovers, gowns, and gloves. Hair is a significant carrier of bacteria; when left uncovered, it collects bacteria. Because bacterial shedding from hair increases surgical wound infection rates, complete hair coverage is necessary. Even when surgery is not in progress, caps and masks should be worn in the surgical suite. Caps should completely cover all scalp and facial hair, and masks should cover the mouth and nostrils (Fig. 15-13). Sideburns and/or beards necessitate a hood for complete coverage. Skullcaps that fail to cover the side hair above the ears and hair at the nape of the neck should not be worn.

Any footwear that is comfortable can be worn in the surgery area. Shoecovers should be donned when first entering the surgical area and should be worn when leaving it to keep shoes clean. New shoecovers are donned when returning to the surgical area. Shoecovers are generally made of reusable or disposable materials that are water repellent and resist tearing.

Masks, constructed from lint-free material containing a hydrophilic filter web sandwiched between two outer layers, should be worn whenever entering a sterile area. Their major function is to filter and contain droplets of microorganisms expelled from the mouth and nasopharynx during talking, sneezing, and coughing. Masks must be fitted over

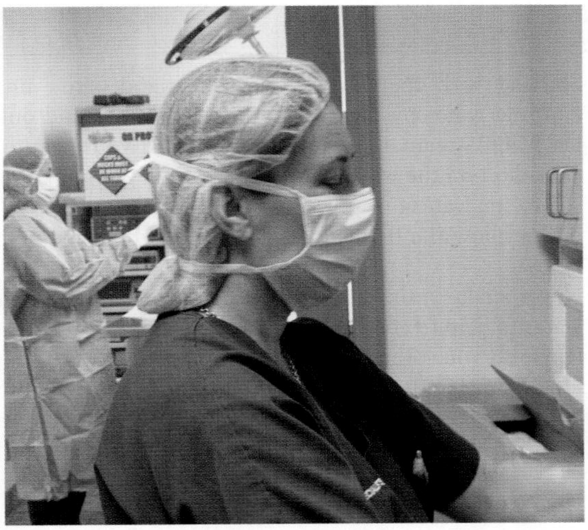

FIGURE 15-13 Hair should be covered by a bouffant-style surgical cap. This is the correct way to tie a surgical mask.

the mouth and nose and secured in a manner that prevents venting. The dorsal aspect of the mask is secured by shaping the reinforcing top edge tightly around the nose.

Surgical gowns may be reusable and made of woven materials (usually cotton), or disposable. Disposable (single-use) gowns are nonwoven and made directly from fibers rather than yarn. Loosely woven cotton is commonly used for reusable gowns. This fabric is instantly permeable to bacteria when it becomes wet. Fewer microorganisms contaminate the surgical environment when disposable (single-use) nonwoven materials are used.

THE SURGICAL SCRUB

Surgical scrubbing cleans the hands and forearms to reduce the numbers of bacteria that come in contact with the wound from scrubbed personnel during surgery. All sterile surgical team members must perform a hand and arm scrub before entering the surgical suite. Objectives of a surgical scrub include mechanical removal of dirt and oil, reduction of the transient bacterial population (bacteria deposited from the environment), and reduction of the skin's resident bacterial population. Relying on latex gloves alone (without a surgical scrub) to prevent microbial contamination is not recommended; up to 50% of surgical gloves contain holes at the completion of surgery. This proportion may increase with long or difficult surgeries.

Antimicrobial soaps or detergents used for scrubbing should be rapid-acting, broad-spectrum, and nonirritating, and they should inhibit rapid rebound microbial growth. They should not depend on accumulation for activity. The most commonly used surgical scrub solutions are chlorhexidine gluconate, povidone-iodine, and hexachlorophene.

Before scrubbing, remove all jewelry (including watches) from your hands and forearms, because they are reservoirs for bacteria. Fingernails should be free of polish and trimmed short, and cuticles should be in good condition. Artificial nails (bondings, tips, wrappings, tapes) should never be worn. More gram-negative bacteria have been cultured from the fingertips of personnel wearing artificial nails than from personnel with natural nails, both before and after handwashing. Fungi residing between an artificial nail and the natural nail can contaminate the surgical wound. Hands and forearms should be free of open lesions and breaks in skin integrity, because such skin infections may contaminate surgical wounds.

Surgical scrubs physically separate microbes from skin and inactivate them via contact with the antimicrobial solution. Two accepted methods of performing a surgical scrub are the anatomic timed scrub (5-minute scrub) and the counted brush stroke method (strokes per surface area of skin) (Procedure 15-3). Recommendations regarding the number of times one should lather and rinse during the scrub, number of strokes per surface area, and time spent on each surface vary. A sequential approach will help ensure that all skin surfaces are properly scrubbed. However, both methods ensure sufficient exposure of all skin surfaces to friction and antimicrobial solutions.

If the hands and arms are grossly soiled, lengthen scrub time or increase brush counts; however, avoid skin irritation or abrasion because this causes bacteria residing in deeper tissues (e.g., around base of hair follicles) to become more superficial, increasing the number of potentially infective organisms on the skin surface. Contact time between the antimicrobial soap or detergent should be based on documentation of product efficacy in the scientific literature. An initial 5- to 7-minute scrub for the first case of the day, followed by a 2- to 3-minute scrub between additional surgical operations is generally adequate.

Once the scrub has been started, nonsterile items cannot be handled without breaking sterility. If your hands or arms inadvertently touch a nonsterile object (including surgical personnel), repeat the scrub. During and after scrubbing, keep the hands higher than the elbows. This allows water and soap to flow from the cleanest area (hands) to a less clean area (elbow). A single scrub brush can generally be used for the entire procedure. No difference has been documented in the effectiveness of a sterilized reusable brush and disposable polyurethane brush/sponge combination.

When the scrub has been completed, dry the hands and arms with a sterile towel. When picking up the sterile towel from the table, take care not to drip water on the gown beneath it and step back from the sterile table. Hold the towel lengthwise and dry one hand and arm, working from hand to elbow with one end of the towel; use a blotting motion (Fig. 15-14). Bend over at the waist when drying the arms so that the end of the towel will not brush against your scrub suit. After one hand and arm are dry, move the dry hand to the opposite end of the towel. Dry the other hand and arm in a similar manner. Drop the towel into the proper receptacle or on the floor if a receptacle is not provided. Do not lower your hands below waist level.

GOWNING

Gowns are another barrier between the skin of the surgical team and the patient. They should be constructed of a

PROCEDURE 15-3 Surgical Personnel Scrub Procedure

1. Locate scrub brushes, antibacterial soap, and nail cleaners.
2. Remove watches, bracelets, and rings.
3. Wet hands and forearms thoroughly.
4. Apply two to three pumps of antimicrobial soap to the hands, and wash the hands and forearms.
5. Clean the nails and beneath the nails with a nail cleaner under running water.
6. Rinse the arms and forearms.
7. Apply two to three pumps of antimicrobial soap to the hand and forearms.
8. Apply two to three pumps of antimicrobial soap to the sterile scrub brush.
9. Proceed with the anatomic timed or counted method.

Following the Chosen Scrub Method

10. When both hands and arms have been scrubbed, drop the scrub brush in the sink.

11. Starting with the fingertips of one hand, rinse under running water by moving your fingertips up and out of the water stream and allowing the rest of your arm to be rinsed off on the way out of the stream.
12. Allow the water to run from fingertips to elbows.
13. Never allow the fingertips to fall below the level of your elbow.
14. Never shake your hands to shed excess water; allow the water to drip from your elbows.
15. Rinse off your other hand similarly.
16. Hold your hands upright and in front of you so that they can be seen, and proceed to the gowning and gloving area.

Anatomic Timed Method

- Start timing; scrub each side of each finger, between fingers, and back and front to the hand for 2 minutes (Fig. 1).
- Proceed to scrub the arms, keeping the hand higher than the arm (Fig. 2).
- Scrub each side of the arm to the elbow for 1 minute.
- Total scrub time is 2 to 3 minutes per hand and arm.
- Rinse the scrub brush well under running water and transfer the brush to your scrubbed hand. Do not rinse the scrubbed hand and arm at this time.
- Repeat the process on your other hand and arm.
- Move to step 10.

Counted Brush Stroke Method

- Apply 30 strokes (one stroke consists of up and down or back and forth motion) to the very tips of your fingers and thumb.
- Divide each finger and thumb into 5 parts (front/back/2 sides/tip) and apply 20 strokes to each surface, including the finger webs (Fig. 1).
- Scrub from the tip of the finger to the wrist when scrubbing the thumb, index, and small fingers.
- Divide your forearm into four planes and apply 20 strokes to each surface (Fig. 2).
- Move to step 10.

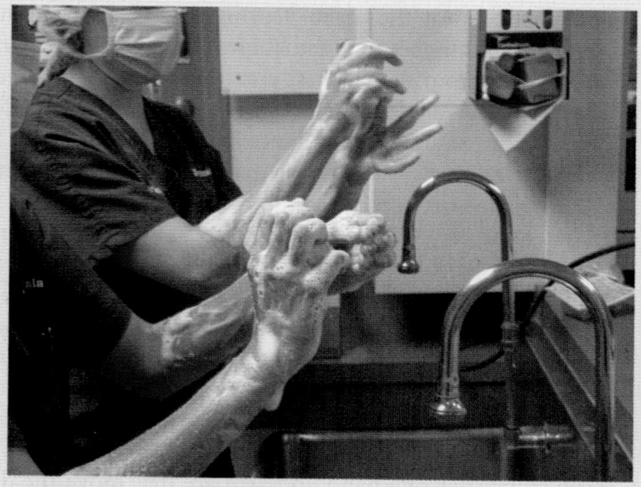

FIGURE 1 Starting with fingers (smallest to thumbs).

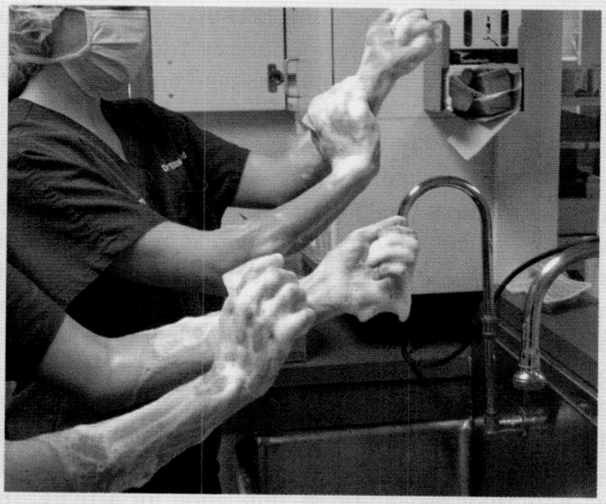

FIGURE 2 Scrubbing forearm (entire circumference).

material that prevents passage of microorganisms between sterile and nonsterile areas. Gowns should be resistant to fluid, lint accumulation, stretching, and tearing (especially at the forearm, elbow, and abdominal areas) and should be comfortable, economical, and fire resistant. Reusable or single-use disposable gowns are available.

Gowning and gloving should occur away from the surgical table and the patient to avoid dripping water onto the sterile field and contaminating it. Gowns are folded so that the inside of the gown faces outward (see Fig. 15-8). Grasp the gown firmly and gently lift it away from the table. Step back from the sterile table to allow room for gowning. Hold

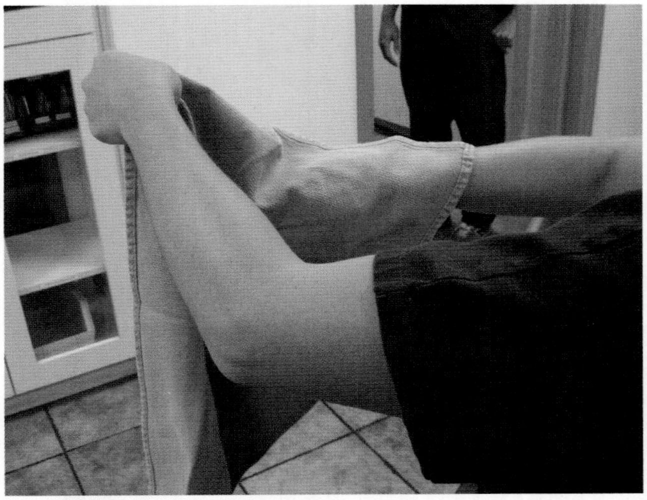

FIGURE 15-14 To dry hands using one towel, one hand picks up the towel from sterile field and drapes the towel over the other hand. One hand and then the forearm is dried at a time, using one half of the towel. The other hand and arm are then dried in a similar manner.

the gown at the shoulders and allow it to gently unfold. Do not shake the gown, because this increases the risk of contamination. Once the gown is opened, locate the armholes and guide each arm through the sleeves. Keep your hands within the cuffs of the gown. Have another person pull the gown up over your shoulders and secure it by closing the neck fasteners and tying the inside waist tie. If a sterile-back gown is used, do not secure the front tie until you have donned sterile gloves.

Latex rubber gloves are another barrier between the surgical team and the patient; however, they are not a substitute for proper scrubbing methods. If the glove of a properly scrubbed hand is perforated during a surgical procedure, bacteria are rarely cultured from the punctured glove. Lubricating agents for latex gloves, such as magnesium silicate (talcum) or cornstarch, allow gloves to slide more easily onto the hand. Unfortunately, these agents cause considerable irritation to various tissues, even if gloves are vigorously rinsed in sterile saline before surgery. Therefore, the surgeon should use gloves in which the inner surfaces are lubricated with an adherent coating of hydrogel.

TECHNICIAN NOTE The only region of gowned and gloved surgical personnel considered sterile is the front of the gown, between the table top and just below the shoulders, down the front of sleeves and the hands.

Closed Gloving

This method ensures that the hand never comes in contact with the outside of the gown or glove. Working through the gown sleeve (your bare hand must not be allowed to touch the cuff of the gown or outside surface of the glove), pick up one glove from the wrapper. Lay the glove palm down over the cuff of the gown, with the thumb and fingers of the glove facing your elbow (Fig. 15-15, *A*). Working though the cuff of the gown, grasp the cuff of the glove with your index finger and thumb. With your other hand still inside the cuff of the gown, take hold of the opposite side of the edge of the glove between your index finger and thumb. Lift the cuff of the glove up and over the gown cuff and hand, bringing the glove cuff below your knuckles. Release and come to the palm side of the glove and take hold of the gown and glove, pulling them toward your elbow while pushing your hand through the gown cuff and into the glove (Fig. 15-15, *B*). Proceed with the opposite hand, using the same technique. Do not allow the bare hand being gloved to contact the gown cuff edge or sterile glove on the opposite hand. Once both gloves are in place, adjust the gown cuffs as needed.

Open Gloving

The open method of gloving is used most commonly for noninvasive procedures (e.g., as for urinary catheterization, bone marrow biopsy, sterile patient preparation). It should not be used routinely for gowning and gloving. To don the first glove, pick up one glove by its inner cuff with the opposite hand (Fig. 15-16, *A*). Do not touch the glove wrapper with your bare hand. Slide the glove onto the opposite hand; leave the cuff down. Using the partially gloved hand, slide your fingers into the outer side of the opposite glove cuff (Fig. 15-16, *B*). Slide your hand into the glove and unfold the cuff; do not touch the bare arm as the cuff is unfolded (Fig. 15-16, *C*). With your gloved hand, slide the fingers under the outside edge of the first cuff and unfold it (Fig. 15-16, *D*).

Assisted Gloving

When gloving another person, the person assisting with the gloving should have on a sterile gown and/or gloves. The assistant's hands should not touch the nonsterile surface of the person being gloved. If both gloves are being replaced, have the assistant pick up one glove and place his or her fingers and thumb under the cuff of the glove (Fig. 15-17, *A*). With the thumb of the glove facing you, have the assistant hold the glove open for you to slip your hand into (Fig. 15-17, *B*). The assistant then brings the cuff of the glove up and over the cuff of your gown and gently lets it go. The assistant picks up the other glove. Assist him or her by holding the cuff of the glove open with the fingers of your sterile hand, while putting your ungloved hand into the open glove (Fig. 15-17, *C*). The assistant keeps his or her thumbs under the cuff while you thrust your hand into it. Ensure that the glove cuff is above your gown cuff before the assistant gently releases it (he or she should not let the cuff snap sharply).

Glove Removal During Surgery

If gloves become contaminated during surgery, they must be replaced. Both gloves may routinely be changed during "dirty" procedures (open GI tract caused by perforation or gastrotomy/enterotomy). Most surgeons are adept at removing gloves themselves, pulling their hands back into surgical

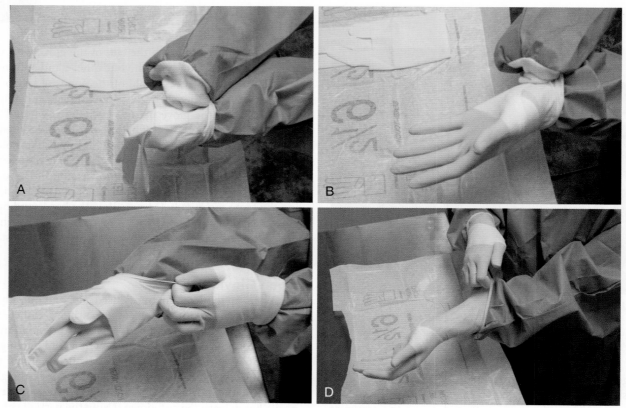

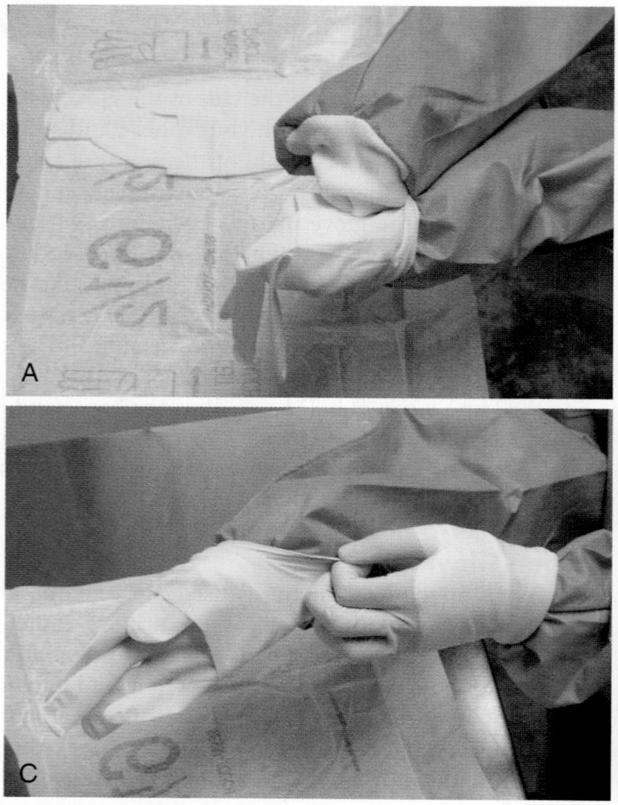

FIGURE 15-15 Closed gloving. **A,** Working through the gown sleeve, pick up one glove from the wrapper, with the glove palm down over the cuff of the gown, the thumb and fingers of the glove facing your elbows, and then grasp the opposite cuff of the glove and bring it up and over the gown cuff. **B,** Release, move to the palm side of the glove, and grasp the gown and glove, pulling them toward the elbow while pushing the hand through the cuff and into the glove. **C,** Repeat steps (**A**) and (**B**) with the opposite glove. **D,** Once both gloves are on, adjust the cuffs as needed.

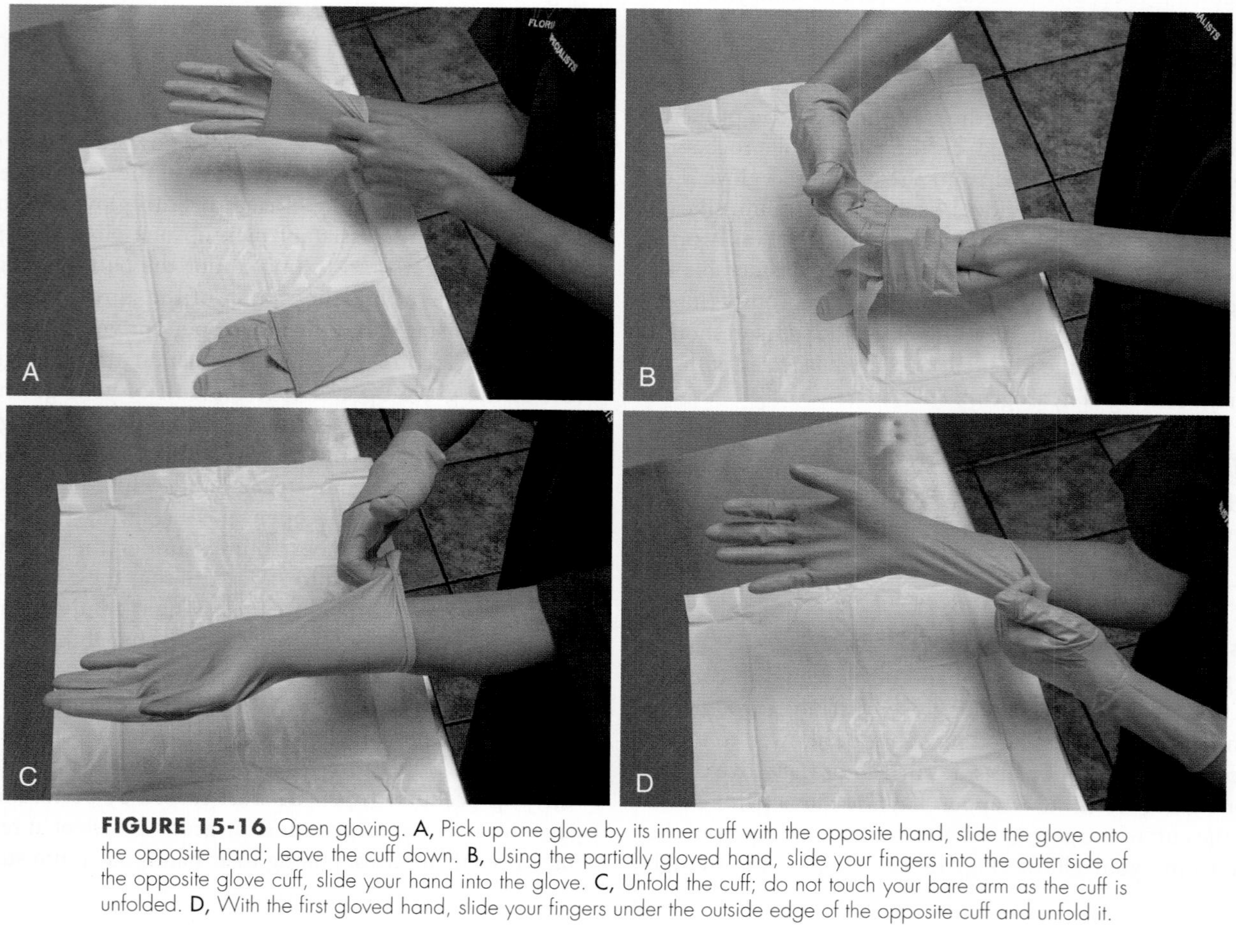

FIGURE 15-16 Open gloving. **A,** Pick up one glove by its inner cuff with the opposite hand, slide the glove onto the opposite hand; leave the cuff down. **B,** Using the partially gloved hand, slide your fingers into the outer side of the opposite glove cuff, slide your hand into the glove. **C,** Unfold the cuff; do not touch your bare arm as the cuff is unfolded. **D,** With the first gloved hand, slide your fingers under the outside edge of the opposite cuff and unfold it.

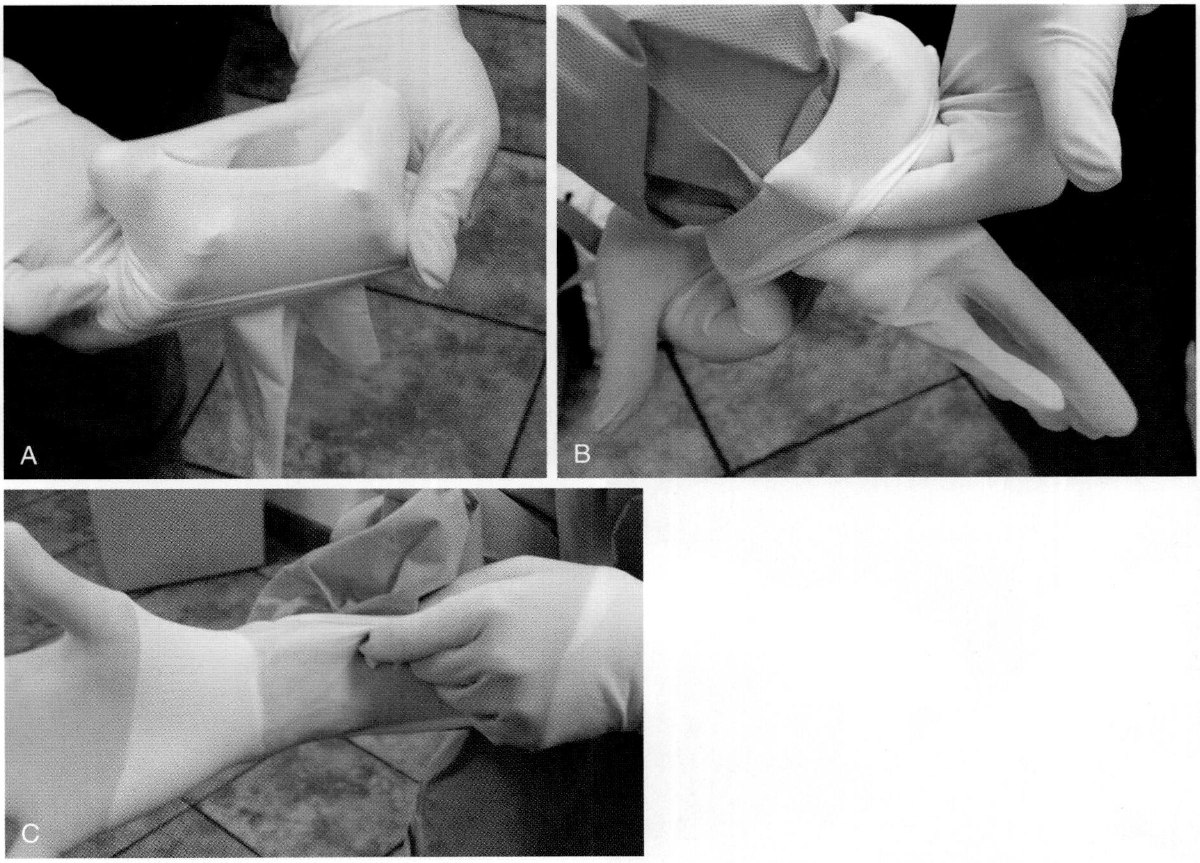

FIGURE 15-17 Assisted gloving. **A,** The assistant holds the glove open for a sterile team member to slip their hand in. Note that the hand remains in the gown cuff until it is within the glove cuff. **B,** The assistant then brings the cuff of the glove up and over the cuff of the gown. **C,** The sterile team member may then adjust the cuff(s).

gown sleeves as they do so. New gloves may be dropped (in their inner, sterile wrapper) on the instrument stand or drape. Then closed gloving may be performed. If only one glove is contaminated, or if the scrubbed personnel needs assistance for any reason, nonsterile personnel may easily help (Fig. 15-18). The cuffs of the gown of the sterile person are grasped through the cuff of the glove. A firm grip is used, but care must be taken not to break the glove or touch the gown. The cuff of the glove is pulled toward the nonsterile assistant, and in turn, the cuff of the gown is pulled back down over the hand of the wearer. The glove is pulled free, and the sterile personnel may again proceed with closed gloving.

SURGICAL ASSISTING

The sterile surgical assistant must don a sterile gown and gloves when entering the surgical suite. Care must be taken to not contaminate the gown by brushing against tables or other individuals when entering the surgical suite.

A circulating assistant (nonsterile) should be available to place needed supplies and equipment onto the Mayo stand. All personnel should have cap and mask on before placing sterile items onto the Mayo stand. Materials should be opened facing away from the body and allowed to fall onto the stand so that the assistant's arms are not directly over the top of the Mayo stand. The sterile surgical assistant should arrange the instruments and supplies on the Mayo stand before the start of surgery. The assistant may also be responsible for operating the surgical suction and passing and holding instruments for the surgeon. A circulating (nonsterile) assistant should be present to provide any additional items that may be needed by the surgeon.

The technician must be familiar with the procedure to be performed and be able to anticipate the instruments and supplies that the surgeon may need. Instruments should be passed to the surgeon by firmly pressing the instrument into the surgeon's hand. Instruments are usually passed so that they will be placed in the surgeon's hand in a ready-to-use position. Curved instruments are passed with their concave side up.

The veterinary technician is also responsible for assuring that the surgical lighting is focused on the surgical site and the site remains dry. Blotting the site gently with gauze sponges or removing excess blood and tissue fluid can be used to accomplish this task. When a body cavity is opened, sponges should be counted at the beginning of the procedure (before the first incision) and before closure to ensure that none have been inadvertently left in the body cavity. Contaminated instruments or soiled sponges should not be placed back on the instrument table. Surgical assistants may

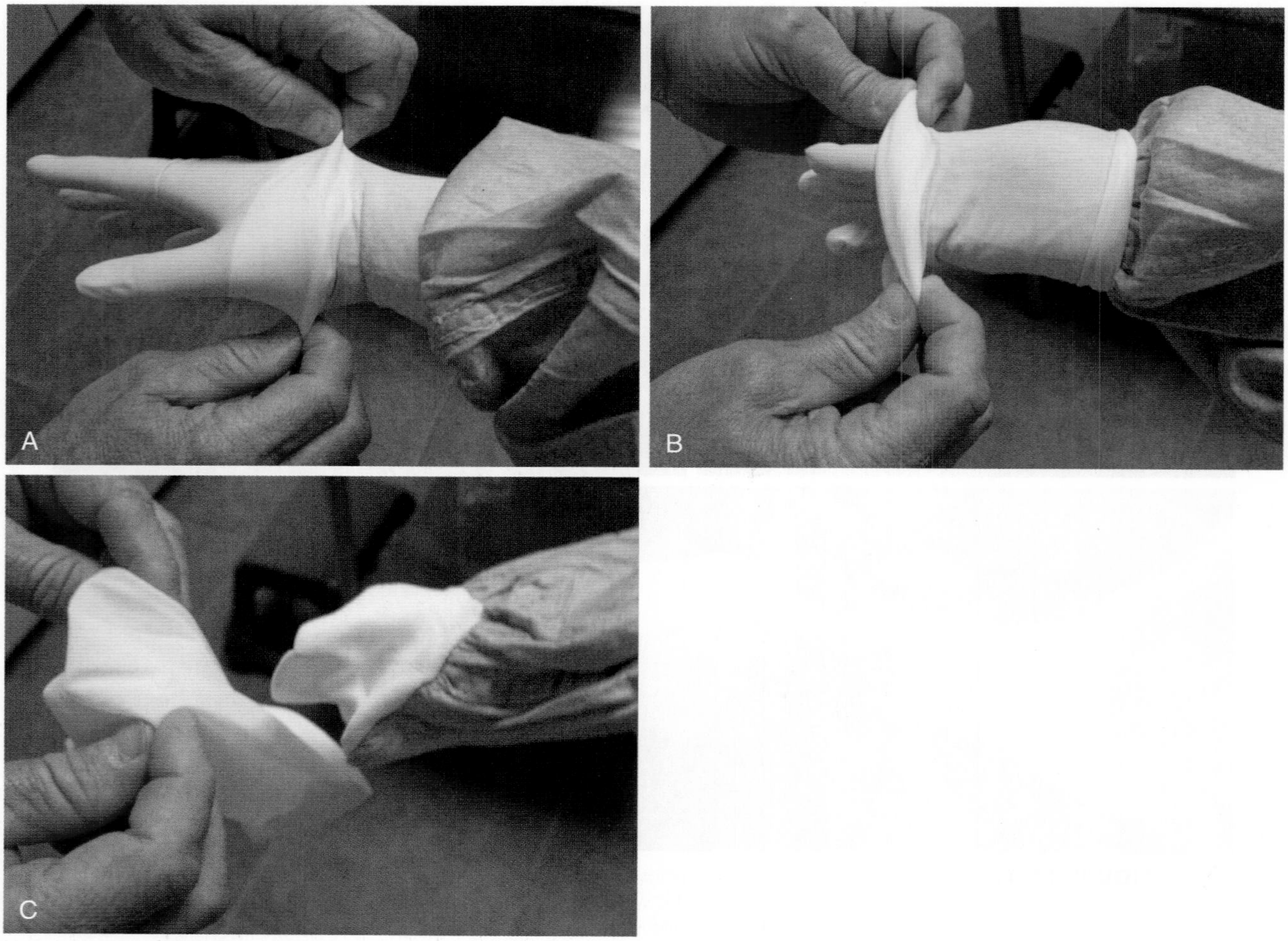

FIGURE 15-18 Assisted glove removal. **A,** Nonsterile assistant grasps the gown cuffs through the glove cuffs. **B,** Both cuffs are pulled toward the assistant together, and the sterile personnel's hand retreats into the gown. **C,** The sterile team member may then proceed again with closed gloving.

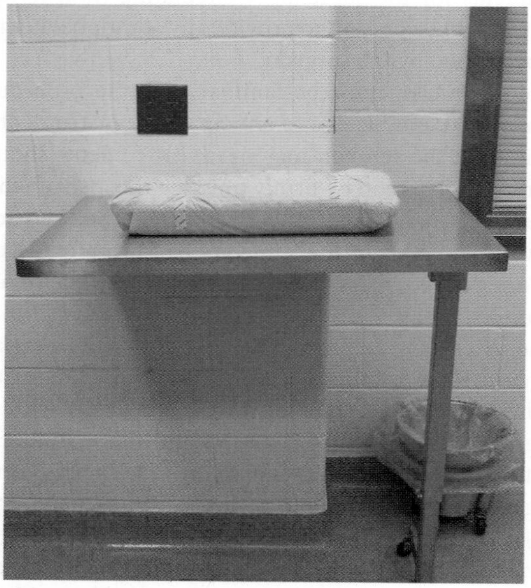

FIGURE 15-19 Mayo stand, or instrument table. (From Tear M: *Small animal surgical nursing*, ed 2, St Louis, 2012, Mosby.)

also be required to hold clamps on tissues or vessels. Always handle tissues gently and keep tissues moistened with sterile saline when they are removed from body cavities.

DRAPING AND ORGANIZING THE INSTRUMENT TABLE

Instrument tables should be height adjustable to allow them to be positioned within reach of surgical personnel. The instrument table should not be opened until the animal has been positioned on the surgical table and draped. Large, water-impermeable table drapes should be used to cover the entire instrument table. To open these drapes, the drape and outer wrap are positioned on the instrument table, the exposed undersurface of the drape is gently grasped, and the ends and then the sides are unfolded. Once the drape has been opened, nonsterile personnel should not reach over it. **Mayo stands** are often used in procedures that require additional instruments (e.g., bone plating); specially designed Mayo stand covers are available to cover these tables. When the instrument pack has been opened, instruments should be positioned so that they can be readily retrieved. The instrument

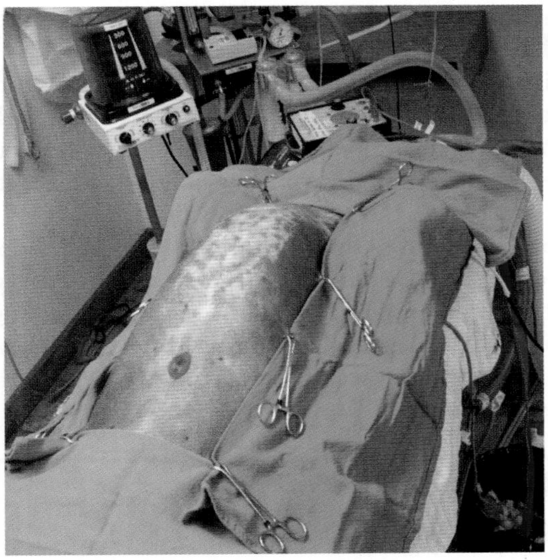

FIGURE 15-20 The patient is positioned for both thoracic and abdominal incisions. Field drapes are secured at the corners and midpoints with towel clamps.

layout is generally determined by the surgeon's preference, but grouping similar instruments (e.g., scissors, retractors) facilitates their use.

DRAPING

Once the animal has been positioned and the skin prepared, the animal is ready to be draped. The drapes maintain a sterile field around the operative site. If electrocautery is being used, sufficient time should elapse between skin preparation and application of drapes to permit complete evaporation of flammable substances (e.g., alcohol) from the skin. If an abdominal incision extends to the pubis in males, the prepuce should be clamped to one side with a sterile towel clamp.

Draping is performed by a gowned and gloved surgical team member and begins with placement of field drapes (quarter drapes) to isolate the unprepared portion of the animal. These towels should be placed one at a time at the periphery of the prepared area. Field (quarter) drapes may be lint-free towels or disposable, nonabsorbent towels. Drapes should not be flipped, fanned, or shaken, because rapid movement of drapes creates air currents on which dust, lint, and droplet nuclei can migrate. Drapes, supplies, and equipment extending over or dropping below the table level should be considered nonsterile because they are not within the surgeon's visual field and their sterility cannot be verified.

Once the towels are placed, they should not be readjusted toward the incision site, because this carries bacteria onto the prepared skin. Towels are secured at the corners with Backhaus towel clamps (Fig. 15-20). The tips of the towel clamps, once placed through the skin, are considered nonsterile and should be handled appropriately. Generally, field towels do not cover the edges of the table; do not brush a sterile gown against this nonsterile field. When the animal and incision site are protected by field drapes, final draping can be performed (Figs. 15-21 and 15-22). A large drape is placed over the animal and entire surgical table to provide a continuous sterile field. Cloth drapes should have an appropriately sized and positioned opening that can be placed over the incision site, while the drape covers the remaining surfaces.

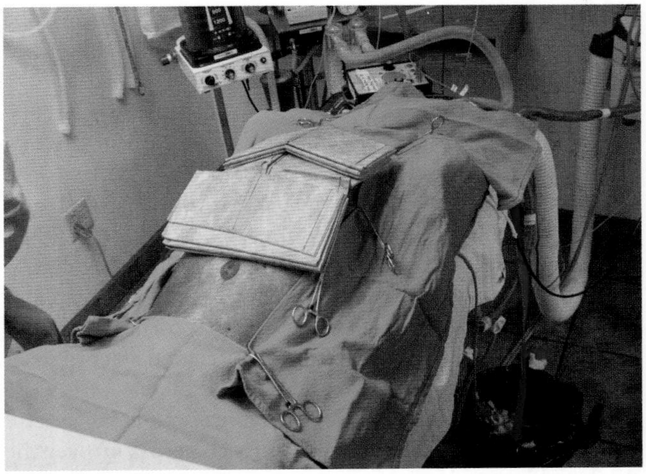

FIGURE 15-21 When the animal and incision site are protected with field drapes, final draping may be performed. Place the large drape with the center or fenestration over the surgical site and unfold it. To avoid contaminating the drape, do not hold it in the air when unfolding it.

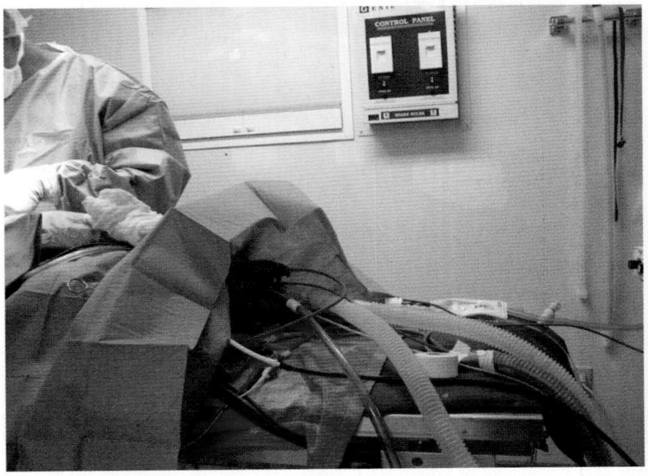

FIGURE 15-22 The patient is positioned and draped in for abdominal surgery. Monitor leads, anesthesia tubes, and a stomach tube can be identified. The technician in charge of anesthesia may access the patient and equipment under the forward edge of the drape.

To drape a limb, place field drapes and secure them as described above to isolate the surgical site or the proximal aspect of the limb, if the leg is hung (Fig. 15-23). The leg can then be wrapped by sterile personnel with sterile Vetrap or a sterile towel. A nonsterile member of the surgical team can cut the tape hanging the leg as the wrap nears the top. The limb should not be released until it is securely held by the sterile surgical team member. The sterile member can wrap the distal (tape) end of limb with the sterile material and continue up the leg again if desired (Fig. 15-24). If a stockinette is used, it should be carefully unrolled down the limb and secured with towel clamps. The end of the stockinette is wrapped with sterile Vetrap. The limb is now ready to be placed through a fenestration of a lap or fanfold drape and the drape secured (Fig. 15-25).

UNWRAPPING OR OPENING STERILE ITEMS

Unwrapping Sterile Linen or Paper Packs

If you are right-handed, hold the pack in your left hand (and vice versa). Using the right hand, unfold one corner of the outside wrap at a time, being careful to secure each corner in the palm of the left hand to keep them from recoiling and contaminating the contents. Hold the final corner with your right hand. When the pack is fully exposed and all corners of the wrap secured (Fig. 15-26), gently pass the pack to sterile personnel, or set the pack onto the table cover, being careful to not allow your hand and arm to reach across or over the sterile field.

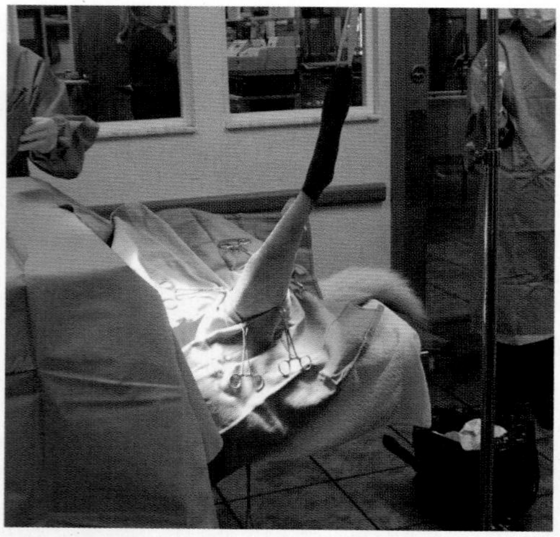

FIGURE 15-23 When performing "hanging leg" preparation, place field drapes around the limb as shown, and secure with towel clamps. The patient is positioned for medial stifle surgery.

Unwrapping Sterile Items in Paper or Plastic or Plastic Peel-Back Pouches

Identify the edges of the peel-back wrapper and carefully separate them. Peel the edges of the wrapper back slowly and symmetrically to ensure the sterile item does not contact the torn edge of the wrapper, which is nonsterile. If the item is small, place it on the sterile area as described, being careful not to lean across the sterile table. If the item is long or cumbersome, have a sterile team member grasp it and gently pull it from the peel-back wrapper (Fig. 15-27), taking care not to brush the item against the peeled edge of the wrapper. Packages containing scalpel blades and suture material are opened similarly.

SURGICAL INSTRUMENTS

SCALPELS AND BLADES

Scalpels are the primary cutting instrument used to incise tissue (Fig. 15-28). Reusable scalpel handles with detachable blades are most commonly used in veterinary medicine; disposable handles and blades are also available. Blades are available in various sizes and shapes, depending on the task for which they are used. Scalpels are usually used in a "slide cutting" fashion, with pressure applied to the knife blade at a right angle to the direction of scalpel pressure.

Laser Scalpel

Laser is an acronym for light amplification by the stimulated emission of radiation. Laser technology has been used to safely and effectively treat patients for nearly two decades. The most commonly used surgical laser is a carbon dioxide laser that produces an invisible beam of light that vaporizes the water normally found in the skin and other soft tissue. Lasers have the unique ability to both coagulate and cut tissue. The technician's role in laser surgery may include practice management duties, client communication, and laser

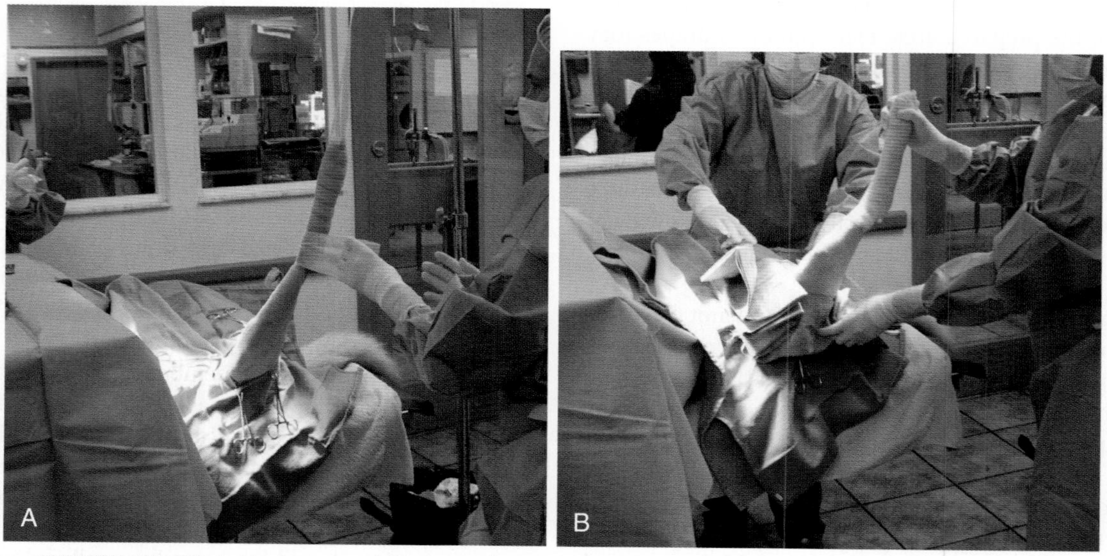

FIGURE 15-24 A, The leg is carefully wrapped with sterile material before being cut down for sterile personnel. B, The leg can then be placed through a fenestrated drape.

safety duties. Although there are a variety of lasers, the most common types used in veterinary practice are carbon dioxide (CO_2) and diode. Diode laser energy is delivered through a quartz fiber instead of being reflected through an articulated arm or waveguide. Quartz fibers are generally more flexible and resilient than waveguides and can be inserted through an endoscope for minimally invasive procedures. Laser-tissue interaction is the other significant difference. The CO_2 laser is completely absorbed by water, which limits the effect to visible tissue. The diode wavelength is minimally absorbed by water and may affect tissue as deep as 10 mm below the surface in the free-beam mode.

Because the laser seals nerve endings and small blood vessels as it cuts, it results in less bleeding and less pain for the patient. Because laser scalpels do not crush, tear, or bruise tissue as traditional scalpels do, swelling is minimized. The laser is ideal for a wide variety of surgical procedures for dogs, cats, birds, reptiles, exotics, horses, and other pets. Laser surgery is commonly used in soft-tissue surgical procedures, such as cat declaws, spays, neuters, amputations, oral/dental procedures, dermatology, and avian and exotic procedures.

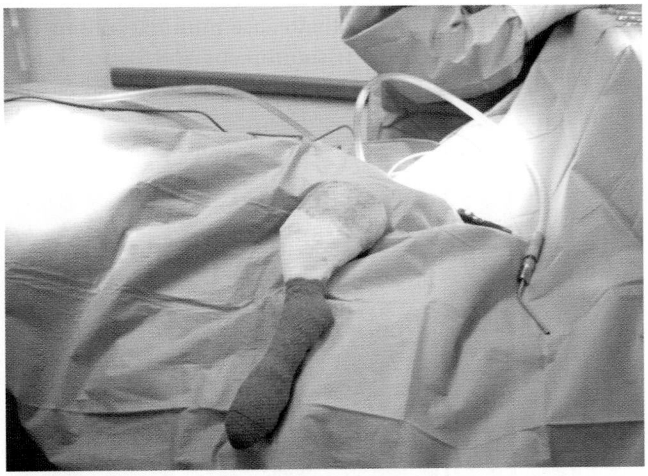

FIGURE 15-25 The patient is positioned for lateral stifle surgery. The limb is positioned through a fenestration of fanfolded drape.

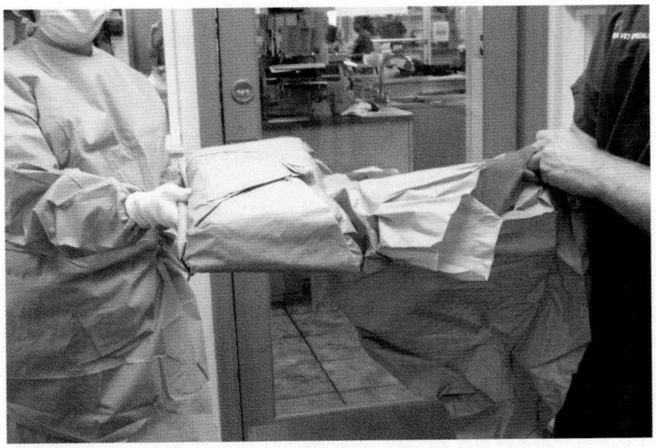

FIGURE 15-26 To unwrap a sterile linen or paper pack that can be held during distribution, hold the pack in your right hand if you are left-handed (and vice versa). Using your right hand, unfold one corner of the wrap at a time, being careful to secure each corner in the palm of your left hand to keep them from recoiling and contaminating the contents. Hold the final corner with your right hand; your hand should be completely covered by the wrap. When the pack is fully exposed and all corners of the wrap secured, it may be grasped and taken by sterile personnel.

Electroscalpel

The electroscalpel functions by passing an electrical current through the unit to the patient's tissues. This causes microcoagulation of tissue proteins as the unit cuts the tissue.

> TECHNICIAN NOTE Every surgical instrument is designed for a specific purpose: holding, clamping, cutting, or retracting.

SCISSORS

Scissors are available in a variety of shapes, sizes, and weights, and are generally classified according to the type

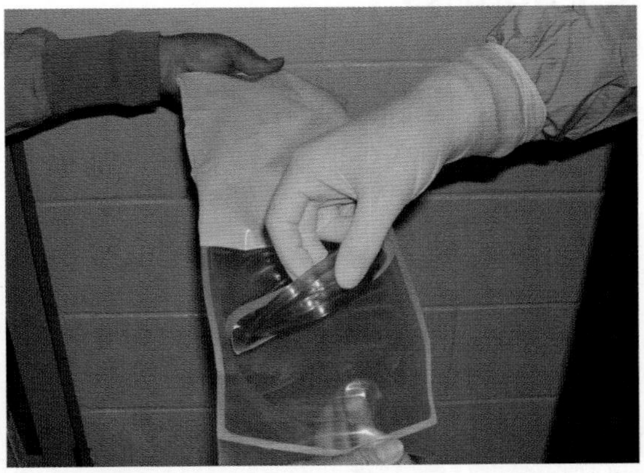

FIGURE 15-27 To unwrap a sterile item in a plastic peel-back pouch, identify the edges of the peel-back wrapper and carefully separate them. Peel the edges of the wrapper back slowly and symmetrically to ensure the sterile item does not contact the torn edge of the wrapper, which is nonsterile. (From Tear M: *Small animal surgical nursing,* ed 2, St Louis, 2012, Mosby.)

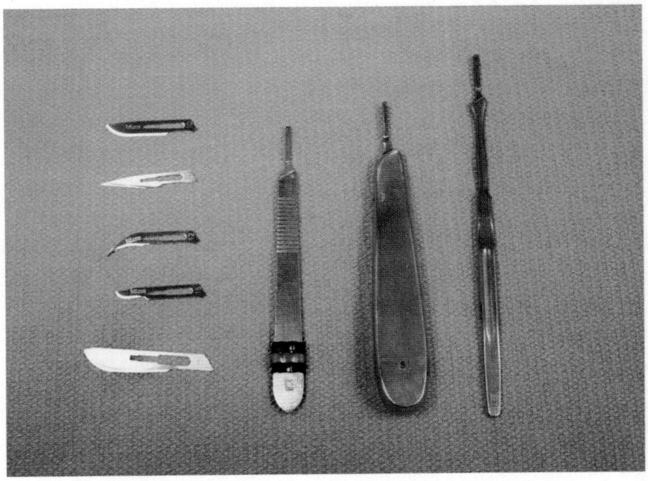

FIGURE 15-28 Scalpel blades *(left),* top to bottom, Nos. 10, 11, 12, 15, and 20. Scalpel handles *(right),* left to right, Nos. 3, 5, and 7.

of points (blunt-blunt, sharp-sharp, sharp-blunt), blade shape (straight, curved), or cutting edge (plain, serrated) (Fig. 15-29). Curved scissors offer greater maneuverability and visibility, whereas straight scissors provide the greatest mechanical advantage for cutting tough or thick tissue. Metzenbaum or **Mayo scissors** are most commonly used in surgery. **Metzenbaum scissors** are more delicate and should be reserved for fine, thin tissues. Mayo scissors are used for cutting heavy tissues, such as fascia. Tissue scissors should not be used to cut suture material; suture scissors should be used. Suture scissors used in the operating room are different from suture removal scissors. The latter have a concavity at the top of one blade that prevents the suture from being lifted excessively during removal. Delicate scissors, such as tenotomy scissors or **iris scissors,** are often used in ophthalmic procedures and other surgeries, where fine, precise cuts are necessary. Bandage scissors have a blunt tip that, when introduced under the bandage edge, reduces the risk of cutting the underlying skin.

NEEDLE HOLDERS

Needle holders are used to grasp and manipulate curved needles (Fig. 15-30). **Mayo-Hegar needle holders** and Olsen-Hegar needle holders have a ratchet lock just distal to the thumb. Castroviejo needle holders have a spring and latch mechanism for locking. Mathieu needle holders have a ratchet lock at the proximal end of the handles of the holder, permitting locking and unlocking simply by a progressive squeezing together of the needle holder handles.

TISSUE FORCEPS

Tissue forceps are used to clamp and hold tissue and blood vessels. Thumb forceps are tweezer-like, nonlocking tissue forceps used to grasp tissue (Fig. 15-31). The proximal ends are joined to allow the grasping ends to spring open or be squeezed together. They are available in a variety of shapes and sizes; tips (grasping ends) may be pointed, flattened, rounded, smooth, or serrated, or have small or large teeth. Tissue forceps with large teeth should not be used to handle tissue that is easily traumatized; smooth tips are recommended with delicate tissue (e.g., blood vessels). The most commonly used type, **Brown-Adson tissue forceps,** have small serrations on the tips that cause minimal trauma but hold tissue securely. Allis tissue forceps and Babcock forceps (Figs. 15-32 and 15-33) are also for tissue grasping and retraction.

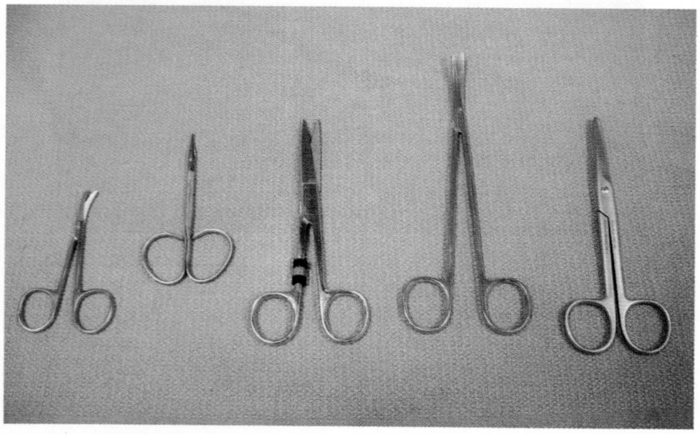

FIGURE 15-29 Scissors *(left to right):* suture removal, tenotomy, sharp/sharp suture, Metzenbaum, and Mayo.

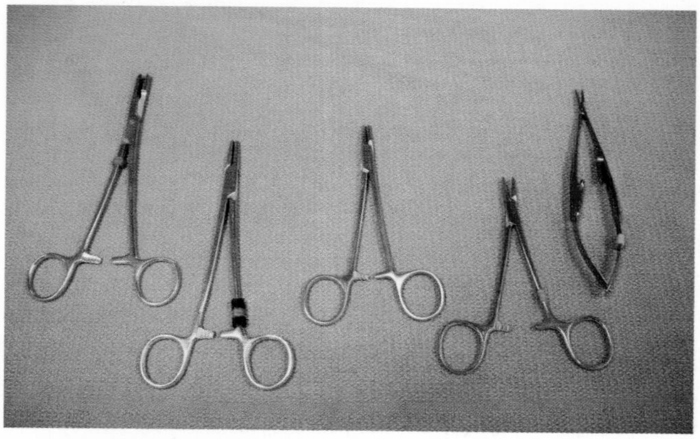

FIGURE 15-30 Needle holders *(left to right):* Olsen-Hegar, Mayo-Hegar, derf, Halsey, and Castroviejo.

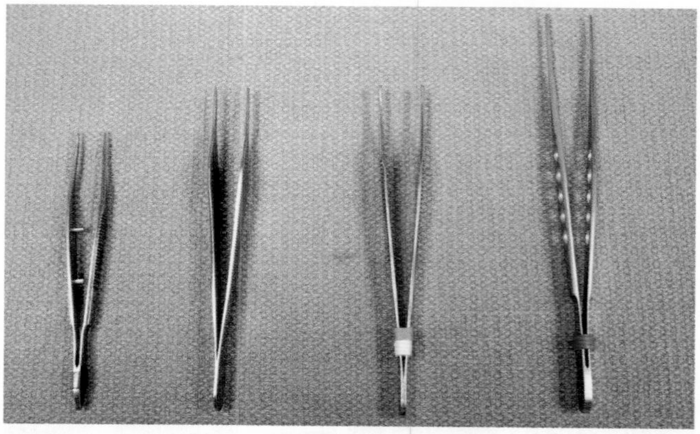

FIGURE 15-31 Tissue forceps *(left to right):* dressing, Adson dressing, Brown-Adson, and DeBakey.

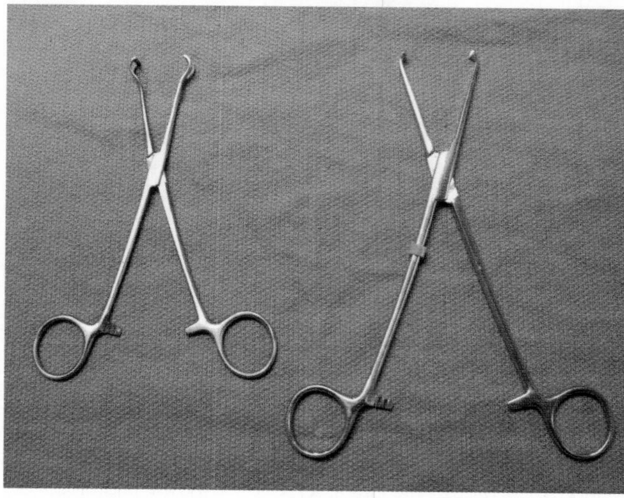

FIGURE 15-32 Tissue forceps: Babcock *(left)* and Allis *(right).*

HEMOSTATIC FORCEPS

Hemostatic forceps, commonly called "hemostats," are crushing instruments used to clamp blood vessels (Fig. 15-34). They are available with straight or curved tips and vary in size from smaller (3-inch) mosquito hemostats with transverse jaw serrations, to larger (9-inch) **angiotribes.** Serrations on the jaws of larger hemostatic forceps may be transverse, longitudinal, or diagonal, or a combination of these. Longitudinal serrations are generally gentler on tissue than cross serrations. Serrations usually extend from the tips of the jaws to the boxlocks, but in **Kelly forceps,** transverse (horizontal) serrations extend over only the distal portion of the jaws. Similarly sized **Crile forceps** have transverse serrations that extend the entire jaw length. Kelly and Crile forceps are used on larger vessels. Rochester-Carmalt forceps are larger crushing forceps, often used to control large tissue bundles (e.g., during ovariohysterectomy). They have longitudinal grooves with cross grooves at the tip ends to prevent tissue slippage.

Curved hemostats should be placed on tissue with the curve facing up. The smallest hemostatic forceps that will accomplish the job should be used to grasp as little tissue as possible to minimize trauma. To avoid having fingers momentarily trapped within the rings of hemostats, fingertips should be placed on the forceps finger rings or your fingers should be inserted into the rings only as far as the first joint.

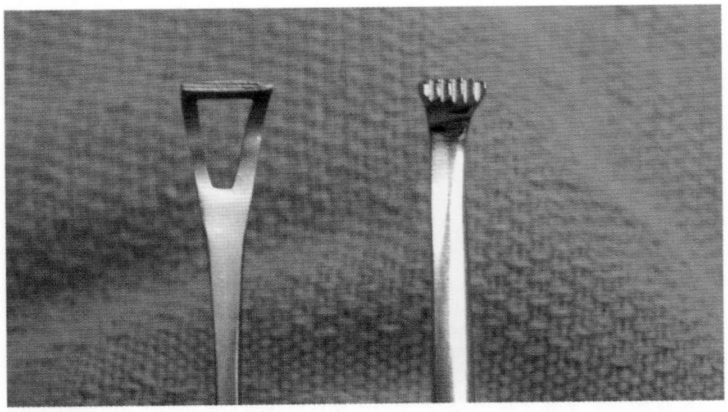

FIGURE 15-33 Tissue forceps close up: Babcock *(left)* and Allis *(right)*.

HEMOSTATIC TECHNIQUES AND MATERIALS

Hemostasis, or the arrest of bleeding, allows visualization of the surgical site and prevents life-threatening hemorrhage. Low-pressure hemorrhage from small vessels can be controlled by applying pressure to the bleeding points with a gauze sponge. Once a thrombus has formed, the sponge should be gently removed to avoid disrupting clots. Large vessels must be ligated (tied off). Hemostatic agents used to control hemorrhage during surgery include bone wax and hemostatic materials made of gelatin or cellulose (e.g., Surgicel, Gelfoam).

Metal clips or staples (Surgiclips, LDS) may be used for vessel ligation (Fig. 15-35). They are particularly useful when the vessel is difficult to reach or multiple vessels must be ligated. The vessel should be one third to two thirds the size of the clip, and the vessel size must be reducible to less than 0.75 mm by the clip or staple to be ligated in this fashion. The vessel should be dissected free of surrounding tissue before the clip is applied and 2 to 3 mm of vessel should extend beyond the clip to prevent slippage.

Electrocoagulation can be used to achieve hemostasis in vessels less than 2 mm in diameter; larger vessels should be ligated. The term electrocautery is often erroneously used in place of electrocoagulation. With **electrocautery,** the needle tip or scalpel is heated before it is applied to the tissue; with **electrocoagulation,** heat is generated in the tissue as a high-frequency current is passed through it. Excessive use of electrocautery or electrocoagulation retards healing.

RETRACTORS

Retractors are used to retract tissue and improve exposure. The ends of hand-held retractors may be hooked, curved, spatula-shaped, or toothed. Some hand-held retractors may be bent (i.e., malleable) to conform to the structure being retracted or area of the body in which retraction is being performed. Senn (rake) retractors are double-ended retractors (Fig. 15-36). One end has three fingerlike, curved prongs; the other end is a flat, curved blade. Self-retaining retractors maintain tension on tissues and are held open with a boxlock (e.g., Gelpi, **Weitlaner**) or other device (e.g., set-screw).

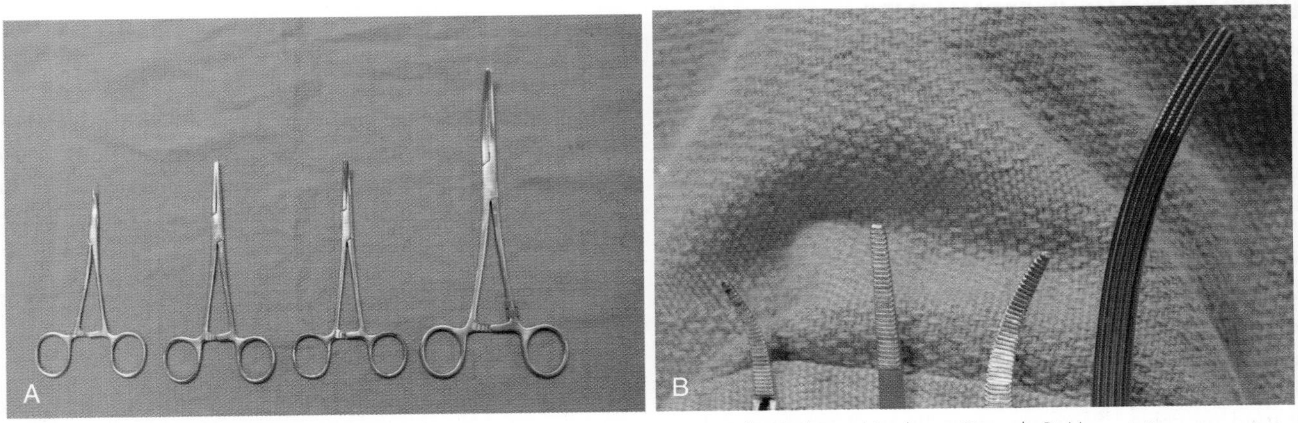

FIGURE 15-34 **A,** Hemostatic forceps *(left to right)*: mosquito, Kelly, Crile, and Rochester-Carmalt. **B,** Hemostatic forceps close up *(left to right)*: mosquito, Kelly, Crile, and Rochester-Carmalt.

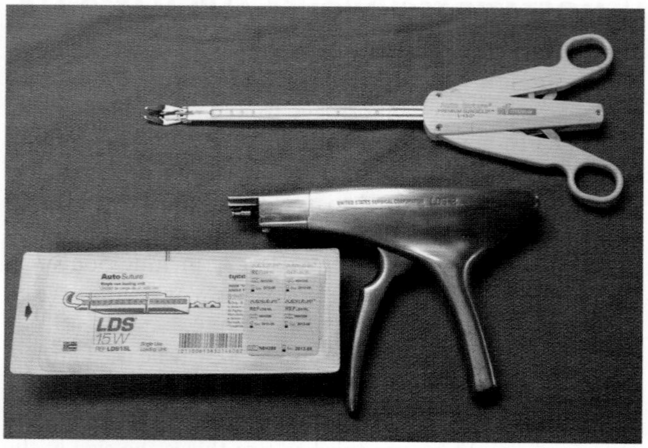

FIGURE 15-35 Ligating clips: Surgi-Clips *(top)*, LDS gun and cartridge *(bottom)*.

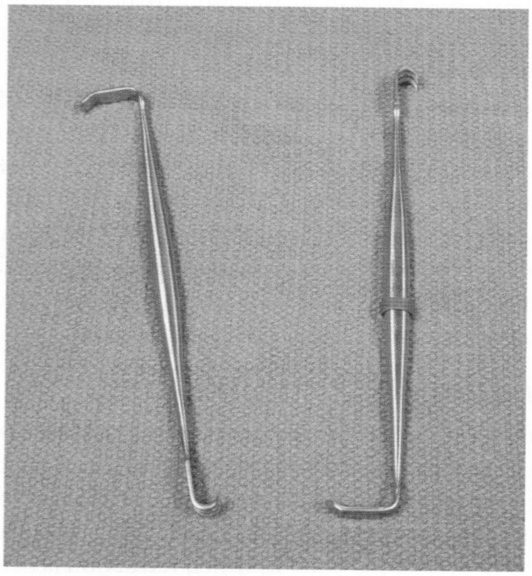

FIGURE 15-36 Senn (rake) retractor.

Examples of the latter are Balfour retractors and Finochietto retractors. Balfour retractors are generally used to retract the abdominal wall, whereas Finochietto retractors are commonly used during thoracotomies.

MISCELLANEOUS INSTRUMENTS

Instruments are available to suction fluid, clamp drapes or tissues, cut and remove bone pieces (**rongeurs**), hold bones during fracture repair, scrape surfaces of dense tissue (**curettes**), remove periosteum (periosteal elevators; Fig. 15-37), cut or shape bone and cartilage (**osteotomes** and chisels), and bore holes in bone (trephines).

INSTRUMENTS FOR LARGE ANIMAL SURGERY

Dehorning Instruments

Various instruments, including gouges and saws, are used to remove horns from cattle (Fig. 15-38). Smaller instruments are used on calves. Saws are generally used to remove the horns of adult cattle.

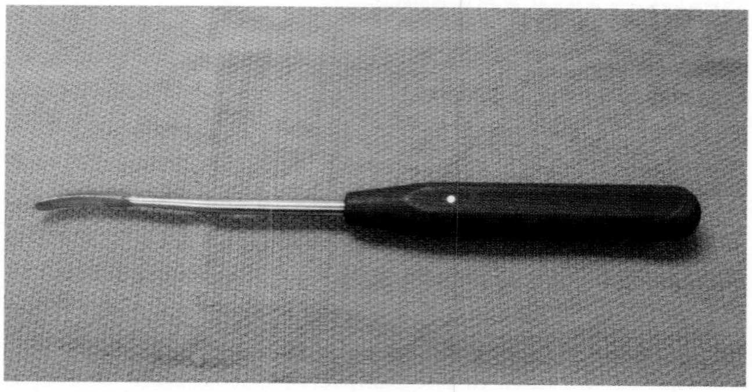

FIGURE 15-37 Joseph periosteal elevator.

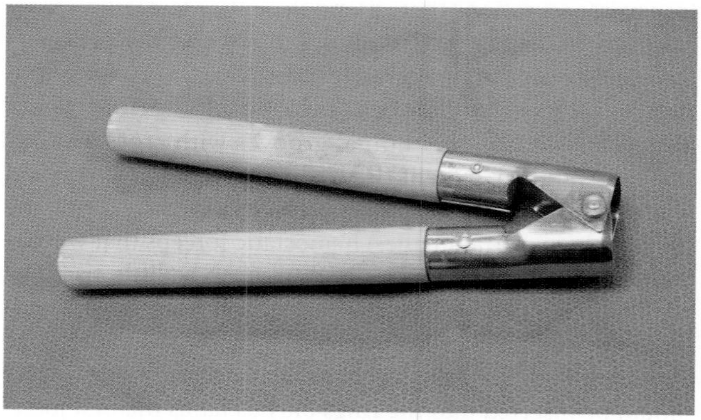

FIGURE 15-38 Barnes dehorner.

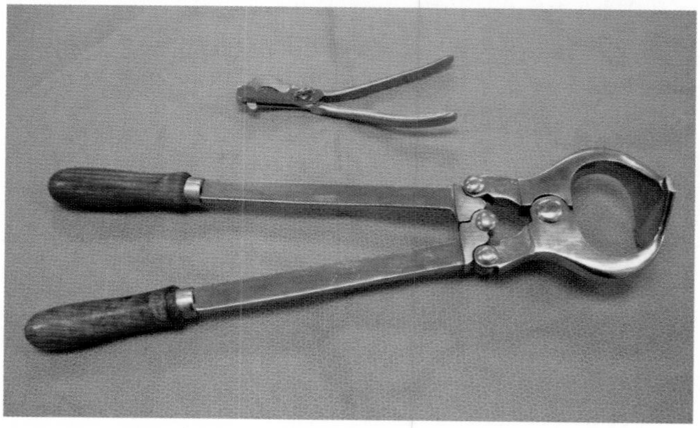

FIGURE 15-39 Castration instruments: emasculatome *(bottom)* and emasculator *(top)*.

Castrating Instruments

An emasculator is used in open castrations to crush and sever the spermatic cord (Fig. 15-39). An emasculatome is used to accomplish the same thing through the intact skin during closed castrations, particularly when fly infestation is likely to be a problem.

SUTURE MATERIALS

SUTURE CHARACTERISTICS

The word **suture** refers to any strand of material that is used to approximate tissues or ligate blood vessels. The ideal suture material is easy to handle; reacts minimally in tissue;

inhibits bacterial growth; holds securely when knotted; resists shrinking in tissues; is noncapillary, nonallergenic, noncarcinogenic, and nonferromagnetic; and is absorbed with minimal reaction after the tissue has healed. Such an ideal suture material does not exist; therefore, surgeons must choose one that most closely approximates the ideal for a given procedure and/or tissue to be sutured.

Monofilament sutures are made of a single strand of material. They create less tissue drag than multifilament suture material and do not have interstitial spaces that may harbor bacteria. Care should be used in handling monofilament sutures because nicking or damaging them with forceps or needle holders weakens them and predisposes to breakage.

Multifilament sutures consist of several strands that are twisted or braided together. Multifilament sutures are generally more pliable and flexible than monofilament sutures. They may be coated to decrease tissue drag and enhance handling characteristics.

The most commonly used standard for suture size is the U.S.P. (United States Pharmacopeia), which denotes suture diameters from fine to coarse according to a numeric scale; size 10-O material has the smallest diameter (finest) and size 7 has the largest diameter (most coarse). U.S.P. uses different size notations for various suture materials (Table 15-4). The smaller the suture diameter is, the lower is its tensile strength. Stainless-steel wire is usually sized according to the metric or U.S.P. scale or by the Brown and Sharpe wire gauge.

ABSORBABLE SUTURE MATERIALS

Absorbable suture materials lose most of their tensile strength within 60 days after placement in tissue, and eventually are absorbed from the site and replaced by healthy tissue during the healing process. Absorbable sutures are used when sutures must be buried within body cavities (Fig. 15-40).

Surgical Gut

Surgical gut is commonly called "catgut." Surgical gut is made from the submucosa of sheep intestine or the serosa of bovine intestine. It comprises approximately 90% collagen. Plain surgical gut is broken down by phagocytosis and elicits a marked inflammatory reaction, as compared with other materials. "Tanning," by exposure to chrome or aldehyde, slows absorption. Surgical gut so treated is called chromic surgical gut. Surgical gut is rapidly absorbed from infected sites or where it is exposed to digestive enzymes. Knots in surgical gut may loosen when wet.

Synthetic Absorbable Materials

Synthetic absorbable materials (e.g., polyglycolic acid, polyglactin 910, polydioxanone, polyglyconate) are generally broken down by hydrolysis. There is minimal tissue reaction to synthetic absorbable suture materials. The rate of tensile strength loss and rate of absorption are fairly constant in different tissues. Infection or exposure to digestive enzymes does not significantly influence their rates of absorption.

TABLE 15-4		Systems Used to Indicate Suture Sizes		
DIAMETER (MM)	METRIC GAUGE	SYNTHETIC SUTURE MATERIALS (U.S.P.)	SURGICAL GUT (U.S.P.)	WIRE GAUGE (BROWN AND SHARPE)
0.02	0.2	10-O		
0.03	0.3	9-O		
0.04	0.4	8-O		
0.05	0.5	7-O	8-O	41
0.07	0.7	6-O	7-O	38-40
0.1	1	5-O	6-O	35
0.15	1.5	4-O	5-O	32-34
0.2	2	3-O	4-O	30
0.3	3	2-O	3-O	28
0.35	3.5	O	2-O	26
0.4	4	1	O	25
0.5	5	2	1	24
0.6	6	3,4	2	22
0.7	7	5	3	20
0.8	8	6	4	19
0.9	0	7		18

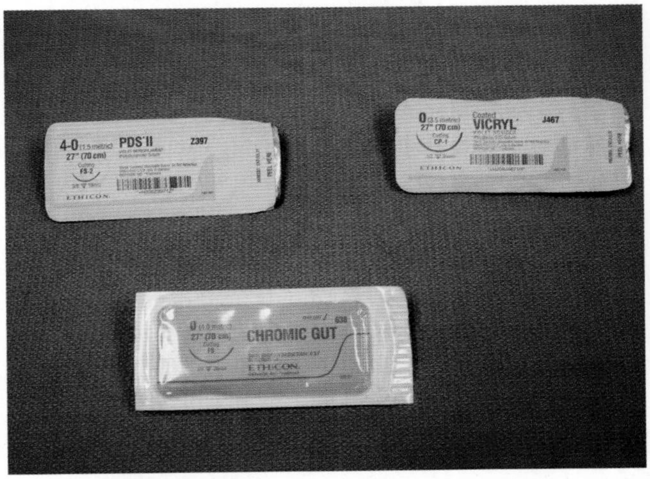

FIGURE 15-40 Examples of absorbable suture material.

NONABSORBABLE SUTURE MATERIALS

There are four basic groups of nonabsorbable suture materials: organic sutures, braided synthetic sutures, monofilament synthetic sutures, and metallic sutures (Fig. 15-41).

Organic Nonabsorbable Materials

Silk is the most common organic nonabsorbable suture material, used as a braided multifilament suture that is uncoated or coated. Silk has excellent handling characteristics and is often used in cardiovascular procedures; however, it does not maintain significant tensile strength after 6 months in tissues and is therefore contraindicated for use with vascular grafts. It also should be avoided in contaminated sites, because it increases the likelihood of wound infection. Cotton suture has less tissue reaction than silk, but supports bacterial growth and is not generally used for skin closure.

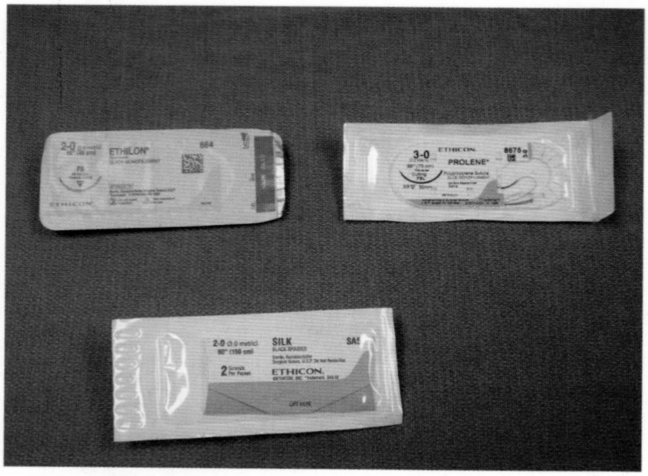

FIGURE 15-41 Examples of nonabsorbable suture material.

Synthetic Nonabsorbable Materials

Synthetic nonabsorbable suture materials are available as braided multifilament (e.g., polyester, coated caprolactam) or monofilament (e.g., polypropylene, polyamide, polyolefins, polybutester) threads. They are typically strong and induce minimal tissue reaction. Nonabsorbable suture materials consisting of an inner core and an outer sheath (e.g., Supramid) should not be buried in tissues, because the outer sheath tends to degenerate, allowing bacteria to migrate to the inner core. This predisposes to infection and fistula formation.

METALLIC SUTURES

Stainless steel is the most commonly used metallic suture. It is available as monofilament wire or twisted multifilament wire. The tissue reaction to stainless steel is generally minimal; however, the knot ends evoke an inflammatory reaction. Wire tends to cut tissue and may fragment. It is stable in contaminated wounds and is the standard for judging knot security and tissue reaction to suture materials.

SUTURE NEEDLES

Suture needles are available in a wide variety of shapes and sizes. The type of suture needle used depends on the characteristics of the tissue to be sutured (penetrability, density, elasticity, thickness), wound topography (deep, narrow), and characteristics of the needle (type of eye, length, diameter). Most surgical needles are made from stainless steel because it is strong and corrosion free and does not harbor bacteria.

The three basic components of a suture needle are the attachment end (swaged or eyed), body, and point (Fig. 15-42, *A*). Suture material must be threaded onto eyed needles. Because a double-strand of suture is pulled through the tissue, a larger hole is created than when a swaged needle is used. Eyed needles may be closed (round, oblong, or square) or French (with a slit from the inside of the eye to the end of the needle for ease of threading) (Fig. 15-42, *B*). Eyed needles are threaded from the inside curvature. With swaged needles, the needle and suture are joined in a continuous unit, minimizing tissue trauma and increasing ease of use.

The needle body comes in a variety of shapes (Fig. 15-42, *C*); tissue type and depth and size of the wound determine the appropriate needle shape. Straight (Keith) needles are generally used in accessible places where the needle can be manipulated directly with the fingers (e.g., placement of purse-string sutures in the rectum). Curved needles are manipulated with needle holders. The depth and diameter of the wound are important when selecting the most appropriate curved needle. One-fourth (¼) circle needles are primarily used in ophthalmic procedures. Three-eighths (⅜) and one-half (½) circle needles are the most commonly used surgical needles in veterinary medicine (e.g., abdominal closure). Three-eighths circle needles are more easily manipulated than one-half circle needles because they require less manipulation of the wrist. However, because of the larger arc of manipulation required, they are awkward to use in deep or inaccessible locations. A one-half circle or five-eighths (⅝) circle needle, despite requiring more wrist manipulation, is easier to use in confined locations.

The needle point (cutting, taper, reverse-cutting; Fig. 15-42, *D*) determines the sharpness of a needle and type of tissue in which the needle is used. Cutting needles generally have two or three opposing cutting edges. They are used in tissues that are difficult to penetrate (e.g., skin). With conventional cutting needles, the third cutting edge is on the inside (concave) curvature of the needle. The location of the inside cutting edge may promote "cut-out" of tissue because it cuts toward the edges of the wound or incision. Reverse-cutting needles have a third cutting edge located on the outer (convex) curvature of the needle. This makes them stronger than similarly sized conventional cutting needles, and reduces the risk of tissue cut-out. Side-cutting needles (spatula needles) are flat on the top and bottom. They are generally used in ophthalmic procedures.

Tapered needles (round needles) have a sharp tip that pierces and spreads tissues without cutting them. They are generally used in easily penetrated tissues (e.g., intestine, subcutaneous tissues, fascia). Tapercut (Ethicon) needles have a reverse-cutting edge tip and a taper-point body. They are generally used for suturing dense, tough fibrous tissue (e.g., tendon) and for some cardiovascular procedures (e.g., vascular grafts). Blunt-point needles have a rounded, blunt point that can dissect through friable tissue without cutting. They are occasionally used for suturing soft, parenchymal organs (e.g., liver, kidney).

OTHER MATERIALS USED IN WOUND CLOSURE

TISSUE ADHESIVES

Cyanoacrylates ("super glue") are commonly used for tissue adhesion during some procedures (e.g., declawing, tail docking, ear cropping). Products advocated for use in vet-

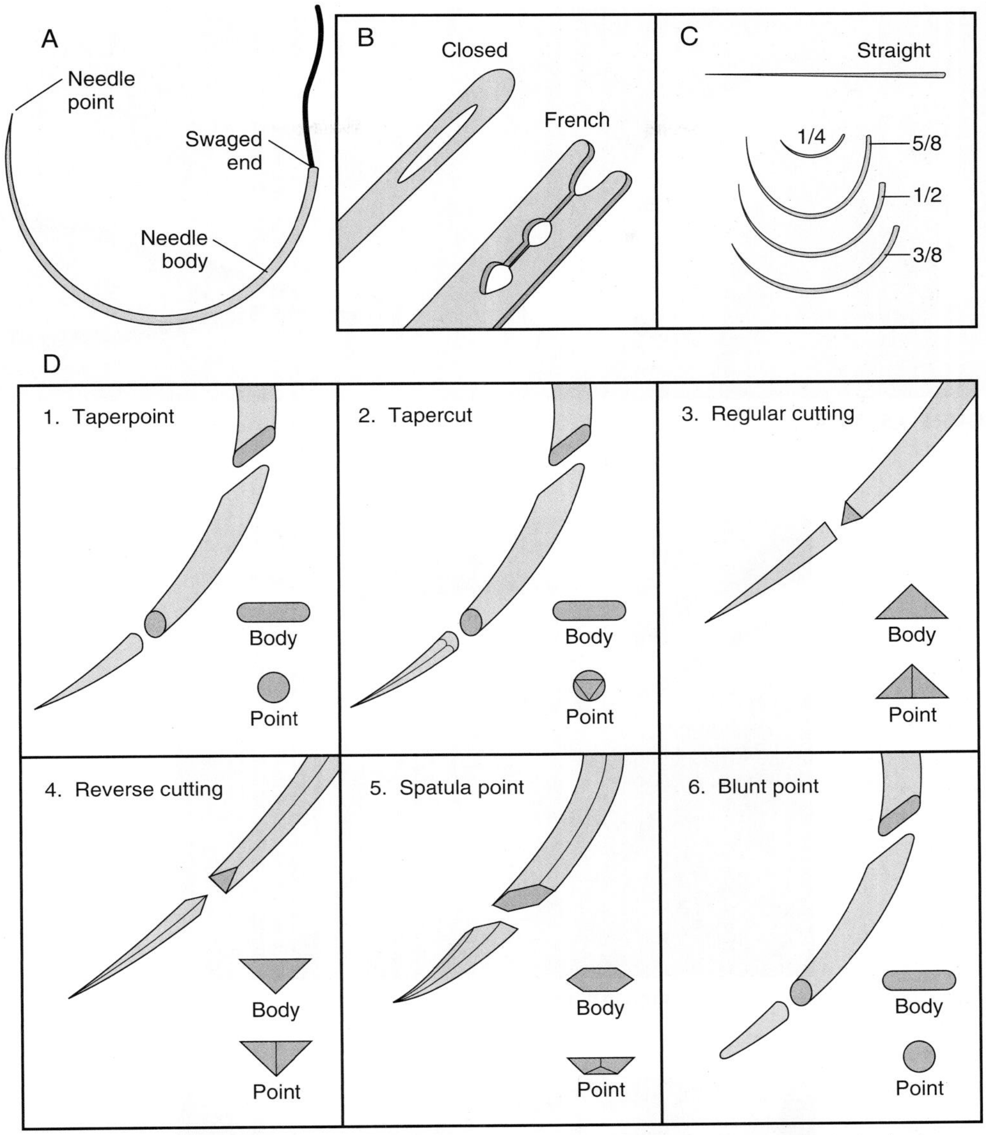

FIGURE 15-42 A, Basic components of a needle. B, Types of eyed needles. C and D, Needle body shapes and sizes. (Adapted from Fossum TW: *Small animal surgery*, ed 3, St Louis, 2007, Mosby.)

erinary patients include Tissueglue (GRx Medical, Gilbert, AZ), Vetbond (3M, St Paul, MN), and Nexabond (Tri-Point Medical). These adhesives rapidly polymerize in the presence of moisture and produce a strong flexible bond. Adhesion of tissue edges generally takes less than 15 seconds, but may be delayed by excessive hemorrhage. Persistence of the glue in the dermis may result in granuloma formation or wound dehiscence, and placement in an infected site may cause fistulation.

SKIN STAPLES

Metal staples (skin staples or Michel clips) are used to appose wound edges or attach drapes to the skin. Care must be used to ensure that the staple is appropriately bent so that, when staples are used for skin closure, they cannot be easily removed by the animal. A special "staple-remover" facilitates clip removal after healing (Figs. 15-43 and 15-44).

SURGICAL MESH

Surgical mesh may be used to repair hernias (e.g., perineal hernias) or reinforce traumatized or devitalized tissues (abdominal hernias). Occasionally it is used to replace excised traumatized or neoplastic tissues. Surgical mesh is available in nonabsorbable (Mersilene, Prelone) or absorbable (Vicryl, Dexon) forms.

SUTURE REMOVAL

Skin incisions are often closed with nonabsorbable suture material. These sutures are removed once healing is sufficient to prevent wound dehiscence, usually after 10 to 14 days.

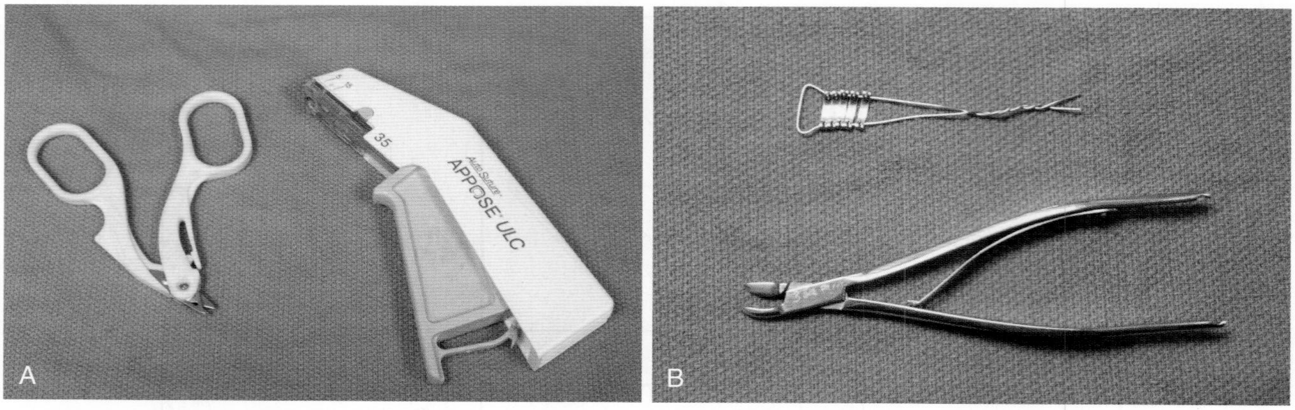

FIGURE 15-43 A, Skin staples (gun, *right*) and staple removal device *(left)*. B, Michel clips *(top)* and applying/removing forceps *(bottom)*.

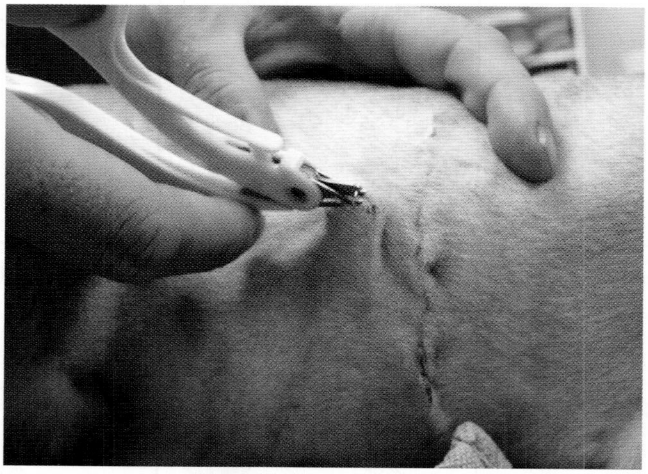

FIGURE 15-44 Skin staple removal.

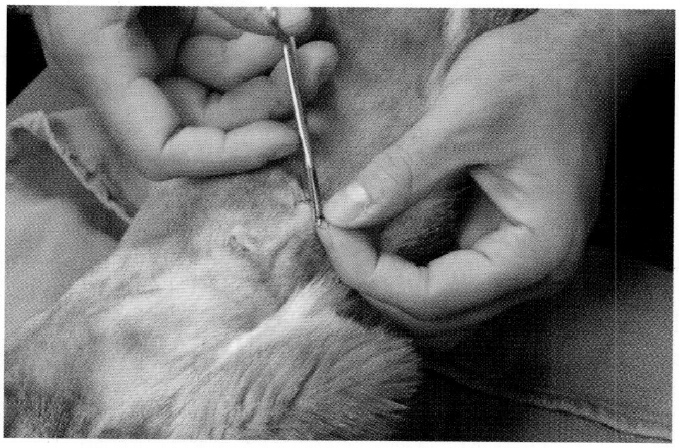

FIGURE 15-45 Suture removal.

However, delayed healing, as in debilitated animals, may require that sutures be left in place for longer periods. Additionally, if fibrosis is desired (e.g., aural hematoma), delayed suture removal may be considered.

Skin suture removal is begun by grasping one or both of the suture ends, which were deliberately left long for that purpose, and pulling the knot away from the skin (Fig. 15-45). Using suture removal scissors, cut one of the two strands of suture beneath the knot at the skin surface, and pull the suture out. It is important that only one of the strands is cut to avoid leaving some of the suture material buried beneath the skin, where it could act as an irritant.

REVIEW QUESTIONS

Matching—Surgical Instruments

Match the following surgical instruments with their primary function:

____1. hemostatic forceps	A. used to incise tissue
____2. needle holders	B. used for cutting tissue
____3. retractors	C. grasp and manipulate curved needles
____4. scissors	D. clamp and hold tissue and blood vessels
____5. scalpels and blades	E. crushing instrument used to clamp blood vessels
____6. tissue forceps	F. used to retract tissue and improve exposure

Matching—Surgical Procedures

Match the following surgical procedures with their definition:

____7. herniorrhaphy	A. incision into the intestine
____8. orchiectomy	B. removal of part or all of one or more mammary gland
____9. gastrotomy	C. incision into the urinary bladder
____10. thoracotomy	D. surgical removal of a claw
____11. enterotomy	E. incision into a simple stomach
____12. cystotomy	F. incision into the abdominal cavity
____13. urethrotomy	G. surgical removal of testes
____14. laparotomy	H. incision into thoracic cavity
____15. mastectomy	I. surgical repair of abnormal opening
____16. onychectomy	J. incision into the urethra

Matching—Surgical Incisions

Match the following surgical incisions with their location or benefit:

____17. flank incision	A. parallel to the last rib
____18. ventral midline incision	B. lateral and parallel to the ventral midline
____19. median sternotomy	C. perpendicular to long axis of body, caudal to last rib
____20. paramedian incision	D. offers excellent exposure of entire abdominal cavity
____21. paracostal incision	E. used when all lung fields need to be visualized

Fill in the Blank

Provide answers to complete the following statements.

1. ____________________ is the term used to describe all precautions taken to prevent contamination or infection of a surgical wound.
2. Surgical procedures are described using ____________________ combined with root words.
3. ____________________ refers to the destruction of all microorganisms (bacteria, viruses, spores) on a surface or object.
4. Hospital-acquired infections are called ____________________.
5. Surgical mesh may be used to repair ____________________ or reinforce traumatized or devitalized tissues.
6. Curved instruments are passed to the surgeon with the ______________ side up.
7. ____________________ ensures that the hand never comes into contact with the outside of the surgical gown or glove.
8. Organic nonabsorbable suture is available made of ______________ or ______________.
9. Surgical instrument manufacturers may recommend rinsing, cleaning, and sterilizing instruments in ____________________, because tap water contains minerals that cause discoloration and staining.
10. Surgical packs may not be completely sterilized if they are ____________________ or improperly loaded in the autoclave or gas sterilizer container.
11. Subcutaneous infections frequently progress to ______ ____________________.
12. Prior to sterilization, surgical drapes are folded so that the ________________ can be properly positioned over the surgical site without contaminating the drape.
13. A ________________ should be available to place needed supplies and equipment on the instrument table or Mayo stand in an operating room.
14. __________ needles have a sharp tip that pierces and spreads tissues without cutting them.
15. Sterile preparation of the surgical site begins after transportation and ____________________ of the animal on the operating table.

RECOMMENDED READING

Fossum TW: *Small animal surgery*, ed 4, St Louis, 2013, Mosby.

Sonsthagen TF: *Veterinary instruments and equipment*, ed 3, St Louis, 2013, Mosby.

Tear M: *Small animal surgical nursing: skills and concepts*, ed 2, St Louis, 2012, Mosby.

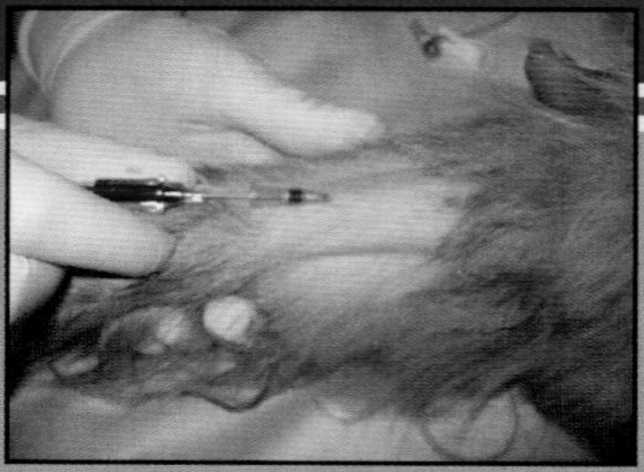

16 Fluid Therapy and Blood Transfusion

OUTLINE

LEARNING OBJECTIVES

After reviewing this chapter, the reader will be able to:

1. Explain the distribution of water throughout the body and the differences in the composition of extracellular fluid and intracellular fluid compartments.
2. Describe how physical exam findings play a role in determining a fluid therapy plan.
3. Differentiate between crystalloid and artificial colloid solutions.
4. List and explain indications for fluid therapy.
5. Identify routes of fluid administration.
6. Compare the different types of intravenous catheters available and the appropriate use of each.
7. Explain the physiology of hemostasis and how it relates to a bleeding patient.
8. Describe the steps necessary in assessing a bleeding patient and identifying the cause of bleeding.
9. List the types of blood products used in transfusion medicine and give examples of when each product would be used appropriately.
10. Describe canine and feline blood types.

LEARNING OBJECTIVES—cont'd

11. Distinguish between the information gathered from a blood type compared to a cross-match.
12. Identify different blood collection methods, giving examples of collection systems available.
13. Calculate blood product dosages.
14. Assess patients receiving blood transfusion support.
15. Identify adverse reactions to blood transfusion.

KEY TERMS

Acidosis	Extracellular fluid	Hyponatremia	Osmotic pressure
Alkalosis	Fibrin	Hypotonic	Packed red blood cells
Balanced fluid solution	Fresh frozen plasma	Insensible water loss	Replacement solutions
Blood cross-match	Fresh whole blood	Intracellular fluid	Secondary hemostasis
Blood type	Hyperkalemia	Isotonic	Sensible water loss
Cryoprecipitate	Hypernatremia	Maintenance solutions	Stored whole blood
Cryosupernatant plasma	Hypertonic	Osmolality	Tonicity
Diffusion	Hypokalemia	Osmosis	Total body water

FLUID THERAPY

Fluid therapy is one of the most commonly used supportive measures in veterinary medicine and is an important aspect of virtually every critical care case. It is primarily used to correct fluid deficits, electrolyte disturbances, and acid-base imbalances. In order to understand the need and value of fluid support, and to recognize and manage patients with fluid and electrolyte disorders, one must have a basic understanding of the physiology of fluid balance.

FLUID DISTRIBUTION

Approximately 60% of lean body weight is composed of fluid, often referred to as **total body water** (TBW). Three major fluid compartments make up TBW: **intracellular fluid** within the cells; interstitial fluid between the cells; and intravascular fluid, or plasma, within the blood vessels. About two thirds of TBW is intracellular fluid (ICF). The remaining third, called **extracellular fluid** (ECF), is composed of interstitial fluid (75%) and plasma (25%) (Fig. 16-1). Some extracellular fluids can collect in various parts of the body secondary to infection, injury, or compromised circulation. These fluids, referred to as third-space fluids, have no functional use (e.g., pleural effusions [fluid between lung pleura], pericardial effusions [fluid within the pericardial sac], ascites [fluid within peritoneal cavity], and generalized edema).

The ECF is in constant motion throughout the body, allowing electrolytes, oxygen, and nutrients necessary for the maintenance of cellular life to reach cells, as well as removal of waste products. These regulatory functions performed by the body contribute to the maintenance of a consistent internal environment, referred to as homeostasis.

The chemical composition of the ECF and the ICF is very different; these differences are extremely important to the life and function of each cell, as well as the regulation of all body systems. Water and electrolytes continually move in and out of cells, working together to maintain water balance. The movement of these molecules (solutes) across a semi-permeable cell membrane from the side with the higher solute concentration to the side with the lower solute concentration until the concentrations equilibrate is called **diffusion.** The diffusion of water, or **osmosis,** occurs when water moves across a cell membrane from a solution with a low solute concentration to the side with the higher solute concentration until the concentrations equilibrate. How much and how quickly osmosis occurs is dependent on the number and size of solutes in the solution and the permeability characteristics of the membrane between the two compartments. A certain amount of pressure is required to stop this process completely and is referred to as the **osmotic pressure.** The concentration of these osmotically active particles (solutes, e.g., sodium and potassium) in solution is called **osmolality** and is expressed as mOsm/kg. The normal serum osmolality in the dog and the cat is approximately 300 mOsm/kg.

ELECTROLYTES

Electrolytes are active chemicals or elements within all body fluids, each playing a specific role that must be maintained in order to ensure normal body functions. In the clinical setting electrolyte balance refers to the maintenance of normal serum concentrations. Measuring the concentration of electrolytes in the ICF is difficult; therefore measuring serum concentrations (i.e., ECF) is used to assess and manage patients with imbalances.

The major extracellular electrolytes are sodium, chloride, and bicarbonate. Sodium is the most abundant and important of the extracellular ions in that the distribution of body water is influenced by sodium more than any other electrolyte. Because sodium attracts water, it is the primary factor responsible for determining ECF volume and osmotic pressure. Maintaining a balance of sodium intake and excretion (via the kidney) is critical in controlling ECF volume.

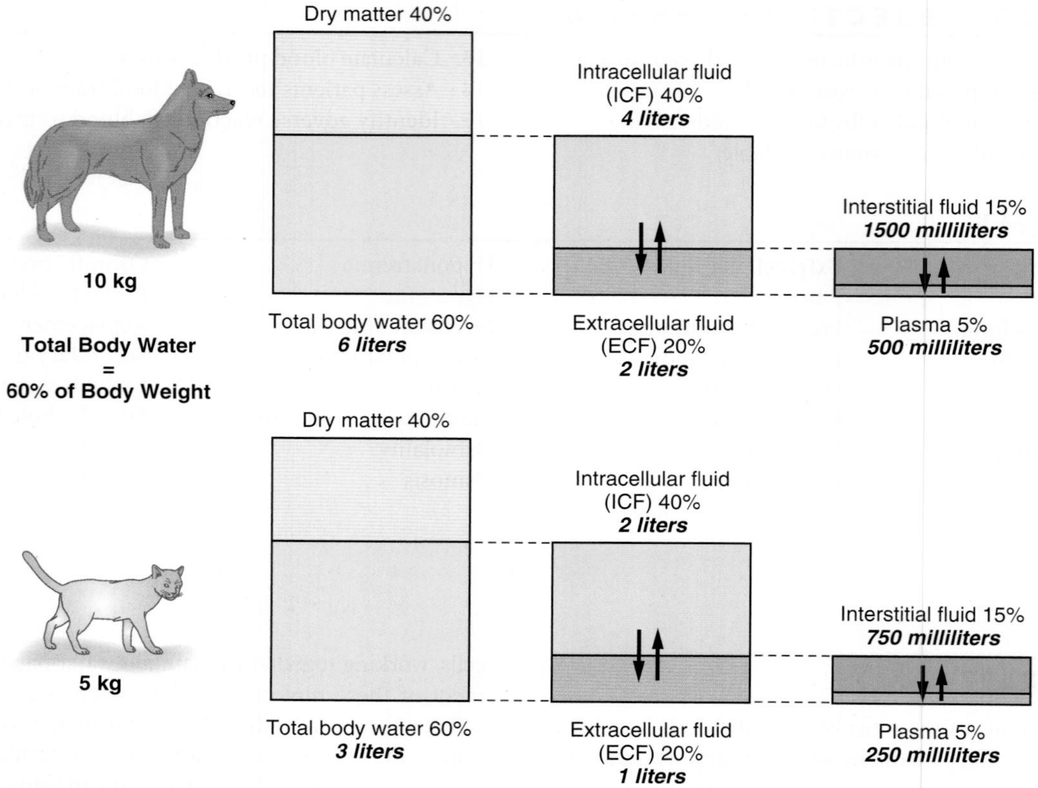

FIGURE 16-1 Compartments of total body water expressed as percentage of body weight and total body water for a 10-kg dog and a 5-kg cat. (From DiBartola SP: *Fluid, electrolyte, and acid-base disorders in small animal practice,* ed 3, St Louis, 2008, Saunders.)

Low extracellular sodium concentration creates a low osmolality and will therefore cause an influx of water into cells. Clinical signs associated with low sodium levels, or **hyponatremia,** are usually neurologic in origin and include generalized muscular weakness, lethargy or mental depression, nausea, inappetence, and hypotension.

Hypernatremia, or sodium excess, can be seen as a result of water loss (dehydration) resulting in an osmotic movement of water out of cells. The clinical signs are also primarily neurologic and include excessive thirst, muscle weakness, disorientation, seizures, and possible coma. In comparison, hypernatremia is a less frequently encountered condition in small animals than hyponatremia.

The major intracellular electrolytes are potassium, magnesium, and phosphate ions. Intracellular fluid also contains sodium but in much smaller amounts than outside the cell. Potassium is the dominant intracellular ion and is responsible for osmotic pressure within the ICF. It plays an important role in normal cell metabolism and is necessary for the maintenance of several body functions, most importantly the generation of electrical potentials in muscles and nerves. Relatively small changes in serum potassium concentration can alter nervous and cardiac functions; therefore serum potassium levels must be maintained within very close limits (Table 16-1).

Abnormal serum potassium concentrations occur frequently in animals with fluid disturbances.

TABLE 16-1 Intracellular vs. Extracellular Electrolytes

FLUID COMPARTMENT	ELECTROLYTES
Extracellular Fluid	Sodium (Na^+)
	Chloride (Cl^-)
	Bicarbonate (HCO_3^-
Intracellular Fluid	Potassium (K^+)
	Magnesium (Mg^{2+})
	Phosphates (HPO_4^{-2}, $H_2PO_4^{-1}$)

Hypokalemia, or low serum potassium, is the most frequently encountered potassium abnormality and usually requires supplementation in hospitalized patients. Causes include decreased intake (e.g., anorexia or restricted diet), excessive loss (e.g., gastrointestinal, urinary, or third-space loss), and movement from extracellular fluid to intracellular fluid (e.g., with alkalosis). The distribution of potassium between ECF and ICF can be affected by serum pH; therefore animals experiencing an increase in pH (**alkalosis**) may become hypokalemic because of potassium being driven into the cells.

When serum levels begin to drop, potassium will leave the cells to increase the serum concentration. Serum potassium will therefore decrease only after a considerable loss of total body potassium. Because we can only measure serum potassium, it is difficult to accurately assess total body deficits. Many animals with hypokalemia have no clinical signs unless depletion is severe. Muscle weakness, polyuria, and polydipsia can be seen in some patients. Also, potassium depletion can impair insulin release, ultimately affecting glucose levels.

Hyperkalemia, or high serum potassium concentration, is less commonly encountered than hypokalemia but can be life-threatening. Potassium is normally excreted by the kidney; therefore hyperkalemia is often encountered in animals where renal excretion is impaired. Hyperkalemia is most commonly seen with urethral obstruction in cats, but also with anuric or oliguric renal failure, Addison's disease, or excess potassium delivery during IV fluid therapy. Given that serum potassium levels are inversely related to serum pH, animals experiencing a decrease in pH (**acidosis**) may become hyperkalemic because of potassium being driven out of cells. Clinical signs of hyperkalemia include classic ECG changes (i.e., tall tented T-wave) representing a weakness in myocardial contractility and bradycardia.

ACID-BASE BALANCE

Acid-base balance is the regulation of hydrogen ion concentration in body fluid. The slightest change in the concentration of this ion can cause marked alterations in chemical reactions in the cells. Because of this, regulation of hydrogen is one of the most important aspects of homeostasis.

Hydrogen ion concentration is expressed as pH. Hydrogen and pH have an inverse relationship: the more hydrogen that is produced, the lower the pH becomes, resulting in acidosis. The less hydrogen that is produced, the higher the pH becomes, resulting in alkalosis. The normal pH of arterial blood is 7.4; the pH of venous blood and interstitial fluid is approximately 7.35. The body must maintain the slightly alkaline pH of blood within this range as major complications in life support can occur if the pH falls below 7.2 or rises above 7.6 for more than a few hours.

The three primary systems that help control acid-base balance are blood buffers, lungs, and kidneys. These systems will be utilized based on the severity of the impending acidosis or alkalosis. The body's first line of defense is blood buffers, most commonly bicarbonate, phosphate, and protein. Within seconds of any small change in hydrogen ion concentration, buffer systems within all body fluids will bind with any excess acid or alkali. Secondly, if the hydrogen ion concentration increases, the respiratory center is stimulated to increase the respiratory rate in order to eliminate carbon dioxide. Similarly, if the hydrogen ion concentration decreases, the respiratory rate decreases in order to retain carbon dioxide. These compensatory processes will ultimately help to return the hydrogen ion concentration to normal (Table 16-2). The respiratory system requires more time (approximately 10 minutes) than the buffer system in readjusting these levels. Finally, the most powerful regulatory system, the kidneys, requires up to several days to readjust the serum concentration of hydrogen through the excretion and/or retention of bicarbonate. The kidneys achieve regulation by readjusting the pH of the urine, and thereby readjusting the pH of body fluid.

TABLE 16-2 Characteristics of Primary Acid-Base Disturbances

DISORDER	pH	[H^+]	PRIMARY DISTURBANCE	COMPENSATORY RESPONSE
Metabolic acidosis	↓	↑	↓ [HCO_3^-]	↓ PCO_2
Metabolic alkalosis	↑	↓	↑ [HCO_3^-]	↑ PCO_2
Respiratory acidosis	↓	↑	↑ PCO_2	↑ [HCO_3^-]
Respiratory alkalosis	↑	↓	↓ PCO_2	↓ [HCO_3^-]

From Rose BD: *Clinical physiology of acid-base and electrolyte disorders*, ed 3, New York, 1989, McGraw-Hill, p. 470, with permission of the McGraw-Hill Companies.

CLINICAL ASPECTS OF FLUID THERAPY

Determining the need for fluid administration requires assessment of the patient's state of hydration and estimation of fluid deficits through subjective patient evaluation. Formulation of a fluid therapy regimen is based on information gathered from an accurate history, a thorough physical examination, and laboratory tests.

HISTORY

A complete history helps to establish the presence of fluid deficits (dehydration and/or hypovolemia). The history should include information on the patient's usual and current food and water intake (i.e., polydipsia, anorexia). Any information regarding urination (i.e., polyuria), defecation (including diarrhea), and vomiting is useful. Ensure that there is no history of trauma or evidence of hemorrhage. To help assess the degree of dehydration, consider exposure to extreme environmental heat, excessive exercise, fever, panting, and the period over which losses have occurred, including the amount and frequency of fluid losses. Information pertaining to medication the animal has been or is currently taking can be useful. Some medications such as diuretics and certain antibiotics can have potentially complicating side effects (e.g., vomiting and diarrhea). These effects cause fluid shifts that impact the fluid status of the patient and should be considered when formulating a fluid therapy plan.

PHYSICAL EXAMINATION

A complete physical examination can help define the avenue(s) of fluid loss. Dehydration and hypovolemia are the most frequently encountered conditions; however, not all dehydrated patients are hypovolemic, and not all hypovolemic patients are dehydrated. Animals should be assessed for signs that will help determine which of these processes or combination thereof is occurring.

Certain physical signs can help estimate hydration status, including dry, tacky mucous membranes, skin turgor, position of the eye in the orbit, body temperature, evidence of decreased peripheral circulation (e.g., poor pulse quality), and changes in body weight (Table 16-3). The cardiovascular and respiratory system should be carefully evaluated. Assessment of perfusion is based on mucous membrane color, capillary refill time, heart rate and pulse rate, pulse strength, and pulse

TABLE 16-3 Clinical Estimation of Degree of Dehydration

	APPEARANCE	EYES	MUCOUS MEMBRANES	SKIN TENT
3%-5%	Normal	Normal	Normal	<2 sec
6%-8%	Mildly depressed	Mildly sunken	Sticky/dry	>3 sec
10%-12%	Depressed	Deeply sunken	Dry ± cold	Persists
>15%	Moribund			

From Table 129-1 in Ettinger SJ, Feldman E: *Textbook of veterinary internal medicine*, ed 7, St Louis, 2010, Saunders.

quality. Most of these assessments are subjective. For this reason, monitoring is more accurate when serial examinations are performed consistently by an experienced member of the healthcare team and results are monitored in relation to one another.

Normal mucous membranes are pink and moist to the touch but can range in color from pale to cyanotic to muddy or injected (dark cherry red). Dry oral mucous membranes may result from panting and should be evaluated in addition to other values or mucous membranes. Also, the degree of dehydration in patients that are vomiting and salivating can be underestimated if one relies solely on mucous membrane assessment. Capillary refill time (CRT) provides an indication of peripheral perfusion. Pressure is applied to the pink mucosa of the gum or the inner lip and then released. The time required for the blanched area to return to pink should be 1 to 2 seconds. Prolonged refill time is suggestive of compromised tissue perfusion and shock. Rapid refill time of less than 1 second is usually associated with tachycardia as a result of the heart's attempt to increase cardiac output when compensating for hypovolemia.

Pulse rate and quality provide information regarding heart rate and perfusion pressure. Veterinary technicians should become proficient at assessment, accurate interpretation, and monitoring of pulse quality. Most easily accessible and palpable are the femoral, dorsal metatarsal, and ulnar arteries. Pulse rate corresponds to and should be synchronous with each beat of the heart. Pulse quality corresponds to the effectiveness of the heart in perfusing the body; a skilled veterinary technician can learn to use pulse pressure in estimating blood pressure when more advanced equipment is not available.

The heart and lungs should be auscultated before the onset of fluid therapy and frequently throughout treatment. Cardiac auscultation allows detection of heart murmurs and arrhythmias. Pulse deficits are detected by palpating a peripheral pulse while simultaneously ausculting the heart. If a compromise in cardiac function is suspected, the approach to fluid therapy may require adjustment. On pulmonary auscultation, crackling sounds indicate fluid accumulation in the alveoli or bronchioles, suggesting edema or overhydration. Wheezing sounds are usually a result of some degree of airway obstruction. When wheezing sounds are detected during auscultation, the stethoscope should always be placed over the trachea to determine whether the same sounds can be heard in this area as those heard over the lung fields. If present, the sounds most likely can be classified as referred upper respiratory noise. Conversely, absence of lung sounds is abnormal and may suggest consolidation of lung tissue, as in pneumonia. The depth of respiration, along with the rate and effort, should also be noted.

> *TECHNICIAN NOTE* The heart and lungs should be auscultated before the onset of fluid therapy and frequently throughout treatment.

Skin turgor is not the most accurate way to detect or estimate dehydration. In addition to tissue hydration, it is affected by the amount of subcutaneous fat and elastic tissue present. The most commonly tested area is over the trunk, avoiding the loose skin of the neck region and the top of the head. The skin is lifted a short distance (tented) and then released, monitoring its return to the initial position. Normal skin returns to its position within 2 to 3 seconds. The skin of dehydrated animals may show varying degrees of slow return to the initial position. The skin turgor of obese animals may appear normal despite dehydration because of excessive stores of subcutaneous fat. Likewise, the skin of emaciated animals lacks subcutaneous fat and elastic tissue and therefore may lead to an overestimation of dehydration.

Obtaining the patient's body weight is an important aspect of the physical exam. An acute decrease in body weight is expected in animals that experience some type of water loss. Dehydration can be more accurately assessed if the patient's current body weight can be compared with a weight obtained before the presenting episode. Frequent, serial body weight measurement is a good monitoring tool for continued fluid loss during treatment. A change in body weight of 1 kg represents a gain or loss of 1 L of fluid. Keep in mind that third-space fluid loss can occur from the ECF into the gastrointestinal tract and thoracic or peritoneal cavities without creating a change in body weight; therefore, concurrent auscultation and abdominal palpation may help determine the presence of third-space losses.

The normal urine output in dogs and cats is 1 to 2 ml/kg/hr. Urine output is a reflection of cardiac function, circulating blood volume, perfusion, and function of the kidneys and lower urinary tract. Urine production should be monitored in patients when abnormalities of these factors are suspected or confirmed. It is very important to monitor the amount of urine being produced as it relates to the amount of fluid being administered. Fluid intake and output records may provide an estimate of the balance between fluid loss and fluid replacement, keeping in mind that they are sometimes inaccurate. Evaluation of hydration status is necessary before proper assessment of urine production; for example, dehydrated patients require fluid replacement before oliguria (urine production of less than 1 ml/kg/hr) is confirmed. Once patients are adequately hydrated and blood pressure is returned to normal, the confirmed presence of oliguria may suggest renal failure.

Hypothermic and hyperthermic patients have complications that require adjustments in fluid therapy and close monitoring during temperature alterations. When a change in body temperature occurs in a previously stable animal, potential causes must be investigated. Spontaneous hypothermia can result from heat loss (e.g., extreme environmental cold, surgery), impaired heat production (e.g., underlying disease), or toxicosis (e.g., ethylene glycol ingestion, drug therapy). In response to decreased cardiac output, hypothermic animals will attempt to conserve heat by shunting blood from the peripheral vasculature and the gastrointestinal tract. Cardiovascular and respiratory support and monitoring must be instituted before initiating warming procedures. A rapid increase in body temperature may lead to peripheral vasodilation and hypotension, further complicating the situation at hand. Spontaneous hyperthermia can be caused by poor environmental ventilation (animals confined in automobiles), heat prostration, inflammatory response, or abnormalities of the thermoregulatory center. Dehydration (as a result of excessive panting) and hypovolemia (secondary to decreased cardiac output) may occur in any of these situations; therefore fluid therapy is a crucial part of the therapeutic plan.

LABORATORY TESTS

Laboratory tests may be vital in establishing the nature and extent of fluid imbalances and in monitoring treatment. Serial determinations of the hematocrit (packed cell volume) and total plasma protein level are important for establishing a trend and adjusting therapy. A decreasing hematocrit and total plasma protein level can suggest acute or chronic bleeding or hemodilution. Patients with a low serum protein level (hypoproteinemia) are in danger of losing fluid from the intravascular space into the interstitium because of low intravascular osmotic pressure (i.e., albumin is essential for maintaining osmotic pressure needed for proper distribution of body fluids between intravascular compartment and body tissues). Once the protein level falls below 3.5 g/dl or the albumin level below 2.0 g/dl, colloid administration should be considered. Although a patient's colloid osmotic pressure (COP) will increase after administering artificial colloids, both the total solids and protein concentrations are no longer an accurate indication of their true oncotic pressure. In addition, the albumin concentration will be lowered because of the dilutional effect of the colloid. An increasing hematocrit and total plasma protein level can indicate fluid loss from the intravascular space, ultimately resulting in dehydration. These two values should routinely be evaluated together to avoid misleading information that could be obtained from evaluation of either value alone. Serum chemistry profiles can be performed to determine the functional status of certain organs (e.g., liver, kidneys, pancreas). The results will assist with patient evaluation, determining the need for electrolyte replacement therapy, detecting complications, and ruling out other diseases.

Urine specific gravity is a measurement of solids in solution and indicates the kidney's ability to concentrate urine. In a normal animal, the specific gravity depends on fluid intake and urine output. An increased urine specific gravity is most likely to occur in animals with decreased water intake. Upon rehydration, the urine specific gravity should decrease. Urine specific gravity should be measured before, during, and after fluid therapy to help evaluate kidney function.

FLUID CHOICES

The goal of fluid therapy is to restore body fluid losses, reestablish normal blood volume, improve tissue perfusion, and facilitate administration of certain drugs and therapeutics. Many considerations are integrated into a fluid choice (e.g., tonicity, amount of glucose, electrolyte balance, acidity, oncotic pressure, oxygen-carrying capability). The choice is based on the composition of fluid lost from the body, abnormalities requiring correction, and the severity and type of fluid depletion that has occurred. There are three main groups of fluids to choose from (i.e., crystalloids, artificial colloids, blood products), and they can be used individually or in a variety of combinations. The choice, composition, and volume of fluid being administered typically require adjustment throughout the course of treatment.

CRYSTALLOIDS

Crystalloid solutions (e.g., lactated Ringer's solution, 0.9% NaCl, Normosol-R) contain small molecules that, when in solution, can pass through a semi-permeable membrane and enter all body compartments. Crystalloid solutions contain sodium as their major osmotically active particle and are categorized as **balanced** if similar in composition to plasma (e.g., lactated Ringer's solution, Normosol-R) or unbalanced if the electrolyte composition differs from that of plasma (e.g., 5% dextrose in water, 0.9% NaCl). For example, lactated Ringer's solution and Normosol-R contain sodium, chloride, potassium, calcium, and lactate in similar concentrations as found in plasma. Although these solutions are comparable with plasma in regard to their electrolyte composition, they do not contain phosphorus, albumin, or other proteins.

Tonicity is the ability of a fluid to change the water content of cells. The tonicity of a solution (defined by its sodium concentration), therefore, will determine the fluid distribution following infusion. A fluid into which normal body cells can be placed without causing either shrinkage or swelling of the cells is said to be **isotonic** (e.g., 0.9% sodium chloride); a solution that causes cells to swell is said to be **hypotonic** (e.g., 0.45% sodium chloride with 2.5% dextrose); a solution that causes cells to shrink is said to be **hypertonic** (e.g., 7% sodium chloride). Crystalloid fluids are available as isotonic, hypotonic, or hypertonic solutions; an isotonic solution will provide no gradient for water movement, whereas a hypertonic solution pulls water into the intravascular space and a hypotonic solution causes movement of water out of the intravascular space. When administering hypertonic solutions intravenously, water is pulled from the intracellular and interstitial space. Conversely, a hypotonic solution will be redistributed to and expand the intracellular space. The decision to use a specific type of crystalloid fluids must be based on the patient's needs and the ultimate distribution of these fluids (Table 16-4).

When using isotonic crystalloid fluid solutions, one must remember that these fluids pass readily through the blood vessel wall. Approximately one-third of the fluid will remain in the vasculature 30 minutes post infusion, whereas two-thirds is redistributed to the interstitium. Although volume restoration can be achieved with crystalloid solutions, effectiveness may be short term. In some cases it is difficult, if not impossible, to administer adequate volumes of crystalloid fluids to reverse the hypovolemic state. If volume depletion does not resolve or recurs, administration of colloid solutions (see below) may need to be incorporated into the treatment plan. Hemodilution is a common concern when utilizing crystalloid therapy only. The addition of a colloid solution has been shown to decrease the volume of additional fluid administration needed to correct the deficit.

Crystalloid solutions can also be classified as to whether they meet replacement or maintenance needs.

TABLE 16-4 Replacement Fluids

SOLUTION	OSMOLALITY (mOsm/L)	SODIUM (mEq/L)	POTASSIUM (mEq/L)	CHLORIDE (mEq/L)	CALCIUM (mEq/L)	BUFFER	TONICITY	INDICATIONS
Lactated Ringer's	273	130	4	109	3	Lactate	Isotonic	Dehydration Hypovolemic shock Vomiting Diarrhea Acute kidney injury Metabolic acidosis
Plasma-Lyte A	294	140	5	98	0	Acetate gluconate	Isotonic	Dehydration Hypovolemic shock Vomiting Diarrhea Acute kidney injury Metabolic acidosis
0.9% NaCl	310	154		154			Isotonic	Dehydration Hypovolemic shock Vomiting Diarrhea Hyperkalemia Metabolic alkalosis
Normosol-R	296	140	5	98			Isotonic	Dehydration Hypovolemic shock Vomiting Diarrhea Hyperkalemia Metabolic alkalosis
Plasma-Lyte M	363	40	13	40			Hypotonic	Replacement/maintenance of extravascular volume
0.45% NaCl	155	77		77			Hypotonic	Maintenance of extravascular volume
5% dextrose in H_2O (D_5W)	253						Hypotonic	Extravascular volume replacement Congestive heart failure Hypernatremia
3% NaCl	1026	513		513			Hypertonic	Hypovolemic shock Intravascular volume expansion
7.5% NaCl	2464	1232		1232			Hypertonic	Hypovolemic shock Intravascular volume expansion
Normosol-M + 5% dextrose	363					Acetate	Hypertonic	Intravascular volume expansion

Modified from Battaglia A, Steele A: *Small animal emergency and critical care for veterinary technicians*, ed 3, St Louis, Saunders, 2015.

Replacement solutions have a composition similar to that of plasma, with high sodium and low potassium concentrations (e.g., lactated Ringer's solution, Normosol-R).

Maintenance solutions differ from plasma in that they contain less sodium and more potassium (e.g., Normosol-M). The most commonly used crystalloid solutions are balanced replacement solutions. When replacement solutions are used for maintenance therapy or in animals with conditions causing loss of potassium, supplementation of potassium may be necessary.

Hypertonic saline solutions can be used in cases where rapid reexpansion of the vascular volume is needed (e.g., hypotensive shock). These solutions (e.g., 7% to 7.5% strengths) provide intravascular volume expansion by recruiting interstitial and intracellular fluid into the intravascular space. The effects are short-lived and can begin to dissipate in as little as 30 minutes; therefore hypertonic saline is often combined with a colloid solution (hydroxyethyl starch) to help prolong its effects. Because the interstitial space and intracellular fluid volumes are utilized by hypertonic saline, this fluid solution should not be used in severely dehydrated animals.

ARTIFICIAL COLLOIDS

The artificial colloid solutions currently available for use are gelatins, dextrans, and hydroxyethyl starches (e.g., Hetastarch). Availability of the various colloid products varies in different countries. These solutions contain large molecules that do not readily pass through a semi-permeable membrane. When colloid solutions are administered intravenously (IV), their distribution is primarily limited to the intravascular compartment, making them more effective than crystalloids at expanding blood volume. Ultimately these solutions increase oncotic pressure and therefore are used in conditions in which the vascular space cannot retain an adequate fluid volume (e.g., hypoproteinemia). Albumin, the molecule responsible for providing osmotic pressure in the natural state, has a molecular weight of 69 kD. Hydroxyethyl starches have a wide range of molecular weights, with an average of 450 kD. Many factors influence the duration of action of artificial colloids, including species of animal, dosage, specific colloid formulation, preinfusion intravascular volume status, and microvascular permeability. The degree of volume expansion is determined by the number of molecules present in the solution; the duration is determined by the size of the molecules in the solution. Although artificial colloids are more expensive, they are more cost effective in that they promote better tissue perfusion and maintain colloid osmotic pressure at a lower infusion volume. As a general rule, colloids should be used in combination with crystalloid solutions to support the fluid shift from the extravascular to the intravascular compartment. Also, crystalloids are held in the vascular space more effectively by the oncotic pressure of the colloids.

One limitation with artificial colloid solutions is their potential to cause bleeding tendencies or aggravate coagulopathies. There are many factors involved in this phenomenon including dilution, decreased activity of certain clotting factors and compromised function of platelets. Dilution occurs as a result of more artificial colloid taking up space in the vascular compartment, leaving less room for plasma, which contains essential clotting factors. Also, colloids have a longer plasma half-life than crystalloids, so their effects are longer in duration. Furthermore, the amount of factor VIII and von Willebrand factor (vWF) has been shown to be decreased even beyond dilutional effects in patients receiving artificial colloids. Factor VIII and vWF form a complex in the circulation that plays a role in platelet adhesion. Hydroxyethyl starches bind to factor VIII and vWF, reducing their availability to platelets. Artificial colloids also inhibit, destroy, and mechanically coat platelets, thereby reducing their functionality. Patients receiving these solutions should have their coagulation status monitored accordingly with potential administration of plasma and plasma products to counteract these adverse side effects.

Note: Blood products are covered in the Whole Blood and Blood Components section.

INDICATIONS FOR FLUID THERAPY

Fluid therapy is an important aspect in the treatment of many hospitalized patients. Dehydration and hypovolemia are the two most common indications for fluid therapy. It is important to understand the differences in these pathologies as well as in their treatments. Dehydration is the loss of total body water (loss of fluid from all three major fluid compartments) with preservation of the intravascular volume. Hypovolemia occurs when the intravascular volume is not large enough to preserve cardiac output. Animals can be dehydrated and have normal intravascular volume, or they can have normal hydration but be hypovolemic. Hypovolemia can be the end result of severe dehydration but is often seen as a separate entity. Similarly, many patients will be dehydrated but not to the extent that intravascular volume is depleted. A good example of hypovolemia is a dog that has been hit by a car and presents with a weak, rapid pulse as a result of intraabdominal hemorrhage. This patient is hypovolemic but initially maintains a normal hydration status; the total body water content is normal but intravascular volume is decreased. An example of dehydration is a cat in chronic renal failure that has lost fluid through increased urination. The kidneys are responsible for conserving the body's water and when not functioning properly, their ability to concentrate urine is impaired and excess fluid is lost via the urine (i.e., polyuria). In this example the patient is dehydrated but maintains adequate blood volume by pulling fluid from the extravascular space. The body has compensatory mechanisms for dehydration but if the dehydration is prolonged, hypovolemia may occur without intervention. Although dehydration can, and must, be corrected slowly so as not to overexpand the intravascular space, hypovolemia requires rapid reexpansion of the intravascular space.

HEMORRHAGE

A significant loss of blood over minutes to hours results in hypovolemia and potential cardiovascular collapse.

The therapeutic goal in the treatment of acute hemorrhagic hypovolemia is to stop hemorrhage and support the cardiovascular system. Aggressive, rapid restoration of vascular volume must be instituted while preventing further blood loss if possible. When choosing resuscitation fluid for intravascular space replacement, volume and composition are critical in determining the effectiveness of volume expansion and duration of its effect.

Following blood loss, the intravascular space is depleted, and only later does interstitial fluid shift from the extravascular into the intravascular space, providing much needed volume. Early in the hemorrhagic situation, focus should be placed on replenishing intravascular space losses. This can be accomplished easily using crystalloid fluid solutions. Crystalloid solutions also enter the extravascular space, and therefore it is necessary to administer two to three times the amount of crystalloid as the volume lost. Risk of fluid overload is of concern when a large volume of crystalloids are administered, especially in geriatric patients or patients with some degree of cardiovascular compromise. Colloid solutions should be considered when there is a need to maintain intravascular oncotic pressure without administering large volumes of fluid. Most often, crystalloid solutions are recommended initially in the treatment of acute blood loss. If blood loss continues and a substantial portion of the blood volume is depleted, colloid solutions can be added to the treatment plan.

The symptoms that occur following hemorrhage are a result of blood volume depletion, not a decrease in red blood cell mass. Unfortunately, volume expansion will further dilute any hemoglobin remaining within the circulation. Although intravascular volume expansion will improve tissue perfusion, patient assessment will help determine whether enough hemoglobin is present to provide oxygenation to vital organs. The need for transfusion should be based on clinical assessment of the signs of anemia, as there is no magic laboratory number at which a patient must be transfused. The aggressiveness of therapy will depend on the volume of blood lost, the rapidity at which it was lost, and the patient's condition. Given that anemia is an extremely dynamic situation, serial laboratory and physical assessments are crucial.

SHOCK

Shock is a condition in which systemic blood pressure is inadequate to deliver oxygen and nutrients to vital tissues and organs. Although the causes of shock vary, the end result of poor perfusion and impaired cellular metabolism are life threatening. Treatment of the patient in shock is directed at identifying the cause, with focus on restoring blood volume and improving tissue perfusion (Table 16-5). Fluid therapy is the foundation of a treatment plan; however, this syndrome affects multiple body systems, and individual patients will respond differently. Thorough patient assessment and continual monitoring is essential for proper adjustment to fluid choice, volume, and rate.

Patients experiencing mild to moderate hypoperfusion usually require crystalloid infusion rates of 20 to 60 ml/kg/hr. Critically ill dogs in shock, severely dehydrated, hemorrhaging, or experiencing poor perfusion may require isotonic crystalloid infusion doses of 60 to 90 ml/kg administered as a rapid intravenous bolus to effect. Cats in these life-threatening situations may require doses of 45 to 60 ml/kg, also as an intravenous bolus to effect. The calculated fluid dose should be divided into 3 or 4 boluses, with patient response monitored following each bolus administration. The total volume of fluid required will be determined by the response of the patient; once tissue perfusion is restored, fluid boluses can be discontinued. Isotonic crystalloids are the only solution that should be used at these recommended doses based on how they redistribute following infusion. Only one-third of the total infused fluid volume will remain in the intravascular space; two-thirds of the total infused fluid volume will redistribute to the extravascular space. Other fluids of varying composition will redistribute differently and can exacerbate dehydration or cause fluid overload.

The maximum rate of fluid administration is usually limited by mechanical ability to administer fluids. In a life-threatening situation, two or more catheters may be used simultaneously to administer large volumes of fluid. In addition, a commercially available pressure infusion cuff allows rapid delivery of fluid, but pressure should not exceed 300 mm Hg. Care should be taken to not introduce air into the system and risk infection or air emboli. In hypoproteinemic animals, caution should be exercised with the rate of administration, even when the patient is severely dehydrated or poorly perfused. Diminished colloid in the vascular space results in less retention of fluid in the circulation, ultimately risking development of edema and respiratory compromise.

DEHYDRATION

Dehydration is the loss of body water, often accompanied by electrolyte imbalances. Excessive loss of body fluid or lack of water intake may occur in any one or combination of conditions (Box 16-1).

The degree of dehydration can be roughly estimated by clinical assessment, and the patient's fluid deficit can be replaced with fluid administration over 12 to 48 hours, depending on the underlying disease process and the severity and duration of the dehydration. Acute fluid losses can be replaced more rapidly than chronic fluid deficits. In general, it is better to overestimate rather than underestimate the replacement volume, unless the patient has some underlying restrictive condition (e.g., cardiac or renal disease).

TABLE 16-5 Clinical Signs of Shock vs. Blood Volume Lost

BLOOD VOLUME LOST	CLINICAL SIGNS
<15%	None
15%-30%	Mild compensatory signs including tachycardia, peripheral vasoconstriction, etc.
>30%	Profound shock: decreased mentation, pale mucous membranes, increased capillary refill time
>40%	Obtunded, imminent death without intervention

Preexisting fluid deficits are usually replaced with IV fluid formulated for replacement (e.g., Normosol-R or lactated Ringer's). Once rehydration has been established in the patient, fluid infusion rates must be recalculated based on maintenance fluid needs and ongoing fluid losses.

MAINTENANCE FLUIDS

In order to maintain body fluid volume, an animal's daily intake of water, nutrients, and minerals must equal the sum of sensible and insensible losses, referred to as maintenance fluid requirements.

Sensible water loss is easy to measure and refers to water lost through the urine and feces.

Insensible water loss is difficult to measure and includes water lost through the respiratory tract (e.g., panting). Normal fluid losses are approximately 40 ml/kg/day in larger animals and 60 ml/kg/day in smaller animals, with urinary losses accounting for approximately 20 ml/kg/day, fecal losses for 5 ml/kg/day, and respiratory and transcutaneous losses for 15 ml/kg/day. These losses are replaced in healthy animals daily by drinking water, water in food, and metabolic breakdown of fat, carbohydrate, and protein. Maintenance requirements are estimated by body weight and are 40 to 60 ml/kg/day, or approximately 2 to 4 ml/kg/hr. Smaller, less active animals have lower calorie, electrolyte, and water requirements than larger, more active animals.

Patients in need of maintenance fluids should be provided with a solution intended for maintenance therapy (e.g., Normosol-M or 0.45% NaCl with KCl). This is especially important for patients receiving maintenance therapy only, given their potassium needs will not be met with a replacement solution. Once patients are returned to a normal state of hydration, maintenance fluids can be administered per os, subcutaneously, intraosseously, or intravenously (PO, SC, IO, or IV).

ONGOING LOSSES

Ongoing fluid losses should be estimated from the daily volume of urine, diarrhea, vomiting, tube drainage, excessive respiratory losses seen with panting, exudative wounds, etc. The calculated amount should be divided over 24 hours and added to the maintenance fluid dose. Replacement solutions are given to compensate for ongoing losses.

Patients receiving fluid support should be closely monitored for signs of overhydration, including restlessness, shivering, tachycardia, serous nasal or ocular discharge, respiratory distress, pulmonary crackles or rales, coughing as a result of pulmonary edema, vomiting, and diarrhea. Fluid administration must then be slowed or stopped, depending on the severity of clinical signs.

BOX 16-1 Possible Causes of Dehydration and Diarrhea

- Prolonged vomiting
- Prolonged fever
- Sequestration of gastrointestinal fluid/fluid-filled bowel
- Sweating/panting
- Exudating burns or open wounds
- Chronic blood loss
- Uncontrolled polyuria (if there is inadequate water intake to compensate for the loss)
- Lack of access to water
- Inability to drink
- Nervous system disturbances
- Systemic illness
- Anorexia

CORRECTING ELECTROLYTE IMBALANCES

Dehydration and known disease processes can cause predictable electrolyte changes in the body. These imbalances are most often corrected through fluid therapy. The fluid choice, additive solutions, and administration route and rate are dependent on the disease, patient status, and laboratory values. If additives of any type are incorporated into the main fluid source, the fluid bag should be labeled to note the additive and its concentration and amount, and the person adding the solution should initial the date and time of addition (Fig. 16-2).

> *TECHNICIAN NOTE* When administering a drug as a constant rate infusion (CRI) in a bag of IV fluids, it is essential to thoroughly mix the supplement once it has been added to the bag, especially potassium. Potassium can settle in the bottom of the fluid bag and be given as an inadvertent but life-threatening bolus if not dispersed well throughout the fluid solution.

Hypokalemia frequently occurs in animals with fluid disturbances, and supplementation is often required. The dosage

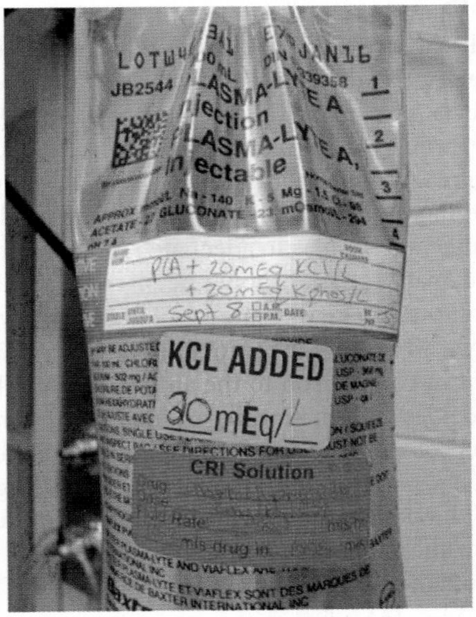

FIGURE 16-2 Fluid bags may contain numerous medications for continuous infusion. Bags should be well-labeled at all times. (From Battaglia A, Steele A: *Small animal emergency and critical care for veterinary technicians*, ed 3, St Louis, 2015, Saunders.)

TABLE 16-6 Guidelines for Intravenous Potassium (K) Supplementation*

SERUM K^+(mEq/L)	mEq K^+ (TO ADD TO 250 ML FLUID)	mEq K^+ (TO ADD TO 1 L FLUID)	MAXIMUM INFUSION RATE OF INTRAVENOUS FLUIDS (0.5 mEq/KG/HOUR)
<2.0	20	80	6
2.1-2.5	15	60	8
2.6-3.0	10	40	12
3.1-3.5	7	28	18
>3.5, < 5.0	5	20	25

*For dogs or cats with hypokalemia or for those with potassium depletion and normal serum potassium levels. This regimen is designed to be infused in maintenance volume of fluids.

From Table 15-5 in Wanamaker BP: *Applied pharmacology for veterinary technicians*, ed 4, St Louis, 2008, Saunders.

and route of potassium supplementation will depend on the cause and severity of the deficiency. Intravenous administration can be used to correct severe potassium deficiencies. The rate of potassium-augmented fluid infusion depends on the amount of potassium added to the fluid. The maximum rate of potassium supplementation in fluids is 0.5 mEq/kg/hr (Table 16-6). Potassium should never be administered in an undiluted form directly into the circulation because of the potential risk of cardiac arrest. When administered as a constant rate infusion (CRI) in a bag of IV fluids, it is essential to thoroughly mix any supplements being added to the bag, especially potassium. As with any CRI, potassium can settle in the bottom of the fluid bag and be given as an inadvertent, but life-threatening, bolus if not dispersed well throughout the fluids. Fluid with potassium in concentrations up to 30 to 35 mEq/L can be administered subcutaneously without discomfort or irritation.

DIURESIS

Certain diseases (e.g., kidney disease) and treatments (e.g., chemotherapy) require diuresis (increased fluid loss through the kidneys) as part of the therapeutic plan. Diuresis is achieved through placement of IV catheters and institution of aggressive fluid therapy. Patients undergoing diuresis should be monitored closely for signs of overhydration. If there is some question as to adequate renal function, an indwelling urinary catheter should be placed and maintained so urine output can be measured and fluid therapy adjusted accordingly. Measuring the amount of fluid administered to the patient in comparison to the amount of fluid being excreted provides information regarding the continued fluid deficits and/or potential fluid overload. It is imperative to continuously monitor the amount of fluid being administered to the patient along with the amount of fluid being excreted by the patient (i.e., "ins" should always be relatively equal to "outs").

TECHNICIAN NOTE Patients undergoing diuresis should be monitored closely for signs of overhydration.

DRUG THERAPY

In medicine today, many drugs are available in IV solution. If medication is administered directly into the circulation, rapid uptake of the drug can have an overall positive or negative effect. Drugs administered via IV will potentially have a much quicker effect with greater impact; therefore IV doses are often lower than those administered by other routes. Most drugs can be vascularly irritating, so dilution to an appropriate and acceptable concentration is important (e.g., antibiotics, chemotherapeutic agents).

TECHNICIAN NOTE Most drugs can be vascularly irritating, so dilution to an appropriate and acceptable concentration is important.

ROUTES OF FLUID ADMINISTRATION

There are many routes through which fluid solutions can be administered. An appropriate route is chosen after careful evaluation of the following several factors:

- Volume of fluid loss
- Rate of fluid loss (acute vs. chronic)
- Fluid solution selected for administration
- Volume and rate of infusion
- Patient status

These factors will be influenced by the cause and severity of the condition. In small animal medicine, medical, practical, and economic considerations may affect the fluid solution chosen and administration route used. A summary of fluid administration routes is in Table 16-7.

ORAL

Oral fluid therapy can be used if the gastrointestinal tract is working properly (no vomiting, diarrhea, or gastrointestinal obstruction). Unfortunately, this route cannot be used to correct severe fluid deficits in critically ill patients in need of rapid fluid and electrolyte delivery. Additionally, severely dehydrated animals have decreased gastrointestinal function and are not able to properly absorb fluids as readily via the gut. If the patient is only mildly dehydrated and will eat and drink and there is no evidence of vomiting, the oral route is an ideal choice for fluid delivery. It should also be the route of choice for animals with maintenance needs only and not requiring replacement fluids or sustaining ongoing losses.

TECHNICIAN NOTE If a patient does not drink fluid voluntarily, it can be offered by syringe into the mouth.

Dogs sometimes voluntarily drink commercially available human electrolyte products. These solutions are not recommended in cats because they lack taurine and other vital nutrients. If the patient does not drink the fluid, it can be offered via syringe into the mouth. A nasoesophageal tube can be placed to administer fluids; however, they are

TABLE 16-7 Routes of Fluid Administration

ROUTE	INDICATIONS	CONTRAINDICATIONS	EQUIPMENT REQUIRED	TECHNICIAN NOTES
Oral	Mild dehydration Short-term illness Small patients Animals with feeding tubes	Hypovolemia Shock Vomiting or nauseous animals Mentally inappropriate patients Decreased to absent gag/swallow reflex	Nasal/esophageal/percutaneous gastrostomy tube Syringes Baby bottles (neonates)	Confirm tube placement in appropriate location before administration of fluids Aspirate tubes before fluid administration/check residual volume
Subcutaneous	Mild dehydration Nonhospitalized animals	Hypovolemia Shock Hypothermia Dermal infection Skin wounds	Bag of sterile IV fluid for injection Administration set Needle (18-20 gauge) Isotonic crystalloid solution	Administer up to 10 ml/kg at each site Do not administer fluids under pressure because it can damage tissues and cause pain New sterile needle for each patient
Intravenous	Dehydration Hypovolemia Anorexia/vomiting/diarrhea of several days' duration Surgical procedures IV drug administration	Patients medically managed at home are not ideal candidates for IV fluid therapy	Sterile fluids for injection Administration set IV catheter and supplies Dial volume set/burette or fluid infusion pump Technical staff	Consider the patient's clinical signs when choosing site for IV catheter When possible avoid areas likely to be contaminated
Intraosseous	Cardiovascular collapse Lack of IV access Neonatal patients Avian patients Short-term use until IV access is obtained	Skin lesions at site of insertion Fractures Osteomyelitis	Hypodermic needle (neonates) Spinal needle IO catheter (various types) Administration set Technical staff	Familiarity with landmarks is essential Fluids safe for IV administration are safe for IO administration

From Battaglia A, Steele A: *Small animal emergency and critical care for veterinary technicians,* ed 3, St Louis, Saunders, 2015.

primarily utilized for nutritional support. Consideration must be given to the amount of stress imposed on the patient during nasoesophageal tube placement.

SUBCUTANEOUS

Subcutaneous fluid administration is frequently employed. Advantages of this method include ease of administration, reduced cost, and avoidance of problems potentially encountered with IV administration. The subcutaneous route is the delivery method of choice when small volumes are needed, such as maintenance requirements in small animals. When animals are being weaned from IV fluid therapy and would recuperate much more quickly at home, owners can be instructed on how to administer subcutaneous fluids to their pet. An implantable subcutaneous catheter is also available and useful for clients to administer long-term fluid therapy at home. Care of this type of catheter requires strict attention to asepsis (Fig. 16-3).

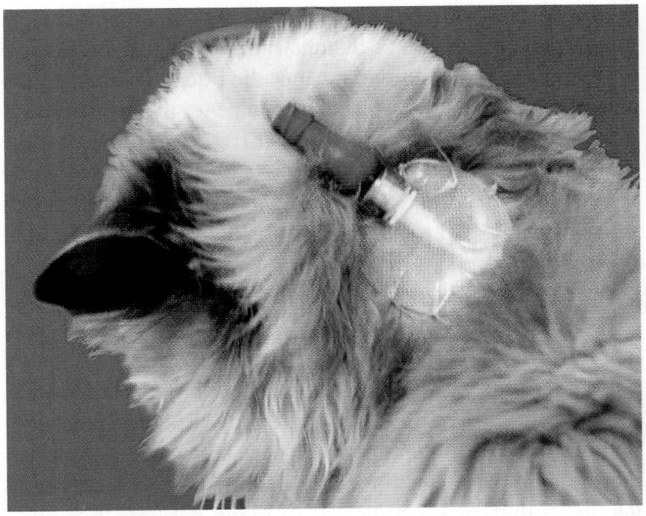

FIGURE 16-3 An implantable subcutaneous catheter can be used by clients to administer long-term fluid therapy at home.

> *TECHNICIAN NOTE* The areas where the limbs join the trunk should be avoided when administering fluid subcutaneously because fluid can gravitate into the limbs and cause discomfort.

Subcutaneous fluid administration cannot be used in animals that require large replacement volumes or in animals that are severely dehydrated or hypothermic. These conditions cause peripheral vasoconstriction, ultimately reducing the fluid absorption rate. Absorption may also be prolonged in animals that are hypotensive. The most effective approach to rehydrate the patient is by initially using the IV route to improve circulation to the subcutaneous tissues, and then incorporating SC fluid administration into the treatment plan.

Fluids are usually administered in subcutaneous space over the dorsal neck and cranial trunk, where loose connective tissue is abundant. The areas where the limbs join the trunk should be avoided, because fluid can gravitate into the limbs and cause discomfort. Warming the fluids before infusion encourages absorption and benefits hypothermic animals. The amount of fluid that can be administered per site is dependent on the elasticity of the skin, size of animal, hydration status, and type (composition) of fluid being used. There are limitations as to the volume that can be mechanically infused under the skin. The volume that can be administered via injection or gravity flow varies from animal to animal. Usually 50 ml or up to a maximum of 10 ml/kg can be infused at each SC site. If larger volumes are required, multiple sites may be used and treatment repeated every few hours.

To avoid skin sloughing, administer nonirritating, isotonic fluids only via the SC route. A solution of 5% dextrose in water (D_5W) should not be given SC as it is devoid of electrolytes; when the fluid is not immediately absorbed, electrolytes from the body can equilibrate into the pooled fluid and potentially initiate or aggravate electrolyte imbalances.

INTRAVENOUS

The IV route of fluid administration is preferable when treating animals that are critically ill, severely dehydrated, hypovolemic, or experiencing some electrolyte or metabolic disorder. Vascular access supplies the most direct route to plasma volume and therefore fluid administered via IV has the most rapid effect on blood volume. If fluid loss is acute, it is important to replace deficits rapidly. If fluid losses have occurred over an extended period, the body has had time to adjust, and slow fluid replacement is generally all that is required. Intravenous delivery allows titration of fluids to meet requirements of the patient. Because of direct access to the venous system, complications are more numerous than with other routes (e.g., infection, phlebitis, hematoma formation, thrombosis).

In a healthy patient, there are many superficial veins that can be easily cannulated. The catheter site selection is determined after careful consideration of many factors: patient status, vascular accessibility, operator experience, therapeutic goals, and risk of infection. The cephalic, medial femoral, and saphenous veins are easy to prepare, catheterize, and bandage for fluid administration. Peripheral venous catheters are sufficient in many patients, but often in critical patients other routes are required. During hypovolemia, peripheral vessels may vasoconstrict or simply not have the blood volume required to distend sufficiently for cannulation; therefore a central venous catheter is the best recourse. Central venous catheters may be placed in the jugular vein and the caudal vena cava (via the femoral vein). Isotonic and hypotonic solutions can be easily administered through any vein, but hypertonic solutions must be delivered through a central vessel. These vessels have higher blood flow and therefore any hemolytic effects of the fluid can be minimized by dilution with the blood. Central venous catheters not only allow for the administration of hypertonic solutions or irritating drugs, but also provide a port for blood sampling and an avenue for direct monitoring of venous pressure.

The size of the catheter is also an important consideration. Rate of flow through a catheter is controlled by three factors: patient's blood pressure, resistance in administration system (e.g., catheter size and placement), and the pressure or height of the fluid source. The resistance to flow of the catheter is dependent on its length and diameter. For rapid fluid administration, the largest gauge, shortest length catheter is best. The maximal fluid flow rate increases as the radius of the catheter lumen is increased. For routine maintenance treatment, the smallest gauge catheter that provides adequate flow should be used.

INTRAPERITONEAL

Intraperitoneal (IP) fluid administration is not often used but is an option available in patients where IV access is difficult to attain. The peritoneum has a large absorptive surface and fluids are absorbed rapidly into the intravascular space if the patient has good perfusion. This route is a good option in the early stages of shock because the blood vessels in the peritoneum do not constrict until later stages. Only isotonic crystalloids may be given into the peritoneal space because hypertonic or colloidal solutions will increase intravascular volume and pull excess water from the peritoneum into the interstitial space. Major complications include accidental puncture of organs and septic peritonitis, so strict aseptic technique should be used when administering fluids via this route. Intraperitoneal fluid administration should be discontinued as soon as IV access can be obtained.

INTRAOSSEOUS

Intraosseous catheters provide excellent access to the peripheral circulation, with absorption equivalent to that of IV infusion. Fluids can be administered via a spinal needle or special intraosseous catheter introduced into the intramedullary space. The bones of choice for placement include the femur, humerus, and wing of the ilium. This is an excellent method for fluid delivery in young animals or in animals where vascular access is a problem. Fluids administered through the intramedullary space are almost immediately available to the general circulation, and all solutions can be given, regardless of their composition. One limitation is the rate at which fluids can be delivered. Also, a major complication associated with this route is the potential for introduction of infection, resulting in osteomyelitis. Secure placement of the intraosseous catheter can be a challenge but is of utmost importance to maintain vascular access and decrease infection risk. These catheters should be temporary and removed once intravenous access can be obtained. If intravenous access cannot be obtained, intraosseous catheters should be replaced every 72 hours (Procedure 16-1).

INTRAVENOUS CATHETER SELECTION

Intravenous access facilitates a direct entryway to the circulatory system and can be accomplished via a number of commercially available catheters or by the use of surgically placed ports. Catheters and ports can be used to administer fluid solutions, medications (including chemotherapeutic agents), and blood products, as well as for blood sampling, hydration status monitoring, and nutritional support.

PROCEDURE 16-1 Intraosseous Catheter Placement

Indications

- Circulatory collapse
- Thrombosed veins
- Edematous states/obesity
- Severe burns
- Very small or pediatric patients

Materials

- 18- to 22-gauge spinal needle (for small or young animals with soft bones) or bone marrow needle (for most adult dogs and cats)
- Clippers with a #40 blade
- Local anesthetic or sedation
- Gauze sponges soaked in chlorhexidine gluconate (Solvahex, Solvay [Abbott], Abbott Park, IL)
- Cotton balls soaked in 70% isopropyl alcohol
- Scalpel blade
- 10 ml syringe
- 1% heparinized saline flushes or saline flush
- Suture material
- Bandaging material

Procedure

The most common access sites include the trochanteric fossa of the femur, the greater tubercle of the humerus, the wing of the ilium, and the medial surface of the tibial crest.

1. Clip and aseptically prepare insertion site.
2. Inject lidocaine into the skin and periosteum.
3. Make a small stab incision into the skin. Advance the spinal or bone marrow needle by rotation and steady pressure into the selected site.
4. Verify that the needle is securely lodged in the bone and that the tip is in the medullary cavity of the bone. Attach the syringe to the needle, and apply gentle suction. A small amount of bone marrow/blood should be aspirated into the barrel of the syringe.
5. Flush the needle with heparinized saline, and observe the site for subcutaneous infiltration.
6. Once the placement is confirmed, suture the needle in place.
7. Apply chlorhexidine to the insertion site and apply a secure tape bandage.

Complications

- Osteomyelitis (rare) related to the use of hypertonic solutions, faulty technique, or prolonged infusion

Intravenous catheters placed in peripheral vessels are intended for short-term use and are suitable for administering nonirritating intravenous medications, fluids, and blood products. Most catheters are generally inexpensive and relatively easy to place. Common sites for peripheral vessel catheterization include the cephalic vein, medial saphenous vein (cat), and lateral saphenous vein (dog). The auricular vein is also utilized in some dog breeds with long ears (e.g., Dachshund, Basset Hound).

Catheters placed in central vessels (e.g., jugular vein) are intended for longer term use and are appropriate for administering multiple drugs and fluids simultaneously, measuring hydration status, providing IV nutritional support, and blood sampling. They are more expensive and require skill to place and secure. Central vessel catheters are directly inserted into a large vein such as the jugular or can be inserted through a peripheral vein, ultimately terminating in the vena cava.

Before placing an intravenous catheter, each patient should be evaluated to determine the best location for insertion. Consideration should include: status of the patient (e.g., critical vs. stable), disease process of patient (e.g., bleeding tendency), why access is needed (e.g., fluid support vs. nutritional support), quality of the patient's vessels, as well as the availability and cost of catheter to be used. For example, if a diabetic patient is critically ill and in need of serial blood glucose monitoring, multiple fluid infusions, several intravenous medications, and nutritional support, a central multilumen catheter (see below) is most likely the best choice. Conversely, a smaller gauge catheter in a peripheral vessel (such as the cephalic vein) is probably a better choice for a mildly dehydrated animal in need of replacement fluids.

There are five recognized categories of catheters: butterfly (winged), over-the-needle, through-the-needle, multilumen, and subcutaneous venous access ports.

BUTTERFLY (WINGED) NEEDLE

Butterfly needle catheters are easy to place and intended for temporary use, given they are difficult to stabilize long term. Butterfly catheters should not be used for long-term fluid administration because of the difficulty in appropriately stabilizing the needle in the vein and potentially causing physical damage to the vessel as well as perivascular leakage of fluid if the animal were to move. These catheters are commonly used for procedures that are short in duration, such as administration of intravenous medications, chemotherapeutic agents, and fluid boluses, as well as collection of blood samples. Butterfly catheters are most often placed in peripheral vessels such as the cephalic and saphenous veins (Fig. 16-4).

OVER-THE-NEEDLE

Over-the-needle catheters are short in length and are commonly used for administering intravenous fluids and medications in patients experiencing acute medical situations. They are inexpensive and relatively easy to place. The catheter is comprised of a plastic tube over a needle-like stylet, used for piercing the skin and keeping the catheter taut during placement (Fig. 16-5). Once placement in the vessel is confirmed by a flash of blood in the hub of the catheter, the stylet is withdrawn and only the plastic catheter remains in the vein. A Luer-lock injection cap or extension tubing is then placed into the hub of the catheter, sealing off the intravascular space to the outside environment. Secure bandaging is applied over the insertion site of the catheter and around the limb. Over-the-needle catheters are frequently positioned in peripheral vessels of larger animals; jugular placement is often required in neonates and very small animals (Procedure 16-2).

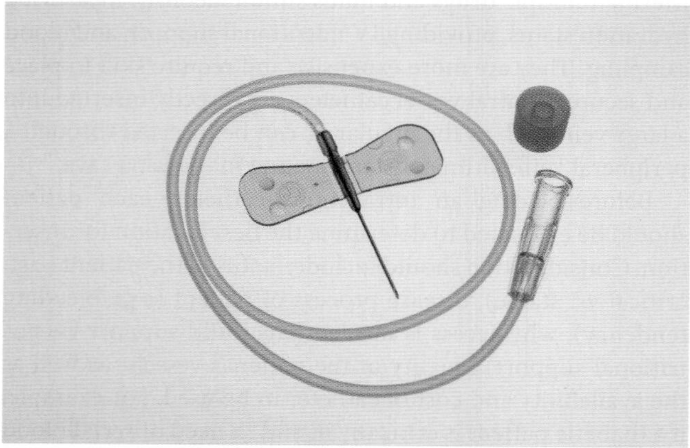

FIGURE 16-4 Butterfly catheter.

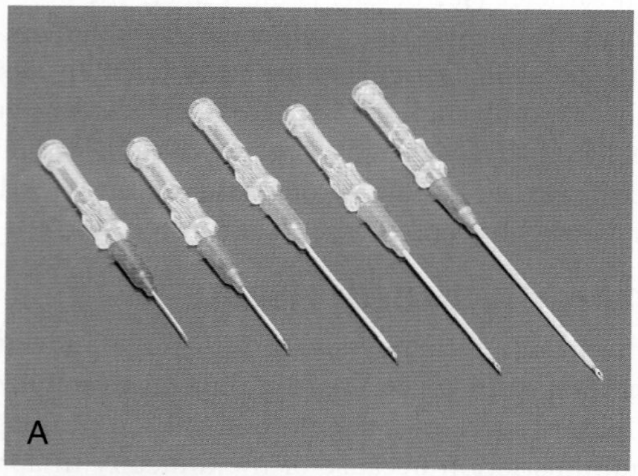

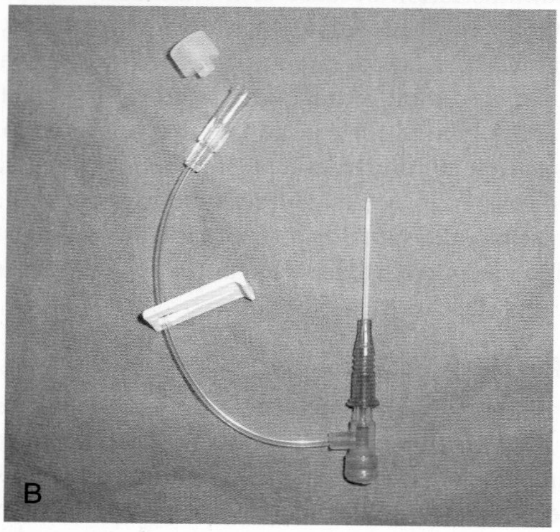

FIGURE 16-5 A, Over-the-needle catheter. B, Over-the-needle catheter with extension set in hub.

THROUGH-THE-NEEDLE

Through-the-needle catheters are longer in length than over-the-needle catheters, so the proper size and length for the patient should be evaluated before placement. Through-the-needle catheters utilize an integrated needle to pierce the vessel, after which the catheter is fed through the center of the needle and into the vein (Fig. 16-6). A plastic sheath covers the catheter to prevent accidental contamination during placement. Once proper placement is ensured via a flash of blood in the hub of the catheter, the needle is withdrawn from under the skin leaving only the catheter remaining in the vessel. The needle is covered with a provided needle guard to prevent severing of the catheter. Because of their length, through-the-needle catheters are usually placed in the jugular vein but can be inserted peripherally through the lateral or medial saphenous vein to terminate in the caudal vena cava, keeping in mind the endpoint of the catheter will depend on the size of the patient. When the end of the catheter is seated in a central vessel (e.g., jugular vein), the catheter is useful for blood sampling, administration of hypertonic solutions, and monitoring of central venous pressure (CVP) (Procedure 16-3).

MULTILUMEN

Multilumen catheters come in a variety of integral lumens, sizes, and lengths. They are costly and require advanced technical skill to place and secure; patient sedation or local anesthetic is needed for placement. They are typically placed in the jugular vein, terminating in the vena cava. A major advantage to these catheters is the ability to administer otherwise incompatible fluids and drugs simultaneously. The locations of exit ports within the catheter lumen are staggered, allowing blood flow to pick up and redistribute the solutions before they have a chance to intermingle. Multilumen catheters can also be used for serial blood sampling, administration of blood products and hypertonic solutions (e.g., total parenteral nutrition), and monitoring of central venous pressure (Fig. 16-7).

PERIPHERALLY INSERTED CENTRAL VENOUS CATHETERS

Peripherally inserted central venous catheters (PICC) are multilumen catheters inserted peripherally via the medial saphenous vein (cat) or lateral saphenous vein (dog). They are placed sterilely and can be maintained in a patient for extended periods of time with proper care. Uses and indications are similar to any other multilumen catheter.

SUBCUTANEOUS VASCULAR ACCESS PORTS

Subcutaneous venous access ports (SVAP) are long-term catheters placed in the jugular vein in dogs and cats for the administration of chemotherapeutic agents. In some instances, the femoral vein is also utilized. SVAP require a short surgical procedure for placement and are comprised of two parts: an indwelling catheter and a subcutaneous injection port or "reservoir," which is completely covered by skin following placement. The center of the port consists of a

PROCEDURE 16-2 Over-the-Needle Intravenous Catheter Placement

Indications
- Facilitate administration of fluids and IV medications
- Administer blood products

Materials
- Catheter of appropriate type, length, and diameter
- Clippers with a #40 blade
- Gauze sponges soaked in chlorhexidine gluconate (Solvahex, Solvay [Abbott])
- Cotton balls soaked in 70% isopropyl alcohol
- Dry, sterile gauze sponges
- 1% heparinized saline solution flushes
- Bandaging material
- Extension set and/or injection cap

Procedure
1. Shave approximately 1 clipper blade width on each side of the vessel, with the shaved length (proximal to distal) approximately twice that of the width. This allows a second attempt at catheterization more proximal than the first (Fig. 1).
2. Prepare the insertion site using a surgical soap and antiseptic (Fig. 2).
3. While an assistant occludes the vessel, grasp the limb with your nondominant hand while your dominant hand holds the catheter with the bevel directed up (Fig. 3).
4. Venipuncture is performed by holding the catheter at a 15- to 30-degree angle over the vein, puncturing the skin, and advancing the catheter needle ¼ inch under the skin into the vessel in a single, quick, smooth motion. Decrease the angle of the needle and slide the catheter off of the needle into the vein. If the catheter does not advance into the vessel, remove the catheter and attempt catheterization with a new catheter more proximal than the first attempt (Fig. 4).
5. Once the catheter is advanced, a flash of blood should be seen in the hub, ensuring placement in the vein. Remove the catheter needle and hold the catheter in place while attaching the injection cap or extension set. Flush a small amount of heparinized saline into the vessel to ensure catheter placement and patency. For very small, pediatric patients, monitor the amount of heparinized saline used to flush the catheter (Fig. 5).
6. Apply chlorhexidine and a secure tape bandage over the catheter and around the limb (Fig. 6).

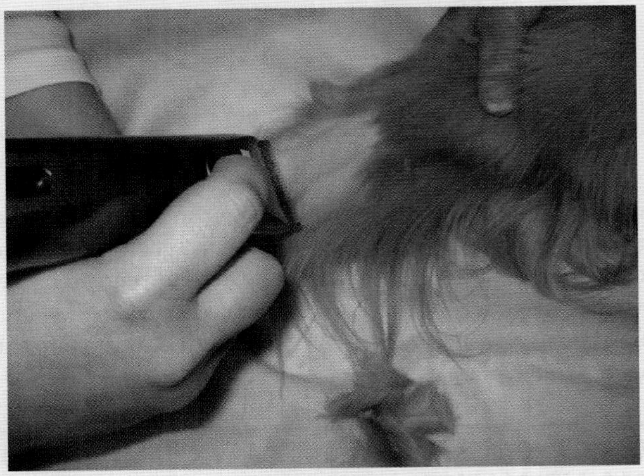

FIGURE 1

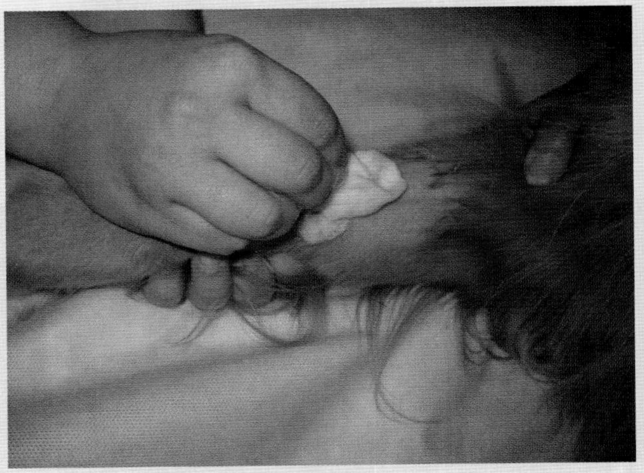

FIGURE 2

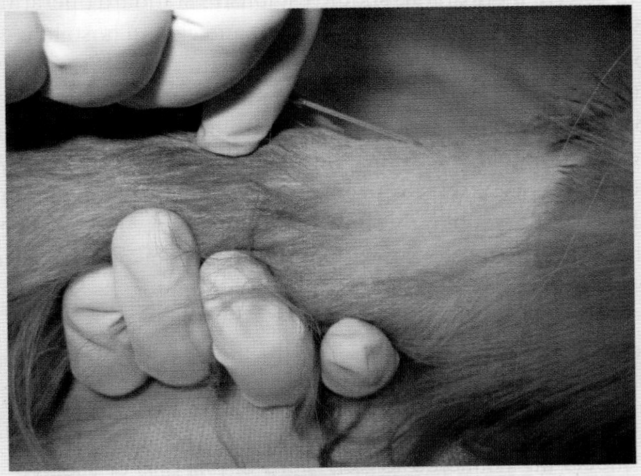

FIGURE 3

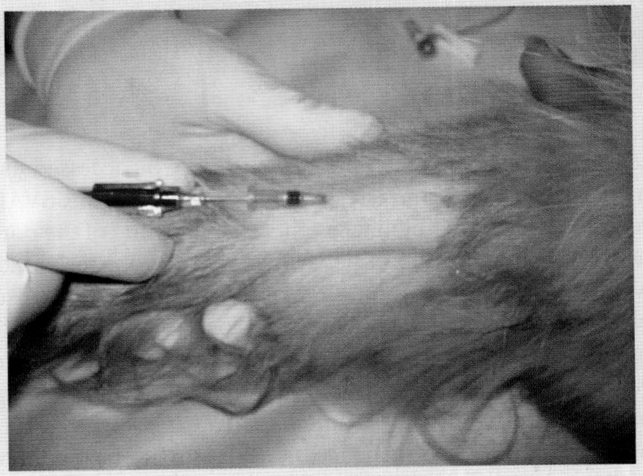

FIGURE 4

Continued

PROCEDURE 16-2 Over-the-Needle Intravenous Catheter Placement—cont'd

Complications
- Sepsis
- Phlebitis
- Thrombosis
- Catheter backs out of vessel
- Catheter clots

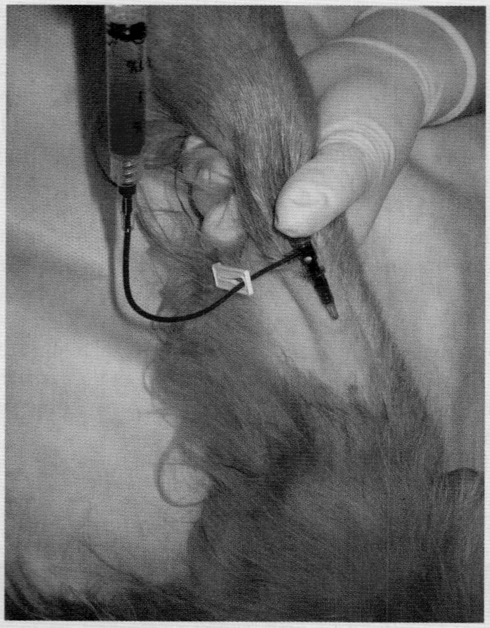

FIGURE 5

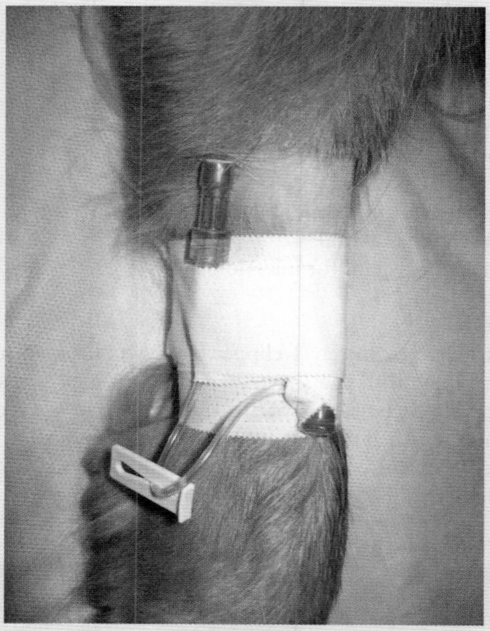

FIGURE 6

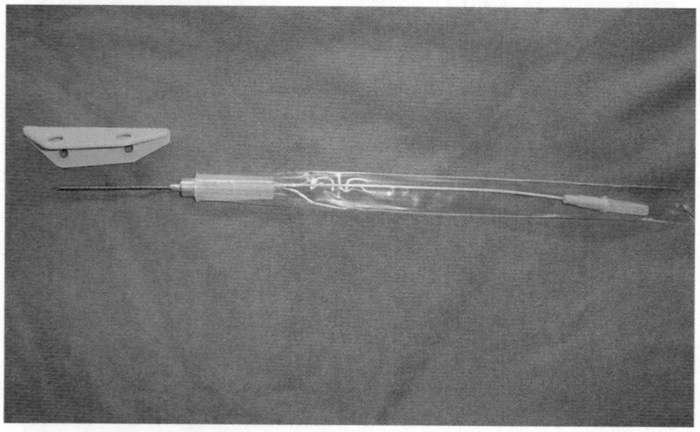

FIGURE 16-6 Through-the-needle catheter.

self-sealing silicone material that must only be accessed using a special noncoring device called a Huber needle. SVAP require minimal maintenance other than flushing of the port with a locking solution of heparin every two to three weeks when not in use to prevent blood clots. Some protocols also place an antibiotic solution into the lock to prevent development of infection. SVAP eliminate the need for multiple venipunctures and catheterizations as well as minimizing patient restraint usually required during treatment. Previously established vascular access decreases the stress normally encountered while administering chemotherapeutics and avoids the risk of extravasation sometimes encountered with normal delivery methods. Minor complications when using SVAP include risks associated with sedation required for placement, localized infection, device clotting, and sore/swollen tissue around the port after placement. Serious complications associated with SVAP are rare, the most common being septicemia.

INTRAVENOUS CATHETER PLACEMENT AND MAINTENANCE

All veterinary hospitals should establish a standard operating procedure for IV catheter placement and care in hospitalized patients. The protocol should include information specifying frequency of patient evaluation and catheter inspection, bandage care and maintenance, length of time a catheter can remain in a patient, and catheter replacement guidelines. A routine fluid check for animals receiving IV fluid therapy should include not only confirmation of proper IV fluids being administered to the patient at the correct rate, but also ensure the patency and integrity of the catheter.

> *TECHNICIAN NOTE* A routine fluid check for animals receiving IV fluid therapy must ensure the patency and comfort level of the catheter. The site proximal to the catheter should be monitored for any signs of phlebitis or subcutaneous fluid accumulation and the toes checked for swelling.

PROCEDURE 16-3 Through-the-Needle Catheter Placement

Indications
- Facilitate the administration of fluids and medications
- Administer blood product transfusions
- Measure central venous pressure
- Facilitate blood sample collection

Materials
- Through-the-needle catheter of appropriate size, length, and diameter
- Clippers with #40 blade
- Gauze sponges soaked in chlorhexidine gluconate (Solvahex, Solvay [Abbott])
- Cotton balls soaked in 70% isopropyl alcohol
- Sterile gloves and drapes
- 5 ml syringe
- 1% heparinized saline solution flush
- Extension set and/or injection cap
- Suture material
- Bandaging material

Procedure
1. Clip a wide area of hair over the catheterization site. (The area should be wide enough to prevent contamination during catheterization procedure.) Prepare the catheterization site just as you would a surgical site. Wear sterile gloves and use sterile drapes if necessary to prevent contamination to either the catheter or catheter site.
2. While an assistant occludes the vessel, grasp the limb with your nondominant hand while your dominant hand holds the catheter with the bevel of the needle directed up.
3. Introduce the needle into the subcutaneous space. Position the needle tip over the vein and align it as close as possible to the longitudinal axis of the vein. Insert the needle tip into the vein. A flashback of blood into the catheter system should be noted when the needle has entered the lumen of the vein. This may not occur if the venous pressure is low. Once the entire needle tip is in the vein, advance the catheter through the needle into the vein. Once the catheter is placed, back the needle out from under the skin and remove the guidewire. Apply pressure over the catheter site and cover the needle with the needle guard. Aspirate the catheter to confirm proper placement and to clear the catheter of air, and then flush with heparinized saline. If blood cannot be aspirated, withdraw the catheter slowly until successful.
4. Cap the catheter with an injection cap or extension set and flush again with heparinized saline. Suture the catheter close to the insertion site. Cover the insertion site and secure the catheter with bandaging material.

Complications
- Sepsis (cellulitis, septicemia)
- Phlebitis
- Thrombosis (vein, catheter lumen)
- Bleeding
- Catheter backs out of vessel

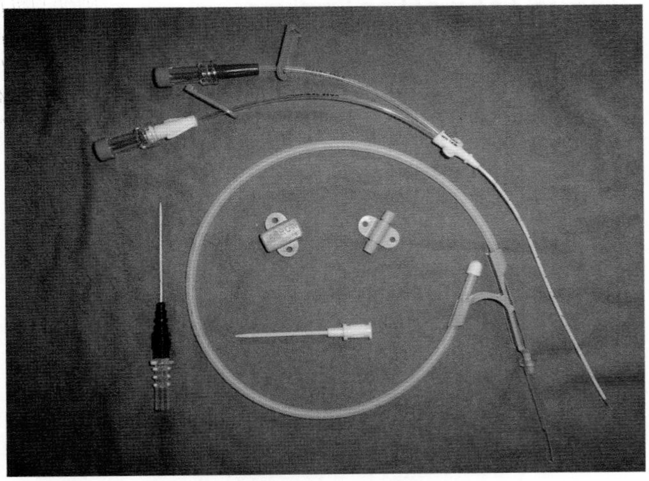

FIGURE 16-7 Multilumen catheter kit.

Proper skin preparation before catheter placement is essential in preventing phlebitis and infection. Strict aseptic technique must be followed during catheterization to avoid sepsis. Proper hand washing is done after clipping and before catheter placement. The individual placing the catheter should wear sterile surgical gloves. All catheters must be secured with tape or sutures and may be covered with a light bandage to protect the insertion site. The Centers for Disease Control and Prevention (CDC) does not recommend routine application of antimicrobial ointment to venous catheter insertion sites because of the potential to promote fungal infections and antimicrobial resistance. Chlorhexidine patches are used as an alternative. The patch slowly releases chlorhexidine, which has been shown in human studies to maintain its bactericidal effects in the presence of bodily fluids over a 7-day period.

Frequent and conscientious care of the catheter is necessary for maintenance and prevention of complications associated with catheterization. Phlebitis (local venous inflammation) can be caused by contamination of the catheter during placement or chemical/mechanical irritation to the vessel while the catheter is in place. Signs of phlebitis include swelling, redness, and pain at the catheter site as well as thickening or irritation of the vessel itself. Phlebitis can lead to the development of thrombosis, a clot that forms in the vessel and potentially obstructs the flow of blood. The signs of thrombosis are similar to that of phlebitis; therefore catheters should be removed at the first sign of phlebitis, thrombosis, or any other catheter malfunction.

The most serious complications associated with all types of indwelling catheters are sepsis and bacterial endocarditis. Bacteria live innocuously on superficial skin. When the skin is punctured at the time of catheter placement, the bacteria are introduced into the bloodstream. Hospitalized patients with compromised immune function may not be able to defend against the bacteremia, ultimately creating the potential for sepsis to occur. If bacteria in the bloodstream lodge on abnormal heart valves or other damaged heart tissue, bacterial endocarditis may develop. Patients with concurrent valvular disease or other cardiac compromise are most at risk for this serious complication. Signs of septicemia and bacterial endocarditis include cardiac arrhythmias, injected mucous membranes, leukocytosis, and fever. Because infection is the most common catheter-associated complication, the patient's body temperature must be monitored daily.

Following IV catheter placement, a closed system should be established by inserting an injection cap into the open end of the catheter. The site proximal to the catheter should be monitored for any signs of phlebitis or subcutaneous fluid accumulation and the toes checked for swelling. The catheter bandage must be kept clean and dry to prevent contamination and changed as soon as possible if it becomes wet or soiled with organic material. At the time of bandage change, the catheter must be evaluated for problems. The catheter bandage may require a plastic covering for protection in incontinent patients. Swabbing the injection port with alcohol or a disinfectant before flushing or injecting medications can help decrease the chance of introducing bacteria into the circulation. Kinked or malfunctioning catheters and extension tubing with blood clots occluding the ports must be replaced immediately. Catheters not in constant use should be flushed several times a day to maintain patency and prevent clotting. Although heparinized saline has traditionally been used to flush catheters, some studies suggest that saline only can be used.

The amount of time a catheter can safely remain in a patient is somewhat controversial. It has been reported in the literature that a short peripheral catheter should be removed and a new catheter inserted in a fresh vessel every 72 hours to prevent phlebitis- and catheter-related infection. If the catheter is properly maintained and patent, it can remain in place as long as needed. Continuous rotation of vascular access sites allows indefinite IV catheterization for therapy. Central catheters may be left in place for longer periods of time with routine bandage changes and insertion site inspections, provided the catheter is still functional.

FLUID ADMINISTRATION

Once vascular access has been achieved, the decision of fluid volume and rate must be made. Fluids are in many ways drugs, and as such have dosages. The difference between drugs and fluids, however, is that the body requires various amounts of fluid in various metabolic states. In patients with ongoing losses, fluid dosages may need to change. Because of this, fluid therapy requires frequent evaluation and adjustments to achieve the proper balance of fluids. There are some basic guidelines to assist in calculating requirements: blood pressure must be maintained, dehydration and ongoing losses must be replaced, acid-base and electrolyte balance must be maintained, and maintenance fluids must be supplied. The fluid volume administered should always be based on lean body weight to avoid fluid overloading a patient because fat has a lower content of water relative to the rest of the body. Box 16-2 shows calculations of fluid requirements for a hypothetical case.

Many factors influence the rate of fluid administration (e.g., disease process, rate of fluid loss, severity of clinical signs, fluid composition and delivery route, cardiac and renal function). Patients with poor perfusion because of severe dehydration or hypovolemia must be given immediate and rapid IV fluid replacements. The goal is to restore intravascular fluid volume and improve tissue perfusion as quickly as possible, as long as the cardiopulmonary and renal systems can handle the fluid load. Animals with marginal cardiovascular function cannot tolerate rapid fluid infusion, so their deficits must be restored with greater care. Patients with brittle cardiovascular systems or compromised renal

BOX 16-2 Calculating Daily Fluid Requirements in a Hypothetical Case

Patient

5-month-old, 20-kg Rottweiler

History

- 3 days of anorexia, lethargy
- 2 days of vomiting and diarrhea, 5 to 6 times/day, becoming bloody
- No vaccinations

Physical Examination Findings

- Depression
- Heart rate: 140 beats/minute
- Pulse: weak to moderate
- Capillary refill time: 1 to 2 seconds
- Tented skin slowly returns to normal position

Replacement Requirements

% dehydration × body weight × 10 = fluid deficit
8 × 20 × 10 = 1600 ml

Maintenance Requirements

Maintenance requirement = 40 to 60 ml/kg/day
50 × 20 = 1000 ml/day

Ongoing Losses

Ongoing losses = losses in diarrhea and vomitus
Estimated diarrhea volume/episode = 100 ml
5 episodes/day = 500 ml
Estimated vomitus volume/episode = 50 ml
5 episodes/day = 250 ml
Ongoing losses 500 + 250 = 750 ml/day

Daily Fluid Requirement

Daily fluid requirement = fluid deficit + maintenance + ongoing losses
= 1600 + 1000 + 750 = 3350 ml/day
= 3350 ml over 24 hr/day
Infusion rate = 140 ml/hr

function are excellent candidates for CVP monitoring. Central venous pressure reflects the heart's ability to accommodate fluid administration. It is regulated by a balance between the ability of the right heart to pump blood to the lungs and the tendency for blood to flow from peripheral vessels back into the right atrium. Valuable information regarding the relationship among intravascular volume, venous return, and right heart function can indirectly be provided with these measurements. CVP monitoring can be useful as a clinical guide for determining rate of fluid administration and monitoring of therapy but not as an indication of fluid volume to be replaced. To perform the CVP measurement, the patient will need to have an IV catheter placed in the cranial vena cava via the jugular vein. A sterile fluid bag with an administration set, an IV extension set, a manometer, and a three-way stopcock are needed (Fig. 16-8). The patient can be in sternal recumbency or lateral recumbency, although lateral recumbency is preferred. The bottom of the manometer is held at the level of the right atrium which is approximately the midpoint between the dorsum and ventrum. Initially the stopcock knob is turned straight up toward the manometer, allowing fluid to flow from the fluid bag to the patient's catheter to ensure the catheter is patent. (If fluid does not flow freely into the patient's catheter, a valid CVP reading will not be obtained.) Then the knob is turned toward the patient and fluid fills the manometer. The manometer should not contain any air bubbles. If air is present in the manometer or fluid line, let the fluids run, overfilling the manometer until all air is purged from the system. Then turn the knob toward the fluids. The level of fluid in the manometer will fall until the height of the fluid column exerts a pressure equivalent to the patient's central venous pressure. The top of the fluid column will slightly oscillate 2 to 5 mm as the animal's heart beats and as the animal breathes. Normal values are 0 to 10 cm of H_2O. A reading less than 5 may indicate hypovolemia while readings greater than 10 indicate fluid overload. Trends in central venous pressure are more informative than single values. Each time a CVP reading is obtained the patient must be in the same position.

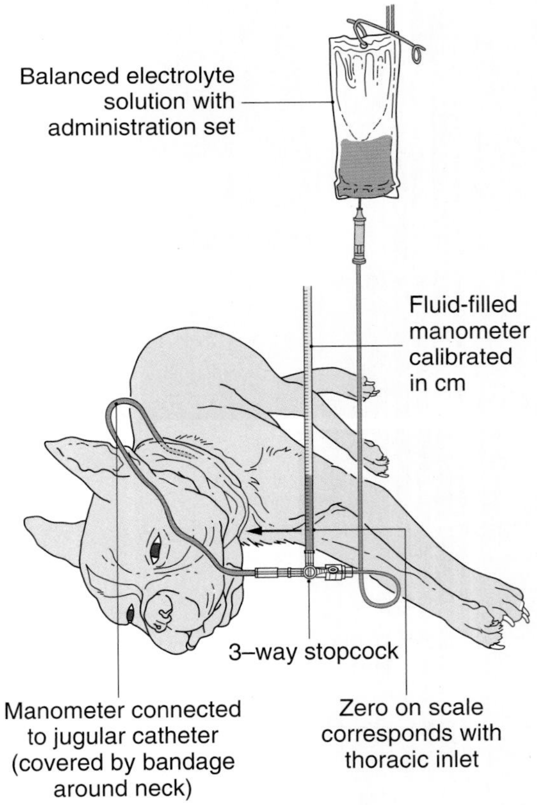

FIGURE 16-8 Diagram of apparatus for measurement of central venous pressure. (From Clarke K, Trim C: *Veterinary anaesthesia*, ed 11, 2016, Elsevier Health Sciences.)

Fluids should either be administered using a fluid pump or by gravity flow (Fig. 16-9A). In either case, the fluid bag should be labeled with a scale indicating the starting fluid level and anticipated fluid levels by the hour so that the volume of fluid administered can be closely monitored (Fig. 16-9B). When fluids are administered, the prescribed rate must be converted into a form that will allow the veterinary technician to program the fluid infusion pump or set the roller clamp on an infusion set. Fluid administration sets can be either the macrodrip or microdrip type. Macrodrip chambers deliver a drop (gtt) size of 15 gtt/ml and are used when infusion rates greater than 100 ml/hr are needed. Microdrip chambers deliver 60 gtt/ml and are used when infusion rates of less than 100 ml/hour are prescribed (Fig. 16-10).

If using a fluid infusion pump, the administration set is placed in the pump and the pump is set to deliver the prescribed rate in ml/hr and total volume to be infused. Most pumps will stop and sound an alarm if an occlusion or air bubble is detected in the line.

> *TECHNICIAN NOTE* The fluid volume administered should always be based on lean body weight because fat has a lower content of water relative to the rest of the body.

TOTAL PARENTERAL NUTRITION

Fluid therapy should be considered as the first supportive measure in reestablishing nutritional balance. Only after the primary goals of rehydration, replacement of electrolytes, and normalization of acid-base balance should parenteral feeding be introduced. As a general rule, animals that have been off food for 3 to 5 days should be considered candidates for total parenteral nutrition (TPN).

Parenteral nutrition is indicated for patients that are severely malnourished and cannot meet nutritional needs adequately using the oral or enteral route. Ideally, nutrition should be maintained via the gastrointestinal tract. If any part of the alimentary tract is nonfunctional, nutrients can be infused IV for some time. Total parenteral nutrition is not an innocuous treatment. Complicating factors associated with TPN include: placement and use of a central catheter dedicated solely to administration of TPN solution; potential

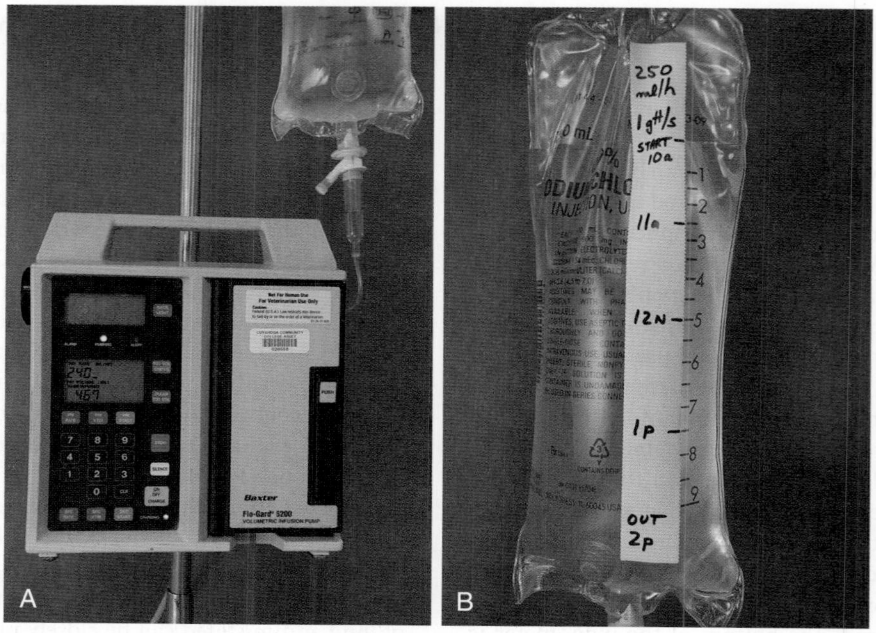

FIGURE 16-9 **A,** Infusion pump. **B,** Tape scale used to monitor the fluid administration rate. The tape should be labeled with the infusion rate (250 ml/hr in this case) and the drip rate (1 gtt/sec in this case) and should have lines drawn indicating the expected fluid level each hour. (From Thomas J, Lerche P: *Anesthesia and analgesia for veterinary technicians,* ed 4, St Louis, 2011, Mosby.)

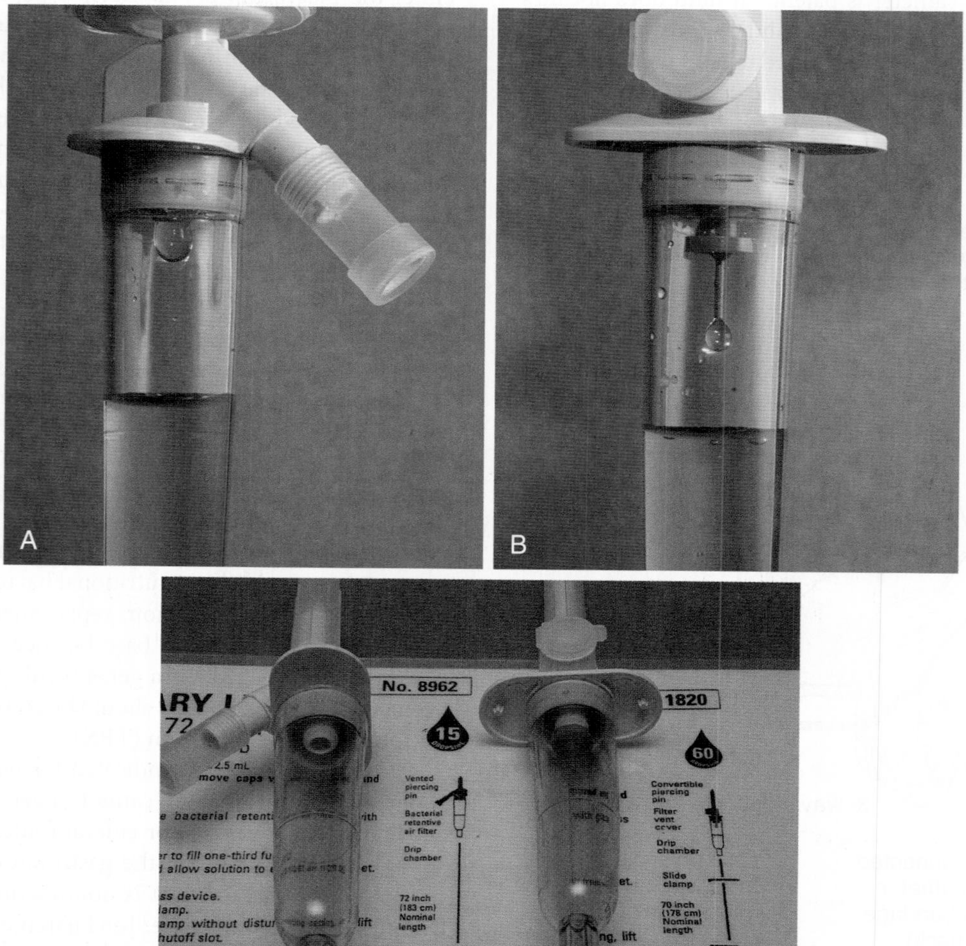

FIGURE 16-10 Fluid administration set chambers, comparing the size of the drops delivered. **A,** Macrodrip set chamber (15 gtt/ml). **B,** Microdrip set chamber (60 gtt/ml). **C,** Macrodrip (15 gtt/ml) and microdrip (60 gtt/ml) fluid administration sets on the left and right, respectively. Note that the delivery rate in gtt/ml is listed on the package. (From Thomas J, Lerche P: *Anesthesia and analgesia for veterinary technicians,* ed 4, St Louis, 2011, Mosby.)

septic and mechanical problems if the catheter is not placed and maintained properly; possible metabolic disturbances as a result of TPN solution composition, concentration, and administration; and expense. The three main ingredients of a TPN solution are dextrose, amino acids, and lipids. Dextrose supplies the calories; amino acids supply protein, nitrogen, and electrolytes; and lipid emulsions serve as a concentrated energy source. Because TPN solutions are hypertonic, they must be infused into a central vein (e.g., jugular, medial, femoral) to allow for rapid dilution of the fluid. Because of the high level of nutrients in TPN solutions, they should be infused slowly to prevent possible rebound hypoglycemia.

TRANSFUSION MEDICINE

Blood products are used in treatment of many patients with hematologic disorders, therefore proficiency in transfusion therapy and blood banking techniques is an invaluable skill for veterinary technicians. Education is clearly the link to ensuring the overall quality of all aspects of blood banking and transfusion services as a safe and adequate supply of blood components for transfusion is indispensable.

CLINICAL EVALUATION OF BLEEDING

When a patient presents with abnormal bleeding, it is important to determine the cause. Although it is the responsibility of the veterinarian to diagnose and choose an appropriate therapy for these patients, the veterinary technician should be knowledgeable and anticipate the needs of the veterinarian and, most importantly, the patient. This requires a basic understanding of the physiology of hemostasis.

HEMOSTASIS

Hemostasis, the body's balancing mechanism of arresting hemorrhage while simultaneously maintaining blood flow within the vascular compartment, occurs through a complex series of events involving the vessels, platelets, plasma coagulation factors and the fibrinolytic system. The role that each component plays in hemostasis is dependent on the size of the vessel and the amount of damage that has occurred. Bleeding in smaller vessels may be controlled by a simple response involving the vasculature and platelets (e.g., normal wear and tear on capillaries), whereas incorporation of the plasma coagulation factors are necessary for hemorrhage control involving larger damaged vessels.

The first response to blood vessel injury is vasoconstriction, which allows for diversion of blood flow around the injured area. Once the endothelial lining of the vessel is disrupted, the subendothelial connective tissue (i.e., collagen fibers) is exposed. Circulating platelets pool to the area of injury and, with the help of certain adhesive proteins (i.e., collagen, fibrinogen, fibronectin, von Willebrand factor), adhere to the endothelial lining to arrest the initial episode of bleeding. This process is known as platelet adhesion. Once the platelets adhere to the subendothelium, they change shape and secrete certain biochemical substances (phosphatidylserine) that enhance platelet layering in the injured area. The platelets form a complete but unstable plug (Fig. 16-11). This portion of the hemostatic process involving the vasculature and platelets is referred to as primary hemostasis and is usually adequate to stop bleeding in smaller vessels.

With greater damage to larger vessels, coagulation factors are needed to form a stable fibrin clot, a process known as **secondary hemostasis.** Blood coagulation involves a complex process by which the multiple coagulation factors contained in blood interact in three major pathways: traditionally referred to as the intrinsic, extrinsic, and common pathways. Although they are discussed separately here, the pathways are interrelated and involve a number of complex processes.

Plasma coagulation factors (denoted by Roman numerals) are produced in the liver, many with the help of vitamin K. They circulate in the blood in the inactive form and become activated only when exposed to certain substances. Initiation of the clotting pathways leads to subsequent activation of all factors in a cascadelike effect. Tissue factor (thromboplastin) is released from the injured vessel wall and helps initiate the coagulation reactions. Factors I through XI serve to amplify the clotting cascade. The coagulation pathways do not operate as independent and redundant pathways. Platelets are essential for secondary hemostasis and the thrombin generated by the coagulation cascade recruits and activates additional platelets and inhibits fibrinolysis

Hemostasis is initiated by interactions of negatively charged phospholipid surfaces of cells and platelets or microparticles. Microparticles are membrane-bound cytoplasmic fragments released from platelets, leukocytes, and endothelial cells and provide an increased surface area on which coagulation complexes can form. Phosphatidylserine-enriched microparticles act as a binding site for the "tenase" (FVIIIa, FIXa, FX) and "prothrombinase" (FVa, FXa, FII) complexes of the coagulation cascade, which activate FX and prothrombin (FVII), respectively. The coagulation factors are assembled into a complex on the surface of platelet

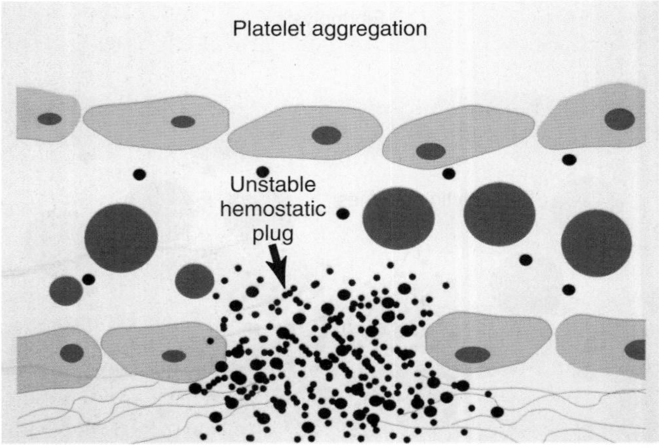

FIGURE 16-11 Platelet aggregation. (Photo courtesy of Dr. David Holt, University of Pennsylvania School of Veterinary Medicine.)

and microvesicles, where they can amplify the coagulation cascade and generate large amounts of thrombin, which converts fibrinogen to fibrin. **Fibrin,** a threadlike protein, forms an insoluble meshwork over the site of the platelet plug, consolidating and stabilizing the clot (Fig. 16-12).

The fourth and final step in the hemostatic process is fibrinolysis. Once the vessel is healed, fibrinolytic enzymes (plasmin) digest the clot that has been formed, restoring normal blood flow (Fig. 16-13). Clot lysis produces small pieces of fibrin, referred to as fibrin split products (FSP) (or fibrin degradation products FDP), which are cleared from circulation by the liver. Small levels of FSP always appear in the circulation as a result of bleeding and clotting secondary to normal wear-and-tear on vessels. FSP levels increase during episodes of excessive bleeding with diffuse coagulation (i.e., disseminated intravascular coagulation [DIC]) and in patients with compromised liver function. Following clot digestion, vessel wall endothelium is reestablished and returned to its original state.

Bleeding disorders can be categorized into three groups: disorders of platelet function or number, disorders of clotting factors, and a combination of both. A working knowledge

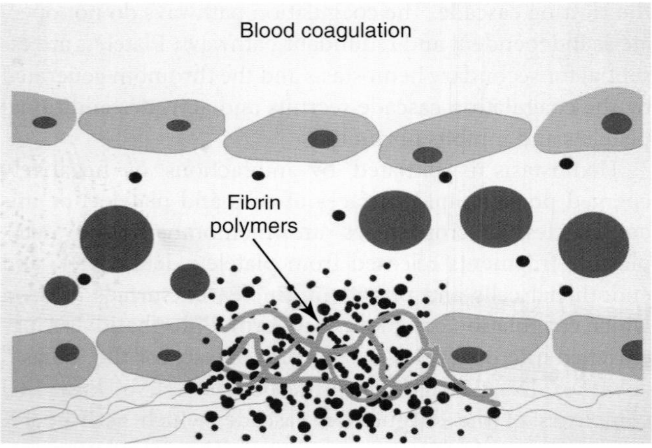

FIGURE 16-12 Blood coagulation. (Photo courtesy of Dr. David Holt, University of Pennsylvania School of Veterinary Medicine.)

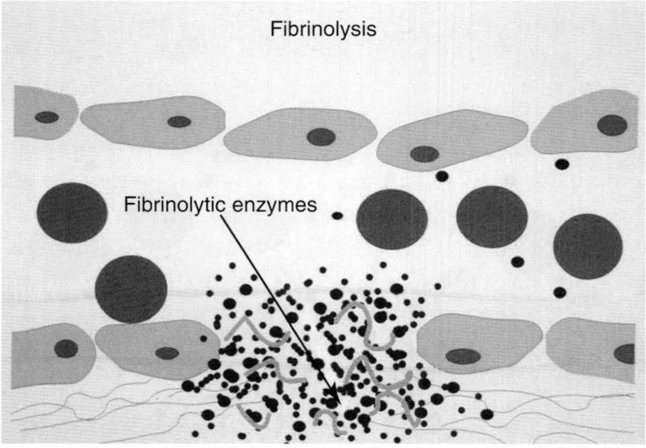

FIGURE 16-13 Fibrinolysis. (Photo courtesy of Dr. David Holt, University of Pennsylvania School of Veterinary Medicine.)

of the hemostatic mechanism along with a complete medical history, thorough physical examination, and specific laboratory tests are integral steps in the diagnostic process. The most appropriate treatment options can only be identified after the cause of bleeding has been determined.

HISTORY

A complete history is critical in beginning a workup for a hemostatic defect. In veterinary medicine, all pertinent information regarding patient history must be gathered from the owners. Obtaining and assessing a complete and detailed history will help define the nature, severity, and duration of clinical signs and aid in making a correct diagnosis. This attention to detail allows the clinician to establish probability for each possible differential early in the diagnostic process.

Questions should be very clear and thought provoking. Devising a list of questions for owners to review will hopefully help stimulate them to think of some very important, most likely not obvious facts. A list of any prescription or over-the-counter medications should be included because many drugs have potentially harmful or complicating side effects, resulting in a toxic effect on red blood cells, white blood cells, and platelets. Complete vaccination history should not be overlooked. The animal's environmental history may suggest potential exposure to toxic or organic substances such as anticoagulant rodenticide poisons or lead. Tick exposure should also be investigated.

It is vital to evaluate the current bleeding episode and characterize the bleed as localized or multifocal. Note whether this is the animal's first bleeding episode, or if there is a history of bleeding tendencies. These facts may help differentiate between an acquired or hereditary disorder. Specific breeds may suggest specific coagulopathies. Any information the owner may have regarding breed history could provide helpful clues.

PHYSICAL EXAM

A complete physical examination and multiple monitoring procedures may be required to properly assess the patient in a bleeding crisis. Optimal assessment cannot be based on the result of a single parameter, but is based on the results of several physical exam findings and monitored parameters that should always be evaluated in relation to one another.

Certain clinical signs found on physical exam may help determine the origin of the bleeding episode. Small surface bleeds (e.g., petechiation, ecchymosis, epistaxis, hematuria) are usually suggestive of platelet or vascular abnormalities (Fig. 16-14). Larger bleeds or bleeding into body cavities (e.g., hematoma formation, hemarthroses, deep muscle hemorrhage) are suggestive of clotting factor deficiencies. A combination of these clinical signs is not uncommon.

> *TECHNICIAN NOTE* Common physical findings in the anemic patient include lethargy, weakness, pale mucous membranes, tachycardia, tachypnea, and bounding pulses.

In anemic patients, the development and progression of clinical signs depends on the rapidity of onset, degree, and cause of anemia, as well as the animal's physical activity. Common physical findings are those associated with a decrease in red cell mass: lethargy, weakness, pale mucous membranes, tachycardia, tachypnea, and bounding pulses. The cardiovascular and respiratory system should be carefully evaluated. Assessment of perfusion is based on mucous membrane color, capillary refill time (CRT), heart rate and pulse rate, strength, and character. In a severe anemic state, a low-grade systolic flow murmur may occur secondary to decreased blood viscosity. Mucous membrane color can be used to monitor the patient's response to therapy or indicate the development of a problem. Prolonged CRT is suggestive of compromised tissue perfusion and shock, but may be difficult to assess in an anemic patient. Weak and rapid pulses suggest severe dehydration and poor perfusion; bounding pulses suggest anemia. Assessment of respiratory rate and effort, as well as careful auscultation, may help differentiate between decreased oxygen carrying capability and possible pulmonary thromboembolism. Monitoring all parameters in unison with one another will lend information regarding bleed severity and potentially life-threatening complications.

LABORATORY TESTS

Although information obtained from the history and specific clinical signs may suggest a diagnosis, certain laboratory tests are necessary for definitive diagnosis. Laboratory tests should be performed as soon as possible and therapy instituted promptly after test samples are obtained.

Serial hematocrit (PCV) determinations may help demonstrate progression or stabilization of bleeding, taking into account the body takes a certain amount of time to equilibrate following an acute bleeding episode. Anemia is suggested when one or more of the red cell parameters are below normal for the age, gender, and breed of the species concerned. Of these parameters, PCV provides a simple, quick, and accurate means of detecting anemia, and allows classification of the anemia as mild, moderate, or severe. Dehydration and splenic contraction may mask anemia, whereas hemodilution may cause a temporary reduction in red cell parameters. Evaluating both PCV and total plasma protein (TPP) levels may help in differentiating these variables. Dehydration is associated with increases in both PCV and TPP, whereas PCV elevation alone is seen with splenic contraction. Decreases in both PCV and TPP are associated with hemodilution following acute blood loss or fluid therapy, whereas a reduction in PCV only is usually associated with hemolytic anemias.

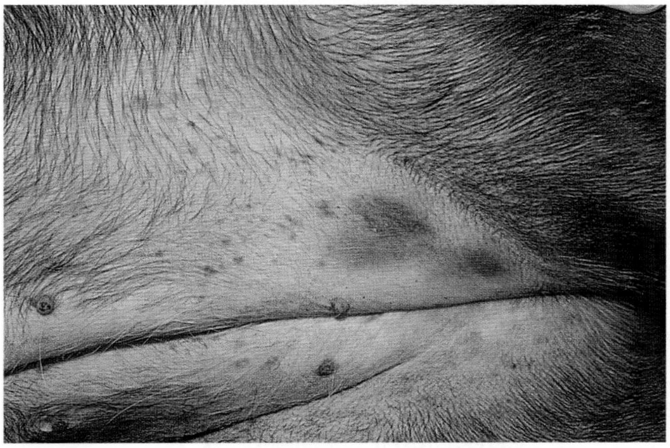

FIGURE 16-14 Petechiae and ecchymotic hemorrhages caused by thrombocytopenia resulting from canine ehrlichiosis infection. (From Rabinowitz PM, Conti L: *Human-animal medicine*, St Louis, 2010, Saunders.)

Normal platelet count is 150,000 to 400,000/μl. While the range is quite large, it does not fluctuate significantly in individual animals that are normal. Abnormal bleeding may occur with platelet counts below 40,000/μl, although each patient varies and some animals may not exhibit clinical signs associated with bleeding with a platelet count of 2,000/μl. The thrombocytopenic patient requires special care (e.g., extra cage padding, avoidance of central vessels for blood collection, extended application of pressure to venipuncture sites). In an animal exhibiting signs of surface bleeding with a normal platelet count, consideration should be given to the function of the platelets.

> TECHNICIAN NOTE One platelet per oil-immersion field represents approximately 20,000 platelets. Approximately 8 to 12 platelets per oil-immersion field is considered normal.

Certain tests are available to monitor coagulation in patients with suspected coagulopathies. Prothrombin time (PT) measures extrinsic and common clotting pathway activity, whereas activated partial thromboplastin time (aPTT) measures intrinsic and common pathway activity. Prolongation of PT/aPTT will be seen when clotting factors are depleted below 30% of normal. PT and aPTT samples must be collected and processed carefully to avoid potential sample errors. Atraumatic venipuncture and smooth blood flow into collection tubes are necessary to avoid extraneous clotting mechanism activation. Samples should be processed immediately after collection and frozen if being sent to an outside laboratory. An in-house analyzer is available for PT and aPTT testing. More information is located in Chapter 7.

Elevation in FSP occurs with excessive bleeding and fibrinolysis, and in animals with severe liver dysfunction. Interpreted in conjunction with the PT, aPTT, and platelet count, elevated FSP levels are useful as a diagnostic indicator of DIC.

Practical Hemostatic Tests

The following are simple, in-house tests requiring no specialized equipment. They are quick, inexpensive, practical tests that allow recognition and characterization of hemostatic defects. These tests are often referred to as "cage-side," in that they provide results almost immediately.

Platelet Estimation. A quick, reasonably accurate estimation of platelet numbers can be made from a stained blood smear. After routine preparation and staining, the blood smear is scanned to ensure even platelet distribution and that there is no evidence of platelet clumping. The average number of platelets in approximately 5 to 10 oil immersion fields is counted to estimate platelet numbers. The count is ranked as very low, low, normal, or high. One platelet per oil-immersion field represents approximately 20,000 platelets. Approximately 8 to 12 platelets per oil-immersion field is considered normal.

Although platelet estimation helps determine the presence of thrombocytopenia in an emergency situation, a true platelet count is necessary to classify the severity of depletion. Ongoing platelet quantitation is helpful in monitoring the course of a disease or the patient's response to certain therapies.

Buccal Mucosal Bleeding Time. Bleeding time is the time it takes for bleeding to stop after severing a vessel. The bleeding time test most often used in veterinary medicine today is the buccal mucosal bleeding time (BMBT).

The BMBT is a screening test used to assess platelet and vascular contribution to hemostasis, thereby evaluating part of the primary hemostatic mechanisms. More information on the BMBT is located in Chapter 7.

Activated Clotting Time. The activated clotting time (ACT) is a simple, inexpensive screening test for severe abnormalities in the intrinsic and common pathways of the clotting cascade. It evaluates the same pathways as aPTT. Prolongation of ACT occurs with severe factor deficiency in the intrinsic and/or common clotting pathway (e.g., hemophilia), in the presence of inhibitors (e.g., heparin, warfarin), or in cases of severe thrombocytopenia caused by the lack of platelet phospholipid (mild prolongation of 10 to 20 seconds). More information on the ACT test is located in Chapter 7.

WHOLE BLOOD AND BLOOD COMPONENTS

The goal in veterinary transfusion medicine is to limit whole blood transfusion and to use component therapy whenever possible. With the availability of variable speed, temperature-controlled centrifuges and the advent of plastic storage bags with integral tubing for collection, processing, and administration, specific blood component therapy is possible.

> *TECHNICIAN NOTE* The use of blood components permits specific replacement therapy for specific disorders, reduces the number of transfusion reactions, and decreases the amount of time needed to transfuse.

Whole blood can be stored or processed into one or more of the following components: red blood cells, platelets, plasma, and cryoprecipitate (Fig. 16-15). The goal in veterinary transfusion medicine is to use component therapy whenever possible. Blood components permit specific replacement therapy for specific disorders, reduce the number of transfusion reactions as a result of diminished exposure to foreign material, and decrease the amount of time needed to transfuse. Most importantly, appropriate therapeutic use of blood

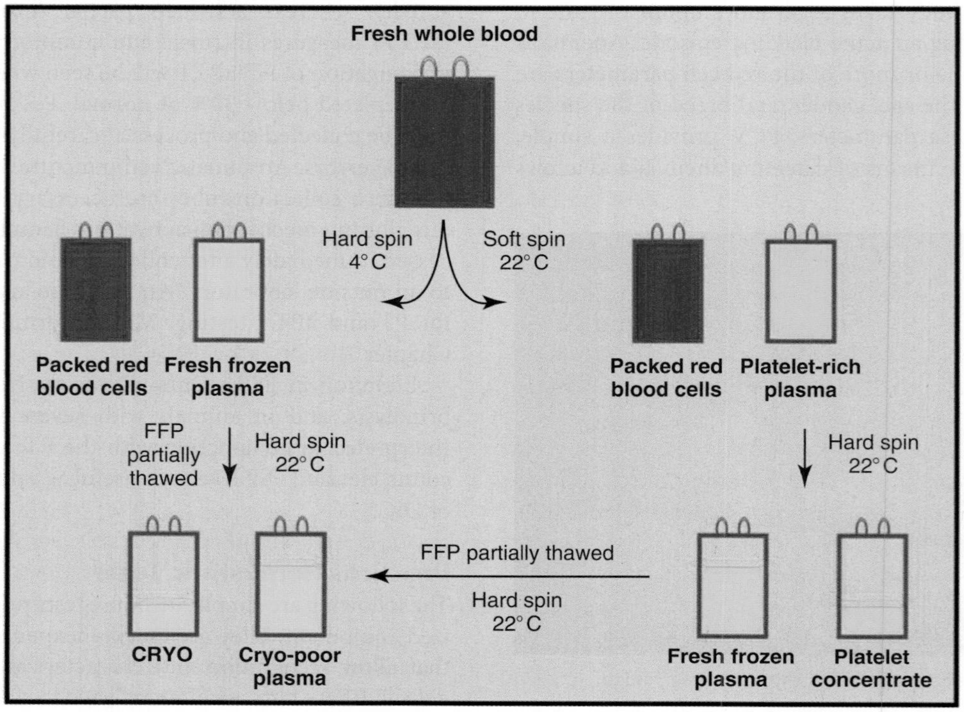

FIGURE 16-15 Blood components.

components increases the number of patients who benefit from this limited resource. Certain disease states will require replacement of one or any combination of components, and the component(s) chosen will depend on the crisis at hand (Table 16-8). The decision to administer any blood product involves a careful balance of anticipated benefit versus risk to the patient (e.g., allergic reaction, infectious disease transmission).

OXYGEN SUPPORT

Transfusion of RBC through whole blood (WB) or packed red blood cells (pRBC) is typically used to augment oxygen-carrying capacity in patients with low packed cell volume (PCV). Nearly all oxygen contained in blood is carried by hemoglobin; therefore RBC transfusions increase the oxygen-carrying capacity of the anemic patient and thus can reverse inadequate delivery of oxygen to tissues. A "transfusion trigger," the PCV at which a red blood cell transfusion is administered, has not been clearly defined in human or veterinary medicine. The point at which a blood transfusion is necessary is based on the summation of clinical assessment and laboratory findings. A PCV of less than 15% to 20% is often considered a threshold at which to provide transfusion support, particularly in ill patients or patients undergoing surgery or other major medical interventions. Low PCV alone, however, is an inadequate parameter for RBC transfusion because there are many additional factors (e.g., cardiac output and oxygen

TABLE 16-8 Blood Component Therapy

CONTENTS	INDICATION	SHELF LIFE	PREPARATION	COMMENTS
Fresh Whole Blood (FWB)				
RBC, plasma proteins, all coagulation factors, WBC, platelets (approx. Hct 40%)	Acute active hemorrhage; hypovolemic shock; thrombocytopenia or thrombopathia with active bleeding	Less than 8 hours after initial collection	Use immediately following collection (temperatures below 20° C compromises platelet viability)	Restores blood volume and oxygen-carrying capacity; may help control some microvascular bleeding in patients with thrombocytopenia/pathia
Stored Whole Blood (SWB)				
RBC, plasma proteins (approx. Hct 40%)	Anemia with hypoproteinemia; hypovolemic shock	Greater than 8 hours old and up to 30 days (dependent on anticoagulant-preservative solution used); refrigerate at 1-6° C	Allow to come to room temperature (temperatures exceeding 37° C will result in hemolysis and bacterial proliferation)	Restores blood volume and oxygen-carrying capacity; WBC and platelets not viable; F V & VIII diminished; not recommended for chronic anemia
Packed Red Blood Cells (pRBC)				
RBC (approx. Hct 80%), reduced plasma	Increase red cell mass in symptomatic anemia	Dependent on anticoagulant preservative solution used; refrigerate at 16° C	Allow to come to room temperature (temperatures exceeding 37° C will result in hemolysis and bacterial proliferation); may reconstitute with 0.9% NaCl before administration	Same oxygen carrying capacity as whole blood but less volume
Packed Red Blood Cells (pRBC), adenine saline added				
RBC (approx. Hct 60%), reduced plasma, 100 ml additive solution	Increase red cell mass in symptomatic anemia	28-30 days; refrigerate at 1-6° C	Allow to come to room temperature (temperatures exceeding 37° C will result in hemolysis and bacterial proliferation)	Additive solution extends shelf life of PRBC by improving storage environment; reduces viscosity for infusion
Platelet-Rich Plasma/Platelet Concentrate (PRP/PC)				
Platelets, few RBC and WBC, some plasma	Life-threatening bleeding due to thrombocytopenia or thrombopathia	5 days at 22° C; intermittent agitation required	Should administer immediately following collection and preparation	Do not refrigerate

TABLE 16-8 Blood Component Therapy—cont'd

CONTENTS	INDICATION	SHELF LIFE	PREPARATION	COMMENTS
Fresh Frozen Plasma (FFP)				
Plasma, albumin, all coagulation factors	Treatment of coagulation disorders/factor deficiencies; liver disease; DIC; anticoagulant rodenticide toxicity	12 months frozen at −18° C or colder	Thaw in 37° C warm water bath (temperatures exceeding 37° C will result in protein denaturation and bacterial proliferation)	Frozen within 8 hours after collection; no platelets; can be relabeled as frozen plasma after 1 year for additional 4 years; must be administered within 4 hours after thawing
Frozen Plasma (FP)				
Plasma, albumin, stable coagulation factors	Treatment of stable coagulation factor deficiencies	5 years frozen at −18° C or colder	Thaw in 37° C warm water bath (temperatures exceeding 37° C will result in protein denaturation and bacterial proliferation)	Frozen after more than 8 hours following collection; no platelets; can be used to treat some cases of acute hypoproteinemia; must be administered within 4 hours after thawing
Cryoprecipitate (CRYO)				
Factor VIII, vWF, fibrinogen, fibronectin	Hemophilia A; von Willebrand disease; hypofibrinogenemia	12 months frozen at −18° C or colder	Thaw in 37° C warm water bath (temperatures exceeding 37° C will result in protein denaturation and bacterial proliferation)	Must be administered within 4 hours after thawing

consumption) involved in tissue oxygenation in each individual patient. Tachycardia, poor pulse quality, pallor, lethargy, weakness, and decreased appetite are important clinical signs that may indicate that a patient is in need of additional oxygen-carrying support.

Whole Blood

Initial collection from a donor yields **fresh whole blood** (FWB) and is defined as FWB for up to 8 hours after collection. FWB provides red blood cells, white blood cells, platelets, plasma proteins, and coagulation factors. Certain components in blood are more fragile than others and will become less effective with time and ambient temperature change. For example, platelet efficacy becomes questionable once whole blood is refrigerated. In order to achieve full benefit of all components when needed, FWB should be administered immediately following collection.

FWB is used in actively bleeding, anemic animals with thrombocytopenia/thrombopathia, anemia with coagulopathies, and massive hemorrhage. In cases of severe hemorrhage, administration of all components may be necessary to support the patient. Massive hemorrhage is defined as a loss approaching or exceeding one total blood volume within a 24-hour period.

Following collection, whole blood must be processed into components or at least refrigerated at 1° to 6° C within 8 hours. After 24-hour storage of whole blood, platelet function is lost and the concentration of labile coagulation factors decreases. The product is then defined as **stored whole blood** (SWB) and provides RBCs and plasma proteins (albumin, globulins). The length of time a unit of WB can be stored under refrigeration is dependent on the anticoagulant-preservative solution used in collection. With the advantages in the use of blood components so well documented in both human and veterinary medicine and the improved availability of these products as a result of commercial blood banks, the use of WB is no longer considered the treatment of choice. However, SWB can be used in patients that require intravascular volume expansion as well as oxygen-carrying support, albumin, or coagulation factors. The use of WB, fresh or stored, is not recommended in severe chronic anemia. Chronically anemic patients most often have increased their plasma volume to maintain a normovolemic state. Rapid administration of WB may expose these patients to the risk of volume overload, especially in patients with preexisting cardiac disease or renal compromise.

> **TECHNICIAN NOTE** Fresh whole blood is used in actively bleeding, anemic animals with thrombocytopenia or thrombopathia, whereas packed red blood cells is the component of choice for increasing red cell mass in patients who require oxygen-carrying support.

Packed Red Blood Cells

Packed red blood cells (pRBC) is the component of choice for increasing red cell mass in patients who require oxygen-carrying support. Decreased red cell mass may be caused by decreased bone marrow production, increased destruction, or surgical or traumatic bleeding. Although it seems logical that blood loss should be replaced with whole blood, replacing blood volume with pRBC and crystalloid or colloid solutions adequately treats most blood loss. This is often adequate therapy for the majority of acutely bleeding patients. Transfusion of pRBC is not recommended in patients who are well compensated for their anemia (e.g., chronic renal failure). The decision to perform red blood cell transfusion should never be based solely on hematocrit or hemoglobin levels. Patients should be properly evaluated, and pRBC administration should be based primarily on clinical status (e.g., tachycardia, poor pulse quality, respiratory distress, lethargy).

Packed RBCs can be harvested from whole blood (fresh or stored) by the use of a refrigerated centrifuge (5000 g for 5 minutes at 4° C). If a refrigerated centrifuge is not available, RBCs can be harvested by allowing whole blood to separate by sedimentation over time. After sedimentation, the plasma is removed and placed in a sterile transfer pack. Ideally, packed RBCs should be reconstituted with a nutrient solution before storage to maintain the cells in a healthier environment. This extends storage time; also, reconstitution of the RBCs reduces viscosity during administration. Packed RBCs can be refrigerated at 4° C, with storage time determined by the anticoagulant-preservative or additive solution used in collection and processing. If a nutrient solution is not used at the time of processing, packed RBCs can be reconstituted with 100 ml of 0.9% NaCl before administration to reduce viscosity. Reconstitution with nonisotonic fluids may cause RBC damage.

HEMOSTATIC SUPPORT

Alterations in primary and/or secondary hemostasis can interrupt normal blood coagulation to varying degrees, putting the patient at risk for hemorrhage. Platelet and coagulation factor replacement is achieved by administering specific whole blood derived components, including platelets, fresh frozen plasma, frozen plasma, cryoprecipitate, and cryosupernatant plasma. Unfortunately, plasma and its derivatives are among the least understood and the most frequently misused of all blood components in both human and veterinary medicine. With the exception of emergencies, the use of plasma without laboratory analysis to verify a suspected coagulopathy is not justified.

Platelets

Of all the primary hemostatic defects seen in small animal medicine, thrombocytopenia is the most common and can result from an increased loss of platelets (i.e., hemorrhage), increased destruction of platelets, increased consumption of platelets (i.e., excessive clotting), or decreased production of platelets (i.e., bone marrow disease). Although rare, qualitative platelet disorders can occur in veterinary patients, including both congenital (e.g., platelet storage pool disease, Glanzmann's thrombasthenia) and acquired (e.g., uremia, drug therapy) disorders. The major indication for platelet transfusion is to stop severe, uncontrolled, or life-threatening bleeding in patients with significantly decreased platelet number and/or function.

Platelets can be harvested from a unit of fresh whole blood (FWB) that is less than 8 hours old and has not been cooled below 20° C; refrigerated platelets do not maintain function or viability as well as platelets stored at room temperature. In human medicine, platelets are routinely stored at room temperature (20-24° C) under constant agitation for up to 5 days. Studies have shown that, even at room temperature, platelet function begins to be compromised after 24 hours and there is greater potential for proliferation of contaminating bacteria within the product. Attempts have been made to freeze platelets to achieve a longer shelf life, but these techniques have yet to be validated for animals. There continues to be interest and research in both human and veterinary blood banking to develop alternative storage options that would increase the shelf-life and availability of platelet products in clinical practice.

Platelet-rich plasma (PRP) is produced from FWB by slow speed centrifugation (referred to as a "soft spin") at 2000g for 3 minutes at 20° C. PRP may be administered following centrifugation, or the platelets may be further concentrated by centrifugation using a "heavy spin" at 5000 g for 5 minutes, also at 20° C. The platelet-poor supernatant is then expressed into a second satellite bag, leaving no more than 50 ml of plasma that will be used for resuspension of the platelet concentrate (PC). Allow the PC to lie undisturbed for 1 hour after processing, followed by gentle resuspension of the platelet button and plasma.

In veterinary medicine, platelet preparation is challenging in regard to the volume needed (and blood donors required) in order to measurably increase platelet numbers in larger breed dogs. Under optimal conditions, platelets prepared from a single unit of FWB administered to a 30-kg dog would be expected to result in an increase in the patient's platelet count of approximately 10,000/µl. Depending on the size of the patient and the severity of bleeding, large volumes of PRP/PC (or FWB) may be required to significantly increase the platelet count, an exercise that is costly and unrealistic for most clinical practices. In some patients, however, cessation of bleeding following platelet transfusion has been achieved without a measurable increase in platelet number. Because of the impracticality associated with production of this component in the required volume necessary for significant impact, specific storage requirements, and the short shelf life, it is common to treat thrombocytopenia/thrombopathia with active bleeding with FWB through which the patient will receive both platelets and red blood cells. In situations of platelet destruction, such as immune-mediated thrombocytopenia, the survival of transfused platelets is a matter of minutes rather than days; however, platelet transfusion may still be warranted if the patient is acutely bleeding into a vital structure (i.e., brain, heart, lung).

In human medicine close to 80% of platelet transfusions are performed with platelets prepared from single donors by apheresis (as opposed to platelets derived from one single unit of whole blood). With plateletpheresis, blood is removed from the donor, anticoagulated, and separated into components by "donor-side" centrifugation, allowing for the concentration of platelets while the plasma, white blood cells, and red blood cells are returned to the donor. Not only is the yield of platelets by apheresis much greater (comparable to 4 to 6 units of single donor platelets), there is also less contamination of both red and white blood cells in the final product. Plateletpheresis is currently being performed at some commercial blood banks and veterinary teaching institutions. However, costly apheresis systems and the need for invasive catheter placement in the donor preclude this process in most veterinary volunteer donor situations.

Plasma

In addition to water and electrolytes, plasma contains albumin, globulins, coagulation factors, and other proteins. Plasma is primarily used for its coagulation factor value; it does not contain functional platelets. Most coagulation proteins are stable at 1° to 6° C, with the exception of factors V and VIII. In order to maintain adequate levels of all factors, plasma must be harvested from a unit of FWB by "heavy spin" centrifugation at 5000 g for 5 minutes at 1° to 6° C. If frozen at −18° C or below within 8 hours from the time of initial collection, the product is referred to as **fresh frozen plasma** (FFP). FFP will retain its coagulation factor efficacy for a period of 12 months, provided it is maintained at the appropriate temperature.

> TECHNICIAN NOTE Fresh frozen plasma is not recommended for blood volume expansion or for protein replacement in animals with chronic hypoproteinemia and should only be administered to patients with compromised hemostatic function who are experiencing hemorrhage or need to undergo invasive procedures.

FFP contains all coagulation factors and can be used to treat multiple coagulation deficiencies occurring in patients with liver disease, anticoagulant rodenticide toxicity, disseminated intravascular coagulation, or massive transfusion. Occasionally, FFP is used to support patients with single factor deficiencies, such as hemophilia A (if cryoprecipitate is unavailable) or hemophilia B, and potentially other conditions (e.g., acute pancreatitis). FFP is not recommended for blood volume expansion or for protein replacement in animals with chronic hypoproteinemia. Alternative products are available for these purposes and do not put the patient at risk for infectious disease transmission or allergic reactions.

Coagulation factor concentrates in a lyophilized form offer a more efficient and effective form of treatment and are the routine mode of therapy in human transfusion medicine, especially for factor VIII deficiency (hemophilia A) and factor IX deficiency (hemophilia B). Factor concentration allows adequate hemostatic function with less than half the plasma volume needed when utilizing FFP. Volume overload is a serious complication of FFP transfusion given it is not a concentrate and has strong colloidal impact.

FFP should only be administered to patients with compromised hemostatic function who are experiencing hemorrhage or need to undergo invasive procedures (e.g., surgery). Coagulation testing should be performed before transfusion support and monitored periodically post transfusion to determine the effectiveness of each transfusion episode. Mild hemostatic abnormalities do not always predict clinical bleeding; therefore the patient's clinical status and invasiveness of impending diagnostics should help determine if FFP transfusion is required.

If FFP is not used within 12 months, it can be relabeled as frozen plasma (FP) and stored for an additional 4 years. Also, plasma may be separated from a unit of whole blood at any time during its recommended storage time (determined by anticoagulant-preservative solution used in collection). When stored at −18° C or less, this component is also called FP and may be kept for up to 5 years from the original date of whole blood collection. If not frozen, it is called liquid plasma (LP) and has a shelf life not exceeding 5 days following the expiration date of the whole blood from which it was harvested. Plasma prepared from outdated whole blood may have higher levels of ammonia than FFP as a result of longer contact with red cells before its preparation.

FP and LP may have varying levels of the more stable coagulation factors, as well as albumin, but they do not contain functional platelets or the labile coagulation factors V and VIII. FP and LP can be used to treat stable clotting factor deficiencies, such as anticoagulant rodenticide toxicity. As with FFP, FP and LP are not recommended for use as a blood volume expander. If animals are severely or chronically protein deficient, plasma must be administered in large volumes in order to have a measurable impact in managing the acute effects of hypoproteinemia (i.e., pulmonary edema, pleural effusion). In this case, synthetic colloid solutions should be considered in that they are readily available and more effective in increasing oncotic pressure.

Cryoprecipitate

Cryoprecipitate (CRYO) is the cold-insoluble portion of plasma that precipitates after FFP has been slowly thawed at 1° to 6° C (refrigerator). This process will take approximately 14 to 16 hours when using a standard blood bank refrigerator. When the product becomes slushy, the unit is centrifuged at 4° C using a "heavy spin" of 5000 g for 7 minutes. Most of the supernatant plasma is expressed into an attached satellite bag, leaving behind a small white mass of precipitated material containing concentrated amounts of von Willebrand factor (vWF), factor VIII, fibrinogen, fibronectin, and factor XIII. Less than 50 ml of the supernatant plasma is left behind to allow for reconstitution of the precipitate before storage.

> **TECHNICIAN NOTE** Cryoprecipitate is used in patients with suspected or diagnosed von Willebrand disease, hemophilia A, or fibrinogen deficiency.

Following production, CRYO must be frozen at −18° C or colder and has a shelf life of one year from the original date of whole blood collection. A delay in refreezing the precipitate or exposure to temperatures above 10° C during processing will significantly decrease the quality of the final product. CRYO should be thawed quickly at 37° C (no more than 15 minutes) to minimize degradation of factor VIII. Thawed CRYO should be administered immediately but can be stored at room temperature for a maximum of 6 hours after thawing.

CRYO is indicated for use in patients with suspected or diagnosed von Willebrand disease (vWD), hemophilia A (factor VIII deficiency), or fibrinogen deficiency. Fresh frozen plasma or fresh whole blood may also be used based on product availability; however, volume overload and greater risk of transfusion reaction is of concern.

Cryosupernatant Plasma

Cryosupernatant plasma, commonly known as cryopoor plasma, contains albumin and immunoglobulins, as well as most coagulation proteins (except for vWF, factor VIII, fibrinogen, fibronectin, and factor XIII). It can be used for patients in need of coagulation support but not those with Hemophilia A or von Willebrand disease. Cryopoor plasma can be used to treat animals with anticoagulant rodenticide toxicity, as it contains functional vitamin K-dependent factors II, VII, IX, and X. When stored at −18° C or colder, this component has a shelf life of 12 months from the original date of whole blood collection.

Alternative Therapies

The shortage of banked blood products in veterinary medicine and the ever-expanding risk of blood incompatibilities and infectious disease transmission sparked interest in developing safe and effective alternatives to red blood cell transfusion. Transfusion alternatives are therapies that reduce the need for allogeneic transfusions. Options for specific pharmacologic intervention do exist (i.e., hemoglobin-based oxygen carrier solutions) and, when indicated, should precede blood transfusion.

Hemoglobin-Based Oxygen Carriers. Synthetic solutions that contain hemoglobin seem to be a logical substitute for RBC transfusion. The ideal red cell substitute would:

- Augment oxygen delivery
- Provide colloidal support
- Be free of infectious agents
- Be universally compatible and safe
- Have room temperature storage and a long shelf life
- Be readily available and reasonably priced

The quest for a hemoglobin-based oxygen-carrying solution (HBOC) led to the development of Oxyglobin, an alternative for delivering oxygen to tissues. Currently, Oxyglobin is available at a limited production rate. Its availability has been inconsistent over the years.

Oxyglobin (OPK Biotech, Cambridge, MA) is a solution of purified, polymerized bovine hemoglobin in a modified lactated Ringer's solution. Under normal circumstances, hemoglobin in RBCs carries 98% of the circulating oxygen, whereas only 2% is carried in plasma. When Oxyglobin is administered, it is the plasma hemoglobin concentration that is increased. It may be more effective than blood at delivering oxygen to tissues because it is carried in the plasma and offloads oxygen more readily than RBCs. Its oxygen affinity is regulated by physiologic chloride concentration, not 2,3-DPG. In addition to providing oxygen-carrying support, Oxyglobin also has a strong colloidal effect, which can be useful in patients who are hypovolemic as well as anemic. Its colloid effects, however, may be associated with circulatory overload in normovolemic and cardiac-diseased animals.

The volume of Oxyglobin to be delivered depends on the patient's degree of anemia and underlying disease. The recommended dosage is 10 to 30 ml/kg intravenously; however, its duration of effect is dose dependent (Table 16-9). At these recommended dosages, the complications associated with volume expansion are minimized as long as the volume status of the patient is such that colloidal solutions can be tolerated.

The best monitoring parameters in the anemic patient are physical examination findings, particularly respiratory and cardiovascular status, as well as hemoglobin concentration. Patients receiving Oxyglobin require measurement of total (RBC and plasma) and/or plasma hemoglobin rather than PCV to assess how much of an impact has been made on oxygen-carrying support. For example, in a patient with a total hemoglobin concentration of 7 g/dl following administration of Oxyglobin, the oxygen-carrying capacity of blood is approximately that of a packed cell volume of 21% (hemoglobin × 3 = PCV). In this patient, if the PCV is 3%, then a PCV equivalent of 18% is due to Oxyglobin.

Side effects can occur with administration of Oxyglobin, including discoloration of the mucous membranes and

TABLE 16-9 Oxyglobin Dose Chart

DOSE (ml/kg)	IMMEDIATE POST-INFUSION PLASMA HEMOGLOBIN (g/dl)	HALF-LIFE (HOURS)	CLEARED FROM PLASMA (DAYS)
10	1.5-2.0	18-26	4-5
15	2.0-2.5	19-30	4-6
20	3.4-4.3	25-34	5-7
30	3.6-4.8	22-43	5-9

sclera, increased central venous pressure, pulmonary edema, vomiting, and diarrhea. Following infusion of Oxyglobin, the patient's serum will appear red, resulting in artifactual increases or decreases in the results of some serum chemistry tests (dependent on type of analyzer and reagents used) (Fig. 16-16). Complete blood count (CBC) results will be valid except for an increase in two RBC indices: mean cell hemoglobin (MCH) and mean cell hemoglobin concentration (MCHC). Total solids measurement will increase because of increased plasma protein in the form of hemoglobin. Oxyglobin does not have an effect on hemostatic function testing (e.g., prothrombin time, partial thromboplastin time, platelet count, D-dimers). Given that a small percentage of the hemoglobin solution is excreted by the kidneys, transient discoloration of the urine will occur, and therefore urine dipstick measurements are inaccurate. It is best to perform a CBC, serum chemistry, and urinalysis before the administration of Oxyglobin.

The most significant limitation of Oxyglobin in comparison to RBC transfusion is its relatively short half-life (30 to 40 hours at the recommended dose of 30 ml/kg) versus RBC survival of approximately 120 and 70 days in dogs and cats, respectively. Additionally, it is recommended as a single-dose administration because antibodies to bovine hemoglobin may be produced after several days, although their significance is unknown. Because of the lack of RBC membranes in Oxyglobin, cross-matching and blood typing are not necessary, and hemolytic transfusion reactions are not a concern.

Xenotransfusion and Autotransfusion

Xenotransfusion is the act of transfusing blood from a member of one species to a member of a different species. This is a treatment of last resort only justifiable if the patient will die without a transfusion and no other option is available. Canine blood has been occasionally used to provide oxygen-carrying capacity for feline patients. Cats do not have naturally occurring antibodies against dog erythrocyte antigens, with first exposure leading to sensitization and a delayed hemolytic transfusion reaction 4 to 7 days later. Subsequent transfusions administered more than 4 to 6 days after exposure result in anaphylaxis.

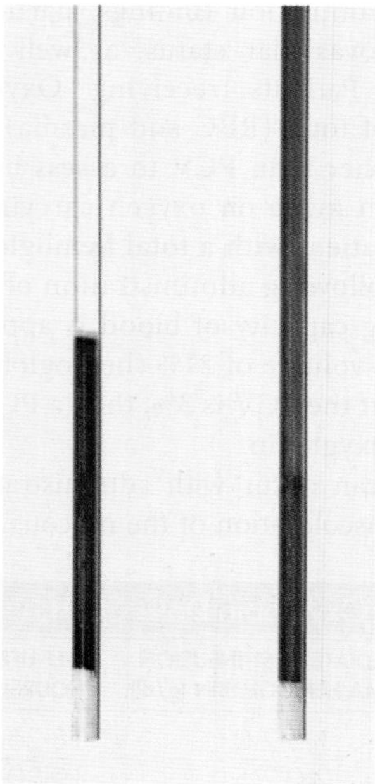

FIGURE 16-16 Feline serum sample before *(left)* and after *(right)* Oxyglobin infusion; red discoloration is visible. (From August JR: *Consultations in feline internal medicine,* vol 6, ed 6, St Louis, 2010, Saunders.)

Autotransfusion is the act of removing blood from a patient and administering it back into the patient's circulation. In emergency medicine, the blood is collected out of a body cavity where hemorrhage has occurred. Salvaged blood may be transfused with a syringe or fluid bag, utilizing blood administration filters. Concerns with autotransfusion lie in potential contaminants to the blood such as bacteria, malignant cells, and thrombi, as well as the potential to induce coagulopathies and systemic inflammation.

BLOOD TYPES

Blood types are genetically determined markers on the surface of red blood cells. They are specific to each species and are antigenic. A set of blood types of two or more alleles makes up a blood group system. More than a dozen blood group systems have been described in dogs. The current nomenclature is listed as Dog Erythrocyte Antigen (DEA) followed by a number. Red blood cells from a dog can either be positive or negative for any blood group system. For example, a dog's red cells can be DEA 3 positive or DEA 3 negative. The DEA 1 system was previously thought to have at least two subtypes, referred to as DEA 1.1 (also known as A1) and DEA 1.2 (also known as A2). However, recent research has documented that these reflected varying degrees of expression of the same gene. Very limited surveys on the frequency of canine blood types have been reported. Some blood types are rare (e.g., DEA 3), whereas others are more common (DEA 4).

Clinically, the most severe antigen-antibody reaction is seen with the DEA 1 antigen. Significant naturally occurring alloantibodies are not seen in the dog, therefore antigen-antibody reactions are not likely to occur on initial transfusion. However, dogs that are DEA 1 negative can develop antibodies to DEA 1 from a mismatched first transfusion. These anti-DEA 1 antibodies can develop within a few days from initial transfusion and can potentially destroy the donor's red blood cells, ultimately minimizing the benefits of the transfusion. However, a previously sensitized DEA 1–negative dog can experience an acute hemolytic transfusion reaction following transfusion of DEA 1–positive blood. Transfusion reactions may also occur after a previously transfused (and now sensitized) dog receives blood that is mismatched for any red cell antigen other than DEA 1. These reactions may occur as early as 4 days after sensitization. For example, a previously sensitized DEA 4–negative dog experienced an acute hemolytic transfusion reaction while receiving DEA 4–positive blood. In an emergency situation, or with specific medical conditions that preclude conclusive typing (e.g., autoagglutination in an IMHA patient), DEA 1–negative blood should be used to avoid sensitization to the DEA 1 antigen.

TECHNICIAN NOTE The most severe antigen-antibody reaction is seen with the DEA 1 antigen.

One blood group system, the AB system, has been well defined in the cat. It contains three blood types: A, B, and the extremely rare AB. Nearly all domestic short hair (DSH) and domestic long hair (DLH) cats in the United States have type A blood. Many purebred cats (and some DSH/DLH) have been identified with type B blood. The proportion of type A and B varies not only among the different breeds, but also geographically. The rare type AB blood has both the A and B antigen on the red cell surface. Many other blood group systems are thought to exist (e.g., Mik blood group antigen), but have not yet been fully characterized.

Cats differ from dogs in that they have significant naturally occurring alloantibodies against the other blood group. Cats with type B blood have very strong naturally occurring anti-A alloantibodies, whereas type A cats have relatively weak anti-B alloantibodies. When administering type B blood to a type A cat, there may not be any obvious clinical reaction, but the transfused red cells have a half life of approximately 2 days. Ultimately, this has no positive effect on the patient. In administering type A blood to a type B cat, the red cell survival can be minutes to hours with severe clinical signs, sometimes fatal. Administration of a small amount of blood to test for incompatibility is not an acceptable procedure given that life-threatening acute hemolytic transfusion reactions can be observed with administration of as little as 1 ml of AB-incompatible blood. These reactions can be avoided by typing donors and patients. If blood typing is not available, a **blood cross-match** should be performed to ensure blood compatibility. The extremely rare blood type AB cat lacks anti-A and anti-B alloantibodies and can be safely transfused with type A packed red blood cells if type AB blood is not available.

CANINE AND FELINE BLOOD TYPING METHODS

Various methods have been developed for blood typing cats and dogs in both the clinical laboratory and practice setting. The principle of blood typing methods is the presence of a hemagglutination reaction that results when a RBC surface antigen binds with known polyclonal or monoclonal antibodies (within seconds to minutes).

Clinical laboratory blood typing methods are slightly more complex and/or require specialized equipment. They include the following: tube and slide method using a polyclonal antibody and agglutination reagent (wheat germ lectin, *Triticum vulgaris*) in the cat, tube assay using polyclonal antisera reagents in the dog, and gel column diffusion technology using monoclonal antibodies in the dog and cat.

Currently, there are two types of commercially available point-of-care assays for canine and feline blood typing: a card-based agglutination test and an immunochromatographic assay. Both of these tests are user friendly and yield reasonably accurate results, making them invaluable in the emergency setting. With both canine and feline blood typing, blood samples must first be evaluated for autoagglutination. If macroscopic autoagglutination is present, washing red blood cells three times with phosphate buffered saline (PBS) (see blood cross-match procedure) may eliminate the problem; otherwise blood typing cannot be performed with these methods.

Card-Based Agglutination Test

RapidVet-H (Canine DEA 1). This blood typing test card is intended for use in classifying dogs as DEA 1 positive or negative (Fig. 16-17). The assay is based on the agglutination reaction that occurs when erythrocytes that contain DEA 1 antigen on their surface membranes interact with a monoclonal antibody specific to DEA 1. Each card has 3 visually defined wells identified as "DEA 1 Positive Control," "DEA 1 Negative Control," and "Patient Test." One drop of whole blood (in EDTA) and one drop of phosphate buffered saline (PBS) are mixed onto lyophilized reagents within each well, being careful to avoid cross-contamination between the wells. In the "Patient Test" well, the monoclonal antibody is reconstituted to form an antiserum and then mixed with whole blood from the patient. DEA 1–positive erythrocytes react with the antiserum causing agglutination. If agglutination is present in the "Patient Test" well, it is then graded from 0 to 4+. The antiserum is completely nonreactive with DEA 1–negative erythrocytes. "Auto-Agglutination Saline Screen" cards are supplied separately if autoagglutination is suspected.

RapidVet-H (Feline). A similar blood typing test card is available to classify cats as type A, B, or AB. The assay is based on the agglutination reaction that occurs when erythrocytes interact with a monoclonal antibody specific for the A antigen and/or an anti-B solution (wheat germ lectin, *Triticum vulgaris*, which causes agglutination of type

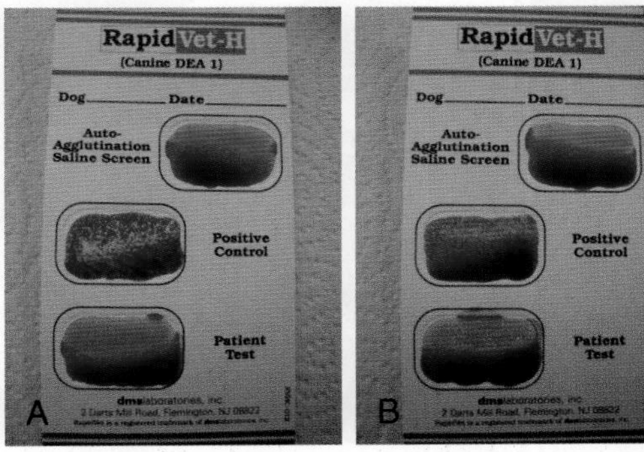

FIGURE 16-17 RapidVet-H blood-typing card for canine DEA 1 antigen showing a negative patient result **(A)** and a positive patient result **(B)**.

B cells). Erythrocytes from type A cats will agglutinate with anti-A monoclonal antibodies (well labeled A on card) and erythrocytes from type B cats will agglutinate with anti-B solution (well labeled B on card). Erythrocytes from type AB cats will agglutinate with both anti-A and anti-B reagents. The third well on the card serves as the autoagglutination saline screen and must be negative in order to interpret results.

Immunochromatography Assay

An alternative method of DEA 1 blood typing for dogs and AB typing for cats is available for use in practice. The technique uses immunochromatography, rather than agglutination. The control band detects a separate antigen on the red blood cells. Autoagglutination does not seem to interfere with this technique.

The canine test uses a monoclonal anti-DEA 1 antibody strip impregnated onto a paper strip and a second control antibody to a universal RBC antigen as a control. An RBC solution diffuses up the strip and if the cells express DEA 1, they concentrate in the area of antibody impregnation. The cells also concentrate in the area of the control antigen, demonstrating that cells have successfully diffused up the length of the strip.

The feline test works in the same way; however, there is an area containing an anti-A monoclonal antibody, an area containing an anti-B monoclonal antibody, and a control antibody against a common feline RBC antigen, allowing determination of blood type A, B, or AB (Fig. 16-18).

SOURCES OF DONOR BLOOD

A safe and adequate supply of blood components for transfusion is indispensable. The American Association of Blood Banks has established acceptable standards for the collection, processing, storage, distribution, and administration of human blood and blood components. Each blood bank and transfusion service strictly follows these standards, as well as certain legal requirements of local, state, and federal governments. Strict compliance with these standards reflects a commitment to providing quality products and appropriate care for patients receiving transfusion support. Although government organizations play less of a role in ensuring quality practices in veterinary medicine, the industry is striving to adhere to similar standards. To that end the American Association of Veterinary Blood Banks and Association of Veterinary Hematology and Transfusion Medicine have established standards in veterinary transfusion medicine and blood banking that guarantee safety and efficacy. Given that blood is a live tissue, adverse events can occur at any time during donor selection and screening, blood collection, component processing, and product storage.

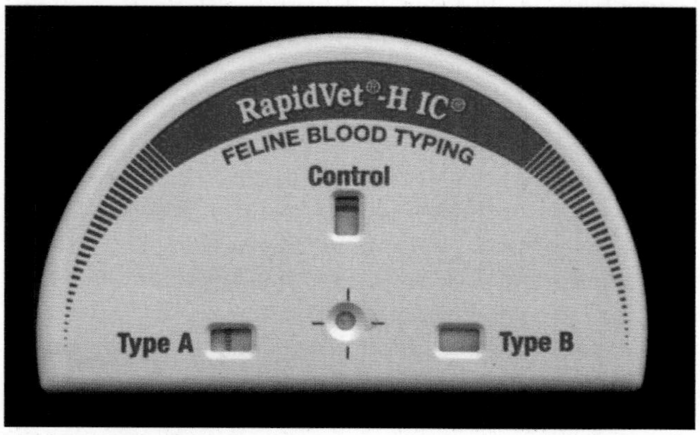

FIGURE 16-18 IC blood-typing test showing a patient result for a type A cat.

Historically, veterinarians have relied on donors living within the hospital facility as a source of blood for transfusion purposes. The cost of an in-house donor is often overlooked, and the charges for a unit of blood are severely underestimated. In the past decade several commercial blood banks have been established to help meet blood transfusion needs in primarily small-animal medicine. Purchasing products from these banks and maintaining an inventory within the facility are much more efficient and cost-effective than maintaining a donor colony within the hospital. Using employee-owned personal pets and healthy client-owned animals as blood donors is a good alternative to maintaining in-house donors. For reasons to be discussed, this type of program is more practical for dogs than cats.

> **TECHNICIAN NOTE** Canine and feline blood donor animals should undergo a complete blood count, serum biochemistry profile, and testing for geographically specific infectious agents each year.

CANINE BLOOD DONORS

Blood donors can be recruited through employee personal pets, client-owned animals, breeders, and organized dog clubs. Many owners are happy to volunteer their animal for periodic blood donation (e.g., three to four times yearly) once they understand the need for blood products in veterinary medicine. Nevertheless, potential donors may carry illnesses that could possibly affect the safety of the donation process and/or the safety and quality of the blood products, thereby further compromising the patient. For this reason, it is important to verify donor health status through a brief history, physical exam, and appropriate laboratory testing, all of which are performed on the day of the donation.

There are specific requirements canine donors must meet before being accepted into a donation program. Donors must be a minimum of one year of age and weigh at least 25 kg to allow for the collection of a full unit (i.e., 450 ml ± 10%). They must be healthy and have a current vaccination status for distemper, hepatitis, parainfluenza, parvovirus, and rabies. A 4-week resting period is required following vaccination before a dog can donate; however, dogs can be safely vaccinated at any point after donation. Dogs are ineligible to donate if they are currently taking any medication (e.g., antibiotics, anti-inflammatory drugs, antihistamines). The majority of infectious diseases in the dog are transmitted by fleas, ticks, and mosquitoes; therefore for the safety of the donor and the blood supply, flea, tick, and heartworm prevention is strongly encouraged. Dogs are also disqualified from the blood donor program if they have ever been diagnosed with any of the following: heart murmur or other cardiac conditions, seizures or seizure-like activity, heartworm disease, chronic illness, or a disease/condition that required a blood transfusion. Intact bitches cannot donate blood if they are in estrus. As canine donors are not sedated for blood collection, donor temperament is critical to the success of the blood donation. The collection process takes approximately five minutes, during which the dog is lying on its side—a very submissive position, and one that many dogs will not tolerate. Any dog that is anxious or fearful will not do well with the blood donation process.

On an annual basis a complete blood count, serum biochemistry profile, and testing for geographically specific infectious agents (e.g., *Ehrlichia canis, Babesia canis, Dirofilariasis immitis*) should be performed (Table 16-10). The hematocrit or hemoglobin concentration should be ≥40% or ≥13.5 g/dl, respectively, before each donation. Blood donor dogs should be typed for DEA 1, and possibly other blood groups. Because of the strong antigenicity of DEA 1, typing of donors and recipients for DEA 1 is strongly recommended. DEA 1–negative blood can be given to DEA 1–negative and DEA 1–positive patients. Dogs positive for the DEA 1 antigen can be accepted as blood donors as long as recipients are typed before administration, with DEA 1–positive blood being given only to patients positive for DEA 1.

FELINE BLOOD DONORS

The approach to the feline donor is much more complicated than with its canine counterpart. At present, there are few commercial feline blood banks. In addition, volunteer programs for cats hold many risks. Although dogs will donate blood voluntarily, the majority of cats must be sedated for blood donation purposes. The legal ramifications associated with sedating personal pets for blood donation is far too great. Another concern is that cats can harbor infectious agents more readily than dogs. Because of this, only 100% indoor cats should be used.

Feline blood donors should be young, good-natured adults. They should be large and lean, weighing at least 5 kilograms. Good health can be verified through a medical history, physical exam, and routine laboratory testing. Donors should have current vaccination status for rhinotracheitis, calicivirus, panleukopenia, and rabies. Annual laboratory screening includes: complete blood count, serum biochemistry profile, feline leukemia virus, feline immunodeficiency virus, *Mycoplasma haemofelis,* and *Mycoplasma haemominutum* (Table 16-11). Before each donation, donor hematocrit (≥35%) or hemoglobin (≥11 g/dl) is checked.

Because of the presence of naturally occurring alloantibodies, there is no universal blood type in the cat. All feline blood donors and recipients must be blood typed, and only typed, matched blood should be administered. The extremely rare blood type-AB cat can be safely transfused with type-A packed red blood cells if type-AB blood is not available.

TABLE 16-10 Canine Infectious Disease Screening Before Blood Donation

DISEASE	CAUSATIVE AGENT	SCREENING
Anaplasmosis	*A. phagocytophylium* *A. platys*	Recommended
Babesiosis	*B. canis, B. gibsoni*	Recommended
Bartonellosis	*B. vinsonii*	Conditional
Brucellosis	*B. canis*	Recommended
Ehrlichiosis	*E. canis,* *E. ewingii,* *E. chaffeensi*	Recommended Conditional
Leishmaniasis	*L. donovani*	Recommended
Lyme Disease	*B. burgdorferi*	Not recommended
Neorickettsiosis	*N. risticic* *N. helminthica*	Conditional
Rocky Mountain Spotted Fever	*R. ricketsii*	Not recommended
Trypanosmiasis	*T. cruzi*	Conditional

BLOOD COLLECTION

The recommended blood collection site in the cat and dog is the jugular vein. Because of this vein's size and increased blood flow, RBC trauma is minimized during collection. Blood should be collected via a single venipuncture to avoid cell damage and excessive activation of coagulation factors. Strict aseptic technique and use of sterile equipment minimize the possibility of bacterial contamination.

> TECHNICIAN NOTE Collection, processing, storage, and administration of blood products must focus on strategies to prevent or delay adverse changes to blood constituents and minimize bacterial contamination and proliferation.

TABLE 16-11 Feline Infectious Disease Screening Before Blood Donation

DISEASE	CAUSATIVE AGENT	SCREENING
Anaplasmosis	*A. phagocytophylium*	Conditional
Bartonellosis	*B. henselae*	Recommended
Cytauxzoonosis	*C. felis*	Conditional
Ehrlichiosis	*E. canis*	Conditional
FIP	Feline enteric corona virus	Not recommended
FIV	Feline immunodeficiency virus	Recommended
FELV	Feline leukemia virus	Recommended
Hemoplasmosis	*M. haemofelis*	Recommended
Neorickettsiosis	*N. risticii*	Conditional
Toxoplasmosis	*T. gondii*	Not recommended

BLOOD COLLECTION SYSTEMS

Whole blood is most often collected into commercially available plastic bags (Fig. 16-19). These sterile bags are considered "closed" collection systems in that they allow for collection, processing, and storage of blood and blood components without exposure to the environment, which diminishes the risk of bacterial contamination to the product. These systems are available in a variety of configurations that will determine blood component preparation and storage. They all meet human blood banking standards and have been tested successfully in veterinary medicine.

A single blood collection bag is used for the collection of whole blood when it is to be administered as whole blood. It consists of a main collection bag containing anticoagulant-preservative solution and integral tubing with a 16-gauge needle attached (Fig. 16-20). This system is not recommended for component preparation in that the bag must be entered to harvest components, risking environmental exposure and potential bacterial contamination. If the bag is entered, the definition of this system then becomes "open," and the product must be used within a 24-hour period. Other collection systems consist of a primary collection bag containing anticoagulant-preservative solution and one, two, or three satellite bags intended for component preparation. One of the satellite bags may contain 100 ml of an additive solution used for red cell reconstitution following plasma removal. Additive solutions (i.e., saline, dextrose, adenine) extend packed red blood cell storage time.

In the dog, blood may be collected using the commercially available human blood collection bags; however, the size of these systems prohibit their use in cats. Currently, smaller closed collection systems are not commercially available. Alternatively, blood can be collected utilizing separate, single syringes. A 19- to 21-gauge butterfly catheter attached to a three-way stopcock and sterile 10- to 30-ml syringes containing anticoagulant may be used (Fig. 16-21). During collection, the syringes should be gently inverted to allow for mixing of blood and anticoagulant, preventing clot formation. Blood collection utilizing this technique is effective, but considered an "open" system. Following collection, blood can be transferred from the syringes into an empty sterile bag, or transfer pack, making delivery more efficient. Products collected via syringe are not intended for storage. Unfortunately, as a result of the lack of closed blood collection systems for cats, the difficulty in preparing blood components from small whole blood units, and limited storage time allowed for blood collected with an "open system," cats in need of transfusion support most often receive fresh whole blood.

Vacuum glass bottles containing ACD anticoagulant-preservative solution have been the most popular collection system used in veterinary medicine for dog. Although blood collection is easier with this system, there are many limitations and disadvantages: this is considered an "open" collection system, the glass activates platelets and certain clotting factors, the foam created during collection will disrupt the red cell surface and cause hemolysis, and component preparation is not possible. For these reasons, vacuum glass bottles are not recommended. Vacuum chambers that allow for more rapid collection into blood collection bags are available.

ANTICOAGULANT-PRESERVATIVE SOLUTIONS

There are several anticoagulants, anticoagulant-preservatives, and additive solutions available for blood collection for transfusion purposes (Box 16-3). The primary goal of preservative solutions is to maintain red cell viability during storage and to lengthen the survival of red cells post transfusion. According to AABB standards, 75% of transfused red blood cells must survive for 24 hours following infusion in order for the transfusion to be considered acceptable and successful. The longer cells are stored, the more viability decreases. Predetermined storage times are based on studies that have

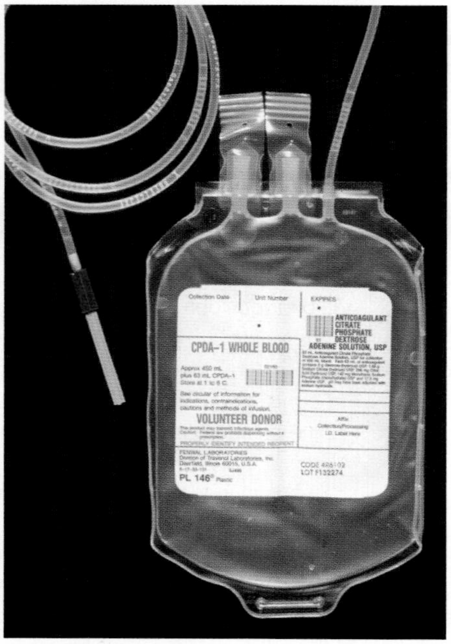

FIGURE 16-19 Whole blood collection bag.

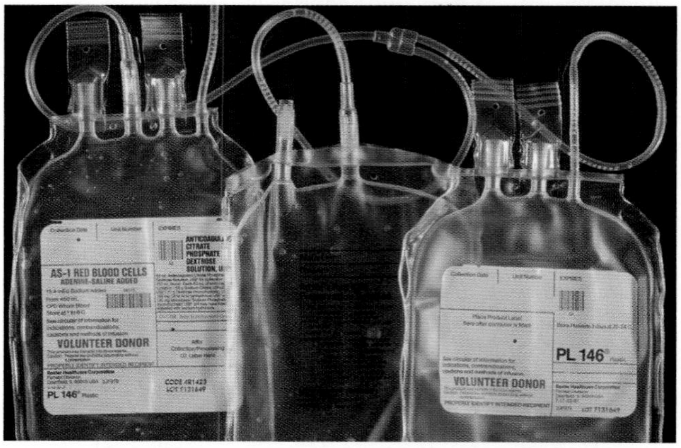

FIGURE 16-20 Component blood collection bag.

investigated adverse biochemical changes that take place during red cell storage. These changes, referred to as the "storage lesion," include a decrease in ATP, pH, and 2,3-DPG (2,3-DPG loss occurs only in dogs) and an increase in the percentage of hemolysis. All of these ultimately lead to a loss of red cell function and decreased viability. Storage time will vary with the anticoagulant-preservative solution used.

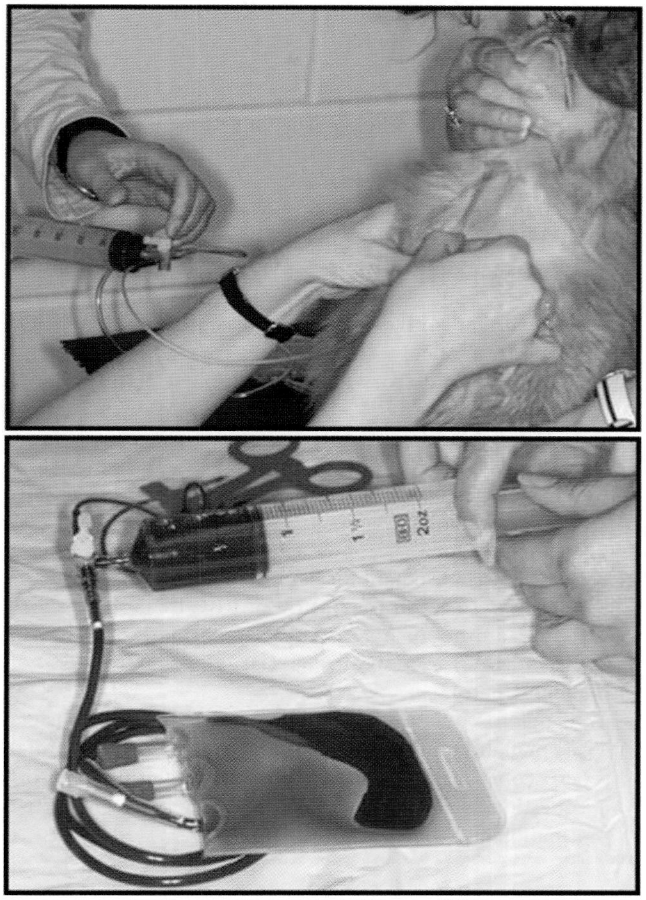

FIGURE 16-21 Feline collection—open system.

BLOOD STORAGE

The shelf-life of blood components is determined by the type of system used for blood collection; the anticoagulant-preservative solution used; the time between collection, processing, and storage; as well as the temperature and conditions under which products are stored. It is critical that appropriate temperatures are consistently maintained in order to secure the quality of both red cell and plasma products. Refrigerators and freezers for blood component storage should be dedicated for this purpose, and evaluation of their temperature performed daily. Commercially-available blood refrigerators and freezers are built to continuously monitor and record temperature, with audible alarm systems that activate before blood products reach unacceptable temperatures.

BLOOD ADMINISTRATION

TESTING FOR COMPATIBILITY

Pretransfusion testing is necessary to ensure the best possible results of a blood transfusion. It includes testing of the donor, selection of appropriate donor units based on the patient's blood type, and blood cross-matching. Although pretransfusion testing will help to determine preexisting incompatibility between the donor and recipient, normal survival of transfused cells in the patient's circulation cannot be guaranteed. Blood samples for initial testing should always be collected from patients before infusion of any donor blood products.

> *TECHNICIAN NOTE* Pretransfusion testing will help to determine preexisting incompatibility between the donor and recipient but does not guarantee normal survival of transfused cells in the patient's circulation.

Dogs lack significant naturally occurring alloantibodies; therefore they may be safely transfused without a blood cross-match (BCM) before the first transfusion. However,

BOX 16-3 Anticoagulant-Preservative Solutions

Citrate-Phosphate-Dextrose-Adenine (CPDA-1)
- RBC 2,3 DPG & ATP better maintained
- Whole blood may be stored for 35 days, pRBCs may be stored for 21 days
- Used at ratio of 1 ml CPDA-1 to 7-9 ml blood

Citrate-Phosphate-Dextrose (CPD)
- Whole blood and pRBCs may be stored for 28 and 21 days, respectively
- Used at ratio of 1 ml CPD to 7-9 ml blood

Acid-Citrate-Dextrose (ACD)
- Whole blood and pRBCs may be stored for 21 days
- Used at ratio of 1 ml ACD to 7-9 ml blood

Heparin
- Dose required for anticoagulation is 0.5 to 2 Units/ml
- Not recommended for transfusion purposes: no preservative qualities, anticoagulant properties neutralized by plasma

Additive Solutions (e.g., *Adsol, Nutricel, Optisol*)
- Protein-free solution added to red cells after plasma removal from whole blood unit
- Increases yield of plasma from whole blood unit
- Provides red cells with adequate nutrients
- Increases volume of red cell component; decreases hematocrit of red cell component, reduces viscosity
- Extends shelf-life of red cell products—additional 7 days storage time

all dogs that have received RBC transfusions more than 4 days previously must be cross-matched before receiving any additional RBC transfusions. Because cats have naturally occurring alloantibodies and may experience a severe reaction to their first transfusion, a BCM should be performed before any blood transfusion if blood typing is not available (Procedure 16-4). A BCM is typically not necessary for a first transfusion if the blood types of the feline recipient and donor are known. As with dogs, feline patients that have received RBC transfusions more than 4 days previously should be cross-matched before receiving any additional RBC transfusions.

A BCM is performed to detect serological incompatibility by identifying antibodies in donor or recipient plasma against recipient or donor red blood cells. The test is composed of three individual tests:

Recipient control → recipient plasma + recipient RBC
Major blood cross-match → recipient plasma + donor RBC
Minor blood cross-match → donor plasma + recipient RBC

An autocontrol sample of recipient RBC and plasma is included because some recipients may have autoagglutination interfering with the BCM. If the recipient control is positive (i.e., agglutination is present), one cannot draw conclusions about blood compatibility between patient and donors. Any hemolysis and/or agglutination in the major or minor BCM (but not the control) indicate an incompatibility and the need to choose a new donor. The minor BCM should be compatible in dogs because canine donor plasma should not contain significant antibodies. Feline patients must be given type-specific plasma products because of the presence of naturally occurring alloantibodies. A blood cross-match kit is also available for in-house use (Fig. 16-22).

> **TECHNICIAN NOTE** A blood cross-match can detect antibodies in donor or recipient plasma against recipient or donor red blood cells.

PROCEDURE 16-4 Blood Cross-Match—Tube Method

1. Collect blood into an EDTA tube from recipient and potential donor(s).
2. Centrifuge (1000 g for 5 min) to separate plasma from RBC. Remove plasma from each sample with a pipette, and transfer plasma to clean, labeled glass or plastic tubes. Note any hemolysis.
3. Wash RBC pellet three times or until supernatant is clear with phosphate buffered saline (PBS):
   a. add 4 to 5 ml of PBS
   b. mix well
   c. centrifuge 1 to 2 minutes
   d. remove saline, leaving pellet of RBC at bottom of tube
4. Resuspend RBC pellet with PBS to make a 3% to 5% RBC suspension.
5. Prepare for each donor 3 tubes labeled major, minor, and recipient control. Add to each tube 2 drops (50 µl) of plasma and 1 drop (25 µl) of RBC suspension as follows:
   - **Recipient control** → recipient plasma + recipient RBC (perform once)
   - **Major blood cross-match** → recipient plasma + donor RBC
   - **Minor blood cross-match** → donor plasma + recipient RBC
6. Mix gently and incubate for 15 to 20 minutes at 37° C in a warm water bath.
7. Centrifuge for 15 seconds at 1000 g.
8. Examine supernatant for hemolysis.
9. Gently resuspend the button of RBC by tapping tube and examine for macroscopic agglutination. Classify as 1+ (fine), 2+ (small), 3+ (large), or 4+ (one large agglutinate).
10. If macroscopic agglutination is not observed, transfer a small amount onto a glass slide and examine for microscopic agglutination (microscopic agglutination is of questionable importance). Differentiate between agglutination and rouleaux formation.

A compatible BCM does not prevent sensitization, delayed transfusion reactions, or non-hemolytic transfusion reactions; it simply indicates that at the present time there are no detectable antibodies against the RBC. Keep in mind that sensitization may develop later from the transfusion of any RBC membrane antigen not produced by the patient. Additionally, there are many types of transfusion reactions not caused by RBC membrane antigen incompatibilities (e.g., febrile non-hemolytic transfusion reactions, transfusion of damaged/lysed blood).

PREPARING BLOOD FOR TRANSFUSION

Refrigerated blood may be gently warmed by allowing it to sit at room temperature for approximately 30 minutes. Properly administered cold blood will not increase the chance of a transfusion reaction, but large amounts of cold blood infused rapidly can induce hypothermia and cardiac arrhythmias. Warming of RBC products is recommended for neonates and patients that require large-volume transfusion. In an emergency situation, the tubing of the blood administration set can be immersed in a warm-water bath (not to exceed 37° C) so that the blood is warmed as it passes through the tubing. The entire unit should not be warmed at one time. Frozen products should be thawed in a 37° C warm water bath. Blood products should not be exposed to temperatures exceeding 42° C; this results in damage to RBCs and denaturation of blood proteins. Warming RBC products or thawing plasma products in a microwave oven is not recommended.

TRANSFUSION VOLUME

The appropriate volume of blood must be administered to each patient. Specific component therapy should be utilized to treat each disorder, and the patient's cardiovascular status should always be assessed before determining the required volume and administration rate. The volume of blood ad-

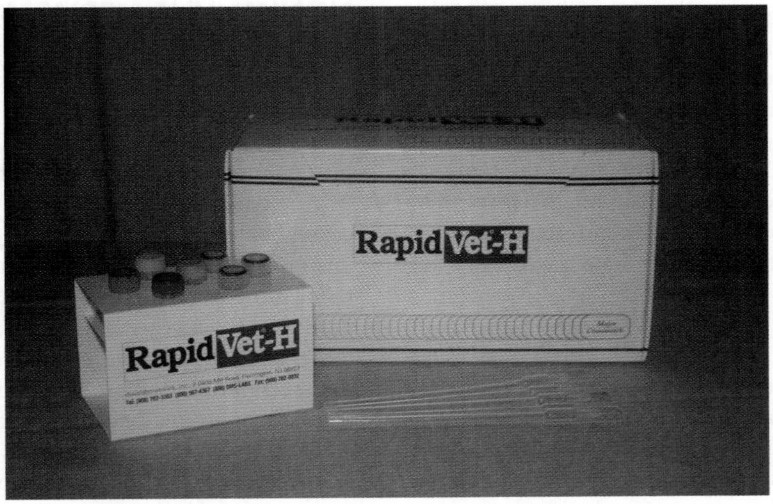

FIGURE 16-22 A blood cross-match kit available for in-house use.

ministered is dependent on the presence of active bleeding, onset and degree of anemia, clinical status of the patient, and body weight. For practical purposes, feline patients initially receive one unit of whole blood (40 to 50 ml) or one unit of pRBC (20 to 25 ml) or one unit of fresh-frozen plasma (20 to 25 ml). Feline patients should be evaluated after each transfusion episode to determine if further blood product support is needed. The following dosages are used to estimate the blood component volume needed per transfusion episode in dogs:

- 20 ml/kg = ml WB needed
- 2 ml/kg WB will raise PCV by 1%
- 10 ml/kg = ml pRBC needed
- 1 ml/kg pRBC will raise PCV by 1%
- 6-10 ml/kg = ml plasma needed

ADMINISTRATION ROUTES

Blood and blood components can be administered via many routes. Intravenous is obviously the most effective route in that the infused red blood cells or plasma products are immediately available to the general circulation. The intraosseous route is utilized in puppies or kittens when vascular access is difficult or unsuccessful. When delivering blood products intraosseously, infused cells and proteins are available to the general circulation within minutes. The most common sites for intraosseous catheter placement are the trochanteric fossa of the femur, the wing of the ilium, and the shaft of the humerus. Care should be taken in the placement of these catheters because of the increased risk of osteomyelitis.

ADMINISTRATION RATES

Blood product administration rates are variable. The desirable rate of infusion depends on the patient's blood volume, cardiac status, and hemodynamic condition. For example, a patient with massive hemorrhage may require a more rapid transfusion than a normovolemic patient with a chronic anemia. The maximum rate of transfusion for a normovolemic patient (where circulatory overload is a potential problem) is 11 to 22 ml/kg/hr, whereas hypovolemic patients can tolerate rates of 22 to 66 ml/kg/hr. If rapid transfusion is needed, blood can be infused as rapidly as the patient's circulatory system will tolerate, within a few minutes, if the rate does not cause the red cells to hemolyze. Animals with cardiovascular compromise cannot tolerate infusion rates that exceed 4 ml/kg/hr. It is recommended for all patients that blood components be infused slowly (e.g., 1 ml/kg) for the first 10 to 15 minutes while closely observing for signs of an acute transfusion reaction. As a rule, the blood product should then be infused as quickly as will be tolerated but should be completed within 4 hours to ensure administration of functional blood components and to prevent growth of bacteria in the event of contamination. Maximum time should not be confused with recommended time; most transfusions are completed within 2 hours. Most feline transfusions may be safely completed in 1 hour, with the exception of cats with heart failure.

All blood products should be filtered in order to help prevent thromboembolic complications. Standard blood infusion sets have in-line filters with a pore size of approximately 170 to 260 microns. A filter of this size will trap cells, cellular debris, and coagulated protein. Trapped debris combined with room temperature conditions may promote proliferation of any bacteria that may be present; therefore blood infusion sets may be used for several units of blood products or for a maximum time of 4 hours. Microaggregate filter systems with a pore size of 20 to 40 microns may be used for low-volume transfusion (i.e., <50 ml whole blood, <25 ml pRBC or plasma).

TRANSFUSION REACTIONS

Animals should be carefully monitored for any adverse reactions during and for several weeks following transfusion. Early recognition of transfusion reactions requires careful and frequent evaluation of the patient. Before infusion, baseline values of attitude, rectal temperature, pulse rate and quality, respiratory rate and character, mucous membrane color, capillary refill time, hematocrit, total plasma protein, and plasma and urine color should be monitored. The majority of these parameters should be checked every 30 minutes throughout the transfusion, and evaluated routinely posttransfusion to ensure the desired effect has been achieved. Transfusion reactions can be classified as immune-mediated or nonimmune-mediated.

IMMUNE-MEDIATED TRANSFUSION REACTIONS

Immune-mediated transfusion reactions can be hemolytic in origin, with either an acute (caused by preexisting alloantibodies or prior sensitization) or delayed (can be exhibited >4 days post transfusion) presentation. Hemolytic transfusion reactions are the most serious but are less common. In acute situations, intravascular hemolysis is caused by preexisting antibodies, as seen in the mismatched transfusion of feline type A blood to a cat with type B blood or in a previously sensitized DEA 1.1–negative dog receiving DEA 1.1–positive blood. Clinical signs include, but are not limited to, fever, tachycardia, weakness, muscle tremors, vomiting, collapse, hemoglobinemia, and hemoglobinuria. Vomiting can be noted with any type of transfusion reaction; therefore patients receiving blood products should not be fed during or just before transfusion.

Non-hemolytic transfusion reactions are a result of antibodies to white blood cells, platelets, or plasma proteins. Clinical signs include urticaria, pruritus, and pyrexia. Present thinking attributes most febrile non-hemolytic reactions to the actions of cytokines, predominantly those produced by leukocytes in the transfused unit. These reactions are most often transient in nature and do not cause life-threatening situations.

NONIMMUNE-MEDIATED TRANSFUSION REACTIONS

There are a variety of factors associated with nonimmune-mediated transfusion reactions. In order to avoid these reactions, careful attention should be given to the collection, processing, storage, and administration of all blood products.

Any type of trauma to the red blood cells will potentially cause hemolysis: (1) overheating red blood cell products (also will cause protein denaturation and may increase bacterial growth during infusion), (2) freezing red blood cell products, (3) mixing red blood cell products with nonisotonic solutions causing cellular damage, (4) warming and then rechilling blood products, and (5) collecting or infusing blood through small needles or catheters.

Bacterial pyrogens and sepsis can be a complication of improperly collected and stored blood. Dark brown to black supernatant plasma in stored blood indicates digested hemoglobin from bacterial growth. Any blood with discolored supernatant should be immediately discarded. Patients experiencing this complication will most often mount a febrile response 15 to 20 minutes from start of infusion.

Citrate intoxication may occur when the citrate/blood volume ratio is disproportionate or in massively transfused patients, particularly in patients with liver dysfunction. Common clinical signs include involuntary muscle tremors, cardiac arrhythmias, and decreased cardiac output. This compromised state can be confirmed by obtaining ionized serum calcium. If citrate toxicity is in question, blood administration should be discontinued and calcium gluconate administered.

Because blood is a colloid solution, vascular overload is a potential complication. Clinical signs include coughing (as a result of pulmonary edema), dyspnea, cyanosis, tachycardia, and vomiting. If volume overload is of concern, blood administration should, at the very least, be temporarily discontinued and supportive care instituted.

REVIEW QUESTIONS

Matching

Match the blood component listed in Column B with the appropriate recipient in Column A.

Column A	Column B
_____1. A hit-by-car dog with a hematocrit of 29 and a total protein of 3.0	a. stored whole blood
_____2. A 17-year-old cat with chronic renal failure; hematocrit 16, total protein 8.0	b. fresh frozen plasma
_____3. A dog that presents with generalized petechia and ecchymosis; hematocrit 18, total protein 4.0	c. cryoprecipitate
_____4. A dog with severe diarrhea; hematocrit 29, total solids 2.5	d. RBCs
_____5. A suspected Doberman with vWF bleeding from a tooth extraction	e. fresh whole blood

True or False

Indicate whether each of the following statements is True or False.

_____1. Some extracellular fluids can collect in various parts of the body secondary to infection, injury, or compromised circulation.

_____2. The movement of solutes across a semi-permeable cell membrane from the side with the lower solute concentration to the side with the higher solute concentration until the concentrations equilibrate is called diffusion.

_____3. Relatively small changes in serum potassium concentration can alter nervous and cardiac functions.

_____4. The capillary refill time can be an important indication of peripheral perfusion.

_____5. Skin turgor is the most accurate way to detect or estimate dehydration.

_____6. Frequent, serial body weight measurement is a good monitoring tool for continued fluid loss during treatment.

_____7. Dehydration is associated with increases in both PCV and TPP, while PCV reduction alone is seen with splenic contraction.

_____8. Prothrombin time (PT) measures extrinsic and common clotting pathway activity, whereas activated partial thromboplastin time (aPTT) measures intrinsic and common pathway activity.

_____9. Fresh frozen plasma does not contain viable platelets.

_____10. Dogs differ from cats in that they have significant naturally occurring alloantibodies against the other blood types.

Choose the Best Response

Choose the best answer to the following questions.

1. Which of the following is the most abundant and important of the extracellular ions in that the distribution of body water is influenced by this electrolyte?
   a. bicarbonate
   b. chloride
   c. sodium
   d. potassium
2. Clinical signs associated with hypernatremia are usually primarily:
   a. neurologic in origin
   b. not detectable
   c. behavioral
   d. weight related
3. What is the normal pH of arterial blood?
   a. 7.0
   b. 7.35
   c. 7.4
   d. 7.45
4. Presence of a cardiac murmur may warrant:
   a. higher fluid rates
   b. lower fluid rates
   c. colloid fluid use only
   d. hypertonic fluid use only
5. A decreasing hematocrit and total plasma protein level suggests:
   a. dehydration
   b. infection
   c. cerebral edema
   d. hemodilution

RECOMMENDED READING

Battaglia AM, Steele A, editors: *Small animal emergency and critical care for veterinary technicians*, ed 3, St Louis, 2015, Saunders.

Devey J: Crystalloid and colloid fluid therapy. In Ettinger SJ, Feldman EC, editors: *Textbook of veterinary internal medicine*, ed 7, St Louis, 2010, Saunders.

DiBartola SP: *Fluid, electrolytes, and acid-base disorders in small animal practice*, ed 4, St Louis, 2011, Saunders.

Oakley DA: Establishing and monitoring central venous pressure in the critical patient, *Vet Tech* 1:40–46, 1987.

Walker RH, editor: *Technical manual of the American Association of Blood Banks*, ed 14, Bethesda, MD, 1996, American Association of Blood Banks.

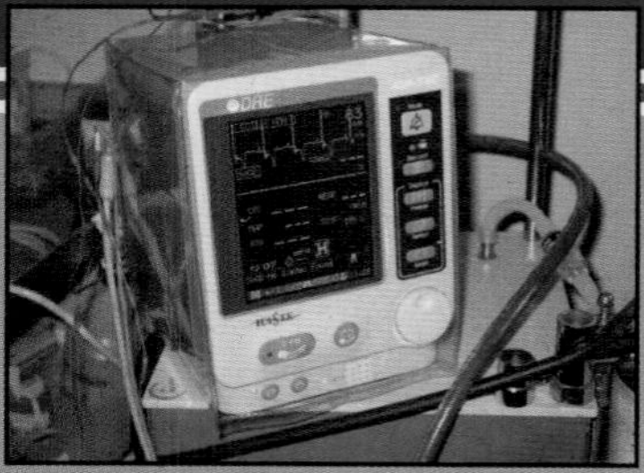

17 Emergency and Critical Care

OUTLINE

LEARNING OBJECTIVES

After reviewing this chapter, the reader will be able to:

1. Describe the role of the veterinary technician on the emergency health care team.
2. List and describe necessary work space and equipment to provide an emergency service.
3. Discuss considerations for rendering first aid to injured or critically ill animals.
4. Describe procedures for performing a systemic evaluation of injured or critically ill animals.
5. Describe procedures used to perform vital functions in injured or critically ill patients.
6. List and describe methods used to monitor the condition of critically ill patients.
7. Describe procedures for placement and care of catheters, chest tubes, and tracheostomy tubes.
8. Describe procedures used in maintaining recumbent patients.
9. Describe procedures used in rendering emergency care in specific medical situations.

KEY TERMS

Aortic thromboembolism
Azotemia
Cardiopulmonary arrest (CPA)
Congestive heart failure
Coupage
Critical care
Cyanosis
Diabetic ketoacidosis (DKA)
Dystocia
Emergency care
Hypoadrenocorticism
Hypovolemic shock
Hypoxemia
Nosocomial infections
Oliguria
Opisthotonus
Perfusion
Pulse oximetry
Pyometra
Saddle thrombus
Triage

Emergency and critical care is an established specialty in veterinary medicine. Although emergencies have always existed in veterinary medicine, the American Veterinary Medical Association recognized emergency and critical care as a distinct specialty in the late 1980s. In January 1996, the North American Veterinary Technicians Association (now the National Association of Veterinary Technicians in America) recognized the Academy of Veterinary Emergency and Critical Care Technicians (AVECCT) as the first specialty for veterinary technicians. There are many similarities between emergency and critical care, but there are also differences. As defined by the Veterinary Emergency and Critical Care Society (VECCS),

emergency care is an action directed toward the assessment, treatment, and stabilization of a patient with an urgent medical problem. **Critical care** is the ongoing treatment of a patient with a life-threatening or potentially life-threatening illness or injury whose condition is likely to change on a moment-to-moment or hour-to-hour basis. Such patients require intense and often constant monitoring, reassessment, and treatment.

The veterinary technician is a front-line member of the health care team. A team approach is mandatory for optimal care of a critically ill patient. For the veterinary technician to excel in emergency and critical care, he or she should have an understanding of the pathophysiology of the disease process in order to understand the patient's current condition and to anticipate developing problems in the patient or the needs of the veterinarian. The technician should be adept at placing a variety of catheters: peripheral and central venous, arterial, and urinary. He or she should also be cognizant of problems involved with the maintenance of asepsis and the patency of such catheters. The technician should be observant and recognize patient deterioration and alert the clinician of the changes, document them, and be prepared to take action. He or she should be familiar with a variety of lifesaving procedures regardless of whether they are performed exclusively by the veterinarian. The technician should be capable of taking diagnostic radiographs and performing basic laboratory tests. He or she must be compassionate and supportive in order to interact with owners under stressful conditions.

In the current age of technology, there is risk in becoming too dependent on monitoring equipment. A carefully performed physical exam remains the best monitoring tool available. Communication between the veterinarian and veterinary technician is also paramount to successful monitoring of patients in the intensive care setting. A written record of all observations, treatments, and events is crucial, particularly if multiple individuals are involved in providing patient care. Patient protocols will allow advanced intellectual thinking, provide effective time use, shorten patient hospital stay, and allow the veterinary technician to play a more active role in patient care.

EMERGENCY READINESS AND PREPARATION

FACILITY AND EQUIPMENT

Clinic facilities should be set up and organized to handle any emergency. This may be an area in the clinic designated for emergency management of patients or a mobile "crash cart" system (Fig. 17-1). When selecting an area, consider the space available; ensure that there is enough room for the emergency team (three or more people) and equipment. An oxygen source should be readily available. Good lighting is essential; it facilitates examination of the patient, endotracheal intubation and visualization of veins, and minor surgical procedures. The area designated for the management of the emergency patient should be centralized and stocked with key emergency supplies and equipment (e.g., ECG, defibrillator, suction). Supplies should be organized for easy accessibility. A crash cart/kit may be as simple as a fishing tackle box or as elaborate as a mobile tool chest. Crash carts/kits make the resuscitation endeavor more efficient. The emergency area should be checked at the beginning of each shift and restocked immediately after each use.

Crash Cart

The crash cart should be stocked with emergency materials stored in a methodical, logical fashion. Typically, the crash cart is a type of rollaway cart that can be moved if needed in an emergency situation, or in a centrally located fixed position in the ICU. The cart should be inventoried on a daily basis by staff members, and restocked immediately after use in a triage situation. The crash cart should contain the following items, as outlined below by drawer.

Drawer One: Airway Items. It is crucial to have proper breathing accessories present and stored in an organized fashion (Fig. 17-2). Large tissue forceps, such as Forrester sponge forceps, should also be located in the drawer, to enable emergency retrieval of airway (perilaryngeal and pharyngeal) foreign bodies, or to swab the airway with gauze if bleeding

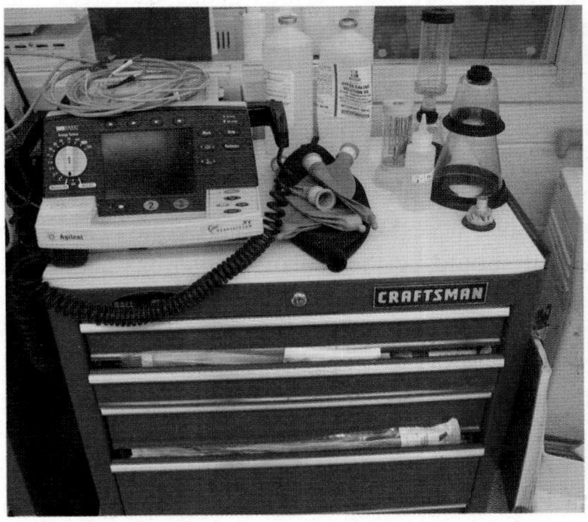

FIGURE 17-1 Mobile crash cart for the emergency patient.

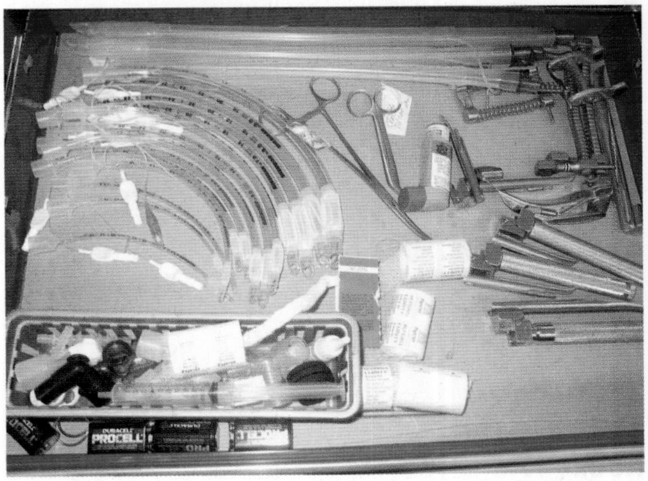

FIGURE 17-2 Airway drawer, typically the top drawer of the emergency cart.

or excessive mucus inhibits intubation. A wide range of sizes of endotracheal tubes should be arranged neatly, with the cuffs checked daily for patency. Clear endotracheal tubes are recommended in order to monitor vapor trails, blood, vomitus, etc. Laryngoscopes with various size blades, as well as wire or plastic stylets, are recommended for difficult intubation. Tie gauze, syringes for cuff inflation, and mouth guards are other necessary items used during intubation.

Other useful breathing gadgets include the "Y" connection pieces, used for simultaneous oxygen insufflation into two nasal cannulas, and the Ambu bag (Fig. 17-3). The Ambu bag is a resuscitator bag with a one-way valve, delivering oxygen through a reservoir bag with each manual compression. When using the Ambu bag, positive pressure ventilation can be used without concern for the pop-off valve, advantageous to patients that have restrictive parenchymal diseases. Other respiratory emergency devices that should be incorporated in the airway drawer include oxygen masks, nasal oxygen catheters and the necessary oxygen tubing (i.e., nonconductive tubing), and asthmatic inhalers for the dyspneic cat (Box 17-1).

Drawer Two: Venous Access Drawer. Items stocked should include not only various gauge catheters, but also catheters that vary in length (Fig. 17-4). Eight- and twelve-inch angiocatheters should be included, for emergency pericardial centesis (note that these catheters must be fenestrated for such procedures). Spinal needles for emergency CSF taps should also be readily available.

Guide-wire central venous catheters are necessary emergency vascular access devices placed by the Seldinger technique and should be located in the venous access drawer. Such catheters include the single- to multi-lumen device catheter systems. Guide-wire catheters are typically soft and flexible and are made of a polyurethane material, which is antithrombogenic and can be maintained for longer periods. Guide-wire central venous catheters are very useful in administration of different fluid types, serial blood sampling, or central venous pressure monitoring. All-in-one catheters that include the dilation and guide wire insertion with one insertion are called Emergency Infusion Devices (Teleflex Medical) (see Fig. 17-5), which are useful in larger patients

BOX 17-1 Airway Items

- Endotracheal tubes: sizes 3.0 to 12 including some half sizes (3.5, 4.5)
  Ensure cuff patency before placing new tubes in drawer
- Laryngoscope with various blades
  Check to see if lights are working
- Wire stylets and polypropylene catheter stylets
- Plastic oxygen connectors
- Mouth guards
- Tie gauze
- Large tissue forceps
- Oxygen masks
- Asthmatic inhaler
- Nasal oxygen catheter and tubing
- Ambu bag

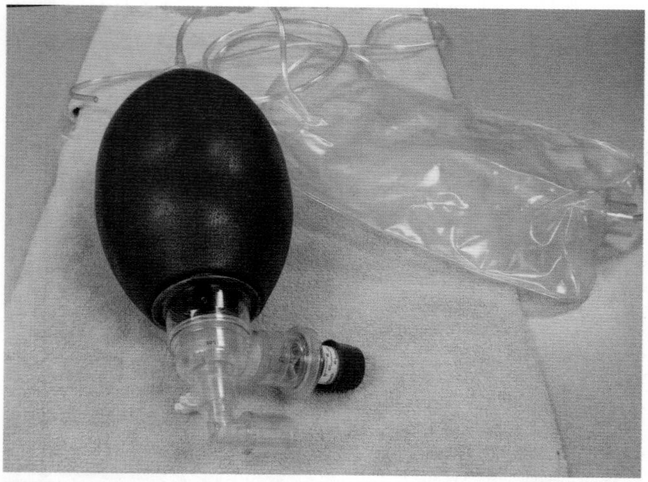

FIGURE 17-3 The Ambu bag is a resuscitator bag with a one-way valve, used to deliver oxygen through a reservoir bag with each manual compression.

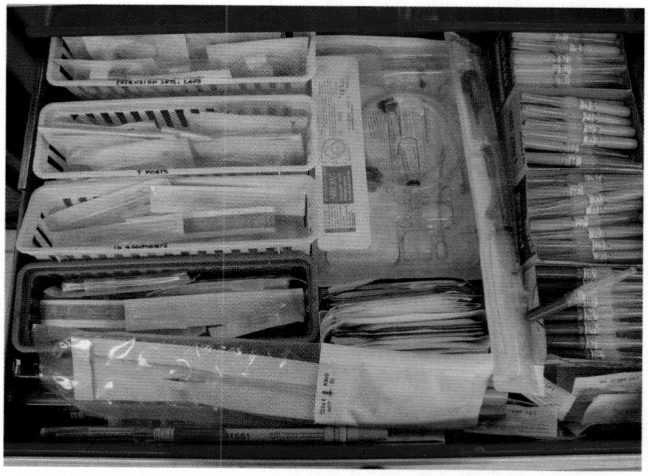

FIGURE 17-4 Venous access drawer; catheters should vary in both diameter and length.

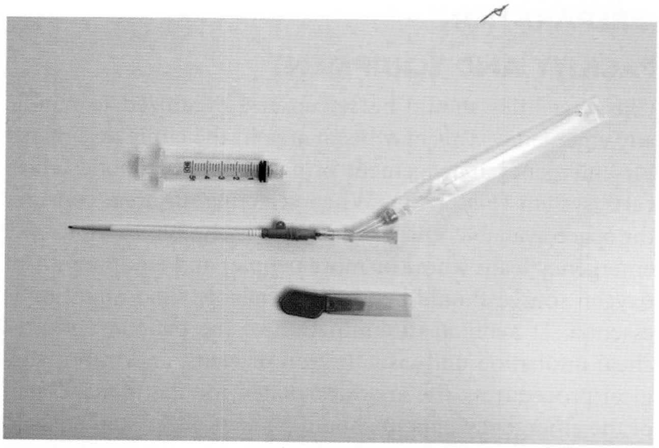

FIGURE 17-5 All-in-one catheters that include the dilation and guide wire insertion with one insertion are called Emergency Infusion Devices (Teleflex Medical), useful in large patients requiring immediate vascular access.

with tough epidermal surfaces. Saline flush, suture material, T-ports, and catheter caps should be included in the venous access drawer, or located within arm's reach, for placement expediency.

Through-the-needle central venous catheters are also useful in establishing emergency venous access. Through-the-needle long catheters are passed through the needle and are typically longer than over-the-needle catheters (8- to 12-inch) and are available in various diameters (Intracath, Becton Dickinson, Franklin Lakes, NJ; Lumed, Santa Ana, CA; Venocath, Abbott Laboratories, Abbot Park, IL). Primarily used in the jugular vein, placement is typically quick and uncomplicated. A plastic sleeve around the catheter prevents contamination during placement. The needle stays with the catheter but is protected by a plastic guard to avoid poking the animal or shearing the catheter itself. Through-the-needle catheters can be placed in a peripheral vessel (canine lateral saphenous or the feline medial saphenous) when the jugular vein is not a feasible option, such as in coagulopathies or severe bite wounds to the ventral cervical region.

Peritoneal catheters should also be readily available to the emergency clinician for diagnostic peritoneal lavage, or for peritoneal dialysis for the acute renal failure patient. Preferred brands include Imperosol (Abbot) or Curl Cath Peritoneal Catheters (Quinton Covidien), both of which have pre-peritoneal cuffs to prevent migration. Box 17-2 contains a summary of emergency vascular access equipment.

Drawer Three: Emergency Drugs. This drawer contains the emergency drugs (Box 17-3). Note that it is important not only to have a dosage chart listed somewhere within or around the crash cart, but also for the technician to ensure that the mg/ml correlate with the particular company brand carried in the hospital (Fig. 17-6). Expiration dates should be checked with frequency. Various size syringes and needles, and saline flush, should be located in the drug drawer in order to not delay delivery. Most emergency drugs are delivered intravenously, although in the absence of venous access, many drugs can be delivered in the intratracheal (IT), intraosseous (IO), or intracardiac (IC) route. The intracardiac route is considered the last resort in cerebral cardiopulmonary resuscitation.

Drawer Four: Emergency Respiratory Equipment. Typically, this drawer is stocked with equipment to help stabilize the patient in respiratory distress (Fig. 17-7). Materials include the Shiley tracheotomy tube, which has both an inner and an outer cannula for easier cleaning. Ensure that tracheotomy tubes have cuffs, necessary for positive pressure ventilation. Other equipment includes a thoracocentesis kit, contained in a box or bin for easy use. Materials in this kit include butterfly

BOX 17-2 Vascular Access Items

- Peripheral IV catheters: 14-24 gauge; 2- and 4-inch
- Angiocatheters, 8- and 12-inch
- Guide-wire central IV catheters: 12-inch and Seldinger, 30 cm and 55 cm, single and double lumen
- Emergency Infusion Devices
- Peritoneal catheters
- T-ports, PRN caps, suture material, saline flush

BOX 17-3 Emergency Drugs

- Epinephrine 1:1000
- Calcium gluconate
- Verapamil
- Glucagon
- Naloxone
- Dexamethasone sp
- Oxytocin
- Doxapram
- Atropine
- Dobutamine
- Dopamine
- Furosemide
- Vasopressin
- Lidocaine 2%
- Protamine sulfate
- Solu-Delta-Cortef 100 mg
- Nitroglycerine ointment
- Diphenhydramine
- Propranolol
- Potassium phosphate
- Bretylium
- Aminophylline
- Procainamide
- Ephedrine
- Sodium bicarbonate
- 50% dextrose
- Solu-Delta-Cortef 500 mg
- Isoproterenol
- Glycopyrrolate
- Solu-Medrol 500 mg
- Yohimbine
- Norepinephrine (Levophed)

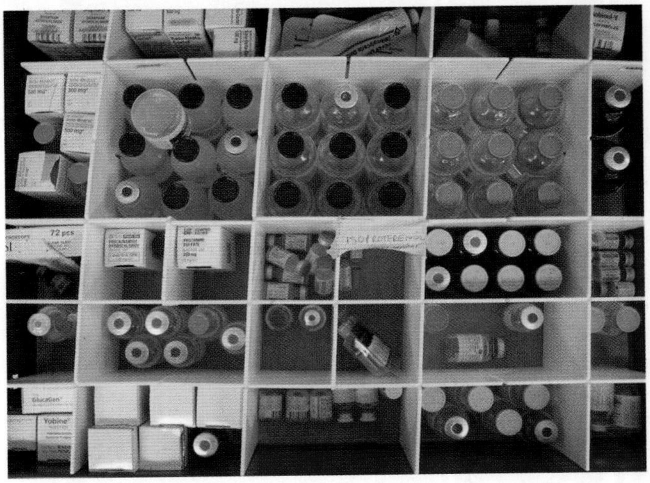

FIGURE 17-6 Emergency drugs should be well organized and separated by compartments. A dosage chart should be nearby for accurate administration.

catheters, three-way stopcocks, and 1.5-inch needles that allow easy penetration into the thoracic cavity.

Chest tubes should also be included in drawer four. Preferred tubes are those with metal trocar for ease of placement, such as the Argyle chest tube. Adapters such as "four-in-one" or Christmas tree connectors should be made available, as well as three-way stopcocks, metal wire to anchor connections, and heavy suture material. C-clamps should also be used to prevent air leakage. Custom-made connectors with three-way stopcocks can also be purchased from Global Vet Products, Inc. Box 17-4 contains a summary of supplies needed for emergency respiratory support.

Drawer Five: Intravenous Fluids. Fluids are kept in the last drawer of the crash cart, typically because of their weight. It is important to keep a combination of both crystalloid and colloid fluid types (Fig. 17-8), as well as both pediatric and adult fluid administration sets. Note that fluid types such as D5W should not be placed in a crash cart, in case of accidental administration. Pressure infusor bags should be kept with the fluids, for rapid fluid administration (Vital Signs, Inc., Totowa, NJ). Such devices are also handy with bleeding appendages. The bag can be placed proximal to or over the site of a large bleeding wound, and then inflated to a sufficient pressure to control active hemorrhage. In small animals, this can be used as an abdominal wrap if abdominal bleeding is suspected. Y-ports should also be used with any multiple fluid administrations. Pump sets, lactated Ringer's solution (LRS) 2 L, Normosol-R 1 L, 0.9% saline 1 L, 0.45% saline/2.5% dextrose 1 L (1), 0.9% saline 250 ml, 6% Hetastarch 500 ml (2), hypertonic saline, and Y-ports should be available.

Miscellaneous Emergency Equipment

Other emergency equipment in or around the crash cart includes suction catheters and suction tubing, large and small reservoir bags, stomach tubes and hand-held pumps, and emergency surgical packs. A blood pressure machine, ECG/defibrillator (Fig. 17-9), patient monitor (Fig. 17-10), a ventilator, warming devices, and intravenous fluid pumps should be in close proximity to the crash cart. Other useful equipment includes a continuous rectal thermometer, easy access laboratory analyzers such as a lactate monitor, coagulation analyzer, blood glucose monitor, and a blood gas machine.

Defibrillators and Monitors. A number of different types of defibrillators are available for clinic use. These vary

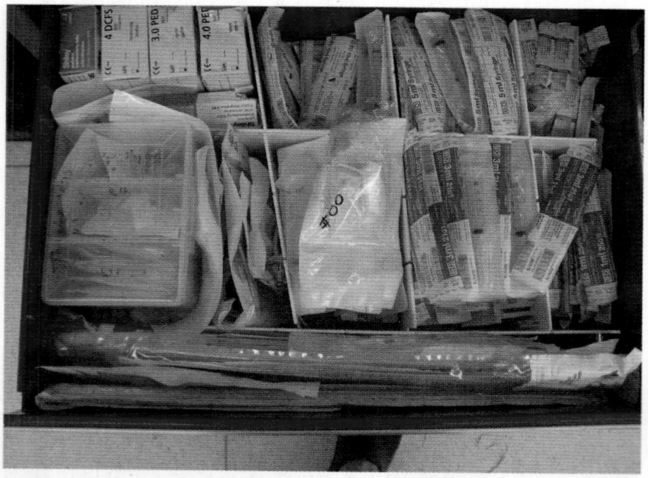

FIGURE 17-7 Respiratory equipment should be logically organized, as time is crucial for the hypoxic patient.

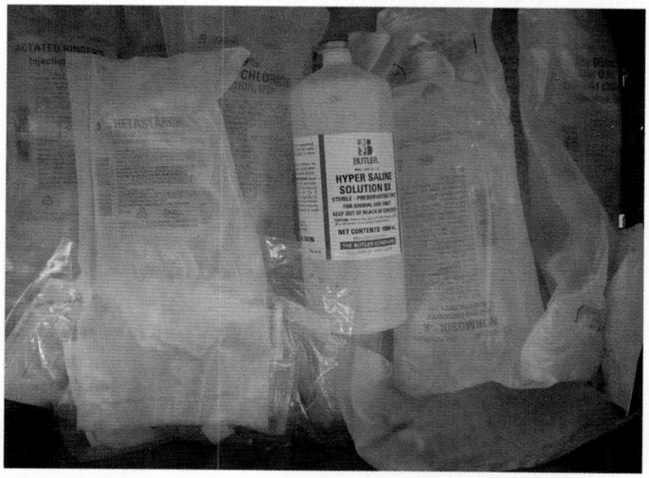

FIGURE 17-8 Intravenous fluids are kept in the last drawer of the crash cart, typically because of their weight. Both crystalloid and colloid solutions are necessary items in the patient with poor perfusion.

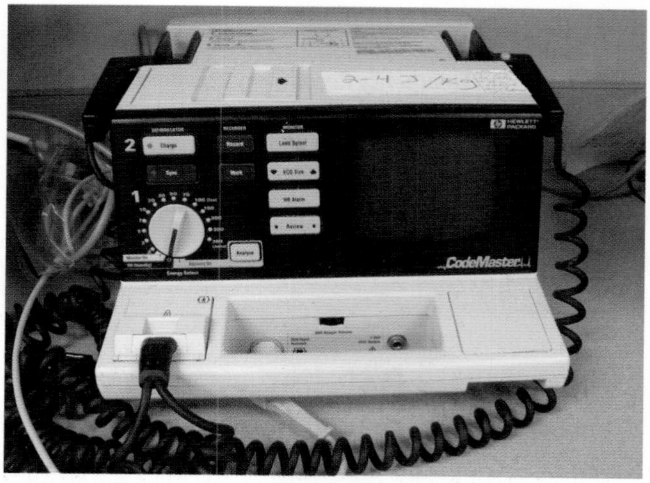

FIGURE 17-9 A lightweight, portable, semi-automated external defibrillator with ECG capability is critical in cardiopulmonary cerebral resuscitation codes.

BOX 17-4 Emergency Respiratory Equipment

- Tracheotomy tubes—Shiley, 4FR-8FR
- Umbilical tape
- Chest tubes (Argyle)
- C-clamps
- Chest tube connectors with three-way attachment
- Thoracocentesis kit to include extension sets, 3-way stopcocks, butterfly catheters (19G, 21G, 23G)
- Syringes, 12-ml, 30-ml, 60-ml

in features with some having multiple modes of operation. Heartstart Defibrillators (Phillips Medical, Andover, MA) are lightweight, portable, semi-automated external defibrillators. Some models also feature analysis of the patient's ECG and advice you whether or not to deliver a shock. Voice prompts guide you through the defibrillation process by providing instructions and patient information. Voice prompts are reinforced by messages that appear on the display.

Patient monitors are a valuable equipment item in an ICU or surgical suite. Most are designed to monitor cardiac and respiratory functions. Some can also monitor continuous ECG with advanced arrhythmia detection, continuous cardiac output waveforms (CVP), continuous direct blood pressure monitoring, continuous pulse oximetry and respiratory rate analysis, and continuous end-tidal CO_2 monitoring. The monitor displays the data on a colored LCD display. Parameters can usually be set for each monitoring component; alarms can notify nursing personnel of patient deterioration, with a function to automatically record a printed strip for clinician analysis. Many are also battery operated, allowing for continuous operation of the monitor even when moving patients between surgery and ICU suites.

Ventilators. The Newport Breeze (Newport Medical Instruments, Inc., Costa Mesa, CA) is a general-purpose ventilator, which can be used for respiratory support of pediatric or adult animals (Fig. 17-11). The ventilator is provided with an air/oxygen mixer to control the F_iO_2 (fraction of inspired oxygen). Controls are provided for the operator to select the function of the ventilator, a transducer monitors peak, mean and baseline pressures, and alarm systems are built-in to alert the clinician to violations of preset limits.

The Breeze can be classified as an electronically controlled, pneumatically powered ventilator with intermittent spontaneous flow (ISF). It can function as a volume controlled, time cycled, constant flow, or a pressure controlled, time cycled, constant flow ventilator. The Breeze operates in seven basic modes. Specifications include tidal volume, trigger level or sensitivity, alarm levels and silencers, indicators for inspiratory effort and apnea, and I:E ratio displays. Gas requirements are oxygen and air (35-70 psi). Accessories include the exhalation valve, reservoir bag cap, and the optional accessory of a heated humidifier.

Bair Hugger Warming Units. The Bair Hugger Total Temperature Management System (Teleflex Medical) (Fig. 17-12) was developed by an anesthesiologist to prevent and/or treat the common but significant problem of hypothermia. The warming unit draws ambient air through a filter and warms the air to the specified temperature. It then delivers the warmed air through a hose to the Bair Hugger blanket, which is placed over the patient. When used properly, the blanket distributes warm air around the patient's body, creating a warm environment. The unit can be mounted on an IV pole or hung on the cage door. Blankets are disposable, but can be reused on several patients before being discarded.

Teleflex Medical also makes a fluid warming set, which allows the Bair Hugger system to warm blood and intravenous

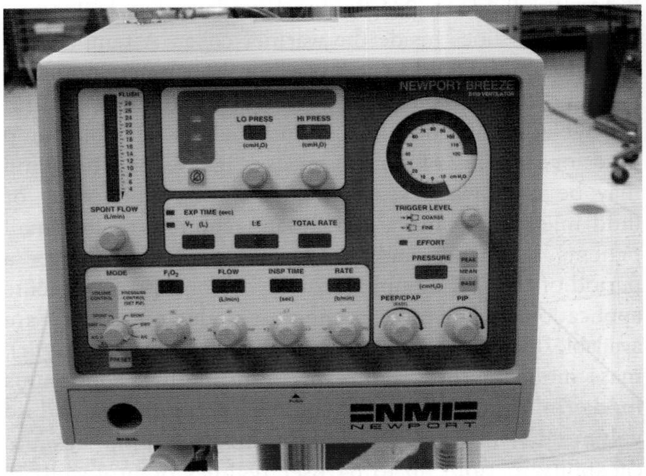

FIGURE 17-11 A general-purpose ventilator can be used for respiratory support of pediatric or adult animals.

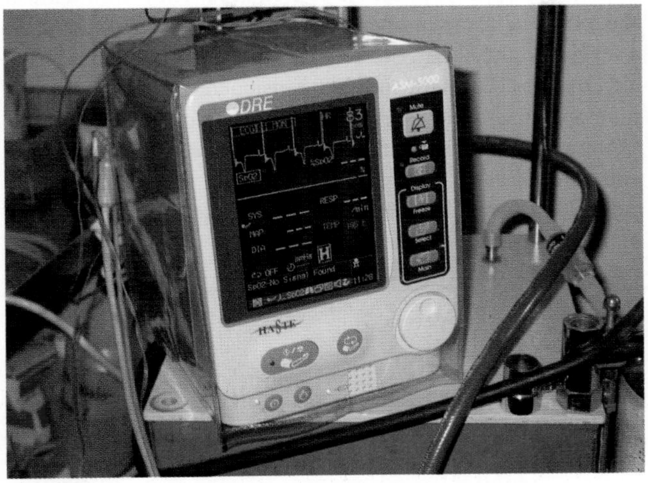

FIGURE 17-10 Patient monitoring systems are useful monitoring devices in any critical or surgical patient.

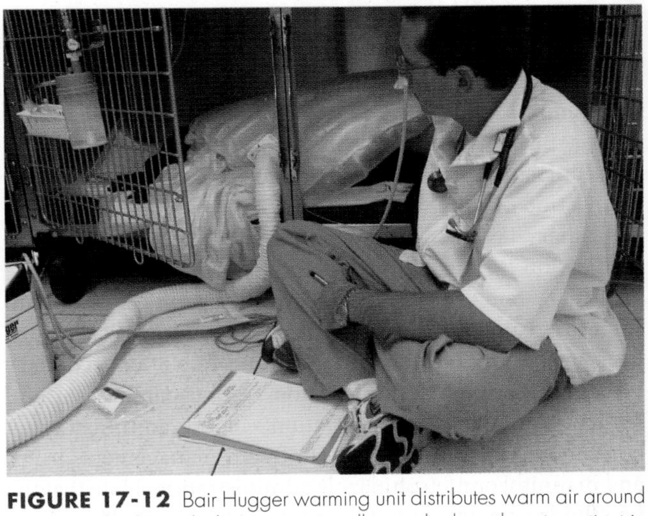

FIGURE 17-12 Bair Hugger warming unit distributes warm air around a patient's body; such devices are excellent in the hypothermic patient in shock or recovering from a surgical procedure.

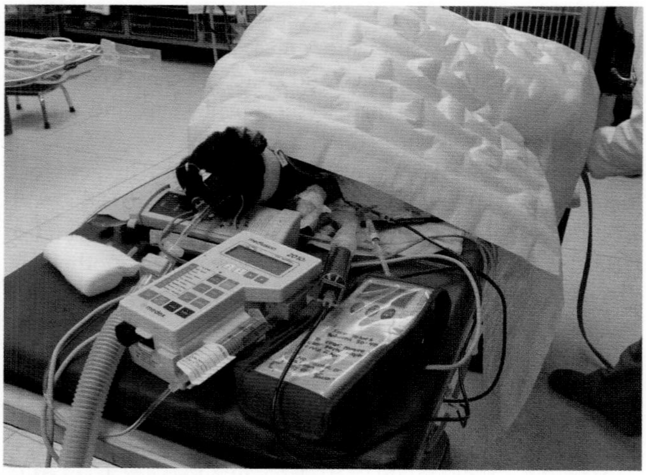

FIGURE 17-13 Syringe pumps may be used whenever meticulous low-volume drug or fluid injections using a syringe are required, or for small patients requiring small fluid volumes delivered over a period of time.

fluids. The fluid set (241 fluid set) is a latex-free coiled system, which slides inside the warmer collar. A temperature indicator on the fluid set will monitor fluid temperature.

Medfusion 2010i Syringe Pump. The Medfusion 2010i Syringe Pump (Medex, Inc., Duluth, GA) is a flexible pump used for a variety of clinical needs (Fig. 17-13). The pump may be used whenever meticulous low-volume drug or fluid injections using a syringe are required, or for small patients requiring small fluid volumes delivered over a period of time. The pumps may be customized for specific applications. Choices of numerous modes of delivery are available, including body weight mode (μg/kg/min, μg/kg/hr), mass mode (μg/min, μg/hr, mg/min, mg/hr), continuous mode (ml/min, ml/hr), and volume over time mode (dose volume/delivery time). In addition, the pump has the capability to store up to 64 user regimes or protocols. A bolus may be programmed then changed or administered at any time before or during drug delivery. Syringe sizes used on the Medfusion range from a 30-ml syringe to a 60-ml syringe.

IV Fluid Pump. The Abbot Plum XLD IV Pump is a device for infusion of both medications/drugs and intravenous fluids (see Fig. 17-14). The pump contains both a primary and a secondary function which enables the clinician to sterilely administer a smaller, secondary medication or fluid type that will be infused into the tubing or primary IV line. The unit will deliver the second fluid or medication through either a syringe or added fluid bag. The secondary rate of infusion is set in ml/hr, with a volume to be infused preprogrammed, which will automatically turn back to the original (or primary) fluid rate after secondary medication or fluid administration. Such capability is useful for chemotherapy administration, blood administration, continuous rate infusion (CRI) of pain management drugs, and mannitol or metronidazole administration. Note that the two fluids or medications cannot be infused simultaneously. A special pump set is required for the Abbot Plum Pump.

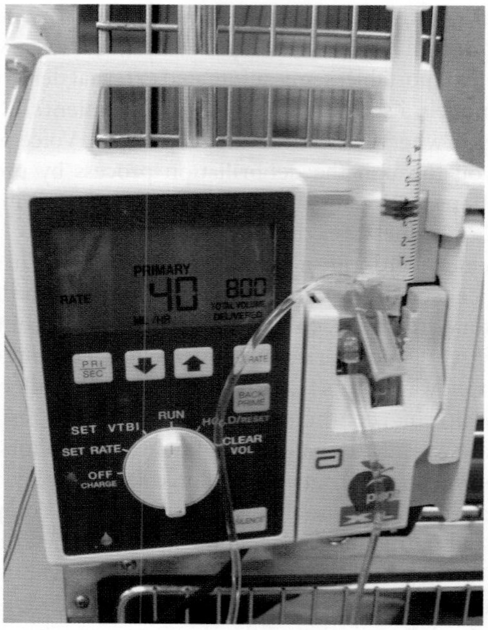

FIGURE 17-14 Many intravenous pumps are now available that contain both a primary and a secondary function enabling administration of medication sterilely infused into the tubing or primary IV line.

STAFF

The emergency team should be composed of at least three people, including veterinarian(s), veterinary technician(s), and other clinic support staff. The team should be prepared to work together. To this end, it is helpful to hold emergency drill sessions so that people can become familiar with specific tasks and procedures. This is also the time to review and update treatment protocols. Treatment protocols or guidelines help maximize efficiency. Protocols should be developed for common problems, but with flexibility to allow modification for specific clinical situations.

CLIENT

Pet owners should be made aware of primary and backup emergency services available in their area. They should know the location, hours of operation, and telephone numbers. As a service to the client, the veterinary staff can hold basic first aid courses. The client should be instructed in recognition of illness/injury, basic care of wounds, foreign bodies, toxins, trauma, and the safe transport of an injured patient. The client should be taught how to put together and use a pet first aid kit. Prehospital care can often influence the final outcome of an emergency.

HOSPITAL CARE

TRIAGE

Triage is the prioritization of treatment based on medical need. On initial presentation to the hospital, the veterinary technician may be the first to receive the patient. It is his or her responsibility to triage the patient(s). While approaching the patient, visually assess ventilation effort, pattern, and any audible airway sounds; the presence of blood, vomitus, or other foreign material about the patient; and the patient's posture and level of consciousness (LOC).

TECHNICIAN NOTE The key to successful triage is organization, teamwork, and remembering to REEVALUATE, REEVALUATE, REEVALUATE. Note that any patient can decompensate despite initial stability.

INITIAL EVALUATION

The initial management of the emergency patient requires immediate assessment and therapy. Therapy often begins before "obtaining" or "making" a diagnosis. Following the initial assessment and resuscitation (primary survey), the secondary survey and plans for definitive management are accomplished.

PRIMARY SURVEY AND RESUSCITATION

The primary survey is an initial brief assessment of the patient (the ABCDEs): A for airway, B for breathing, C for circulation, D for dysfunction or disability of the central nervous system, and E for whole-body examination. When a life-threatening problem is identified during the primary survey, resuscitative action should be instituted immediately.

AIRWAY/BREATHING

First, airway and adequacy of ventilation should be assessed by visualization, palpation, and auscultation. Life-threatening airway/breathing problems may be caused by apnea, airway obstruction, open chest wounds, severe pneumothorax, or hemothorax. Clinical signs associated with inadequate ventilation vary depending on severity of respiratory compromise. They include stridor, intercostal retraction, decreased breath sounds, restlessness and/or anxiety, minimal or absent chest wall motion, cyanosis (late sign), absence of air exchange from the nose or mouth, abnormal body stance (orthopnea), and labored use of accessory muscles of respiration. (Refer to Chapter 22 for physical examination techniques.) Normally the patient should have a free, easy, and regular ventilatory pattern. The patient should not be exerting an extraordinary amount of effort. The mucous membrane color should be pink; cyanotic or blue mucous membranes indicate hypoxemia, which is a decrease in blood oxygen content. Cyanosis is an unreliable indicator of hypoxia; it is always a late sign and does not occur in severe anemia. The chest wall should be palpated for integrity and wounds. Normal lungs should sound clear over a large area of the lung fields. Suspect large airway obstruction (e.g., foreign body, laryngeal paralysis) in patients with loud sonorous or squeaking sounds on inspiration or expiration or if the chest wall retracts severely during inspiration. Suspect a lower airway obstruction (e.g., asthma) if you hear wheezes or if the patient exhibits a prolonged expiration. Pleural filling defects (pneumothorax, pleural effusion, diaphragmatic hernia) should be considered if the breath and heart sounds are diminished or absent. Crackles suggest fluid-filled airways (pulmonary edema, pneumonia, tracheobronchial fluid, pulmonary contusions) and can be auscultated on either inspiration or expiration. (Refer to Chapter 22 for common abnormal lung sounds.) Any abnormal lung sounds with an increased respiratory effort warrants oxygen delivery in the least stressful route. The patient should be placed in sternal recumbency to facilitate lung expansion.

BOX 17-5 Clinical Signs of Poor Perfusion

- Altered mental state
- Abnormal temperature
- Abnormal heart rate
- Tachypnea, irregular breathing pattern
- Pale gray or brick red mucous membranes
- Prolonged capillary refill time
- Urine production <1 ml/kg/hr
- Weak or irregular pulses
- Cool extremities

If an upper airway obstruction is suspected, the mouth and pharynx should be examined for easily removable foreign bodies. If the patient will not permit the examination, or the foreign body cannot be removed, preoxygenation and rapid safe anesthetic induction may be indicated. If the obstruction cannot be removed, the patient should be intubated (oral or tracheostomy) in an attempt to bypass the obstruction. If the patient is apneic, mechanical or manual ventilation will be required. Initial ventilatory requirements are as follows:

- Rate: 10 to 15 breaths per minute
- Inspiratory time: approximately 1 second
- Proximal airway pressure: 15 to 20 cmH_2O, or a tidal volume of 10 to 20 ml/kg
- End-Tidal CO_2: 25 to 35 mm Hg

If the patient has an open chest wound, it can be temporarily closed manually or by placing a generous globule of ointment and a sterile dressing over the wound. Thoracocentesis or thoracostomy tube placement should be quickly performed to relieve respiratory distress resulting from pleural filling defects.

CIRCULATION

Circulation is assessed by visualization, palpation, and auscultation. The signs of inadequate perfusion include abnormal level of consciousness (LOC), increased heart rate (an effort to increase cardiac output), abnormal pulse quality (bounding pulses indicates early compensatory shock, followed by poor pulse pressure or stroke volume), pale mucous membranes, prolonged capillary refill time, and decreased appendage temperature (indicators of poor peripheral perfusion) (Box 17-5). Inadequate perfusion may be caused by hypovolemia as a result of external or concealed blood loss (loss into body cavity or limb). It may also be caused by pump failure (e.g., intrinsic heart failure, arrhythmias, cardiac tamponade), toxicity, anesthesia overdose, severe hypo/hyperthermia, or severe electrolyte abnormalities. Quick laboratory testing such as blood lactate levels can help determine perfusion status.

DYSFUNCTION/DISABILITY

Dysfunction/disability of the nervous system is assessed via visualization and palpation. The patient's LOC, pupillary light reflex, menace reflex response, posture, and response to pain (superficial and/or deep) are particularly important.

The terms normal, obtunded, stupor, and comatose are used to characterize the LOC but are not specific for a particular type of neural lesion. Pupils are normally equal in size and respond quickly to light. Pupillary constriction, dilation, or anisocoria with a diminished pupillary light reflex, in the absence of ocular trauma, is indicative of neurological involvement. Hyperesthesia (patients exhibit abnormal, exaggerated responses to touch or sound) may also indicate a nervous system abnormality.

Abnormal postures such as decerebrate, decerebellate rigidity, and Schiff-Sherrington should be noted. Decerebrate and decerebellate rigidity are characterized by extensor rigidity in the front limbs and opisthotonos. The rear limbs are in extensor rigidity in the decerebrate posture and flexed or extended in decerebellate. The decerebrate patient is unconscious, whereas the decerebellate patient exhibits varying levels of obtundation. Decerebellate rigidity progressing to decerebrate rigidity suggests an extension of the damage to the brain stem. The Schiff-Sherrington posture is extensor rigidity of the forelimbs with flaccid hind limbs (Fig. 17-15). This posture indicates a lesion at T2-L4. It is also a poor prognostic sign when a patient does not perceive pain. Pricking or pinching the skin will test superficial pain. Applying a strong noxious stimulus to the toes or a joint will test deep pain. The patient should show some visible response indicating conscious recognition of the stimulus, such as vocalizing, turning and looking, or turning and biting. This is important because the withdrawal of the appendage alone is a spinal reflex and does not warrant against a more proximal spinal cord lesion.

FIGURE 17-15 The Schiff-Sherrington posture is extensor rigidity of the forelimbs with flaccid hind limbs.

> **TECHNICIAN NOTE** Pinch toes with hemostats to assess deep pain. The patient should vocalize or respond by turning and looking. Important: Withdrawal of the limb is considered a reflex and does not necessarily indicate deep pain!

Nonambulatory traumatized patients should be treated as spinal or head trauma patients until proven otherwise (e.g., avoid spinal flexion or twisting, use a board for patient transfer, use tape, use drugs only if necessary to keep patient calm, get a lateral spinal radiograph only after stabilization, and avoid jugular compression). Swab each ear canal and nasal cavity with a cotton-tipped applicator to detect the presence of bleeding, which could indicate head trauma.

EXAMINATION

During this final phase of the primary survey, a rapid whole-body examination is performed. Major lacerations may be uncovered and areas of bruising noted. Areas of bruising that appear to be worsening may be indicative of active bleeding. Abdominal girth should also be measured if intra-abdominal bleeding is suspected, as well as serial monitoring of the packed cell volume and total protein. Any signs of abnormal breathing or poor perfusion should warrant oxygenation in the least stressful route.

> **TECHNICIAN NOTE** If abdominal bleeding is suspected, a snug "belly bandage" should be applied to limit ongoing hemorrhage. Ensure that the bandage does not compromise respiration.

SECONDARY SURVEY

The secondary survey is the timely, systematic, and directed evaluation of each body system for injury or other signs of illness, after initial stabilization. The ABCDEs are quickly reevaluated to ensure that no new problems have developed. A thorough head-to-tail physical examination and history are completed. Finally, a comprehensive plan of diagnostics and monitoring is developed.

DEFINITIVE MANAGEMENT

A review is made of the initial ancillary diagnostics that were performed (e.g., radiographs, ECG, lab data), and a management plan is developed. The plan may result in emergency surgery or temporary stabilization of fractures and continued monitoring.

EMERGENCIES

CARDIOVASCULAR EMERGENCIES

Cardiac Arrest

Cardiopulmonary arrest (CPA) is the cessation of functional ventilation and effective circulation. Sudden gasps may occur, but this action does not produce effective ventilation or mean that the patient is breathing. Similarly, cardiac

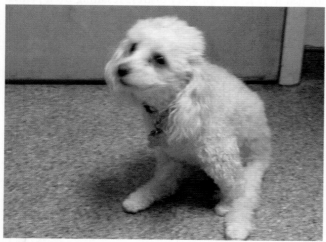

electrical or muscle activity may persist, but effective tissue perfusion does not occur. Clinical signs of CPA include absence of auscultable heartbeat, lack of palpable pulse, apnea or agonal gasping, absence of bleeding, loss of consciousness, and pupillary dilation.

When an arrest occurs, the veterinary team must respond with urgency, but not with panic. Successful CPR is dependent on several factors, the most important factor being the true cause of the arrest. Patients who were healthy before and whose arrest was initiated by pharmacologic causes or problems easily identified (e.g., kinked endotracheal tube, improper anesthetic depth, or allergic reactions) have the best chance of survival. Conversely, patients who experience an arrest as a result of disease or traumatic injury, yet are successfully resuscitated, are still considered extremely critical and unstable. The likelihood of rearrest is typically 65% to 68% for dogs and 22% to 38% for cats, and usually occurs within 4 hours of the initial arrest. Outcomes following CPA in human medicine were significantly improved with the institution of evidence-based guidelines for resuscitation along with mandatory comprehensive training of healthcare personnel. The veterinary industry undertook a campaign, referred to as the Reassessment Campaign on Veterinary Resuscitation (RECOVER), to develop similar guidelines. The guidelines were published in 2012 as a series of articles in a special issue of the *Journal of Veterinary Emergency and Critical Care.* Five domains were identified and a total of 101 clinical guidelines were developed as part of the RECOVER initiative. A summary of some of the guidelines is in Table 17-1. Each of the guidelines was assigned a class and level based on risk-benefit analysis and the quantity and quality of research that is available to support the specific guideline. Class I refers to those specific guidelines in which the benefit greatly outweighs the risk, and the intervention should be performed. A Level A guideline is one that is supported by a large number of studies performed in multiple populations. The RECOVER initiative also developed specific practice tools, such as a chart of recommended emergency drug dosages and an algorithm for use while performing CPR. Review the additional detailed information regarding the RECOVER initiative and guidelines on the website of the Veterinary Emergency and Critical Care Society at www.veccs.org.

Patients that regain spontaneous heart rhythm need to have continuous care in order to support normal organ function. Initial efforts should be directed at supporting normal body physiology to protect the cerebral tissue, identifying and correcting any electrolyte and acid-base disturbances, and initiating aggressive pulmonary support. The underlying cause of the arrest should be quickly identified and the primary disease treated accordingly. Managing the post-arrest patient is labor intensive and is dependent on clinical and technical aptitude.

Hypovolemic Shock

Hypovolemic shock can be a sequela to a variety of problems such as protracted vomiting/diarrhea, trauma, sepsis, or gastric dilatation volvulus caused by a decreased intravascular volume. As a result of the decreased intravascular volume, venous return to the heart is decreased, which results in decreased ventricular filling (preload). This causes a decreased stroke volume (amount of blood ejected by the ventricle with each contraction) and cardiac output (product of stroke volume and heart rate; the volume of blood ejected by the heart per unit of time). The end result is inadequate tissue perfusion and oxygenation. Peripheral vasoconstriction, in an attempt to maintain arterial blood pressure, further compromises peripheral tissue perfusion.

Fluid therapy must be initiated to improve tissue perfusion and return cardiovascular parameters to normal. Intravenous (IV) catheter(s) are placed; preferably first a short, large-bore cephalic catheter for rapid fluid resuscitation, followed by the placement of a jugular catheter to measure central venous pressure, beneficial in guiding fluid resuscitation. If difficulty is encountered in placing the catheter percutaneously, consider performing a cut-down (Procedure 17-1) or placing an intraosseous catheter (see Procedure 16-1). Absorption of fluids via the bone marrow is rapid. In addition to fluids, some drugs may also be administered via this route.

> **TECHNICIAN NOTE** First, place a large-bore cephalic catheter in patients with hypovolemic shock for rapid fluid administration, followed by a central line for CVP monitoring only after the patient is more stable.

Fluid resuscitation is the cornerstone of shock therapy. Fluid options for fluid resuscitation include isotonic, polyionic crystalloids (solutions with electrolyte concentrations similar to plasma [lactated Ringer's, Normasol R, Plasmalyte 148, Normal Saline]), and colloids (plasma, Dextran 70 [6% Gentran: Baxter], Hetastarch [6% Hetastarch: Abbott, Oxyglobin, Hemopure], and whole blood). Initially, crystalloids are used in the treatment of shock. The shock dose of crystalloids is 80 to 90 ml/kg and 50 to 55 ml/kg in the dog and cat, respectively (equivalent to one blood volume). It may be necessary to administer 0.5 to 1.5 times the blood volume to resuscitate the patient. In about 30 minutes, 75% to 80% of the crystalloids shift from the intravascular space into the interstitial space. Colloids are better blood volume expanders, producing nearly twice the plasma volume as crystalloids. By definition, colloids are large-molecular-weight substances that are restricted to the intravascular space. Colloids are generally useful in resuscitation from shock and when albumin in plasma is less than 2.0 g/dl. Examples include septic shock or massive extravasation of fluid through leaky, vasodilated capillaries. Use of colloid solutions help prevent peripheral constriction by retaining intravascular volume and can prevent pulmonary edema. Colloid therapy can also be used to increase albumin levels and can correct oncotic pressure. Note that colloid administration volumes are much smaller than crystalloid volumes in resuscitation scenarios. In addition, cats are much more susceptible to fluid overload from colloid use; subsequently, administration rates are much less.

TABLE 17-1 Overview of the RECOVER Guidelines

DOMAIN/ISSUE	SUMMARY OF GUIDELINE/TOPIC ADDRESSED
Preparedness and Prevention	
Equipment and Training	• Use of a standardized crash cart and/or pre-stocked CPA station • Comprehensive staff training, including simulations and assessment • Cognitive aids available for use during CPR (worksheets, checklists, algorithms, dosage charts)
Education and Leadership	• Refresher training every 6 months • Leadership training • Debriefing after CPR
Basic Life Support (BLS)	
Recognition of CPA	• Do not delay CPR; begin on initial recognition of suspected CPA due to apnea or unresponsiveness

Chest Compressions (Figures 1 and 2)	• In dogs and cats, chest compressions should be done in lateral recumbency.
	• In dogs and cats, chest compression depth of between $\frac{1}{3}$ and $\frac{1}{2}$ the width of the chest is reasonable.
	• Chest compression rate of 100–120 compressions/min are recommended for both dogs and cats.
	• Allow full chest wall recoil between compressions and avoid leaning on the chest during recoil. Alternate with abdominal compressions.
	• Position of hands:
	  • In large and giant breed dogs, the hands should be placed over the widest portion of the chest.
	  • In keel-chested dogs, the hands should be placed directly over the heart.
	  • In barrel-chested dogs, sternal chest compressions in dorsal recumbency may be considered.
	  • In cats and small dogs, circumferential compressions rather than lateral compressions may be considered.

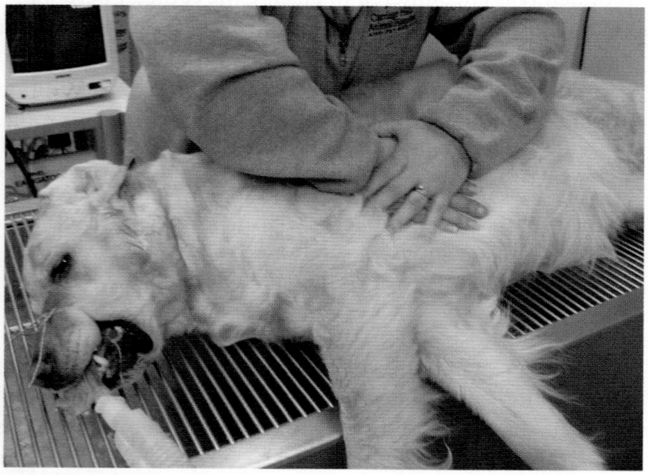

FIGURE 1 Chest compressions performed by bending elbows, placing palm-over-palm, and leaning into the patient.

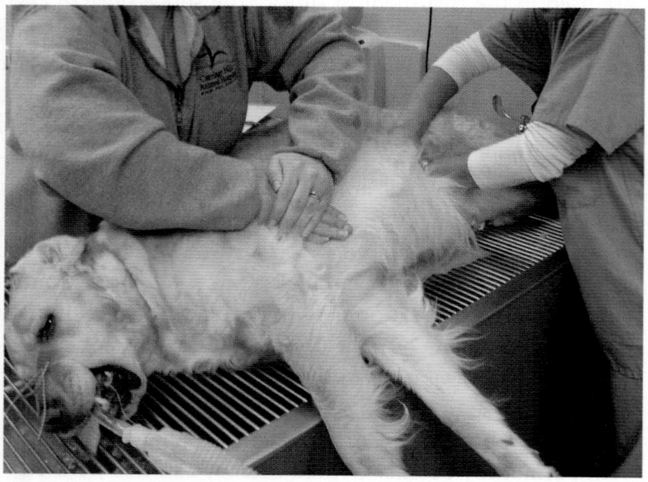

FIGURE 2 Counter compressions will improve venous return; rhythmically alternate abdominal compressions with chest compressions.

TABLE 17-1 Overview of the RECOVER Guidelines—cont'd

DOMAIN/ISSUE	SUMMARY OF GUIDELINE/TOPIC ADDRESSED
Ventilation	• Rate of 10 breaths per minute with a tidal volume of 10 ml/kg and an inspiratory time of 1 sec • In nonintubated dogs and cats or single-rescuer CPR, use a C:V ratio of 30:2 • Ventilation with 100% oxygen is preferred, room air is acceptable using an Ambu bag • In single-rescuer CPR, mouth-to-snout ventilation is recommended, with 2 breaths delivered after every 30 compressions • In intubated, multiple-rescuer CPR, use continuous chest compressions with simultaneous ventilation
CPR Cycles	• Perform CPR in 2-minute cycles without interruption • Rotation of team members performing chest compressions every 2 minutes to reduce potential for compromise of compression efficacy due to fatigue
Advanced Life Support (ALS)	
Emergency Drugs	The specific uses of epinephrine, atropine, vasopressin, and other medications are addressed
Defibrillation	• Use a biphasic defibrillator • Defibrillation dosing should start at 2-4 J/kg with a biphasic defibrillator • Administer a single shock rather than 3 stacked shocks with immediate resumption of CPR in the case of nonsuccessful defibrillation • In cases of VF, immediate defibrillation is recommended with energy increased if initial shock is not successful
Other Procedures (Figure 3)	Use of supplemental oxygen therapy, intratracheal administration of specific medications, open chest CPR, and IV fluid therapy are addressed

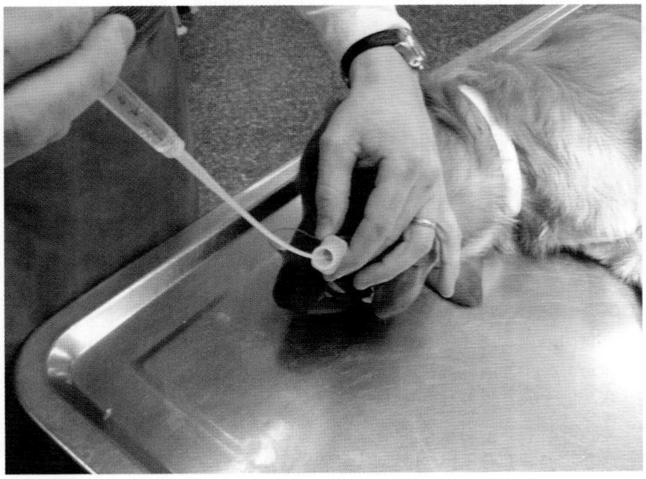

FIGURE 3 Intratracheal drug delivery during CPR.

DOMAIN/ISSUE	SUMMARY OF GUIDELINE/TOPIC ADDRESSED
Monitoring	
End-tidal CO_2	• In intubated and ventilated dogs and cats, the use of $EtCO_2$ is recommended in patients at risk of CPA • Use $EtCO_2$ monitoring during CPR as an early indicator of ROSC

Continued

TABLE 17-1 Overview of the RECOVER Guidelines—cont'd

DOMAIN/ISSUE	SUMMARY OF GUIDELINE/TOPIC ADDRESSED
Pulse Palpation (Figure 4) 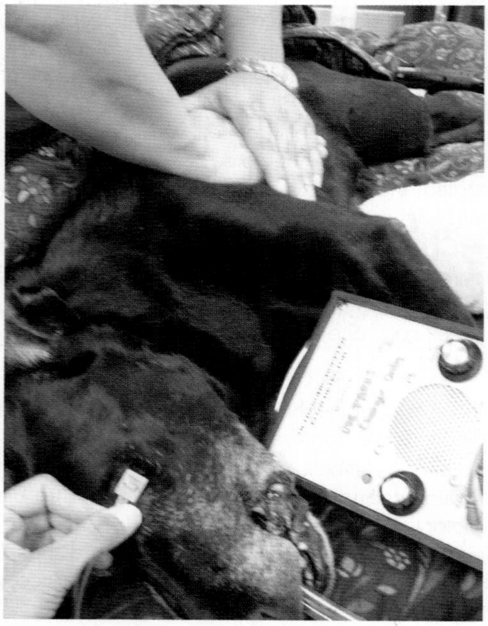 **FIGURE 4** Detection of a retinal pulse during CPR chest compressions.	• Do not interrupt chest compressions specifically to palpate the pulse or check the ECG • Palpation of the pulse for detection of ROSC during pauses in CPR cycles should not delay resumption of chest compressions
Doppler	In dogs and cats at risk of CPA, use continuous Doppler monitoring of peripheral arterial blood flow for early identification of CPA
ECG	• Evaluation of the ECG during intercycle pauses in CPR is recommended, but should not delay resumption of chest compressions • Use rapid assessment of the ECG to determine if VF has resolved immediately after defibrillation but ensure that the delay in resumption of chest compressions is minimal
Blood Gases and Electrolytes	Routine monitoring can be considered
Post-CPA Care	
Fluid Therapy	Not generally recommended unless hypovolemia is strongly suspected or confirmed
Oxygenation	• After ROSC, inspired oxygen should be titrated to maintain normoxia (PaO_2 = 80-100 mm Hg, SpO_2 = 94-98%) • Avoid hypoxemia and hyperoxemia
Medications	• Vasopressors and positive inotropic agents are acceptable • Administration of corticosteroids is not recommended • Administration of barbiturates as a seizure preventative measure is acceptable
Referral	Referral of the patient that has been successfully resuscitated to a 24-hour specialty care practice is recommended

CPA, cardiopulmonary arrest; ROSC, return of spontaneous circulation.

Colloids should be administered when crystalloids are not improving or maintaining blood volume, or if the patient has low total protein or albumin. Blood and/or plasma are given in sufficient quantities to maintain the packed cell volume above 25% and a total protein above 4.0 mg/dl. Colloids are dosed at 10 to 40 ml/kg and 5 to 20 ml/kg in the dog and cat, respectively.

> *TECHNICIAN NOTE* Avoid excessive crystalloid fluids in patients with a history of (or suspected) cardiac disease, pulmonary contusions, or head trauma.

Hypertonic saline (7.0% Sodium Chloride Injection USP: Sanofi Animal Health, Berlin, MD) has been recommended

PROCEDURE 17-1 Peripheral Venous Cut-Down

Indications

- Unable to visualize cephalic or lateral saphenous vein for accurate percutaneous placement
- Need to establish IV access with certainty on first attempt

Materials

- Clippers
- Peripheral catheter
- Surgical prep (Povidine or Nolvasan)
- 20-gauge or 18-gauge hypodermic needle
- 1-inch tape
- Triple antibiotic ointment
- T-port
- Catheter cap
- Saline flush

Method

- Surgical prep of catheter site as for routine percutaneous catheter placement
- Use edge of bevel of 20-gauge or 18-gauge hypodermic needle as "scalpel"
- Cut over vein across skin tension line; i.e., craniomedial to caudolateral direction at 15 to 30 degrees off horizontal
- Visualize vein and insert catheter
- Dissect vessel further as needed using needle as "mini-scalpel" with bevel directed parallel to vein
- Place triple antibiotic over cut-down site
- Tape in catheter as normal and place sterile dressing

Care

- Change bandage and disinfect site daily while catheter is in place
- When catheter is removed, cover with antibiotic ointment and sterile dressing and allow to heal by second intention
- Culture catheter tip if indicated

for use in shock therapy for cases in which it is difficult or contraindicated to administer large volumes of fluids rapidly enough to resuscitate the patient (e.g., head trauma victims). Hypertonic saline causes fluid shifts from the intracellular space to the extracellular (including intravascular) space, resulting in improved venous return and cardiac output. Hypertonic saline may have other beneficial cardiovascular effects as well. The recommended dose range is 4 to 6 ml/kg over 5 minutes. Crystalloids should be administered at 50% of the shock dose when synthetic colloids or hypertonic saline is used to avoid fluid overloading of the patient. Additional information on fluid therapy can be found in Chapter 16.

> **TECHNICIAN NOTE** Hypertonic saline is contraindicated in dehydrated patients.

Sympathomimetics, such as dopamine (Dopamine HCL Injection: Abbott) and dobutamine (Dobutrex: Eli Lilly) are indicated when the patient is unresponsive to vigorous fluid therapy and when blood pressure, vasomotor tone, and tissue perfusion have not returned to acceptable levels. These drugs support myocardial contractility and blood pressure with minimal vasoconstriction. Blood pressure monitoring is important for the knowledgeable administration of these drugs. The effects of dopamine are dose-dependent: 1 to 5 μg/kg/min for the dopaminergic effect (dilate renal, mesenteric, and coronary vascular beds). Cats, as opposed to people and dogs, do not appear to have renal dopaminergic receptors. Beta-1 activity (positive inotropic) is seen at a dose range of 5 to 10 μg/kg/min, and dosages greater than 10 μg/kg/min cause alpha-receptor stimulation (vasoconstriction). Dobutamine has primarily beta activity. It has minimal effect on heart rate and peripheral vascular resistance except at higher dosages. Dobutamine is the preferred drug for cardiogenic shock or myocardial depression secondary to sepsis. The dose range is 5 to 15 μg/kg/min. Sympathomimetics should not be used as a substitute for adequate volume restoration. Dopamine and dobutamine can also be used to increase glomerular filtration rate (GFR) if anuria or oliguria is present despite aggressive fluid therapy.

> **TECHNICIAN NOTE** If either dopamine or dobutamine is used as a constant rate infusion, blood pressure and heart rate should be monitored.

Congestive Heart Failure

Heart failure is the inability of the heart to supply adequate blood flow to meet the body's metabolic needs. **Congestive heart failure** occurs when increased pulmonary (left side) or systemic venous (right side) and capillary pressures increase, causing fluids to leak from the capillary beds resulting in edema (peripheral and pulmonary) or effusions (ascites, pleural, and pericardial). General protocol for patients with suspected heart disease includes oxygen, IV catheter placement, and judicious fluid therapy (in order to avoid overhydration).

Left-sided congestive heart failure (LCHF) manifests dyspnea, tachypnea, orthopnea, cough (cats rarely), the appearance of a pink frothy serosanguinous fluid at the nostrils, cyanosis, and weakness. Tachycardia, heart murmurs, and arrhythmias resulting from myocardial pathology may be noted. The clinical manifestations of right-sided congestive heart failure (RCHF) include jugular distention, pleural effusion, hepatomegaly, hepatojugular reflux (sustained pressure is applied to the abdomen with one or both hands, causing the jugular veins to be distended), ascites, and peripheral edema (Fig. 17-16).

> **TECHNICIAN NOTE** Dogs with heart failure are usually tachycardic; cats may be bradycardic and hypothermic.

Radiographs, echocardiography, and electrocardiography are useful aids in diagnosing heart failure. Radiographically, chamber enlargement, evidence of pulmonary edema, and pericardial and pleural effusions support the diagnosis of heart failure (Fig. 17-17). Echocardiography is useful in diagnosing valvular disease, chamber size, atrial and ventricular function, and the recognition of pulmonary vascular distention. Fluid in the pericardial sac is an excellent contrast medium for assessing cardiac structures during ultrasound. Electrocardiography changes in wave-form amplitude, axis deviation, rhythm, and electrical alternans can further support the diagnosis of heart failure, but their absence does not rule out heart failure.

Minimizing stress should be part of the therapeutic plan when treating heart failure patients, especially patients that are hemodynamically unstable. In some instances of patient excitement, sedation may be beneficial. Oxygen therapy improves oxygenation and decreases the work of breathing. Oxygen may be administered via mask, nasal catheter, or oxygen cage. The patient should not be stressed or excited by the oxygen administration technique.

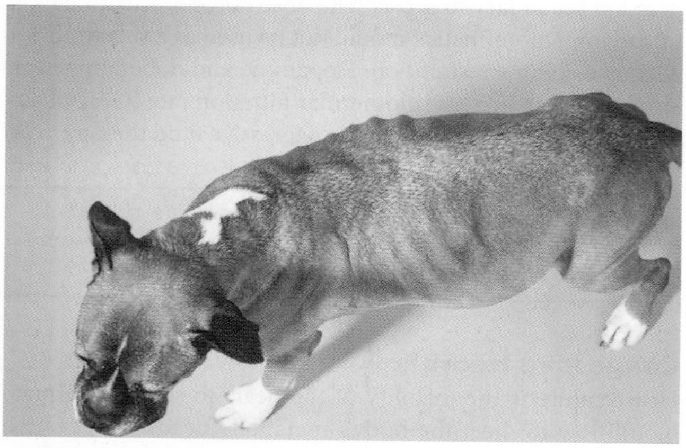

FIGURE 17-16 Ascites is a common clinical manifestation of right-sided congestive heart failure. (From Nelson RW: *Small animal internal medicine*, ed 4, St Louis, 2009, Mosby.)

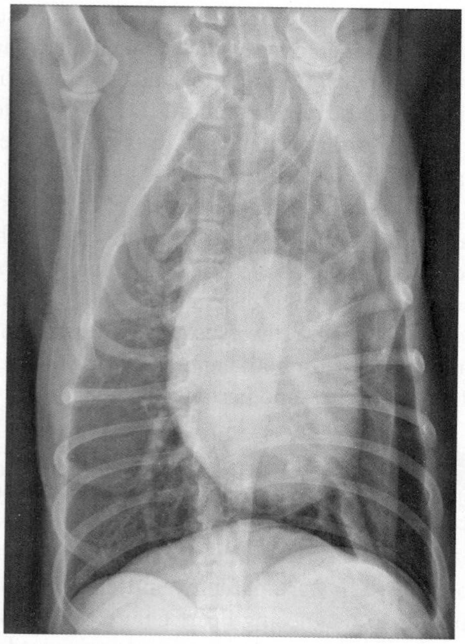

FIGURE 17-17 Cardiomegaly (enlarged heart) secondary to congestive heart failure; pulmonary edema is a typical sequela to cardiac insufficiency.

In the case of LCHF, the goal is to reduce preload (the end-diastolic ventricular volume) and/or afterload (the arterial blood pressure resistance against which the heart has to pump). Administration of vasodilators such as nitroglycerine (venodilator), and nitroprusside (venous and arteriolar dilator) reduce preload. Hydralazine (arteriolar dilator) is used to decrease afterload. ACE inhibitors (arterial and venous dilator) do not act quickly enough to be useful in the emergency treatment of heart failure patients. In addition to its ability to clear pulmonary edema, furosemide also reduces venous pressure or preload. Drugs such as dopamine, dobutamine, and amrinone can be used to increase contractility of the heart. Therapy in RCHF may be directed at removing pleural fluid (commonly in cats) and/or pericardial fluid and ascites (rare in cats). A thoracocentesis has both diagnostic and therapeutic value and is indicated when there is a significant thoracic fluid accumulation.

TECHNICIAN NOTE Ensure adequate blood pressure before administering nitroglycerin; wear gloves before application in the ear pinnae.

Abdominocentesis is indicated when fluid accumulation impairs ventilation or venous return, or causes patient discomfort (Fig. 17-18). Pericardiocentesis should be performed when pericardial effusion impairs cardiac output. If cardiac output is severely compromised in the face of pericardial effusion, shock doses of fluids should be administered. The fluids increase cardiac filling pressure.

Repeated physical examinations determine the effectiveness of therapy in the patient with heart disease (Box 17-6). Patients with respiratory distress secondary to heart failure often appear anxious and unwilling to sit or lie down. They will also be tachypneic and may have cyanotic mucous membranes. If therapy is effective, resolution of the respiratory distress will be evident as a decrease in respiratory rate and effort and an improvement in attitude and mucous membrane color.

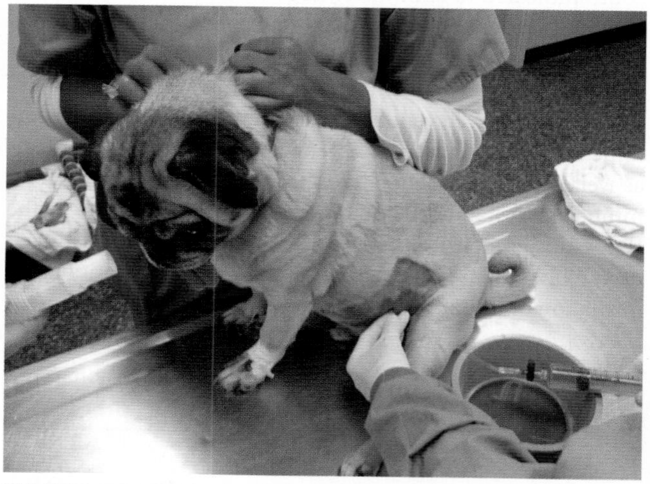

FIGURE 17-18 Abdominocentesis is indicated when fluid accumulation impairs ventilation, perfusion, or causes extreme patient discomfort.

The use of vasoactive drugs necessitates the monitoring of systemic blood pressure. The ECG is useful in monitoring heart rate and rhythm. The use of furosemide should result in increased urine production and a decrease in respiratory effort. Urine output should be documented and/or serial body weights obtained. Furosemide can alter acid-base and electrolytes; therefore, they should also be monitored. Excessive furosemide-induced dehydration can lead to prerenal azotemia, severe hypokalemia, and alkalosis. Packed cell volume/total solids, urine specific gravity, and blood urea nitrogen (BUN) or creatinine should be monitored. All patients receiving furosemide should have access to fresh water at all times, unless intake is restricted because of vomiting.

> **TECHNICIAN NOTE** If an ECG is not available, a Doppler can be used to monitor heart rhythm. Tape the probe on the ventral aspect of the dorsal plantar surface; monitor the heart rhythm by listening for any abnormal patterns.

Aortic Thromboembolism

Aortic thromboembolism occurs when an aggregation of platelets and fibrin with entrapped cells migrates and lodges at a distant site in the circulatory system. In feline aortic thromboembolism, the thrombus usually resides within the lumen of the left atrium or is attached to the endocardial surface of the left atrium. The embolus can break loose and occlude one or more branches of the aorta at the aortic trifurcation. This condition is referred to as a **saddle thrombus.**

Clinical signs associated with aortic thromboembolism vary with the location of the embolus. In the case of a saddle thrombus, pain, pallor, paresis, poikilothermy, and lack of pulses in one or both of the hind limbs may be observed. The muscles of the rear limb may be affected and are commonly swollen and turgid, particularly the gastrocnemius. Cats with aortic thromboembolism commonly have myocardial disease. Blockage of the aorta can cause hypertension and an increase in afterload to the left ventricle, resulting in increased left heart filling pressure and pulmonary edema. Consequently cats may present with dyspnea. Body temperature is also used as a prognostic indicator; severe hypothermia (<98° F) generally indicates a worse prognosis. Warming procedures should be implemented immediately.

BOX 17-6 Clinical Signs of Heart Disease

- Injected, pale, or cyanotic mucus membranes
- Dull lung sounds on auscultation
- Crackles, wheezes
- Labored breathing
- Tachycardia
- Poor pulse quality
- Pulse deficits
- Jugular venous distension
- Ascites

> **TECHNICIAN NOTE** Assess both femoral pulses simultaneously in cats to determine if there is some degree of flow obstruction as seen with saddle thrombus. Inspect the rear toe pads and look for an abnormal bluish color.

Diagnostic tests should be directed at determining the underlying cause that led to the thromboembolic event. This may include the standard minimum database (CBC, chemistry, and UA), cardiac workup (ECG, echocardiography, chest radiographs), and coagulation profile. Tests that might be considered specific and sensitive for thromboembolism include Doppler flow studies, ultrasound to visualize the thrombus, and angiography (selective and nonselective). Compare the toenail bed color of the rear paws with the front paws. The rear paws may be cyanotic (Fig. 17-19). In some cases, cutting the toenail of the affected limb to the quick may be helpful in diagnosing the problem (there is no bleeding). Cats with severely compromised blood flow will ooze black-colored blood from the cut nail.

Emergency therapy is directed at treating the underlying cause. In some instances the patient will present with heart failure, which will certainly need to be addressed. If fluid therapy is given, care should be exercised not to aggravate or produce heart failure. If pain is present, analgesia will be required. Analgesic options include butorphanol and oxymorphone. Thrombolytic and anticoagulant therapy may be considered to lyse the thrombus and prevent further thrombi formation, respectively.

COMMON NON-CARDIAC EMERGENCIES

Acute Abdomen

The "acute abdomen" is not a specific entity, but refers to any disease or disorder that causes the rapid onset of abdominal distress. The primary sign is abdominal pain. One may also see lethargy or collapse, anorexia, fever, dehydration, vomiting, diarrhea, abdominal distension, dysuria, or unusual posturing.

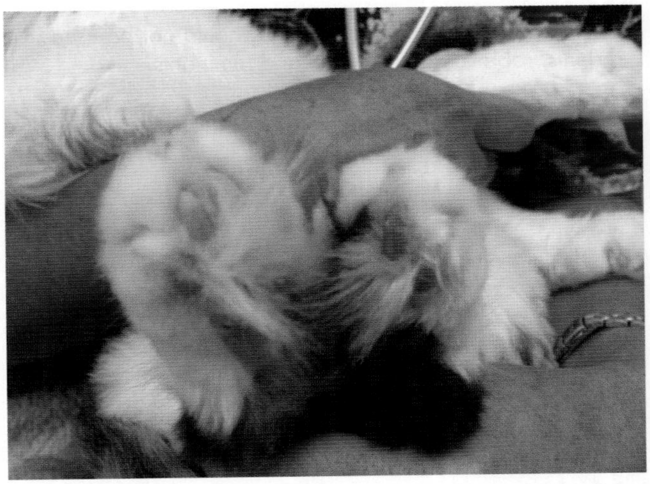

FIGURE 17-19 Cats with saddle thrombus will have poor perfusion to the rear limbs; femoral pulses will be weak or absent. Inspect toe pads for a bluish color, indicating poor blood flow.

Causes of an acute abdomen include the following: intestinal obstruction/overdistention (e.g., gastric dilatation/volvulus, foreign body, and intussusception); organ displacement (e.g., diaphragmatic/abdominal hernias, uterine/splenic torsion); infection/inflammation (e.g., parvovirus, pancreatitis, peritonitis, and pyometra); and trauma (e.g., visceral perforation, bladder rupture). In addition to initial evaluation and stabilization, additional diagnostics may be required such as repeated physical examinations, radiographic procedures (plain and contrast), laboratory testing (CBC, chemistry, blood gases, and electrolytes), and diagnostic peritoneal lavage. Therapy is directed at the cause of the acute abdomen (Box 17-7).

Poisonings and Intoxications

Diagnosis is based primarily on history and clinical signs. Once the veterinarian is reasonably confident that a toxin is involved, efforts are made to identify the type of toxin, prevent further exposure and absorption, treat the symptoms, and give the specific antidote. National or local animal poison control centers should always be called once the toxin has been identified in order to correctly treat the patient. Human poison control centers are also very helpful in determining the toxin's effects on various organs. Clinical signs of a poisoning or intoxication are diverse and overlapping because of the variety of such agents to which an animal may be exposed. General, nonspecific signs may include such findings as obtundation and weakness, anorexia, and gastrointestinal signs such as vomiting and diarrhea. CNS excitation (e.g., nervousness, apprehension, hypersensitivity, and seizures) may be seen with common poisons such as strychnine, metaldehyde, moldy food products, ivermectin in Collie breeds, chocolate, cocaine, marijuana, amphetamine, toxic mushrooms, and vitamin D-analog rodenticides. Hemorrhage may be seen with vitamin K antagonist rodenticides. Miosis and muscle tremors may be seen with organophosphate, carbamate, pyrethrins, or nicotine intoxication. Salivation may be seen with CNS excitants or with irritating or corrosive ingestions such as household cleaning products or muriatic acid. Commonly encountered toxins are presented in Box 17-8.

> *TECHNICIAN NOTE* Emetics should not be used in rodents, rabbits, birds, horses, and ruminants.

BOX 17-7 Clinical Signs of Acute Abdomen

- Fever
- Dehydration
- Depression
- Polyuria/polydipsia
- Abdominal pain
- Shock
- Vomiting
- Hematemesis
- Diarrhea
- Melena
- Abdominal distension

If the animal has the toxin on its skin, it will need to be bathed to diminish further exposure. Vacuum or towel off powder-based products; bathing with water may exacerbate toxic effects. Induce vomiting (Box 17-9) if it has been 2 hours or less since the ingestion. Do not induce vomiting if the patient has CNS depression or seizure activity, decreased gag reflex, breathing difficulty, or has ingested caustic substances such as petroleum distillates. Dilution with milk or water in combination with demulcents is recommended in cases of corrosive ingestion. Perform gastric lavage (see Procedure 17-2) following induction of anesthesia and endotracheal intubation. A stomach tube is passed, and several cycles of warm water are injected and aspirated until the return fluid is clear. Following emesis or lavage, the patient is given activated charcoal to absorb the remaining toxin in the stomach and intestines; it is also not uncommon to administer activated charcoal both before and after lavage.

If the toxin is identified, then a specific antidote may be given. The technician will play a vital role in the supportive care of the patient. It will be necessary to maintain respiratory and cardiovascular function, body temperature, acid-base balance, and control of the CNS. Some toxins may result in hyperactivity or seizures, requiring the need for sedation or anesthesia.

BOX 17-8 Commonly Encountered Toxins

Plants
- Lilies
- Oleander
- Laurel
- Foxglove
- Lily of the valley
- Cycad (Sago) palm
- Castor beans

Foods
- Grapes
- Raisins
- Currants
- Onions
- Caffeine
- Chocolate
- Xylitol

Pesticides and Rodenticides
- Permethrins
- Pyrethroids
- Organophosphates
- Anticoagulant rodenticides
- Cholecaliferol
- Zinc phosphide

Environmental Toxins and Pharmaceuticals
- Ethylene glycol
- Acetaminophen
- Ibuprofen
- Naproxen
- Meloxicam
- Zinc
- Lead

> **TECHNICIAN NOTE** Try mixing canned cat food or blenderized dog food with activated charcoal before gastric tube delivery in conscious patients. Many patients willingly eat such a concoction.

BOX 17-9 Emetic Agents

3% Hydrogen Peroxide
- Effective in the dog, pig, ferret, and cat.
- Dosage is 1 teaspoon (5 ml) per 5 lbs (1 teaspoon per 2.5 kg), not to exceed 3 tablespoons (45 ml).
- Vomiting usually occurs within minutes and the treatment can be repeated once if not initially successful.

Apomorphine Hydrochloride
- Use cautiously in cats.
- Administer conjunctivally; rinse eyes after vomiting has occurred.
- Side effects such as CNS and respiratory depression, ataxia, excitement, and protracted vomiting may occur.
- If severe side effects are seen, apomorphine can be reversed with naloxone (Narcan).

UROGENITAL EMERGENCIES

Azotemia

Azotemia is an increase in nitrogen-containing waste products in the blood (BUN and creatine). Azotemia is categorized as prerenal (inadequate renal blood flow), renal (renal disease), and postrenal (urinary tract obstruction or perforation). Patients with prerenal azotemia show an increase in BUN and creatinine but maintain the ability to concentrate urine to a specific gravity greater than 1.035. Conditions that may predispose the patient to prerenal azotemia include dehydration, hypotension (low blood pressure), hypovolemia, and congestive heart failure. Acute renal failure (ARF) is a clinical syndrome that results in a rapid decline in renal function. In renal failure the kidneys are unable to adequately excrete metabolic waste and regulate fluid, electrolyte, and acid-base balance. Causes of renal azotemia include toxins (e.g., aminoglycoside, ethylene glycol, grapes, envenomization), renal hypoperfusion (anesthesia), and infectious agents (e.g., *Leptospira* spp). Postrenal azotemia occurs when the urinary pathway is obstructed, preventing adequate urine flow, or from rupture of the urinary tract causing spillage of urine into the abdomen. Causes of postrenal azotemia include urethral plugs (common emergency in the male cat), bladder or urethral tumors, and urolithiasis (urinary stones).

PROCEDURE 17-2 Gastric Lavage

Indications
- Elimination of toxins from the stomach within 2 hours of ingestion
- Gastric dilatation
- Gastric dilatation-volvulus

Materials
- Endotracheal tube and syringe for cuff
- Sterile lubricant
- 1-inch white tape or marker
- Stomach pump or large syringes
- Warm water (syringes or bucket)
- Empty bucket or garbage pail
- Activated charcoal

Procedure
- If possible, perform under anesthesia or with inflated endotracheal tube in place.
- Endotracheal tube should extend 2 inches rostral to the teeth.
- Obtain a stomach tube roughly 2.5 times the diameter of the endotracheal tube.
- Measure the stomach tube from the mouth to the 12th-13th rib.
- Place a mark or piece of tape on tube to monitor length.
- Lubricate the end of the tube and advance slowly. (Do not force if resistance is met.)
- Visualize gastric contents within the tube.
- Administer activated charcoal before and after lavage.
- Attach the stomach pump to the tube.
- Tilt the patient's head down to minimize risk of aspiration.
- Place the stomach pump in bucket of warm water; instill water appropriate for patient size; large syringes of water can be used if a stomach pump is not present (Fig. 1).

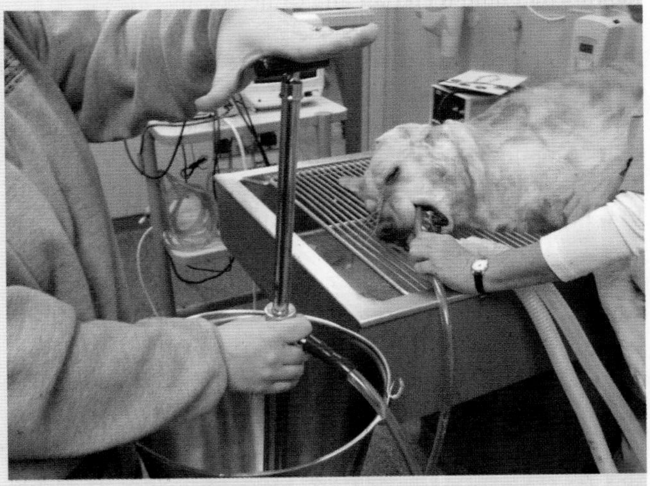

FIGURE 1 Gastric lavage performed using a stomach pump.

- Remove stomach pump and allow gastric contents to be evacuated into a bucket. An assistant may gently press on the stomach to assist elimination.
- Repeat lavage with water until stomach content is clear.
- Repeat administration of activated charcoal.
- Kink the tube before removal.
- Extubate at the last possible moment, keeping the patient sternal and head down.

Acute Renal Failure

Clinical signs of ARF include lethargy, anorexia, dehydration, vomiting, diarrhea, dysuria (difficult urination), **oliguria** (decreased urine production), and anuria (lack of urine production). Additional diagnostics may be required such as repeated physical examinations, laboratory testing (CBC, chemistry, urinalysis, blood gases and electrolytes), radiographic procedures (plain and contrast), and ultrasonography. The objectives of treatment of ARF are to minimize further renal injury, promote diuresis if oliguria exists, and combat metabolic consequences of uremia. Hemodialysis has been used successfully to treat ARF resulting from toxic and infectious agents. Hemodialysis uses an artificial kidney to reduce azotemia and correct fluid, electrolyte, and acid-base imbalances. There are several hemodialysis units in the United States for animal use.

Peritoneal dialysis is an alternative that can be accomplished in most practice settings. Like hemodialysis, it is technically demanding, expensive, and labor intensive. The peritoneum is used as a semipermeable membrane. A peritoneal dialysis catheter is placed in the abdomen (Fig. 17-20). A fluid (dialysate) is infused into the abdomen and allowed to dwell for 30 to 60 minutes. The dialysate is drained, and along with it comes solutes such as urea. The technician should be familiar with urinary and IV catheter placement and management. Measurement of central venous pressure may help guide the delivery of the fluid therapy plan. Nursing care includes monitoring fluid inputs and outputs. It is helpful to weigh the patient several times per day. Acute changes in body weight are usually related to fluid gains or losses. Strict aseptic technique should be used when handling all fluid materials and catheters.

Feline Lower Urinary Tract Disease (FLUTD) With Obstruction

Dysuria, anuria, hematuria, inappropriate voiding, incessant grooming of the perineum, vocalizing, vomiting, bladder distention, and abdominal pain are signs consistent with FLUTD with obstruction. The narrow urethra of the male cat becomes obstructed with a mucoproteinaceous plug and/or urothroliths. In addition to postrenal azotemia, urinary obstruction leads to impaired excretion of potassium and hydrogen ions, resulting in hyperkalemia and metabolic acidosis. Vomiting and anorexia may cause volume depletion.

> **TECHNICIAN NOTE** Hyperkalemia is a common sequela to urinary obstruction. Clinical signs include bradycardia. Warning! Any excessive stress may cause cardiac arrest if serum potassium is significantly elevated.

The immediate therapeutic goal is to relieve the obstruction and correct the metabolic abnormalities. The patient's condition will dictate treatment priorities. Relieving the obstruction is required for resolution of azotemia and hyperkalemia. In cases in which hyperkalemia and hypovolemia are life threatening, cardioprotective treatments and fluid resuscitation become top priorities. Therapeutic options to protect the heart from toxic effects of hyperkalemia include administration of calcium and/or insulin and 50% dextrose. The administration of calcium antagonizes the effects of potassium on the heart. Regular insulin and dextrose administration causes potassium to shift from the extracellular fluid (ECF) to the intracellular fluid. The insulin dextrose combination has a slightly slower onset of action when compared to calcium administration but a longer duration of action. In addition to volume restoration, fluid therapy with crystalloids will dilute potassium in the ECF.

Very sick cats with urethral obstruction probably will not require sedation to relieve the obstruction. The obstruction may be relieved by gently massaging the penis or by passing an open-ended tomcat catheter and flushing (retropulsing) the urethra with saline (Figs. 17-21 and 17-22). Once the obstruction is relieved, a soft urinary catheter is placed until it is determined that it can be removed. The catheter should be attached to a closed urinary collection system to prevent infection and to monitor urine production. Cats commonly

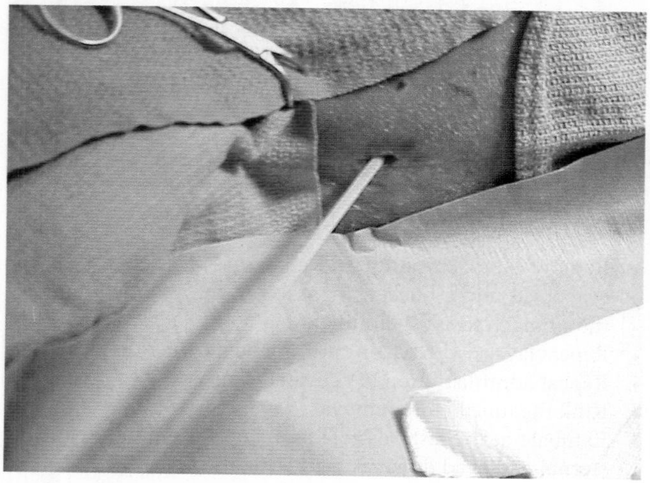

FIGURE 17-20 Peritoneal catheter placement for the treatment of acute renal failure.

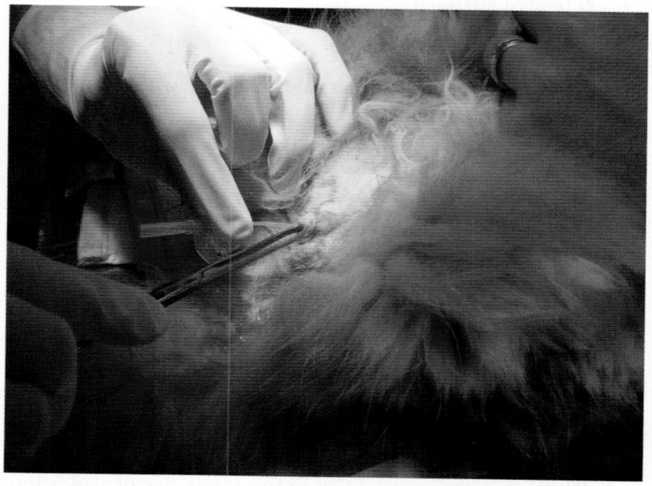

FIGURE 17-21 An open-ended tomcat catheter can be inserted into the urethra to relieve an obstruction.

exhibit a postobstructive diuresis; a high fluid administration rate will be required to meet urine losses. Fluids are given to correct dehydration and to meet normal maintenance requirements as well as to match urine output. Potassium supplementation is necessary because of the potential development of hypokalemia secondary to the postobstruction diuresis. Eventually, fluids will be tapered off.

> **TECHNICIAN NOTE** After relieving a urinary obstruction, the urine may be hematuric and still full of debris. Monitor urine production not only by emptying the collection bag, but also by palpating the bladder every 4 to 6 hours to ensure that the urinary catheter does not get plugged. The catheter and/or the line may be flushed with sterile saline.

Dystocia

Dystocia is rare in the queen but not uncommon in the bitch. The two primary causes of dystocia are either maternal (poor straining effort [uterine inertia], anatomic abnormalities) or fetal (fetal oversize, malposition). Dystocia can be characterized as any of the following:

- Active straining for more than 30 to 60 minutes without delivery of a fetus
- Resting, without straining for more than 4 hours between deliveries with known retained fetuses
- Intermittent weak contractions for more than 2 hours

Diagnosis and the mode of therapy are based on thorough history and physical examination. Radiography and, if available, ultrasonography, may aid in the decision-making process. Three options are available for the management of the dystocia patient; they include medical intervention (use of oxytocin, calcium, and glucose), manual manipulation, and surgery.

> **TECHNICIAN NOTE** Labor should begin within 12 to 24 h after temperature decline (<99° F) for both the dog and cat.

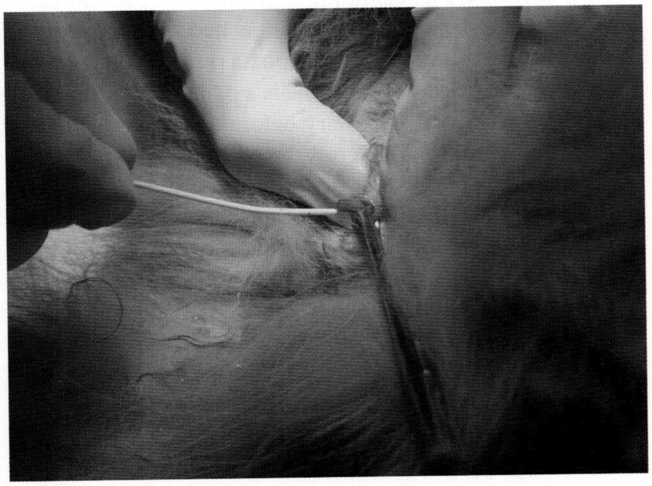

FIGURE 17-22 After relieving the obstruction, a softer and more flexible urinary catheter may be placed for indwelling use.

Pyometra

A pyometra is an infection in the uterus. It is caused by hormonally induced changes in progesterone or exogenous estrogens. Patients may be depressed and septic or clinically normal. Clinical signs include lethargy, anorexia, dehydration, vomiting, injected (brick-red) mucous membranes, diarrhea, polyuria, polydipsia, and vaginal discharge (with open pyometra). Laboratory tests (CBC, chemistry, urinalysis, cytology and culture, blood gases, and electrolytes) and imaging (radiographs and ultrasonography) aid in the diagnosis of the disease. Pyometras may be surgically or medically managed. Surgery is the treatment of choice. Treatment choice is based on the condition, age, and breeding value of the animal. The patient will need to be supported with intensive fluid therapy and good basic nursing care.

ENDOCRINE SYSTEM EMERGENCIES

Diabetic Ketoacidosis

Diabetic ketoacidosis (DKA) is one of the more common endocrine emergencies. A patient presenting with DKA is glucosuric, hyperglycemic, ketonuric, ketonemic, typically hypovolemic, and acidotic. DKA is the result of altered carbohydrate, protein, and fat metabolism because of insulin deficiency. Clinical signs include polyuria (PU), polydipsia (PD), polyphagia (excessive ingestion of food), weight loss, depression, dehydration, weakness, tachypnea, vomiting, and sweet acetone odor to the breath (Box 17-10). The goals of initial therapy are to correct ketonemia and acidosis, blood glucose, hyperosmolality, dehydration, and electrolyte abnormalities (through insulin and fluid therapy).

Hypoadrenocorticism (Addisonian Crisis)

Hypoadrenocorticism (Addison's disease) is a deficiency in the production of mineralocorticoid and/or glucocorticoid steroid hormones. Hypoadrenocorticism occurs in the dog and is rare in the cat. Addison's disease is nicknamed "The Great Pretender" because clinical signs are nonspecific and often mimic other diseases. Owner's complaints may include anorexia, lethargy, vomiting, weakness, weight loss, and diarrhea, with waxing and waning signs. Physical findings may include mental depression, weakness, collapse, decreased body temperature, and bradycardia (Box 17-11).

BOX 17-10 Diabetic Ketoacidosis

Clinical Signs

- Early—polydipsia, polyphagia, polyuria
- Weight loss, sudden onset of cataracts (dogs)
- Later—vomiting, anorexia, depression, tachypnea

Physical Exam Findings

- Dehydration
- Hepatomegaly
- ± Abdominal pain
- Acetone breath
- Tachypnea

BOX 17-11 Clinical Signs of Addison's Disease

- Anorexia
- Vomiting
- Diarrhea (± melena)
- Weight loss
- Polyuria/polydipsia
- Weakness
- Ataxia
- Tremors

Many of the signs may be attributed to decreased tissue perfusion and electrolyte abnormalities. Diagnosis is confirmed by performing an ACTH stimulation test. Other laboratory findings may include hyperkalemia, hyponatremia, sodium/potassium ratio less than 27:1 (and usually less than 20:1), azotemia, metabolic acidosis, and normocytic normochromic anemia. The Addisonian crisis is a medical emergency; supportive therapy is often begun before a definitive diagnosis is made. Therapy includes fluid resuscitation, usually with normal saline. If the patient is hypoglycemic, hyperkalemic, or has metabolic acidosis, the appropriate therapy is undertaken. Monitoring entails repeated physical examinations, ECG monitoring, blood pressure and central venous pressure measurements, and acid-base and electrolyte measurements.

EMERGENCY PROCEDURES

Technicians should be familiar with the variety of lifesaving emergency procedures available. The technician should be prepared to render the procedures they are allowed to perform, or be prepared to assist the veterinarian. The technician should know the indications for each procedure, what equipment will be necessary, how the procedure is performed, potential complications, and nursing implications of the procedure whether it goes well or not.

EMERGENCY ENDOTRACHEAL INTUBATION

Endotracheal intubation is a basic but important technique that can easily be mastered with practice. Successful intubation is verified by direct visualization of the tube entering glottis and/or palpation of the tube in proper position between arytenoids cartilages (Procedure 17-3).

PROCEDURE 17-3 Emergency Intubation

Indication

- Nonpatent airway

Materials

- Laryngoscope
- Endotracheal tube
- Syringe for cuff inflation
- Suction if airway occluded

Procedure

- Always intubate patients in shock in lateral or dorsal recumbency; elevating the head may cause a precipitous decline in blood flow to the brain and a cardiac arrest.
- Use laryngoscope because manipulation of the larynx can cause vagal stimulation, which may lead to cardiac arrest.
- If intubating in lateral recumbency, hold laryngoscope in standard fashion.
- If intubating in dorsal recumbency, grasp laryngoscope so that the handle is upward and the curved blade is facing the patient, curve pointing upward.
- Insert blade into the mouth; use the tip of the blade to push the epiglottis ventrally.
- Use laryngoscope as lever; use end of blade closest to operator to push hard palate dorsally at same time as epiglottis is elevated.
- Visualize arytenoid cartilages alongside the blade.
- Insert tube through the cartilages and secure in standard fashion.

TRACHEOSTOMY TUBE PLACEMENT

Ideally, an endotracheal tube is placed first to control the airway and stabilize the patient. Then preparation is made to place the tracheostomy tube under controlled, aseptic conditions (see Procedure 17-4). The veterinary technician should set up for the procedure, prepare the patient, assist in the placement, and provide pre- and post-tracheostomy wound and tube care.

There are many types of tracheostomy tubes available. Shiley adult (see Fig. 17-23) and pediatric tracheostomy tubes are recommended. The adult tube consists of an outer tube with fixation flanges and an inner cannula. The tube is soft and pliable, and is nonirritating to the tissues. It has a high-volume, low-pressure cuff. The inner cannula is removed for cleaning. An obturator is included to assist in the smooth placement of the tracheostomy tube. The pediatric tube is cuffless and does not have an inner cannula. An endotracheal tube can be substituted for a tracheostomy tube and is often cut to decrease dead space and resistance.

Nursing management of the tracheostomy tube is critical to the patient. Sterile technique is indicated to prevent nosocomial infection. Suctioning will be necessary to prevent tube occlusion and subsequent hypoxia (see Procedure 17-5). Suctioning the tracheostomy tube is a painful procedure; analgesic agents may be necessary before this procedure. During suctioning, the character of the secretions should be observed (Fig. 17-24). If the secretions are minimal or thick, approximately 0.2 ml/kg of saline is injected into the trachea, the lungs are again hyperinflated several times with oxygen, and the suctioning is repeated. It is important to oxygenate the patient immediately before and immediately after each suctioning attempt. The suctioning procedure should be stopped immediately if the patient displays excessive discomfort, restlessness, or changes in cardiac or respiratory rhythm. The site around the tracheostomy tube should be inspected for signs of infection every 8 hours. In addition, the site should be cleaned with hydrogen peroxide or dilute chlorhexidine and covered with a gauze pad.

PROCEDURE 17-4 Tracheostomy Tube Placement

Indications

- Airway obstruction
- To facilitate long-term access to the airway and positive pressure ventilation

Materials

- Several tracheostomy tubes (one size smaller and larger than the estimated size)
- Surgical kit
- Suction
- Sterile suction catheters
- Sterile drapes
- Bandage material
- Sandbags (to aid in patient positioning)

Procedure

- Sedate the patient if necessary. Place the patient in dorsal recumbency and position as straight as possible. Place a sandbag or roll of towels underneath the neck to cause dorsiflexion of the cervical region. Make a wide clip over the region of the incision site and prepare the skin antiseptically.
- The clinician will make a midline skin incision from approximately the first to the fourth tracheal ring. Blunt dissection is continued until the trachea is clearly exposed. Three types of tracheal incisions have been used: transverse, tracheal flap, and vertical. It may be helpful to place sutures around a tracheal ring, above and below the opening (in the transverse incision). The suture is left in place for the duration of the tracheostomy. Sutures help to manipulate tracheal rings during intubation and reintubation if the tube becomes dislodged.
- Clean the trachea of blood and mucus before intubation.
- Insert the tracheostomy tube and inflate the cuff. Suction if necessary using sterile technique.
- Close the skin incision (not tightly around the tube), and tie the tube securely around the patient's neck with umbilical tape or other material.
- Drape a sterile 4-by-4 gauze around the tube to absorb serum and secretions from the surgical site.

Complications

- Tube obstruction with mucus
- Tube dislodgement from the trachea
- Infection of the incision site
- Tracheal stenosis as a result of an oversized tracheostomy tube, torqued tube positioning, excessive tracheal tube movement, or excessive cuff inflation

THORACOCENTESIS

Thoracocentesis is useful for collection of pleural fluid to obtain samples for diagnostic laboratory evaluation or for alleviation of respiratory distress. This procedure may be used for patients with respiratory distress and decreased to absent lung sounds. In an emergency situation, a technician can perform the procedure (see Procedure 17-6).

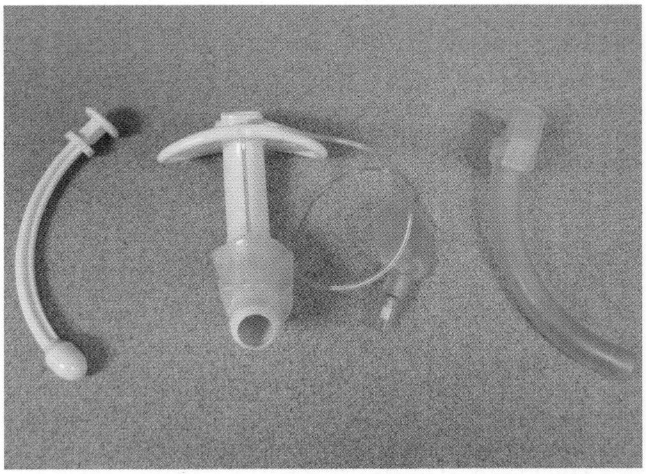

FIGURE 17-23 Shiley tracheostomy tube *(center)* with obturator *(left)* and inner canula *(right)*. The inner cannula fits into the tracheostomy tube.

CHEST TUBE PLACEMENT

Chest tubes are placed through the chest wall into the pleural space to remove fluid or air from around the lungs, allowing the lungs to expand maximally (see Procedure 17-7). The chest tube must be securely attached (sutured) to the patient to prevent inadvertent leakage of air into the chest by accidental removal of the chest tube. More than one clamp (e.g., hemostats with padded jaws) and a three-way stopcock should be placed on the chest tube to prevent leakage of air into the pleural cavity between aspirations. Aseptic removal of fluid or air from the chest will facilitate effort of breathing and prevent secondary infection (see Fig. 17-25).

Commercial chest tubes come in a variety of sizes with and without trocars. Recommended sizes are 14- to 16-French tubes for cats and very small dogs; 18- to 22-F tubes for small dogs; 22- to 28-F tubes for medium to large dogs; and 28- to 36-F tubes for very large dogs. If necessary, red rubber or Foley catheters may be used; however, it may be necessary to add a few more holes to the chest tube for maximum efficacy.

Once the chest tube has been placed and anchored, a bandage should be applied. The bandage securing the chest tube in place should be tight enough (or attached to the patient with tape) to prevent slippage but loose enough to allow the patient to breathe. Always cover the jaws of the hemostat and the three-way stopcock with an easily removed layer of tape. This will prevent the hemostats or the stopcock from catching on anything and becoming dislodged. If the patient is left unattended with a chest tube in place, an Elizabethan collar should be placed to prevent tube removal by the patient. Nursing responsibilities include evaluation of the bandage and the chest tube for security when aspirating, and inspection for any subcutaneous emphysema, indicating possible tube migration.

> TECHNICIAN NOTE Mark any tube at the point of entry into the patient (e.g., thorax, stomach, or nares) with a permanent marker in order to monitor for migration. Palpate daily for the presence of subcutaneous emphysema.

PROCEDURE 17-5 Tracheostomy Tube Maintenance

Indication
- Prevent tube occlusion

Materials
- Oxygen
- Sterile suction catheter
- Suction unit
- Sterile saline
- Sterile gloves
- Dilute chlorhexidine solution
- 4×4 gauze sponges

Procedure
- Preoxygenate patient.
- Instill 1 to 2 ml sterile saline down trach tube.
- Connect suction catheter to suction source; use as low suction pressure as possible.
- Gently insert sterile suction catheter down trach tube until resistance is met (Fig. 1).
- Suction quickly.

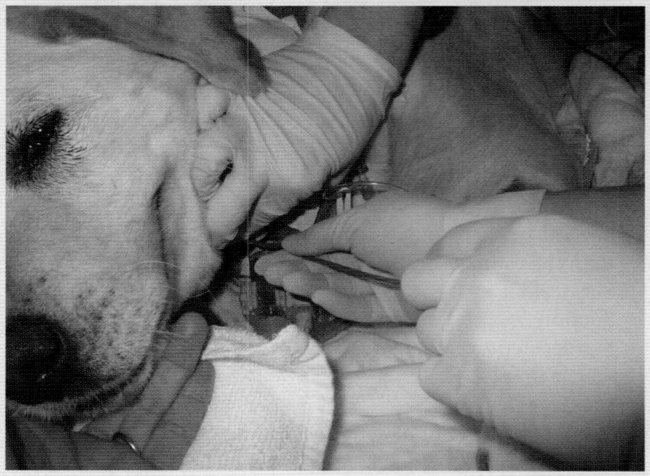

FIGURE 1 Sterile suctioning of tracheostomy tube.

- Give oxygen after suctioning for several minutes.
- Wipe area around stoma with dilute chlorhexidine.

OXYGEN THERAPY

OVERVIEW

Hypoxemia is defined as deficient oxygenation of the blood. Hypoxemia is a result of impaired gas exchange caused by small airway and alveolar collapse, an excessive ventilation/perfusion mismatch, or both. Oxygen therapy may be beneficial. The goal of oxygen therapy is to provide adequate blood oxygenation, using the lowest possible inspired oxygen concentrations. The best method for assessing oxygenation is analysis of arterial blood gases. Pulse oximetry (SpO_2) can also be used to assess oxygenation. Clinical signs of hypoxia include cyanosis, dyspnea, tachypnea, orthopnea, tachycardia, and anxiety. Indications for oxygen administration include hypoxemia ($PaO_2 < 60$ mm Hg) or increased effort of breathing.

METHODS OF OXYGEN ADMINISTRATION

There are a variety of methods of oxygen delivery. The method selected depends on expected duration of therapy, demeanor of the patient, and equipment availability. Available methods include face mask, oxygen hood, oxygen cage, and nasal insufflation.

Face Mask

Face masks are readily available and easy to use. An oxygen mask placed over the mouth and nose provides the patient with 100% oxygen. Care must be taken not to use excessive restraint while administering oxygen. Because some patients may not tolerate a mask, flow-by oxygen may provide temporary respiratory support. Masks are only good for short-term use. High-inspired oxygen concentrations can be obtained if a properly fitted face mask is used. Unfortunately, patients often fight the face mask (unless obtunded), thereby increasing oxygen consumption and diminishing the effects of the oxygen therapy. The patient's face and nose should fill the mask as much as possible to reduce the amount of dead space in the mask. Increased dead space will increase the work of breathing. Sometimes it is helpful to remove the rubber diaphragm from the face mask to achieve a better fit and achieve better patient cooperation, or remove the mask altogether and provide flow-by oxygen by holding the hose near the patient's face (Fig. 17-26).

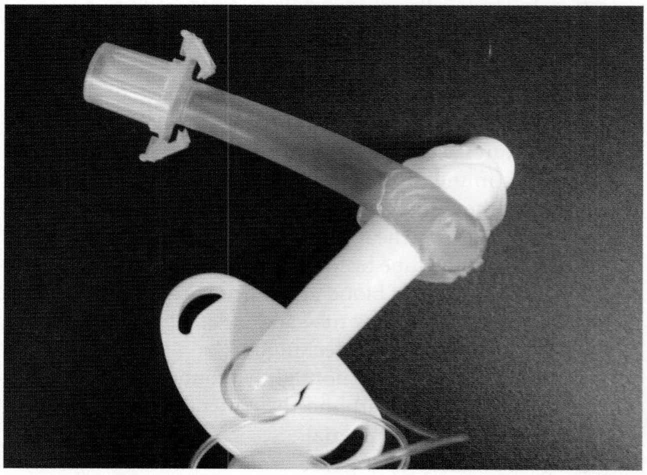

FIGURE 17-24 Partial obstruction of tracheostomy tube with dried airway secretions and mucus.

Oxygen Hood

An alternative to the face mask is a clear plastic bag placed over the head of a patient with an oxygen hose placed near

PROCEDURE 17-6 Thoracocentesis

Indications
- Pneumothorax
- Hemothorax
- Pleural effusion

Materials (Fig. 1)

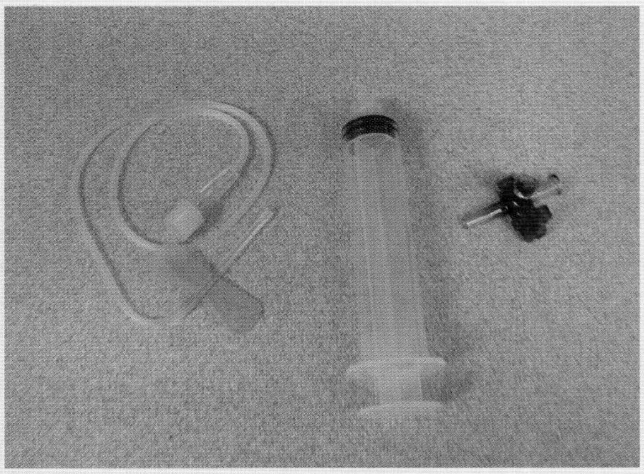

FIGURE 1 Materials needed for thoracocentesis.

- Butterfly catheter, hypodermic needle, or over-the-needle catheter
- Three-way stopcock
- 3-ml syringe (if procedure is done to obtain diagnostic sample)
- 35- or 60-ml syringe (if procedure is done to remove a substantial amount of fluids)
- IV extension set
- Clippers, surgical prep solution and scrub

Procedure
- Place patient in sternal recumbency and administer oxygen (Fig. 2).

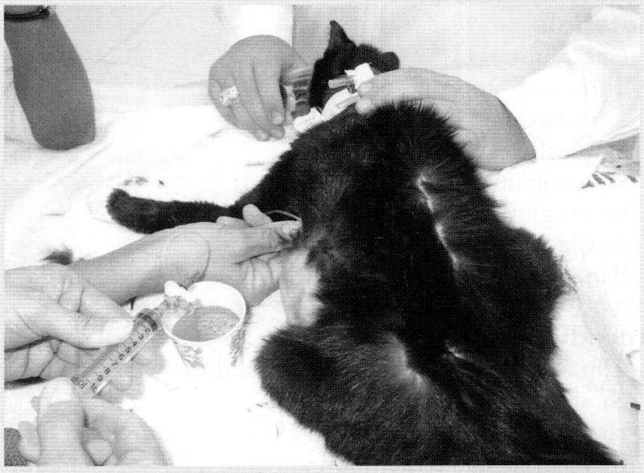

FIGURE 2 Patient position should be sternal if possible.

- Clip and prep area where thoracocentesis is to be performed (dorsally for the collection of air or ventrally for fluid).
- After putting on sterile gloves, assemble catheter, needle or butterfly, stopcock, and syringe.
- Palpate anterior edge of rib.
- Insert needle into the pleural space so that it comes to lie on the pleural surface of the palpated rib; the bevel is directed away from the rib.
- Aspirate using gentle pressure.

Complications
- Iatrogenic lung trauma and pneumothorax
- Iatrogenic hemothorax

the animal's nose. The bag remains open along the animal's neck to allow the gas to escape. A flow rate of 5 to 8 liters per minute is used. It has been reported that animals tolerate this bag/hood method when they resist the oxygen mask. Use caution with this method, as the patient may become hot, stressed, and has an increased potential to aspirate if vomiting occurs. Make sure oxygen is always flowing into the hood.

Oxygen Cage

Patients in acute respiratory distress can be temporarily placed in an incubator or oxygen cage. The cage provides an environment with stable temperature, humidity, and oxygen. The temperature should be adjusted to make the patient comfortable and the humidity kept at 40% to 60%. Oxygen is delivered to provide 40% oxygen in the environment (normal room air contains 20.9% oxygen). A major drawback to using the oxygen cage is limited access to the patient. If the cage is opened, the percentage of oxygen in the air immediately drops and the patient may become dyspneic. Use pillows to prop the patient in sternal recumbency in the oxygen cage. The oxygen cage should be used only until other means of oxygen delivery can be provided, if possible.

A good oxygen cage should have the following features: It must have a system for eliminating carbon dioxide; deliver a known amount of oxygen in a concentration beneficial to the patient (40% to 50%); and a mechanism for controlling temperature (70° F) and humidity (50%). The disadvantages of oxygen cages are: expense to purchase and operate, minimal access to the patient by caregivers, patient hyperthermia, and difficulty accommodating large patients.

TECHNICIAN NOTE A temporary, make-shift oxygen cage may be created by covering a cage door with plastic wrap (Fig. 17-27). Leave small holes for carbon dioxide escape. Monitor patient temperature frequently to avoid hyperthermia.

PROCEDURE 17-7 Chest Tube Placement

Indications
- To relieve progressive pneumothorax
- To relieve progressive pleural effusion

Materials
- Chest tube
- Three-way stopcock, C-clamp, or hemostats
- 2% lidocaine
- Surgical kit
- Suture material
- Sterile gloves
- Sterile drapes
- Bandaging material

Procedure
- Clip and surgically prepare caudal dorsal quadrant of the chest wall.
- Have an assistant grasp skin along the entire lateral chest wall just caudal to the elbow and pull it forward and downward.
- Locate an intercostal space about 8 or 9 high on the chest wall (about junction of upper one third and lower two thirds of the chest wall).
- Inject lidocaine along path of the skin and intercostal muscle incision.
- Make a skin incision 1½ times the length of the tube diameter.
- Make an intercostal relief incision, but do not penetrate the pleura.
- Penetrate the pleura with a blunt object so as not to lacerate the lung.
- Insert the chest tube through the chest wall and into the pleural space. Guide the tube in a cranial ventral direction at about a 45-degree angle. If a trocar is used, pull it back from the tip of the chest tube as soon as the pleura is penetrated. When the tube is in the desired location, remove the trocar and clamp the tube.
- Have an assistant release the skin, creating a tunnel that prevents air from entering the pleural space.
- Verify the position of the chest tube with the trocar on the outside of the chest.
- Secure the chest tube to the chest wall, and apply a triple antibiotic dressing. Attach a C-clamp (or hemostats) and a three-way stopcock.
- A chest radiograph may be taken to verify the position of the tube. This is not necessary if the tube is draining properly, but must be done if the tube is not draining properly. Mark the entry point into the chest with a permanent marker to allow for visible evaluation of potential migration.
- Place a light bandage around thorax to help prevent tube migration.
- Place an Elizabethan collar on the patient before fully awake.

Complications
- Infection
- Laceration of intercostal artery
- Lung trauma/pneumothorax
- Trauma to heart and great vessels/hemorrhage
- Subcutaneous emphysema

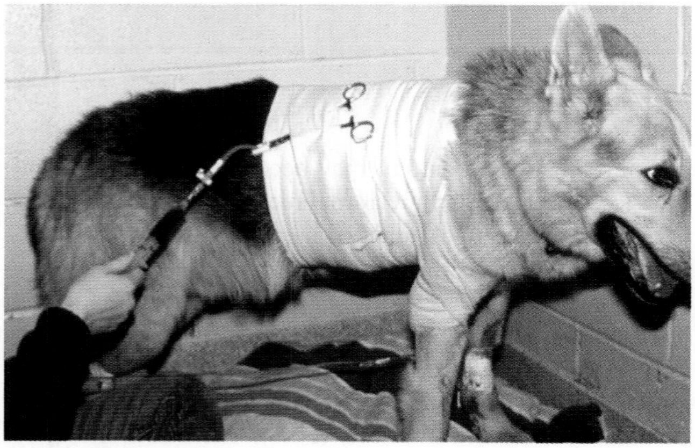

FIGURE 17-25 Aspiration of chest fluid or air from chest tube will improve patient respiration. The patient should be sternal during aspiration.

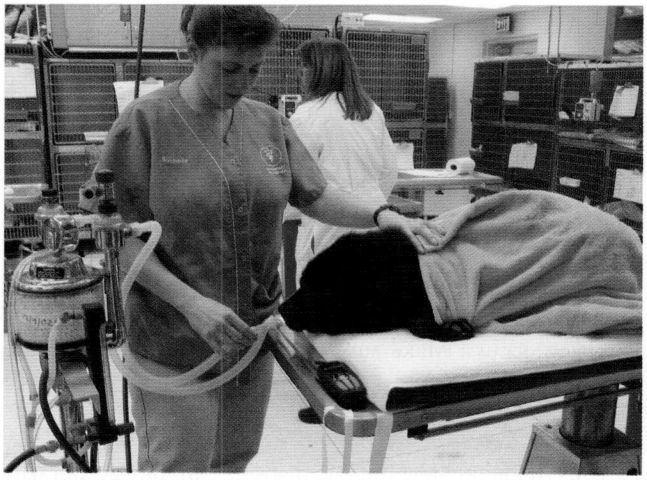

FIGURE 17-26 Oxygen administration via flow-by method. Always provide oxygen using the least stressful route.

Nasal Oxygen
Nasal oxygen is an easy way to provide oxygen without causing undue stress to the patient, and is considered superior to oxygen cages, hoods, or flow-by methods of providing oxygen. An oxygen flow rate of 100 ml/kg/minute provides approximately 40% oxygen to the patient. Nasal insufflation allows full access to the patient without decreasing or stopping the flow of oxygen during treatment procedures (Procedure 17-8).

Some patients may not tolerate a nasal insufflation tube and require an Elizabethan collar to prevent removal of the

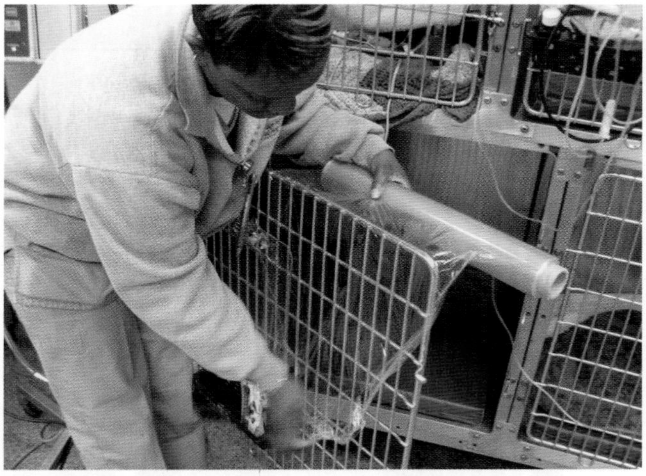

FIGURE 17-27 A temporary, make-shift oxygen cage may be created by placing plastic wrap around a cage door; ensure small holes in the corners to allow carbon dioxide to escape.

tube. Oxygen administered through a tube placed in the nasal cavity must be humidified to prevent drying of the respiratory mucosa. A humidification unit can be attached to the flow meter. A Y-connector piece can be used to increase flow through a single or double catheter. Contraindications to nasal oxygen include patients with suspected coagulopathies, nasal tumors, head trauma, or suspected increased intracranial pressure.

DIAGNOSTIC PERITONEAL LAVAGE

Diagnostic peritoneal lavage is useful in diagnosing some abdominal disorders when other diagnostic tests are equivocal. It is not indicated when there is historical, physical, or radiographic evidence of the need for an exploratory laparotomy. Fluid is infused into the abdomen via a peritoneal lavage catheter. The fluid is recovered and analyzed. This procedure is helpful in diagnosing abdominal hemorrhage, ruptured bowel, peritonitis, and bladder rupture (see Procedure 17-9).

CRITICAL CARE

Once the patient has made the transition from the crisis or emergency care phase, critical care nursing may be required. Critical care patients require moment-to-moment monitoring and nursing care. The technician should be able to monitor, reassess, and respond to the patient's needs in an appropriate manner as the condition changes. In addition, the veterinary technician should be knowledgeable in fluid therapy (Chapter 16) and critical care nursing protocols.

PATIENT ASSESSMENT AND MONITORING

A great deal of the veterinary technician's responsibility involves patient monitoring during the definitive management phase. Communication between team members is crucial; documentation of procedures, vital signs, and hemodynamic measurements are imperative in improving patient outcome.

Cardiovascular System

Assessment of the cardiovascular system should begin with the heart rate. A normal heart rate for a dog is 100 to 140 beats per minute. For a cat it is 110 to 140 beats per minute. There are several reasons for tachycardia (e.g., hypovolemia, fever, excitement, exercise, heart disease in the dog, and pain) and bradycardia (e.g., high vagal tone, severe electrolyte disturbances, heart disease in the cat, and atrioventricular conduction blocks). If arrhythmias are auscultated, then an ECG is indicated. The ECG measures electrical activity; it does not measure mechanical activity. Indicators of peripheral perfusion include mucous membrane color, capillary refill time (normal CRT 1 to 2 seconds), urine output, and appendage temperature. A full strong pulse indicates a good pulse pressure and stroke volume. Refer to Chapter 24 for additional patient nursing care techniques.

> **TECHNICIAN NOTE** Simultaneously palpate the femoral pulse and auscultate the heart to check for asynchronicity. Any heart beat without a palpable femoral pulse, or variable pulse strength differences, warrants an ECG measurement.

Arterial blood pressure is the product of cardiac output, systemic vascular resistance, and blood volume. Normal systolic, mean, and diastolic blood pressure are approximately 100 to 160 mm Hg, 80 to 120 mm Hg, and 60 to 100 mm Hg, respectively. Noninvasive methods of measuring blood pressure include ultrasonic Doppler and oscillometric devices.

> **TECHNICIAN NOTE** When taking a blood pressure, the patient should be in lateral recumbency. Place the BP cuff on the down limb as close to the dorsal pedal artery as possible. Record cuff size used to ensure consistent readings.

Central venous pressure (CVP) measures the ability of the heart to pump the quantity of blood returned to it. CVP is also an estimate of the relationship between blood volume and blood volume capacity. Normal CVP ranges between 0 and 10 cm H_2O. A CVP less than 0 suggests that the patient is vasodilated or hypovolemic. A CVP greater than 10 cm H_2O may indicate fluid overload, right heart failure, venoconstriction, cardiac tamponade, presence of pleural effusion, or is indicating the effects of positive pressure ventilation. Central venous pressure, like other hemodynamic markers, can be a useful tool only when used in combination with other parameters to assess the critical patient.

CVP measurements require the placement of a jugular catheter, such that its tip lies in the anterior vena cava; the catheter is then attached to a water manometer or transducer.

PROCEDURE 17-8 Nasal Catheter Placement

Indications
- Hypoxia
- Decrease effort of breathing
- Materials
- Red rubber urinary catheter or 5-F infant feeding tube (for cats and small dogs) or 8-F tube (for medium to large dogs)
- 2% lidocaine
- Lubricating jelly
- Suture material or surgical stapler
- ½-inch tape
- Unheated bubble humidifier
- Extension tubing
- Oxygen source
- Elizabethan collar

Procedure
- Place a few drops of 2% lidocaine in the nostril. Wait 30 to 60 seconds, and repeat.
- Select a catheter of appropriate size. Measure the distance from the tip of the nose to the medial canthus of the eye. Mark the catheter at the tip of the nostril.
- Lubricate the catheter with sterile lubricating jelly. Insert and direct the catheter ventromedially into the nostril until you reach the mark on the catheter.
- The catheter can then be brought out around the alar notch and sutured to the skin at that point (Fig. 1). Position the catheter back over the head, and suture it to the top of the head. Place an Elizabethan collar on the patient.

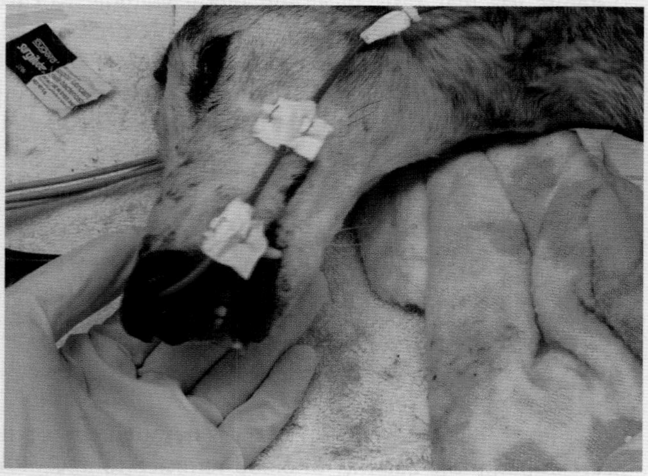

FIGURE 1 Nasal oxygen is a highly effective route for oxygen administration.

Oxygen Administration
- Fill a bubble-through humidifier with sterile water, and attach it to an oxygen source (Fig. 2).
- Attach this to the nasal catheter. (Flow rates of 50 to 200 ml/kg per minute are usually effective in increasing inspired oxygen concentration to 40% or greater. The goal is to see improved mucous membrane color, decreased anxiety, decreased breathing and/or heart rate, decreased magnitude of respiratory distress, and improved PaO_2 or SPO_2 to an acceptable level.)
- A second nasal catheter can be placed if the patient does not respond positively to the oxygen flow. A Y-connector piece can be used and the oxygen flow increased through

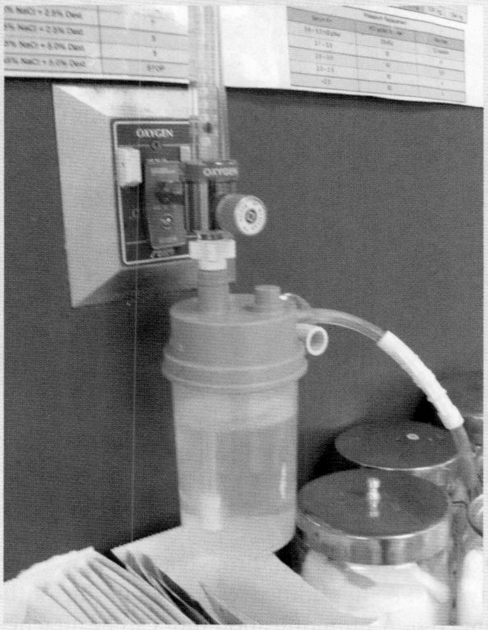

FIGURE 2 Humidification is necessary for nasal oxygen administration to prevent drying of the nasal mucosa.

one single oxygen line (Fig. 3). Nasal-tracheal oxygen may be indicated for patients that do not respond to nasal oxygen, such as the brachycephalic breeds.

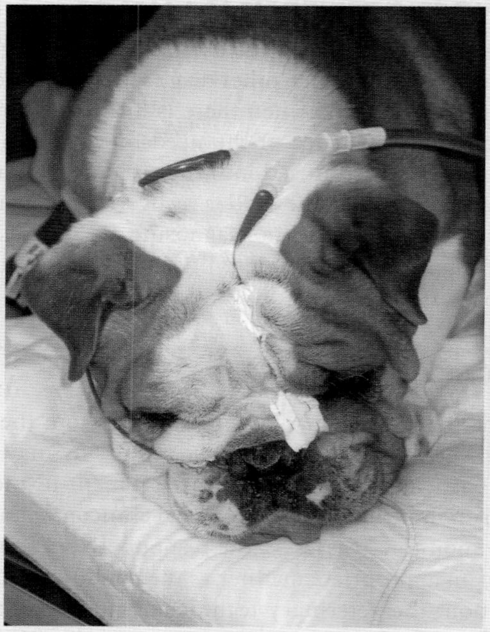

FIGURE 3 Use of a Y-connector piece in order to increase oxygen flow through a single or double nasal catheter.

Complications
- Gastric distension
- Epistaxis
- Serous or mucoid nasal discharge
- Decreased mucus clearance without humidification
- Patient discomfort

PROCEDURE 17-9 Diagnostic Peritoneal Lavage

Indications
- Diagnosis of abdominal hemorrhage, ruptured bowel, peritonitis, and bladder rupture

Materials
- Peritoneal lavage catheter or over-the-needle catheter
- Warm lactated Ringer's or normal saline
- IV administration and/or extension sets
- Surgical kit
- Sterile gloves
- Lab collection tubes
- Clippers
- Surgical prep

Procedure
- After the bladder is emptied, clip and prepare the skin caudal to the umbilicus.
- Infiltrate the skin and abdominal wall with lidocaine.
- Make a small incision through the skin, subcutaneous tissue, and superficial abdominal fascia.
- Insert the catheter through the incision, and direct it caudally and dorsally.
- Infuse 20 ml/kg of warmed lactated Ringer's or normal saline into the abdomen. Gently rock the patient from side to side for a few minutes.
- Collect the fluid aseptically as it flows freely from the catheter; fluid removal may require gentle aspiration.
- Remove the catheter if the fluid is clear; otherwise, suture it in place and use as needed.
- If necessary, perform gross, cytologic, and biochemical analysis on the sample.

Complications
- Infection
- Iatrogenic hemorrhage or viscous perforation

To measure the CVP, it is recommended to place the patient in right lateral recumbency without stressing the patient. The water manometer is then filled three-quarters of the way full. The fluids are then allowed to flow from the manometer into the patient (Fig. 17-28). Small fluctuations in the fluid meniscus synchronous with heart beat and ventilation should be evident. The zero reference point is established by drawing an imaginary horizontal line from the thoracic inlet to the manometer. Once the fluid level stabilizes, the difference between the actual fluid level in the manometer and the zero reference point is the CVP measurement. For example, if the fluid level in the manometer is 12 and the zero reference point is 5, the CVP is 7 cm H_2O. A fluid bag and IV administration set can be used in the absence of a water manometer (Procedure 17-10). CVP trends in response to intravenous fluids are more important than a single number. Methodology should be consistent; it is recommended that the patient be placed in right lateral recumbency and to clearly note on the patient's record the zero reference point.

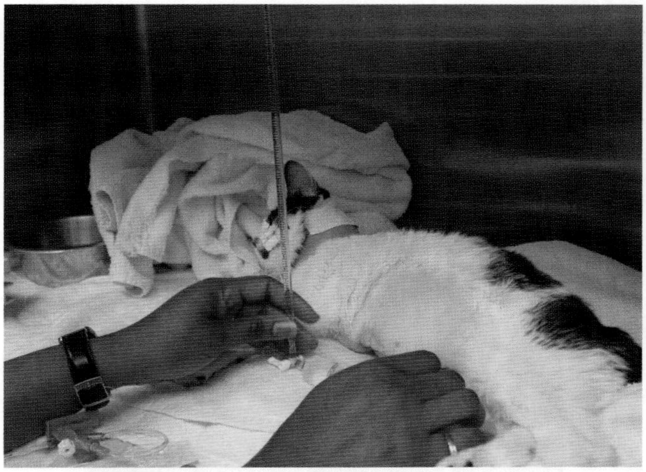

FIGURE 17-28 Measurement of central venous pressure using a manometer.

> **TECHNICIAN NOTE** When measuring CVPs, first ensure the catheter tip is in correct position by taking a lateral radiograph if the patient is stable; otherwise, CVP readings may be inconsistent and provide false data.

Respiratory System

Assessment of the respiratory system includes answering questions such as the following:

- Is the rate increased?
- Is the breathing effort smooth and easy, or labored?
- Is the breathing pattern regular?
- Are you able to auscultate normal breath sounds? Abnormal breath sounds may be described as crackles, wheezes, squeaks, muffled, or quiet.
- Is the patient able to meet its ventilation and oxygenation requirements?

Arterial blood gases (ABG) are an excellent way to assess ventilation and oxygenation. $PaCO_2$ (normal: 35 to 45 mm Hg) tells how well the patient is ventilating. PaO_2 (normal: 80 to 100 mm Hg breathing room air) tells how well the patient is oxygenating. Sometimes arrangements can be made to run ABGs through a local human hospital. Recently new inexpensive portable blood analyzers have been developed (Fig. 17-29). Most blood gas analyzers can also run electrolytes. It is financially and technically feasible for use in private practice. The sample should be collected into a lithium-heparinized syringe, with all visible air expelled from the syringe following sample collection. If the sample is not going to be analyzed immediately, it should be capped and placed on ice until analyzed.

Pulse oximetry is a noninvasive technique that continuously measures arterial oxygen saturation in the blood (normal SpO_2 is greater than 95%). Corrective measures should be undertaken when the SaO_2 is 90% or less. An SaO_2 of 90% equates to a PaO_2 of 60 mm Hg that indicates severe hypoxemia. There are a variety of pulse oximeters that work well in the veterinary patient (Fig. 17-30). The pulse oximeter should never replace a physical exam; always monitor mucous membrane color, respiratory effort, and lung sounds.

PROCEDURE 17-10 Central Venous Pressure Monitoring Using IV Fluid Bag Method

Materials
- Centimeter ruler
- IV fluid line and IV fluid bag

Method
- Place patient in right lateral recumbency (Fig. 1).

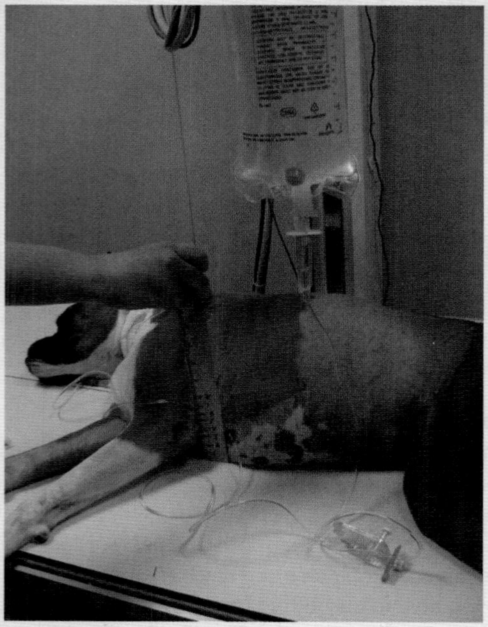

FIGURE 1 Measurement of central venous pressure using a fluid bag.

- Place ruler perpendicular to patient.
- Identify "zero" point on the ruler, typically at the midline.
- Attach IV fluid line to central catheter.
- Open up fluid clamp.
- Lower IV fluid bag until drops stop forming.
- If drip chamber is vented, measure CVP as height from level of right atrium to level of fluid in drip chamber.
- If drip chamber is not vented, CVP is distance from fluid line in IV fluid bag to level of right atrium.
- Subtract zero point on the ruler from the measured number.

TECHNICIAN NOTE Warning! The pulse oximeter measures oxygen saturation and not oxygen content. Pulse oximetry must be used in conjunction with other hemodynamic markers and not used solely to determine a patient's respiratory stability.

Central Nervous System

Assessment of mental status (level of consciousness or LOC) includes observing whether the patient is conscious, unconscious, or somewhere in between. The Modified Glasgow Coma Score (MGCS) can be used in an effort to grade the severity of neurologic injury. The MGCS was developed in 1983 in an effort to monitor patient progress over time by first establishing a baseline, in addition to predicting prognosis (see Table 17-2). A score is given in each of the categories (motor activity, brain stem reflexes, and level of consciousness) and then the scores are totaled. A score of 3 to 8 suggests a grave prognosis; 9 to 14 suggests a guarded prognosis; and 15 to 18 suggests a good prognosis.

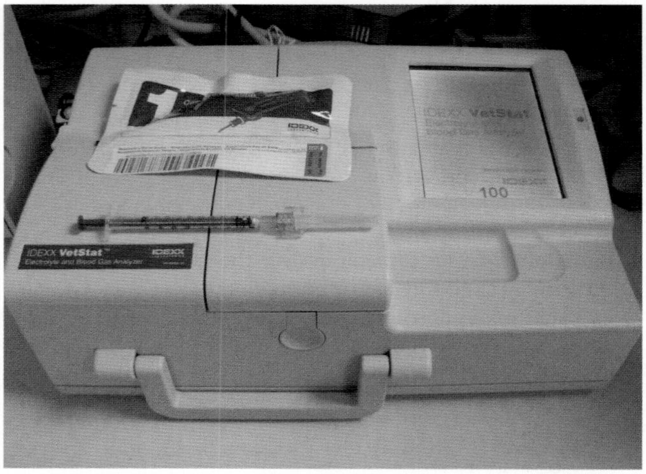

FIGURE 17-29 Blood gas machines are useful in determining oxygen content, acid-base status, and serum electrolytes.

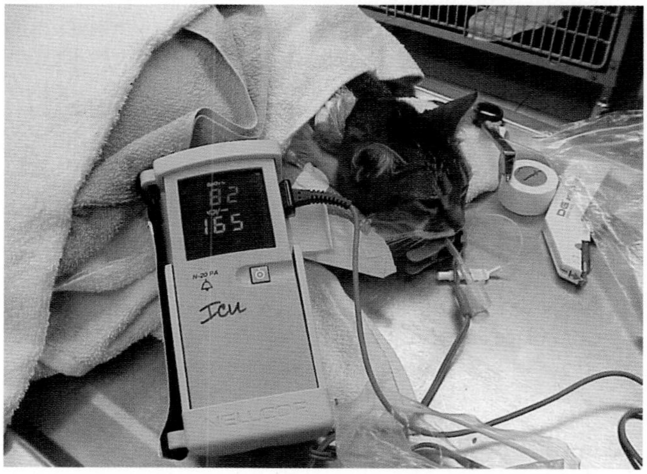

FIGURE 17-30 Pulse oximetry is a noninvasive technique that continuously measures arterial oxygen saturation in the blood.

Patients that are conscious on presentation should be monitored to ensure that their level of consciousness does not change for the worse. Pupils should be equal in size and reactive to light. Pupils are considered abnormal if they show any combination of unresponsiveness, dilation, constriction, or asymmetry in the absence of ocular trauma. Irregular breathing patterns indicate brain stem disease or high cervical trauma. The patient should be observed for abnormal postures such as **opisthotonus.** Patients that are unconscious should be intubated and ventilated immediately. Refer to Chapter 24 for additional nursing care protocols.

TABLE 17-2 Modified Glasgow Coma Scale

MOTOR ACTIVITY	
Normal gait, normal spinal reflexes	6
Hemiparesis, tetraparesis, or decerebrate activity	5
Recumbent, intermittent extensor rigidity	4
Recumbent, constant extensor rigidity	3
Recumbent, constant extensor rigidity with opisthotonus	2
Recumbent, hypotonia of muscles, depressed or absent spinal reflexes	1
LEVEL OF CONSCIOUSNESS	
Occasional periods of alertness and responsive to environment	6
Depression or delirium, capable of responding but response may be inappropriate	5
Semicomatose, responsive to visual stimuli	4
Semicomatose, responsive to auditory stimuli	3
Semicomatose, responsive only to repeated noxious stimuli	2
Comatose, unresponsive to repeated noxious stimuli	1

Fluids In and Fluids Out

Urinary output is a reflection of tissue perfusion. If the kidneys are producing urine, then other organs are probably also being perfused. The normal urinary output is 1 to 2 ml/kg per hour. Ideally, it is important to quantitate the urine output. (Refer to Chapter 16 for additional information on urinary output and patient hydration.)

In addition to quantitation of urine, it is also helpful to quantitate defecation and emesis; this can provide you with a better picture of your total fluid balance. Weight gains and losses should be monitored on a daily basis, as well as frequent auscultation to monitor for fluid overload. Acute changes in weight are usually a result of fluid changes as opposed to muscle mass. Patients receiving large amounts of intravenous crystalloid fluids should be monitored for pitting edema, typically found on the distal limbs. Patients with low albumin are also susceptible to limb edema (Fig. 17-31).

Any fluid loss should be compared to fluid intake; they should just about balance out. Any large discrepancy in the inputs and outputs may be significant.

Temperature

A deep rectal or esophageal thermometer monitors core temperature. Early recognition of hypothermia or hyperthermia and establishing trends in the patient's status are also important. Frequent temperature monitoring is also critical on all patients receiving blood products. Refer to Chapter 24 for temperature monitoring.

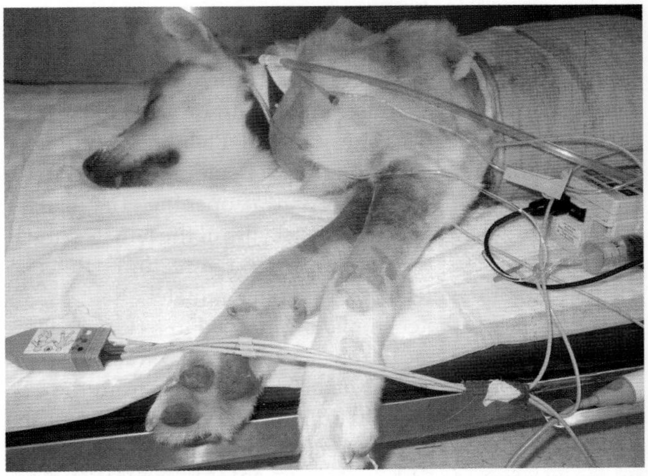

FIGURE 17-31 Pitting edema may be caused by fluid overload and/or low albumin.

Charting

It is important to monitor trends. Use a charting system to help you keep track of the trends. It need not be elaborate, but it should allow you to see all parameters measured.

CRITICAL CARE NURSING PROTOCOLS

Veterinarians and technicians should hold rounds at the beginning of each day or shift. Rounds give you the opportunity to talk about the patients.

The technician should perform a basic physical examination on each patient as soon as possible at the start of the day or shift. This will give you a baseline for comparison regarding the patient's progress throughout the day. In addition to temperature, pulse, and respiration, the lungs should be auscultated, the bladder should be palpated, and mentation should be noted. Also check the operation of all IV and urinary catheters, other monitoring apparatus, and the cleanliness of the patient and bedding.

> *TECHNICIAN NOTE* Discuss the patient's scheduled diagnostic procedures daily with the veterinarian in order to ensure an organized, efficient process.

Check emergency supplies and equipment to be sure that all emergency drugs are present and have not expired, and that the equipment is functional. Pay special attention to airway supplies such as endotracheal tubes and cuffs, suction, and oxygen supply.

IV Catheter Care

IV catheter care should be performed 24 hours or on an as-needed basis. The catheter dressing should be removed and the site inspected. Refer to Chapter 24 for detailed care of all IV catheter types.

Urinary Catheter Care

Urinary catheter care is performed every 8 hours. It entails cleaning the prepuce or vulva and its surrounding area with a mild soap and water rinse. The sheath or vestibule is then flushed with either weak tea-colored Betadine solution or 0.05% chlorhexidine solution. Apply Betadine ointment with a cotton swab to the sheath or vulvar opening. The urinary catheter should be kept clean, especially in the female patient where the catheter is in proximity to the rectum. (Refer to Chapter 24 for detailed care of urinary catheters.)

The urinary catheter should be attached to a closed collection system to decrease the chance of a urinary tract infection (UTI). Do not disconnect the urinary catheter from the collection system. The system is drained every 2 to 4 hours. Urine collection bags may be obtained commercially, or you can use an empty, sterile fluid bag (Fig. 17-32). The addition of 3% hydrogen peroxide to the urinary collection system has been shown to decrease the incidence of UTI. Add 5 to 10 ml of hydrogen peroxide to the urinary collection system to minimize bacterial growth in the collection bag. Hydrogen peroxide is contraindicated when the patient has gross hematuria (blood in the urine). The hydrogen peroxide reacts with the red blood cells causing a gas to form and preventing urine flow.

> TECHNICIAN NOTE When using an IV set attached to a sterile fluid bag, ensure that the roll clamp is taped open to avoid accidental restriction of urine flow.

Respiratory Care

Nebulization therapy is used to promote bronchial drainage with minimal irritation by depositing large quantities of bland substances such as saline. Nebulization promotes bronchial drainage by liquefying thick respiratory secretions. Nebulization can be accomplished by use of ultrasonic or jet (updraft) nebulizers. Ultrasonic nebulizers increase the water content of inspired gas; jet nebulizers either pass a high-velocity gas stream across the top of a capillary tube that is immersed in saline, or pump air through a vapor chamber containing saline. Ultrasonic nebulizers are electrically driven units that convert electric energy into high-frequency vibrations that are, in turn, transmitted to the nebulizer reservoir. A fine, dense, cool fog with a particle size less than 5 microns in diameter is produced. Refer to Chapter 24 for more information on nebulizer therapy.

The latest approach to the management of inflammatory airway disease is via inhalation therapy with metered-dose inhalers, wherein high drug concentrations can be delivered directly to the lungs and subsequently avoid systemic side effects. Administration of medications via metered-dose inhaler (MDI) is now commonplace in the treatment of human asthma and appears beneficial in the management of veterinary patients (e.g., feline asthma).

Coupage is a technique that may be used in conjunction with nebulization to promote removal of respiratory secretions. The patient should always be in sternal recumbency if possible to avoid choking on pulmonary excretions. The hands should be slightly cupped with the fingers and thumbs together. In this position, the hands are placed on the chest wall, clapping the chest wall over the involved lung. Coupage is delivered primarily by flexion and extension of the wrist and elbows. Coupage should be maintained for 3 to 5 minutes in a steady even fashion. (Refer to Chapter 24 for detailed therapy.)

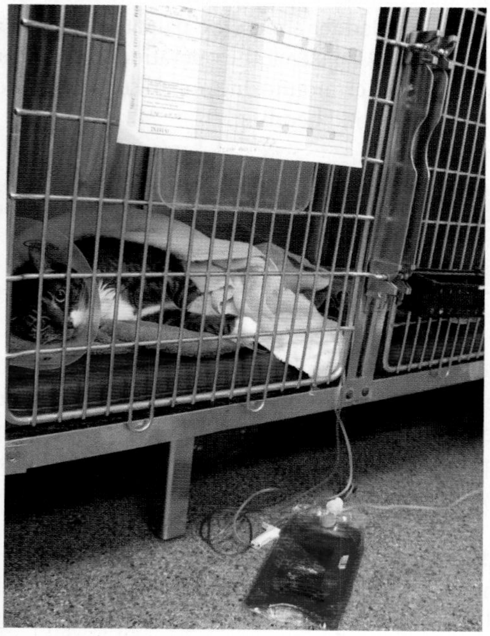

FIGURE 17-32 Tape clamp open to prevent accidental occlusion when using IV fluid sets as collection systems.

Blood Transfusion

Transfusions with whole blood or its components are indicated in acute blood loss, chronic anemia, thrombocytopenia, hypoproteinemia, and coagulopathies. Transfusions are not an innocuous procedure; there are several complications that can occur. The patient may be subject to either an immune-mediated reaction or a nonimmune-mediated reaction. Refer to Chapter 16 for additional blood transfusion therapy techniques.

Monitoring the patient during a blood transfusion is crucial. A baseline TPR should be obtained and the patient should be NPO during the transfusion. Whole blood or its components is usually administered at a rate of about 5 to 10 ml/kg/hr but may be administered much faster in severely hypovolemic patients. The first hour of the transfusion should be given at half of the desired rate. This will allow for observation of incompatibility reactions. If no problems occur during this test period, the rate of the transfusion may be increased to the desired rate. The drip rate should be checked frequently; intravenous fluids pumps are recommended over gravity drip infusions in order to control the administration rate more accurately. The intravenous fluid pump should not be a "through the door" pump where the fluid line is crushed or compressed. Refrigerated blood has a high viscosity and will infuse slower. All blood products should have a blood filter as close to the IV catheter as possible, in order to prevent clots from being infused into the patient. The patient should be observed continuously for a transfusion reaction and the TPR performed hourly. The earlier a reaction occurs in the transfusion, the more severe the reaction. In the event of a mild reaction (vomiting, fever, restlessness), the transfusion should be slowed down. Antihistamines, steroids, and supportive care may be indicated. With severe reactions, the blood transfusion should be stopped.

Care of the Recumbent Patient

Patients suffering neurological, orthopedic, or traumatic problems can be recumbent for prolonged periods of time. The recumbent patient should be turned every 2 to 4 hours. Turning the patient prevents the formation of decubital ulcers and atelectasis of the lungs. Refer to Chapter 24 for detailed care of the recumbent patient.

Nosocomial Infection

Nosocomial infections are hospital-acquired infections. Factors that predispose a patient to a hospital-acquired infection include age (geriatric or neonate), immunosuppression, diagnostic and therapeutic invasive procedures, antimicrobial therapy, and long-term hospitalization. Examples of nosocomial infections include *Escherichia coli, Klebsiella, Salmonella,* canine parvovirus, and feline panleukopenia.

Ways to help reduce the chance of hospital-acquired infection include the following:

- Diligent handwashing by staff before handling medications, fluids, and IV lines, and between patients
- Swabbing injection ports with alcohol before administering IV medication
- Use of disposable thermometer sheaths
- Disinfection of patient care equipment (clipper blades, ECG leads and clips, endotracheal tubes, and breathing circuits)
- Disinfection of environmental surfaces
- Aseptic technique in catheter/tube placements (IV, urinary, and chest)
- Treating patients with known infections last when doing treatment rounds

Patient's Mental Well-Being

Take the time to make friends with the patient before treatment (poking, sticking, and prodding). This may set the tone for further encounters. It is helpful to talk and pet the patient when treatments are not due. Then the patient will not assume that every time you open the cage door it means poking and prodding.

Taking a patient out on a walk can do a lot to lift its spirits. Because many dogs do not like to urinate in their cage, this will give them the opportunity to urinate outdoors. With cats, try to position their cage near a window so they can get some sun.

It is important for patients to have time to rest. In a 24-hour ICU, a patient may have treatments every hour. If at all possible, treatments should be grouped so that the patient has some time to rest. During slow periods in the ICU, dim the overhead lights to induce a more peaceful, quiet environment.

If a patient will not eat, it may be helpful to find out what the patient likes to eat normally. Also, it may be helpful to find out what time the patient eats when at home.

SUMMARY

Veterinary technicians will find that the responsibilities in emergency and critical care nursing are challenging and diverse. The technician must have a thorough understanding of emergency conditions to better meet the needs of the patient. The technician is the vital link between the veterinarian and the patient. Competent nursing care will increase the odds for patient recovery.

REVIEW QUESTIONS

Matching—Clinical Signs of Disease

Match the clinical signs from Column A with the correct disease in Column B.

Column A	Column B
___1. ascites, jugular distension	A. acute renal failure
___2. lethargy, vomiting, anuria	B. left-sided congestive heart failure
___3. cough, dyspnea	C. saddle thrombus
___4. pulselessness, paresis	D. right-sided congestive heart failure

Matching—Procedure Indications

Match the procedure needed to be performed in Column A with clinical signs in Column B.

Column A	Column B
___1. central venous pressure	a. muffled heart sounds, poor pulse quality, tachycardia
___2. pericardiocentesis	b. severe abdominal pain in a patient with pancreatitis
___3. Diagnostic peritoneal lavage	c. pulmonary crackles in a patient in renal failure

Fill in the Blank

Choose from the following list of words to supply answers to the statements below.

Dyspnea	Sterile	Nebulization	ACTH stimulation	thoracocentesis	hyperkalemia
Hypoxemia	fluid	brain stem	pulse oximetry		

1. Indications for oxygen administration include_____, or a $PaO_2 < 60$ mm Hg.
2. ___________ is a simple, useful procedure for collection of pleural fluid to obtain samples for diagnostic evaluation or for alleviation of respiratory distress.
3. ______ technique is indicated to prevent nosocomial infection in all invasive procedures.
4. Clinical signs of hypoxia include cyanosis, tachycardia, and ____________.
5. Diagnosis of hypoadrenocorticism is typically by an __________ test.
6. __________is a common sequela to urinary obstruction.
7. __________promotes bronchial drainage by liquefying thick respiratory secretions.
8. Acute changes in weight are usually a result of_____ changes as opposed to muscle mass variations.
9. Irregular breathing patterns may indicate _____ disease or high cervical trauma.
10. _______is a noninvasive technique that continuously measures arterial oxygen saturation in the blood.

RECOMMENDED READING

Battaglia A, Steele A, editors: *Small animal emergency and critical care*, ed 3, St Louis, 2015, Saunders.

Dewey C: *Canine and feline neurology*, ed 2, Ames, IA, 2008, Wiley-Blackwell.

Macintire DK: *Manual of small animal emergency and critical care medicine*, Philadelphia, 2005, Lippincott Williams and Wilkins.

Matthews KA: *Veterinary emergency and critical care manual*, Guelph, Ontario, Canada, 2006, Lifelearn Publication.

Murtaugh RJ, editor: *Quick look series in veterinary medicine: critical care*, Jackson Hole, WY, 2002, Teton NewMedia.

Plunkett SJ: *Emergency procedures for the small animal veterinarian*, ed 3, St Louis, 2012, Saunders.

Veterinary Emergency and Critical Care Society: Reassessment campaign on veterinary resuscitation, *evidence and knowledge gap analysis on veterinary CPR (special issue)* 22(s1):S1–S131, 2012.

Winfield WE, Raffe MR, editors: *The veterinary ICU book*, Jackson Hole, WY, 2002, Teton NewMedia.

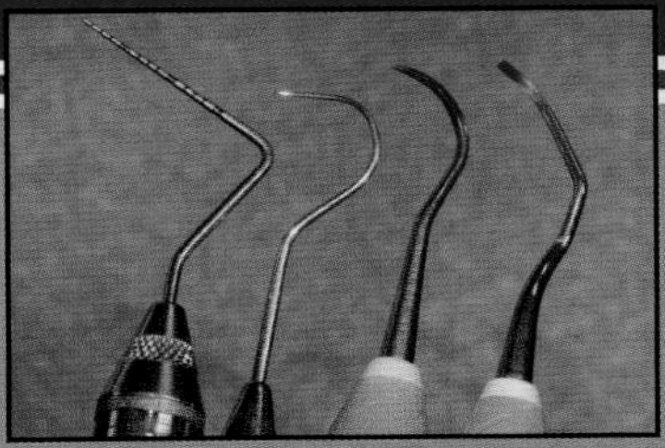

18 Small Animal Dentistry

OUTLINE

LEARNING OBJECTIVES

After reviewing the following chapter, the reader will be able to:

1. Describe the normal anatomy of a tooth and the surrounding structures.
2. List the dental formulas of companion animals.
3. List and describe the instruments and equipment used during a routine dental prophylaxis.
4. List and discuss the steps involved with a dental prophylaxis.
5. Differentiate between the most common charting systems.
6. Describe procedures used in basic dental radiology.
7. Discuss common dental care home care products.

KEY TERMS

Alphanumeric system
Bisecting angle technique
Brachycephalic
Brachygnathism
Buccal
Calculus
Cementoenamel junction
Cementum
Crossbite
Crown
Deciduous teeth
Delta foramina
Dentin
Dolichocephalic
Enamel
Furcation
Gingival margin
Gingival sulcus
Gingivitis
Mesaticephalic
Mucogingival line
Occlusion
Parallel technique
Periodontal ligament
Periodontium
Periodontitis
Plaque
Prophylaxis
Prognathism, maxillary
Pulp cavity
Rete pegs
Rostral
Subgingival
Supragingival
Triadan charting system
Wry bite

Dentistry can be one of the most rewarding areas of veterinary medicine for technicians, and the benefits to the practice and patients are numerous. A veterinary practice that invests in the training of staff and in good quality equipment can see a profitable return quickly. A patient that receives a good quality cleaning and a home care program will stay healthier. Owners can play an active role in their pets' health and by keeping their pets healthier, they will have them in their lives longer. The veterinary technician becomes even more valuable to the practice when knowledgeable and skilled at dentistry. Veterinary technicians receive instant gratification from dentistry. They see the patient's mouth before and after. It is usually very obvious that you have made a difference and helped the patient.

ORAL ANATOMY

Before a dental cleaning can be done, the dental technician will need to be familiar with oral anatomy. The oral cavity consists of the teeth, tongue, cheek and lip area, gingival and mucosa, palates, and the face. As with physical examinations, it is important to develop a pattern when performing a dental examination. Begin by looking at the patient's face. Look for eye and nasal discharge. Lacrimal glands and the nasal cavity can drain into the oral cavity. Infections, fistulas, or foreign bodies may cause a blockage or drainage from these areas. Look for any swelling. Abscessed roots, especially the fourth upper premolars, may be seen as lumps on the face. The shape of the head may be noted and bite can be recorded. There are common malocclusions and tooth conditions associated with different head shapes and bites.

SKULL TYPES AND MALOCCLUSIONS

There are three recognized skull types in dogs and cats (Table 18-1). By recognizing these types, you can identify the problems that are inherent with their dentition and ideally pretreat them (Table 18-2).

Mesaticephalic

Mesaticephalic is the most common skull type. Poodles, Labradors, and shorthair cats best illustrate this skull type. One problem seen in the toy breeds is loose incisors. This is because of the fact that there is less bone in the **rostral** jaw because of the small size of the mouth. Thus gingival recession, tooth mobility, and the potential for fractured jaws occur more quickly in these breeds.

TABLE 18-1 Skull Types

TYPE	DESCRIPTION	BREED EXAMPLES
Mesaticephalic	Muzzle is a medium length and width	Poodles, Labradors, Shorthair Cats
Dolichocephalic	Muzzle is long and narrow	Collies, Greyhounds
Brachycephalic	Muzzle is short and wide	Boxers, Pugs, Persians

Brachycephalic

Boxers, Pugs, and Persian cats best illustrate the **brachycephalic** skull type. They have short, wide heads that lead to increased tooth crowding, causing the teeth to rotate or overlap. This in turn causes a higher incidence of periodontal disease.

Dolichocephalic

The long, narrow skulls of the Collie and Greyhound best illustrate the **dolichocephalic** skull type. The genetic abnormality called posterior **crossbite** can be found in these breeds. Performing a routine cleaning on their teeth often seems endless because of the length of the jaw.

It is important to check the bite status of your patient before administering anesthesia because the placement of an endotracheal tube will prevent you from evaluating the bite once the tube is placed.

VISUAL ORAL ANATOMY

Some patients may be experiencing mouth pain or dislike having their mouth handled. Lift up the lip area on one side then the other. You will be able to visualize the outside area of the teeth. Be sure to pull back on the lip to see the molars and caudal premolars. When you open the patient's mouth, look at the inside of the teeth, the palates, tongue, and the caudal oral cavity. If you are able to, look under the patient's tongue (Fig. 18-1). Record your findings. This is a brief oral examination; a thorough examination will be done under anesthesia and your findings charted.

As with every other body system, it is essential to know the normal anatomic structures of the oral cavity and how they function. Knowing this, one can determine whether a certain condition is abnormal and if further assessment is necessary.

TOOTH ANATOMY

Teeth are the primary functional structures of the oral cavity. A mature tooth can be divided into the exposed **crown** and the submerged root portions that join at the neck of the tooth (**cementoenamel junction,** or CEJ) (Fig. 18-2).

TABLE 18-2 Common Occlusal Abnormalities

ABNORMALITY	DESCRIPTION
Maxillary Prognathism (Overbite)	Maxillary arcade is longer than the mandibular arcade
Maxillary Brachygnathism (Underbite)	Mandibular arcade is longer than the maxillary arcade
Anterior Crossbite	Maxillary incisors are caudal to mandibular incisors
Posterior Crossbite	Mandible is wider than the maxilla
Wry bite	Right and left, mandible and maxilla are different lengths and widths
Base Narrow/Wide Canines	When the angle of the canine growth is directed inward (narrow) or outward (wide) from a normal occlusion

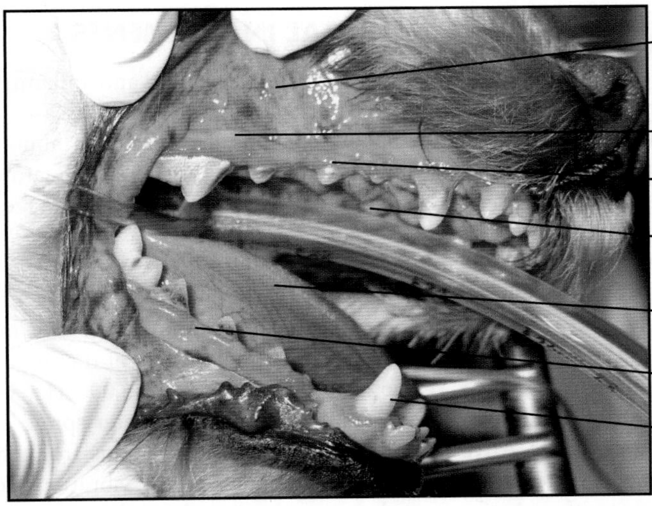

FIGURE 18-1 Gingival and mucosal areas of the mouth. (Photo courtesy Coleen Johnston, DVM.)

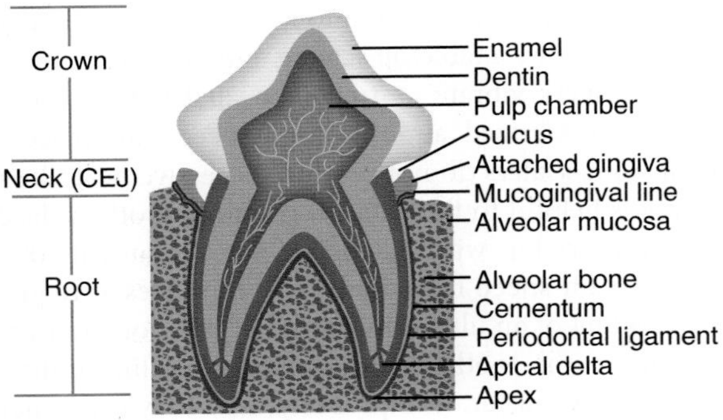

FIGURE 18-2 Dental anatomy and supporting structures.

The **enamel** covering of the crown is the hardest substance in the body (96% inorganic) and is made of hydroxyapatite crystals. A layer of **cementum** covers the root. Cementum is closer in composition (45% to 50% inorganic) to bone than enamel. Because cementoblasts also participate in the initial formation of cementum, cementum also regenerates, unlike enamel. Underlying the enamel and cementum for the entire length of the tooth is a layer of **dentin** (70% inorganic, 30% organic collagen fibers and water). Although the dentin layer is very thin in immature teeth, odontoblasts from pulpal tissue continue to manufacture dentin in a tubular pattern throughout the life of the tooth. This makes the dentinal walls progressively thicker and the canal space of the tooth narrower as the tooth matures.

PERIODONTIUM

The supporting structure around the teeth, or **periodontium,** maintains the stability of the teeth in the oral cavity. The periodontium includes the gingiva, the cementum of the root, the **periodontal ligament** (goes from the cementum to the alveolar socket), and the alveolar bone or socket. The mandible and maxilla have a series of depressions, or sockets, in the alveolar ridge to house the root structures. The periodontal ligament stabilizes the tooth within the socket and absorbs some of the shock of the occlusal forces generated during chewing. The cementum must remain healthy to maintain attachment of the periodontal ligament to the tooth. Covering all of these structures is the gingival mucosa.

The specialized tissue of the attached gingiva immediately adjacent to the tooth structure provides the first line of defense against bacteria for the rest of the periodontium. The attached gingiva is histologically different from the looser alveolar mucosa. Interdigitations of connective tissue (**rete pegs**) provide firm attachment to the underlying periosteum of the alveolar bone. Without this specialized keratinized epithelium, bacteria can readily attack the underlying periodontal ligament and bone. A minimum of 1 to 2 mm of attached gingiva is necessary to provide this protection and can be measured from the **mucogingival line** that delineates its connection to the alveolar mucosa. This mucogingival line is most readily apparent on the facial or **buccal** surfaces of the teeth.

The free edge, or **gingival margin,** of this epithelial collar is often not directly attached to the tooth, although it can be very close to the teeth in a cat's mouth. The space between the tooth and the free gingiva is termed the **gingival sulcus.** At the depth of the sulcus, the junctional epithelium attaches to the tooth. A sulcus depth of up to about 2 to 3 mm is considered normal in dogs (depending on patient size); sulcus depth should not be more than 0.5 to 1.0 mm in cats without a concurrent disease process. Any variation in sulcus pocket depth should alert the technician to potential problems (see Periodontal Disease section).

The internal canal space surrounded and protected by the dentin is called the **pulp cavity** for the entire tooth; the pulp chamber, including pulpal horns, for the crown; and the root canal for the root. This internal space, or pulp cavity, houses the blood vessels, nerves, and connective tissue that serve the tooth. These pulpal structures enter the tooth in small animals at the apical, or root tip end, often through the **delta foramina** or apical delta, a formation with many small openings. These pulpal tissues provide oxygen and nutrients through the blood vessels, contain cells instrumental in laying down and removing dentin (odontoblasts and odontoclasts), and have nerves to conduct impulses in response to various stimuli. The junction where multiple roots join the neck of the tooth is known as the **furcation.**

Although teeth can sense a variety of stimuli from cold to heat (depending on the health or sensitivity of the teeth) and pressure, the animal only feels the sense of pain. This is a good defense mechanism, because if a tooth is compromised to the extent that it is sensitive to cold or heat, the resulting pain may alert a client to the denture problem.

Both **deciduous** (primary) and permanent (adult) teeth arise from a ridge of dental laminar epithelium. In a young animal with deciduous teeth, the permanent tooth buds are located adjacent to them underneath the gingiva (gum). Any stimulus, from generalized infection (distemper) or fever to a local infection from an abscessed deciduous tooth, can affect development of the permanent tooth, much like a developing fetus in the uterus. Deciduous teeth are often shed in sequence as the permanent teeth erupt. This sequence can be influenced by many factors, including genetics, nutrition, and trauma. If a deciduous tooth is still present when a permanent tooth is erupting, the deciduous tooth should be carefully extracted to avoid deflection of the adult tooth into an abnormal position.

DENTAL FORMULAS

A dental formula (Table 18-3) is a way of expressing the normal number and arrangement of deciduous and permanent teeth in a species. By knowing the dental formula for a species, you can determine when there are an inappropriate number of teeth or a variation in tooth eruption times.

TABLE 18-3 Dental Formulas for Cats and Dogs

CATS		
Deciduous	I3/3, C1/1, P3/2	= 26 teeth
Permanent	I3/3, C1/1, P3/2, M1/1	= 30 teeth
TIME OF ERUPTION		
	DECIDUOUS:	***PERMANENT:***
Incisors	2 to 3 weeks	3 to 4 months
Canines	3 to 4 weeks	4 to 5 months
Premolars	3 to 6 weeks	4 to 6 months
Molars		4 to 6 months
DOGS		
Deciduous	I3/3, C1/1, P3/3	= 28 teeth
Permanent	I3/3, C1/1, P4/4, M2/3	= 42 teeth
TIME OF ERUPTION		
	DECIDUOUS:	***PERMANENT:***
Incisors	2 to 3 weeks	3 to 4 months
Canines	3 to 4 weeks	4 to 5 months
Premolars	3 to 6 weeks	4 to 6 months
Molars		4 to 6 months

DENTAL INSTRUMENTS

Although antibiotics and anti-inflammatory drugs have their place in treating periodontal disease, mechanical removal of plaque, calculus, bacteria, and abnormal tissue with dental instruments is the focus of treatment. A wide variety of equipment is available to help manage periodontal disease.

POWER SCALING UNITS

The most commonly used scaling unit in veterinary dentistry is the ultrasonic scaler. The magnetostrictive scaler works through vibrations of the metal stacks that cause the tip to rotate at around 45,000 Hz, with continuous emission of an aerosolizing water spray. This vibration helps to remove the tartar or calculus from the teeth. Piezoelectric ultrasonic scalers use the vibrations generated from electrical current running through a quartz crystal. Newer ceramic models show promise with potentially less damage, but these are more expensive. Ultrasonic scalers produce heat, and a constant water flow is essential to keep the instrument cool. Figure 18-3 shows a tabletop scaling and polishing unit.

Sonic scalers vibrate at 16,000 to 20,000 Hz generated from the pressurized air of a high-speed handpiece. Although sonic scalers do not produce excessive heat, the water spray is helpful to flush debris from the tooth surface. A soft steel rotary bur with six cutting flutes rotates at 300,000 rpm on a high-speed handpiece. This produces a frequency similar to that of an ultrasonic unit, but it is potentially very damaging to the tooth. Although power scaling units can quickly remove tartar, if improperly used they can generate excessive heat, even with adequate water flow, and can damage the tooth structure inadvertently (Fig. 18-4).

HAND-SCALING INSTRUMENTS

Although power equipment is certainly faster, at times hand-scaling instruments may be a better choice. The dental technician will find it necessary to know what the basic hand instruments are and how to use them (Table 18-4). Hand instruments used for scaling include scalers and

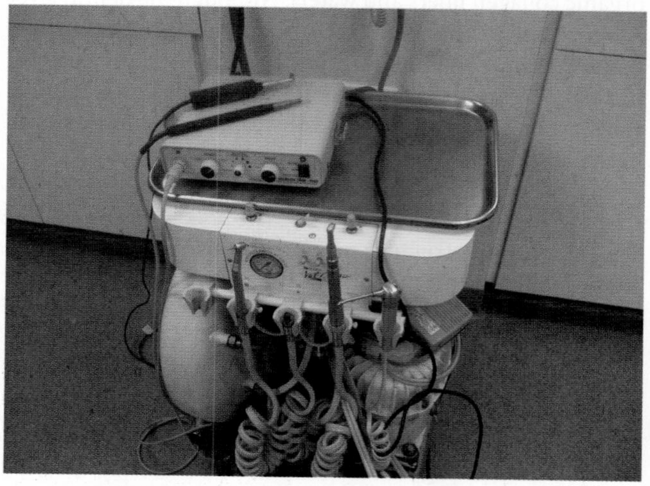

FIGURE 18-3 Tabletop scaler and polishing unit.

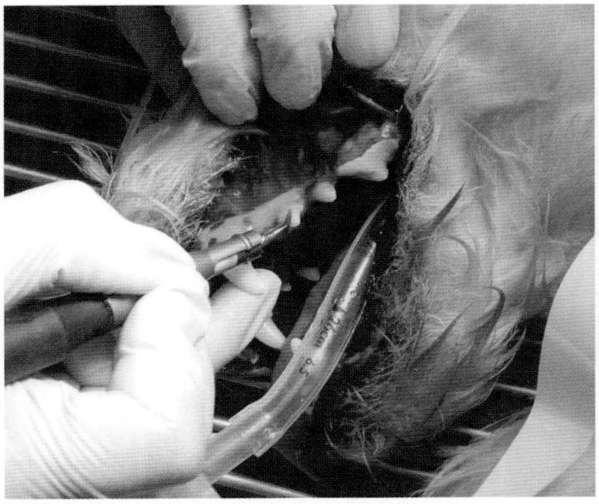

FIGURE 18-4 Proper handling of ultrasonic scaler.

TABLE 18-4	Hand Instruments
INSTRUMENT	**USES**
Scaler	Used to remove calculus and plaque from the surface of the crown of the tooth. Supragingival use only.
Curette	Used to remove subgingival deposits from the root surface and debride tissue lining
Probe	A measuring device used to assess the tooth and its surrounding anatomy
Explorer	Used to detect softened areas and defects in the enamel
Calculus forceps	Used to remove heavy calculus from the surface of the tooth
Extraction forceps	Used to grasp the tooth and extract it from the socket
Elevators	Used to elevate the root of the tooth from the periodontal ligament

curettes (Fig. 18-5). Although hand-scaling instruments are available in various types, the most typical form is a sickle scaler. These instruments, with their sharp tip and triangular cross-section, can be used to scale calculus off the crown of the tooth. Sickle scalers should never be used subgingivally because of the potential for gum damage.

The instrument of choice for removing **subgingival** deposits is the curette, with rounded toe and back. With small to moderate subgingival pockets less than 5 mm deep, the curette can be gently introduced into the pocket and used to scale the root surface and debride the lining of the soft tissue.

The working end of scalers and curettes must be sharpened after every use; dull instruments only burnish the calculus instead of removing it. Although the face of the instrument can be sharpened with a conical sharpening stone, it is usually best to use an oiled flat stone, drawing the working edge across at a 110-degree angle to approximate the angle of the head.

Other hand instruments that are essential in evaluation of periodontal disease are periodontal explorers and probes. A periodontal explorer has a sharp, thin tip, often curved into a "shepherd's crook." This tactile instrument is used in human dentistry to detect softened areas of enamel that are starting to decay. Carious lesions are not as common in dogs and cats because of fewer occlusal surfaces in the mouth. The instrument is used to detect roughened areas or residual calculus on the tooth surface; resorptive areas (feline or canine odontoclastic resorptive lesions called CORLS or FORLS); and open canals in broken teeth.

The periodontal probe is an even more important tool in assessment of periodontal disease. Probes are marked in varying millimeter increments, with either notches or color changes on the working end, which can be round or flat. A probe can be gently introduced into the gingival sulcus to determine the depth of any pocket (Fig. 18-6). Measurements at up to six sites around a tooth's circumference give an indication of any increased pocket depth, which can then

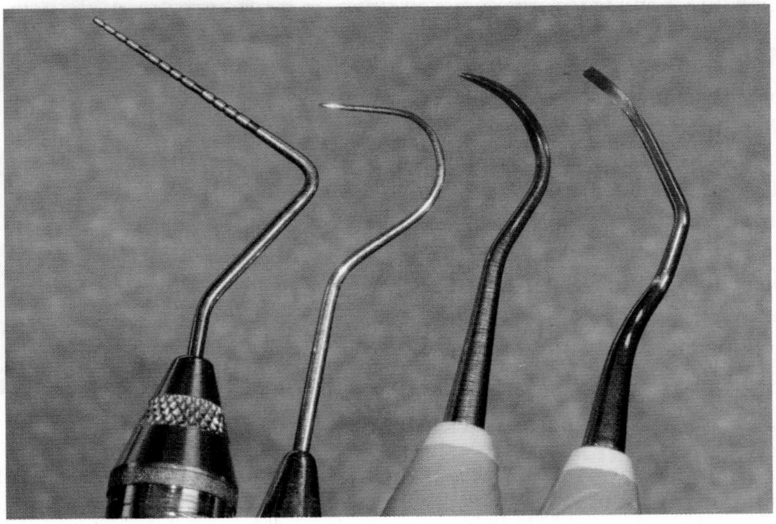

FIGURE 18-5 Hand instruments. Periodontal probe, Shepherd's hook, scaler, and curette. (From Holmstrom SE: *Veterinary dentistry: a team approach*, ed 2, St Louis, 2013, Saunders.)

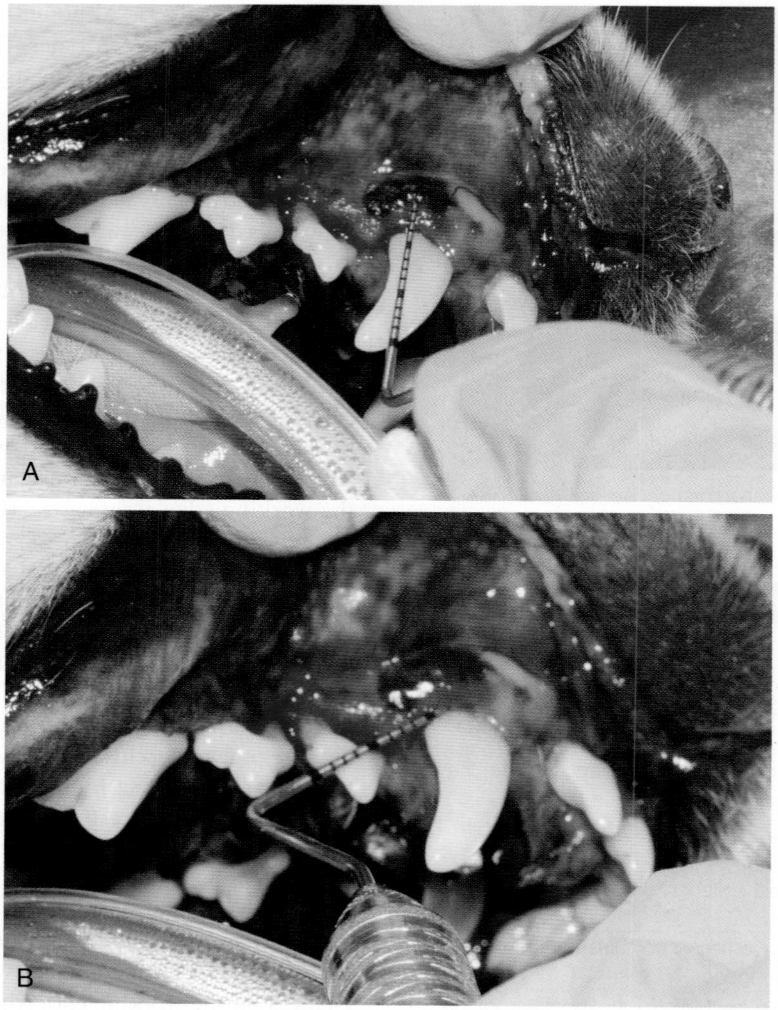

FIGURE 18-6 Probing a canine tooth. (From Holmstrom SE: *Veterinary dentistry: a team approach,* ed 2, St Louis, 2013, Saunders.)

be noted on the record. Careful attention should be made to place this tool gently into the sulcus as the operator can create a "pocket" if too much pressure is applied.

POLISHING EQUIPMENT

Polishing equipment is another essential tool in treatment of periodontal disease (Fig. 18-7). Scaling roughens the enamel surface of a tooth; this must be polished to produce a smooth surface that slows accumulation of plaque. Battery-operated polishing instruments can be used, but these typically do not last long. Rotary hand tools (Dremel-type) can be used to power the polishing handpiece, but rotational speed must be controllable and maintained at less than 3000 rpm. Micromotor units often have the option of using a prophy angle, or the slow-speed handpiece of an air-driven unit can be used.

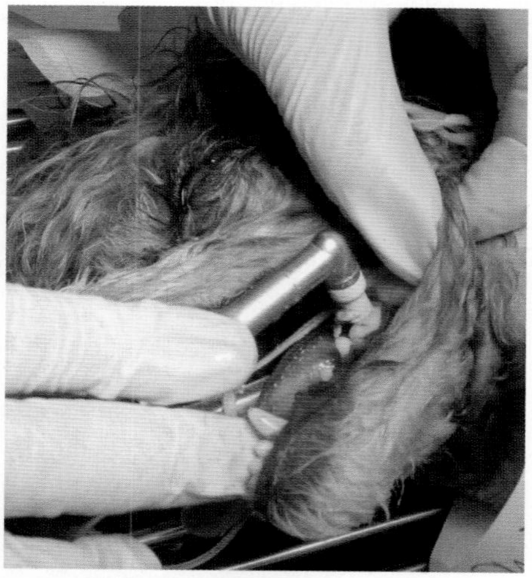

FIGURE 18-7 Polishing a tooth.

PREPARATION FOR DENTAL PROCEDURES

Before anesthesia can be administered and a dental cleaning can begin, the patient should be given a complete physical examination. This allows for the opportunity to repeat any lab work, address any additional issues that may be found, and record a starting set of values for monitoring anesthesia. This is a good time to take a photo of the patient's mouth. Photos are a good way to document the condition of the patient's oral condition both before and after the dental prophylaxis.

ANESTHESIA AND PAIN MANAGEMENT

Preparation of your patient before beginning the dental prophylaxis can make the difference between a successful dental and an unsuccessful dental (Box 18-1). Anesthesia is required for proper dental cleaning. The length of time a patient is under anesthesia can vary greatly during a dental procedure. The condition of a patient may determine if a dental procedure can be completed or if the patient will have to undergo anesthesia a second time. Body temperature can greatly affect the body's response to anesthesia; warming your patient is of the utmost importance. This can be done several different ways. There are forced warm air devices, towels or blankets, IV fluid warmers, warm water bottles, and circulating water pads. All warming methods have positive and negative aspects. Caution should be used with any warming method. It is possible to overheat or burn a patient. If a patient has a low body temperature before anesthesia, the veterinarian may request that you begin warming the patient ahead of time. This may include using a heat lamp or warm water bottles. Extra care should be given to keeping a patient dry. A wet pet can become cold quickly and will contribute to burning a patient if a warming device should come in contact with the wet area. Placing an intravenous catheter in all patients that will receive anesthesia can serve three main purposes. The first is venous access if an anesthetic emergency should occur. During an emergency every second counts. The next is to allow the patient to receive intravenous fluids. A patient that is receiving anesthesia has not been able to eat or drink for several hours and may become slightly dehydrated. Some anesthetics may cause an initial drop in blood pressure upon induction and fluids will help to correct this. Many patients undergoing anesthesia for a dental prophylaxis are older and many have health concerns. An older patient's liver, kidney, heart, and endocrine system may be compromised and therefore have a difficult time eliminating the anesthesia from the body. Intravenous fluids will rehydrate and ease the burden on these body systems. By metabolizing and eliminating the anesthesia more quickly from the body, recovery may be a smoother process.

Pain management is an important component to consider for the dental patient. Preemptive analgesia is ideal, although it will not substitute for post-procedure pain management. There are a variety of methods that can be used for analgesia. Many clinicians prefer to administer local anesthetics to block pain prior to performing dental procedures and will often also include an opioid medication as part of the premedication before anesthesia. Nonsteroidal anti-inflammatory medications can be administered post-procedure and additional local anesthesia can be administered at the end of the procedure to provide continuing pain management during recovery.

EQUIPMENT SETUP

Any patient that has anesthesia administered will require monitoring. Monitoring your patient will depend greatly on the type of equipment your hospital possesses. Veterinarians are beginning to invest in equipment that keeps track of everything from heart rate to blood pressures. These monitoring devices add a secondary level of safety, especially if you are responsible for monitoring your patient, as well as completing the dental prophylaxis. If your clinic does not possess a monitor, most parameters can be evaluated with a stethoscope and a thermometer. It is vital that you monitor your patient.

Prepare your anesthesia and dental equipment ahead of time. Be sure to perform a safety check of your anesthesia machine and leak test the endotracheal tubes ahead of time. It is equally as important as testing your dental equipment. Hand instruments should be laid out. Dental packs can be prepared ahead of time and should include a probe and explorer, a curette, a hand scaler, tartar removal forceps, and the ultrasonic scaling tip. These packs can usually be autoclaved but it is recommended to follow the manufacturer's recommendations. There should be one pack per patient. The number of extraction packs will vary depending on the number of procedures performed each day. A minimum of two extraction packs should exist. If the need arises for more extraction packs, the used packs may be "flash" sterilized between patients.

BOX 18-1 Pre-Dental Procedure Checklist

Patient Preparation

Preanesthetic examination
Pre-dental photo
Place camera nearby for any photographs during and post dental
Preanesthetic diagnostic and lab work
Preanesthetic patient preparation
Intravenous catheter
Intravenous fluids
Warm patient

Equipment Preparation

Safety check the anesthetic machine
Test the ultrasonic scaler, the drill, the water/air pic
Lay out the necessary number of dental packs
Prepare dental radiographic supplies
Enter the patient's information into the computer for digital dental systems

Dental Accessories

Suture and blade
Gauze and cotton tip applicator
Disclosing liquid
Fluoride
Prophy paste
Prophy cups for each patient
Oravet
Water rinse
Chlorhexidine rinse
Charting supplies

Personal Protective Equipment

Mask
Gloves
Splash goggles or face shield

Lay out your work area with other necessary dental accessories (Fig. 18-8). Items include:

- Absorbable suture for extraction site closure and a surgical blade if the veterinarian would need to perform a gingivectomy or make a gingival flap for easier extraction site closure.
- Gauze and cotton-tipped applicators for drying the mouth if necessary and holding the tongue for intubation.
- Prophy paste for polishing the teeth after scaling. If your hospital uses disposable prophy angles, a new one should be used for each patient.
- Some hospitals use disclosing liquid on their patients after scaling to look for any remaining plaque that may have been missed.
- A fluoride gel or foam should be used if the water in your area is not supplemented. The fluoride should be allowed to stay in contact with the teeth for 1 to 4 minutes depending on the manufacturer's recommendations.
- Water and a chlorhexidine rinse in a bottle that allows you to flush or rinse the patient's mouth
- Oravet.
- Place your chart on a clipboard with a working pen.
- A camera can be used to document pre-dental cleaning and post-dental cleaning condition of the teeth (Fig. 18-9). These can be shown to the owner at the time the patient goes home.

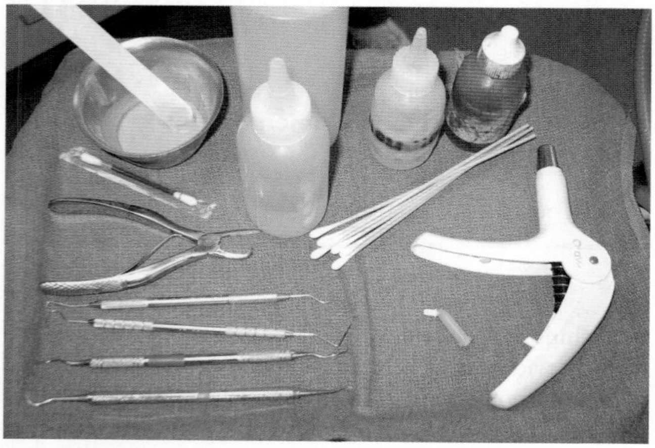

FIGURE 18-8 Pre-dental instrument setup. (Photo courtesy of Coleen Johnston, DVM.)

PERSONAL PROTECTIVE EQUIPMENT

The dental technician will need to prepare the necessary PPE (personnel protective equipment) (Fig. 18-10). It is required that the dental technician wears gloves, splash goggles or face shield, and a mask. Choose gloves that fit your hands to allow you to feel the tooth or gingival and allow you to easily handle the equipment. During a dental cleaning, plaque and calculus are aerosolized. This plaque and calculus contains bacteria. Your mask will prevent you from breathing in the bacteria. Your eyes are equally at risk from the bacteria, and splash goggles or a face shield will protect you. Eye protection will protect you from any flying debris. Safety glasses and prescription glasses are not acceptable for eye protection because they will not protect you from water, which may spray around your face. Ergonomics have played a large part in the comfort level of the technician. Many dental stations are set up to allow a technician to sit during the dental process. Choose a chair that allows for easy movement around the table and a relaxed angle over the patient.

PERIODONTAL DISEASE

Periodontal disease is the most common oral disease in pets and is probably the most common infectious process in the body. Bacteria are normally found in the oral cavity as a component of plaque. **Plaque** is a soft mixture of bacteria and mucopolysaccharides (carbohydrates) that adheres to the tooth. These carbohydrate molecules are very sticky and act as a matrix. The bacteria and associated endotoxins in the plaque initiate the inflammatory process in the gingival tissue (**gingivitis**). The inflammation may start as a mild gingivitis with edema and redness of the free gingival margin. If the inflammation is limited to this region and there is no attachment loss, it can be reversible with appropriate therapy (stage I periodontal disease: gingivitis). A slight increase in sulcus depth is typically attributable to swollen gingival margins and usually resolves when the edema subsides.

More extensive involvement of the periodontal ligament without intervention leads to **periodontitis** and subsequent attachment loss, as evidenced by an increased pocket depth and bone loss (stage II periodontal disease: periodontitis). Stage II periodontal disease consists of pockets up to 5 mm

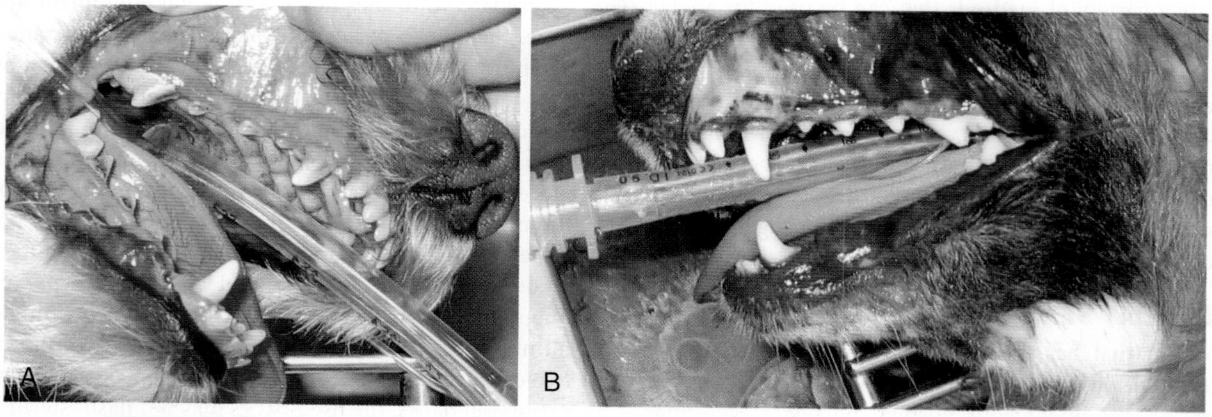

FIGURE 18-9 A, Pre-dental photograph. B, Post-dental photograph. (Photo courtesy of Coleen Johnston, DVM.)

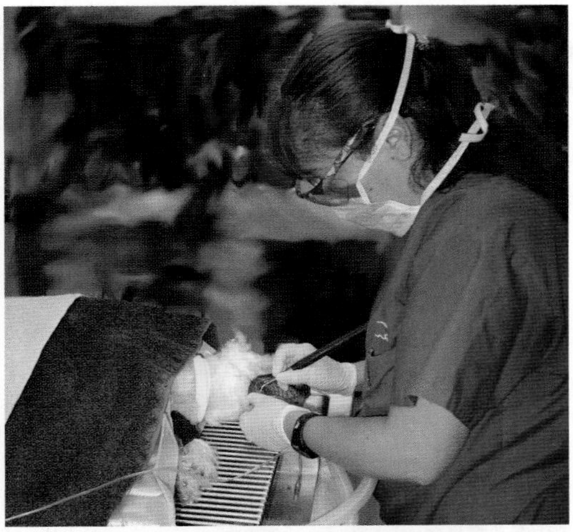

FIGURE 18-10 Technician wearing personal protective equipment. (Photo courtesy of Coleen Johnston, DVM.)

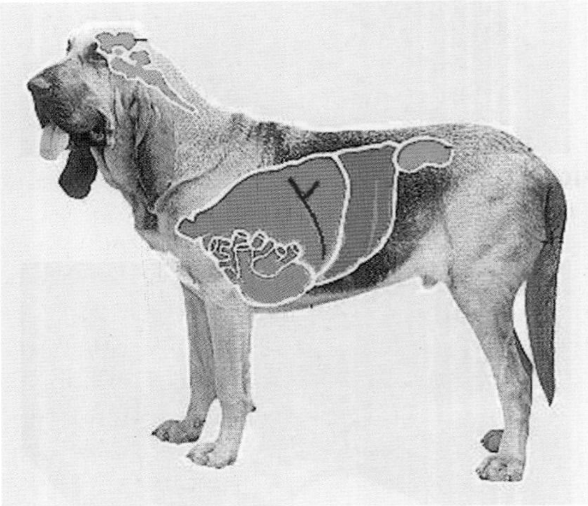

FIGURE 18-11 Organs affected by periodontal disease include the liver, kidneys, and heart. The lungs and nervous system can also be affected. (From "How to prevent tooth loss"; courtesy Pharmacia Animal Health.)

deep in dogs (1 mm in cats) or up to approximately 25% attachment loss. Pockets up to 9 mm deep (1.5 mm in cats) and 50% attachment loss are characteristics of stage III periodontal disease. Stage IV periodontal disease shows greater than 9-mm pocket depth and over 50% attachment loss. Often there are different stages of periodontal disease in different areas of a patient's mouth.

The bacteria associated with reversible gingivitis are generally located above the gumline (**supragingivally**) and tend to be aerobic, gram-positive, nonmotile cocci. As the disease progresses, the periodontal pockets enlarge, and bacteria work their way into the deeper structures. The bacterial flora in these deeper tissues tends to be more anaerobic, gram-negative, motile bacilli. The damage from bacteria and associated toxins can be significant, but the body's response with influx of many neutrophils, lymphocytes, and plasma cells can cause as much or more tissue destruction than the bacteria. Therefore the primary goals of treating periodontal disease are controlling bacterial populations, minimizing pocket depth, and maintaining healthy attached gingiva.

With advanced periodontal disease, owners usually notice how their pet's breath begins to smell and eventually the pet's refusal to eat because of the pain involved.

If left untreated, periodontal disease has serious implications of canine health. Besides breath odor and unpleasant appearance of teeth, periodontal disease inevitably leads to tooth loss. There can be a loss of appetite leading to weight loss. The problems of periodontal disease can affect the liver, kidneys, and heart (Fig. 18-11). Less commonly, the lungs and nervous system can be affected by persistent invasion of toxins and bacteria into the bloodstream. Periodontal disease is a progressive disease (Table 18-5).

All pets are at risk for developing periodontal disease but there are several factors that may increase an animal's risk. Home care is just as important with animals as it is with humans. If a pet is lucky enough to have its teeth brushed every

TABLE 18-5 Stages of Periodontal Disease

STAGE	DESCRIPTION
Stage1: Gingivitis	• Scattered plaque covers less than one third of the buccal tooth surface and mild inflammation appears as a redness of the gingiva with no attachment loss. • There is slight to no bleeding when probed.
Stage 2: Early Periodontitis	• Plaque covers between one third and two thirds of the buccal tooth surface and scattered calculus covers less than one third of the buccal tooth surface. • Gingiva shows moderate inflammation and edema with less than 25% of attachment when probed. • There is mild bleeding when probed. • Tooth mobility is less than 1 mm when an instrument is applied to the crown.
Stage 3: Moderate Periodontitis	• Plaque covers greater than two thirds of the buccal tooth surface and calculus covers between one third and two thirds of the buccal tooth surface with mild to moderate subgingival deposits. • Advanced gingivitis with severe inflammation clinically reaching the mucogingival junction usually with ulceration. • There is a moderate loss of attachment or moderate pocket formation with between 25% and 50% support loss. • Mild to moderate furcation exposure. • The tooth is still firmly attached in the alveolus but moves greater than 1 mm laterally.
Stage 4: Advanced Periodontitis	• Calculus covering greater than two thirds of the buccal tooth surface and extending subgingivally and there is a breakdown of support tissues with severe (>50% support loss) pocket depth or gingival recession. • Furcations are moderately to severely exposed and the tooth freely moves in the alveolus laterally and apically.

day, the owner will be removing most of the soft plaque from the surface of the tooth before it has a chance to build up and harden into **calculus.** They will also be reducing the amount of plaque that is being pushed subgingivally. Smaller breeds and pure breed cats have increased prevalence of dental disease. Many smaller breed dogs have normally occurring malocclusions, which lead to overcrowding and rotated teeth. Supernumerary or missing teeth commonly occur. It becomes difficult to remove plaque and calculus from the teeth if there are malocclusions present. The types of diets fed to smaller breeds and purebred cats may increase the plaque buildup. Although studies have been inconclusive, feeding hard foods seems to contribute less to plaque build-up than soft or human foods. Smaller breeds and purebred cats are frequently fed soft food. As the pet ages, its body systems may become affected by conditions or diseases that may weaken its immune system, or require dietary changes or medications that impinge on other body systems. The body may be unable to fight off the infections as easily as it could when it was younger.

PROPHYLAXIS OR DENTAL CLEANING

The process by which the teeth are cleaned is referred to as **prophylaxis.** By definition prophylaxis means to prevent or protect from disease. By removing plaque and calculus, the dental technician is removing harmful bacteria and minerals that cause gingivitis and decay of the tooth and bone, or periodontal disease.

The dental prophylaxis should be approached in a systematic manner (Box 18-2) to avoid missing any portion of the cleaning process. Because a brief examination was performed while the patient was awake, a complete examination may be performed once the patient is stable under anesthesia. Reexamine the face and entire oral cavity.

Using calculus forceps, gross tartar should be removed from the crowns (Fig. 18-12). If an ultrasonic scaler is available, the remaining calculus should be removed (Fig. 18-13). It is important to note the tip of the ultrasonic scaler is continuously vibrating, which can develop heat and injury to tooth and the soft tissue surrounding it. Do not use the tip or point of the scaler directly on the tooth or subgingivally. Adjust the power and water settings on your scaler properly to avoid injury. Once the calculus has been removed, it will be easier to probe and chart any findings. Hand scaling should be used to remove calculus from difficult areas supragingivally (Fig. 18-14). Technicians may or may not be

BOX 18-2 Systematic Approach to Dental Prophylaxis

1. Examine
2. Ultrasonic scaling
3. Hand scaling
4. Subgingival curette
5. Disclosing liquid and flush
6. Probe/explore
7. Radiographs
8. Extractions
9. Polish
10. Sealants
11. Charting/recording treatment

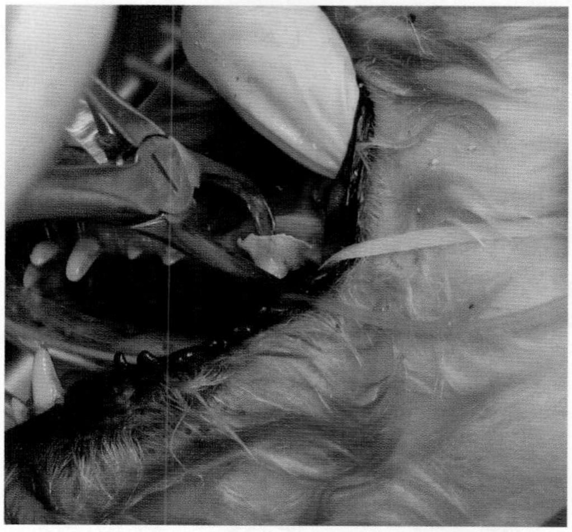

FIGURE 18-12 Gross tartar removal with calculus forceps.

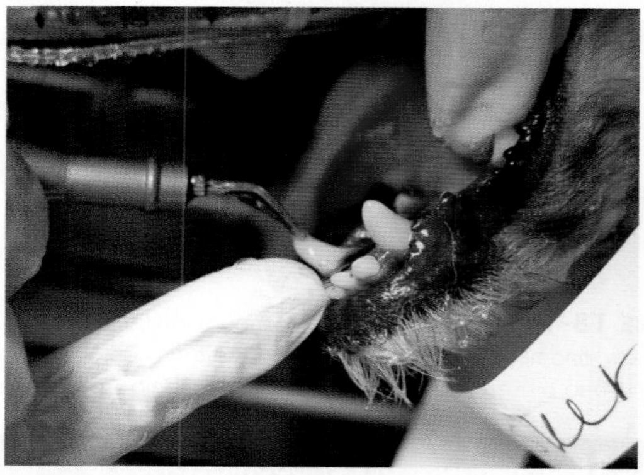

FIGURE 18-13 Power scaling a tooth.

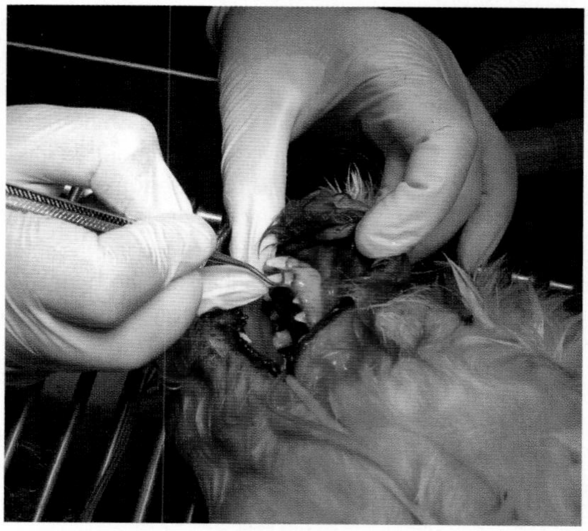

FIGURE 18-14 Hand scaling a canine tooth.

allowed to remove debris from the subgingival area. Some states consider this oral surgery that must be performed by the veterinarian.

The purpose of subgingival curettage, or root planing, is to remove any plaque, calculus, foreign material, and diseased tissue from below the gumline. Curettes are inserted to the bottom of the sulcus, or pocket, with the curved side directed toward the gingiva and the rounded tip aimed toward the root. The curette is rotated to allow the cutting edge to rest against the surface of the tooth and withdrawn from the pocket. This is repeated from various directions in a cross-hatched pattern.

The next step would be to flush the entire mouth, including the subgingival area, thoroughly with saline or dilute chlorhexidine. Subgingival irrigation can be done by using a blunt tip needle inserted into the sulcus. This removes all the loose debris that may settle into pockets and cause irritation or infection. Once the mouth has been rinsed, the probe and explorer can be used to examine the teeth and their surrounding tissue more closely and take measurements of pocket depth, furcation exposure, mobility, and inflammation. When measuring sulcus depth, it is necessary to measure the depth around the entire tooth (Fig. 18-15). Explorers detect subtle defects in the tooth surface. This is a good time to chart your findings. Some technicians prefer to use a plaque-disclosing liquid that highlights any plaque as a bright pink color (Fig. 18-16). This is a quick and inexpensive way to ensure a thorough cleaning has been achieved. Keep in mind, this step is one of personal preference and these products may stain the hair of your patients.

When radiographs are to be taken, it is best to do them before any stains, sealants, or polish has been applied to the teeth. Dental radiographs are usually performed after a closer examination has been done with the probe and explorer (Fig. 18-17). Additional films may be necessary to focus on areas of concern. In Figure 18-18, although the oral exam on this patient did not indicate a large sulcus area, there was gingival recession noticed and bifurcation exposure and radiographs indicated a tooth abscess. Most states consider extractions oral surgery that must be performed by the veterinarian (Fig. 18-19). There are some states that have made exceptions to this. In those states the technicians are allowed to extract single rooted teeth, like incisors and deciduous teeth.

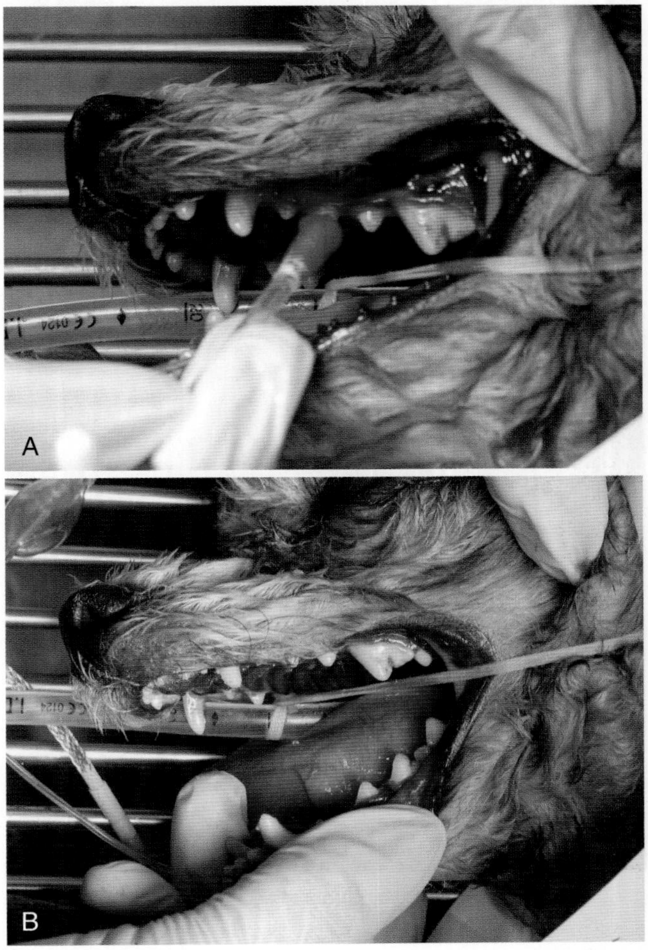

FIGURE 18-16 A, Applying disclosing solution. B, After rinsing, disclosing solution colors remaining plaque a bright pink color.

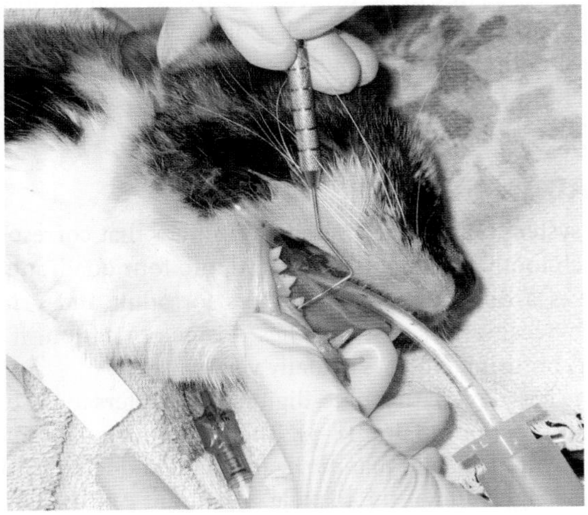

FIGURE 18-15 Using the explorer/probe to measure sulcus depth.

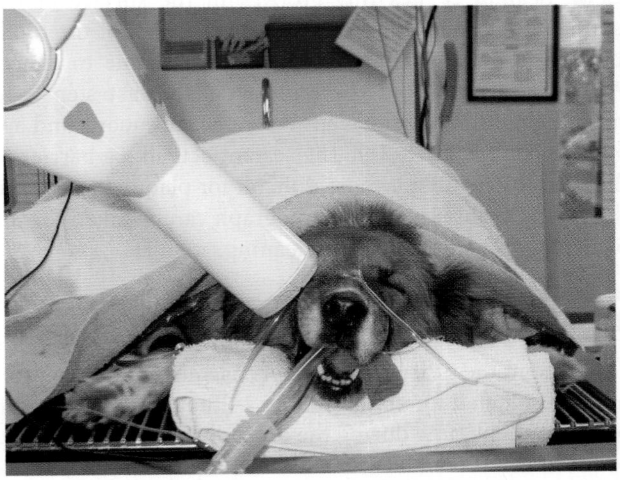

FIGURE 18-17 Dental x-ray positioning for 4th upper premolar.

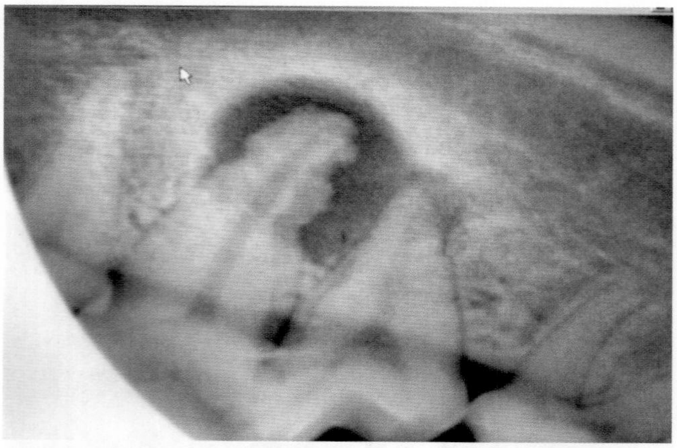

FIGURE 18-18 Radiograph of abscessed 4th upper premolar.

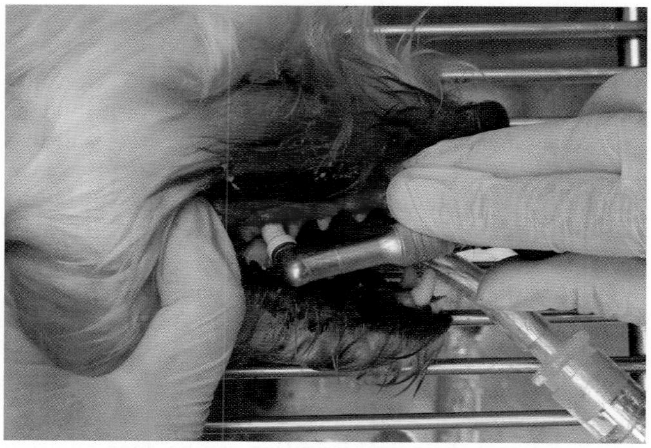

FIGURE 18-20 Polishing a carnassial tooth.

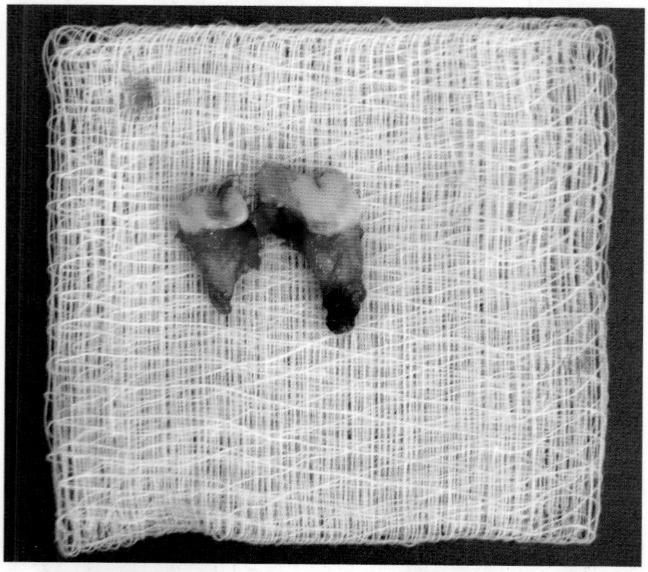

FIGURE 18-19 Extracted abscessed 4th upper premolar.

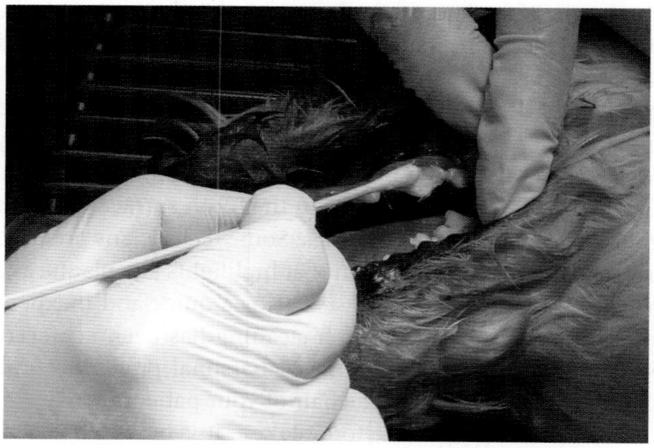

FIGURE 18-21 Applying a sealant.

After the extractions are finished, the technician can resume the dental prophylaxis by polishing the teeth (Fig. 18-20). It is necessary to polish each surface of the tooth. Scaling creates tiny grooves in the surface of the enamel. The grooves increase the surface area of the tooth and create better contact conditions for plaque to attach. Polishing smooths out these grooves. The last step is to rinse the mouth, dry the teeth with a gauze square, and apply a sealant (Fig. 18-21). The sealant acts like a barrier to the tooth by making it more difficult for plaque to attach to the tooth. A post-cleaning photograph can be taken for the owner to see before and after cleaning.

DENTAL RECORDS

Throughout the process of prophylaxis, the mouth is continuously evaluated for abnormalities. Although notations can be made at any time during the procedure, it is often best to review the entire oral cavity after the prophylaxis and ensure that all items are noted on the record. Recording observations in the dental chart should follow a systematic order to avoid missing any details. Many forms of dental records are available, including complete record sheets, stickers to affix to the records, and even ink stamps (Fig. 18-22). Any variations in tooth appearance, pocket depth, or other abnormalities should be recorded, along with the appropriate treatment. Individual teeth can be described using several techniques. For consistency, your hospital should choose one charting system and everyone should use it. There are two systems commonly used—the **Triadan system** and the alphanumeric system.

TRIADAN SYSTEM

This system relies on a three-digit number that corresponds to each tooth. The mouth is divided into four quadrants and there is a different set of numbers for adult and primary teeth. Because this system relies on memorization, it may seem confusing, but it is actually very simple.

The first digit of the three-digit number refers to the quadrant of the mouth (Box 18-3). There are four quadrants divided by maxilla and mandible, and right and left. Quadrant 1 is the right side of the maxilla. Quadrant 2 is the left side of the maxilla. Quadrant 3 is the left side of the mandible.

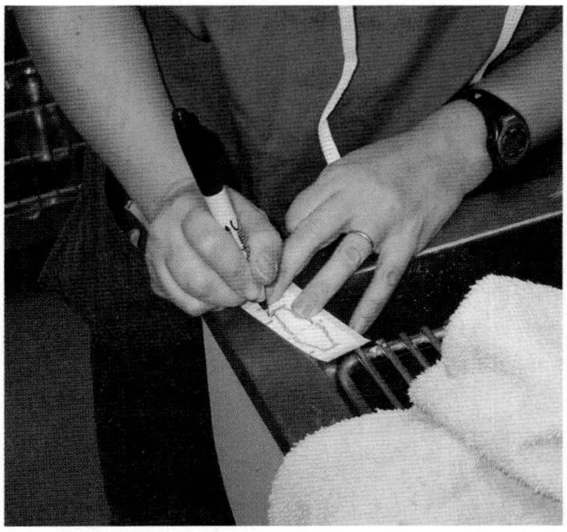

FIGURE 18-22 Charting on a dental sticker. (Photo courtesy of Coleen Johnston, DVM.)

BOX 18-3 Triadan Charting Quadrants

Adult Teeth		Primary Teeth	
1	2	5	6
4	3	8	7

Quadrant 4 is the right side of the mandible. The quadrants are in a clockwise pattern.

The second two digits refer to the actual tooth. The teeth within each quadrant are set up the same way. They start with the incisors, then the canine, the premolars, and finally the molars. To number them, begin with the first incisor counting toward the last molar are the numbers 01-11. An easy-to-remember reference is the rule of 4's and 9's. All canine teeth are numbered 04 and all first molars are numbered 09. These are easily recognized teeth at a glance. Once you have memorized these teeth, just count forward or backward to number everything else.

The primary teeth are numbered the same way with the exception of the quadrants. Instead of 1 through 4, the quadrants are 5 through 8, as follows. Quadrant 5 is the right side of the maxilla. Quadrant 6 is the left side of the maxilla. Quadrant 7 is the left side of the mandible. Quadrant 8 is the right side of the mandible.

TECHNICIAN NOTE **"The rule of 4's and 9's"** All number 4 teeth (e.g., 104, 204, ...) indicate canine teeth. All number 9 teeth (e.g., 109, 209, ...) are the first molars. Remembering this reference point will allow you to quickly count forward or backward to identify a tooth.

ALPHANUMERIC SYSTEM

The **alphanumeric system** can be easier to learn because there is a direct correlation with the abbreviations used to the type of tooth, for instance: incisors (I), canine (C), premolar (PM), and molar (M). The quadrants of the mouth are sectioned the same as in the Triadan system, but the way the quadrant is recorded will be different. Each tooth has a number, such as 1-3 for the incisors, 1 for the canine, 1-4 for the premolars, and 1-3 for the molars. These numbers are placed around the abbreviation depending on the location of the tooth. The right maxillary canine would be recorded as ^{1}C. The left maxillary canine would be recorded as C^{1}. The left mandibular canine would be recorded as C_1. The right mandibular canine would be recorded as $_{1}C$.

Adult teeth are recorded using capital letters for the abbreviations and deciduous teeth are recorded as lowercase abbreviations.

MODIFIED ALPHANUMERIC SYSTEM

The modification to the alphanumeric system came about because of different charting software and difficulties reading handwriting. Instead of circulating numbers around the abbreviation, more abbreviations were added. The abbreviations are as follows: Maxilla is upper (U). Mandible is lower (L), right (R), and left (L). Instead of using capital and lowercase, a lowercase d is used after the tooth abbreviation to delineate a primary tooth.

Figure 18-23 is an example of a reference sheet that combines both the Triadan and modified alphanumeric systems. It identifies normally missing teeth in adult canines and felines as well as their primary teeth. The pictures of the teeth show how many roots are associated with each tooth. Directional terms and tooth anatomy are listed as well as the common symbols.

CHARTING SYSTEM OVERVIEW

Charting is essential for proper documentation and monitoring of the oral cavity. Charting can be confusing with so many methods to choose from. The method that your hospital chooses to use will depend on the experience, training, and medical record system (computer vs. paper) that it uses. A comparison of the different methods is shown in Table 18-6.

TECHNICIAN NOTE To allow for easier and quicker charting, a diagram can be printed out and laminated. This can be taped to the back side of your dental clipboard for a quick reference.

OTHER SYMBOLS AND ABBREVIATIONS

Once a tooth can be identified on the chart, there are many symbols and abbreviations that can be used to distinguish specific problems (Box 18-4). Of these symbols and abbreviations, many are ranked in order from 0 (Normal) through 3 (Severe) (Table 18-7).

ORAL RADIOLOGY

Radiographs are an important part of dentistry. There are many abnormalities, diseases and traumatic events that may affect the tooth subgingivally. Survey films have been a part

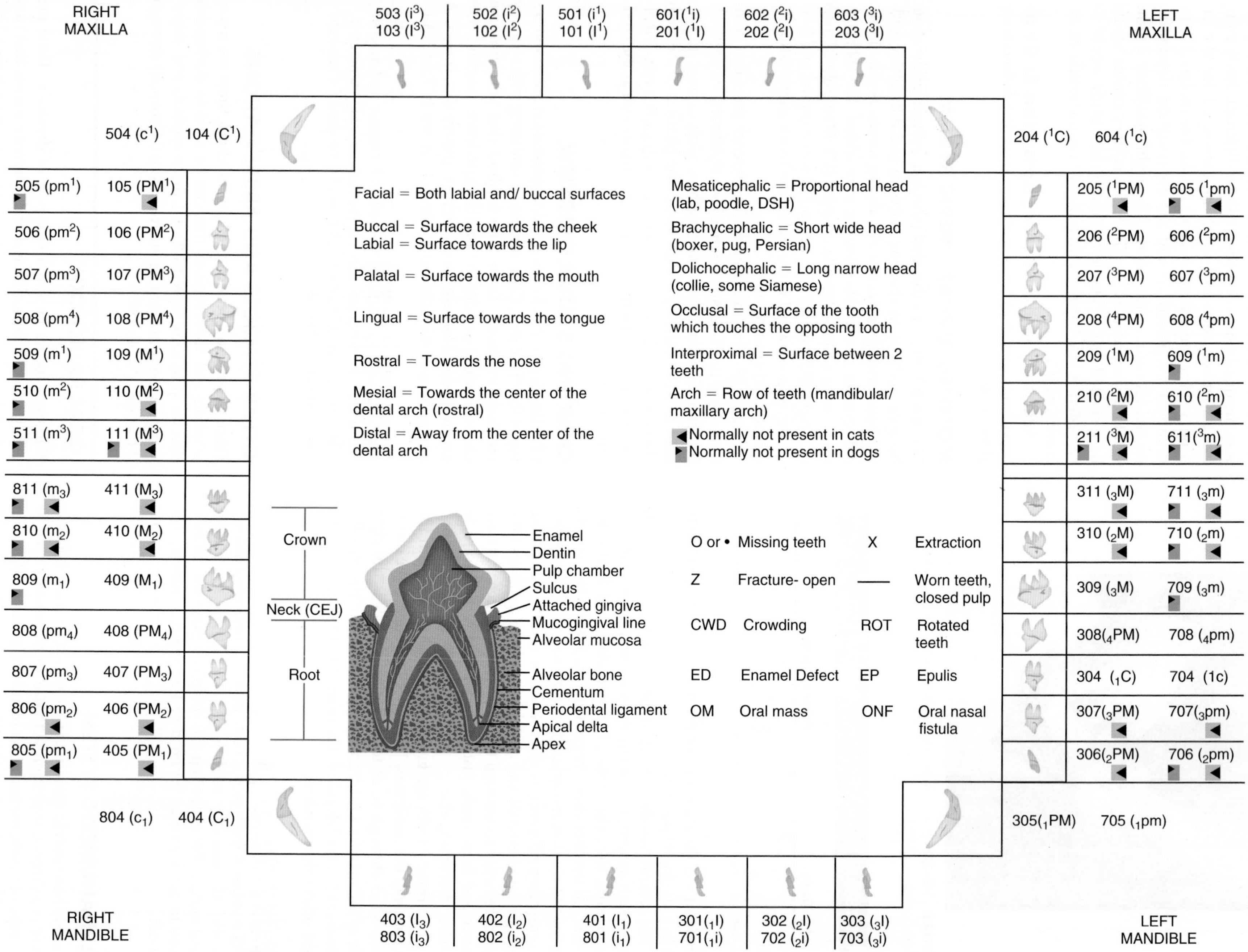
RIGHT MAXILLA
LEFT MAXILLA
503 (i^3) 103 (I^3)
502 (i^2) 102 (I^2)
501 (i^1) 101 (I^1)
601 (^{1}i) 201 (^{1}I)
602 (^{2}i) 202 (^{2}I)
603 (^{3}i) 203 (^{3}I)
504 (c^1) 104 (C^1)
204 (^{1}C) 604 (^{1}c)
505 (pm^1) 105 (PM^1)
506 (pm^2) 106 (PM^2)
507 (pm^3) 107 (PM^3)
508 (pm^4) 108 (PM^4)
509 (m^1) 109 (M^1)
510 (m^2) 110 (M^2)
511 (m^3) 111 (M^3)
205 (^{1}PM) 605 (^{1}pm)
206 (^{2}PM) 606 (^{2}pm)
207 (^{3}PM) 607 (^{3}pm)
208 (^{4}PM) 608 (^{4}pm)
209 (^{1}M) 609 (^{1}m)
210 (^{2}M) 610 (^{2}m)
211 (^{3}M) 611(^{3}m)
811 (m$_3$) 411 (M$_3$)
810 (m$_2$) 410 (M$_2$)
809 (m$_1$) 409 (M$_1$)
808 (pm$_4$) 408 (PM$_4$)
807 (pm$_3$) 407 (PM$_3$)
806 (pm$_2$) 406 (PM$_2$)
805 (pm$_1$) 405 (PM$_1$)
311 ($_3$M) 711 ($_3$m)
310 ($_2$M) 710 ($_2$m)
309 ($_3$M) 709 ($_3$m)
308($_4$PM) 708 ($_4$pm)
304 ($_1$C) 704 (1c)
307($_3$PM) 707($_3$pm)
306($_2$PM) 706 ($_2$pm)
804 (c$_1$) 404 (C$_1$)
305($_1$PM) 705 ($_1$pm)
403 (I$_3$) 803 (i$_3$)
402 (I$_2$) 802 (i$_2$)
401 (I$_1$) 801 (i$_1$)
301($_1$I) 701($_1$i)
302 ($_2$I) 702 ($_2$i)
303 ($_3$I) 703 ($_3$i)
RIGHT MANDIBLE
LEFT MANDIBLE
Facial = Both labial and/ buccal surfaces
Buccal = Surface towards the cheek
Labial = Surface towards the lip
Palatal = Surface towards the mouth
Lingual = Surface towards the tongue
Rostral = Towards the nose
Mesial = Towards the center of the dental arch (rostral)
Distal = Away from the center of the dental arch
Mesaticephalic = Proportional head (lab, poodle, DSH)
Brachycephalic = Short wide head (boxer, pug, Persian)
Dolichocephalic = Long narrow head (collie, some Siamese)
Occlusal = Surface of the tooth which touches the opposing tooth
Interproximal = Surface between 2 teeth
Arch = Row of teeth (mandibular/ maxillary arch)
Normally not present in cats
Normally not present in dogs
Crown
Neck (CEJ)
Root
Enamel
Dentin
Pulp chamber
Sulcus
Attached gingiva
Mucogingival line
Alveolar mucosa
Alveolar bone
Cementum
Periodental ligament
Apical delta
Apex
O or • Missing teeth
X Extraction
Z Fracture- open
—— Worn teeth, closed pulp
CWD Crowding
ROT Rotated teeth
ED Enamel Defect
EP Epulis
OM Oral mass
ONF Oral nasal fistula

FIGURE 18-23 A dental charting system that combines both the Triadan and the modified alphanumeric systems.

TABLE 18-6 Charting Comparison

TOOTH	TRIADAN	ALPHANUMERIC	MODIFIED ALPHANUMERIC
Right maxillary first incisor tooth	101	^{1}I	RUI1
Left mandibular fourth premolar tooth	308	PM_4	LLPM4
Left maxillary deciduous canine tooth	604	c^{1}	LUC1d

BOX 18-4 Symbols Used on Dental Charts to Designate Specific Problems

O or •	Missing teeth	*Z*	Fracture—open
X	Extraction	—	Worn teeth, closed pulp
CWD	Crowding	OM	Oral mass
EP	Epulis	ONF	Oral nasal fistula
ED	Enamel Defect	ROT	Rotated teeth

TABLE 18-7 Charting Index

DESCRIPTION AND SYMBOL	GRADING SCALE
Plaque Index (PI#) Refers to the amount of plaque (soft material) on a tooth.	**PI 0** No observable plaque **PI 1** Scattered plaque covering less than one third of the buccal tooth surface **PI 2** Plaque covering between one and two thirds of the buccal tooth surface **PI 3** Plaque covering greater than two thirds of the buccal tooth surface
Calculus Index (CI#) Refers to the amount of calculus on a tooth.	**CI 0** No observable calculus **CI 1** Scattered calculus covering less than one third of the buccal tooth surface **CI 2** Scattered calculus covering between one third and two thirds of the buccal tooth surface with minimal subgingival deposition **CI 3** Calculus covering greater than two thirds of the buccal tooth surface and extending sub-gingivally
Gingivitis Index (GI#) Is the number assigned to designate the degree of gingival inflammation.	**GI 0** Normal healthy gingival with sharp non-inflamed margins **GI 1** Marginal gingivitis with minimal inflammation and edema at the free gingival. Slight–No bleeding on probing **GI 2** Moderate gingivitis with a wider band of inflammation and mild bleeding upon probing **GI 3** Advanced gingivitis with inflammation clinically reaching the mucogingival junction usually with ulceration. Periodontitis will usually be present.
Periodontal Disease (PD#) (Stage #) is the graded or staged number on the dental chart. Healthy gingiva can be graded PD0.	**PD1** Stage 1: Gingivitis appears as a redness of the gingival and no attachment loss. **PD 2** Stage 2: Early periodontitis shows increases in inflammation and edema. Less than 25% of support when probed. **PD 3** Stage 3: Moderate periodontitis occurs when there is a moderate loss of attachment or moderate pocket formation with between 25% and 50% support loss. Furcation exposure and mobility may be present. **PD 4** Stage 4: Advanced periodontitis occurs when there is a breakdown of support tissues with severe (>50% support loss) pocket depth or gingival recession.
Mobility (M#) of teeth exists from trauma, endodontics, and/or periodontal disease. Mobility can be graded.	**M 0** Indicates no mobility. **M 1** Indicates the tooth moves less than 1 mm when an instrument is applied to the crown. **M 2** Exists when the tooth is still firmly attached in the alveolus but moves greater than 1 mm laterally. **M 3** Occurs when the tooth freely moves in the alveolus laterally and apically.

Continued

TABLE 18-7 Charting Index—cont'd

DESCRIPTION AND SYMBOL	GRADING SCALE
Furcation Involvement/Exposure (F#) The furcation is the area where multiple roots diverge from the tooth. Furcation involvement or exposure occurs secondary to periodontal disease. The degree of furcation disease can be recorded in grades.	**F 1** Furcation Involvement Is a depression in the furcation area that extends less than halfway under the crown in a multi-rooted tooth. **F 2** Furcation Involvement Exists when a depression in the furcation area extends greater than halfway under the crown but not through and through. **F 3** Furcation Exposure Exists when a periodontal probe extends "through and through" from one side of the furcation and out the other side.
Feline Odontoclastic Resorption Lesions (RL#) There are five stages (based on clinical and radiographic findings), and two types (based on radiographic findings) of feline resorption lesions. AKA: neck lesions, FORL, cervical line lesion	**RL 1** Stage 1 Extends into cementum only on the root surface. **RL 2** Stage 2 Has destroyed a significant amount of dentin and cementum but has spared the pulp. **RL 3** Stage 3 Enters the pulp cavity without extensive crown destruction. **RL 4** Stage 4 has extensive root and crown damage. **RL 5** Stage 5 lacks a clinical crown but root fragments remain on radiographs. **Type I** lesions arise in the cervical area of the tooth and extend inward and/or up or down the root. Type I lesions are inflammatory in nature and radiographically have a relatively normal root structure. **Type II** More common lesions begin subgingivally. Radiographically, roots appear to be resorbing. Periodontal ligament will not be readily recognizable due to ankylosis.
Dental Fracture Classification (Fxo OR Fxc)	**Fxo** Open fracture involving the pulp cavity. **Fxc** Closed fracture not involving the pulp cavity. **Fxslab** o/c Common fracture of the 4th upper premolars usually involves the pulp cavity and extends from the crown to below the gumline.
Malocclusion Types	**Type I:** Base narrow canines; Posterior crossbite; Crowded or rotated teeth; Lance (partially erupted) teeth **Type II:** Distoocclusions (mandibular brachygnathism, maxillary prognathism) **Type III:** Mesiocclusion (mandibular prognathism, brachycephalic) **Type IV:** Mesiodistocclusion (wry bite)

of human dentistry as part of a regular oral examination. Until recently survey films were considered costly and unnecessary for animals. Many veterinarians have begun to see how they can better monitor and diagnose oral conditions with survey films. Dental radiography is now considered the standard of care and should be included as part of the diagnostic and treatment plan for every patient. There are a few situations where it is especially vital to take dental radiographs (Box 18-5).

RADIOGRAPHIC EQUIPMENT

Radiographic equipment is essential for a quality dental practice. Although one may purchase expensive dental radiographic equipment, it is possible to do oral radiography using standard equipment with intraoral films and rapid developer/fixer solutions. There are a variety of digital systems available that are dedicated for use in dentistry. These vary in complexity and price but many are reasonably priced.

BOX 18-5 Reasons for Using Dental Radiographs

- Gingival pockets greater than 1 mm in a cat
- Gingival pockets greater than 3 mm in a dog
- Areas of facial swelling, especially below the eye
- Periodontal disease, grade 2, 3, or 4
- Chronic discharge from one or both nares
- Evaluation of a tooth undergoing root canal or pulp capping procedure
- Evaluating fractured tooth or jaw
- Oral bony or soft growths
- Malocclusion/supernumerary or deciduous teeth
- Malformed teeth

Extraoral films and oblique projections can be used for survey films, but these generally produce some degree of superimposition of other oral structures over the area to be viewed. Small, flexible intraoral films can be used with the standard radiographic unit with few variations. Intraoral films provide excellent detail, and superimposition of other oral structures is rarely a problem, unless positioning was incorrect. The unit can be used with the radiographic head positioned at a 36- to 40-inch focal distance for $\frac{2}{5}$ to $\frac{3}{5}$ of a second at 100 mA. It is preferable if the radiographic head is mobile, however, to decrease the focal distance to 12 inches and the exposure time to $\frac{1}{10}$ to $\frac{1}{15}$ of a second to minimize distortion and exposure. Depending on the equipment, the kVp may vary from 65 for a small dog or cat up to 85 for a large breed (Fig. 18-24).

The intraoral films come in a variety of small sizes (0, 1, 2, 3, 4); No. 2 film (periapical) is most commonly used. No. 4 film (occlusal) measures 2 by 3 inches and can be used to view a larger area of the incisors and canines or the nasal cavity (also for small rodents, birds, and cat feet). These non-screened, double-emulsion films are encased in a black paper sleeve with a lead foil back sheet that helps prevent back scatter produced by x-rays bouncing back off the table. A paper or plastic covering protects the films until after exposure, when they are removed before developing.

Dental films can be developed in standard tanks or automatic processors (taped to the lead end of a larger film). They take the same amount of time and volume of developing solutions as for a larger film. These smaller films can sometimes be lost in standard developing tanks. As an option, rapid dental developer and fixer solutions can be used in individual containers, either in the existing darkroom or in a chairside developer at the dental station. After rehydrating the emulsification of the film in water for 3 to 5 seconds, developing time ranges from 15 to 30 seconds, using fresh developing solutions. After a water rinse, fixing time is in the same range, so a film can be developed in less than 1 minute. This makes use of dental films very convenient. Rapid development time is particularly important when multiple films must be made.

RADIOGRAPHIC TECHNIQUES

The difficulty of oral radiography lies in positioning the film and the patient to obtain an image with the least distortion.

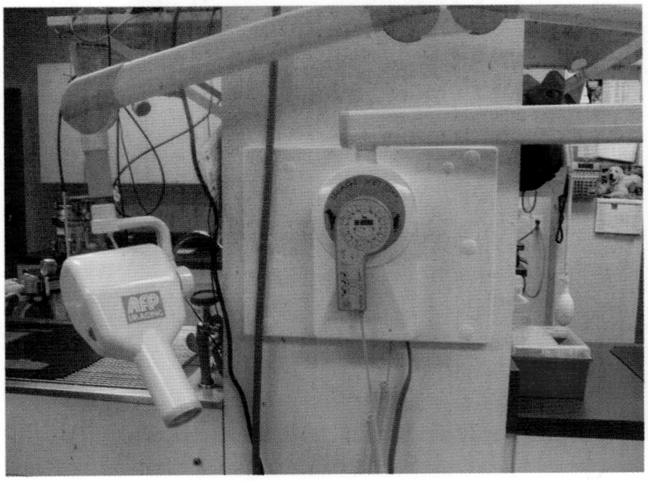

FIGURE 18-24 Digital dental unit.

A **parallel technique** is used only with the mandibular premolars/molars, when the film can be placed parallel to the teeth, with a corner pressing down into the intermandibular space. With the film so positioned, the x-ray head can then be aimed perpendicular to the parallel items. Elsewhere in the oral cavity, the film cannot be positioned directly against the object to be viewed, particularly in the maxilla, because of the shape of the palate. To accommodate for this obstacle, the **bisecting angle technique** can be used to minimize distortion that is inherent when the film cannot be placed parallel to the tooth.

If the x-ray beam is aimed perpendicular to the film, the tooth image will be shortened; if it is aimed perpendicular to the long axis of the tooth, the image will be elongated. Therefore if the beam is aimed midway between the two positions, the image should approximate the size of the tooth itself. One way to visualize this is to imagine an angle formed by the line of the film and the line of the long axis of the tooth or its root. Once this angle is assessed, a line that would bisect this angle is determined. By aiming the beam perpendicular to this bisecting line, the image will closely approximate the tooth size. To better visualize the angle when working on the buccal teeth, one should stand facing the nose of the animal. To determine the angle of the rostral teeth, stand at the patient's side. Sometimes better visualization is achieved by working with models or using three cotton-tipped applicator sticks to elongate each axis until you are more familiar with the technique. Certain corrections must be made when taking x-rays of the maxillary premolars and molars in the cat. Because of its prominent zygomatic arch, if one followed the standard bisecting angle rule there would be superimposition of the arch over these teeth. In order to avoid this, the operator must come in at a steeper angle, thus creating elongated teeth but no interference from the cat's zygomatic arch.

PATIENT POSITIONING AND FILM PLACEMENT

Although dental radiographs may be taken from a variety of positions, for consistency, all the patients should have their hard palates or nose parallel to the table. Positioning devices such as wedges, fluid bags, and towels can be helpful maintaining the patient's position. When placing the film in the mouth, always center the film under the area of interest. To hold the film into position gauze and tape rolls are commonly used. Rubber bands can be used but tend to bend the film, which distorts the picture.

Patient positioning for maxillary incisors and canines of the dog and cat will be ventral recumbency. Place the film centered below the incisors and canines and over the endotracheal tube. If the canines are too large to be included in the same film as the incisors, the film will be centered under the desired canine. Film will be parallel to the hard palate. If the film is placed as far back as the third premolar, the roots of the canines will be included in the x-ray.

Patient positioning for maxillary premolars and molars of the dog and cat will be in ventral recumbency. The film is placed along the hard palate near the tongue side of the opposite teeth (film will be mostly over the hard palate). The long end of the film is parallel to the muzzle.

Patient positioning for mandibular incisors and canines of the dog and cat will be in dorsal recumbency. The film will be placed centered below the incisors and canines and over the endotracheal tube. If the canines are too large to be included in the same film as the incisors, the film will be centered under the desired canine. The film will be parallel to hard palate. If placed as far back as the third premolar, the roots of the canines will be included.

Patient positioning for the mandibular premolars and molars will be in lateral recumbency. The film is placed in the vestibule (space) between the tongue and teeth. Long end of the film is parallel to the muzzle. Film can be slightly folded. Center the film under the area of interest.

The dimple on the film is a permanent marker. It will be useful in determining which side of the mouth you are viewing once the film is developed. Positioning the dimple on the film can be confusing. Remember the up side of the dimple points toward the cone of the x-ray machine (Table 18-8). When the film is placed lengthwise in the patient's mouth, the dimple remains on the outside of the mouth. When the film is place parallel to the canines, the dimple is positioned to match the right side of the mouth (Fig. 18-25).

TABLE 18-8 Dimple Placement in the Mouth

VIEW IN MOUTH	DIMPLE PLACEMENT
Right Maxilla	Toward molars
Left Maxilla	Toward canine
If film is parallel to canines	Toward molar on right side of face
Left Mandible	Toward molar
Right Mandible	Toward canine
If film is parallel to canines	Toward canine on left side of face

CONE PLACEMENT

Cone position is the angle in which you place the cone of the x-ray machine to acquire the view you desire. To set the cone you will need to position two angles—the perpendicular (up and down) angle and the lateral (side to side) angle. This can be the most difficult part of dental radiology because the shape and position of the patient's head will affect the position of the cone. Table 18-9 provides some guidelines on cone placement. Minor adjustments should be made once you are able to visualize the placement.

HOME DENTAL CARE

A necessary and often overlooked part of dental health is the continued care a pet receives at home. Owners play a pivotal role in their pets' oral hygiene. The veterinary technician is often responsible for educating the client about the different products available as well as how to use the products. The veterinary technician should become familiar with the different products available from the veterinary hospital as well as the surrounding pet stores (Table 18-10).

HOME DENTAL CARE PRODUCTS

There are a few things to remember about the different products. The means by which a tooth is cleaned would include toothbrushes, finger brushes, gauze and gauze pads, and sponge applicators. Some pets will allow owners to use electric toothbrushes. An ultra soft toothbrush works the best in most cases. The other devices will work but may not provide a thorough cleaning. Many owners will start with gauze or finger brushes to help the pet become accustomed

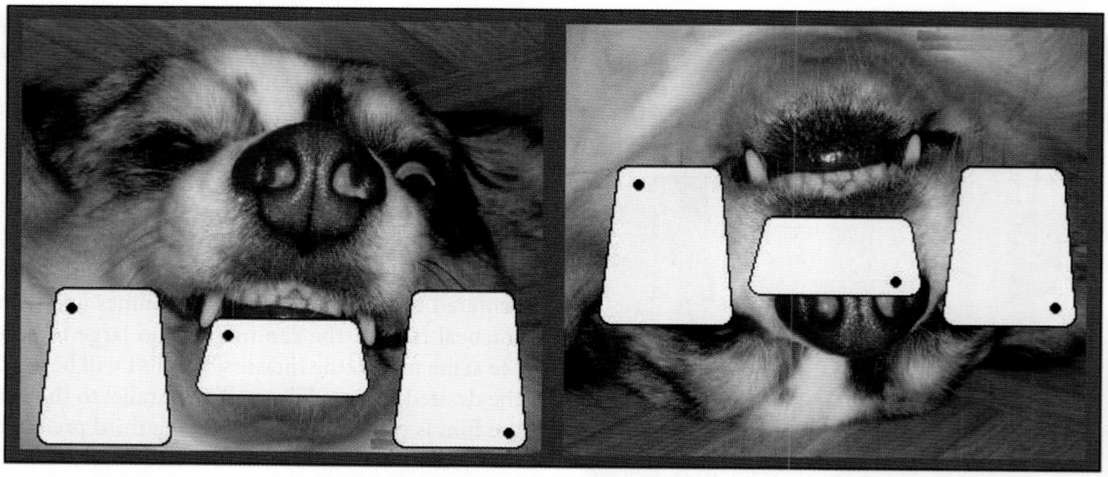

FIGURE 18-25 Dimple placement in the mouth.

TABLE 18-9 Cone Placement for Dental Radiographs

CANINE MAXILLARY INCISORS

Center beam over the nose. Aim cone downward at a 50- to 60-degree angle to hard palate.
OR
Aim beam at the dorsal midline, perpendicular to the bridge of the nose. Then tip the tube so the beam is angled at 20 degrees caudally.

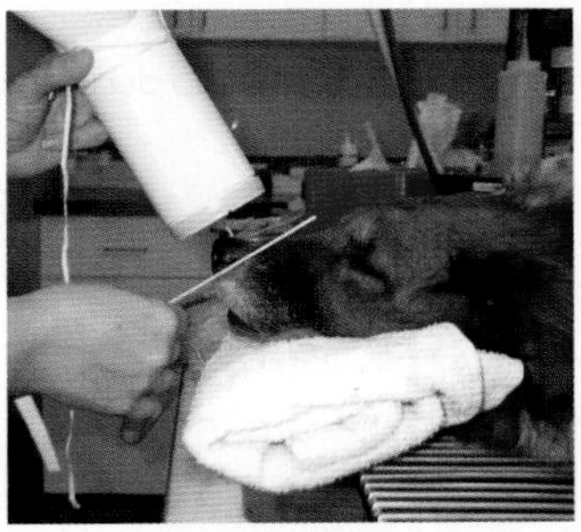

CANINE MAXILLARY CANINES

Lateral: Cone is centered over canine and adjacent to PM2. Aim cone about 80 to 90 degrees to the midline and tipped down at a 45-degree angle to the hard palate. Beam directed canine to canine.
OR
Aim beam dorsally over the top canine, similar to the upper incisor view. Then tip the tube so the beam is angled at 20 to 30 degrees caudally and 20 to 30 degrees toward the midline.

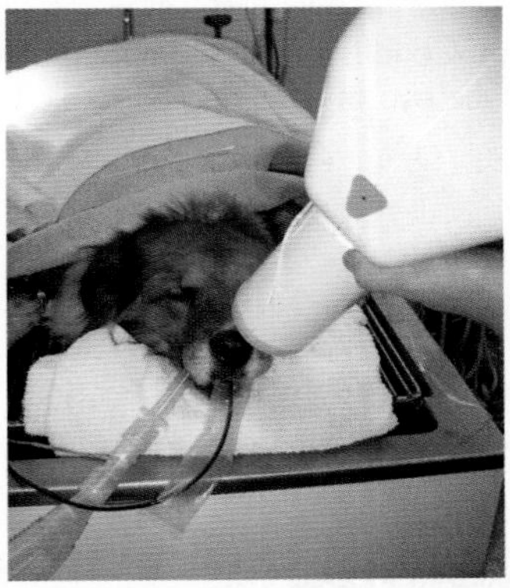

CANINE MAXILLARY PREMOLARS

PM1-3: Position cone over desired premolars. Aim cone from a lateral direction at a 45-degree angle to hard palate.
OR
Aim cone dorsally over the top of the target teeth. Tip the tube so the beam is angled ≈45 degrees toward the midline.

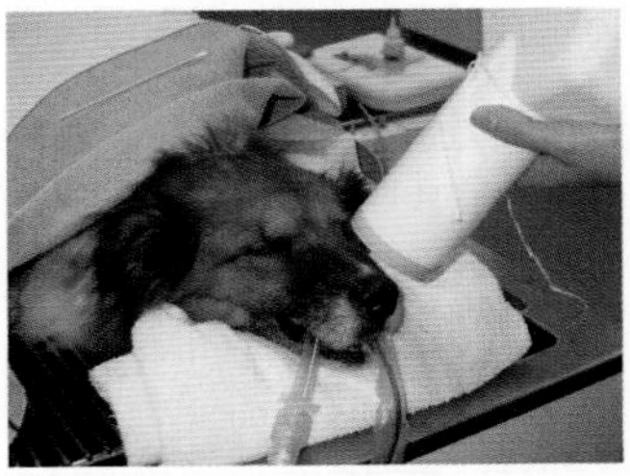

CANINE MAXILLARY 4TH UPPER PREMOLAR

Lateral: Cone is positioned over premolars and molars. Aim cone (perpendicular the head) at lateral canthus of the eye at a 45-degree angle to the hard palate.

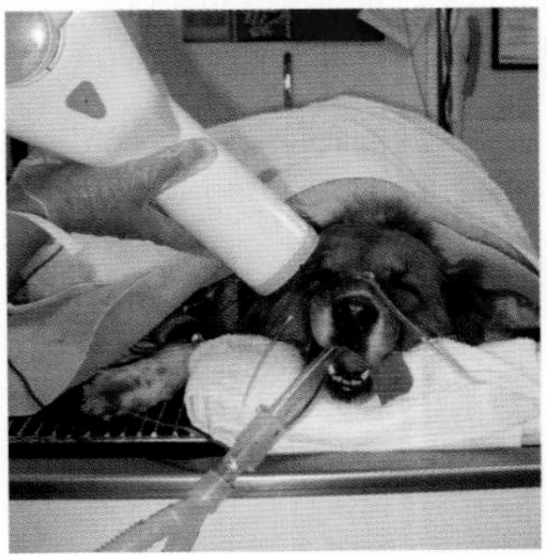

Continued

TABLE 18-9 Cone Placement for Dental Radiographs—cont'd

CANINE MAXILLARY 4TH UPPER PREMOLAR

Mesiolateral: Cone is positioned over premolars and molars. Aim cone vertically at lateral canthus of the eye at a 45-degree angle to the hard palate.

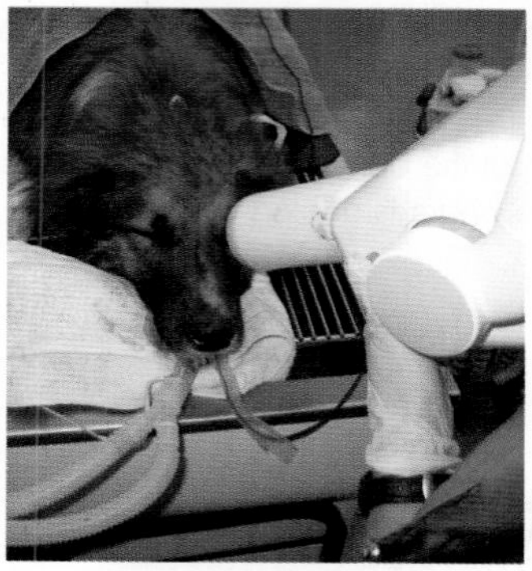

Distolateral: Cone is positioned over premolars and molars. Aim cone distally at lateral canthus of the eye at a 45-degree angle to the hard palate.

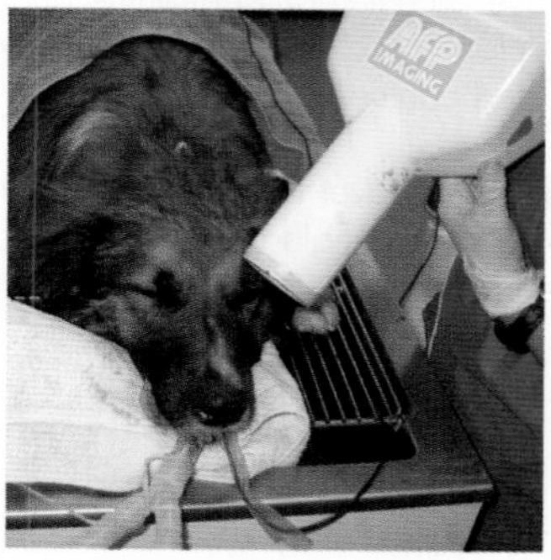

CANINE MAXILLARY MOLARS

Cone is positioned over premolars and molars. Aim cone (perpendicular to the head) at lateral canthus of the eye at a 45-degree angle to the hard palate.
OR
Aim cone dorsally over the top of the target teeth. Tip the tube so the beam is angled ≈45 degrees toward the midline.

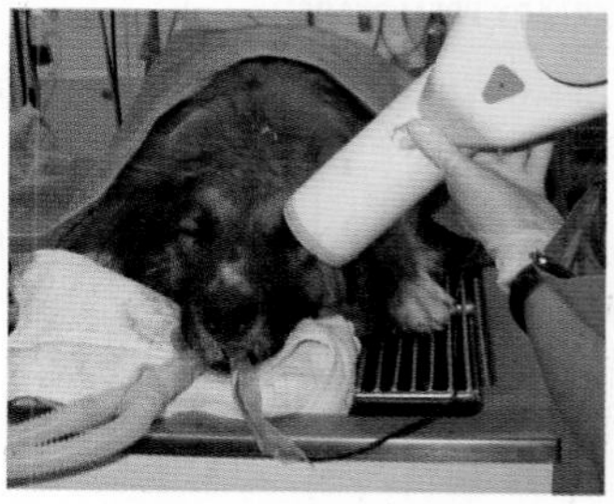

CANINE MANDIBULAR INCISORS

Center beam over the lower incisors. Aim cone downward at ≈60-degree angle to hard palate.
OR
Aim beam on the ventral midline, perpendicular to the mandible. Then tip the tube so the beam is angled at 20 degrees caudally.

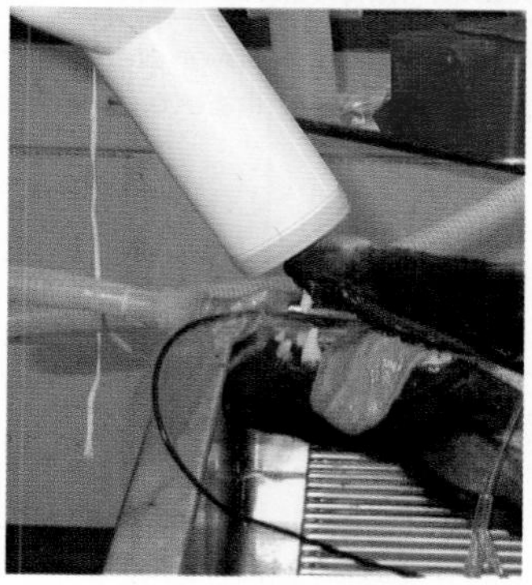

TABLE 18-9 Cone Placement for Dental Radiographs—cont'd

CANINE MANDIBULAR CANINES

Center over lower canines to PM2. Aim cone laterally at interproximal space between canine and I3. Tip down at 45- to 60-degree angle to hard palate. Beam directed canine to PM3-4.

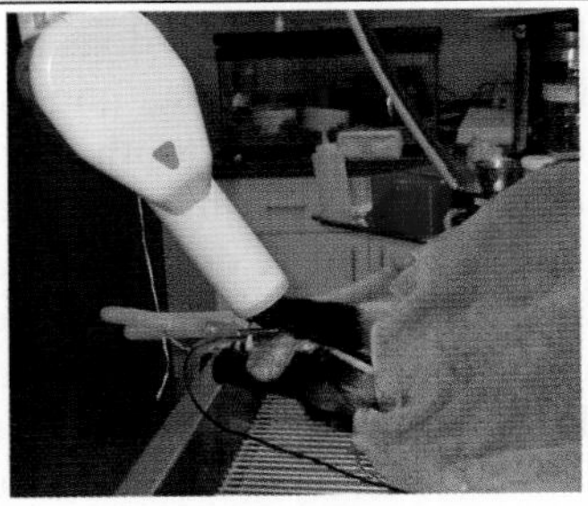

CANINE MANDIBULAR PREMOLARS AND MOLARS

PM1-2: Same as PM3-4. Can be viewed in canine x-ray also.
PM3-4: Center beam over target tooth at a 90-degree angle (perpendicular) to the film. And a 60-degree angle to table top. Use gauze to stabilize film in mouth.
M1-3: Same as PM3-4.

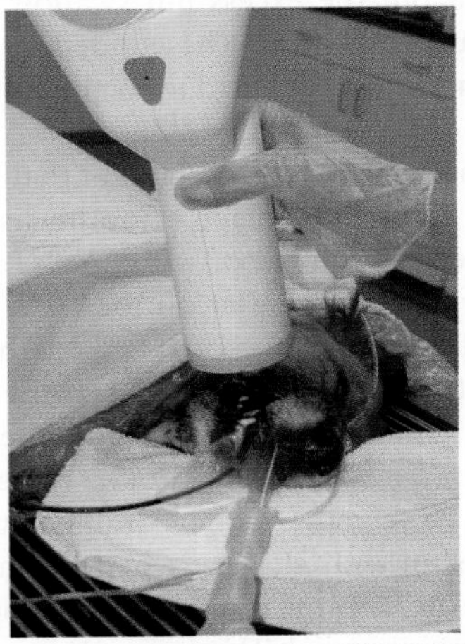

TABLE 18-10 Home Care Products

PURPOSE	MANUFACTURER
BRUSHING	
Ultra soft toothbrushes, Finger brushes, or Gauze pads	Marketed by various companies
Mechanical toothbrushes	Marketed by various companies
Dentifrices	CET Toothpaste (Virbac, St Louis, MO)
GELS/RINSES/WIPES	
Mechanical Water Picks	Marketed by various companies
Oral Wipes	Dent-Acetic (Derma pet)
Chlorhexidine Rinse	CET product line (Virbac)
Zinc Ascorbate Gel	Maxiguard Gel (Addison Biological Laboratory, Inc., Fayette, MO)
Plaque prevention system	OraVet (Merial)
DENTAL DIETS	
T/D	Hill's Science Diet
Dental Defense	IAMs/Eukanuba
DENTAL DD	Royal Canin
TARTAR CONTROL BISCUITS	
Rawhide Chewing Products	Tartar Shield
Non-Rawhide Chewing Products	Greenies (Franklin, TN)
Toys	Kong

to their mouths being handled. An electric toothbrush may work well except most animals do not like the vibrating and the noise. Choose a toothbrush that fits your pet's mouth. There are brushes marketed for dogs and smaller ones for cats. A children's toothbrush is a good alternative. Brushing removes plaque from the tooth surface before it has a chance to calcify. Tooth brushing is an effective way to remove plaque and should be done on a daily basis. To make the brushing experience complete and more palatable, many companies manufacture toothpaste that is formulated especially for animals. The toothpastes can be found in a variety of flavors. Human toothpaste should not be used because of the fluoride and detergent content. Most patients do not spit out the excess but swallow it instead. Baking soda mixtures should also be avoided for older patients and those with cardiac issues due to the potential for sodium overload.

There are a variety of products that owners can use if their pets refuse to accept a toothbrush and toothpaste. They come in the form of wipes, gels, and rinses. Wipes, gels, and rinses are gentler on the teeth and tissues in the mouth. It is generally accepted that tooth brushing is better (because it is able to reach between the teeth and slightly under the gumline), but the use of these other products is better than no home care at all. Wipes, gels, and rinses would be preferred products immediately after a dental prophylaxis or oral surgery when the mouth is the most sensitive. After a professional dental prophylaxis, a sealant may be recommended. The sealant is a waxy type substance that significantly reduces plaque and tartar formation by creating an invisible barrier that helps prevent bacteria from attaching to the pet's teeth.

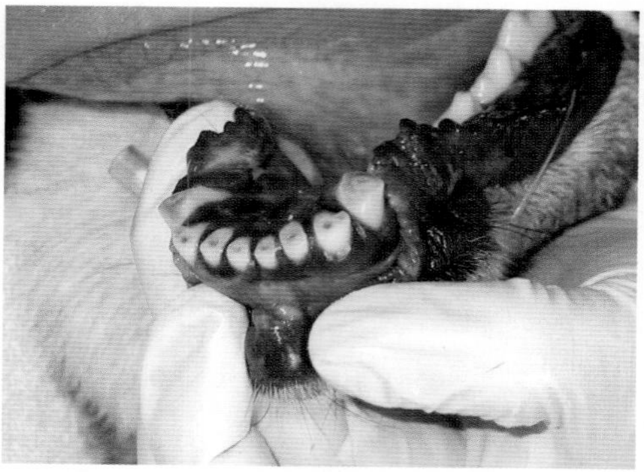

FIGURE 18-26 Worn incisors and canines.

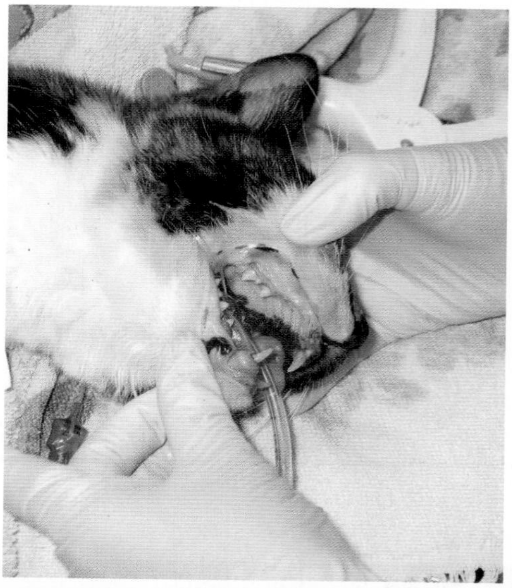

FIGURE 18-27 Cat missing canine tooth.

INGREDIENTS IN DENTAL PRODUCTS

There are several common ingredients found in the products available to the clients. Some products may combine several of these ingredients to achieve a synergistic effect.

Fluoride promotes remineralization of decalcified enamel, and inhibits cavities caused by the bacteria in plaque. Chlorhexidine comes in two forms: acetate and gluconate. It is a nonspecific bacteriostatic and bactericidal antiseptic. It acts by causing a separation of the cytoplasmic contents of the bacterium. Although chlorhexidine has been shown to reduce plaque and gingivitis, it can increase the rate of calculus formation. Frequently chlorhexidine is combined with some of the other products listed below. A "dual-enzyme system" was designed to be activated by saliva and oxygen to produce hypothiocyanite ions. These ions eliminate plaque-forming bacteria. The enzyme/substrates consist mainly of glucose oxidase and lactoperoxidase, which are capable of activating or supplementing naturally occurring peroxidase systems. Zinc ascorbate–based products are a combination of three parts—zinc, ascorbic acid, and taurine. The zinc component is antibacterial and important for healthy epithelium. The ascorbic acid or vitamin C component is important in the production of collagen, which is the main structural protein in gingiva. The taurine component reduces halitosis by binding to the sulfur compounds produced by oral pathogens and oxidizing volatile fatty acids in the mouth. Cetylpyridinium chloride is an antiseptic that is effective against most bacteria, some fungi (including yeasts), and protozoa. It has been shown to be effective in preventing dental plaque and reducing gingivitis. Hexametaphosphate (HMP) is a sequestering agent, which binds salivary calcium effectively, inhibiting the transformation (mineralization) of dental plaque into calculus. It has no direct effect on oral bacteria or plaque.

There are specially formulated diets that incorporate a specialized fiber formula that help clean the teeth as the food is chewed. In addition, some diets contain ingredients to discourage mineralization of plaque. The tartar control biscuit formulas may be similar to that of the food. Chew toys and rawhides can help reduce the accumulation of plaque and calculus. Extremely hard objects like calves' hooves and bones, ice, and tennis balls can cause serious wear of the teeth and even fractures (Figs. 18-26 and 27). These products

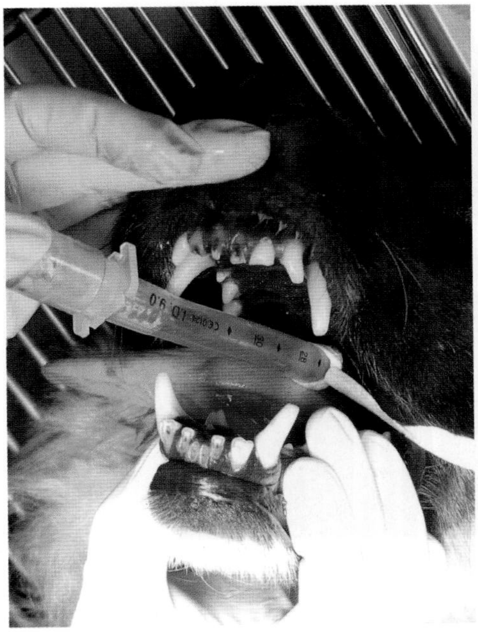

FIGURE 18-28 Broken incisors.

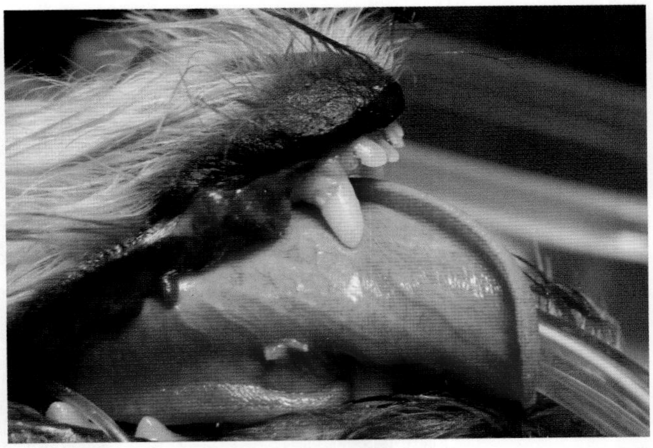

FIGURE 18-29 Enamel defect.

should be avoided. Chew toys may be designed to add pastes into crevices and rawhide chewing products may be impregnated with some of the ingredients found in the gels, rinses, and wipes. Finding the right toy or chew product can be difficult. When choosing a product, keep in mind that some toys can fracture teeth if they are too hard (Fig. 18-28). Rawhides become soft and flexible and may become a choke hazard if not sized appropriately for the pet. Some soft toys and tennis balls can wear down the enamel of the tooth (Fig. 18-29). The wrong material will lead to wearing or bad habits (shoes, ropes, etc. should be avoided because any rope, shoe, etc. will be viewed as a chew toy). The right chew toy will exercise the jaw, be enjoyable or stimulating mentally, and be able to rub plaque from the tooth surface without wearing or damaging the enamel.

AT-HOME BRUSHING PROCESS

It may take some training to accustom a patient and client to routine brushing, so a gradual, gentle beginning is recommended. Teaching a young animal to tolerate brushing is much easier for both client and pet. Encourage new puppy and kitten owners to make toothbrushing part of their pet's daily routine care, so the animal becomes used to the task and the client succeeds. Working with older pets requires more diligence, but it can also have a successful outcome.

The client can begin by touching the pet more around the mouth and head, gently keeping the mouth closed with one hand and lifting the lips with the other. A soft washcloth or gauze can be used to carefully wipe the outer surface of the teeth. Once the patient accepts the initial attempts, a soft toothbrush can be introduced to the regimen.

Depending on the individual, the patient may immediately accept flavored toothpaste, or it may have to become accustomed to the toothpaste.

It is important that the process remain stress free. Choose a time during the day where everyone has plenty of time and can be relaxed. If a pet follows the owner and seeks attention during a particular time of the day, begin acclimating the pet to having its mouth handled at that time. Offer positive attention or play time following the tooth brushing. The recommended minimum frequency of brushing is three times per week. Just as human dentists recommend brushing after every meal, pets would benefit from the same frequency. The average owner can usually brush his or her pet's teeth once every day (Fig. 18-30).

Even the most conscientious owners who schedule their pets for regular professional cleanings by their veterinarian will find that this regimen will not prevent every problem. The reason is simple. Each time a dog eats, plaque forms around its teeth. In 1 to 3 days, the plaque hardens into tartar that irritates gums, and opens the door to painful and damaging diseases. Regular cleaning is needed to prevent tartar buildup and dental problems.

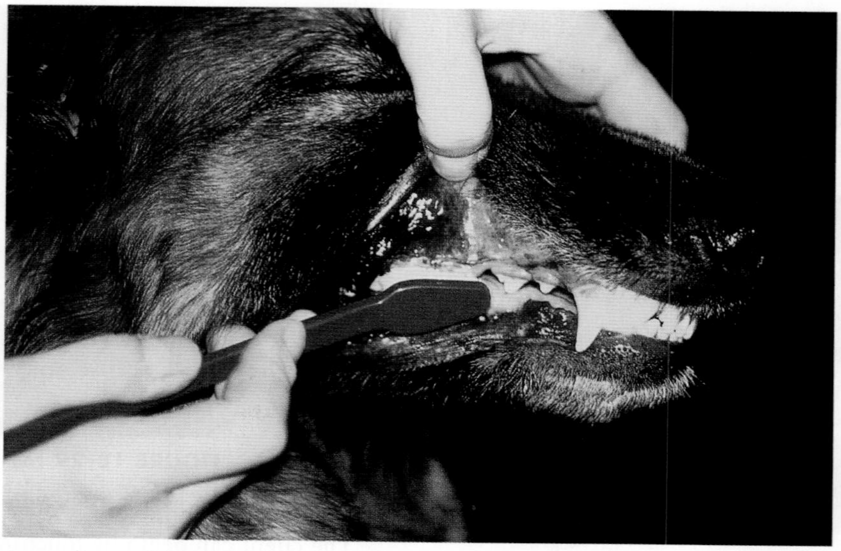

FIGURE 18-30 Toothbrushing technique. To remove plaque from the gingival sulcus, the toothbrush is angled at 45 degrees to the tooth surface, which allows the bristles to enter the sulcus. Even with optimal technique, toothbrushing will not clean more than 1 to 2 mm below the gingival margin. Consequently, the best way to prevent plaque accumulating in the sulcus is meticulous supragingival plaque control. (From Gorrel C: *Veterinary dentistry for the general practitioner*, ed 2, St Louis, 2013, Saunders, 2013.)

REVIEW QUESTIONS

Matching

1. Match the stage of periodontal disease with its description.

___**A.** Stage 1
___**B.** Stage 2
___**C.** Stage 3
___**D.** Stage 4

a. pocket depth of 9 mm (dog)/1.5 mm (cat) and 50% attachment loss
b. pocket depth >9 mm(dog)/1.5 mm (cat) and >50% attachment loss
c. inflammation, mild gingivitis, no attachment loss
d. pocket depth of 5 mm (dog)/1 mm (cat), 25% attachment loss

2. Match the correct number of teeth to the correct tooth type and species.

___**A.** Feline deciduous
___**B.** Feline permanent
___**C.** Canine deciduous
___**D.** Canine permanent

a. 30
b. 26
c. 28
d. 42

3. Match the skull type with the description.

___**A.** Mesaticephalic
___**B.** Brachycephalic
___**C.** Dolichocephalic

a. long narrow face
b. short wide face
c. average, proportional face

4. Match the skull type with a common breed example.

___**A.** Mesaticephalic
___**B.** Brachycephalic
___**C.** Dolichocephalic

a. Labrador
b. Collie
c. Boxer

5. Match the dental hand instrument to the correct purpose.

___**A.** Sickle scaler
___**B.** Probe
___**C.** Explorer
___**D.** Curette

a. used to determine depth of sulcus or pocket
b. used to detect softened areas in enamel
c. used to scale calculus off the crown of the tooth
d. used to remove calculus subgingivally

6. Match each adult tooth quadrant with its corresponding number.

___**A.** 1
___**B.** 2
___**C.** 3
___**D.** 4

a. left mandible
b. right mandible
c. left maxilla
d. right maxilla

7. Match each primary tooth quadrant with its corresponding number.

___**A.** 5
___**B.** 6
___**C.** 7
___**D.** 8

a. left mandible
b. right mandible
c. left maxilla
d. right maxilla

8. Match the Triadan tooth number with the correct tooth.

___**A.** 01
___**B.** 06
___**C.** 10
___**D.** 04

a. canine
b. second premolar
c. first incisor
d. second molar

9. Match the Triadan tooth number with the correct tooth.

___A. 03		a. first premolar
___B. 07		b. third premolar
___C. 09		c. third incisor
___D. 05		d. first molar

10. Match the Triadan tooth number with the correct tooth.

___A. 11		a. fourth premolar
___B. 02		b. third molar
___C. 08		c. canine
___D. 04		d. second incisor

RECOMMENDED READING

Dupont G: *Atlas of dental radiography in dogs and cats*, St Louis, 2008, Elsevier.

Eisner C: *Dentistry: creating a profit center*, Lakewood, CO, 1999, AAHA Press.

Gorrel C: *Veterinary dentistry for the general practitioner*, ed 2, St Louis, 2013, Elsevier.

Holmstrom SE: *Veterinary dentistry: a team approach*, ed 2, St Louis, 2013, Saunders.

Holmstrom SE, Front P, Eisner E: *Veterinary dental techniques for the small animal practitioner*, ed 3, St Louis, 2006, Saunders.

Kesel ML: *Veterinary dentistry for the small animal technician*, Ames, IA, 2000, Iowa State University Press.

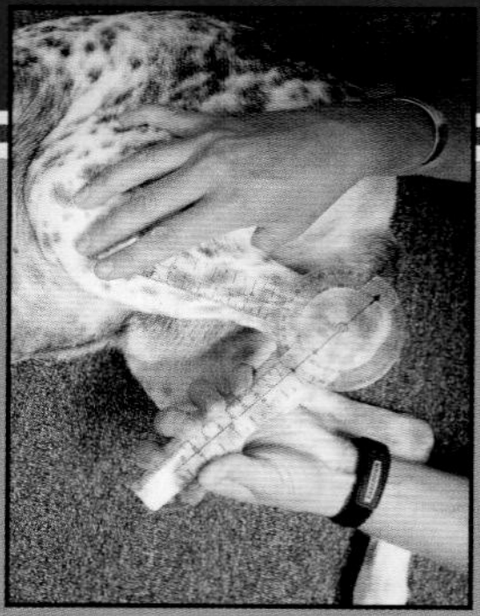

19 Physical Therapy, Rehabilitation, and Complementary Medicine

OUTLINE

LEARNING OBJECTIVES

After reviewing this chapter, the reader will be able to:

1. Differentiate between vibrational hands-on and manipulation hands-on therapies.
2. Describe the benefits of physical therapy and rehabilitation.
3. Discuss appropriate uses for thermal therapy.
4. Describe the differences in massage types and variations of applications.
5. Describe the concepts of passive range of motion therapy and active exercise for rehabilitation.
6. Define allopathic medicine.
7. Differentiate between alternative and complementary therapies.
8. Discuss similarities in various cultural philosophies of energy and healing modalities.
9. List and describe commonly used veterinary complementary therapies.
10. Describe the concepts of traditional Chinese medicine.
11. List and describe the theories, techniques, and uses of acupuncture.
12. Describe contraindications and adverse reactions to acupuncture.
13. Describe the cultural origins and uses of herbal therapy and define terms used in herbal therapy.
14. Discuss concepts of aromatherapy and list therapeutic uses of aromatherapy in veterinary medicine.
15. Discuss flower essences history, theories, and uses.
16. Describe the uses and procedures for laser therapy in veterinary medicine.

KEY TERMS

Acupressure
Acupuncture
Allopathic medicine
Alternative therapies
Aromatherapy
Ayurveda
Chiropractic
Complementary therapies
Compress
Cranial sacral
Dosha
Effleurage
Fomentation
Friction massage
Hands-on therapy
Healing crisis
Herbal therapy
Homeopathy
Hydrosols
Hydrotherapy
Integrative Veterinary Medicine
Meridians
Mother tincture
Passive exercise
Petrissage
Poultice
Qi
Reflexology
Reiki
Rescue Remedy
Samuel Hahnemann
Stretch pressure massage
Subluxations
Tellington TTouch
Thermal therapy
Tincture
Tisane
Traditional Chinese Medicine (TCM)
Yang energy
Yin energy

HANDS-ON THERAPY

Hands-on therapy covers a wide range of practices including massage, physical therapy and rehabilitation, chiropractic, acupressure, cranial sacral, and reiki. Practitioners use their own hands or body to move, adjust, or manipulate the patient to facilitate the healing process. **Hands-on therapy** can be vibrational or energy modalities such as cranial sacral and reiki, or manipulation therapies such as massage, physical therapy and rehabilitation, chiropractic, and acupressure.

Energy or vibrational modalities such as cranial sacral or reiki transfer healing energy from the practitioner to the patient.

Cranial sacral uses subtle manipulation of the skull and spine to relax and align the body for optimal energy flow. Stagnant energy is transferred to the practitioner who then expels it. Cranial sacral can be used in conjunction with other complementary therapies or as a stand-alone treatment.

> TECHNICIAN NOTE Cranial sacral can be used in conjunction with other modalities or as a stand-alone treatment.

Reiki is a Japanese hands-on energy healing practice that promotes the flow of chi ("Ki" in Japan) or life force energy to aid in the healing process. The practitioner enters the therapy session with healing intention and transfers this energy to the patient. Reiki can be practiced from a distance for wild or fractious animals.

> TECHNICIAN NOTE Reiki can be practiced from a distance for wild or fractious animals.

PHYSICAL THERAPY AND REHABILITATION

Physical therapy and rehabilitation are complementary therapies that have been proven to accelerate recovery and healing from surgeries and acute injuries as well as chronic conditions.

Rehabilitation is an extremely important part of medical management. Patients that receive some form of rehabilitative treatment recover faster than those who do not. The type of therapy used depends on the severity of the problem and condition of the patient. Rehabilitation therapy can prevent decubital ulcers, enhance blood and lymphatic circulation, prevent muscle contracture, maintain muscle tone and joint flexibility, produce relaxation, and reduce pain.

Although some types of rehabilitation can be expensive, most are not. Many are easy to perform so that the owners can do it at home, if needed. This helps keep costs down, or, if done in the clinic, does not require much overhead. Types of rehab therapy include **thermal therapy**, passive exercise, and active exercise.

Cryotherapy

Hypothermia is most effective during the first 24 to 48 hours after surgical procedures and after acute soft tissue contusions, muscle/tendon strains, and ligament sprains or lacerations. The cold decreases the tissue temperature, which decreases pain perception and reduces nerve conduction and muscle spasms. Local vasoconstriction also helps decrease edema.

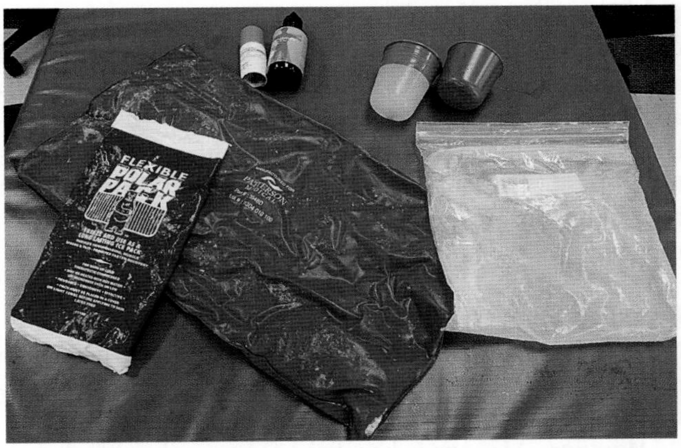

FIGURE 19-1 Cryotherapy options *(clockwise starting top right):* Popsicle-type molds for ice massage, alcohol-water slush plastic bags, cotton wraps, commercial cold wraps, fluoromethane cold spray. (From Millis D, Levine D: *Canine rehabilitation and physical therapy,* ed 2, St Louis, 2014, Saunders.)

A variety of options are available for providing cryotherapy (Fig. 19-1). Local hypothermia can be as easy as applying an ice pack to the affected area. These can be the cold packs used for shipping by drug companies, ice cubes wrapped in a towel, or continuous surface cooling blankets. Cold packs should be covered with a towel; ice should be placed in a plastic leak-proof bag wrapped in a towel. Applications should be for 5 to 10 minutes, two to four times a day. Treatment should not last longer than 30 minutes. Edema may become more severe if treatments exceed 30 minutes. Open wounds must be protected with a sterile, water-impermeable dressing to avoid contamination; use light pressure and avoid excessive cold. If the condition worsens at any point, discontinue treatment.

Local Hyperthermia/Heat Therapy

Hyperthermia is applied 48 to 72 hours after injury. Caution should be used when applying heat. Patients with sensory nerve involvement and those recovering from anesthesia could sustain thermal injuries. Before applying hot packs or a hot towel to any patient, some form of insulation, such as a towel, should be placed on the skin. The hot pack should be 104° to 113° F and applied for 10 minutes, two to four times a day. Every 1 to 2 minutes, the skin should be checked to see if it is overly hot. If so, another towel should be placed over the treatment area.

The therapeutic benefits of hyperthermia include muscle relaxation, pain relief, localized vasodilation, and localized increase in metabolic rate. This form of treatment is contraindicated for acute injuries, because it increases edema. Some of the different forms of heat treatments are radiant heat (applied with infrared lamps), ultrasound, and some forms of warm-water hydrotherapy.

Combination Therapy

Combination therapy is used in the later stages of healing and can be used with other forms of physical therapy. Heat applied before massage or exercise can improve muscle relaxation and circulation. Cold applied to the injured area after exercise helps decrease swelling and pain. If the patient has just had surgery, it is best to wait 2 to 3 days before beginning physical therapy.

Passive Exercise

No voluntary muscle activity is required by the patient in passive exercise. Two forms of passive exercise include massage and range of motion (ROM).

Massage. Massage is beneficial for animals with chronic health issues, limited mobility, or recovery after injury or surgery. Massage can be administered within a few days post surgery. The patient that is treated medically also can receive massage, but care should be taken to prevent aggravating the existing lesion. Massage also can be done after a session of active therapy is performed (combination therapy). Massage enhances muscle tone and range of motion, reduces stress, promotes relaxation, and stimulates lymph flow and immunity. Deeper forms of massage can decrease the chances of fibrosis. Massage contraindications include acute inflammation of soft tissue, bones, and joints, recent fractures, sprains, foreign bodies under the skin, hemorrhage or lymphangitis, advanced skin diseases, fever or heat stroke, round incision sites, and torn muscles. State regulations vary as to who can practice animal massage and under what level of supervision.

> TECHNICIAN NOTE State regulations vary as to who can practice animal massage and under what level of supervision.

There are five factors to consider when administering massage: the direction of the massage (which should always be toward venous return); amount of pressure to use (start with superficial pressure and gradually work to deeper muscles); duration of massage; rate and rhythm of massage (which depends on the type used); and frequency of massage.

In effleurage, strokes are given with the palm and fingers, slowly and lightly, just like petting. Gradually increase the pressure of the strokes. This produces a calming effect, which allows the animal to relax. This also allows the animal to become accustomed to the therapist. With light strokes, apply fifteen per minute; with heavy strokes, apply five per minute. Give 5- to 10-minute sessions of effleurage. Use a distal to proximal motion. This type of massage enhances draining of veins and lymph channels (Fig. 19-2).

With fingertip massage, use two or three fingers and keep them close together. Do not lose contact with the skin. Massage slowly and gently in a circular motion, increasing the pressure as the animal relaxes. This massages underlying muscles. Massage for 5 to 10 minutes.

Petrissage or deep massage is used on the back, flank, and chest. The skin is lifted, pulled, and rolled between the fingers and thumb, like rolling dough. For the shoulder, thigh, and limbs, the deeper muscles and tendons can be kneaded between the thumb and fingers of the right hand, while the left hand holds the limb and occasionally flexes and extends it. The kneading movements should be slow and rhythmic. Muscle is compressed from side to side and always in the direction of venous return. Deep massage enhances circulation, stretches muscles and tendons, and prevents adhesions and contracture.

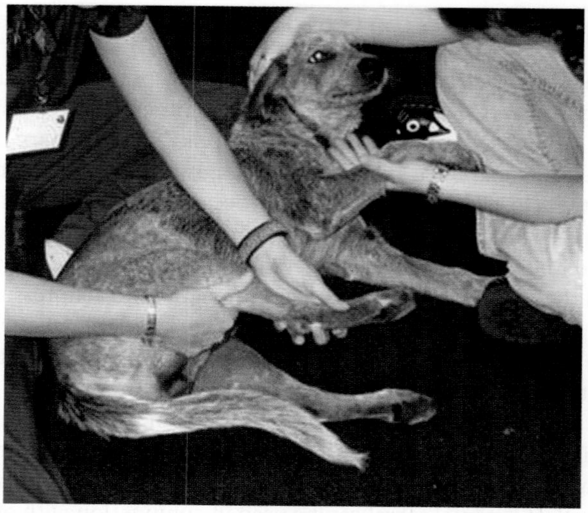

FIGURE 19-2 Massage, specifically effleurage, performed distally to proximally on the hind limbs of a dog with pelvic fractures repaired surgically. (From Millis D, Levine D: *Canine rehabilitation and physical therapy*, ed 2, St Louis, 2014, Saunders.)

Friction massage is fast, invigorating, circular massage given with the first two or three fingers. Massage at a rate of one circular motion every second, gradually increasing to twice that rate. This massage helps loosen superficial scar tissue and adhesions, as well as remove loose hair from the coat.

Stretch pressure massage combines pressure on a muscle with a stretching motion. This type of massage provides mechanical deformation of the skin and elongation of underlying muscle fibers and spindles. It helps maintain skin compliance and benefits muscle.

Tellington TTouch. Tellington TTouch is a gentle manipulation therapy based on the theory that animals can learn new responses quickly if their old habit patterns are disrupted in a nonthreatening way. Even though massage techniques are used, it is considered to be a realignment technique. A Tellington TTouch practitioner will use his or her fingers to massage in a circular pattern and in a clockwise direction. Tellington TTouch allows the body to relax into a more natural pattern, disrupting old learned behavior. Tellington TTouch also borrows technique and practice from auricular medicine with ear massage and manipulation.

> TECHNICIAN NOTE Even though massage techniques are used, Tellington TTouch is considered to be a realignment technique.

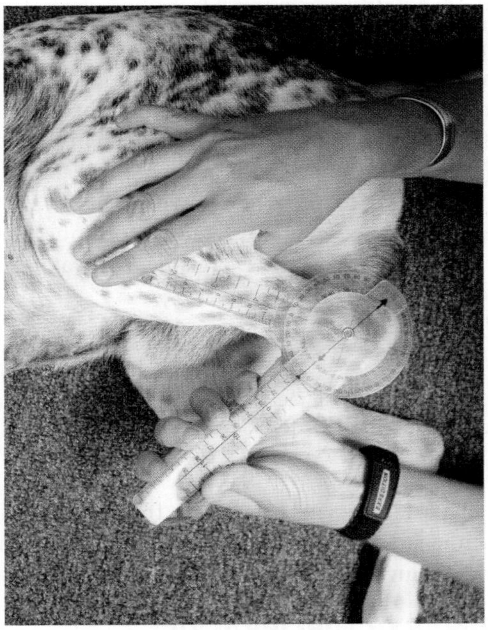

FIGURE 19-3 Joint angles of flexion and extension are measured using a goniometer. (From Millis D, Levine D: *Canine rehabilitation and physical therapy,* ed 2, St Louis, 2014, Saunders.)

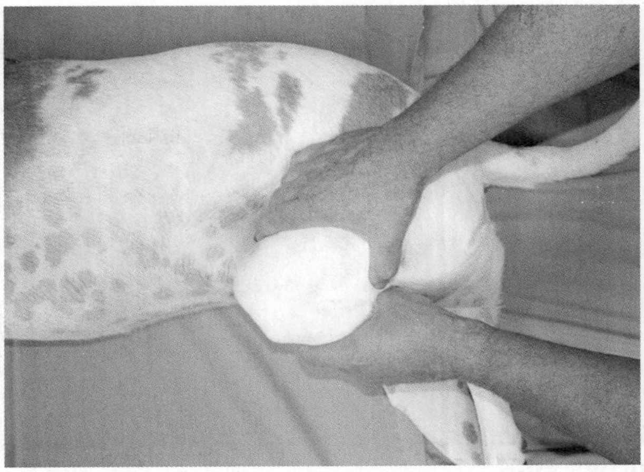

FIGURE 19-4 Placement of hands for passive range of motion to a dog's stifle. (From Gaynor J, Muir W: *Handbook of veterinary pain management,* ed 3, St Louis, 2015, Mosby.)

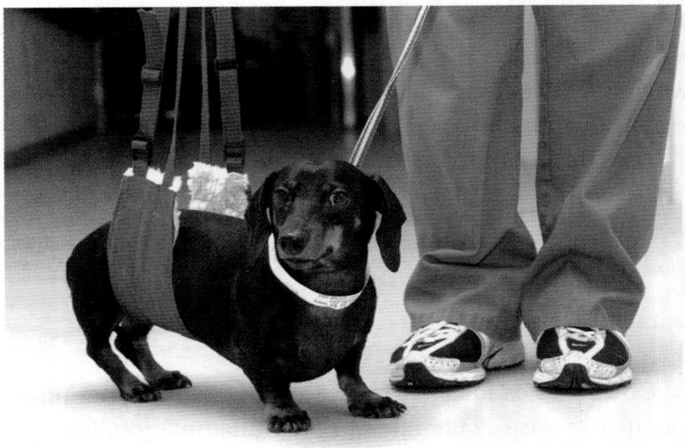

FIGURE 19-5 An assistive device, such as an abdominal sling, can be used to help a thoracolumbar patient stand and ambulate. (From Millis D, Levine D: *Canine rehabilitation and physical therapy,* ed 2, St Louis, 2014, Saunders.)

Acupressure and Reflexology. **Acupressure** uses finger pressure instead of needles to stimulate acupoints. Clients can be taught acupoints and proper technique in order to practice acupressure at home. **Reflexology** uses hand and finger pressure to massage and stimulate pressure points located in the feet or paws.

Range-of-Motion Therapy. Range-of-motion therapy helps maintain the proper range of motion of a limb by minimizing muscle and joint contraction from disuse. Measuring the animal's comfortable range of motion involves slowly flexing the joint until the first indications of pain are evident. The quantity of extension and flexion is measured with a goniometer (Fig. 19-3). Take the affected limb and slowly move it through its normal range, making sure not to hyperextend the limb (Fig. 19-4). Treatment should be for 5 or 10 minutes, two to four times a day. Range of motion can be combined with other forms of rehabilitation.

For patients with orthopedic injuries/conditions and muscle contractions, a slow controlled movement should be applied. Caution should be used not to over-stress the limb, because this may loosen fixation devices or cause muscle/tendon/ligament damage.

Active Exercise

The intent of active exercise is to stimulate as much voluntary activity as possible. Voluntary muscle contraction is the most beneficial form of therapy. Many patients must be supported with a sling or supporting them at the base of the tail (Fig. 19-5). Exercise carts and hoists can also be used to help the patients walk. These exercises should be done on textured surfaces, because most patients slip or slide on tile floors. Treatment time depends on the patient. Once you notice the patient becoming tired, treatment should end. This may be as short as 1 to 2 minutes. Within the first few weeks, treatment should not extend past 20 minutes.

Standing exercises are done when the patient starts supporting weight. Allow the animal to do so for as long as possible. It may be only a second or two in the beginning. After the patient sinks back down, pick it up and repeat for as long as possible. As the patient becomes stronger and can support its total weight, gently apply downward pressure over the hips or shoulders. This helps strengthen the muscles as the animal attempts to resist.

Walking exercises are performed when patients start to regain voluntary muscle movements or with paraplegic patients. Although the patients may only have function of their forelimbs, they must start exercising them again as soon as possible. A leash should always be used to restrict their activity.

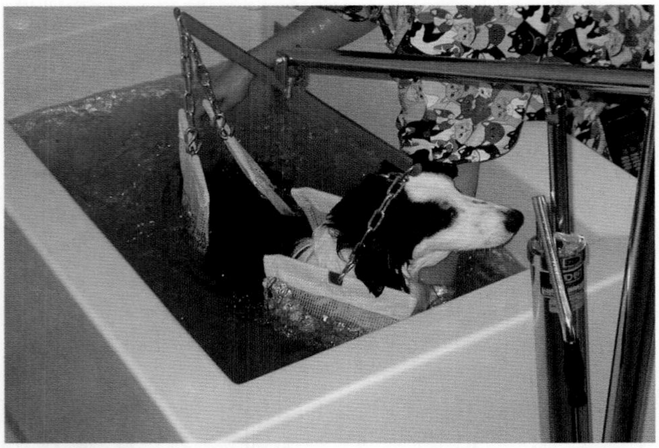

FIGURE 19-6 Whirlpool with hydraulic hoist and sling. (From Millis D, Levine D: *Canine rehabilitation and physical therapy*, ed 2, St Louis, 2014, Saunders.)

Hydrotherapy

Hydrotherapy provides passive and active therapy. Passive hydrotherapy is provided with the whirlpool (Fig. 19-6), whereas active hydrotherapy is swimming (underwater exercise). Animals may be fearful of the water; time should be allowed to acclimate the animal to the water.

> TECHNICIAN NOTE Animals may be fearful of the water; time should be allowed to acclimate the animal to the water.

Contraindications of hydrotherapy include peripheral vascular disease, acute injury, acute inflammation, fever, recent surgery, hemorrhage, cardiac disorders, and respiratory disorders. Hydrotherapy should not commence until at least 5 days after surgery. In animals treated medically, wait 10 to 30 days. Before placing an animal in the tub, water temperature should be checked to be sure it is appropriate. The patient should never be left alone in the tub!

An animal with an elevated temperature should not be treated with warm-water therapy until its temperature has been normal for 72 hours. Animals with respiratory or cardiac insufficiency should not be treated.

Whirlpool therapy provides a vigorous hydromassage. This massaging effect helps in removing dirt, necrotic tissue, and purulent exudates, and can also help fight infection if povidone-iodine is added. It speeds wound healing, reduces hyperesthesia of the skin, and may facilitate urination and defecation.

Before putting the animal in the whirlpool, remove all bandage material. During treatment, the water surface should be skimmed to remove hair and other debris. The water temperature should be 102° to 105° F. Caution should be taken not to scald the animal. For the first treatment, the animal should just sit in the tub for 5 minutes to become accustomed to immersion. Each treatment should increase in duration, ending up with a 20-minute treatment after several days.

Swimming is an excellent form of physical therapy. Buoyancy and hydrostatic pressure in a pool provide support and allow voluntary exercise with a minimum of effort. Animals with paresis must be helped through the motions of walking or swimming. Weights can be added to the animal's legs to build strength and endurance. Water also creates resistance to movement, which helps strengthen weakened muscles as exercise sessions continue. Because a patient produces heat while exercising, the water temperature should be 80° to 90°.

> TECHNICIAN NOTE During active exercise in the water, the animal will be producing heat, so water temperature should be 80° to 90° F.

Veterinary technicians can pursue training and advanced certification in physical therapy, rehabilitation, massage, reiki, and Tellington TTouch.

VETERINARY CHIROPRACTIC

Chiropractic is based on the theory that misalignment of vertebrae (**subluxations**) cause compensation in posture or movement, resulting in compromised function of the spine, which in turn can lead to secondary subluxations and various diseases and disorders. Chiropractors perform spinal adjustments (usually a short, rapid thrust on the affected vertebrae) to reverse a variety of nerve, muscle, and motion problems.

Only human chiropractors or licensed veterinarians can become certified in veterinary chiropractic through the American Chiropractic Association. Veterinary technicians can act as restrainers and can be essential to a vet chiropractor with client education.

> TECHNICIAN NOTE Only human chiropractors or licensed veterinarians can become certified as veterinary chiropractic practitioners.

ALTERNATIVE AND COMPLEMENTARY MEDICINE

The Western approach to veterinary medicine (sometimes referred to as **allopathic medicine**) is considered to be the "traditional" approach because it is the type of medicine that is commonly practiced by veterinarians and veterinary technicians in the United States and Canada. The term **alternative therapies** is often used to describe practices that deviate from the Western approach, but for veterinary medicine, the more accurate term would be **complementary therapies** because they often are used in conjunction with, or as a complement to, Western veterinary medicine. Complementary and Alternative Veterinary Medicine (CAVM) is also known as **Integrative Veterinary Medicine** (IVM) because it combines natural and holistic therapies with conventional veterinary therapies such as radiographs, blood work, surgery, etc.

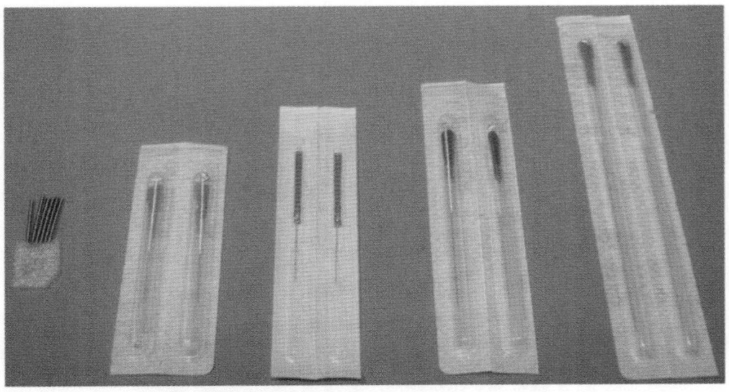

FIGURE 19-7 Acupuncture needles.

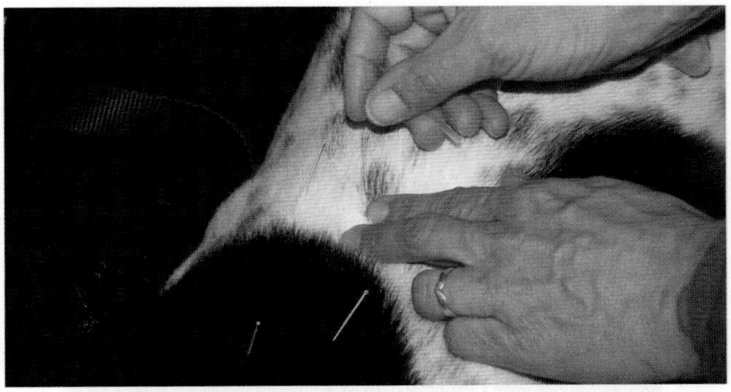

FIGURE 19-8 Acupuncture needle placement.

Many CAVM modalities can only be practiced by licensed veterinarians, but veterinary technicians can be vital members of the CAVM team by assisting with restraint, accurately recording history and treatment plans, dispensing pharmaceuticals, and providing client education. It is the responsibility of the veterinary technician to know state regulations as they pertain to CAVM and to practice within the scope of the laws. AVMA recently published guidelines for the recognition and practice of CAVM, which helps to clarify accepted areas of CAVM.

TECHNICIAN NOTE Veterinary technicians can be vital members of the CAVM team by assisting with restraint, accurately recording history, dispensing pharmaceuticals, and providing client education.

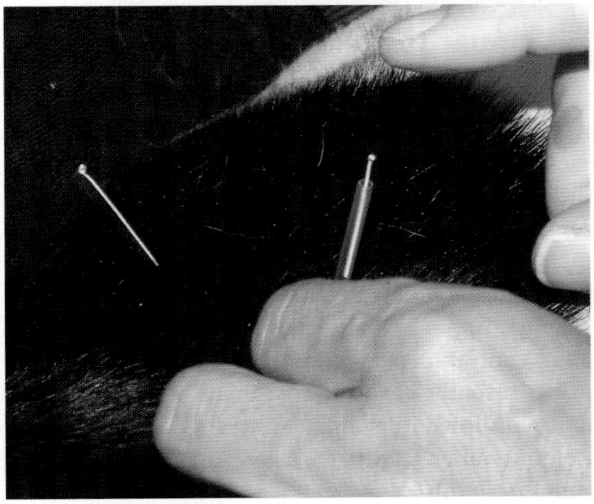

FIGURE 19-9 Acupuncture needles in place.

TRADITIONAL CHINESE MEDICINE

Traditional Chinese medicine (TCM) is the use of small, sharp needles (Fig. 19-7) placed into specific points on the body (**acupuncture**) and select herbs to facilitate energy movement through the body. TCM is based on the philosophy that energy imbalances cause illnesses and correcting these imbalances cures the disease.

TCM focuses on **Qi** (pronounced "chee"), the central life force, or energy that is found in all living beings. Qi travels through the body along **meridians,** which are described as rivers or channels that connect and regulate different body parts and organs. In a healthy body, Qi travels freely along the meridians and enters and leaves the body through points near the skin surface known as acupoints.

Qi has distinct qualities that are known as yin and yang. **Yin energy** is referred to as female energy. It is calm and yielding and represents stillness, darkness, water, and the moon. **Yang energy** is referred to as male energy. It is insistent and unyielding and represents activity, brightness, fire, and the sun. Yin and yang complement each other and should be balanced. Each is incomplete without the other. TCM herbs are often used to balance yin and yang.

Acupuncture

Acupuncture is the placing of small, sharp, sterile needles into acupoints along meridians (Fig. 19-8). TCM practitioners believe that needles help unblock stagnant energy or draw energy into deficient areas. Free-flowing energy is required for healing and continued good health. Western practitioners observe that the acupoints are close to nerve endings and therefore the needles act to stimulate nerves and trigger the release of endorphins and cortisol. The needles also increase blood circulation and relieve muscle spasms, all assisting the body in healing.

Veterinary acupuncture has been used to successfully treat a variety of illnesses including:

- Skin problems such as lick granulomas and allergic dermatitis
- Feline asthma and other respiratory disorders
- Diarrhea, colic, and other intestinal disorders
- Arthritis and other joint disorders
- Inflammation, burns
- Trauma and shock

Animals tolerate acupuncture very well (Fig. 19-9). Most show minimal discomfort as the needles are being placed. Cats tend to react to needle placement more than dogs, and large animals may show some discomfort because the needles have to be larger in order to prevent the needles from bending as they pass through the skin. The amount of time the needles stay in place varies from 10 seconds to 30 minutes. Once the needles are placed, most

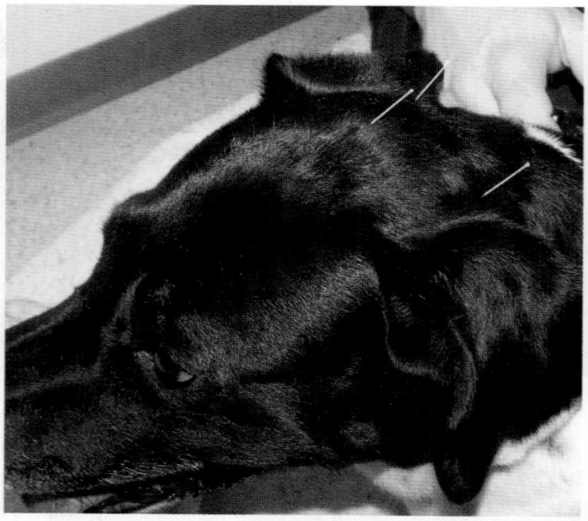

FIGURE 19-10 Acupuncture needles in place.

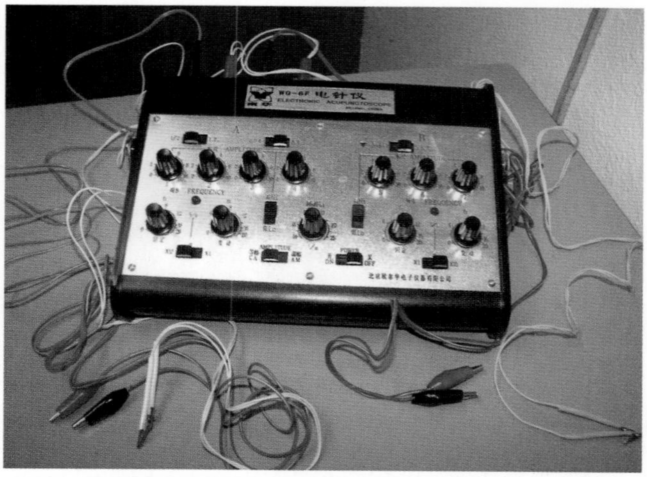

FIGURE 19-11 Electroacupuncture controller.

animals become very relaxed or sleepy (Fig. 19-10). Acute injuries may just need one treatment, whereas chronic conditions often require several treatments before improvement is observed. Once peak effect is reached, maintenance of two to three treatments a year may be required to maintain the benefits.

Acupuncture is considered to be a very safe modality; but it is contraindicated for pregnant animals or animals that have recently been bred, animals with high fevers, or animals with infectious diseases. It is recommended to wait 3 to 4 hours after feeding or exercising before performing acupuncture.

> TECHNICIAN NOTE Acupuncture is contraindicated for pregnant animals or recently bred animals, animals with high fevers, or animals with infectious diseases.

Adverse reactions to acupuncture are rare, but can occur. They include:

- Muscle spasms
- Excessive licking or chewing
- Yawning or stretching
- Breath changes
- Leg stretching

Owners should be cautioned that the pet may be tender after treatment.

There are a variety of methods and techniques for acupuncture. Depending on the individual case and the individual practitioner, treatment may include:

- Electroacupuncture: Needles are placed, then stimulated with an electrical current (Fig. 19-11).
- Sonapuncture: Ultrasound is used to stimulate the acupoints (usually 10 to 30 seconds/point) instead of needles.
- Aquapuncture: Sterile liquid (Vitamin B_{12} is commonly used) is injected into acupoints; the pressure of the liquid stimulates the point instead of a needle.
- Moxibustion: Use of heat to stimulate acupoints.
- Acupressure: Using finger pressure instead of needles, clients can be taught beneficial points and techniques for treatment at home.
- Auricular medicine: Acupuncture to the ears—ears contain energy points that correspond to all parts of the body—this practice can be used in conjunction with other acupuncture techniques, or as a stand-alone practice.
- Reflexology: Energy points found in the feet of humans and the paws of animals; uses hands to manipulate feet and stimulate points.

In the United States, veterinary acupuncturists are licensed veterinarians. Because acupuncture is considered to be a surgical procedure, veterinary technicians are prohibited from practicing acupuncture. The International Veterinary Acupuncture Society (IVAS) offers accredited certification for veterinarians, and veterinary technicians can be instrumental to the acupuncturist as restrainers as well as history takers because the TCM history is very detailed and complex.

> TECHNICIAN NOTE Acupuncture is considered to be a surgical procedure, so veterinary technicians are prohibited from practicing acupuncture in the United States.

Herbal Therapies

Herbal therapy is the use of specific plant leaves, roots, and or flowers to assist healing (Fig. 19-12). Every culture has some form of herbal therapy, many dating back centuries. Some herbal practices originated through zoopharmacognosy (the observance of animals instinctively choosing healing plants) and using those plants to benefit humans. Modern Western medicine is in part based on plants and herbs and is founded on a rich oral history.

The strength of herbs lies in their unique and complex properties of being an original natural substance. Herbs exhibit slower and deeper actions than modern Western medications and assist in the healing process—they are not always considered to be the cure. Herbs can work in a variety of

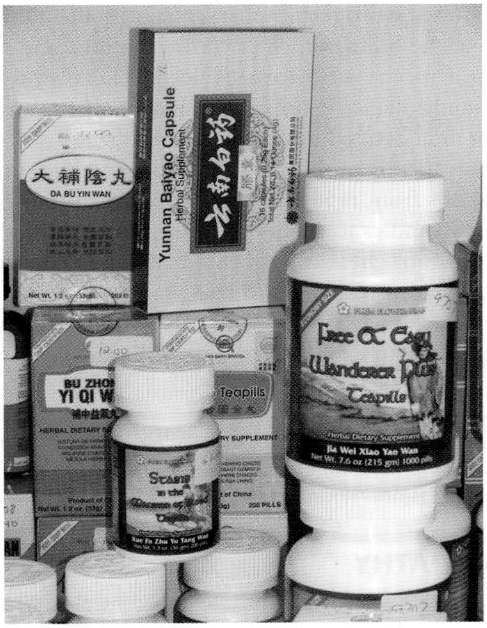

FIGURE 19-12 Herbal remedies.

ways: Some eliminate wastes and detoxify organs; others act as tonics, or help to strengthen the immune system. All herbs are nutritious and contain vitamins and minerals. Table 19-1 shows herbal remedies used in veterinary medicine.

> **TECHNICIAN NOTE** Herbs are not always considered to be a cure.

In Traditional Chinese Medicine (TCM), herbs are used in conjunction with acupuncture to regulate Qi in the body. Building on the TCM philosophy that disease is caused by Qi stagnation or blockages, herbs help to promote Qi movement through the body. TCM practitioners classify herbs based on certain qualities. Some herbs are chosen based on their thermal properties (hot, warm, cold, cool, neutral), their directional properties (upward, downward, or outward), or their functional properties (sweating herbs, harmonizing or tonifying herbs). TCM herbs are often used in combinations known as formulas.

East Indian herbal therapies are an integral part of the Ayurvedic tradition, a combination of diet, herbs, and exercise used to promote health and vitality.

Ayurveda uses **doshas,** the metabolic body type of an individual, to determine balances and imbalances. Herbs are used to bring the constitution of the individual back into harmony and in balance with the mind, body, spirit, and environment.

Western herbalism includes European traditional plants, New World herbs (Native American), and the more recent folk herbs of the United States. Western herbalism is based on scientific findings of plant medicine combined with the energetic and spiritual elements of each unique herb. Great value is placed on the rich history and the traditional uses

TABLE 19-1 Herbal Remedies Used in Veterinary Medicine

HERB	ORIGIN	FORM	USE
Aloe vera	Egyptian/Greek	Juice/gel; oral/topical	Skin irritation; arthritis; digestive aid
Arnica	Europe	Topical	Bruises, sprains, inflammation
Ashwagandha	India	Oral	Increase stamina and endurance
Astragalus	China	Oral	Immune system strengthener; diuretic; antiviral
Boswellia	India	Oral or Topical	Improves circulation; joint disorders
Burdock root	Northern U.S. and Europe	Oral	Blood cleanser; kidney tonic
Echinacea	U.S.	Oral	Stimulates immune response; upper respiratory infection; wound healing
Feverfew	Europe	Oral	Pain reliever
Fo-Ti or Ho Shou Wu	China	Oral	Longevity; liver tonic; diuretic; kidney strengthener
Ginger	India, China, West	Oral	Upper respiratory infection; kidney disease; nausea; improves circulation and digestion

of herbs. Regardless of the culture, herbal practitioners focus on balance in the body and the integration of all living things.

Herbs can be prepared and administered in a variety of ways. Single herb remedies are known as simples; combinations of herbs are known as blends. Any herb known for its effectiveness in the treatment of a particular condition is known as a specific. Herbs can be administered orally in the form of teas or **tisanes** (herbal infusions), **tinctures** (liquid extracts usually preserved with alcohol or vegetable glycerin), capsules, tablets, or tea pills. Topical applications include **poultices** (wet herbal packs), **compresses** (cold herbal tea on a cloth), **fomentations** (hot compresses), washes, rinses, and salves.

AROMATHERAPY

Aromatherapy is the therapeutic use of pure essential oils derived from aromatic plants to help balance and heal the mind, body, and spirit (Fig. 19-13). Essential oils are extracted from the leaves, flowers, roots, or bark of select plants through a distillation process. In steam distillation,

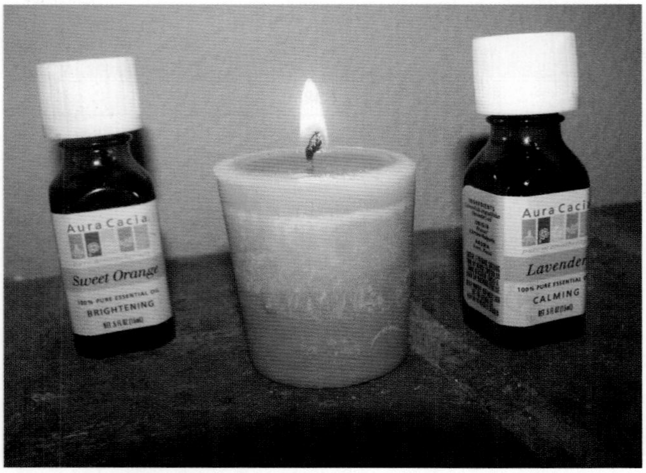

FIGURE 19-13 Materials used for aromatherapy.

TABLE 19-2 Uses for Essential Oils in Veterinary Medicine

ESSENTIAL OIL	USE
Chamomile	Calming, anti-inflammatory
Clary Sage	Calming
Eucalyptus	Antiviral, anti-inflammatory, expectorant
Geranium	Antifungal, tick repellent
Lavender	Antibacterial, antipruritic, calming
Sweet Marjoram	Calming, antibacterial, insect repellent
Niaouli (Related to Tea Tree Oil)	Antihistamine, antibacterial, used for skin allergies and ear infections
Oregano	Antibacterial
Peppermint	Stimulating, increases circulation, used for car sickness, insect repellent
Thyme	Relaxing, antibacterial, antifungal
Valerian	Calming, used for separation anxiety and fear of loud noises
Sweet Orange	Calming, tonic, flea repellent

the plant matter is placed over boiling water in a closed container. The steam condenses at the top into essential oils, which are non-oily, extremely concentrated, and very aromatic. The water left over from the distillation process becomes **hydrosols,** which are dilute, gentle, and only subtly aromatic.

There are a variety of uses for aromatherapy in veterinary medicine (Table 19-2). Many plants used in aromatherapy have antibacterial, antifungal, and other therapeutic qualities. If administered topically, essential oils can aid the physical healing process. For topical use in animals, always dilute essential oils in nongreasy carrier oils such as sesame or sweet almond. Topical applications include massage oils, ear washes, insect repellents, shampoos, and cleansers.

> TECHNICIAN NOTE Always dilute essential oils in nongreasy carrier oils for topical use in animals.

The aromatic properties of essential oils affect the limbic portion of the brain, which governs emotions and feelings. Scenting a room can help pets sleep, relieve stress, speed healing, and enhance energy levels. Essential oils can be used in sprays or added to humidifiers or nebulizers.

For therapeutic purposes, it is important to use only pure essential oils from reputable sources. Use caution with aromatherapy candles to ensure they are scented with pure essential oils, not chemically scented with perfume or other additives. Hydrosols are considered safer to use in animals, but caution should be used with cats. Aromatherapy is not recommended for exotics.

> TECHNICIAN NOTE Hydrosols are considered safer to use with animals, but use caution with cats. Aromatherapy is not recommended for exotics.

HOMEOPATHY

In the early 1800s a German physician, **Samuel Hahnemann,** began research based on his observation that "like cures like." He found that medications given to a healthy person caused that person to exhibit certain signs and symptoms. Pairing those medications with people sick with identical symptoms successfully treated the illness. Dr. Hahnemann's research tested a variety of remedies by administering them to a healthy volunteer and observing their reactions (a method known as proving). During his research, Dr. Hahnemann discovered that the more a remedy is diluted and agitated, the more potent the remedy becomes.

Homeopathic remedies are created when a natural source (vegetable, mineral, or animal) is combined with alcohol, creating a **mother tincture.** The mother tincture is diluted and vigorously shaken (successed) several times to create various potencies. The potency of homeopathic remedies is measured according to the number of dilutions and successions. Homeopathic dosages are based on potency (strength) and frequency of doses. As soon as symptoms improve, the treatment is discontinued and the body is allowed its natural healing process.

Homeopathic remedies should be stored at room temperature and kept dry and clean. When administering a remedy do not touch it directly or it can contaminate the dose. Administer doses at least 30 minutes before food and water or wait for 1 hour after food and water.

> TECHNICIAN NOTE To avoid contamination homeopathic remedies should not be touched.

Homeopathy remedies should never be combined because combinations tend to only relieve symptoms, not cure the disease, and may actually mask deeper disease issues. When using homeopathy, clients need to be aware of a potential **healing crisis:** a temporary worsening of symptoms followed by overall improvement. A healing crisis can be alarming, but if the remedy is working, the healing crisis shouldn't be severe or last long.

TABLE 19-3 Used of Common Homeopathic Remedies in Veterinary Medicine

HOMEOPATHIC REMEDY	USES
Arnica	Physical and emotional shock; injury
Ledum	First aid; trauma; puncture wounds; reported success against Lyme disease
Nux vomica	Vomiting, diarrhea; urinary tract infections

Veterinary homeopathy requires advanced training offered through the Academy of Veterinary Homeopathy. Homeopathy is a stand-alone therapy and is contraindicated in conjunction with Western therapy, acupuncture, and aromatherapy. Homeopathy is compatible with nutritional therapy, chiropractic, and flower essences (Table 19-3).

TECHNICIAN NOTE Homeopathy is considered to be a stand-alone therapy and is contraindicated in conjunction with Western therapy, acupuncture, and aromatherapy.

FLOWER ESSENCES

Flowers have special meaning and significance throughout time and in most cultures. In the Victorian era, the "language of flowers" was in vogue, complete with proper etiquette and meaning behind the gift of flowers. In modern times flowers are still given as tokens of affection, as mood lifters, and to signify important occasions.

In the 1930s a physician named Edward Bach recognized a link between stress, emotions, and illness. Close observation of a variety of clients led Dr. Bach to believe that individual personalities govern how a person reacts to stress and that unbalanced moods can lead to illness. Through the study of flower color, texture, and growth patterns, Dr. Bach observed that flower and plant characteristics mirrored personality traits. He recognized that flowers have qualities that can counteract negative emotions, balancing moods and stress levels and allowing for natural healing. Dr. Bach extensively studied flowers and their effects, creating 38 essences and a 5-flower combination formula known as **Rescue Remedy**. Flower essences (Fig. 19-14) have been used therapeutically throughout Europe and Australia since Dr. Bach's time and different essences have been created, but Bach Formulas tend to be the recognized name in the United States.

Flower essence therapy falls into the category of vibrational therapies, which are based on the concept that there is vital energy in all living things. This energy is essential to the health of an individual and is interrelated and interacts with the energy of other living beings. Flower essence therapy is related to homeopathy in that it is the energy signature of the flower that is therapeutic, not the flower itself. The process of creating flower essences requires fresh flowers, pure spring water, a clear glass bowl, and sunlight. The energy signature of the flower is transferred to the water and the sunlight facilitates the energy transfer, making the essence more potent.

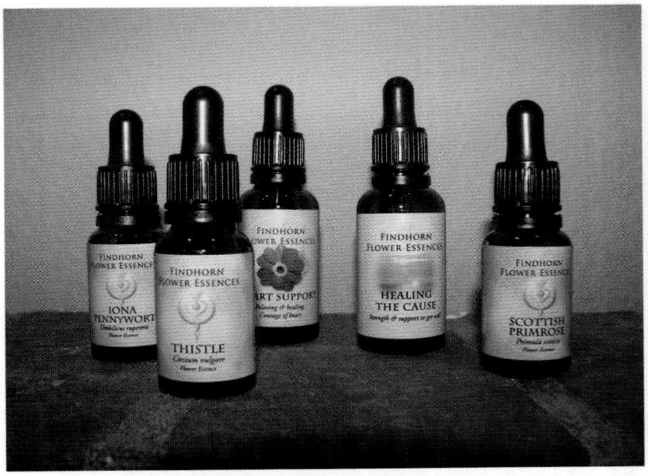

FIGURE 19-14 Flower essences.

The energized water is then added to brandy and is stored in amber-colored bottles. This mixture is known as the mother tincture. The mother tincture will keep for several years and is used to prepare stock bottles of the essence (spring water plus two drops of the mother tincture). Common uses of flower essence therapy are listed in Table 19-4.

TECHNICIAN NOTE Flower essences are compatible with other modalities and are safe to use with animals.

Flower essences are compatible with other modalities and are safe to use with animals. There are no contraindications. When administering flower essences to animals, drops can be given directly into the mouth, or they can be added to drinking water, placed on food, or massaged into the skin. Typically, flower essences are given several times a day for several weeks. The potency is increased by giving the remedy more often, not by adding drops to the dosage.

TECHNICIAN NOTE The potency of flower essences is increased by giving the remedy more often, not by adding drops to the dosage.

Rescue Remedy (Fig. 19-15) is a combination of five flower essences (Table 19-5) and is used to calm an individual experiencing shock, trauma, panic, or mental paralysis. This formula helps give relaxation and reassurance in stressful situations and can be helpful in a veterinary clinic for both patients and staff members.

LASER THERAPY

The term laser is an acronym that stands for light amplification by stimulated emission of radiation. Lasers are devices that produce or amplify electromagnetic radiation. Lasers are categorized into different classes based on their potential to cause change in biological tissues. Class I lasers are used in laser printers; Class II lasers are the type used by product bar code readers.

TABLE 19-4 Common Uses of Flower Essence Therapy

FLOWER ESSENCE	USES
Borage	Depression and grief—companion loss
Chestnut bud	Encourages positive behavioral changes
Cosmos	Enhances communication (for both humans and animals)
Dill	Hypersensitivity—builds inner strength and tranquility—good for travel; new environments
Holly	Fosters trust—introducing new animals or family members
Mariposa Lily	Maternal issues—abandoned animals (needy, not aggressive or hostile)
Mimulus	Fear and anxiety—helps build courage and confidence in animals that startle easily or are nervous and anxious
Oregon Grape	Hostility—suspicious animals—aggressive or abused
Quaking Grass	Develops group bonding—multiple pet households, introductions
Red Clover	Trauma—promotes calm, helps prevent panic—good for trapped wild animals and pets afraid of thunder or fireworks
Self-Heal	Overall remedy for sick animals in recovery—stimulates self-healing
Snapdragon	"The mouth remedy"—created specifically for animals—nipping dogs, chewers, constant vocalization
Tiger Lily	Encourages cooperation—good for feral cats, wild animals, difficult to train dogs
Walnut	Eases transitions. Develops courage; good for traveling animals, moving to new home, cats that spray territory

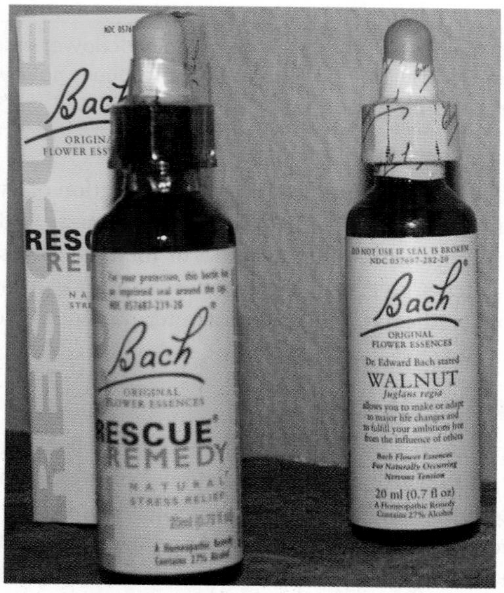

FIGURE 19-15 Rescue Remedy.

TABLE 19-5 Components of Rescue Remedy

RESCUE REMEDY ESSENCES	USES
Impatiens	Impatience, irritability, agitation
Clematis	Unconsciousness, faintness
Rock Rose	Terror, panic, hysteria, great fear
Cherry Plum	Loss of mental or physical control
Star of Bethlehem	Mental and physical trauma

BOX 19-1 Some Conditions Treated With Therapeutic Lasers in Veterinary Medicine

- Acral Lick Dermatitis
- Burns
- Indolent Ulcer
- Pyoderma
- Hip Dysplasia
- Aural Hematoma
- Snake Bites
- Mastitis
- Pancreatitis
- Trauma/Fractures
- Intervertebral Disc Disease
- Arthritis
- Gingivitis
- Otitis

Some low-level therapy lasers are categorized as Class III and are capable of output power of less than 500 milliwatts. Output power and the wavelength emitted by the laser influences the depth to which the laser can penetrate tissue. Class IV lasers are high-energy lasers with healthcare applications and emit electromagnetic radiation primarily in the near infrared spectrum. Surgical and therapeutic lasers generally produce output power of 4 to 12 watts. Class IV surgical lasers are used to cut tissue while Class IV therapy lasers are used in tissue healing. The application of that form of laser therapy is referred to as photobiomodulation therapy or photostimulation therapy.

Class IV therapeutic lasers have been used to stimulate acupuncture points in lieu of needles. They are commonly used to treat pain and often incorporated into the intra-operative and post-operative management of patients undergoing surgery, including elective surgery and dental procedures. Some additional conditions that have been successfully treated with therapeutic lasers are summarized in Box 19-1.

Tissue repair and cell growth are enhanced as a result of numerous biological effects of the laser, including increased cellular production of ATP, increased rate of cellular mitosis and collagen synthesis, activation of fibroblasts, osteocytes, and other regenerative repair cell types, accelerated tissue granulation and epithelialization of wounds, increased leukocyte and macrophage activity, and stimulation of capillary formation. Therapeutic lasers reduce the perception of pain by increasing the release of tissue endorphins and suppressing nociceptors. The therapeutic laser also enhances lymph

BOX 19-2 Dose Guidelines for Various Therapeutic Laser Uses in Dogs

Analgesic Effect
- Muscle pain: For acute pain apply 2-4 J/cm^2; for chronic pain, apply 4-8 J/cm^2.
- Joint pain: Apply 4-6 J/cm^2 for acute pain, and 4-8 J/cm^2 for chronic pain.

Anti-inflammatory Effect
- Acute and subacute: Apply 1-6 J/cm^2.
- Chronic: Apply 4-8 J/cm^2.

Open Wounds
- Acute wounds: Apply 2-6 J/cm^2 sid for 7-10 days.
- Chronic wounds: Apply 2-8 J/cm^2 sid.
- Laser head should not be applied directly to the wound.
- Clean laser head before and after treatment.
- Do not apply laser to wounds following removal of neoplasia.

Postsurgical Wounds
- A daily dose of 1-3 J/cm^2 is recommended for the first 7 to 10 days if possible, followed by a 1- to 2-day break, continued until the wound is healed. If daily treatment is not possible, then treatment three times per week may be performed.

Lick Granulomas
- Administer 1-3 J/cm^2, directly over the entire granuloma and at least 1 cm from the periphery. Depending on the size of the granuloma, the wound should be treated as frequently as possible; daily to a few times a week is beneficial. The granuloma should be treated until the wound is healed and hair growth has resumed.

Osteoarthritis
- Administer 8-10 J/cm^2.
- Treat along the joint lines and surrounding area.
- Hip: Start treatment at the greater trochanter, then direct around the cranial, medial, and caudal surfaces of the hip in a circumferential pattern.
- Stifle: Start at the patella. The joint line may then be followed either medially or laterally to complete the full circumference.
- Hock and digits: Start below the point of the hock and circle around the hock while applying treatment. It is important that the anatomy of the tarsus be considered, with its distal extent at the tarsometatarsal junction, to be certain that the appropriate areas are treated. The calcaneal tendon may also be treated. Individual toes may be treated but it is recommended that a small laser apparatus be used.
- Shoulder: Start at the greater tubercle, continuing circumferentially around the joint. Because of the tissue depth in this area, a longer wavelength laser source is necessary. If the biceps tendon or other tendons are involved, the treatment should include the length of the tendon.
- Elbow: Start below the olecranon process and continue around the entire joint in a circumferential manner. Treating distally and proximally from the elbow also benefits the surrounding soft tissue.
- Carpus and digits: Start at the accessory carpal pad and then treat in a circumferential manner. Sweeping motions may be performed distally and proximally to cover the distal and proximal aspects of the joint as well as the surrounding soft tissue. The digits may be approached the same way, although it is sometimes difficult to move in a circumferential manner. The dorsal and palmar aspects of the digits may be treated.
- Cervical spine: Treat the entire cervical spine from the suboccipital area down to the upper thoracic region. The laser may be applied directly over the dorsal cervical spine, and then moved over the epaxial musculature on both sides. Do not apply the laser for a prolonged period over the carotid arteries.
- Thoracic and lumbar spine: Treat directly over the area as well as the epaxial and surrounding musculature.
- Tendon conditions (biceps tenosynovitis, supraspinatus tendonitis, patellar tendonitis, and other tendon inflammatory conditions): The length of the superficial aspect of the tendon should be treated along with the surrounding soft tissues.

sid, Once daily.
From Millis D, Levine D: *Canine rehabilitation and physical therapy,* ed 2, St Louis, 2014, Saunders.

drainage, producing rapid reduction of edema. Inflammation is reduced due to the vasodilating effects of the laser.

The dosage needed for therapeutic effect varies depending on location and severity of the injury and the total size of the treatment area. Therapy is measured in joules administered to the specific area measured in cm^2. Most conditions require application of 1 to 8 joules/cm^2. The time needed to administer the dose must also be calculated. For example, for a 250 mW laser, 4 seconds is needed to deliver 1 joule (J) of energy:

$$0.250\ \text{W} = 1\ \text{J} \div x\ \text{seconds}$$
$$0.250\ \text{W} \times x\ \text{seconds} = 1\ \text{J}$$
$$x\ \text{seconds} = 1\ \text{J} \div 0.250\ \text{W}$$
$$x = 4\ \text{seconds}$$

A variety of companies market laser therapy equipment to veterinary practices. Many of these are reasonably priced and treatments can be performed by the veterinary technician. Most have preset controls for treatment of specific conditions that will provide a specific number of joules, thus minimizing the need to calculate time required. Once the total dose is calculated, it is usually administered daily for three days and then twice a week as needed until the desired effect is achieved. However, the dosages and frequencies have been extrapolated from research that is not specific to these conditions in veterinary species and should be used with caution. Box 19-2 contains dosage guidelines for a variety of conditions.

Safety concerns in the use of therapeutic lasers are primarily related to protection of the eyes of those in the room during the procedure, including the patient. Laser light can be reflected off a variety of surfaces (e.g., exam tables, jewelry) and cause indirect exposure to the eyes. Safety goggles designed to filter out the specific

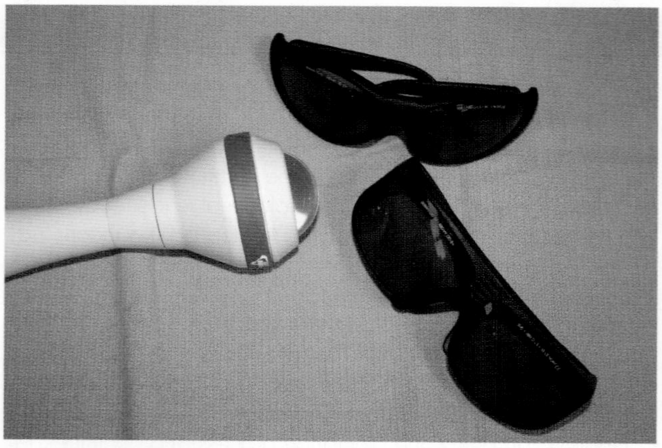

FIGURE 19-16 Protective eyewear should always be used when using a laser therapy. (From Millis D, Levine D: *Canine rehabilitation and physical therapy*, ed 2, St Louis, 2014, Saunders.)

wavelengths emitted by the laser device must be worn by all individuals involved in the therapy (Fig. 19-16). The patient's eyes should also be shielded with eye goggles or a thick piece of cloth.

Prepare the patient by clipping the hair over the treatment area; 50% to 99% of the light may be absorbed by hair. If the treatment area contains dark pigmentation, it is recommended that the dose be increased by 25%. Any iodine or povidone iodine should be washed off the area. Any topical medications, especially corticosteroids and other photosensitizing agents, should be removed. Be sure that the patient and all individuals in the area have protective eyewear.

Laser therapy is administered with a handheld probe; most probes have a small beam area that is useful for treating small surfaces (Fig. 19-17). Other lasers have several beam sizes in the same unit to treat larger areas. For most treatment applications, the laser is applied with the probe in contact with the skin. With the noncontact method, it is necessary to hold the probe perpendicular to the treatment area to minimize wave reflection and beam divergence. Noncontact application is recommended for wound treatment. The appropriate dosage may be applied to larger areas by administering the calculated dose to each individual site in a grid fashion, or by slowly moving the probe over the entire surface, being certain to evenly distribute the energy to each site. A coupling medium is not necessary, as in ultrasound, because the laser beam is not attenuated by air. A summary of a protocol for application of laser therapy is in Box 19-3.

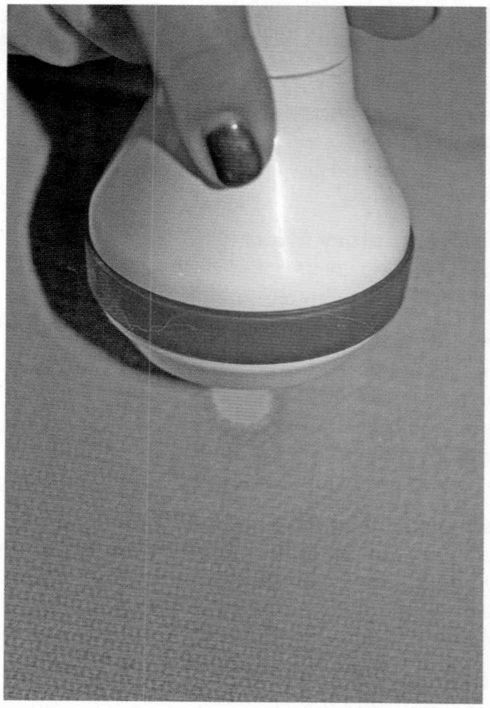

FIGURE 19-17 Laser therapy is generally administered with a handheld probe; most probes have a small beam area that is useful for treating small surfaces. (From Millis D, Levine D: *Canine rehabilitation and physical therapy*, ed 2, St Louis, 2014, Saunders.)

BOX 19-3 Key Points for Laser Use in Dogs

1. Clip hair.
2. Measure area to be treated (a playing card is 57 cm^2).
3. Determine treatment dose.
4. Increase dose for dogs with dark skin by 25%.
5. Determine the number of J/cm^2, total joules, and the length of treatment time for laser application. If treating an area the size of a playing card with 10 J/cm^2, the total treatment is 600 J. If using a 10-W laser, the treatment time is 60 seconds.
6. Place safety goggles on all in the immediate area.
7. Hold laser perpendicular to the skin (direct contact minimizes laser light reflection; noncontact application is recommended for wounds).
8. Apply laser treatment using an overlapping grid technique to be certain that the treatment is applied equally to all areas.

From Millis D, Levine D: *Canine rehabilitation and physical therapy*, ed 2, St Louis, 2014, Saunders.

REVIEW QUESTIONS

Matching—Traditional Chinese Medicine (TCM)

Match the TCM term with its description or definition.

_____ **1.** qi
_____ **2.** meridians
_____ **3.** yin
_____ **4.** yang
_____ **5.** moxibustion
_____ **6.** acupuncture
_____ **7.** acupressure
_____ **8.** sonapuncture

A. calm, dark, moon
B. placing of needles into acupoints
C. use of heat to stimulate acupoints
D. channels found throughout the body
E. unyielding, active, sun
F. use of ultrasound to stimulate acupoints
G. using fingers to stimulate acupoints
H. life force energy

Matching—Herbal Therapies

Match the herbal therapy term with its definition.

_____ **1.** single herb remedies
_____ **2.** herb combinations
_____ **3.** an herb known for effectiveness in treatment of a particular condition
_____ **4.** herbal infusion
_____ **5.** liquid herbal extract preserved with alcohol
_____ **6.** wet herbal pack
_____ **7.** hot herbal compress

A. blends
B. tisane
C. simples
D. poultice
E. fomentation
F. tincture
G. specific

Matching—Massage

Match the type of massage with its definition.

_____ **1.** enhances lymph drainage
_____ **2.** stretches muscles and tendons
_____ **3.** helps loosen superficial scar tissue
_____ **4.** helps maintain skin tone

A. petrissage
B. stretch pressure massage
C. effleurage
D. friction massage

Short Answer/Fill in Blank

Complete the following statements or answer the questions.

1. What is the primary safety equipment required for laser therapy?
2. How many joules can a 1 Watt laser deliver in 1 second?
3. To minimize wave reflection and beam divergence, the laser probe must be held ___ to the skin.
4. In pigmented areas, how is the laser therapy dose modified to achieve the desired result?
5. Most conditions require application of ____ joules/cm^2.

RECOMMENDED READING

Bell KL: *Holistic aromatherapy for animals*, Forres, Scotland, 2002, Findhorn Press.
Fulton E, Prasad K: *Animal reiki*, Berkeley, CA, 2006, Ulysses Press.
Gaynor G, Muir W: *Handbook of veterinary pain management*, ed 3, St Louis, 2015, Elsevier.
Graham H, Vlamis G: *Bach flower remedies for animals*, Forres, Scotland, 1999, Findhorn Press.
Harvey C: *The new encyclopedia of flower remedies*, London, 2007, Watkins Publishing.
Mills D, Levine D: *Canine rehabilitation and physical therapy*, ed 2, St Louis, 2014, Elsevier.
Morgan D: *Ayurvedic medicine for dogs*, Forres, Scotland, 2007, Findhorn Press.
Puotinen CJ: *The encyclopedia of natural care*, Los Angeles, 2000, Keats Publishing.
Riegel R: *Laser therapy in companion animal practice*, Newark, DE, 2008, LiteCure, LLC.
Schwartz C, Schwartz ME: *Four paws, five directions: a guide to Chinese medicine for cats and dogs*, Berkeley, CA, 2004, Celestial Arts.
Selby A: *Ayurveda*, Minneapolis, MN, 2001, Creative Publishing International.
Soisti-Mattelon K, Mattelon P: *The holistic animal handbook*, Hillsboro, OR, 2000, Beyond Words Publishing.
Tellington-Jones L, Taylor S: *The Tellington TTouch*, New York, 1993, Penguin Books.

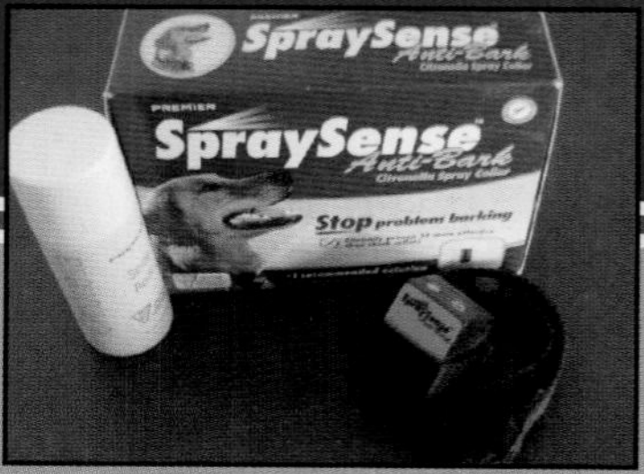

20 Animal Behavior

OUTLINE

LEARNING OBJECTIVES

After reviewing this chapter, the reader will be able to:

1. Describe the processes by which behaviors develop.
2. Differentiate between positive and negative reinforcement and punishment.
3. List and describe types of aggressive behavior that may be seen in dogs and cats.
4. Describe the role of veterinary professionals in preventing behavior problems.
5. List the steps in house training a puppy.
6. Describe proper litter box care.
7. List the different options cats look for in scratching posts.
8. Describe the role of veterinary professionals in managing behavior problems.
9. List and give examples of various behavior modification techniques.
10. Describe the procedure for referring clients to professionals for resolution of behavior problems.

KEY TERMS

Aggression	Elimination	Pheromone	Socialization
Agonistic	Ethology	Punishment	Stimulus
Anthropomorphism	Imprinting	Queen	Substrate
Behavior	Operant conditioning	Reinforcement	Veterinary behaviorist

Experts agree that behavior problems are common and a leading cause of death in dogs and cats. Often, the "problem" is normal dog and cat **behavior** that the owner finds inappropriate and then makes worse in attempts to correct it (Fig. 20-1). This may start at a young age with house training and continues with attention-seeking behaviors, destruction, barking, and aggression. Often, the pet owner does not know where to go for advice, and it is here that the veterinary practice can provide an important service to its clients and their pets. There are now many books and continuing education (CE) programs on this topic, which allow technicians and veterinarians to gain advanced training in behavior. The Society of Veterinary Behavior Technicians provides information on CE opportunities for technicians in behavior. In 2007 the Academy of Veterinary Behavior Technicians was approved by NAVTA to provide a Veterinary Technician Specialty credential for technicians in behavior.

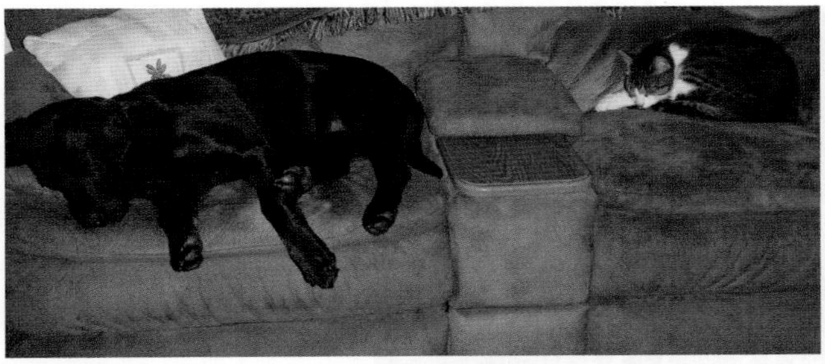

FIGURE 20-1 Owners need to decide whether a particular behavior is a problem, because the animal rarely recognizes it as such. For example, barking may be a desirable behavior for one owner, but a problem for another.

WHAT IS BEHAVIOR AND WHERE DOES IT COME FROM?

Behavior is any act done by an animal. An animal does not exhibit a behavioral act without a reason, although the reason may not be obvious to humans. For any behavior to occur, there must be a **stimulus,** some internal or external change that exceeds a threshold causing stimulation of the nervous and/or endocrine systems. This receptor and cellular stimulation and integration of information requires a number of chemical messengers in the animal's body, including epinephrine, acetylcholine, dopamine, serotonin, and many others. Some problem behaviors are caused by increased or decreased amounts of these neurotransmitters. This has led to the development of veterinary psychopharmacology.

The study of animal behavior is referred to as **ethology.** Most ethologists agree that animal behavior is both genetically programmed (instinctive) and learned (conditioned response). There are two general categories of conditioned responses: classical conditioning and operant conditioning. Classical conditioning refers to the association of stimuli that occur at approximately the same time or in roughly the same area. **Operant conditioning** refers to the association of a particular activity (the operant) with a punishment or reward.

The pattern of behaviors that bonds animals to their caretakers occurs in early life and is referred to as **imprinting.** In wild animals, this is the process that allows a newborn animal to recognize and follow its parents. In domestic animals, the imprinting process usually involves other animals and humans that the animal encounters during a specific period of time in early life. The most important time period for behavior development in dogs and cats is from 3 to 12 weeks. At this young age, the animal learns about its environment, how to interact with others, and what not to fear. What occurs during this habituation or socialization period can affect the animal for the rest of its life. For example, animals that are not socialized during this period can develop lifelong phobias (Fig. 20-2). Although veterinary professionals have little effect on genetics (other than to recommend that an animal not be bred or help a client choose a specific breed to adopt), they play an important role by educating clients about the correct way to raise and interact with their pets. Of course, it is important to remember that disease also plays a role in animal behavior problems such as in hypothyroidism in dogs, hyperthyroidism in cats, and cognitive dysfunction in older animals. Sometimes aggression or even house soiling may be caused by a medical problem.

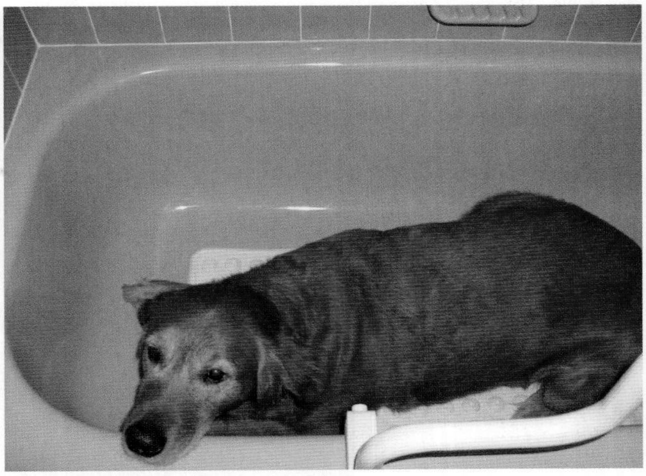

FIGURE 20-2 This dog was frightened by thunder when it was 10 weeks old and became afraid of thunder and then loud noises for the next 14 years. For years, it exhibited destructive behavior trying to escape the noise. The dog finally found refuge in the bathtub.

Animals also must learn how to interact with one another. Many households have more than one dog or cat and often have both. Introducing young animals is usually easier than introducing adults. Being social animals, dogs have a hierarchy or pecking order that determines which one gets first access to coveted resources such as food, toys, owners, and resting spots (Fig. 20-3). These relationships can fluctuate and are not to be confused with the more structured hierarchy relationships between nondomestic species, such as wolves.

Operant conditioning can be used to reinforce a desired behavior or punish an undesirable one, although the latter is not recommended. Positive **reinforcement** refers to any immediate pleasant occurrence that follows a behavior. For example, if a dog receives a treat or immediate praise when it sits on command, that behavior is reinforced with a pleasant experience. Negative reinforcement refers to any immediate unpleasant occurrence used to create a desired behavior. An example of negative reinforcement is the use of electric fences to help a dog learn the boundaries it may navigate. This differs from punishment in that **punishment** is used to remove or decrease a behavior. For example, depending on how they are used, shock collars and citronella collars designed to reduce barking behaviors is a form of positive punishment (Fig. 20-4). Positive punishment involves adding an undesirable occurrence to decrease a behavior. Negative punishment involves removing a desirable occurrence to decrease a behavior. Withholding affection when a dog jumps up to greet you or not giving treats when a dog is begging are examples of negative punishment. It is more difficult to use punishment to influence a dog's behavior and it may cause the dog to become fearful or aggressive. Many trainers and behaviorists use a combination of positive reinforcement and negative punishment.

FIGURE 20-3 The dog on the ground is exhibiting submissive behavior to its sibling. It is important for owners to recognize and respect the canine hierarchy in the home, or interdog aggression may result. (From Beaver BV: *Canine behavior: insights and answers*, ed 2, St Louis, 2009, Saunders.)

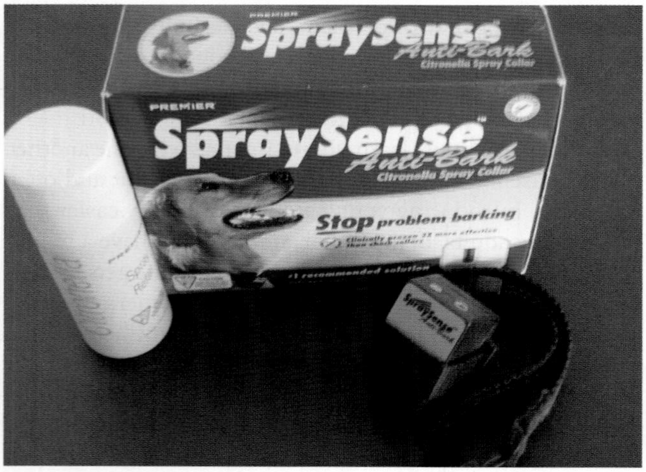

FIGURE 20-4 Citronella collars may be used to reduce barking behavior in dogs.

PREVENTING BEHAVIOR PROBLEMS IN COMPANION ANIMALS

Most behavior problems are easier to prevent than to correct. Aggression is the most common problem for which owners seek guidance, but many pet owners are annoyed when their animals damage household belongings and exhibit house soiling behavior. Techniques based on scientifically valid ethologic and learning principles minimize such behaviors. However, much of the information to which owners have easy access does not always meet these criteria. Thus, veterinary technicians are an important source of scientifically accurate information on preventing behavior problems.

Although many clients consider their pets to be part of the family, it is especially important that clients be provided with basic information on animal behavior to avoid the unrealistic expectations that develop when clients "anthropomorphize" their pets. **Anthropomorphism** refers to the attribution of human characteristics and emotions to animals. Pet owners often misinterpret their pet's behavior as spite, jealousy, or guilt, when the pet is in fact reacting based on learned behaviors. For example, a pet that an owner describes as "looking guilty" when the owner returns home to discover a house training "accident" is more likely exhibiting fear as a result of learning that the owner becomes angry in the presence of house soiling, not that the pet caused the anger by having an accident.

HOUSE TRAINING

House training is one of the most important and first behaviors that young pets are expected to learn. Many owners use outdated methods to attempt to house train their pets. These methods often interfere with success or damage the relationship with the pet. Problems related to house training may result in the animal being turned loose, isolated in a yard or tied, or relinquished to a shelter. Dogs and cats can be encouraged to eliminate reliably in locations that are acceptable to their human owners. Cats, dogs, pigs, ferrets, and rabbits can learn to use litter boxes. Other species of domestic companion animals are either caged or kept outside because their **elimination** behavior is not restricted to specific locations.

Dogs

People have probably been training dogs not to eliminate in the house for almost as long as dogs have been domesticated. You might assume that thousands of years of practice have resulted in good house training techniques. Surprisingly, this is not always the case.

House training requires that the dog be taken out frequently, especially when it wakes up, after it eats, and whenever it appears to be sniffing around the house. When a puppy cannot be monitored, it should be confined to a crate (Fig. 20-5). Most "accidents" occur when the puppy is left alone. There are different types of crates, including collapsible ones, and those made of wire, plastic, and wood. Crate training is also useful for preventing destructive behaviors such as chewing. The use of the crate should not be excessive,

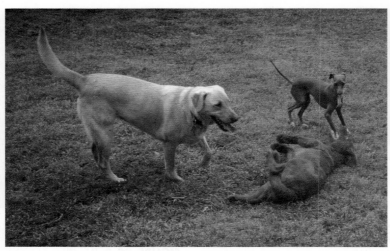

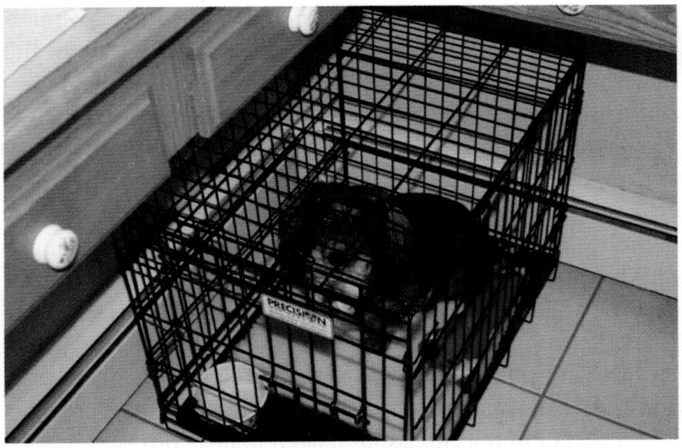

FIGURE 20-5 The crate is a useful tool to manage a puppy when it cannot be supervised in the home. This helps with house training as well as preventing destructive behavior. (Courtesy Donna Harris.)

because 8-week-old puppies cannot hold their bowels longer than 4 to 6 hours. Puppies will soil in the crate if they cannot get out when they need to eliminate or if the crate is too large. Crates can be purchased for the pet's adult size and many now come with partitions to subdivide it when the puppy is small.

TECHNICIAN NOTE Help clients select a crate that is easy to clean and the correct size for the puppy when it is an adult.

Owners must be made aware of several important points when house training their dog. First, a dog's confinement to a crate must not exceed the time the animal can control its bladder and bowels. For young puppies, this can be as little as 1 hour, or sometimes as much as 2 or 3 hours at a time. In addition, many puppies need to eliminate at least once during the night.

Second, the dog must be actively taught, by reinforcing correct behavior, the desired location for elimination. Owners should reward elimination outside with verbal praise and petting, and possibly a special tidbit. The timing of this reward, however, is critical. Research in animal learning suggests that a delay of longer than 0.5 seconds between the behavior and the subsequent reinforcement significantly decreases the effectiveness of the reinforcement. For example, if the owner waits by the door to reinforce the puppy at the door as it returns from eliminating in the yard, the behavior that has been reinforced is coming to the door. In these cases, owners often complain that all the puppy does when taken out is to attempt to go back in or to stand by the door. This should come as no surprise because going to the door is what the puppy has inadvertently been rewarded for doing. To reinforce the elimination behavior, the owner must go outside with the puppy and provide reinforcement immediately following elimination at the location where it occurs. Clicker training may also be useful in house training of puppies (Box 20-1).

BOX 20-1 House Training Puppies: Clicker Method

1. Use a collar and leash to take the puppy outside.
2. Go to the same spot in the yard each time.
3. Cue the puppy to "go potty."
4. Click and treat the puppy as the puppy passes urine or stool.

Finally, use of physical punishment in house training is never appropriate. Interactive punishment that involves the owner (even if delivered at the time of house soiling) may cause the dog to become reluctant to eliminate in the owner's presence at other times or may even result in the dog becoming afraid of the owner. This interferes with the owner's attempts to appropriately reinforce elimination outside. Calmly saying "oops" or calling the puppy should be sufficient to temporarily interrupt the behavior. The dog can then be taken outside in a positive, nonthreatening manner and rewarded if it eliminates. The use of aluminum cans containing pennies or other loud noises, even when not associated with humans, can startle the puppy and further inhibit learning.

In an ideal house training program, the dog's environment and behavior should be so well managed that correct behavior is reinforced with 100% consistency, and opportunities for inappropriate behavior never occur. In reality, this ideal is seldom met, but if owners are made aware of it through your educational efforts, it may give them a much more accurate perspective on the time and effort required for house training.

Educating owners about house training dogs should be much more detailed than simply telling them to "get a crate and put the dog in it when you can't watch him." Handouts on this important process should also be provided.

Cats

One of the reasons people choose cats as pets instead of dogs is because they can be readily trained to use a litter box for elimination and do not need to be walked. The process of encouraging cats to consistently use litter boxes is based on different developmental events than is house training dogs. It is normal instinctual behavior for kittens and cats to use a **substrate** for elimination. Kittens do not need to observe the **queen** eliminating or have the owner demonstrate part of the process by raking the cat's paws in the litter. Providing a clean, easily accessible litter box with an acceptable substrate is sufficient. However, the accessibility of the litter box and suitability of the substrate must be examined from the kitten's or cat's perspective. The major complaint owners have is that their cats stop or inconsistently use the litter box and choose to eliminate somewhere else in the house. If this problem is not corrected, these cats may be confined to the outdoors or relinquished to shelters. Because there are many reasons for a cat to stop using its litter box, a detailed history is needed to determine the cause.

Because kittens are physically and behaviorally immature, a litter box should be within easy access at all times. This may mean providing several litter boxes at strategic locations in the house or initially limiting the cat's access to only portions of the house. The litter box should be easily accessible but also should afford some privacy. High-traffic areas are not a good choice, but neither is locating the box in a basement with a cold cement floor. Proximity to appliances that make unexpected, startling noises, such as the washer, furnace, or hot water heater, should also be avoided.

Studies have found that cats prefer the softer texture of fine-grained substrates. Thus, a cat is less likely to develop an aversion to a clumping litter composed of very small particles. However, cats develop idiosyncratic preferences for substrates and locations for elimination for reasons that are not well understood. These changing preferences are often the basis of many inappropriate elimination problems in cats. Sometimes these preferences can be influenced by the condition of the litter material. Cats may avoid litter that is consistently dirty, too deep, or scented (Fig. 20-6). One study found that cats with elimination problems were more likely to have scented than unscented litter as compared with cats without such problems.

Owners are sometimes under the impression that the more litter they put in the box, the less often they need to clean it. General guidelines are to keep the litter depth at no more than 2 inches, remove feces and urine clumps daily, and change the litter frequently enough to prevent odors from developing and ensure that the majority of the litter is always dry. **Veterinary behaviorists** recommend that the litter box be changed once a week. Changing the litter should include disposing of dirty litter and washing the box with warm soapy water.

> TECHNICIAN NOTE Covered litter boxes may appeal to owners but from a cat's point of view it is difficult to see who may be lurking outside. When collecting a history on an inappropriate elimination case always ask for the type and location of litter box in addition to the substrate.

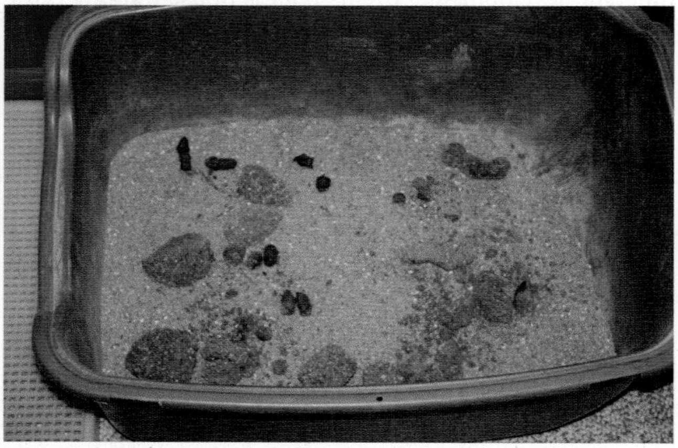

FIGURE 20-6 Cats are fastidious, and one reason they stop using the litter box is that it is too dirty for them. Litter boxes should be cleaned daily, and there should be one litter box per cat in the household plus one extra.

Another consideration influencing the cat's perception of litter box accessibility is the presence of other cats in the household. A litter box may be temporarily unavailable because another cat is either using it or "guarding" it. Thus, advise owners to provide one litter box per cat, plus one extra, and to keep the boxes in different locations so that a single cat cannot block another cat's access to the litter box area. In addition, the litter box location should allow the cat using it to be aware of the presence of other cats so as to prevent any surprise attacks that may occur during elimination. The owner must also understand that if the cat learns to associate the litter box with punishment such as catching it there in order to administer medication, it may stop using it. Box 20-2 provides a checklist of important issues related to litter boxes.

PREVENTING DESTRUCTIVE BEHAVIOR BY CATS

Probably more owners recognize the need to provide their cats with litter boxes than to provide scratching posts. Because cats scratch for a variety of reasons, cats may want to scratch in different locations for different reasons. One of the most important motivations for cats scratching objects with their front claws is territorial marking. Scratching leaves a visual as well as an olfactory mark that serves as an indication of the cat's presence. In addition to marking, scratching also serves to stretch the muscles and tendons of the legs and remove the worn outer sheaths from the claws. It may also be used as a greeting or play behavior.

Scratching objects should be provided in locations in which the behavior is likely to be triggered. Even if the cat scratches objects when allowed outdoors, it still should have access to an acceptable object indoors. Merely providing a scratching object does not guarantee the cat will use it preferentially to carpet, drapes, or furniture. The scratching objects must match the cat's preferences for desirable locations, and with regard to height, orientation, and texture (Fig. 20-7).

If a new cat is encouraged to use its own scratching post, it may avoid exercising its claws on furniture or drapes. Owners must understand that they should discourage cats from clawing their possessions. They can do this by distracting the cat caught in the act or preventing its access to the items. Many clients merely resort to having the cat declawed as a preventive measure or solution to the problem behavior. Technicians are in the best position to educate owner about all of the options surrounding nail care and scratching behavior.

BOX 20-2 Checklist for Litter Boxes

1. Place the box in a quiet location.
2. Make sure the location is accessible from the cat's perspective.
3. Use fine-grained unscented litter.
4. The litter depth should be approximately 2 inches.
5. Scoop daily, empty, and wash the litter box once a week.

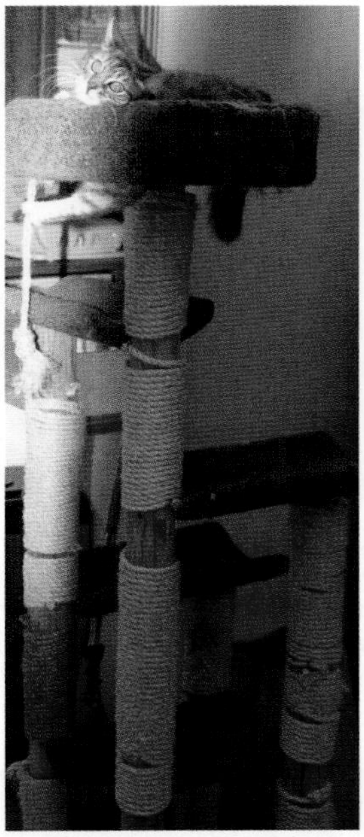

FIGURE 20-7 Cats normally exercise their claws, and it is important to provide them with scratching posts that are large and sturdy enough to support their weight. The scratching posts must also be located in appropriate places in the home. (Courtesy Donna Harris.)

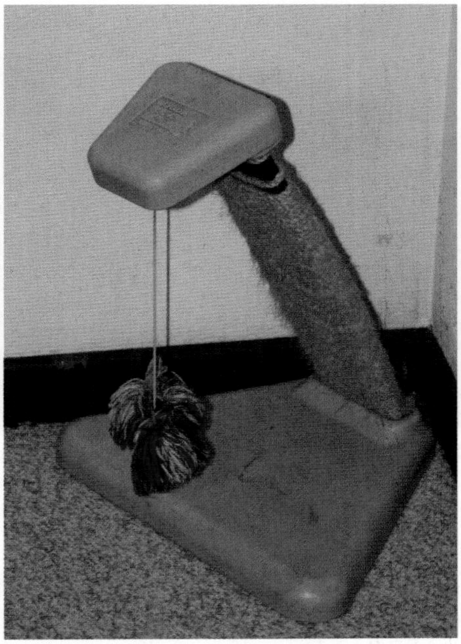

FIGURE 20-8 This scratching post is not tall enough to allow the cat to stretch to its full height while using it. This may result in the cat finding more suitable objects to use, such as the couch or the curtains. (Courtesy Donna Harris.)

SCRATCHING POSTS

Many scratching posts available commercially do not permit the cat to reach vertically to its full height to scratch, as many cats like to do (Fig. 20-8). Also they are not sturdy enough to support the cat's weight and readily fall over, frightening the cat. For larger cats using relatively short posts, this means they are scratching almost with their abdomen on the floor. It may be a good idea to talk to owners about the desirability of taller or even floor-to-ceiling scratching poles. If the back of the couch allows the cat to reach to its full height to scratch but the scratching post does not, it is easy to guess which surface the cat will prefer.

Orientation

Not all cats scratch vertically all of the time. Some cats may prefer to stretch their legs out in front and rake backward in a horizontal motion. If this is the case, the cat may be more likely to use a flat, horizontal object (Fig. 20-9) than a vertical post. Some cats may use both, depending on where, when, and why they scratch. One unusual cat was reported to only scratch upside down by pulling herself along on her back as she scratched the underside of the couch.

Texture

This may be the most frequently overlooked aspect of providing an acceptable scratching object. As with other aspects of the behavioral pattern of scratching, cats vary in textures they prefer. Cats that like to rake their claws in long, vertical motions may be more likely to use an object with a texture that permits this. If the cat scratches vertically and the texture is not conducive to those motions, the cat may not use the object. Other cats use more of a "picking" motion and may prefer items covered with sisal, wrapped horizontally. It has been proposed that an object that has been scratched repeatedly, with the result that the covering is somewhat shredded and holds the cat's scent, will be preferred over a new, unused object. This suggests that owners should not replace well-worn scratching posts, even if they appear unsightly.

> *TECHNICIAN NOTE* Remind clients to save scraps of material off favorite scratched items to use on scratching posts when purchasing new furniture. Scratching posts of the same material can help protect new furniture.

The scratching object should be placed in a location where the cat is likely to be motivated to scratch, or adjacent to an unacceptable item the cat is already using. To encourage the cat to use the desirable object, it can be scented with catnip or a commercial **pheromone** (Feliway, CEVA Animal Health, St. Louis, MO), or a toy can be attached to the top to entice the cat to reach high up the post. Raking the cat's feet up and down the post is not necessary and may actually have adverse effects. The most reliable way to discourage scratching of inappropriate objects is to first provide an appropriate substitute and then change the texture of the "off-limit" items. Owners can change the texture by covering it with plastic, sandpaper, or another covering with an unpleasant (from the cat's perspective) texture.

PREVENTING DESTRUCTIVE BEHAVIOR BY DOGS

Destructive behavior is a classification of behavior based more on the owner's view of the result (destruction) than on the actual behavior that caused it. Digging, chewing, tearing,

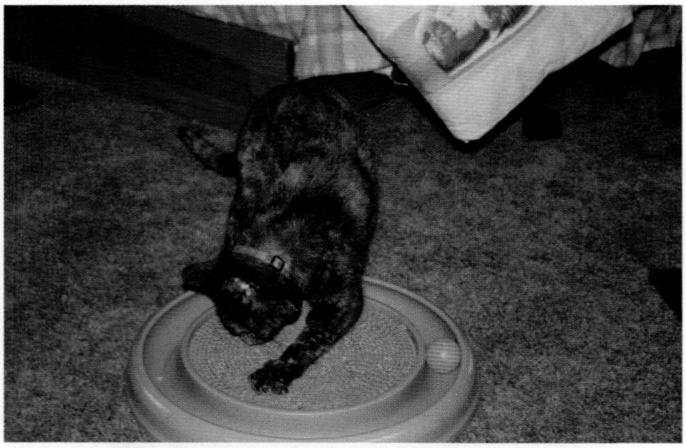

FIGURE 20-9 Horizontal scratching objects such as this pad scented with catnip may be preferred over vertical objects. (Courtesy Donna Harris.)

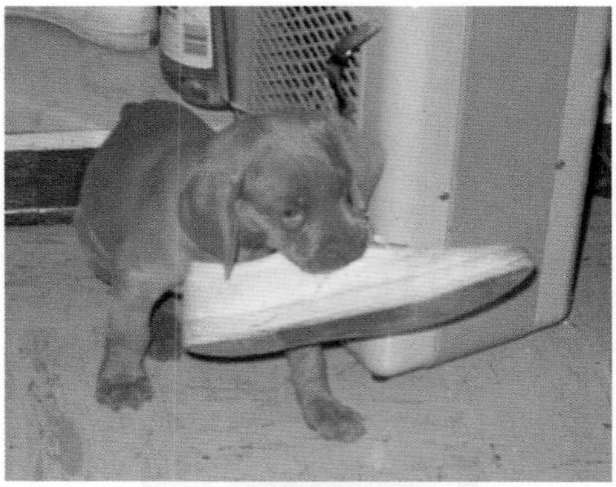

FIGURE 20-10 Chewing is normal dog behavior and needs to be directed to acceptable objects. Owners should remove their things from the dog's mouth and replace them with the dog's own toys. A dog cannot tell the difference between an old shoe and a new one. (From Beaver BV: *Canine behavior: insights and answers*, ed 2, St Louis, 2009, Saunders.)

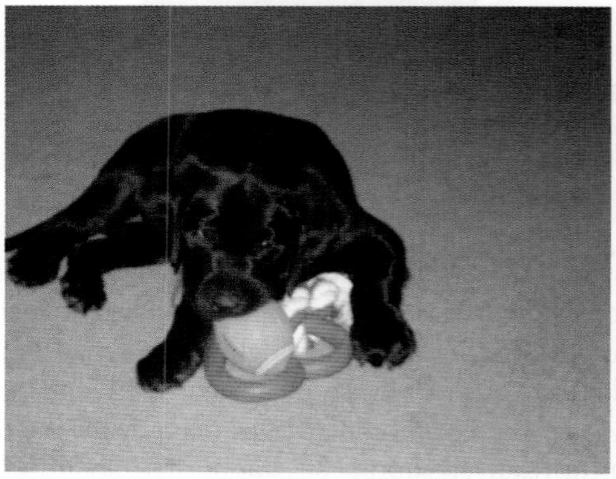

FIGURE 20-11 This puppy did not even notice that a different item had been placed in its mouth. It is best to introduce puppies to suitable toys when they are young and encourage them to play with the toys.

scratching, moving objects from one place to another, and removing the contents from the trash are all considered destructive behavior and are self-rewarding.

Dogs show these behaviors for a variety of reasons. Destructive behavior that is the symptomatic manifestation of other problems, such as separation anxiety or noise phobias, can be treated but may not be prevented. In these cases, the underlying problem must be resolved, rather than trying to treat the symptom. However, destructive behavior that occurs as the result of a normal developmental process, such as teething, play, and investigative behavior, can often be prevented or at least minimized.

Dogs vary in their need for physical activity and play. Some dogs are content to lead relatively inactive lives, whereas others seem to be on the move constantly. Just as with cats' scratching, the goal in minimizing problem destructive behavior resulting from teething, play, and investigative behavior is not to eliminate the behavior, but to direct it toward acceptable objects by making acceptable toys more attractive than household items. This must be done on a consistent basis or some items may be destroyed.

APPEALING TOYS

Dogs should be exposed to suitable toys when they are young. The attractiveness of acceptable toys can be maximized by first rewarding the dog every time it plays with them. Toys should also elicit the play patterns that the dog is likely to exhibit. For example, dogs that like to shake toys may be more satisfied with one made of lambskin than with a tennis ball. Toys should be available for chewing and tearing, as well as for carrying and chasing, if the dog displays both patterns of play behavior. It may be helpful to establish a toy rotation so that different toys are available each day to make them more appealing.

If the dog is caught chewing an unacceptable item, the item should be taken away and replaced with one that is acceptable (Figs. 20-10 and 20-11). To decrease the dog's interest in household items, even when the owner is not present, attempts can be made to lessen their appeal. Commercial products, such as Bitter Apple, are available to give objects a bad taste. Motion detectors or Snappy Trainers (modified mousetraps that do not harm the animal) can discourage animals from bothering specific items or areas, or items can be "booby-trapped" in other creative ways. Remind owners of the advisability of "dog-proofing" the house just as they would for a young child.

Dogs that insist on digging outside can be provided with their own area in which to do so. This area should consist of loose soil or sand to facilitate digging. Owners can shallowly bury enticing items in this area to attract the dog.

PREVENTING AGGRESSIVE BEHAVIOR PROBLEMS

Aggression is the most common type of behavior problem reported in dogs and occurs in cats as well. Aggressive behavior is normal behavior for most species of animals, including companion animals. **Aggression,** defined as behavior that is intended to harm another individual, is an aspect of agonistic behavior. **Agonistic** behaviors are behaviors that animals show in situations involving social conflict. Submission, avoidance, escaping, offensive and defensive threats, and offensive and defensive aggression are all part

TABLE 20-1 Common Type of Aggressive Behavior in Dogs and Cats

TYPE OF AGGRESSION	COMMENTS
Conflict-related	Result of unpredictable environment or inconsistent/inappropriate use of punishment
Fear-induced	Fearful situations, e.g., noises, veterinary office
Predatory	Instinctual stalking and pouncing with no warning growl
Pain-induced	Protective instinct
Intermale	Natural instinct usually eliminated by castration
Territorial	Dogs: usually directed toward humans that are not members of their household Cats: usually directed toward other cats
Maternal	Normal protective instinct

of the agonistic behavior system. There are many different types of aggression displayed by dogs and cats (Table 20-1). Aggression may be directed against people, family members or strangers, children, or other dogs and species. Different types of aggression include fearful, territorial, maternal, intermale, interfemale, predatory, play-related, redirected, and others. It is important to determine which type is present so as to treat it. The most common complaint from dog owners is aggression toward people, whereas the most common complaint from cat owners is aggression toward other cats. Because the factors that determine when and where an animal will display aggressive or threatening behavior are not fully understood, it is unlikely that preventing problems will be a simple process. In some cases, owners inadvertently reinforce aggressive behavior by withdrawing from the pet when it acts aggressively.

Aggression directed at children is considered the number one public health problem in children. The statistical group reporting the highest number of bites is young boys, 5 to 9 years of age. More than 50% of children have sustained a bite injury before the age of 18. Dogs must be socialized to children when they are young, and children must be taught how to behave around dogs, particularly strange ones. Parents also often worry about dog aggression toward infants. It is important to advise new parents about how to introduce their new baby to their dog.

> *TECHNICIAN NOTE* Aggression is the most common type of behavior problem reported in dogs.

PUPPY TESTS

One way to prevent aggression problems in animals would be to select pets that are unlikely to develop such problems. Popular literature describes a variety of "puppy tests" that supposedly predict a puppy's likelihood for dominant behavior or aggression problems as an adult. This information can be used to suggest behavioral tendencies and match puppies and new owners. Current research suggests that temperament testing may be too subjective to truly aid in matching puppies with owners. When selecting a new pet it is far more advisable to match activity and lifestyle. An active puppy living in a small apartment with a sedentary family is more likely to develop behavior problems than a puppy with an active family who receives daily exercise.

CASTRATION

Castrating male animals clearly reduces some forms of aggressive behavior in many species, including dogs, cats, and horses. Postpubertal castration seems to be as effective as prepubertal. Reports on dog bite statistics show that intact male dogs are more often involved in dog bites (70% to 76% of dog bite incidents reported). The sex of dogs in unreported dog bite incidents is not known. Therefore, selection of female animals as pets may reduce problems with aggressive behavior. All male dogs should be castrated unless they are purebreds that are to be used in a breeding program. In addition to aggression, castration prevents other potential problems such as roaming, urine marking, and prostate problems.

SOCIALIZATION

Many species of mammals and birds have sensitive periods of development of normal species-typical social behavior. This sensitive period in dogs has been well studied, and to a lesser degree in cats and horses. The sensitive socialization period usually occurs fairly early in life. For example, in dogs it is from 3 to 12 weeks of age and in cats from 2 to 7 weeks.

Companion animals must have a variety of pleasant experiences with different types of people, other animals, and environments during these sensitive periods so that they are able to accept humans as their social peers later in life. Poorly socialized animals are typically fearful of people or may attach strongly to one or two individuals but are unable to generalize this acceptance to unfamiliar individuals. It is also important to habituate the puppy and kitten to a variety of environmental situations (Fig. 20-12). Fear of people or specific situations can sometimes develop into defensive aggression problems (Fig. 20-13). Because many young animals are seen in the veterinary hospital, it is important that these experiences be pleasant to avoid fear and aggression problems. Veterinary technicians should encourage dog owners to enroll puppies in puppy classes and expose both puppies and kittens to a variety of gentle handling and play sessions with people outside the family.

> *TECHNICIAN NOTE* Training and educational material for veterinary technicians on running puppy or kitten kindergarten classes is widely available.

BEHAVIOR IN THE CLINIC

Pets brought into the veterinary clinic may exhibit behaviors unique to that situation. A normally pleasant dog may become fearful and aggressive. A normally outgoing pet may

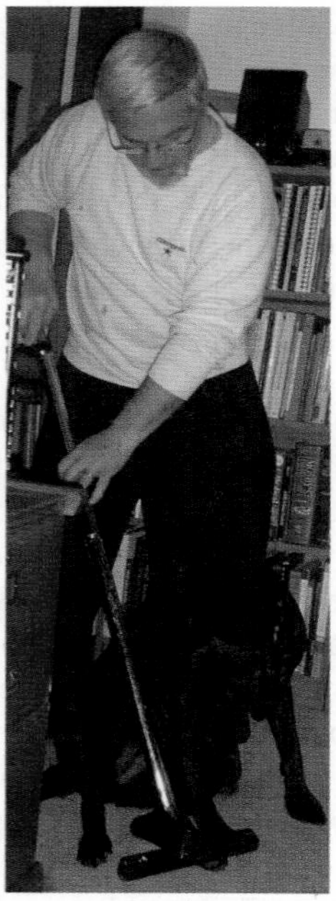

FIGURE 20-12 This dog was well socialized to loud noises during the sensitive socialization period and shows no fear of the vacuum cleaner.

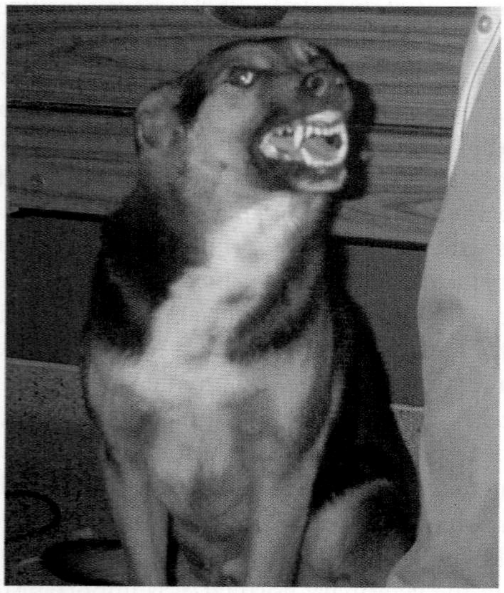

FIGURE 20-13 Aggression is a common owner complaint. Sometimes the aggression occurs only in the veterinary hospital and is related to fear. Veterinary health professionals should strive to prevent this from occurring and attempt to find ways to alleviate this behavior in hospitalized animals. (From Beaver BV: *Canine behavior: insights and answers,* ed 2, St Louis, 2009, Saunders.)

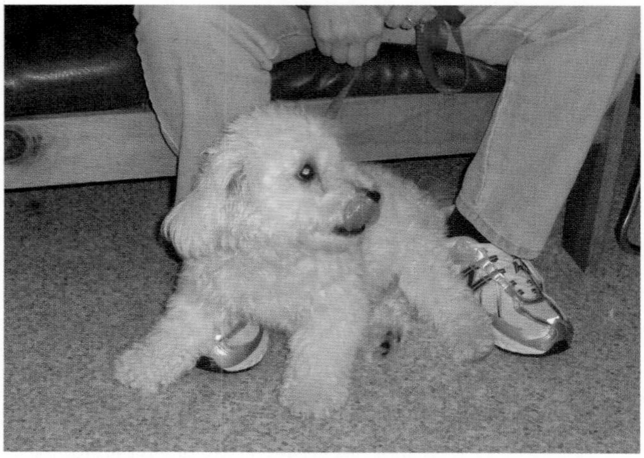

FIGURE 20-14 Licking may be a sign of conflict that very often passes unnoticed by both owners and professionals. (From Landsberg G, Hunthausen W, Ackerman L: *Behavior problems of the dog and cat,* ed 3, Philadelphia, 2013, Saunders.)

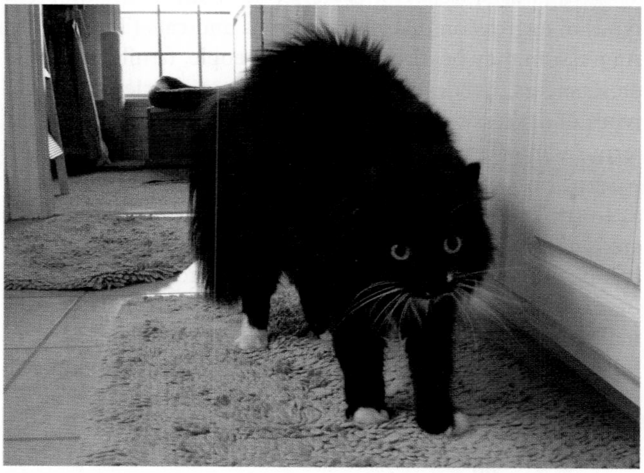

FIGURE 20-15 Fearful cat: arched back, dilated pupils, piloerection. (From Landsberg G, Hunthausen W, Ackerman L: *Behavior problems of the dog and cat,* ed 3, Philadelphia, 2013, Saunders.)

become withdrawn. In recent years, the focus in veterinary medicine is to adopt procedures that reduce fear in pets that come to the veterinary clinic. This was partly driven by survey data that revealed that many pet owners perceive veterinary visits as too stressful for their pet and too much of a hassle for themselves. The Fear Free initiative was developed to address these concerns.

The fear-free approach involves a variety of techniques that are used both at home by the client and in the veterinary practice by the veterinary health care team. This begins with educating new pet owners about methods that can be used to keep their pet calm when preparing for and traveling to the veterinary practice. Common signs of fear in dogs include panting, pacing, licking the lips, furrowed brows, and yawning (Fig. 20-14). Fearful cats will often try to hide and may exhibit signs of agitation or aggression such as dilated pupils, piloerection, and hissing (Fig. 20-15). More details on the Fear Free approach to low stress handling is located in Chapter 21.

PROVIDING PROBLEM PREVENTION SERVICES

Knowing what to tell clients to prevent problems is a separate issue from finding sufficient time to do so. It may not be realistic to expect the veterinary professional to do so during a 15-minute office visit when the time is allocated to addressing the presenting medical concern, or in a brief telephone call while also greeting clients at the front desk or searching for a client record. Veterinarians and technicians must purposely decide how the valuable information regarding problem prevention can be disseminated. One obvious way is to make it a policy to schedule extra time for appointments involving new animal examination and to charge accordingly. These are often new puppy and kitten appointments, but not always. The fee structure for new animal appointments can include an extra 15 to 20 minutes of staff time, even if the problem prevention discussion takes place separately from the medication examination and vaccination time. Talking to clients about these issues is preferable to relying on videos and written materials alone. However, written materials can be of value because they reinforce what was said and allow clients to read them as often as needed and at their convenience. It can also be argued that the expenses for the time required for problem prevention, even if not charged directly as a fee, may be recouped indirectly. Problem prevention sessions can improve the chances that the animal will remain in the home and thus continue being a patient. Also, the owner's perception of the clinic is enhanced, making word-of-mouth referral of new clients more likely.

PROVIDING PROBLEM RESOLUTION SERVICES

Problem resolution is almost always a more complex process than is problem prevention. It requires first arriving at a behavioral diagnosis for the type of problem. The presenting complaint, whether excessive barking, house soiling, or aggression, can be thought of as behavioral signs similar to medical signs, such as vomiting, limping, or a poor haircoat. Each of these signs can potentially be related to a variety of problems. In the case of behavior problems, medical conditions that may account for the behavioral signs should be evaluated first. This is especially important with aggression and house soiling. Once this is done, arriving at a behavioral diagnosis requires obtaining a complete behavioral history and ideally observing the animal and its environment. For some types of problems, such as feline elimination problems, seeing the animal in its home environment may make it possible to identify physical features of the environment that are contributing to the problem. Behavioral diagnosis sometimes requires several hours to interview the owner and observe the animal. In some cases, the owner may need to return home and maintain a log or even videotape the behavior.

Once the type of problem has been narrowed down to one or a few possibilities, a behavior modification plan must be devised. The type of problem dictates the specific procedures used. A variety of methods are used to treat behavior problems (Table 20-2). Time is required to explain these procedures to the owner, provide written handouts, demonstrate them if necessary, and have the owner practice them, if appropriate. Keep in mind that severe behavior disorders that involve aggression or intense fear often require referral to a behavior specialist. Once treatment begins, the case must be followed up with either additional in-home or clinic visits or regularly scheduled telephone calls. These follow-up contacts may be relatively brief (sometimes less than 15 minutes) or longer in more complex cases.

A number of pharmaceuticals are used to treat animal behavior problems such as aggression, house soiling, and various phobias. Medications used to treat behavioral problems may be FDA approved or off-label use (Fig. 20-16). The purpose of drug therapy is often to relieve symptoms and allow the patient to learn new behaviors. There are many different human tranquilizers and antianxiety drugs that have shown promise as an adjunct in treating problem behaviors. A variety of nutritional and herbal remedies also have been used for certain behavioral problems (Fig. 20-17). Clients must be aware of the limitations of these products in behavioral therapy, including the fact that the problem may return when the drug therapy is stopped, the dosages may need to be adjusted to see the desired effect, and side effects may occur. Some form of behavior modification is needed to accompany drug therapy to increase the chances of a successful resolution of the problem. The goal is to ultimately wean the animal from the drugs and correct the problem.

The process of problem resolution cannot be collapsed into "25 words or less" solutions. This oversimplified approach to problem solving trivializes the importance of the problem and omits the scientific knowledge required to successfully modify behavior. Because technicians often have the opportunity to solve behavior problems, but may not have the time or expertise to do so, it is important to be aware of the veterinary practice's policies regarding referrals and become proficient in referring cases to behavior specialists.

REFERRING CASES TO BEHAVIOR SPECIALISTS

Before referral of an animal to a behavior specialist, evaluate medical conditions that could contribute to the problem behavior. Behavior referrals should be based on the same model of professionalism as are medical case referrals (Box 20-3). This includes determining the qualifications of the referral resource, learning the preferred method of referral, facilitating contact between client and specialist, and informing the client of what type of services to expect from the referral.

EVALUATING REFERRAL RESOURCES

Many types of professionals offer to assist pet owners with animal behavior problems. These can range from self-taught dog trainers to academically trained, degreed, and certified behavior specialists. Veterinarians who meet the established criteria may become board certified by the American College of Veterinary Behavior and are considered veterinary behavior specialists. The Animal Behavior Society, the largest organization in North America dedicated to the study of animal behavior, offers two levels of certification to individuals holding a master's or doctoral degree in the behavioral sciences and who meet educational, experiential, and ethical criteria. Although veterinary behaviorists can be

TABLE 20-2 Types of Behavioral Modification Programs

METHOD	DESCRIPTION	EXAMPLE(S)/POSSIBLE USES
Command-response-reward	Involves giving a command and immediately rewarding the desired response every time it is performed	Giving the command to sit and providing praise and/or treats as soon as the pet sits
Clicker training	Use of a sound to signal to the animal that it performed the right behavior and will receive a reward	Clicking when a puppy eliminates outside and immediately giving a treat
Extinction	Elimination of a problem behavior by completely removing the reinforcement for the behavior	Not providing food when a pet is begging
Aversion therapy	Associating an unpleasant stimulus with an object	Spraying an object with something that has a foul odor or taste to keep a pet from chewing it
Avoidance therapy	Associating an unpleasant stimulus with a behavior	Using a citronella collar to minimize barking behavior
Habituation	Involves surrounding the animal with the stimulus at low levels until the animal becomes acclimated to the stimulus and is no longer afraid of it	Playing recordings of thunderstorms or vacuum cleaners to a litter of puppies so that they become accustomed to the sound
Counterconditioning	Replacing an undesirable behavior with a desirable one	Using rewards to teach a pet to pull a bell on a string rather than scratching at the door to be let inside
Desensitization	Often used in combination with counterconditioning and involves diminishing a particular behavior by gradually exposing the animal to the stimulus that produces the inappropriate response	Exposing a pet that is afraid of children to children using increased periods of time and decreasing distance
Environmental modification	Changing one or more environmental parameters	Placing pet in crate when unsupervised; changing the location of a litter box
Surgery	Anatomic alteration	Castration of male pets to decrease aggressiveness and territorial urine marking
Medication	Sedatives, hormonal agents, herbal remedies	Canine cognitive dysfunction; as an adjunct to other behavioral therapies in aggressive or extremely fearful animals

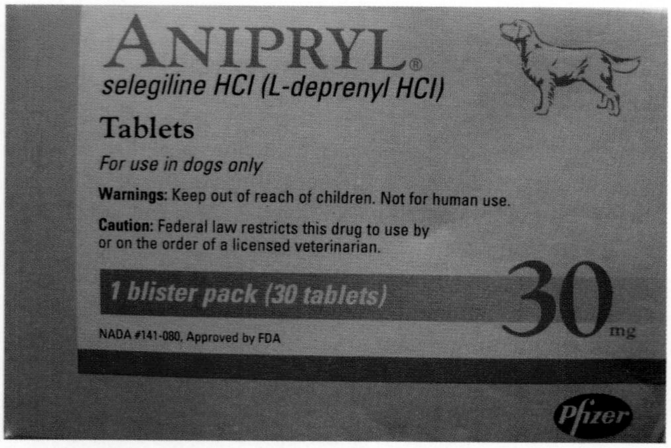

FIGURE 20-16 Anipryl is an FDA-approved pharmaceutical product used to treat behavioral changes related to canine cognitive dysfunction.

board certified, and applied behaviorists can be certified by the Animal Behavior Society, anyone, regardless of academic training, can legally use the professional title of animal behaviorist.

The National Association of Dog Obedience Instructors (NADOI) and the Association of Pet Dog Trainers (APDT) are two professional organizations that dog trainers can join. NADOI membership is open only to trainers who meet the organization's qualifications. APDT, which recently developed its own certification program, encourages and promotes use of positive reinforcement in training, but its membership is open to anyone who trains dogs.

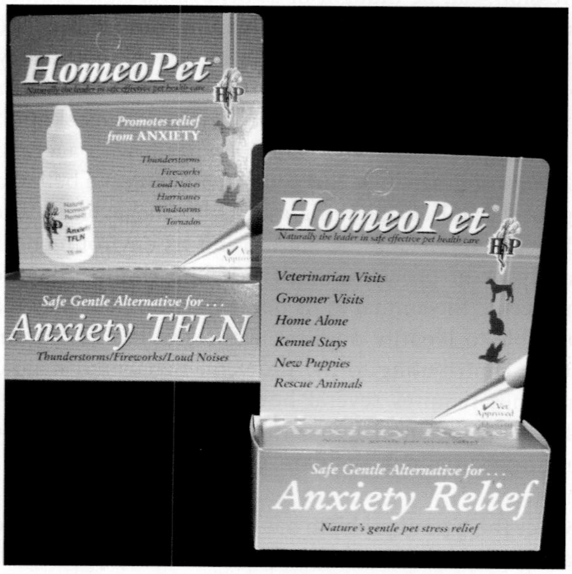

FIGURE 20-17 A variety of homeopathic remedies may be used to calm an individual experiencing shock, trauma, or panic.

It is the referring professional's responsibility to evaluate the credentials, knowledge, competence, and philosophies

BOX 20-3 Referring Behavior Cases

Treat behavior cases just like a surgical or medical case. Include:
1. Physical exam
2. CBC, profile, urinalysis and fecal results
3. Past and current medical history

of individuals considered as potential referral resources for the clinic. This is because certification does not guarantee competence, and professionally trained and some qualified people may not be certified. This may include interviewing these individuals and also observing their classes and/or behavior consulting sessions. Gathering information about the individuals from others who offer behavioral assistance can be a valuable service the technician can perform for the clinic.

When choosing a referral resource for behavior cases, technicians should be aware that obedience or command training does not resolve behavior problems. Teaching a dog sit, down, and/or stay does not address aggression, separation anxiety problems, house soiling problems, or other types of problems unrelated to obedience performance. However, training classes can be a useful tool in helping dog owners to establish a more consistent relationship with their dogs. You may want to identify referral resources for dog training classes as well as for behavior counseling for whatever species of animal the clinic provides medical care. You may need to select several individuals. Certified behavior specialists consult only on those species with which they have experience. Thus, a behaviorist may work with cats and dogs but not birds or horses. Every veterinary hospital should refer all of their puppy owners to an educated trainer. Some practices offer training classes in the hospitals, which may even be taught by staff members.

MAKING THE REFERRAL

Handle behavior referral cases as you would medical referrals. When referring a client to a veterinary medical specialist, such as a cardiologist or oncologist, a veterinary professional probably would not instruct the client to call the specialist for "tips" or "advice." Unfortunately, all too often this is the way clients are referred to behavior specialists. Find out whether the behavior specialist prefers the initial contact to be from the client or the veterinary medical professional. If contact from the veterinary professional is preferred, be prepared to provide a pertinent medical and behavioral history during the initial conversation.

Give the client a reasonable set of expectations about the referral. Discuss information about the fee structure, where the consultation will take place, how to schedule the appointment, and the amount of time required. You can also encourage the client to seek behavioral help without giving false expectations. Although most animal behavior problems can benefit from professional assistance, not all problems can be completely and permanently resolved.

Dealing with behavior referrals in a professional manner may help clients to view the behavior consulting process as a legitimate aspect of health care and overcome some of their embarrassment about seeking "psychological help" for their pets. It may also help them to better understand why behavior specialists charge fees for professional services, just as veterinarians do. The veterinary clinic can facilitate referrals by having business cards, brochures, and other information about the behavior specialist available to give to clients at the clinic.

BEHAVIOR PROBLEMS IN EXOTIC AND FARM ANIMALS

Avian and small mammal species are commonly seen in companion veterinary practice. In addition, large animals, especially horses, may develop behavior problems. The basic mechanisms for behavioral development are similar in these species as those described for dogs and cats. The sensitive periods for socialization vary considerably among different species. The most common problem behavior seen in pet birds and small mammals is biting. Often, this is aggression directed toward humans as a result of fear. Horses may exhibit a number of problem behaviors, commonly referred to as stereotypical behaviors. These are generally repetitive type abnormal activities such as cribbing. Cribbing refers to a repetitive action in which a horse grasps a solid object with its incisors and produces a distinct grunting noise. Stereotypical behaviors of horses are generally regarded as arising from a combination of environmental and genetic factors and treatment requires a multifactorial approach that also addresses husbandry-related causes of problem behaviors. Additional information on avian behavior is located in Chapter 27.

REVIEW QUESTIONS

Circle the Best Answer

Circle the answer choice that best completes each of the following statements.

1. Kittens do / do not (circle one) need to observe the queen eliminating in the litter box in order to know how to use it properly.
2. Studies have found that cats with elimination problems were more likely to have scented / unscented (circle one) litter as compared with cats without such problems.
3. It is recommended that in multiple cat households there should be one litter box per each / every two cat(s) (circle one) plus one extra.
4. The average age of young boys / girls (circle one) bitten by dogs is 5 to 9 years old.
5. Male / Female (circle one) dogs are reported to be involved with 70% to 75% of all reported dog bites.

Fill in Blank

Provide the best answers to complete the following statements.

1. For any behavior to occur, there must be a _______________.
2. Some problem behaviors are due to _______________ or _______________ amounts of neurotransmitters.
3. The study of animal behavior is referred to as _______________.
4. _______________ conditioning refers to the association of a stimulus that occurs at approximately the same time or in roughly the same area as the behavior.
5. _______________ conditioning refers to the association of a particular activity with a punishment or reward.
6. The most important time period for behavior development in dogs and cats is from ______ to ______ weeks.
7. Genetics can play a role in behavior problems but also _______________ can cause inappropriate behavior.
8. _______________ reinforcement refers to any immediate pleasant occurrence that follows a behavior.
9. _______________ reinforcement refers to any immediate unpleasant occurrence used to create a desired behavior.
10. _______________ is used to remove or decrease a behavior.
11. Positive punishment involves adding an _______________ occurrence to decrease a behavior.
12. _______________ punishment involves removing a desirable occurrence to decrease a behavior.
13. A delay of longer than ______ seconds between the behavior and the subsequent reinforcement significantly decreases the effectiveness of the reinforcement.
14. _______________ refers to the attribution of human characteristics and emotions to animals.
15. Eight-week-old puppies cannot hold their bowels for longer than _____ to ______ hours.
16. One of the most important motivations for cats scratching objects with their front claws is _______________ marking.
17. The most common complaint from dog owners is aggression toward _______________, while the most common complaint from cat owners is aggression toward other _______________.
18. The sensitive socialization period in dogs is from ______ to ______ weeks of age and in cats from ______ to ______ weeks.
19. When assessing a case of behavior problems, medical conditions that may account for the behavioral signs should first be evaluated; this is especially important with _______________ and _______________ behaviors.
20. Behavior modification is needed to accompany _______________ to increase the chances of a successful resolution of the problem.

RECOMMENDED READING

Beaver BV: *Feline behavior: a guide for veterinarians*, ed 2, St Louis, 2003, Saunders.

Beaver BV: *Canine behavior: insights and answers*, ed 2, St Louis, 2008, Saunders.

Crowell-Davis S: *2007 Veterinary psychopharmacology*, Indianapolis, IN, 2007, Wiley-Blackwell.

Hetts S: *Pet behavior protocols: what to say, what to do, when to refer*, Denver, 1999, AAHA Press.

Horwitz D, Neilson J: *Blackwell's five-minute veterinary consult clinical companion canine and feline behavior*, Indianapolis, IN, 2007, Wiley-Blackwell.

Landsberg G, Hunthausen W, Ackerman L: *Behavior problems in the dog and cat*, ed 3, Philadelphia, 2014, Saunders.

Miklosi A: *Dog behaviour, evolution, and cognition*, Oxford, UK, 2009, Oxford University Press.

Mills D, Nankervis K: *1999 Equine behavior: principles and practice*, Oxford, UK, 1999, Blackwell Science.

Overall K: *Clinical behavioral medicine for small animals*, St Louis, 1997, Mosby.

Pryor K: *Don't shoot the dog*, ed 3, Lydney, UK, 2002, Ringpress Books.

Rodan I, Heath S: *Feline behavioral medicine: prevention and treatment*, St Louis, 2015, Elsevier.

Shaw J, et al.: *Companion animal behavior for veterinary technicians and nurses*, Indianapolis, IN, 2010, Wiley-Blackwell.

Society of Veterinary Behavior Technicians: *Getting started in behavior*, SVBT Publication (pdf), 2003.

Turner D, Bateson P: *The domestic cat: the biology of its behavior*, ed 2, Cambridge, UK, 2000, Cambridge University Press.

Yin S: *Low stress handling*, Davis, CA, 2009, CattleDog Publications.

BEHAVIOR ORGANIZATIONS

Academy of Veterinary Behavior Technicians: www.AVBT.net.

American College of Veterinary Behaviorists: www.veterinarybehaviorists.org.

American Veterinary Society of Animal Behavior: www.avsabonline.org.

Animal Behavior Society: www.animalbehavior.org.

Society of Veterinary Behavior Technicians: www.SVBT.org.

21 Physical Restraint

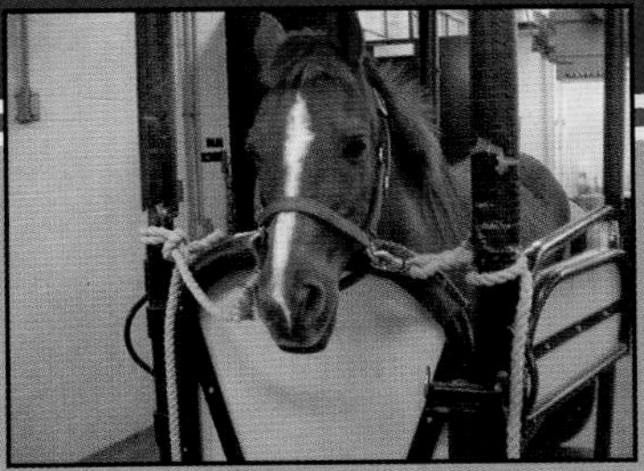

OUTLINE

LEARNING OBJECTIVES

After reviewing this chapter, the reader will be able to:

1. Describe the psychological principles underlying physical restraint techniques.
2. Explain and implement the safety precautions taken before and during physical restraint.
3. Restrain dogs, cats, small mammals, birds, horses, cattle, goats, sheep, and pigs for routine procedures such as physical exams, nursing care, and sample collection.
4. Give examples of behavior responses of animals to physical restraint.
5. Correctly identify and use restraint equipment.

KEY TERMS

Catchpole
Distraction technique
Dorsal recumbency
Flanking
Gauntlets
Hobbles
Hog snare
Lateral recumbency
Muzzle
Snubbing
Squeeze chute
Sternal recumbency
Stock
Tail jacking
Twitch

BASIC ANIMAL BEHAVIOR

FLIGHT OR FIGHT

All animals, including humans, operate on the flight or fight principle, which means that when threatened they will try to get away. If they are restrained from doing so, whether by physical methods or perceived containment, they will often resort to fight. For this reason care must be taken not to corner animals or push them into the fight mode by using cruel or extremely restrictive restraint techniques.

PROTECTIVE MOTHERS

Most mothers are protective of their young when they are approached by people. Their reaction can range from mild concern to full-fledged attack. Sows and cows are the most dangerous and should be handled extremely carefully when there are young at their side. Sows in particular will come through fencing and doors if their piglets are screaming within hearing distance. Horses will fret and try to be reunited with a baby at all costs if it is moved out of sight. Sheep often reject their lambs if not allowed to bond with them before they are handled.

FEAR FREE PRACTICE AND LOW STRESS HANDLING

In recent years, the number of veterinary visits has been declining. Studies indicated that this was due in large part to pet owners' perception that veterinary visits were too stressful for their pet and too much of a hassle for them. In many cases, this was true. The Fear Free initiative is a movement within the veterinary industry to transform practice so that the experience is positive for both the client and pet. The fear-free approach involves a variety of techniques that are used both at home by the client and in the veterinary practice by the veterinary health care team.

Educate new pet owners about methods that can be used to keep their pet calm when preparing for and traveling to the veterinary practice. Cats should be allowed daily access to their carrier so that they become acclimated to it and it becomes a comfortable resting spot. Allow pets to become accustomed to car rides as a positive experience. Always place cat carriers on the floor of the car or secure them with a seat belt and cover the carrier with a towel to minimize visual stimuli during the car ride. Consider the use of calming pheromones before car rides and veterinary visits.

Have the client withhold food the day of the veterinary visit so that treat rewards used by the veterinary practice team will be more effective. Ideally, a separate waiting area should be used for each species. Visual barriers such as plants or informational brochure racks can be used to create separate areas within the exam room. Place cat carriers on a shelf or chair so that they are not subject to investigation by dogs and others that pass by. Waiting room time should be kept to a minimum. Fearful patients should be moved to an exam room immediately. If an exam room is not immediately available, the client and pet should be instructed to wait outside or in their car until a room is ready.

Separate exam rooms for each species are also preferred. Pheromones can be used in the exam room to help the patient remain calm. Allow the patient to approach staff members on its own. Stand sideways rather than directly in front of the patient and toss some small treats to entice the patient to approach you. Do not look directly at the patient until the patient chooses to interact. Cats should be left in their carriers until they choose to come out. Removing the top of the carrier and replacing it with a towel may make the cat feel more comfortable.

Although long considered a last resort, sedation should be considered for any patient that shows signs of fear. Common signs of fear in dogs include panting, pacing, licking the lips, furrowed brows, and yawning. Fearful cats will often try to hide and may exhibit signs of agitation or aggression such as dilated pupils, piloerection, and hissing.

When preparing to restrain for specific procedures, work with the pet to find a position in which it is comfortable while still secure enough to safely perform the procedure. Avoid forcing a pet into a specific position. If signs of fear become evident, stop the procedure and consider sedation. If sedation is not an option and the procedure is not an emergency, consider rescheduling the procedure for another day.

RESTRAINT AND HANDLING OF DOGS

CANINE BEHAVIOR

Dogs exhibit a number of personalities that can be identified by their body language. This is important to note before attempting to restrain them. The majority of dogs are happy to be with people and enjoy interacting with others. The body language can be straightforward or somewhat submissive. They greet you with wagging tail and a slightly lowered and cocked head and initiate affection. These dogs rarely bite, but can retaliate if handled too harshly or cornered. The second common personality is the nervous or fearful dog. If a fearful dog is cornered it feels threatened and often bites. The last personality type is the aggressive dog. Aggressive dog body language is head lowered between the shoulders, a level stare, tail straight out (possibly wagging), and perhaps a grimace or growl. These dogs take offense at anyone's improper body language, such as a direct look into their eyes or a frontal approach. Aggressive dogs and nervous or fearful dogs should be handled with the knowledge that they will bite, and appropriate steps, such as a muzzle and sedation, should be considered before working with this type of dog. Regardless of the personality, never expose your face to an unfamiliar dog; approach the dog with your body turned slightly, avoid direct eye contact, and extend your hand with the fingers curled in with the palm up.

> *TECHNICIAN NOTE* Study the body language of every dog you meet to enable you to identify its personality at a glance.

DANGER POTENTIAL

A dog's main means of defense is retreat, but it will fight if cornered. Dogs are equipped with formidable teeth that are designed to crush and tear. Regardless of personality, if a dog is curling its lips, showing its teeth, growling, or raising its hackles, it is imperative to control its muzzle to avoid being bitten.

A lesser weapon is a dog's toenails. They rarely cause severe injuries, but can inflict painful scratches that can become infected.

MECHANICAL DEVICES

Leash

The rope leash is a standard tool for restraining dogs. It can be made of a rolled or flat nylon rope with a handle at one end and a slip ring to form a sliding loop at the other. The loop is easy to keep open and can be flipped over the head and/or body of a dog to bring it out of a cage or run (Fig. 21-1). It is easy to remove by allowing the loop to loosen and the dog to slip its head out. It fits easily into a pocket and can be used on cats just as effectively as dogs.

Gauntlet

Gauntlets are heavy leather gloves designed to protect the hands and forearms (Fig. 21-2). Even though they are made of thick leather, most dogs, cats, and birds can pinch or actually bite through the leather. However, it slows them down enough that you can usually escape the worst of it. One way to use them is to place one partially on your nondominant hand and hold it in front of the animal as a distraction. The animal will usually bite the empty fingers of the glove, allowing you to reach in and scruff or leash it with the other hand. If you restrain an animal with the gloves on, take care not to exert too much pressure because the gloves reduce your sense of touch and strength. Once the animal is out of the kennel and placed on a table, another person can grasp the animal, or you can wrap your hand and arm around the animal's neck or head, get rid of a glove, or switch hands and get rid of the gloves. This allows you to restrain the animal with your bare hands. If this is not possible because the animal is too aggressive, then keep the gloves on and monitor that the animal is not turning blue from the pressure you are exerting.

Muzzle

Many commercially manufactured **muzzles** are available and should be fitted to the dog by the owner. Before coming to the clinic, the client should muzzle an aggressive or nervous dog. A muzzle can also be made with a length of roll gauze, a nylon sock, or a length of rope (Procedure 21-1).

To remove the gauze muzzle, untie the bowknot, and gently pull the ends back and forth and forward. Often the dog will help with a paw. Be careful that the dog does not bite as the muzzle is removed; have people cleared out or have the head restrained carefully. Also note that this muzzle is only used for short-term procedures, because the dog cannot pant and will overheat if the muzzle is left on for extended periods. Keep scissors close by in case the muzzle must be quickly cut off.

Catchpole

Many types of catchpoles are available commercially. A **catchpole** is used to move an aggressive or fearful dog to or from a run or cage. The rigid pole separates the restrainer and dog, and a quick-release handle is used to prevent strangulation. The loop at the end of the pole is placed around the dog's neck and tightened (Fig. 21-3). This allows the restrainer to move the dog in and out of a run or cage. Care should be taken not to choke the dog, while ensuring that the loop is tight enough that its head does not slip out. Often another person can approach the rear of the dog and administer a sedative or vaccination without fear of being bitten.

Voice

Dogs often respond to voice commands and tones. The voice can be a very useful tool to comfort and soothe or direct an animal to obey. When using it to direct an animal, make the tone of your voice deep and commanding. Avoid the uplift inflection of a question because it is similar to "puppy talk," the high-pitched yelping and barking that is used for play or atten-

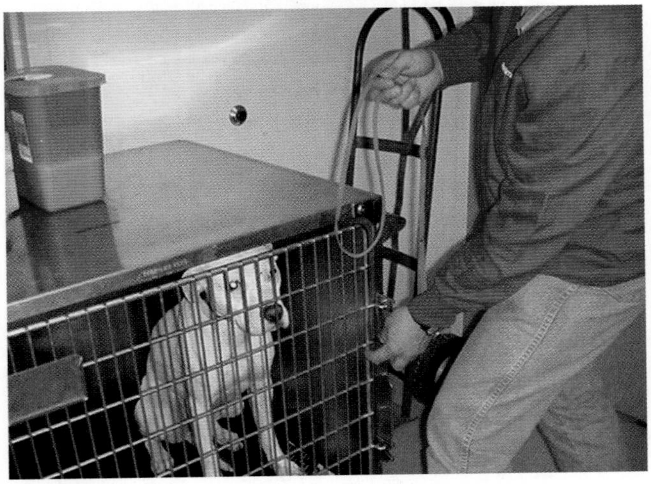

FIGURE 21-1 Using a rope leash to remove a dog from a cage.

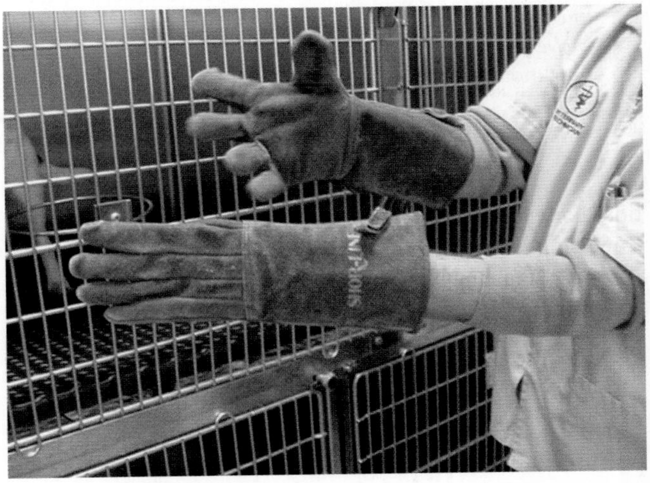

FIGURE 21-2 Gauntlets or restraint gloves.

PROCEDURE 21-1 Applying a Gauze Muzzle

1. Tear off a 4-foot-long piece of gauze.
2. Make a loop by tying an overhand knot that is not tightened down (Fig. 1).

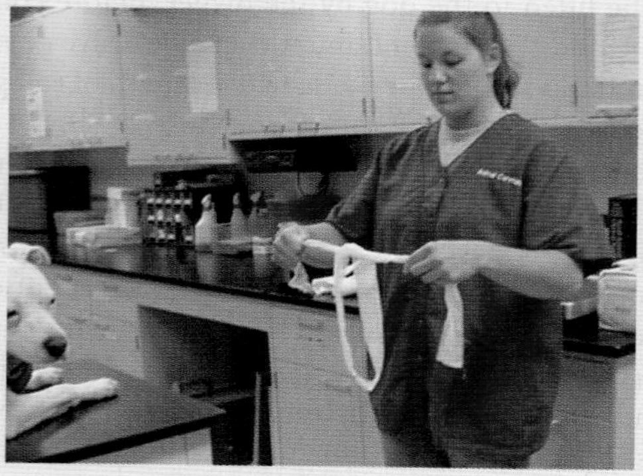

FIGURE 1

3. Have the dog either restrained by the scruff of the neck or a capture pole.
4. Stand slightly to the left or right of the dog's head, just out of its reach, and slide the loop around the dog's muzzle (Fig. 2).
5. Quickly tighten the gauze down around the muzzle by pulling on the ends of the knot (Fig. 3).

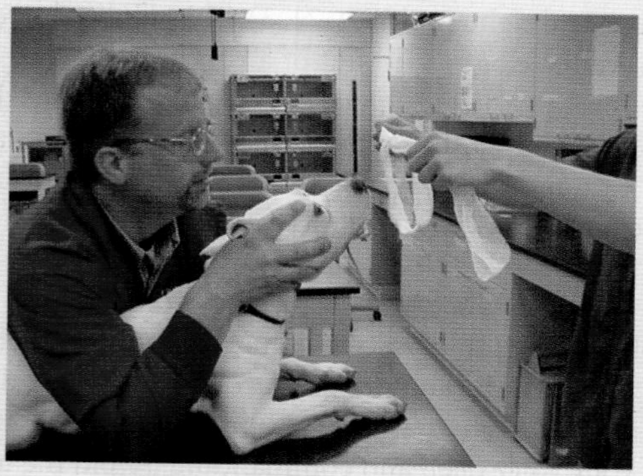

FIGURE 2

6. Bring the ends under the muzzle and tie another overhand knot under the chin (Fig. 4).
7. Move in closer, and pass the ends behind the ears and tie a bowknot (Fig. 5).

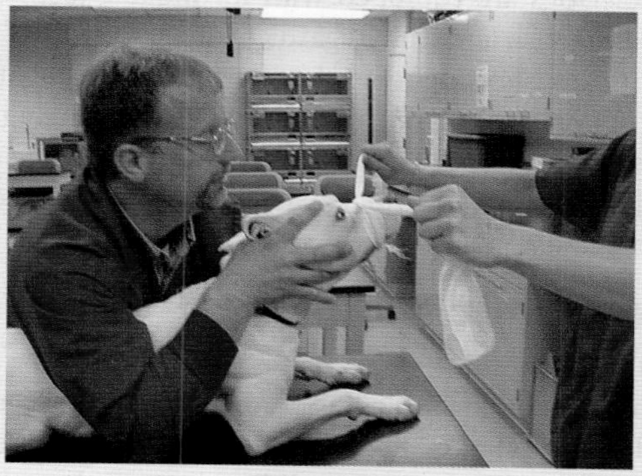

FIGURE 3

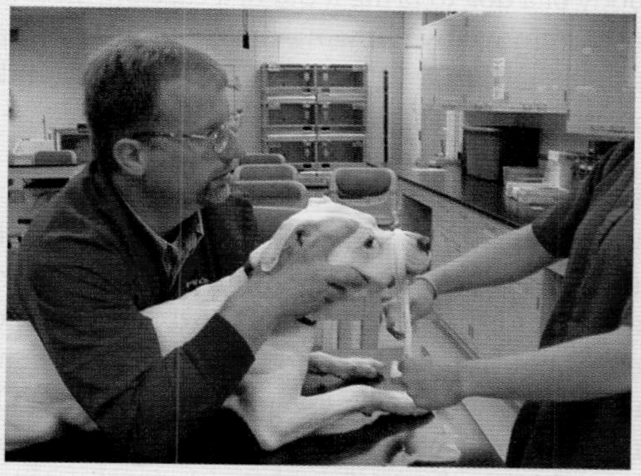

FIGURE 4

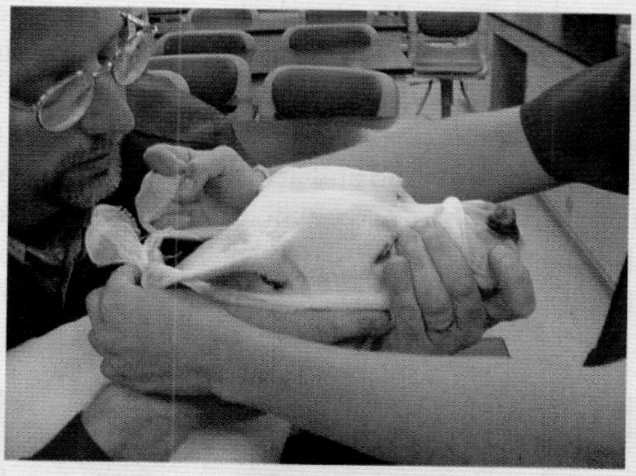

FIGURE 5

tion. For example, a sit command is given as a command, not a question. However, almost all animals respond to a soothing croon or "shushing" noise as a distraction, so do not be afraid of sounding silly when comforting an animal.

RESTRAINT TECHNIQUES

Removing Dogs From Cages or Runs

Because many dogs bolt out from kennels if given the opportunity, make certain that all escape routes are closed before opening any kennel door. To prevent this, the handler should block the door with a knee or forearm in the door opening (Fig. 21-4).

> **TECHNICIAN NOTE** To keep a dog from bolting out of the cage, place your knee or body in the open space between the door and frame.

Nonaggressive Nonfearful Dogs. Small dogs usually can be grasped gently by the scruff or under the chin and then

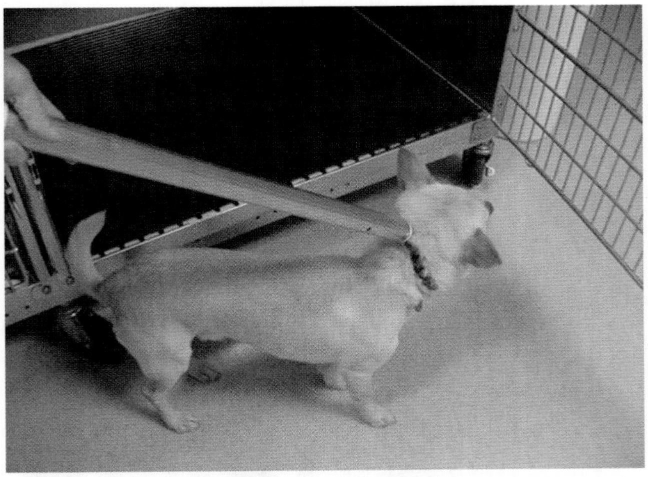

FIGURE 21-3 Using a capture pole on a dog.

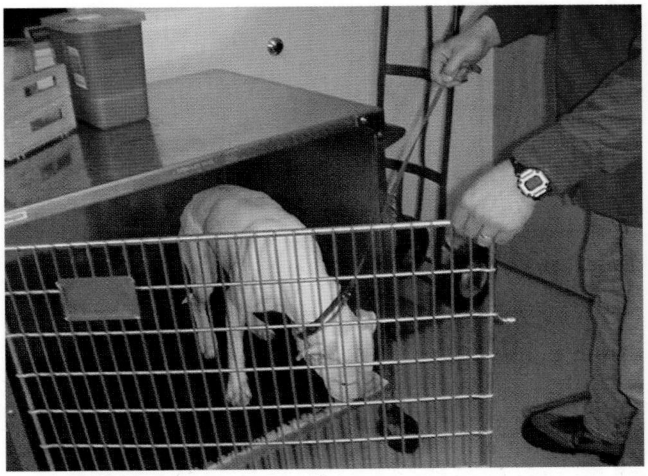

FIGURE 21-5 Slip the leash around a dog's head and allow it to step out of the cage.

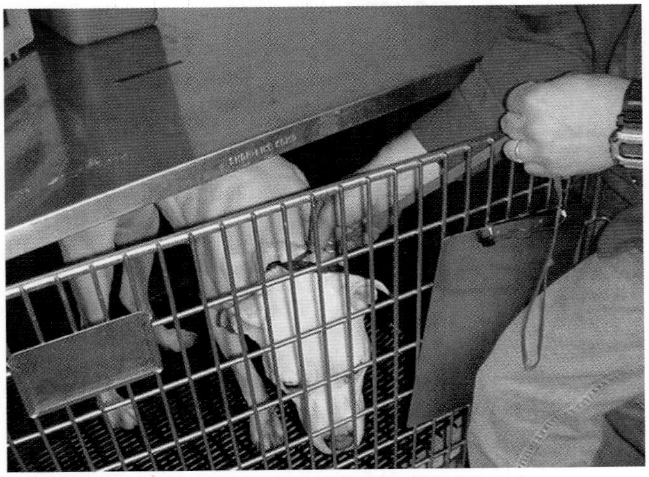

FIGURE 21-4 Blocking a dog from bolting out of a cage.

PROCEDURE 21-2 Removing a Dog From a Cage

1. Open the kennel door and slip a leash over the dog's head if possible.
2. Walk the dog out of the run or floor-level kennel if it is a medium-sized dog.
3. With a small dog, capture it with the leash, and then pull it to the edge of the kennel, retaining a steady pressure on the neck with the leash.
4. Reach in with a gloved hand and grasp a hindquarter.
5. Quickly lower it to the ground or place it on a table, holding the leash tight around the neck and the leg with the other hand.
6. Never pull a dog out and let it drop to the floor. You can cause severe injury to the legs, joints, back, and neck.

lifted out of the cage with one hand around and under the dog's thorax. Snug its body close to yours, or place a leash around its neck and place the dog on the floor. Medium-sized to large dogs are usually led out with a leash from a floor-level cage (Fig. 21-5).

Never pull a dog out of a cage, allowing it to jump to the floor. Most are not ready for the jump, and the height of the cage can cause injury to legs and joints as well as the neck if it is jerked.

Fearful and Aggressive Dogs. It takes practice and sensibility to remove fearful or aggressive dogs safely from cages or runs (Procedure 21-2). Ideally, dogs that are likely to bite should be muzzled, sedated, or both before they are placed in a cage or run. If this is not possible, proceed with caution. Do not corner the dog by stepping into the run or leaning into a cage. Calmly encourage the dog verbally with praise and comfort.

An alternative with a dog in a run or floor-level cage is to narrowly open the door, stepping behind the door to allow the dog to exit. As the dog's head comes through the doorway, quickly flip a leash over its head and move out with it. Most dogs actually calm down once they are "out of their territory" and will come along willingly. Remain on guard, as these animals can turn nasty without much notice.

If a dog is attacking the leash or the front of the kennel, the use of a capture pole is warranted, regardless of whether the dog is small, medium, or large.

Lifting a Dog

Small dogs are draped over a forearm, with the other hand holding onto the head just below the mandible. Medium-sized dogs are held around the neck with one arm and around the rear end or under the abdomen with the other. Carry both sizes close to your body until they can be placed in a kennel or an exam table (Fig. 21-6).

Large dogs of 50 pounds or more should be lifted by two people, one with an arm around the neck and thorax, the other with an arm around the abdomen and rear quarters. A count or signal should be given to lift in concert. Most large dogs get quite nervous on a table; procedures may be done on the floor if possible. If this is not possible, be sure to have enough people to hold the dog securely on the table.

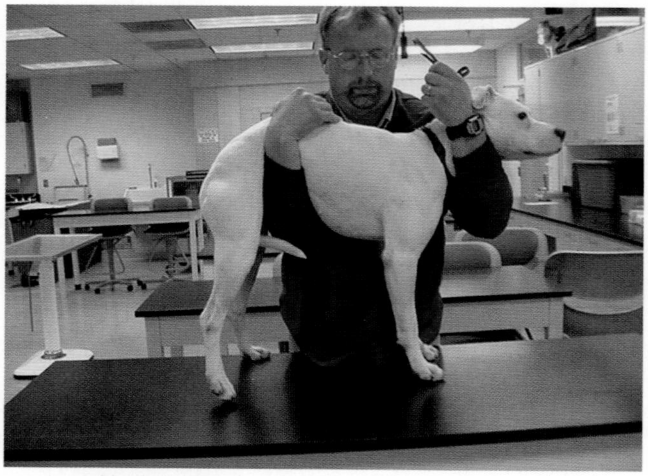

FIGURE 21-6 Lift and hold a medium to large dog.

Standing Restraint

This technique is used for such procedures as physical exams, anal sac expression, rectal temperature, and obtaining vaginal smears. Place one arm around the dog's neck or muzzle and the other around the abdomen, and hug it close to your body. If the dog is very large, you may have to have another person help as described for lifting a large dog. A gentle hold and some soothing words are often all that is necessary to keep the dog still. Be ready to strengthen your grip if the dog starts to struggle or tries to bite.

Crowding

This technique may be used with very large dogs. Place the dog in a sitting position close to a corner of the room. Gently slide the dog's rear into the corner so it cannot back away. Then straddle the dog and restrain the head with both hands, gripping the mandibles, or kneel to the side and wrap an arm around the neck and steady the front legs with the other hand. Do not make it appear that you are cornering the dog; otherwise, it may become frightened and retaliate.

Sitting or Sternal Recumbency

Sternal recumbency is usually used on the examination table and sometimes on the floor with large dogs (Procedure 21-3). This technique is useful for blood collection from the cephalic or jugular vein, intravenous injection, nail trimming, oral and ophthalmic exam or medication, and some radiographs.

One difficulty with this hold is keeping the dog from scratching you with its front paws. Instead of holding on to the rear, move your arm into the same position as you would for a venipuncture procedure, but grasp both legs, with a finger in between the legs, just above the carpals (Procedure 21-4). This will keep the dog from scratching you or the person performing the procedure.

Lateral Recumbency

Lateral recumbency is usually used on the examination table, but also can be used on the floor. It is useful for urinary catheterization, radiographs, suture removal, ECGs, access to the lateral saphenous vein, nail trims, and other short procedures (Procedure 21-5).

PROCEDURE 21-3 Restraining a Dog in Sitting Position

1. Ask the dog to sit or place the dog in a sitting position (Fig. 1).

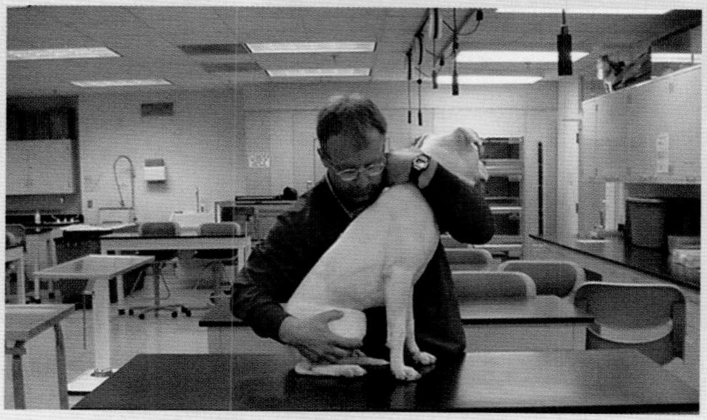

FIGURE 1 Sitting restraint.

2. Place one arm around the dog's neck or hold onto the muzzle and put the other arm around the rear of the dog. This will prevent it from biting and backing away.
3. Pull the dog close to your body to provide added security. Lean your body onto the dog's body to keep it from backing up.
4. If you need to abduct one of the dog's forelegs for venipuncture, move the arm that normally holds onto the rear across the shoulders and grasp the leg opposite from your body.
5. Hold the leg by placing the elbow into the palm of that hand and push the leg forward. To occlude the vein, place your thumb on top of the leg, squeeze, and rotate laterally. This occludes and helps stabilize the vein.

Dorsal Recumbency

Dorsal recumbency is used for procedures such as radiography, cystocentesis, and blood collection from the jugular vein. It sometimes requires two persons, depending on how restless and how wide the dog is. Place the dog in lateral recumbency, and then roll it onto its back. If it is a very deep-chested dog, a V-trough or foam wedges may be necessary to keep the dog from rolling. The forepaws are stretched cranially, and the back paws are stretched caudally, exposing the thorax and abdomen.

Snubbing

Snubbing can be used to administer an IM injection if you are alone, and it can be used to prevent an aggressive dog from getting too close to the restrainer. In one variation, one end of the leash is run through the wires on a kennel door. The leash is then pulled so the restrainer is on one side of the door and the dog on the other, again tying with a quick-release knot. This allows another technician to vaccinate or give an injection to the dog.

PROCEDURE 21-4 Sternal Restraint for a Cephalic Venipuncture

1. For sternal recumbency restraint, say "down" or gently pull the front legs out until the dog rests on its sternum.
2. Hold the neck or muzzle as described in Procedure 21-3, and use your free hand to either steady the rear or hold the foreleg out for venipuncture (Fig. 1).

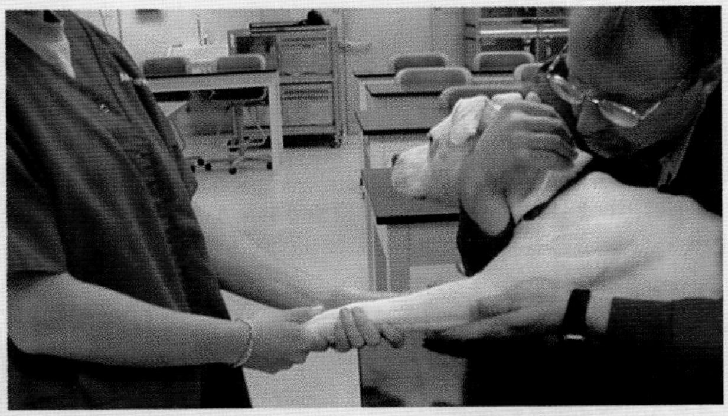

FIGURE 1 Sternal restraint for a cephalic venipuncture.

3. Lean some of your body weight on top of the dog to keep it in the down position.
4. This technique can also be used for jugular venipuncture. One hand reaches over the shoulders under the chin and wraps around the muzzle, raising the head to expose the neck.
5. The other hand grasps both front legs and stretches them over the edge of the table.
6. Put a finger between the legs and grasp around the carpal area, which will allow you to hold on better. Again, lean your body on top of the dog.
7. This is a very uncomfortable position for you and the dog. Do not apply this hold until the phlebotomist is ready to begin.

PROCEDURE 21-5 Restraining a Dog in Lateral Recumbency

1. Place the dog on its left or right side by reaching over the dog and grasping the legs closest to you and pulling them out from under the dog.
2. Hold onto the legs touching the table (left legs in left recumbency, right legs in right recumbency), lifting them slightly.
3. Put one wrist or arm across the dog's neck and the other across the flank. This prevents the dog from getting up (Fig. 1).

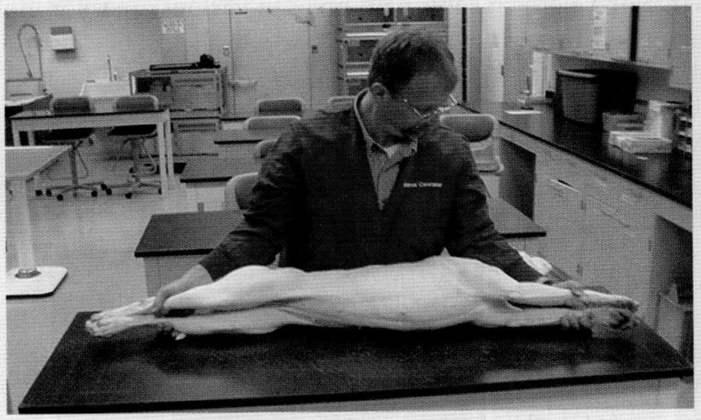

FIGURE 1 Lateral recumbency.

4. If you need one hand free, the only hand available is the one holding the rear legs. Lift the front legs slightly so the dog's weight is shifted onto its shoulder, then you can release the rear legs. Maintain pressure on the dog's neck with your forearm.
5. For a more secure hold on the legs, place a finger between them, above the carpal joint on the front legs and the tarsal joint on the back.

RESTRAINT AND HANDLING OF CATS

FELINE BEHAVIOR

Always begin with a minimum amount of restraint and perform the procedure as fast as possible. Many procedures can be accomplished by barely holding on, but you need to be ready to tighten the hold as necessary. If the cat begins to resist, tighten your grip so no one gets hurt. However, if the cat vigorously resists the restraint, release it and consider use of chemical restraint after it has calmed. Before releasing the cat, make sure the person doing the procedure knows that you are going to let go. Rough handling, extreme physical restraint, and a hot temper are counterproductive and have no place in cat restraint. Keep in mind that it is a good idea to make friends before placing a cat in any restraint hold. Relax the cat by petting it, speaking to it gently, and finding its favorite "itchy" spot.

TECHNICIAN NOTE Cats do NOT like to be held tightly or for very long. Start with a gentle hold, but be ready to tighten your hold if necessary.

DANGER POTENTIAL

Cats will also try to get away from a scary or painful procedure; most of the time a cat will try to scare you off by batting at you with its front feet and/or hissing. If you are foolish enough to keep coming, it will resort to bringing out its formidable weapons. Their canine teeth are sharp but small in diameter, and if they bite you, the result is a deep puncture wound that often becomes infected. They also defend themselves with very sharp claws. Hanging onto a cat is very difficult, because they are agile and strong enough to bring into use all four feet as well as their teeth in defense. Remember, the idea is to not push a cat into fighting "for its life."

MECHANICAL DEVICES

Towel and Blanket

A large towel is one of the best tools to keep around to assist in restraining a cat. It can be used to wrap the cat's body snugly, thus controlling the feet and body. A front or back leg can be pulled out for a cephalic or femoral vein exposure, or for an IM injection, the cat can be rolled onto its back for a jugular venipuncture, and oral or ophthalmic medicines can be given without fear of being scratched. Also, covering the head with the towel often calms the cat down. Procedures 21-6 and 21-7 provide details on two techniques that can be used to wrap a cat.

Both methods are useful if you have to give an oral or ophthalmic medication by yourself, or can be used for a jugular, cephalic, femoral, or saphenous venipuncture. Most cats submit to procedures when wrapped up, so it is less traumatic for the cat (Fig. 21-7).

Feline Restraint Bags

Feline restraint bags or cat bags work like towels (Procedure 21-8). They are made of canvas or heavy nylon and have zippered or Velcro closures with holes in various areas for limb exposure. They are available in a variety of sizes, because one size does not fit all.

PROCEDURE 21-6 "Burrito" Technique for Wrapping a Cat for Restraint

1. The towel is placed flat on the table, and the cat is placed at about one third of the way from one end of the towel.
2. Taking the short end or the end closest to the cat, wrap it very snugly around its body.
3. Once that is in place, quickly wrap the long end around and around its body.
4. This covers everything but the head, and a front or back leg can be extracted or the cat rolled onto its back and the head extended for a jugular venipuncture (Fig. 1).

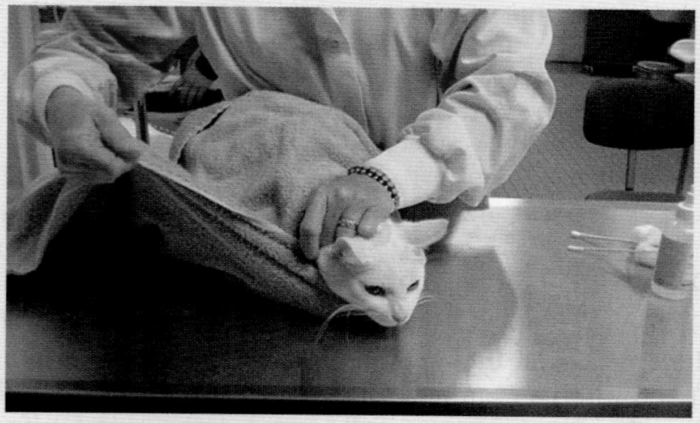

FIGURE 1 "Burrito" wrapping of a cat.

PROCEDURE 21-7 "Taco" Technique for Wrapping a Cat for Restraint

1. Drape a towel over the cat so the middle of the towel is directly over the cat's back.
2. Quickly sweep the sides of the towel together and lay the cat on its side.
3. Continue to wrap the two ends of the towel completely and snugly around the cat.
4. As with the "burrito" wrap, it completely encircles the legs, but allows access to the head and rear.
5. This technique is especially useful for getting angry cats out of a cage.

Never leave a cat on a tabletop in a cat bag, because it can roll over and fall off the table. To remove the cat, unzip the zipper, either all or part of the way, and then loosen the neck strap. Most cats will walk straight out. However, if the cat is terribly upset, be ready to pull your hands back quickly when loosening the neck strap. Also, it is not always easy to put an upset cat into a restraint bag, especially by yourself. If given the option, a towel is much easier to use to control an upset cat.

Muzzle

Commercial muzzles are available for cats. Most are designed to cover the cat's eyes, but leave a fairly small hole for breathing, which often upsets the cat even more. If a situation calls for a muzzle, sedation may be a better alternative.

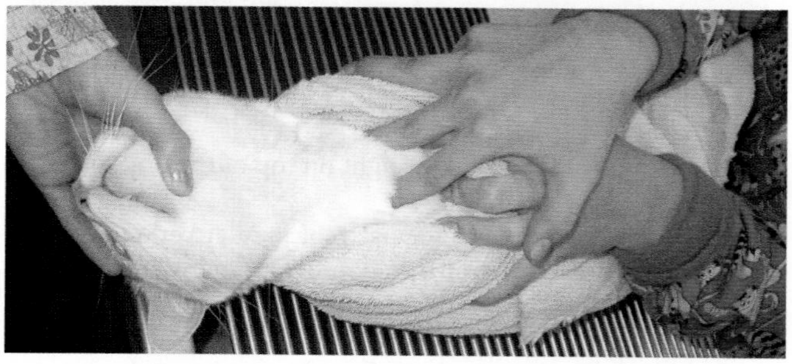

FIGURE 21-7 Position for a jugular venipuncture.

PROCEDURE 21-8 Restraining a Cat Using a Cat Bag

1. To insert a cat into a cat bag, you must have the bag laid out and opened wide.
2. Place the cat in the middle of the bag and quickly wrap the neck strap around the neck, fastening it snugly, but not so much that it occludes the airway.
3. Then with a hand on its back or over its shoulders and hip, have another person zip the zipper, being careful not to zip hair or skin.
4. The legs can be brought through zippered openings for injections or venipunctures (Fig. 1).

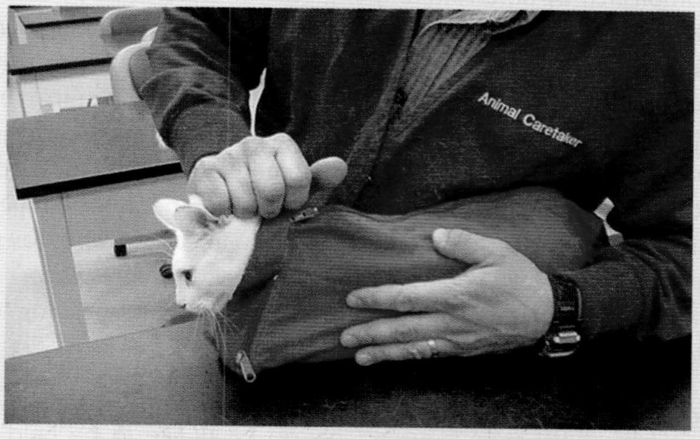

FIGURE 1 A cat in a feline restraint bag.

Gauntlet

Refer to the dog restraint section; these gauntlets are used in the same manner. The only difference is that you may use them more for cats than dogs.

DISTRACTION TECHNIQUES

Cats can often be distracted from procedures by the restrainer. The following are some distraction techniques that work well with cats.

Caveman Pats

Caveman pats are exaggerated heavy but gentle pats or rubbing on the head. They can be rapid or slow and steady or somewhere in between. The idea is to get the cat to concentrate on what you are doing and ignore the procedure being performed. Varying the pressure and stroke is usually more successful than a continuous pattern. Some people tap a cat's nose with their finger. This is not recommended, because the cat may not be able to resist biting such a tempting target.

Puffs of Air

Blowing or puffing air into a cat's face is another way to redirect its interest. Again, vary the speed and force of the puff to obtain better results.

RESTRAINT TECHNIQUES

Removal From a Carrier

Be sure all routes of escape are closed before restraining. Most cats will not willingly walk out of a carrier on demand. Therefore it is a good idea to open the carrier door as soon as the client is escorted into the exam room. While you are talking to the client, the cat may decide to walk out and explore. If not, you can assess the temperament of the cat. If the cat is friendly, reach in, gently grasp the scruff, and bring it forward until you can get a hand around its midsection. Most cats do not object to this; however, most clients do not understand this and may think you are hurting their cat. Always explain that scruffing is a natural hold for them because it is how their mother carried them. However, never lift an adult cat up by grasping the scruff.

If the cat resists, elevate the rear of the carrier and allow the cat to slide out. Do not raise it so high that the cat drops from the carrier. If you are not successful, you can dismantle most carriers quickly. This is much safer than reaching into its territory and trying to grab it.

Removal From a Cage

If the cat is friendly, reach in across its shoulders, grasp the front feet, quickly lift it out of the cage, and snug its body against yours. Your elbow can gently pin the cat's body against yours, thereby controlling the back legs. Cradle the chin or encircle the neck with the other hand.

If the cat is upset, you can try a number of things. Throwing a large beach towel or small blanket over the cat and then scooping it up works well to get it out of the cage. Once out of its "territory," it will usually calm down and allow you to work with it. It is also recommended that you wear gauntlets while getting it out of the cage. You can also try lassoing a cat with a rope leash; you usually end up getting the leash around its chest, which is not all that bad. If that does occur, you can pull the cat to the front of the cage and with a gloved hand reach in for a back leg and quickly transport it to an exam table. If the cat is terribly upset, there are a number of devices designed to trap and/or pin it to the floor of a cage or inside a device so a sedative can be administered. A dose of ketamine can be given by squirting it into the eyes or open mouth if hissing. It is absorbed through the mucous membranes, and the cat will quickly become sedated.

Sitting or Sternal Recumbency

This procedure can be used for physical exams, oral and ophthalmic exams and medications, and cephalic or jugular venipuncture. For a routine physical examination, have the cat sit and place one hand in front of its chest while the other steadies its back. Gently talk to and stroke the animal as it is being examined. When it is time to examine the head or perform more invasive procedures, encircle the neck holding the mandibles with one hand (Fig. 21-8); with the other hand reach across the back and grasp the front feet. Snug the cat up against your body. If necessary, lean a bit over the cat to keep its back legs in place.

A very gentle grip is a must to keep the cat from getting worried and struggling. If the procedure is almost finished and the cat starts to struggle, it is a simple matter to tighten your grip and hang on until the procedure is completed. If at all possible, do not let go. However, if you are losing your grip and the cat is trying to bite and/or scratch, alert the person performing the procedure and let go when she or he steps away. This works well, and most cats do not object unless they are being held too tightly.

If the procedure is a cephalic venipuncture, you can hold the cat in the same manner as described for a dog. Some people are dexterous enough to tuck the other foot between their little finger and ring finger and hang onto it so the cat cannot reach up and scratch (Fig. 21-9).

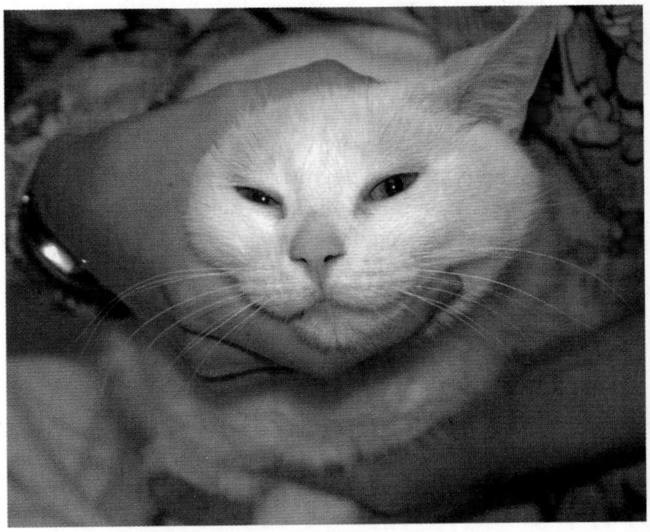

FIGURE 21-8 Head restraint for procedures.

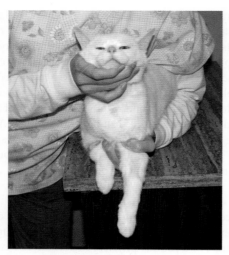

FIGURE 21-9 Sternal restraint.

The jugular venipuncture hold is also similar to the way you hold dogs. However, a cat's neck is a lot shorter, which results in having to hold onto the head and mandibles, usually with just a few fingers, as you stretch it up. It can be quite difficult to keep the cat's head under control; however, there is one method of adding support to the hold. As you stretch the head up, jut your chin out and place it against the top of the cat's head. This sounds dangerous, but it really gives you added stability, and you can quickly move out of the way if the cat starts to escape. It bears repeating: Perform this hold in a very gentle manner. Most students learning to restrain cats grip them too tightly right from the start. This will cause the cat to resist almost immediately, even before it has been poked. Hold a cat gently, talk to it, and only tighten as necessary. Another mistake sometimes made is putting the cat into a hold before everything is ready to perform the procedure. Do not start until you are sure everything is prepared and all personnel are in place.

Lateral Recumbency

Cats can be restrained in lateral recumbency just as for a dog. However, they are very agile and can often maneuver their heads around and bite. This should be reserved for very placid cats and noninvasive procedures. If you need them in lateral recumbency for a femoral venipuncture, placing them in a cat bag or burrito towel wrap is the safest way to accomplish the task.

A fetal hold or scruffing technique is more useful for giving subcutaneous or intramuscular injections or placing a rectal thermometer (Procedure 21-9).

Small cats can be lifted off the table, and a back leg can be moved up toward the neck and be hooked by the thumb of the hand holding the scruff. This presents the biceps femoris muscle into which an intramuscular injection can be given by the restrainer with the other hand (Fig. 21-10).

Do not use this on cats more than 7 pounds, because it can cause a lot of damage to tissues and vertebrae. Another precaution when using this technique is to have the injection ready to go and the cotton ball full of alcohol before placing the cat into position. The cat should not be held in this position longer than 5 to 6 seconds; otherwise even a small cat can suffer some injury. However, it is a real timesaver if you are alone and an injection must be given.

PROCEDURE 21-9 Restraining a Cat in Lateral Recumbency

1. As the cat sits, grasp the scruff of the neck, gathering as much of the skin as possible in one hand.
2. Lift the cat slightly off the table and grasp both back legs with the other hand.
3. Stretch the cat's back against the forearm, holding the scruff.
4. If the cat is stretched out fully, a reflex causes the cat's tail to curl ventrally toward its abdomen and the legs tend to be relaxed (Fig. 1).
5. The person doing the intramuscular injection can either take the top back leg or both back legs, which then allows the restrainer to grasp the front legs.

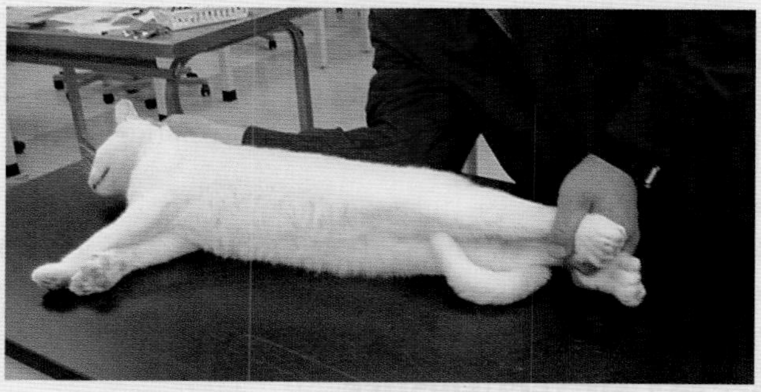

FIGURE 1 A lateral restraint for injections.

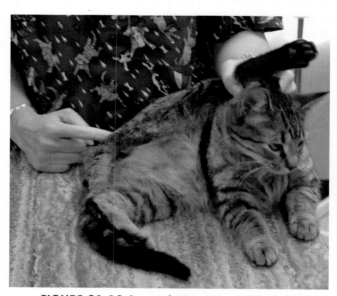

FIGURE 21-10 Restraint for IM injections when alone.

Dorsal Recumbency

This technique is used for blood collection from the jugular vein, radiography, and cystocentesis. It sometimes requires two persons. However, with practice one person can usually accomplish the hold alone (Procedure 21-10).

PROCEDURE 21-10 Restraining a Cat in Dorsal Recumbency

1. Scruff the cat, grasp the rear legs with the other hand, and roll it on its back.
2. Coming from the rear with the other hand, palm up, gather the back legs and then the front legs between the fingers of that hand.
3. Try to grasp the back legs above the hocks and the front legs above the carpals. This gives you more purchase on the legs.
4. Continue to scruff the head, or switch your hold so that you are hanging onto the mandibles from the back of the head.
5. The phlebotomist can hold off the jugular vein with one hand and insert the needle with the other.
6. Often it is easier to insert the needle pointing toward the chest versus the traditional insertion point.
7. If the procedure is for a radiograph or cystocentesis, you will most likely need two people.

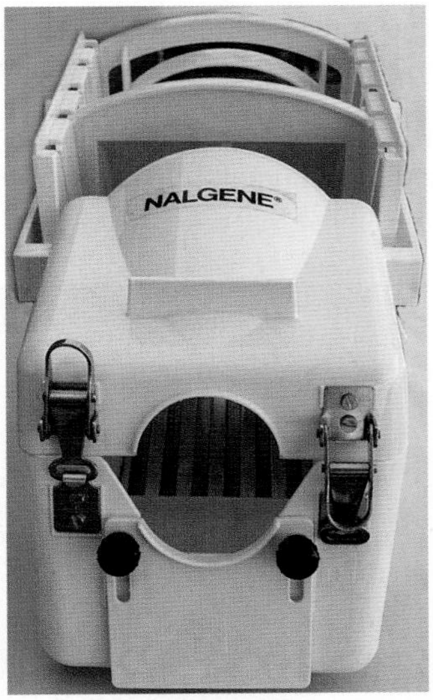

FIGURE 21-11 Rabbit restraint box.

RESTRAINT AND HANDLING OF SMALL MAMMALS

If small mammals (e.g., rabbits, gerbils, guinea pigs, rats, mice, ferrets) are restrained correctly and humanely, the chances of being bitten are minimal. Many of these "pocket pets" are frequently played with by children and do not resent being handled. If, however, the restrainer is fearful and mishandles the animal, it may become fearful as well.

DANGER POTENTIAL

Flight is the main means of defense, and if these little critters cannot get away they will use very sharp incisors to give you a good bite as well as using their toenails for scratching. Rabbits in particular can cause deep scratches with their toenails.

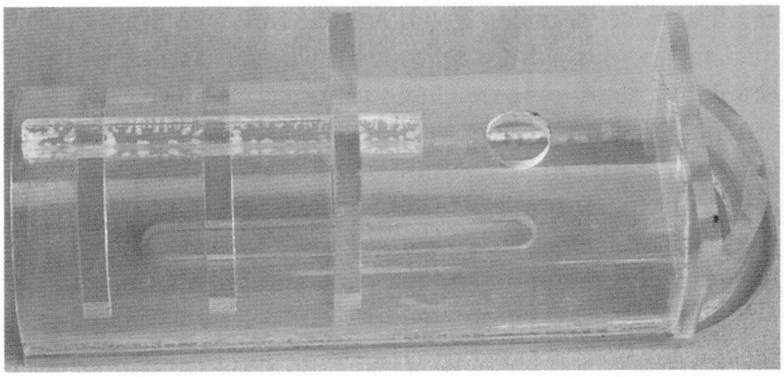

FIGURE 21-12 Mouse and rat restraint chamber.

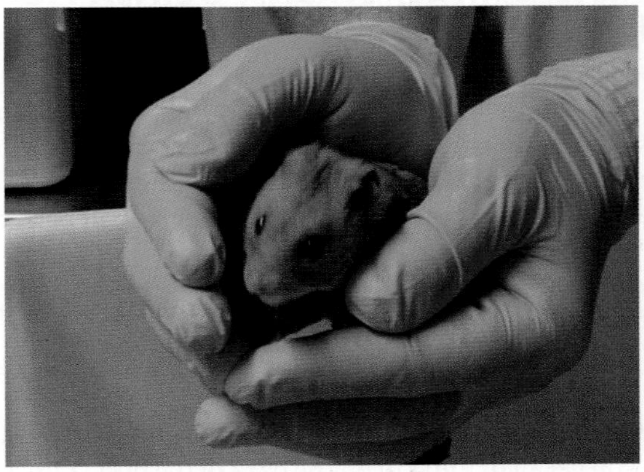

FIGURE 21-13 Capturing a hamster.

MECHANICAL DEVICES

A rabbit restraint box is used to securely hold a rabbit for venipuncture or injection using the ear veins. There is a head gate that allows you to adjust it firmly around the neck, and there is a back panel that is used to squeeze the rabbit forward. This prevents the rabbit from hopping and possibly causing a fractured spine (Fig. 21-11).

Mouse and rat restraint chambers are plastic holders that allow you access to the head, tail, and body (Fig. 21-12). The only difficulty is getting them into it. They grab onto the edges of the chamber with their front feet as they are lowered into it and stop their forward motion. You often have to twirl them around by the base of the tail to make them dizzy enough to miss the edges. Once you get the hang of getting them into the chamber, use of the restraint chamber can prevent a lot of bites. A tail can be extracted and used for venipuncture.

Capture

There are three ways to capture small mammals. The first method is scooping them up with both hands. Quickly and without hesitation, cup your hands with palms pointing down and cover their bodies; then bring your hands together under the animal and scoop up the critter (Fig. 21-13). This works well for hamsters, gerbils, and guinea pigs.

The second method is to grasp the base of the tail (Fig. 21-14). Quickly raise it out of the cage and place it on a grate or near an edge, gently pull back on the tail. The animal will hang onto the bars or edge with the front feet while you scruff it with your nondominant hand. This works well for rats and mice. Transfer the tail to that hand by pinning it or a back leg to your palm with your little finger. This allows your dominant hand to be free hand for injections or gavaging.

The third method is to quickly reach in and grasp the animal over the shoulders and wrap your fingers around and under the neck or scruff (Fig. 21-15). Lift the body out of the cage and support the rear end with the other hand. This works well for rabbits, guinea pigs, and ferrets. As you lift, face the rabbit away from you to prevent scratching and gently curl the body inward. Tuck its head into the crook of your arm for transporting.

HAMSTERS, MICE, GERBILS, GUINEA PIGS, AND RATS

Restraint

The most common method to securely hold mice, rats, hamsters, and gerbils is by the scruff of the neck, as previously described (Procedure 21-11). Procedures such as gastric lavage and injections other than venipunctures can be accomplished using this procedure. The key to a good hold is to be sure you get all of the skin on the back of the neck. Otherwise the rodent will be able to turn its head and bite. However, you must be careful not to impede the trachea. You will know you are doing this when the rodent turns blue.

> **TECHNICIAN NOTE** Make sure you have all the skin on the back of the neck when scruffing rodents.

Hamsters are nocturnal rodents that tend to be grumpy when handled in the daylight hours. It is always a good idea to knock on their cage to wake them up and give them a moment to get their eyes open before reaching in to capture them. Another thing to avoid doing with hamsters is poking your finger through their cage bars. Most will oblige and give you a good solid bite. Hamsters have huge pouches on either side of their head and necks that need to be kept in mind when scruffing a hamster. Be sure you have all of the skin.

Mice require you to move fast or twirl them around while grasping the base of the tail because many are able to climb up their tails and bite. Move them quickly to the grate or edge

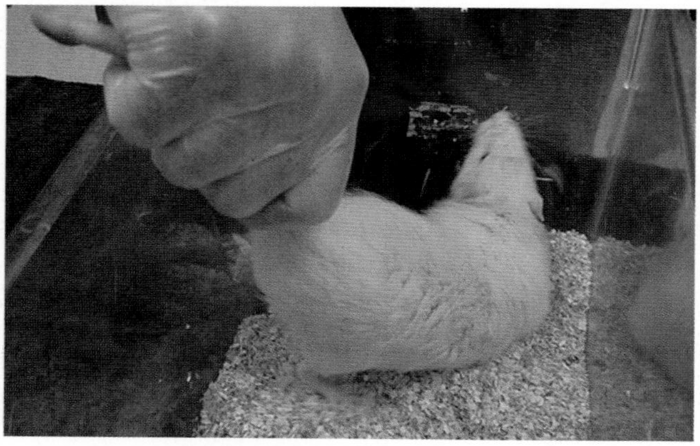

FIGURE 21-14 Capturing a rat.

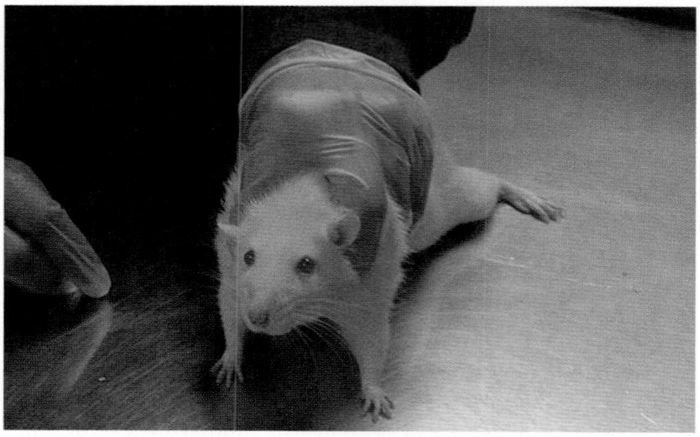

FIGURE 21-15 Capturing a rat.

PROCEDURE 21-11 Restraint of Rodents

1. Scruffing is accomplished by placing the animal on a grated surface.
2. Poise your index finger and thumb over the neck region, and gently push down and grasp the skin at the same time. The downward pressure keeps the animal from scooting away.
3. Once you have the animal scruffed, a tail or back leg can be restrained by pinning it to your palm with your little finger (Figs. 1 and 2).

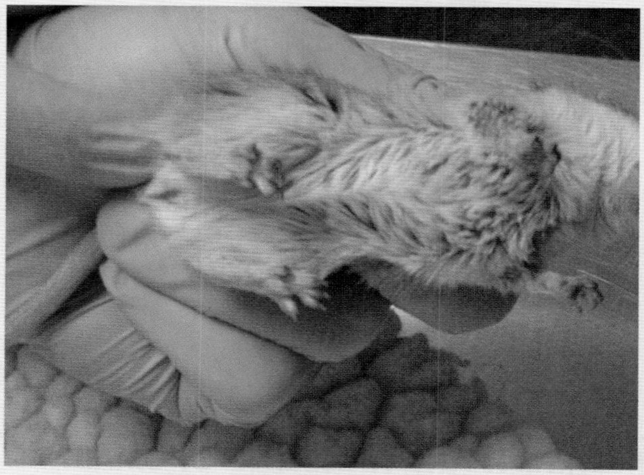

FIGURE 1 Scruffing a gerbil.

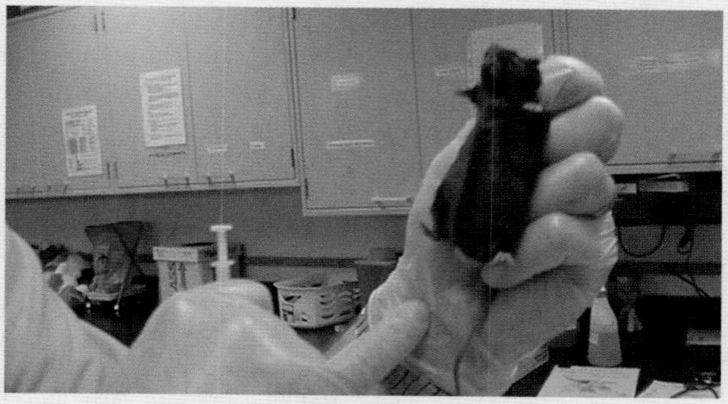

FIGURE 2 Scruffing a mouse.

and firmly press down when scruffing them; otherwise, they will turn and bite you. This restraint will allow you to perform gastric lavage and injections (see Procedure 21-11).

Gerbils are great jumpers and hard to catch if they are loose on the floor. They are prone to epileptic-like seizures that can occur if startled or handled too harshly. Because a gerbil has a long tail, some people try to use it to capture the animal. Because they are so quick, you usually end up grasping the end of the tail as they run away. When grasping just the tip of the tail, it is possible for the entire tip to come off in your fingers, leaving a few vertebrae and a very sore gerbil. It is better to use the scoop method to capture them and then scruff them if an invasive procedure needs to be done.

Guinea pigs are one of the easiest animals to restrain, because they rarely bite, do not move as quickly as smaller rodents, and tend to remain still when frightened. Capture the guinea pig by scooping it up with both hands under the thorax. Take care not to exert pressure on the chest, as it can restrict breathing. Quickly transfer one hand to support the hindquarters. Most procedures can be done with the guinea pig standing, with just the restrainer's hands surrounding its body (Fig. 21-16).

They can also be scruffed, set up on their rear, or wrapped in a towel for various procedures.

Rats enjoy attention and generally do not require much more restraint than distraction and simple holding. However, for examinations, injections, and gastric lavage you hold them as described for mice, guinea pigs, or ferrets. Rats can be wrapped in a towel, allowing the tail to be exposed for venipuncture or placed in a rat restraint chamber.

RABBITS

Rabbits can be difficult to restrain; they can be nervous and fragile. Rabbits have been known to struggle and kick violently, breaking their own spines. When very frightened, rabbits emit high-pitched screams.

Do not use the ears or scruff to lift an adult rabbit. Using the scruff for handling damages the subcutaneous tissues; this is painful and can devalue the animal. Young rabbits can be scruffed for a very short time, although a better method is to pick them up like a ferret or guinea pig. Placing a rabbit back into a cage requires you to set it down and continue to hold it for a second. The rabbit will give a little jump and then walk out of your hold. If you let go as you set it down, it may jump forward and either bang into the cage wall or out the door. You may also turn the rabbit so it is facing toward you as you place it in the cage.

Sternal Recumbency

Rabbits can be restrained in sternal recumbency for most procedures. Pad an exam table with a nonslip mat, place the rabbit on the mat, and encircle the rabbit's body with your forearm, or hold the head with one hand (Fig. 21-17). Examinations and medication applications can be performed using this technique.

Wrapping

Like cats, rabbits can be wrapped in towels for venipuncture. When using this method, watch that the rabbit does not overheat.

Dorsal Recumbency

Place a thick towel on the table and place the rabbit on the towel. Lay the rabbit in lateral recumbency as you would for a dog or cat. Gently roll the rabbit over on its back. Transfer one hand to the head, and gently flex the neck back until the rabbit goes limp and enters a hypnotic-like state. Maintain the position with the head, and add a gentle rub on its stomach. This works for radiographs or examinations of the stomach; it does not work for a painful procedure.

FERRETS

Ferrets are rather easygoing animals. They may "hiss" as a warning sign, but they usually do not bite unless distressed. Ferrets can easily become hyperthermic. Panting is an indication of overheating; and these animals must be cooled quickly. Always talk to the ferret to reassure it.

When a ferret bites, it may not let go. If this happens, put the ferret under running water. This is the best way to get the ferret to release its grip.

Distraction works well with ferrets. Place a dab of liquid treat on the ferret's lips, stomach, or forepaws for nonpainful

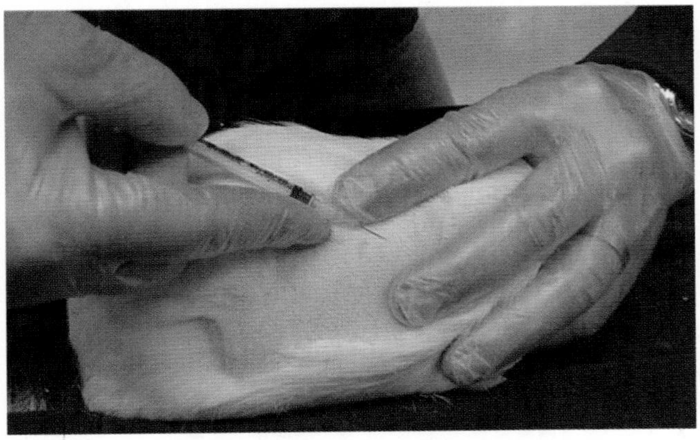

FIGURE 21-16 Restraining a guinea pig.

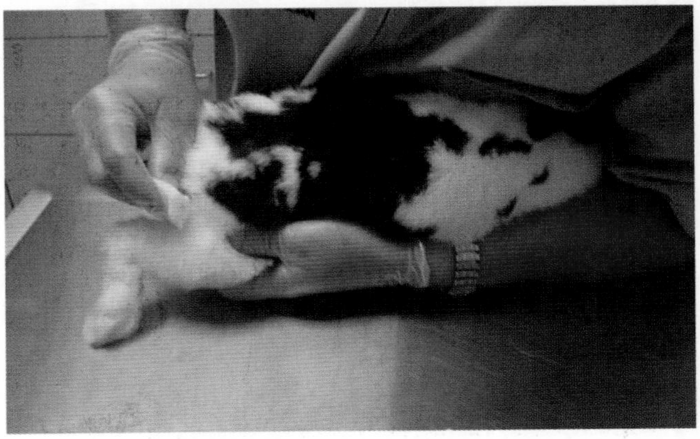

FIGURE 21-17 Restraining a rabbit.

procedures, such as nail trimming, physical examination, vaccination, auscultation, or rectal temperature. The ferret will become engrossed in cleaning it off.

Scruffing

Scruffing can be applied for restraint during procedures that require no movement, such as radiography or cystocentesis. Use the same technique for cats. This method is recommended for dental examinations, vaccinations, rectal temperature, venipuncture, and injections. Do not use scruffing for oral drug administration, because the ferret cannot swallow when held by the scruff (Fig. 21-18).

Wrapping

Towels can be used to wrap a ferret for eye or ear procedures. If the ferret struggles and begins to pant, this indicates overheating. Quickly unwrap the animal if this occurs.

RESTRAINT AND HANDLING OF BIRDS

Birds can be a challenge to restrain, which requires very careful planning and execution. Before applying restraint, carefully check to be sure that all potential escape routes are closed. Restraint of birds is covered in Chapter 27.

RESTRAINT AND HANDLING OF HORSES

EQUINE BEHAVIOR

Horses are herd animals that feel safer when in a group. Because there is safety in numbers, a herd of horses develops strong social relationships. They use numerous vocal sounds and a variety of body language to communicate with offspring, indicate social position in the herd, and signal fear and nervousness. If separated from its herd mates, a horse can become nervous, agitated, distracted, and uncooperative. They have well-developed senses to detect possible threats and when combined with a strong sense of self-preservation they can become very jumpy. By recognizing these signs we can often use our voice to calm them down or move them away from the stimulus.

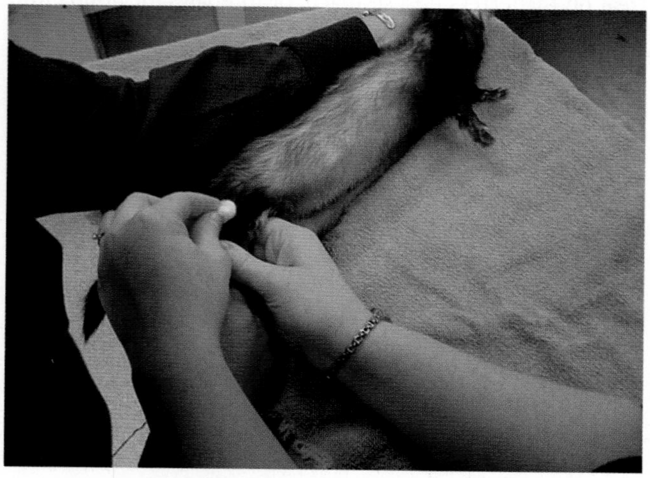

FIGURE 21-18 Restraining a ferret.

Horses have keen binocular, stereoscopic vision. Their eyes are situated on the sides of their heads (as in most prey animals) to see in two directions at once. However, they have small "blind spots" directly behind them and a short distance laterally from their rear flanks. Although this is very advantageous for horses, it also makes them shy away from objects located in their blind spot. The horse's depth perception is good if it is using both eyes, meaning it has to look directly at the object, such as a jump or a hole in the ground. Horses can distinguish the colors yellow, red, and green but have trouble with blue and purple.

> TECHNICIAN NOTE Always call out or announce yourself when approaching a horse, especially one that seems to be sleeping.

Horses have excellent hearing and can recognize each others' calls from great distances. By watching a horse's ears, you can locate the origin of sounds. Although most domestic horses are accustomed to certain amounts of noise, sudden loud sounds can startle a horse into flight.

The sense of touch is well developed in the horse. The body surface of a horse is very sensitive, especially under the belly in the flank area.

If a horse cannot run away from a threatening situation, it will resort to jumping, kicking, bucking, rearing, and biting. Although unprovoked aggression is rare in horses, defensive biting and kicking are relatively common.

BODY LANGUAGE

A horse's temperament and intentions are often signaled by its body language. A combination of signals should be taken into account for the most accurate "reading" of that body language.

Ears

Pinned-back ears indicate aggression or, if working, thinking hard. Forward-pointing ears indicate listening or attentiveness. One ear pointed forward and the other pointed backward indicates listening in two directions. Drooping or relaxed ears can indicate a sleeping, tired, or unwell horse.

Mouth

An open mouth with teeth exposed may signal attack. Lifting of the upper lip to expose the gums, with teeth together, is the Flehmen response, a type of sexual behavior in males. A tightly clamped mouth with a grimace can indicate pain.

Head

A lowered head and pinned-back ears are threatening gestures, as in a mare protecting its foal. An elevated head with eyes widely opened and ears moving in all directions signals attention and/or fright.

Feet

Pawing at the ground indicates impatience. Lifting of a rear foot with slight kicking motion indicates a possible defensive kick. Elevation of both front feet off of the ground signals the intent to rear defensively. Standing on three legs usually indicates a sleeping horse or one that has a sore leg. Shifting from leg to leg or rocking back on the heels can indicate pain in the legs or feet.

Tail

Tucking of the tail tight against the hindquarters signals fear or pain. Swishing or circling the tail signals agitation.

DANGER POTENTIAL

The main defense of horses is accurate kicking with the rear feet. The safe zones for passing behind a horse are 10 to 12 feet away or in direct contact with the rear of the horse. Most horses have a range of 6 to 8 feet, with the apex of the kick being the most deadly. You can be kicked when in close contact with the horse, but it does not have the power of the full leg.

Front legs can be used to paw at you or come down on you from rearing up, or both. That is why it is so important not to stand directly in front of a horse at any time.

Horses have very strong jaws. If a horse does not want to let go, it is nearly impossible to remove yourself from its jaws. A horse can lift an adult off the ground and shake it like a rag doll. A horse can cause horrible bruising and dislocations by biting and shaking. Most horses do not bite, but those that bite or try to bite should be disciplined. If a horse tries to bite, an immediate sharp rap to the muzzle is a must to get them to stop. Once they start biting, it is very hard to get them to stop.

MECHANICAL DEVICES

Halter

A halter is the main tool of restraint used on horses. Check your halter and lead rope for worn spots that could tear if the horse bolts. Make sure the lead rope is attached to the center ring at the bottom of the halter and that it is at least 6 feet long. Hold the halter open; if it is tangled, untangle it so that a smooth application of the halter can be accomplished. If the equipment checks out, proceed to halter the horse (Procedure 21-12).

Twitch

A **twitch** is a mechanical device that is attached to a horse's upper lip (muzzle) to distract its attention from a procedure being performed elsewhere on its body by exerting mild pain. It can be a flat chain that is wound around the lip

PROCEDURE 21-12 Applying a Horse Halter

1. Standing on the left side of the horse, tie the end of the lead rope around the neck of the horse with just an overhand throw. This convinces most horses into believing they've been caught. It also gives you something to grasp if the horse decides to move off.
2. Hold the neck strap of the halter in your left hand. Reach your right hand over the neck close to the poll and grasp the long end of the neck strap from your left hand.
3. With your left hand, grasp the buckle for the neck strap and allow the halter to fall open.
4. Pull the nose band over the bridge of the nose, and then buckle the neck strap (Fig. 1).
5. The halter should fit snugly, with two fingers easily slipping under the nose band.
6. Untie the lead rope from around the neck, and loosely gather the lead so it can be grasped in the left hand.
7. Position the right hand approximately 6 inches from where it is connected to the halter.
8. Stand to the side and slightly ahead of the front feet, facing the same direction as the horse (Fig. 2).

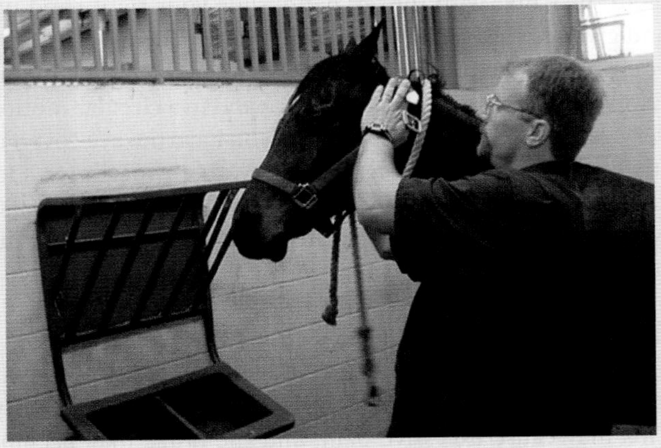

FIGURE 1 Connecting the neck strap on a horse halter.

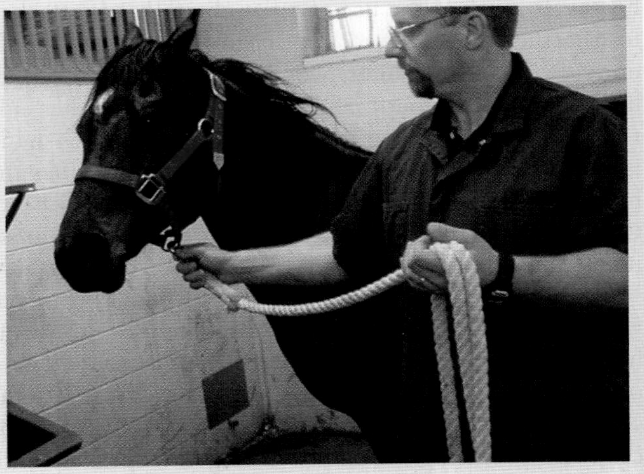

FIGURE 2 A haltered horse.

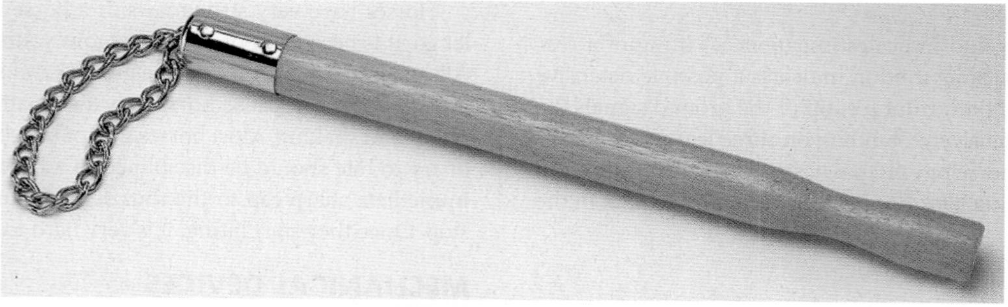

FIGURE 21-19 Chain twitch.

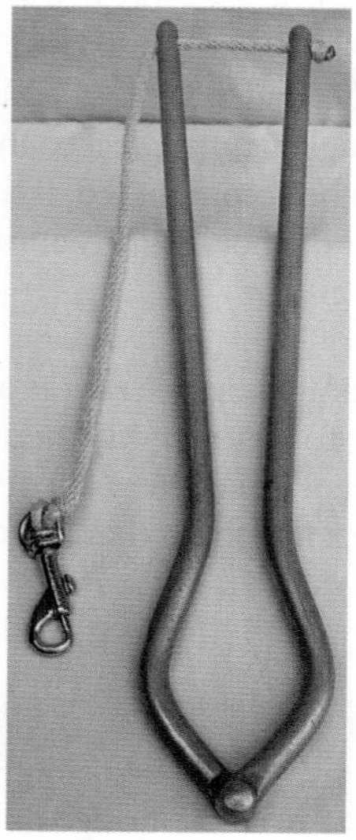

FIGURE 21-20 Humane twitch.

(Fig. 21-19) or a clamp that is closed and tightened over the lip or an aluminum bar that has curves to accommodate the horse's muzzle (Fig. 21-20). Procedure 21-13 shows how to apply a twitch.

Chain Shank

A chain shank is actually more of a discipline technique than a form of restraint. Think of it as a choker collar for horses. It involves the use of a flat chain that is attached to a leather or rope lead. The chain shank is run from one side ring of the halter, over the nose, under the upper lip or inside the mouth, and connected to the other side ring (Fig. 21-21). When the horse misbehaves, the shank is popped or tightened. This immediately disciplines the horse and often results in getting it to lower its head. Quickly loosen the tightened shank and comfort the horse if it settles down.

Some people put the shank beneath the horse's chin; but when popped or tightened, it causes the horse to throw its head up. The higher the head is, the less control you have over the horse. Only an experienced person should use the chain shank, as it can cause a great deal of harm both physically and psychologically. By watching and speaking with an experienced person, you will be able to learn this useful technique.

Stocks

Stocks are the ideal piece of equipment for procedures such as floating teeth, eye treatments, cleaning superficial wounds, changing head bandages, nasogastric intubation, and rectum or uterine examinations. Stocks usually have solid panels on the sides and a gate on either end. The panels are often removable or repositionable to allow access to trunk, legs, and feet (Procedure 21-14).

DISTRACTION TECHNIQUES

Distraction techniques are most useful for examinations, suture removal, injections, radiography, hoof work, and oral administration of paste dewormers. The person holding the halter usually applies the distraction techniques. If the horse is really uncooperative, a second person may be called in to help.

Skin Twitch

A horse's sensitivity to touch is used to distract its attention away from procedures such as injections or venipunctures. The restrainer stands on the same side as the person performing the procedure. Grasp a handful of loose skin on the lateral aspect of the neck or shoulder. Roll the skin under and give it a little shake or jiggle. You may also have the person giving the injection do the skin twitch. After the procedure is completed, release, scratch, and pet the area.

Eyelid Press

Hold the halter with the left hand, slide your right hand up, and give the base of the ears a nice scratch. Then gently move your cupped hand down and cover the eye closest to you. Exert a mild pressure or move your hand in a circular motion very gently. Talk to the horse while you have the eye covered. It will focus on you and ignore most other procedures. Occasionally lift your hand away from the eye and the horse will concentrate on focusing; then cover it back up until the procedure is completed.

Ear Hold

Grasp the very base of the ear, and gently move it in a small circular pattern. Do not bend it over or move too vigorously. This may cause excessive pain, and the horse may become head shy. You can also tie a light rope around the ear. Fold the edges in, and tie it closed with a piece of baling twine

PROCEDURE 21-13 Applying a Twitch

1. Start with the horse haltered; with the right hand hold the lead rope, halter, and twitch.
2. Reach the left hand through the opening in the twitch and grasp as much of the upper lip as possible, curling the lips in to protect the mucous membranes (Fig. 1).
3. Slide the twitch down around the bunched lip with your right hand, and tighten on the lips.
4. If the twitch has been applied properly, the horse should begin to look drowsy.
5. Slightly loosening and tightening the chain twitch or gently squeezing and releasing the humane twitch will keep the horse focused on the twitch (Fig. 2).
6. After the twitch has been released, gently massage the lip.
7. The maximum time for the twitch to be applied is 20 minutes; after that the muzzle loses feeling.

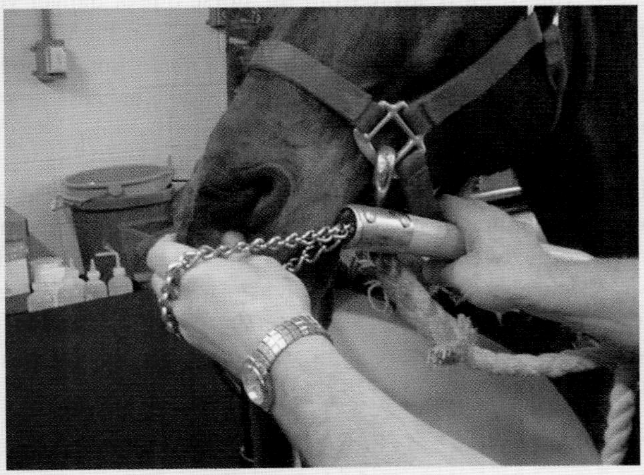

FIGURE 1 Applying chain twitch.

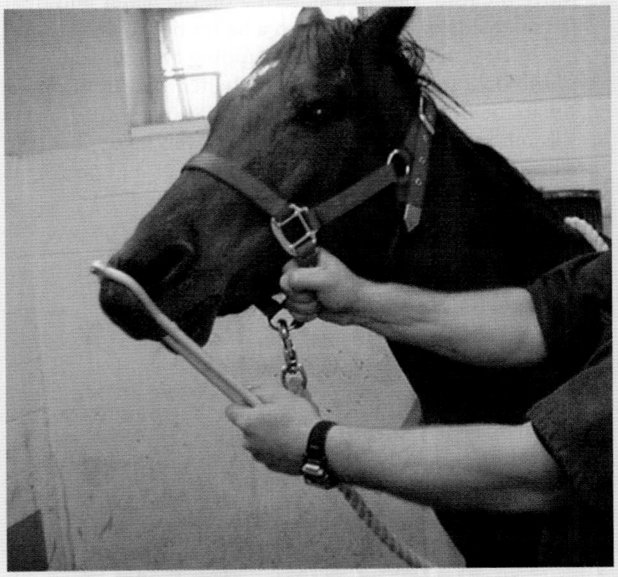

FIGURE 2 An applied humane twitch.

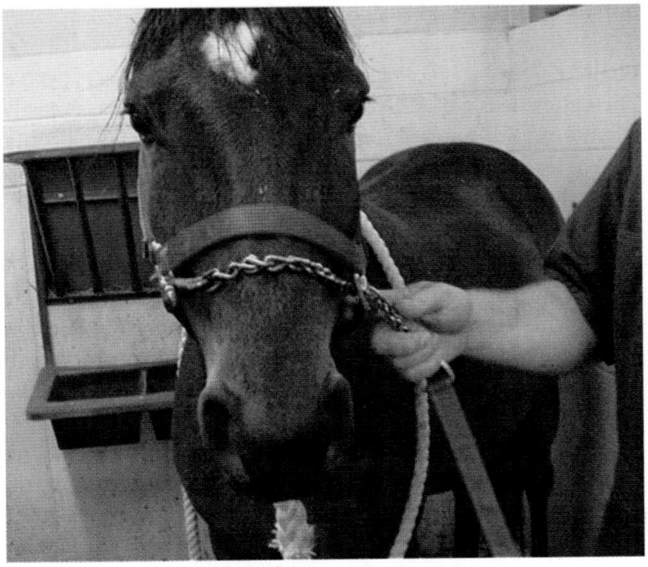

FIGURE 21-21 Chain shank in place.

or cotton rope. Again it causes the horse to focus on the ear and not what is going on elsewhere. Once the procedure is finished, release the ear and give a good scratch all over so the horse knows that every time you reach for an ear it is not going to be painful.

Blindfolding

Horses often become docile when blindfolded with a soft towel, jacket, or other large piece of clean cloth. Halter the horse; do not tie it. Stand on the same side as the person performing the procedure, slip the cloth underneath the halter and over the eyes, and then secure it to both sides of the halter. Make sure the horse cannot see around the blindfold. If you do this, talk to the horse continually and move slowly; the horse will depend entirely on you to keep it safe.

RESTRAINT TECHNIQUES

Horses are prey animals and therefore have a strong flight or fight response to danger. To restrain a horse, the handler must first convince the horse that it is not being threatened, and then win its trust and therefore its cooperation.

Approaching a Horse

If possible, try to approach a horse from the left or "near" side. Most horses are trained to be bridled, saddled, and mounted from the left side, so they are accustomed to people working from that side. Call out its name and wait for it to look at you. Approach, gently pat it lower down on the neck, and wait for it to smell you. At that time you can offer it a treat such as grain or an apple or carrot. Then you can proceed to halter or bridle it. If possible, do not approach the

PROCEDURE 21-14 Placing a Horse in a Stock

1. To place a horse into a stock, lead it up to the stock, allow it to go into the stock, and walk outside, passing the rope around the posts.
2. Close the tail and head gates as the horse reaches the front of the stocks.
3. Move the lead rope to a side ring on the halter and tie it to either side of the stock with a halter tie. You can cross-tie the head for added security, adding another lead rope to the opposite side ring on the halter, and tie it opposite to the first lead rope (Fig. 1). You can cross-tie horses without being in stocks as well. However, remember that a horse can still paw at you with its front legs, swing its body, and kick with its back legs.
4. Adjust any parts, such as side rails, as necessary to accommodate the horse.

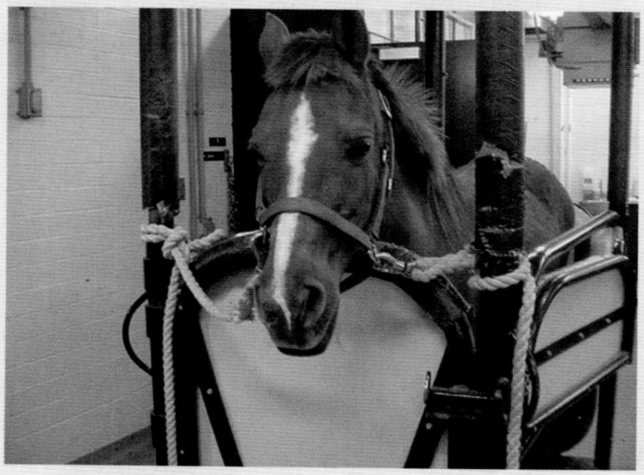

FIGURE 1 A cross-tied horse in a stock.

horse from the rear. If it is in a stall, it is best to persuade the horse to turn until its head is facing you. Call out to it and offer a treat. If it will not face you, carefully move into the stall paying close attention to the animal's body language. If a rear foot is cocked into the kicking position, try to approach on the other side of the horse. Move close in so that your body is in close contact to its body. This minimizes the strength of a kick if it is coming. Continue to move up to the front of the horse and halter it.

Leading a Horse

Never wrap the lead rope around your hand. This is extremely dangerous because of the possibility of injury if the horse bolts. The rope will tighten down around your hand, and you will be dragged with the horse. Loosely loop the lead rope, and then grasp it in the middle; it should look like you have a handful of "eights."

Standing on the left side of the horse just slightly ahead of the front left leg, give the lead rope a forward tug and ask the horse to move out. This can be a clicking sound made with your mouth or "giddy-up." Watch the front feet so they do not step on you, and watch where the horse is looking and listening. Be very alert to things that may frighten or startle the horse.

If the horse tries to pull ahead, pull back on the lead rope and say, "whoa." Sometimes you may have to jerk the lead rope sharply to get the horse to pay attention to you. If the horse refuses to be led, turn its head toward the right and push on its neck. This forces the horse to move its front feet and usually will get it to move off. Keep the horse's head level with your eye or lower. If the head is allowed to go above your shoulders, it is almost impossible to control the horse if it should bolt. If the horse is startled, the long lead rope allows you to move away from the horse out of danger yet maintain some control. Talk to the horse, and try to work your way back to the original position. Some technicians will use an even longer lead rope, allow the horse to settle down on its own, and then regain control.

If the horse is being uncooperative, it is important to discipline it immediately. Every time a horse gets loose by being bad tempered it learns the behavior and can become even more bad tempered. Not allowing the horse to act this way teaches it to behave and listen to you. This can be accomplished with sharp tugs on the halter with a command to whoa or stop. Sometimes you will have to use a chain shank to really get its attention.

Tying a Horse

Because a horse tends to frighten easily, never tie it to anything that could be torn loose and dragged behind it. Always tie the lead rope with a quick-release knot around a vertical post or pole. Never pass under the neck of a tied horse to get to its other side. Many people have been injured because a horse was frightened and jumped forward.

Halter Tie

The halter tie is a quick-release knot. The knot releases easily when you pull on the free end of the lead rope. The proper type of lead rope is also important; heavy braided, round cotton is the best (Procedure 21-15).

Picking up Feet

Have someone hold onto the horse on the same side as you. If the horse decides to bolt, it will then go in the opposite direction from you and your helper. To prepare to lift either foot, face toward the rear of the horse with a hand placed firmly on the horse so it knows you are there. Front feet are picked up by first placing your hand at the top of the leg near the shoulder. Firmly run your hand down the front of the leg until you reach the fetlock joint (Fig. 21-22).

With one hand on the front of the joint, reach around opposite to you and grasp the back of the joint. Lean against the horse, lift on the joint, and say "up" or "give me your foot." The other hand can grasp the front of the hoof and tip the foot in a flexed position. If the horse begins to resist, flex the foreleg a bit more. Place the hoof between your legs and above your knees (Fig. 21-23).

PROCEDURE 21-15 Halter Tie

1. Select a stout vertical post and place the free end of the lead rope around it (Fig. 1).
2. The rope should be at least wither height, with approximately 2½ feet of slack in the lead rope. More slack than this may allow the horse to put its foot over the rope and become entangled.
3. Make a loop in the free end of the rope and set it over the standing part of the rope (the part attached to the horse) close to the post (Fig. 2).
4. Make another loop with the free end, pass it underneath the standing part, and push it up and through the first loop (Fig. 3).
5. Pull the loop to tighten it. This traps the long end of the rope and forms a quick-release knot.
6. Test the knot by pulling the free end of the rope. It should release easily.
7. Some horses have learned to pull on the free end of the rope, thus freeing themselves. To thwart them, place the free end of the rope into the loop formed in the knot. Do not tighten the rope; just leave it hanging loosely. The horse will pull on the end of the rope but will not release or tighten the knot.

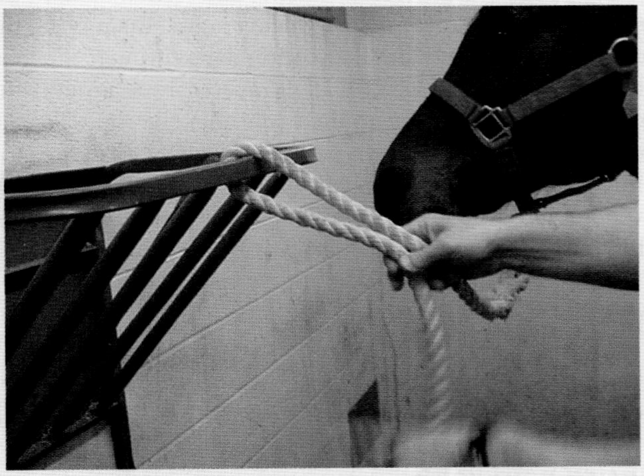

FIGURE 1 Place rope around sturdy object or post.

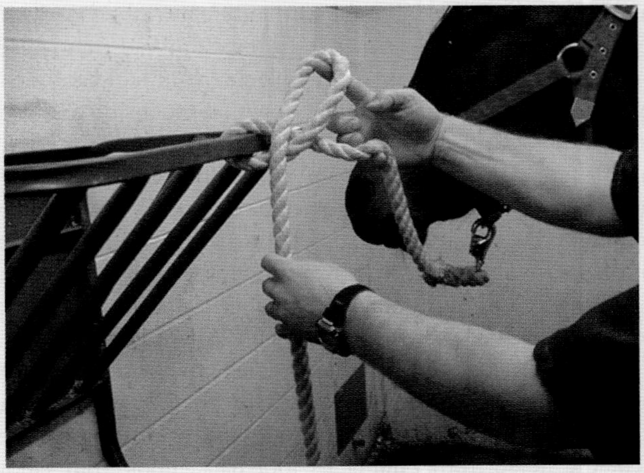

FIGURE 2 Make a loop and place it on top of the standing part of the rope close to the post.

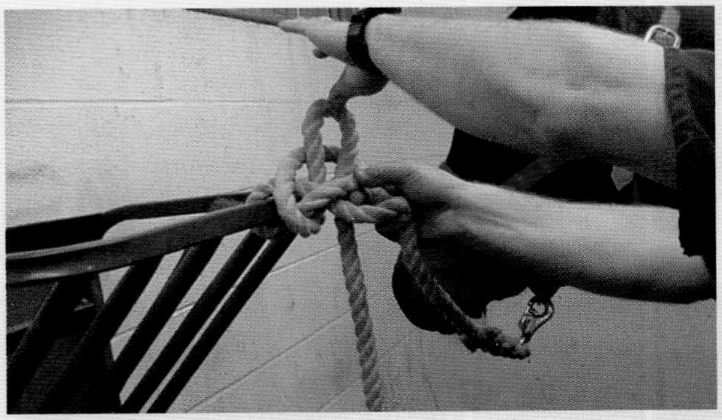

FIGURE 3 Make another loop and pass it under the standing part and through the first loop. Pull up on the loop to tighten.

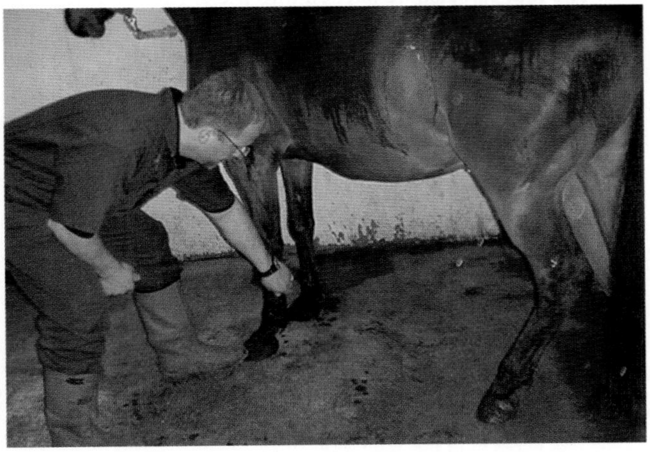

FIGURE 21-22 Start at the shoulder and slide your hand down to the fetlock joint.

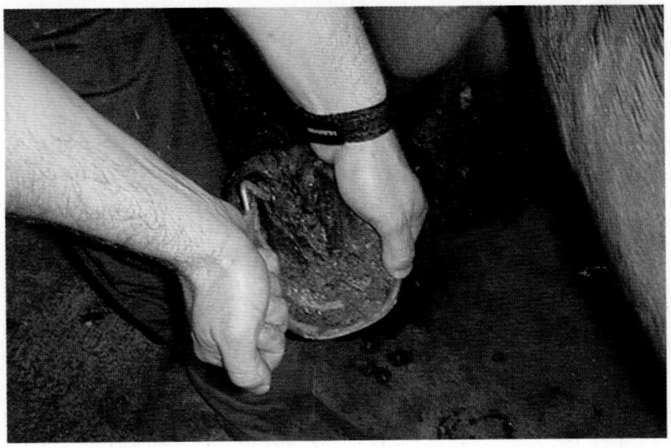

FIGURE 21-23 Placing the front hoof between your knees.

This allows both hands to be free for cleaning, bandaging, or checking for soft spots. When you are finished, hang onto the hoof until your leg is out of the way and then set the foot down. Do not let it drop, as it can startle the horse and cause it to jump.

Rear feet are picked up by first placing your hand at the top of the rump and firmly sliding it down on the inside of the leg until you get to the fetlock joint. Lean into the horse, pull up on the fetlock joint, give the "up" command, and start to walk forward. This brings the leg out to the rear of the horse. Keeping the foot extended prevents the horse from gathering a lot of power in which to kick. It can still kick out but without the force of coming from the ground. Once the foot is extended, rest the hoof on top of your thigh (Fig. 21-24).

Do not place it between your legs like the front foot. If the horse kicks back, the leg simply moves away from you; if the foot was between your knees it would send you flying. To prevent the horse from pulling its foot back, hook your elbow around the hock and take another step forward. This "locks" the leg, and it has a harder time moving it. However, if a horse is really adamant about moving its leg, go ahead and set it down so you do not get hurt. The person restraining the head can aid this process by performing distraction techniques, talking to the horse, and watching it for signs that it is going to move or jump. He should alert others if the horse starts to show signs of moving or jumping. This is usually indicated by an anxious look in the horse's eye, and the muscle is bunched before a leap.

Tying a Leg

This technique has a very powerful psychological effect on a horse. By taking away its ability to flee, the horse must rely on you to be its protector. The first time this procedure is done, a horse may panic and hop around. Eventually, the horse will relax and allow you to work with it.

The technique involves tying up one front leg in a flexed position. The horse should not be tied to an inanimate object because it may struggle and injure itself. Have someone hold the head while you tie up the leg. Pick the front leg up as you would for any other procedure, but instead of placing the leg between your knees, fold it so the leg is in a flexed position. Using a soft cotton rope or a leather strap with a buckle, wrap it around the leg several times and secure it with either two half-hitches or by buckling the strap.

Release the leg and step away from the horse. Once the horse has accepted its fate, you can perform radiographs, bandaging, or other fairly noninvasive procedures. This is not recommended for painful procedures, because the next time to you try to pick up one of its legs, the horse may remember the procedure and react violently.

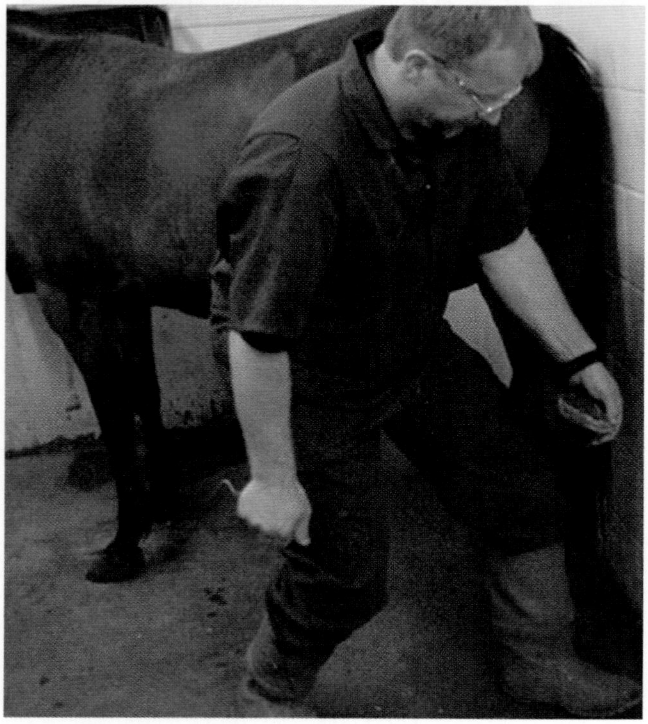

FIGURE 21-24 Placing rear hoof on top of the knee.

Tail Tie

When the tail is tied up, a horse cannot swish it or tuck it under. Procedures such as rectal palpation, Caslick's surgery, and artificial insemination can be performed on the hindquarters. Grasp the tail in one hand, and form a bend in the hair just distal to the last coccygeal vertebra. Then bring the loose end of a heavy braided cotton rope through the loop from the bottom (Fig. 21-25). Wrap the rope around the horse's tail, and then bring the end under the rope. Pull up on the short end and down on the long end. Grasp the long end, and tie it to the front leg with a quick-release knot. If you preplaced a rope around the neck and tied with a nonslipping knot, you can attach it to that rope.

> *TECHNICIAN NOTE* When tying a rope to any animal's neck, make sure you use a bowline knot, which is a nonslipping knot.

Restraining Foals

Newborn foals can be restrained by placing one arm in front of the foal's chest and the other behind the foal's hindquarters. The foal can also be backed into the corner of a stall and gently held in position with an arm placed in front of the chest. Foals are always kept in their mother's view because both foal and mother will do almost anything to be reunited.

Once the foal is up and moving around, a small halter can be fitted to the head. A loop is made in a lariat and placed over the foal's rump. A tug on the lead rope with the appropriate command and a tug on the lariat are usually all that is needed to get the foal to move forward. Praise is appropriate when the foal is walking along with no tugs on the lariat.

RESTRAINT AND HANDLING OF CATTLE

BOVINE BEHAVIOR

Rough or inappropriate handling of cattle can reduce conception rates, weight gain, the immune response, and rumen function. Understanding cattle behavior will help you predict how they are likely to respond to handling and can facilitate handling, reduce stress on the animal, and improve handler and animal safety.

Remember too that dairy cows are usually used to having humans around and do not need a lot of physical manipulation to get them to go where you want. They are often treated either in their stanchions or haltered and tied to a post. Dairy bulls can be very unpredictable in their behavior and should not be handled by a novice. Beef cattle of both sexes can be very shy of humans and should be handled via the use of alleyways and chutes.

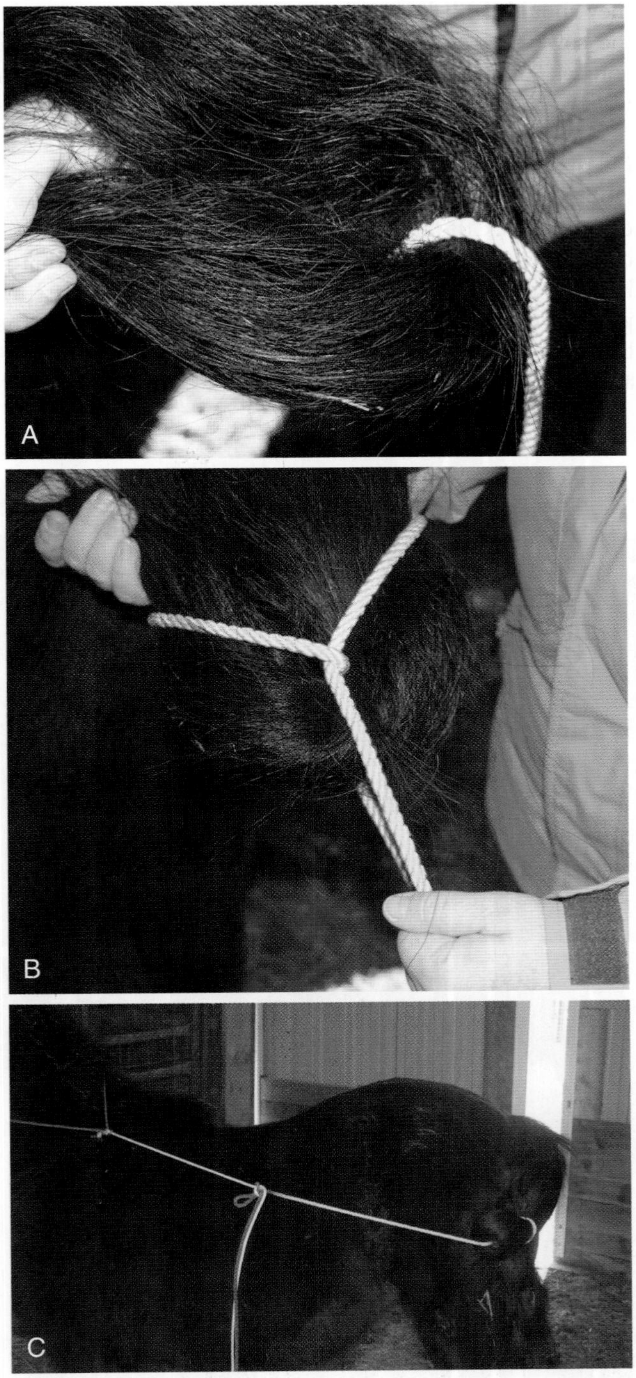

FIGURE 21-25 A, Bend the hair of the tail at the end of the vertebrae and pass a rope through the resulting loop. B, Pass the rope around the tail and then under the rope and tighten using both ends. C, Tie the long end to the end of the rope tied around the neck with a quick release knot.

DANGER POTENTIAL

The most common means of defense for cattle are kicking and butting. When cattle kick, it is usually with one leg at a time. Their kick is an arch starting forward, moving off to the side, and then straight back. Some cattle kick straight out, but that is usually not the case. Also note that they are very accurate.

Cattle will slam into you with their heads, and once you are on the ground or against a wall or fence they will continue to hold you there. Some will even grind you into the ground. If that should happen, try to curl up and protect your head as much as possible and lie still. Most cattle will back off if you stop moving, but be aware that if you move and they are still watching you they will come back and attack again. This usually occurs when a cow has a calf at her side, although bulls have been known to do this as well. They are very protective of their young and will defend them aggressively no matter how tame they are. Many people have lost their lives while working on a calf and not paying attention to the whereabouts of its mother.

MECHANICAL DEVICES

Squeeze Chute

The **squeeze chute** is a restraint device used almost exclusively on beef cattle (Fig. 21-26). Nearly all medical procedures can be facilitated by use of a properly constructed chute. A chute usually has three mechanical working parts: the head gate, tailgate, and squeeze. An animal is run into a chute by means of an alleyway (Procedure 21-16).

Cows will usually settle if they feel they are confined in this way. The head gate is closed tight enough so that the animal cannot put a foot through, but not so tight as to clamp the cow's neck to occlude the airway. There are side panels

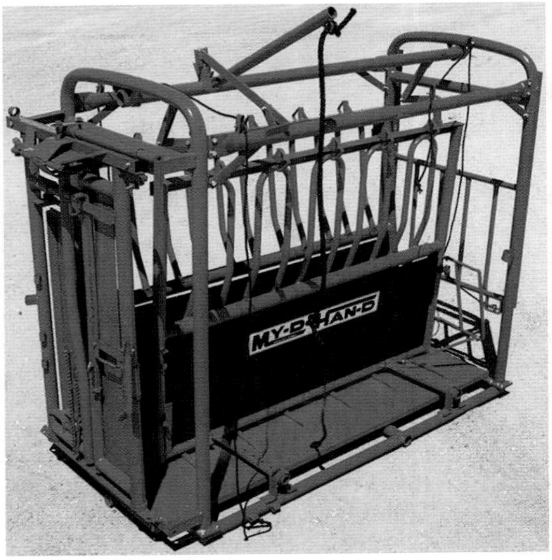

FIGURE 21-26 Cattle squeeze chute.

that can be opened to allow access to the cow's side or feet. The tailgate acts as a barrier between you and the cow's rear legs. This allows access to the perineal area for pregnancy checking, tail bleeding, or assistance during calf delivery. The head gate allows you to approach the cow to place a halter or administer oral medications.

Be aware that a cow can still stretch its neck quite a way out and can move it from side to side. The danger is being butted with the head, which is usually not fatal, unless there is direct contact to your head. If the cow's head needs to be controlled, a halter should be applied.

Halter

The halter used on cattle is usually a rope halter that can be adjusted to fit any sized cow or bull. Two things to remember when applying a halter are that the part that tightens when the lead is pulled goes around the nose and the lead comes off the left side of the cow's head. Before applying the halter, be sure the head stall is large enough to go behind the ears, but not so large that you have to make major adjustments while standing close to the cow's head. Most people slip the nose band on first, then the headstall behind the ears (Fig. 21-27).

Pulling the lead will cause the halter to tighten up, and the cow's head can be tied to the side of the chute. Make sure that you adjust the side straps so they are not resting over the eyes. Halter and tying the head to the chute allows jugular venipuncture or injections, ear tag placement, and ophthalmic procedures to be performed.

Stanchions

A stanchion usually consists of a head gate without sidebars to restrict lateral movement (Fig. 21-28). Dairy cattle are often placed in stanchions and are comfortable being worked on in them. They are usually not substantial enough to handle beef cattle. The handler must be aware that even though the head is secured, the cow can kick you.

Electric Prod

Battery-powered prods are sometimes used to deliver a shock to the animal, and if used correctly will only be applied to the hindquarters (Fig. 21-29). These instruments should be used sparingly if at all. Keep the prod directly behind the animal; prodding on the top line confuses the cow because in its mind it cannot go down. Indiscriminate use of the cattle prod is cruel and often unnecessary if the handler slows down and allows the cow to figure out what it is being asked to do.

PROCEDURE 21-16 Placing Cattle in a Squeeze Chute

1. Close the head gate securely behind the head. This can be an automatic system or a manual lever that is pulled by a person.
2. Slide the tail gate closed at virtually the same time so another cow does not run in behind the captured cow. This also prevents the captured cow from backing out of the head gate and into the alleyway.
3. Squeeze the animal snugly, but not so tightly against the cow's sides that it impedes breathing.

Whips

Whips are also used sparingly to make cattle move. If used, they should be flicked at the heels or hindquarters to make the cow move forward. You can also use a whip to make yourself "bigger." This can help when guarding an opening or walking behind them to move them forward.

Hobbles

Hobbles are usually used on dairy cattle that have tendency to kick the milkers. Hobbles can be either a metal clip that is placed on each hock or a padded strap that is buckled around the lower leg. With both types, it is important to keep the cow's legs squared under her. If the back legs are brought in too close, she could lose her balance and fall.

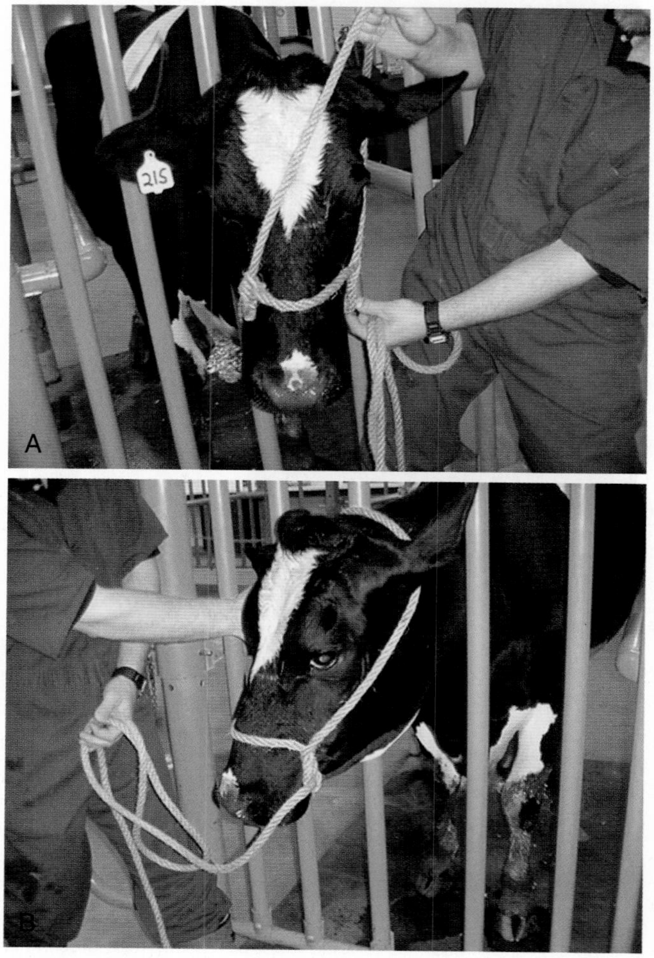

FIGURE 21-27 A, Placing a halter on a cow. B, Halter in position on a cow.

Tilt Table

Cattle, especially bulls, often need their feet trimmed. This can be done in a chute, but it is easier to do on a tilt table (Fig. 21-30).

Lead the animal or use an alleyway to put the animal near the table in its vertical upright position. Then sedate the animal and strap it to the table. Tilt the animal so it is in lateral recumbency. This allows access to all four feet at a comfortable height.

RESTRAINT TECHNIQUES

Approaching and Moving

Cattle have the same wide-angle vision as horses. This can be used to the handler's advantage when getting them to move in a desired direction. Cattle have a "pressure point" at the shoulders. If you move past the shoulder going toward the rear of the cow it prompts the cow to move forward. If you move toward the head it will make the cow stop. Use this information to move cattle into a pen or down an alley without a lot of prompting with a whip or paddle (Fig. 21-31).

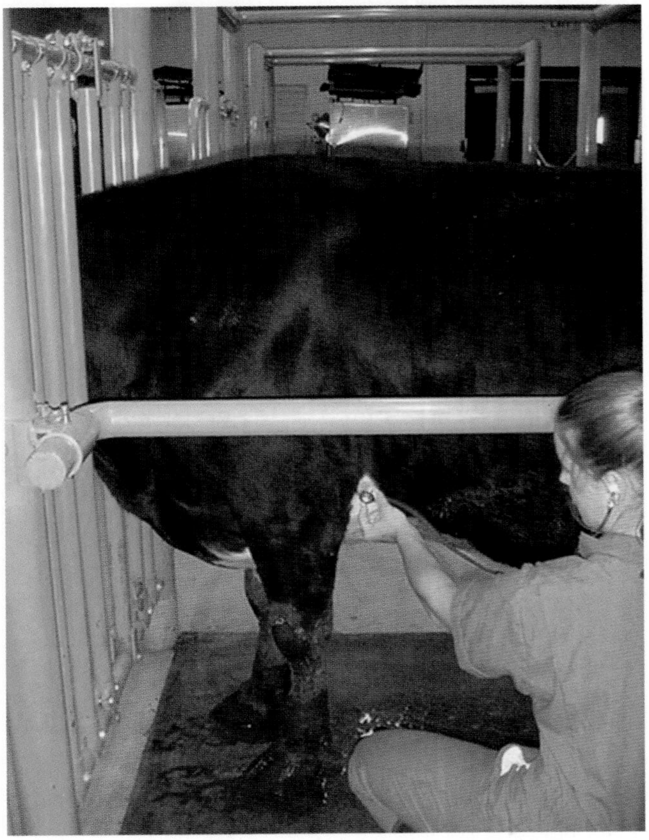

FIGURE 21-28 Cow stanchion—used with dairy cows.

To move a herd or group of cattle into a pen or alley, do not push them too hard. Rather, allow them to look inside and inspect the area. If you do not allow them to look the place over, they will either scatter in every direction or move in a circle and will not enter the enclosure. Place one person toward the opening of the gate and one behind the group you need to move. The person in the back puts pressure on the group by stepping forward; the person toward the front puts pressure on the group by walking toward the rear of the group from directly behind their shoulders toward the rear. As the cattle start to move into the pen, the person at the front of the group continues the forward motion by stepping behind the group as he or she moves in that direction. Be aware that cattle will kick if frightened or pushed too hard. They seldom kick straight out, having an arch from front to back. This is important to remember because you can get kicked standing to the side of a cow as well as behind it. Either stand right next to the rear of the cow or back at least 6 to 8 feet. You can be kicked standing next to the animal, but it will not be as deadly as inside the 6-foot range.

Sometimes it is difficult and even dangerous to separate a cow and her calf away from the herd. Instinctively they try to remain with the herd for protection. The best scenario is to move a small group, containing the intended cow and calf, into a pen that has a gate into another pen. One person operates the gate, opening and closing it as the appropriate animal approaches. Two other people are placed in the same positions as described for pushing a group into a pen. Move the mother and her calf along the fence opposite to the person at the gate. This allows the gate to close behind the cow and calf.

Remember that mothers are very protective of their calves and may chase after you if they feel threatened. Have escape routes in mind and watch the cattle carefully. Do not turn your back on the group. Many people have lost their lives to upset cows.

It is also important to lock up any dogs that may be around, even if they are trained cattle dogs. Cows with young at their side will get very upset when a dog is in the pen with them and often charge the dog. Unfortunately, the dog often looks to people for protection and will run behind the closest person. The cow will not differentiate between you and the dog.

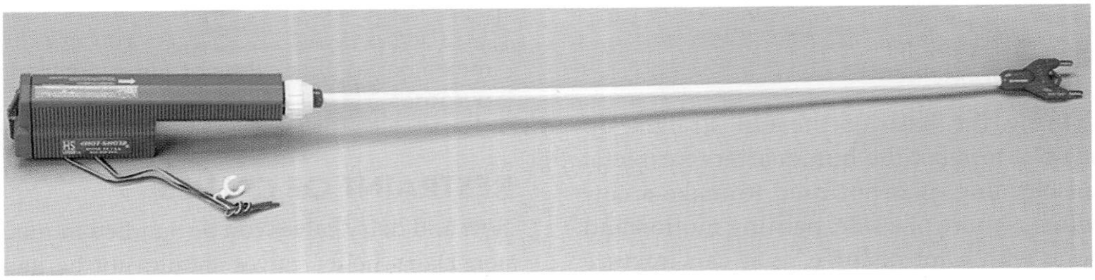

FIGURE 21-29 Cattle prod.

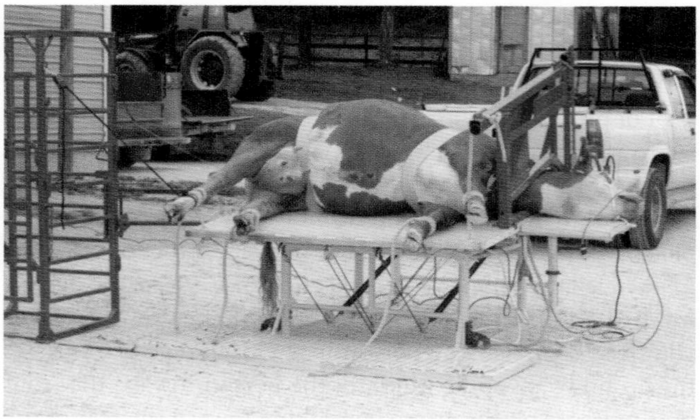

FIGURE 21-30 Tilt table for hoof trimming.

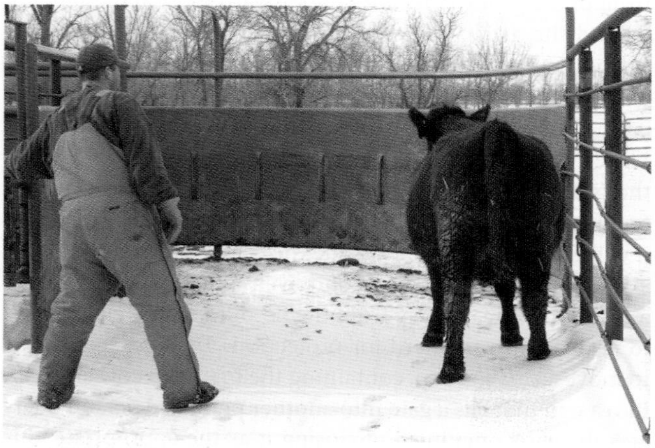

FIGURE 21-31 Moving a cow forward.

Oral Medications

Oral medications are delivered by a balling gun, a drenching bottle or gun, and a stomach tube, which requires a speculum. To open the mouth for placement of a balling gun or mouth speculum, stand to the side of the cow's head opposite to your dominant hand. Hold the balling gun or speculum in your dominant hand; reach over the bridge of the nose with the opposite hand. Slide your fingers into the animal's mouth at the commissure of the lips to gently open the mouth, by lifting up on the soft palate (Fig. 21-32). Quickly slide the balling gun or speculum down the center of the throat. You will feel some resistance as the balling gun or speculum bumps over the esophageal groove. If you direct both instruments down the center of the tongue it goes a lot easier. After the speculum is in place, the stomach tube can be passed down the center of the speculum.

Tail Jacking

Tail jacking is lifting the base of the tail straight up (Fig. 21-33). It is used to relax the hindquarters for rectal palpation and tail bleeding. It is not used to make a cow move forward, which is more of a side-twisting motion and should not be done with a lot of force, as it can fracture the vertebrae in the tail. With both techniques, you must

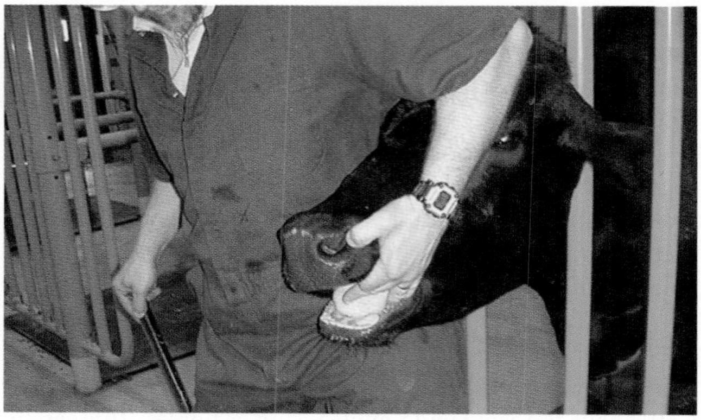

FIGURE 21-32 Opening the cow's mouth for oral medications.

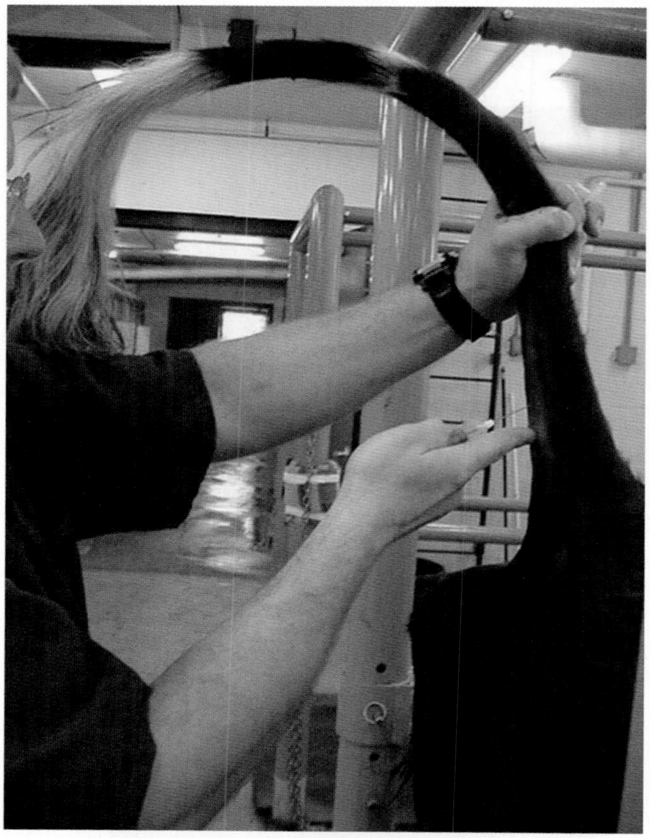

FIGURE 21-33 Tail jacking.

be prepared for the cow to kick. Always make sure the tail gate or a bar is placed directly behind the cow's back legs to prevent serious kicks.

> *TECHNICIAN NOTE* As you are drawing samples, remember to check the ear tag on cattle for identification purposes.

RESTRAINT OF CALVES

Beef and dairy calves can be handled in much the same manner. Dairy heifer calves should not be handled roughly, as this may result in a bad-tempered adult cow.

If the cow is with her calf, move the cow in the desired direction and the calf will follow. Once separated from the dam, as previously described, move the calf by wrapping one arm around the front of the calf's chest and the other hand around the rear quarters and walking it forward. A larger calf can be led by using a rope halter, but this often results in a tug of war. It is easier to treat larger calves like adults and simply herd them to the desired area.

> TECHNICIAN NOTE Always be aware of the dam when working with a calf.

Flanking

Flanking, or placing a calf in lateral recumbency, is easy if you position yourself properly (Procedure 21-17).

PROCEDURE 21-17 Flanking a Calf

1. Place the calf's body so its left side is parallel to your legs.
2. Position your right knee into the calf's flank and reach around the calf's body to grasp the opposite flank with the right hand (Fig. 1).
3. With the left hand, grasp the loose skin just behind the shoulder.
4. Push into the calf with your knee and lift up with both hands at the same time, letting the calf slide down your legs to break the fall.
5. Follow the calf down and place one knee on the neck. Raise the front leg that is closest to the ground to keep the calf down.

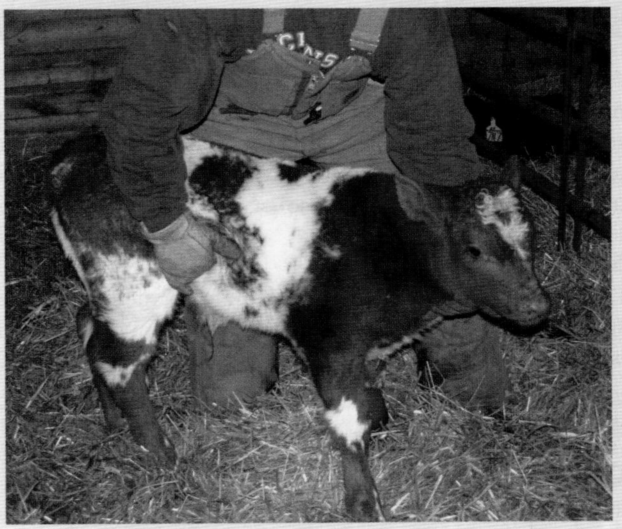

FIGURE 1 Flanking a calf.

RESTRAINT AND HANDLING OF GOATS

CAPRINE BEHAVIOR

Goats are gregarious, ruminant animals. Although they are herd animals, they do not move together as easily as sheep. Also, goats become very vocal when separated from herd mates. It is usually easier for all involved if a companion goat is kept near the patient during a procedure. Goats that are used to being handled are docile and enjoy attention and petting.

Goats cannot be treated like sheep or controlled by force. They are much more agile and resistant to restraint. Although goats can withstand more stress than sheep, rough handling is unnecessary. Goats also tolerate heat fairly well. Goats become agitated and tend to struggle against restraint after a certain point. When handling goats, it is best to keep untrained dogs away, because goats make a game of attacking dogs. Although goats do not bite or kick, they do rear and charge humans and dogs, especially to defend their kids. Goats are also excellent escape artists and have been known to unlatch gates, climb, and jump more than 6 feet.

> TECHNICIAN NOTE Goats are gluttons, and can easily be lured into a pen with grain.

RESTRAINT TECHNIQUES

Catching and Holding

When you work with a herd of goats, the ideal restraint is to use a small pen. Lure them into the pen with grain or some other treat. Chasing goats rarely works, as they scatter to the four winds.

Goats can be crowded into a pen, and then an individual goat can be caught and moved out to a work area. You can catch a goat by placing an arm around its neck and the other hand on its tail, much like a foal, and then direct its movements with forward or backward pressure. Goats that are handled frequently may have a collar that can be used to lead it to the work area. If the goats are in a panic and you cannot get an arm around the neck, grasp a front leg and hold it off the ground. Most goats will stop and allow you to encircle them with your arms or place a collar or halter on them. Some may throw themselves to the ground and cause a disturbance. Be careful not to wrench the leg if this happens.

Once caught, place the goat's rear end in a corner to prevent it from backing up, and press its body against a wall to prevent lateral movement. Hands can be wrapped around either side of the face to lift the head for medications, IM or SC injections, or jugular venipuncture (Fig. 21-34).

Small goats can actually be handled much like a dog; they can be put in lateral recumbency and straddled.

Never grab hold of a goat's horns; they resent this and will resist violently. They will either run at you and butt you or shake their heads vigorously. This is especially true of billy goats. Also it is advisable not to grasp the beard on intact male goats. They urinate on their beards as a means of attracting females and the musky scent is difficult to remove. Goats also remember people and rough handling, so be kind. Their payback can be an unpleasant knock with their heads.

Halter

A halter that is similar to a horse halter but cut to size can be used on a goat. The flat chain collar or a leather collar is most often seen. Goats that are milked or shown usually can

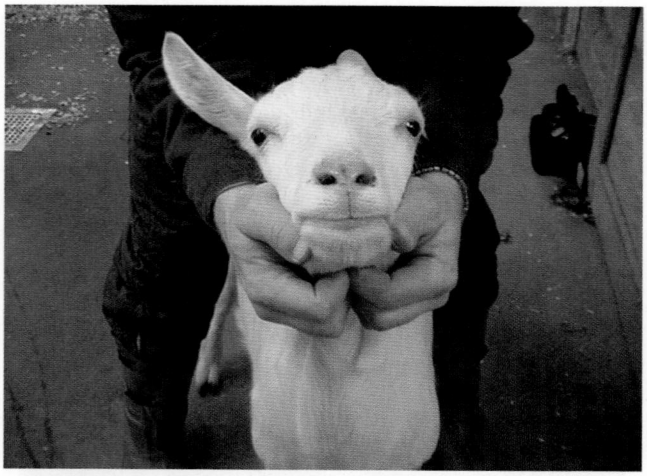

FIGURE 21-34 Holding the head for jugular venipuncture.

be led easily. A goat will stand quietly for short periods if tied securely to an object using a collar or halter and lead. These techniques can be used for such procedures as hoof trimming, vaccination, and blood collection.

Stanchion

Dairy goats that are accustomed to a stanchion can be restrained easily for most procedures in this manner. Grain can be fed as a distraction.

RESTRAINT AND HANDLING OF SHEEP

OVINE BEHAVIOR

Sheep depend on their speed and flocking instinct as defense against predators. By moving as a group they confuse predators so the predator cannot pick one out of the group. If one keeps that in mind, the amount of handling, which causes sheep a good deal of stress, can be minimized. Sheep become hyperthermic easily because of their wool and normally high body temperature (102° to 104° F). Use caution when working with sheep in ambient temperatures greater than 50° F and high humidity. Working in the early part of the morning with good ventilation is a must to keep sheep from overheating.

Sheep have a frail skeletal system and can be injured easily if they are chased into fences. Rough handling can break their back and legs. Never grab sheep by the wool; it is easily pulled out and the skin tears easily, causing bruising, which devalues the carcass and pelt.

Although uncommon, a sheep may charge and butt a person. Ewes protecting lambs and other adult sheep sometimes charge dogs. Usually sheep that are behaving defensively face the assumed "predator" and stamp their feet. Sheep can bound over obstacles or people when feeling threatened; however, they are not good jumpers, and usually catch a person in the mid-chest.

RESTRAINT TECHNIQUES

Catching and Holding

One of the easy things about sheep is that once one goes they all go. This can work very well if they are going in the direction you want them to, but not if they are escaping. Sheep should be moved as a group into a small containment pen. This can be built with portable 4′ × 4′ wooden panels or gates. Set them up in a funnel-like configuration to get them into a smaller pen. Once they are in the pen, single out the sheep that needs treatment.

FIGURE 21-35 Moving a single sheep into position.

To capture a single sheep, place one hand around the tail and the other under the jaw (Fig. 21-35). A forward or backward pressure with the hands will direct the sheep. Be careful not to choke the sheep by placing your hand on its throat. Alternatively, use a shepherd's crook to catch a sheep by the hock, and then hold it as mentioned. Move the sheep out to a work area, but not out of sight from the other sheep. This will keep the sheep calmer.

Jugular venipuncture, oral medications, and physical exams can be accomplished using the same technique as described for a goat.

Setting Up

Sheep are often set on their hindquarters for shearing and other procedures, such as hoof trimming and subcutaneous injections (Procedure 21-18).

> TECHNICIAN NOTE Do not try to muscle a sheep to set it up. Use its weight to throw it off balance.

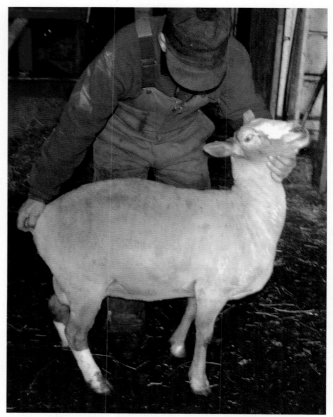

PROCEDURE 21-18 Setting Up a Sheep

1. Stand with your legs against the sheep's shoulder and flank.
2. Push the sheep's head laterally to its shoulder. After a few moments, the sheep will begin to slowly sag (Fig. 1).
3. At this point, lift up on the flank, step back with the leg closest to the flank, pivot on the other leg to throw the sheep off-center, and set the sheep on its rump (Fig. 2).
4. Rock the sheep back so that it is resting on the top of the pelvis versus directly on the rear. This keeps the sheep off-balance, and it will cease to struggle.
5. Rest the back between your legs, freeing both hands for other work (Fig. 3).

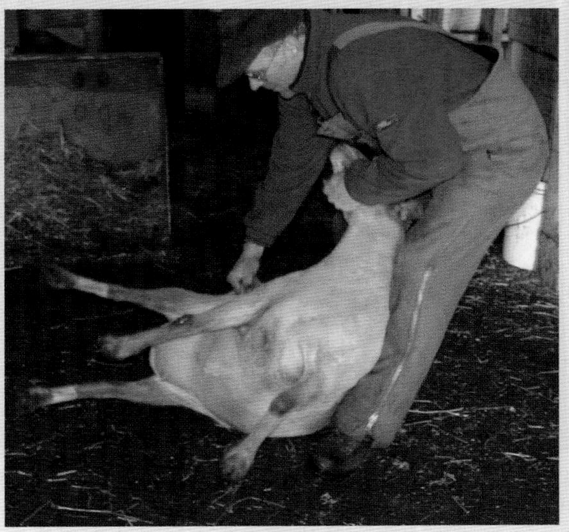

FIGURE 2

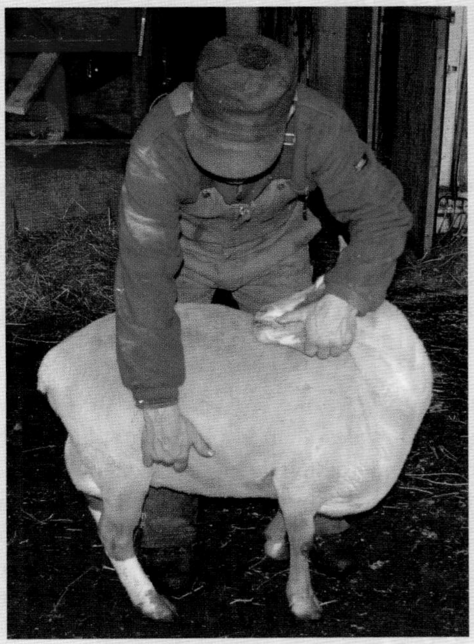

FIGURE 1 Setting up a sheep.

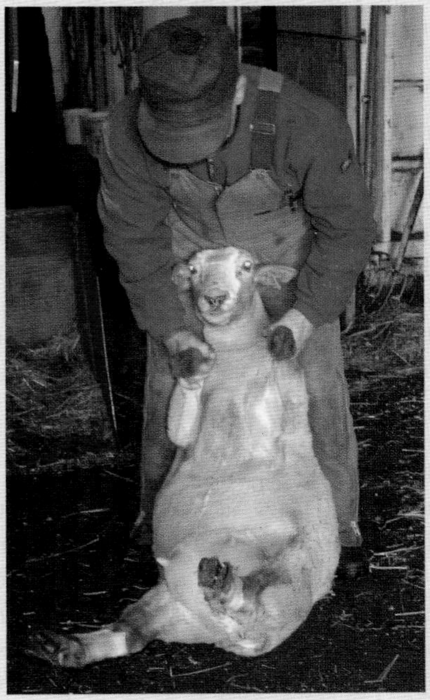

FIGURE 3

Halter

If a sheep restraint table is not available, apply a sheep halter after it has been caught. Take care not to occlude the nostrils with the nose band. Show sheep are trained to be led using a halter, whereas others must be coaxed and pushed from behind.

RESTRAINT AND HANDLING OF PIGS

PORCINE BEHAVIOR

Pigs are not herd animals, but they tend to follow other pigs. When one pig becomes distressed and screams, the others may react as a group and panic, or they may come to the rescue of the "injured" pig. Pigs are extremely protective of their young and will come running if a piglet cries out. Pigs are also extremely stubborn, which can be used to advantage with various restraint procedures, particularly the hog snare.

Pigs can become hyperthermic if chased or roughly handled even in cool weather. Overheated pigs must be cooled immediately or they are likely to die of heat stroke.

DANGER POTENTIAL

Pigs' main defensive weapons are their teeth. They can tear flesh easily and have very strong jaws; the tusks of boars can be very dangerous. Enter all adult swine enclosures with

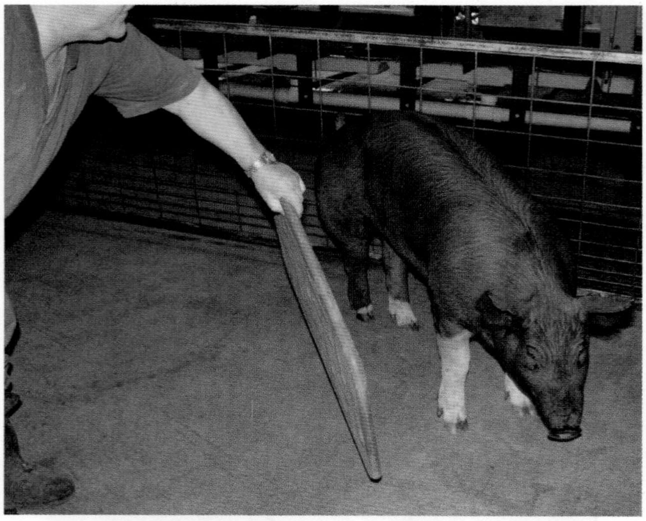

FIGURE 21-36 Moving a pig with a hurdle.

caution and be prepared to exit quickly. Sows are very dangerous when there are piglets at their side; a handler should never get into the same pen with a sow and piglets.

RESTRAINT TECHNIQUES

Driving and Catching

Pigs can be difficult to drive in an open pen. Solid-paneled hurdles work well to move pigs, as well as pieces of PVC piping or a cane. Pigs stop when confronted with a solid barrier, such as hurdles, and pigs will move along when tapped on the rear quarters. Pigs should be driven into a small pen with solid walls at least as high as a pig's shoulder. They can be separated from the group again using the hurdles and pipe or cane.

Directing a Single Pig

When moving a single pig, walk behind it with a hurdle in front of you (Fig. 21-36). Use a cane or paddle to direct the pig by tapping it on the flank to move it forward or on the shoulder to move it right or left. If it turns and moves toward you, set the edge of the hurdle on the ground and tilt it forward. This prevents the pig from getting its snout under it and lifting, allowing it access to or through your legs. The solid barrier will make the pig turn around.

Hog Snare

A **hog snare** is used for restraining pigs for venipunctures or other injections. The snare is usually a metal pipe with a cable loop on one end. The free end of the cable runs through the hollow pipe, so the size of the loop can be controlled (Procedure 21-19).

Excessive tightening can injure the pig's snout. A snare should be in place for a maximum of 20 to 30 minutes. A rope can be used in place of the pipe and cable snare. If using a snare on a boar with tusks, it is important to get the snare behind the tusks. However, this creates a possible hazard if the snare gets hung up on the tusks as it is removed. The pig is strong enough to jerk the snare from your hands and then swing it around. If the snare hits you or becomes airborne, someone is going to get hurt. Be advised that once a pig has experienced a snare, it is difficult to capture it again.

It is advisable to wear ear protection when using a hog snare, as they scream the entire time they are held. Even employing a hog snare for the short time it takes to complete one procedure can cause your ears to ring for the rest of the day.

PROCEDURE 21-19 Applying a Hog Snare

1. Hold the loop in front of the pig. Most will investigate it in case it is something to eat.
2. When the pig mouths the loop, quickly move the loop into the mouth and over the snout and tighten the loop.
3. Lean or pull back on the snare (Fig. 1). The pig will lean back from the snare and emit a loud scream, which it will keep up until released.
4. When releasing the snare, push down on the handle. Do it quickly and step out of the way.

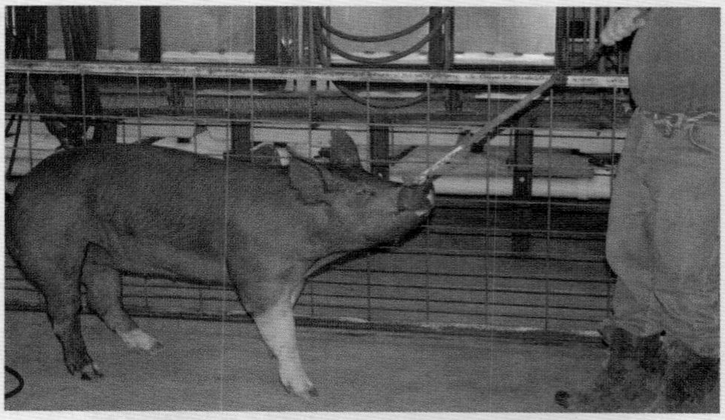

FIGURE 1 A hog snare applied to a pig.

Restraining Piglets

Baby pigs weighing less than 50 pounds are captured by grasping a back leg and holding the pig upside down until it can be held on your forearm close to your body or placed in a holding pen. If removing piglets from a sow, do it quickly and move to a different room to perform the procedure so you do not agitate the sow. Many farms have a cart to place the piglets in so they can be together, which makes them quiet down faster. Another way to quiet a piglet while holding it is to cradle its body against yours. This gives it a sense of security and it will not squeal.

Piglets can be restrained by holding both hind legs (Fig. 21-37) or placing them in a V-trough for such procedures as castration, ear notching, and cutting needle teeth. Piglets weighing more than 30 pounds can be held the same way, but it may take two people to hold them upside down by their hind legs.

Restraining Potbellied Pigs

Potbellied pigs are usually kept as pets and have a docile temperament; however, some potbellied pigs may show aggression. Small pet pigs tend to squirm, jump, and climb on whomever is trying to restrain them. Ear protection is important for the handler because they can squeal as loud as a full-sized pig. Chemical restraint is sometimes the best choice.

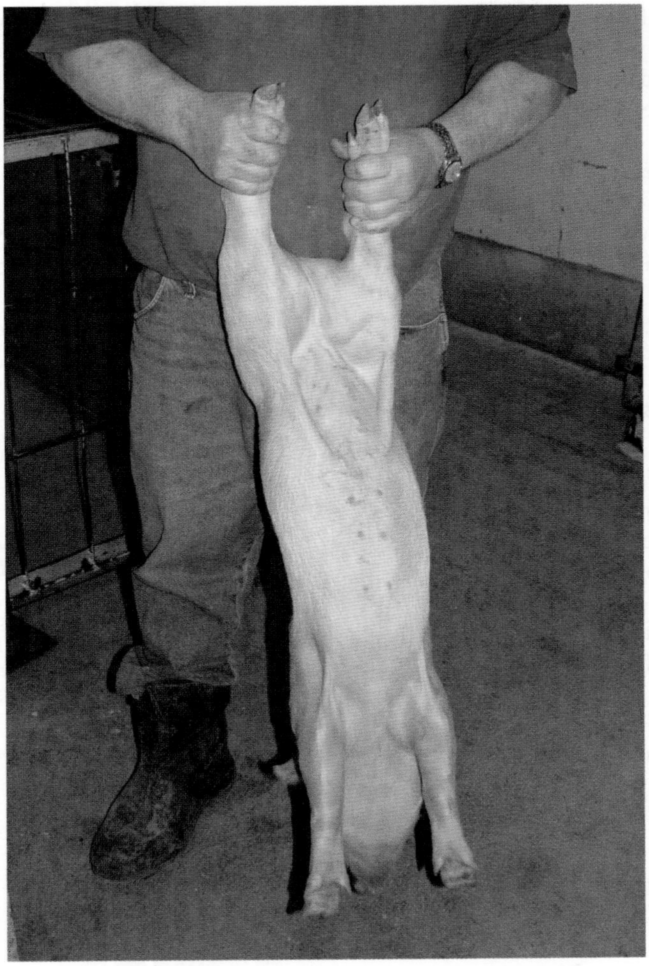

FIGURE 21-37 Holding a pig for transportation.

REVIEW QUESTIONS

Matching—Danger Potential

Match the animal to the body part or action that presents a danger potential. You may use an answer more than once or not at all. Some questions may have more than one correct answer.

_____ **1.** dogs	**A.** hooves
_____ **2.** cats	**B.** toenails
_____ **3.** horses	**C.** tusks
_____ **4.** cattle	**D.** head
_____ **5.** sheep	**E.** flight or running away
_____ **6.** pigs	**G.** teeth and toenails
_____ **7.** rodents	**H.** teeth
_____ **8.** ferrets	**I.** hooves and teeth
_____ **9.** goats	
_____**10.** rabbits	

Matching—Animal Characteristics

For each statement, select the animal being described.

_____**1.** The males can be very unpredictable and a novice should not be handling them.

_____**2.** Always work with the young of this animal in sight of its mother.

_____**3.** Agile and vocal and will resist restraint if harsh.

_____**4.** Bruising and carcass damage can occur if animal is grabbed by wool.

_____**5.** Solid-paneled hurdles can be used to hold and move them.

A. bovine
B. porcine
C. caprine
D. equine
E. ovine

_____ 6. Tail jacking is a useful distraction technique.
_____ 7. Feet are extremely dangerous; either walk up close or out 10-12 feet.
_____ 8. Able to unlock ropes and gate latches.
_____ 9. Never get into a small pen with this mother and her offspring.
_____10. Has an extremely strong flocking instinct.

Matching—Instruments for Restraint

Select the instrument that could be used to help restrain an animal for the specific procedure or circumstance.

_____1. Remove a shy or cowering dog from a cage
_____2. Tail venipuncture on a beef cow
_____3. Agitated, angry cat that is hiding under the refrigerator
_____4. A horse that is throwing its head and needs to be tubed
_____ 5. Gentle dairy cow for a jugular venipuncture
_____ 6. Scruff an angry Cocker Spaniel (in the back room)
_____ 7. Rabbit for an ear vein injection
_____ 8. Moving several pigs from one place to another
_____ 9. Getting a blood sample from the femoral vein on a cat
_____10. Moving a horse from one place to another

A. leash
B. gauntlet
C. capture pole
D. muzzle
E. restraint bag
F. towel
G. twitch
H. hurdles
I. halter
J. chute
K. stanchion

RECOMMENDED READING

Sheldon CC, Sonsthagen T, Topel JA: *Animal restraint for veterinary professionals*, St Louis, 2006, Mosby.
Tully T, Mitchell M: *A technician's guide to exotic animal care*, Lakewood, CO, 2001, AAHA Press.

22 Patient History and Physical Examination

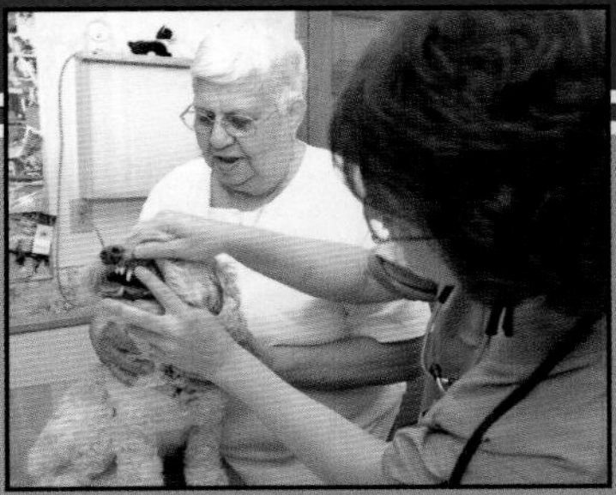

OUTLINE

LEARNING OBJECTIVES

After reviewing this chapter, the reader will be able to:

1. Discuss the importance of clear communication with the client.
2. List and describe the components of the patient's history.
3. Discuss appropriate ways to elicit information from the client.
4. Describe approaches used for performing the physical examination.
5. List and describe the components of a physical examination.
6. Describe methods used to assess patients in emergency situations.

KEY TERMS

Alopecia	Ectropion	Nystagmus	Strabismus
Arrhythmia	Entropion	Posture and gait	Symmetry
Auscultation	Homeostasis	Presenting complaint	Systole
Ballottement	Hyperresonance	Pulse deficit	Tachycardia
Bradycardia	Hyperthermia	Sensory nerves	Thorax
Bronchial sounds	Hypothermia	Signalment	Triage
Capillary refill time	Ileus	Sinus arrhythmia	Vesicular sounds
Cyanosis	Mentation	Spinal nerves	
Dyspnea	Motor nerves	State of nutrition	

A patient's history and physical examination are the foundations on which sound medical and nursing interventions are based. Animal patients cannot verbally communicate the ailments or discomforts caused by disease. Therefore you must pay meticulous attention to the observations and concerns voiced by the client, who provides information from which you may formulate the patient's history. Astute observation from both the veterinarian and the nursing staff is crucial when performing the physical examination.

TECHNICIAN-CLIENT INTERACTION

COMMUNICATING WITH CLIENTS

Communication is the key to successful history taking. The interviewer must be able to ask questions that are easily understood and are geared toward the animal's owner. If necessary, slang words describing certain conditions may be used to facilitate communication and avoid misunderstanding.

The interview is most successfully conducted when the technician is professional but cheerful, friendly, and genuinely concerned about the patient (Fig. 22-1). A dry, inquisitional approach, consisting of rapid-fire questions, is typically less effective in unearthing important details of the history.

The best clinical interview focuses on the patient. When speaking with the client, determine the primary medical problem (presenting or chief complaint) as well as the way the animal is manifesting the illness. An important interviewing technique uses reflective listening methods that incorporate active listening, infrequent interruption,

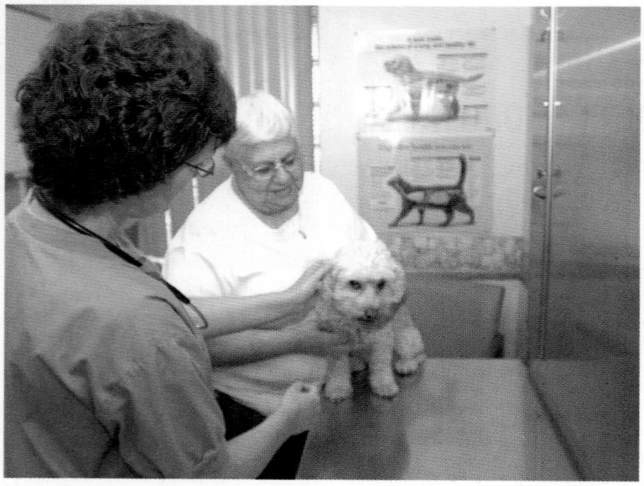

FIGURE 22-1 The interview should be conducted in a professional yet friendly manner, while displaying genuine concern for the patient and client. The appearance, attire, and attitude of the veterinary staff set the tone of the visit and convey an impression of the quality of veterinary services being rendered.

BOX 22-1 Five Vowels of a Good Interview

1. Audition: listening carefully to the client's story
2. Evaluation: sorting data to determine which is important and which is irrelevant
3. Inquiry: probing into the significant areas requiring more clarification
4. Observation: observing nonverbal communication, body language, and facial expressions, regardless of what is said
5. Understanding the client's concerns and apprehensions enables the interviewer to play a more emphatic role.

limited speaking, and asking for clarification when needed (Box 22-1). Interrupting an animal owner may disrupt his or her train of thought and prevent the client from reporting important facts.

Allow the client to control the interview, at least in part. Once the client has reported the facts, repeat important information, indicating that you have heard him or her and understand the concern. If the history given is vague, use direct questioning. Asking "how," "where," and "when" is generally more effective than asking "why."

The technician's appearance influences the success of the interview. Neatness counts. An untidy interviewer wearing a soiled smock will be viewed as unprofessional, careless, or incompetent. Some clients may view a sloppy appearance as a sign of not caring, and as such will taint their expectations and impressions of the entire veterinary team. The physical setting of an interview can enhance or hinder it. A key to successful history taking is to put the client at ease (Box 22-2).

Obtaining a thorough history by a medical interview depends on the technical knowledge and communication skills of the interviewer. The interview should be flexible and spontaneous, not interrogative. The major goal of the interview is to sort through the reported signs associated with the illness to better understand the pathophysiology of the disease in question. Although the novice may have limited knowledge of the signs associated with various diseases, with experience and education, one can learn to recognize the history and signs as they relate to various injuries and illnesses.

BOX 22-2 Ideal Physical Setting of an Interview

- Quiet, properly lighted room or lighting adjusted to produce optimal illumination; may not be possible in field situations.
- Make the client feel as comfortable as possible. You and the client should be seated on an even level, allowing for direct eye contact.
- Maintain a distance of 3 to 4 feet between you and the client. Distances greater than 5 feet are impersonal; distances less than 3 feet intrude on the client's comfort zone.
- Sit in a relaxed position. Avoid crossing your arms across your chest, which projects an attitude of superiority and may interfere with communication.

OBTAINING A HISTORY

The information gathered when obtaining a history should alert the veterinary team to potential problems and direct the technician's attention to some of the patient's body areas during the examination.

Diseases tend to be characterized by a certain group of signs. With only one isolated clinical sign, do not jump to conclusions or allow premature assumptions or preconceptions to affect your objectivity when making additional assessments.

The Introductory Statement

For example, you might say: "Good morning, Mrs. Schwartz. My name is Joe Smith. I'm a veterinary technician and I'll be obtaining a history and performing a preliminary examination on Buffy. Can you please tell me the reason for Buffy's visit today?" You can then validate the preliminary data if needed and go on to obtain the history for the presenting complaint (Box 22-3).

Some technicians prefer to address the presenting complaint first, and then validate or confirm the preliminary data. Regardless of which approach you prefer, develop a consistent routine that is comfortable for you and the client and that obtains the necessary data (Box 22-4).

Patient Characteristics

The receptionist can obtain certain preliminary data and **signalment** (e.g., age, breed, gender, reproductive status, markings). The technician should verify that the patient's age, breed, sex, and reproductive status have been correctly recorded and note any changes since the patient's last visit (e.g., if patient has been spayed or castrated).

BOX 22-3 Introduction to the Client

- Review the preliminary data (e.g., animal's name and sex) before introducing yourself to the client.
- If the patient is a new animal to the household or farm or a geriatric patient not seen recently, or if the owner is a new client, note the medical record.
- Greet the client by name, make eye contact, shake hands firmly, and smile.
- Always address the client by an honorific title (e.g., Mrs., Mr.) and his or her last name.

BOX 22-4 Checklist for Physical Examination

Introduction to the Client

Patient History

- Patient characteristics
- Geographic origin
- Current environment
- Diet
- Previous medical history and vaccination status
- Presenting complaint(s)
- History of chief presenting complaint
- Conclusion

Physical Examination

- General observation
- Recording vital signs
- Level of consciousness
- Respiratory rate and effort
- Heart rate and rhythm
- Indications of perfusion

Systematic Physical Examination (Visual Inspection, Palpation, Percussion, Auscultation)

- Examination of head and neck
- Examination of trunk and forelimbs
- Examination of thorax
- Examination of abdomen
- Examination of skin and lymph nodes
- Examination of hind limbs
- Examination of external genitalia and perineum

Pay close attention to the patient's age. Congenital and infectious diseases, parasitism, ingestion of foreign bodies, and intussusceptions are usually predominant in young animals. Degenerative diseases and neoplasia are more common in adult animals.

Certain species or breeds are predisposed to particular problems. For example, toy breeds of dogs (e.g., Chihuahuas, Pomeranians) are predisposed to patella luxation and hydrocephalus. Brachycephalic (short-nosed) dogs are predisposed to respiratory problems. Combined immunodeficiency affects Arabian horses. These predispositions are considered when the veterinarian formulates a list of differential diagnoses (diagnostic possibilities).

TECHNICIAN NOTE The initial medical history often helps guide the diagnostic plan.

The patient's gender and reproductive status are important, because certain conditions are gender-specific and determine what areas should be given special attention in patient evaluation. For example, in a 10-year-old intact (not spayed) female dog with a history of excessive water consumption and urination, vomiting, and lethargy, pyometra (uterine infection) would be an important differential diagnosis. In a 5-year-old spayed female with the same history, however, diabetes mellitus would be an important differential diagnosis. The incidence of some diseases decreases markedly as a result of ovariohysterectomy (spay) or castration. Dogs spayed at an early age are less likely to develop mammary tumors, and castrated male dogs are at lower risk of developing perianal adenomas.

Origin, Prior Ownership, and Current Environment

Questions concerning geographic origin and prior ownership may indicate exposure to infectious or parasitic diseases. Information on the pet's current environment, including information about the patient's diet, is also needed to help identify risk factors for specific diseases. For example, free-roaming or pastured animals are at higher risk of exposure to toxins or trauma; multiple-cat households and catteries have a higher prevalence of infectious respiratory diseases and feline leukemia virus infection. Box 22-5 lists some common questions used to obtain this information from the client.

Past Medical History

Past medical history provides information about the patient's health before the current illness. Carefully inquire about and record the dates of previous illnesses and treatment, hospitalization, and surgeries, followed by a brief description of each problem, how it was managed, and how the patient responded to treatment. Ask the client to describe any allergies (environmental, ingestible, or drug-related) and how these were diagnosed. Note any medications the patient is currently receiving. It is important to determine if the client is giving medications as prescribed.

Vaccination Status

Question the client about the patient's vaccination status and when any vaccinations were given. Some clients are not familiar with vaccination schedules and may simply report that their animal "has been vaccinated." It is easy to presume that the patient is up-to-date on vaccinations, when in fact the vaccinations may have been given several years ago. Be aware of recommended intervals for vaccinations and diagnostic tests. For example, inquire when a cat was last assessed for exposure to feline leukemia virus and feline immunodeficiency virus. Ask if a dog has been checked for heartworm infection in the past year, and if and what type of preventive is being used.

BOX 22-5 Commonly Used Questions for Obtaining Patient Environmental Information

Geographic Origin and Prior Ownership

1. Where the patient originated (e.g., home, breeder, pet shop, animal shelter, neighboring farm, livestock auction)
2. Where it has recently traveled
3. If it was recently boarded or shown

Environment and Activities

1. Is it an indoor or outdoor animal?
2. Is the pet free-roaming or confined to a yard or house?
3. Is the animal housed in a pasture or stable?
4. Does the patient share the environment with other animals?

Dietary Questions

1. Can you describe the pet's appetite?
2. Has there been any noticeable weight loss or gain?
3. What type of diet is fed? (e.g., dry, moist, or table food)
4. Does the pet receive any dietary supplements?
5. What is the brand name of food that is fed?
6. How often is the pet fed? (free choice or individual meals)
7. How much food is consumed daily?

BOX 22-6 History of Presenting Complaint

The History of the Current Complaint Helps Determine

- When the animal was last normal
- If the condition is acute or chronic
- What medications and dosages were used previously
- How the patient responded to previous therapy
- Duration and progression of clinical signs

The Presenting Complaint

The **presenting complaint** is the reason the client has sought veterinary care for the animal. For example, the client may say a cow has had diarrhea for three days, is not eating, and is depressed. It is important to remember that the presenting complaint is what the client perceives the patient's problem to be. Although the client's fears or anxieties may influence your observations of the animal, pay attention to these concerns. Allow the client to communicate these observations, and then continue with the interview. This tends to relieve a client's anxieties about the animal.

Another important interviewing skill is the ability to assess the source and reliability of the information obtained. A history obtained from second parties presenting the animal for evaluation (friends, neighbors, children) may lack important information that only the client can provide.

It is also important to determine if the client understands the meaning of the medical terms he or she uses to describe the problem. Ask the client to define such terms. For example, "What do you mean when you say the cat regurgitated?" A client may bring in a dog and say that it "just had a stroke." To an experienced veterinary professional, the patient's ataxia, incoordination, head tilt, and horizontal nystagmus may indicate vestibular disease rather than a cerebrovascular accident (stroke). It is important to record the clinical signs observed and not the client's presumptive diagnosis. Be aware that the client's comments, observations, and conclusions are based on his or her experience. We must interpret their comments, observations, and conclusions in light of our professional experience.

Once the presenting complaint is listed, record the information gathered in chronologic order to clarify areas of possible confusion. Separate the client's **observations** from his or her conclusions, and amplify certain portions of the complaint that may be important.

History of Presenting Complaint. The history is best recorded by chronology (i.e., in the order in which events occurred). This provides a better understanding of the sequence and development of the problem (Box 22-6). Begin with the first sign of illness observed by the client, and follow its progression to the present time.

It is important to determine when the client first noticed the presenting complaint, apart from any other health problems. Some patients might have other ongoing health problems (e.g., flea-bite dermatitis, food allergies) unrelated to the current complaint. Ask for specific information that describes the signs observed (e.g., color, odor, consistency, and volume of vomitus or diarrhea). When the client uses such terms as somewhat, a little, sometimes, or rarely, ask for clarification. Remember, precise communication is important.

Some clients simply cannot remember when the signs first developed. You may be able to help the client relate the onset of signs to some event. For example, ask, "Was the horse's lameness evident around the Thanksgiving or Christmas holidays?" When obtaining information on the presenting complaint, use open-ended questions that allow the client to describe the problem, rather than simple yes or no questions. Table 22-1 illustrates a series of open-ended questions that elucidate the sequences of events and the nature of the problem.

Concluding the History

If any part of the history needs further clarification, it should be done after all of the initial information has been gathered. At this point, you may wish to summarize for the client the most important parts of the history. Encourage the client to correct any misinterpretations, and discuss any additional concerns. Allow the client the final say. At the conclusion of the interview, thank the client and say that you will now perform a physical examination of the patient.

TABLE 22-1 Examples of Open-Ended Questions

QUESTIONS	PURPOSE
Why is Buffy being presented?	Identifies the presenting complaint.
When did you first notice the problem?	Determines the onset of the problem.
What was the first sign that you observed? What did you notice after that initial sign?	Helps establish progression of the problem.
Can you describe in detail the signs you observed?	Helps identify clinical signs observed, rather than the client's diagnosis.
Was there any change in routine or anything new, unusual, or different in Buffy's routine at the time of onset?	Helps determine precipitating events.
Has Buffy been treated for this problem before? How did she respond?	Determines the response to previous treatment.

REPORT OF PHYSICAL EXAMINATION

ABC Animal Clinic
South Beach Street
Sunshine FL

Patient Name Gandalf Abbott
Description brown
Microchip ID 183469
Date 12/12/15
Gender M **Breed** Boxer **Age** 3yrs

(1) General	(2) Integument	(3) M/S	(4) Circulatory	(5) Respiratory	(6) Digestive
☑ WNL ☐ Abn ☐ NE	☐ WNL ☑ Abn ☐ NE	☑ WNL ☐ Abn ☐ NE	☑ WNL ☐ Abn ☐ NE	☑ WNL ☐ Abn ☐ NE	☑ WNL ☐ Abn ☐ NE
(7) Genitourinary	**(8) Eyes**	**(9) Ears**	**(10) NS**	**(11) Lymphatic**	**(12) Mucosa**
☑ WNL ☐ Abn ☐ NE	☑ WNL ☐ Abn ☐ NE	☑ WNL ☐ Abn ☐ NE	☑ WNL ☐ Abn ☐ NE	☑ WNL ☐ Abn ☐ NE	☑ WNL ☐ Abn ☐ NE
Temp (F) 102	**Pulse** 140	**Resp** 18	**Weight** 41kg	WNL = no abnormalities; Abn = abnormalities noted; NE = not examined	

Temperament / Behavioral Assessment
Playful; curious; doesn't walk well on leash

Describe Examination Findings Below:

1. BAR; very playful
2. No evidence of alopecia, rashes, lesions; skin turgor reveals adequate hydration; sl flea dirt at base of tail
3. No evidence of joint swelling; full range of motion on manipulation of limbs; no evidence of pain, limping, guarding, or tenderness; overall muscular symmetrical/well fleshed
4. No evidence of arrhythmia on cardiac auscultation; No pulse deficit detected; CRT < 2 secs.
5. No evidence of crackles or wheezes on auscultation; no postural signs of dyspnea; no evidence of nasal discharge
6. No evidence of diarrhea on or around rectum' no evidence of vomitus in/around oral cavity' sl tenderness on palpation – caudal 1/3 of abdomen
7. Kidneys palpate firm; bladder palpates full; no evidence of penile discharge; testicles present in scrotal sacs
8. Characteristic pupillary light response; no evidence of ocular abrasions or discharge
9. Characteristic odor; moderate cerumen; no evidence of parasites or tenderness
10. No evidence of head tilt or tremors; characteristic gait
11. Lymph nodes not palpable
12. Mucosa – pink; no evidence of periodontal disease

FIGURE 22-2 Completed physical examination form.

PHYSICAL EXAMINATION

The physical examination assesses the animal's current state of health. It is crucial that all observations be recorded accurately using standardized terminology. Figure 22-2 shows an example of a properly recorded comprehensive physical examination. The four primary techniques used during physical examination are inspection, palpation, percussion, and auscultation.

TECHNICIAN NOTE Accurate and detailed recording of observations and results of palpation and auscultation is vital to proper performance of the physical examination.

PRIMARY TECHNIQUES FOR PHYSICAL EXAMINATION

Inspection

Inspection begins with the technician's first contact with the patient and continues throughout the data collection. Early in the physical examination, the technician visually examines the patient's entire body for structure and function, paying close attention to deviations or abnormalities. Inspection is an active process, not a passive one. The technician must know what to look for and where. It should be done in a systematic manner so that nothing is missed.

Palpation

Palpation involves using the hands and the sense of touch to detect tenderness, altered temperature, texture, vibration, pulsation, masses or swellings, and other changes in body integrity (Fig. 22-3). The sense of touch is most acute using light, intermittent pressure; heavy, prolonged pressure causes loss of sensitivity in the hands of the examiner.

The fingertips are highly sensitive to tactile discrimination. The pads of the fingertips are used to assess skin turgor, texture (e.g., hair), position, size, consistency, mobility (e.g., mass or organ), distention (e.g., urinary bladder), pulse rate and quality, tenderness, and pain (Table 22-2). Temperature of a skin area is best assessed using the dorsum (back) of a hand or finger. The palm of the hand is more sensitive to vibrations, allowing one to feel such abnormalities as crepitus (grinding) in a joint.

TECHNICIAN NOTE Use the tips of your fingers when assessing the condition of the skin and hair and palpating internal organs.

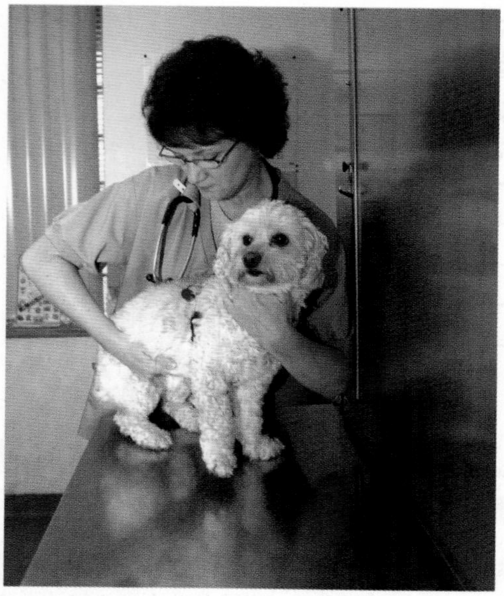

FIGURE 22-3 Because of patient size and personal safety, abdominal palpation is used more commonly in small animals than in large animals. In cats and small dogs, one hand can be used to restrain the animal while the other is used for palpation.

Palpation can be classified as light or deep. Light palpation of structures such as the abdomen is performed primarily to detect areas of tenderness. Deep palpation is used to assess underlying organs (e.g., liver), while giving careful consideration to the discomfort the procedure may cause the patient.

Percussion

Percussion is tapping of the body's surface to produce vibration and sound. The sound reflects the density of underlying tissue and size and position of organs (Table 22-3). Percussion is most commonly used on the thorax for examining the heart and lungs. It helps determine if a tissue is fluid-filled, air-filled, or solid.

The area referred to as the **thorax** is located between the neck and the diaphragm. Normally there is negative pressure (partial vacuum) in the thorax. Combined with the elasticity and pliable nature of the lungs, this causes the lungs to conform to the size and shape of the thoracic cavity. A small amount of pleural fluid lubricates the lung surfaces and the thoracic (pleural) lining.

Thoracic percussion in the standing patient can be used to detect a fluid line, as found in hydrothorax. Percussion ventral to the fluid line produces a dull thud, whereas percussion dorsal to the fluid line produces a resonant or **hyperresonant** sound.

Abdominal percussion can detect large volumes of air or fluid in the peritoneal cavity. Rhythmic palpation of a fluid-filled abdomen elicits a fluid wave that is transmitted to the opposite side.

TABLE 22-2 Terms Used to Describe Structures Palpated

TERM	MEANING
Doughy	Soft, malleable
Firm	Normal texture of organs
Hard	Bonelike consistency
Fluctuant	Soft, elastic, undulant, as with a cyst or abscess
Emphysematous	Air or gas in tissue planes

TABLE 22-3 Types of Sound Elicited by Percussion

TERM	SOUND	SOUND PRODUCED BY:
Flatness	Extremely dull	Very dense tissue, i.e., muscle or bone
Dullness	Thudlike	Encapsulated tissue, i.e., liver or spleen
Resonance	Hollow	Air-filled lungs
Hyperresonance	"Booming"	Gas-filled area, i.e., an emphysematous lung (always abnormal)
Tympany	Musical or drumlike	Air-filled organ, i.e., such as with gastric dilatation-volvulus

Auscultation

Listening to sounds produced by the body is termed **auscultation.** Auscultation may be direct (with the ear and no instrument) or indirect (using a stethoscope to amplify sounds). The stethoscope allows auscultation of specific areas within a body cavity for assessment of the cardiovascular, respiratory, and gastrointestinal systems (Fig. 22-4).

Abnormal sounds can be recognized only after one has learned to identify the types of sounds normally arising from each body structure and the location in which they are most commonly heard. Proficiency at auscultation requires good hearing, a good-quality stethoscope, and knowledge of how to use a stethoscope correctly. The technician should become familiar with this instrument before attempting to use it with the patient.

The stethoscope's chestpiece should have a stiff, flat diaphragm and a bell (Fig. 22-5). The diaphragm is the flat, circular portion of the chestpiece covered by a thin, resilient membrane. It transmits high-pitched sounds, such as those produced by the bowel, lungs, and heart. The bell is not covered by a membrane. It facilitates auscultation of lower-frequency sounds, such as third and fourth sounds of the heart, or what is most commonly termed a gallop rhythm. Some types of stethoscopes incorporate both the diaphragm and bell into a single head.

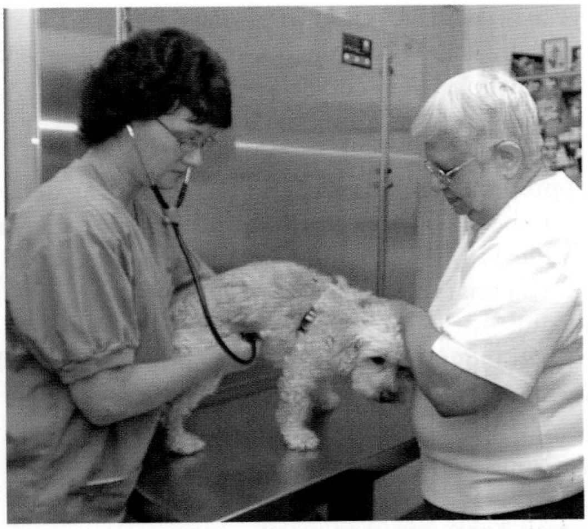

FIGURE 22-4 Thoracic auscultation should be performed systematically, evaluating the lungs first and then the heart. The abdomen can also be auscultated to evaluate gastrointestinal sounds.

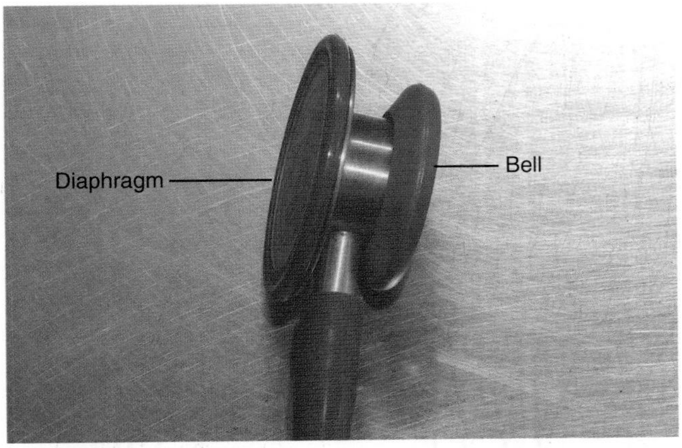

FIGURE 22-5 The diaphragm of the stethoscope is used to detect high-pitched sounds, such as heart, bowel, and lung sounds. The bell is used to detect lower-frequency sounds, such as the third and fourth heart sounds.

Heart. The heart is a muscular two-way pump that propels blood around the body and receives it back. It consists of dense accumulations of cardiac muscle cells and connective tissue organized into two side-by-side pumps that together are composed of four chambers (two atria and two ventricles) and four one-way valves.

- Right atrium: The right atrium lies just above the right ventricle and receives CO_2-rich blood from cranial and caudal venae cavae.
- Left atrium: The left atrium lies just above the left ventricle and receives oxygenated blood from pulmonary veins. It is separated from the right atrium by an interatrial septum.
- Right ventricle: The right ventricle receives blood from the right atrium through the right atrioventricular opening (A-V opening), which is guarded by a tricuspid valve. The pulmonary artery originates from the right ventricle, and its opening is guarded by pulmonary semilunar valves.
- Left ventricle: The left ventricle receives blood from the left atrium through the left atrioventricular opening, which is guarded by a bicuspid valve or mitral valve. The aorta originates from the left ventricle, and its opening is guarded by aortic semilunar valves.

Cardiac Cycle. The cardiac cycle is the series of events happening during one heartbeat. It includes relaxation of heart chambers (diastole) to receive the blood and contraction of heart chambers (**systole**) to pump the blood into body tissues and lungs.

The receiving chamber of the right side of the heart is the right atrium. Blood flows into it from the vena cavae, the large systemic veins. When the right atrium contracts, it pumps blood through a large one-way valve, the tricuspid valve, into the right ventricle. The tricuspid valve gets its name from its three flaps, or cusps. When the right ventricle contracts, the tricuspid valve closes and blood flows out through the one-way pulmonary valve into the pulmonary artery, which carries blood to the lungs. When the right ventricular contraction is complete, the pulmonary valve closes, preventing blood from flowing back into the right ventricle.

The dynamics are similar on the left side of the heart. Blood flows into the left atrium from the pulmonary veins. When the left atrium contracts, it pumps blood through the mitral valve into the left ventricle. The mitral valve is named for the resemblance (in an ancient anatomist's eye) of its two cusps to the miter worn by high-ranking Catholic clergy. When the left ventricle contracts, the mitral valve closes and blood flows out through the aortic valve into the aorta, the beginning of systemic circulation. When left ventricular contraction is complete, the aortic valve closes to prevent flow of blood back into the ventricle (Fig. 22-6).

Specialized areas and bundles of cardiac muscle cells initiate each heartbeat, but the rate of heartbeat is controlled by the autonomic nervous system. By its nature, cardiac muscle contracts without needing external stimuli, but the activity of the many millions of individual cardiac muscle cells must be coordinated for the heart to contract in an organized, efficient manner.

On auscultation, the first heart sound represents the closure of the tricuspid and mitral valves. The second heart sound represents the closure of the pulmonary and aortic valves. Most heart sounds are best heard by placing the stethoscope on the left side of the animal near the apex of the heart, which is approximately at the level of the elbow. The tricuspid valve sound is best heard on the left side of the animal (Fig. 22-7).

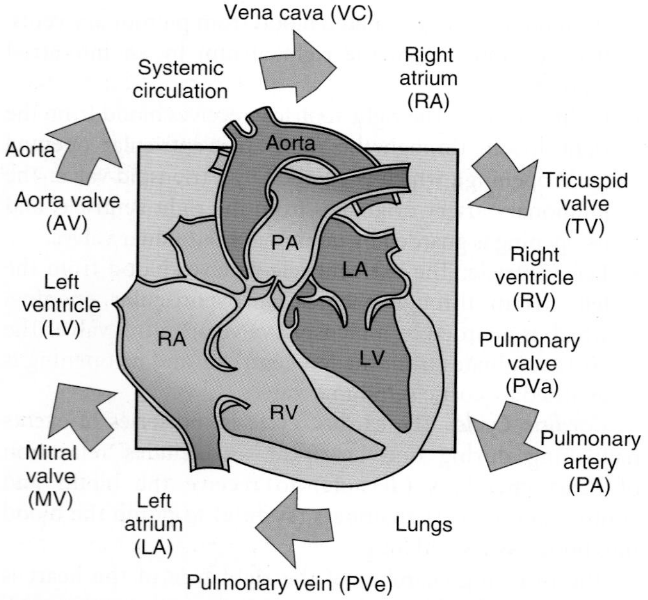

FIGURE 22-6 Schematic depiction of blood flow. (From Colville TP, Bassert JM: *Clinical anatomy and physiology for veterinary technicians,* ed 2, St Louis, 2008, Mosby.)

TECHNICIAN NOTE Evaluation of mentation, general appearance, state of nutrition, symmetry, and posture and gait are part of the general survey performed during physical examination.

GENERAL SURVEY

The physical examination begins from the moment the client and the patient enter the examination area. While obtaining the history, the technician should generally observe the patient to note certain characteristics. These are **mentation,** general appearance, **state of nutrition, symmetry,** and **posture and gait.**

Mentation and Level of Consciousness

The patient's attentiveness or reaction to its environment provides a basis to evaluate the degree of consciousness, depression, excitement, or overreaction to stimuli. The patient's ability to walk or avoid objects can be used to assess vision and balance. A declining level of consciousness suggests progressive brain damage and a worsening prognosis (Box 22-7). A patient might be conscious yet have abnormal mentation (mental function). Mentation changes can include:

- Slow but appropriate responses to stimuli (suggesting severe depression)
- Inappropriate responses to stimuli (suggesting dementia)
- Bizarre behavior may also be seen (e.g., biting at imaginary flies)
- Slow responses and unaware of stimuli (suggesting mentally dull)

Any pathologic change can lead to brain edema or hemorrhage and result in increased intracranial pressure (Box 22-8). When this occurs, the brain is compressed and it malfunctions.

General Appearance

Assess the patient's facial expression, size and position of the eyeballs, general body condition (flesh and haircoat), response to commands, and temperament.

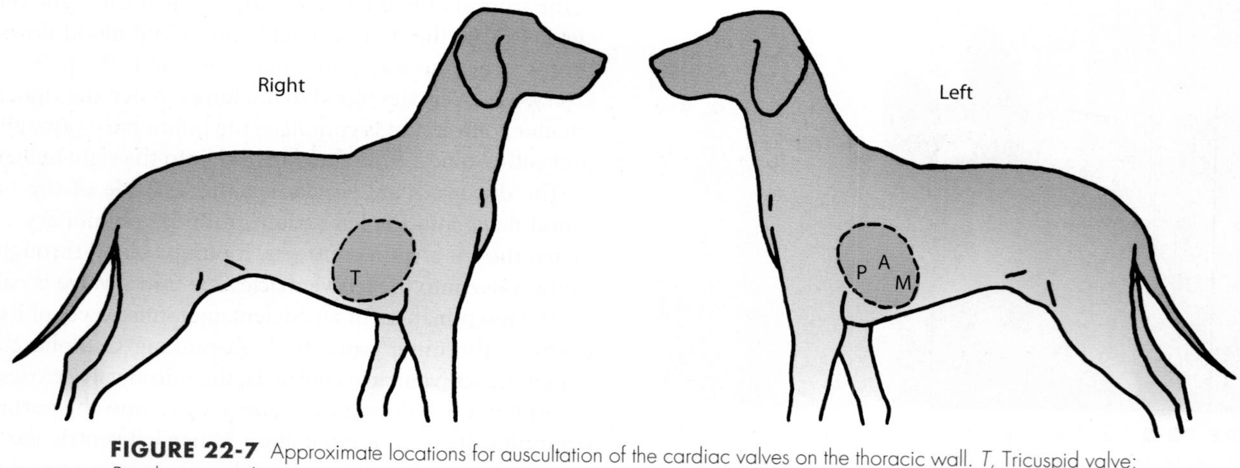

FIGURE 22-7 Approximate locations for auscultation of the cardiac valves on the thoracic wall. *T,* Tricuspid valve; *P,* pulmonary valve; *A,* aortic valve; *M,* mitral valve. (From Figure 14-18 in Colville T, Bassert J: *Clinical anatomy and physiology for veterinary technicians,* ed 3, St Louis, 2016, Mosby.)

State of Nutrition

Note if the patient appears in normal body condition, is thin and frail, or is obese. Most patients with chronic disease appear cachexic (wasted). Sunken eyes, temporal muscle atrophy, and excessively loose skin turgor are signs of poor nutrition in chronically ill patients. Long-standing disease, such as renal failure, hyperthyroidism, and cancer, can result in marked wasting. A body condition score should be assigned using a scale such as those found in Chapter 23.

BOX 22-7 Levels of Consciousness in Order of Declining Consciousness

1. Alert and responsive
2. Depressed: patient is conscious but slow to respond to stimuli
3. Uncontrolled hyperexcitability
4. Stupor: semiconscious patient that can respond to noxious (painful) stimuli
5. Coma: unconscious patient that does not respond to any stimuli. Coma warrants the worst prognosis.

BOX 22-8 Possible Causes of Changes in Level of Consciousness or Mentation

Changes in Level of Consciousness or Mentation Can Be Caused by

- Metabolic problems (e.g., liver failure, portacaval shunts, hyperglycemia, hypoglycemia, hypernatremia, hyponatremia)
- Hypoxia
- Hypotension
- Iatrogenic rapid elevation in serum osmolality (e.g., mannitol overdose, total parenteral nutrition)
- Trauma
- Toxicity (e.g., ethylene glycol)
- Brain damage (e.g., tumors, infection, inflammation)
- Drugs (e.g., sedatives, anesthetics)

Symmetry

The body is normally symmetric; note any asymmetry. Observe closely for complementary (balanced) or noncomplementary conformation of the thorax and abdomen. Note any difference in size or shape of the extremities.

Posture and Gait

Walking requires coordination and integrity of the nervous and musculoskeletal systems. Note if the patient can walk and describe any abnormalities in the gait. Proprioception (sense of body part position), soundness (lack of lameness), and coordination can be quickly assessed.

VITAL SIGNS

Vital signs include the respiratory rate and effort, heart rate and rhythm, and indications of perfusion. These reflect overall patient status; changes in any vital sign can warn the medical team of impending complications. Vital signs are monitored at regular intervals. The initial findings are used as the baseline, and subsequent findings help establish trends indicating improvement or deterioration. To identify abnormalities, technicians must know the normal ranges for each species, age group, and sometimes breed (Table 22-4).

TECHNICIAN NOTE Respiratory rate, effort heart rate and rhythm, and evaluation of perfusion are assessed and recorded at regular intervals.

Vital signs should be evaluated in relation to the presenting complaint, history, and current health status. Technicians must know the normal ranges for each vital sign and understand which variations might be considered "normal" with regard to a particular patient's status. Remember that vital signs reflect function of various body systems. For example, when assessing the level of consciousness, pupillary light response, and eye position, to some degree we are assessing the nervous system. All body systems (e.g., neurologic, cardiovascular, and respiratory) contribute to overall function of the individual; failure of one system can lead to compromise of others.

TABLE 22-4 Normal Ranges of Heart Rate, Respiratory Rate, and Rectal Temperature in Adults of Some Domestic Species

	HEART RATE (BEATS/MIN)	RESPIRATORY RATE (BREATHS/MIN)	RECTAL TEMPERATURE
Dogs	70-160	8-20	37.5°-39° C
Cats	150-210	8-30	38°-39° C
Hamsters	250-500	35-135	37°-38° C
Guinea pigs	230-280	42-104	37.2°-39.5° C
Rabbits	130-325	30-60	38.5°-40° C
Horses	28-50	8-16	37.5°-38.5° C
Cattle	40-80	12-36	38°-39° C
Sheep	60-120	12-72	39°-40° C
Pigs	58-100	8-18	38°-40°C

For example, in patients with heart disease, a drop in blood pressure can compromise kidney function.

The Senses

The senses are the means by which the body monitors its internal and external environment. Sensory receptors are specialized nerve endings that convert mechanical, thermal, electromagnetic, and chemical stimuli from the environment into nervous impulses. When sensory impulses reach the central nervous system, they are perceived as such sensations as smell, taste, or sight.

Various sensations are received and interpreted by the central nervous system. The five senses we usually think of (hearing, smell, taste, touch, and sight) are not the only sensations perceived by the central nervous system.

The general senses (tactile, temperature, kinesthetic, pain) are so named because they are distributed generally throughout the body or over the entire skin surface. Their receptors are fairly simple modified nerve endings. The tactile sense, or the sense of touch, perceives mechanical contact with the surface of the body. The temperature sense is a thermal sense that perceives hot and cold. The position of the limbs is monitored by the kinesthetic sense, a mechanical sense that provides information on the position of joints and the relative force exerted by muscles and tendons. The sense of pain can be set off by overloads of mechanical, thermal, or chemical stimuli.

The special senses (gustatory, olfactory, auditory, vestibular, visual) are so named because their sensory receptors are concentrated in certain areas, rather than being generally distributed. All receptors for special senses are located in the head. Also, in several cases, the sensory receptor cells are aided by sophisticated accessory structures.

The gustatory sense, the sense of taste, is a chemical sense. It detects chemical substances in the mouth and dissolved in saliva. The olfactory sense, the sense of smell, is also a chemical sense. It detects chemical substances in inhaled air. The auditory sense is the sense of hearing. Through a complex set of auditory passageways and ear structures, mechanical vibrations of air molecules are converted into impulses that the brain decodes as sounds. The vestibular sense, also a mechanical sense, monitors balance and head position. The visual sense (sight) is the only well-developed electromagnetic sense of mammals. Its receptor organ, the eye, has a complex organization of component parts that function together to gather and focus light rays on photoreceptor cells.

Changes in behavior, the response to stimuli, or posture may be significant. Unconscious patients can be tested by toe pinching to detect their response to this painful stimulus. Any decline in the level of consciousness suggests worsening pathologic changes and warrants immediate neurologic examination and medical or surgical intervention.

Neurologic Evaluation

The nervous system is a complex communication system in the animal body. It detects and processes internal and external information and formulates appropriate responses to changes, threats, and opportunities that the animal continually faces. Nearly all conscious and unconscious functions of the body are controlled or influenced by the nervous system.

The basic structural and functional unit of the nervous system is the nerve cell, the neuron. Neurons are specialized cells that respond to stimuli and conduct impulses from one part of a cell to another. Two types of fiberlike processes extend from the cell bodies of neurons: dendrites and axons. Dendrites are often multiple, and they conduct impulses received from other neurons toward the nerve cell body. Axons are usually single, and they conduct impulses away from the cell body, to other neurons or the effector organs, such as muscle cells. The junction of an axon with another nerve cell is called a synapse.

The branched end of an axon is called the telodendron. When a nerve impulse reaches the telodendron, it causes release of tiny sacs of chemicals called neurotransmitters into the narrow synaptic space. When neurotransmitter molecules diffuse across the synapse to contact the cell membrane of the adjacent nerve cell, they induce a change in the other nerve cell. Enzymes in the synaptic space then quickly inactivate the neurotransmitter molecules.

Neurons have three unique physical characteristics: they do not reproduce, their processes are capable of limited regeneration if damaged, and they have an extremely high oxygen requirement. Their lack of reproductive ability means that any loss of neurons, as from disease or injury, is permanent. Their dendritic and axonic processes sometimes regenerate if the nerve cell body is intact; this may restore function of reattached digits or limbs under some circumstances.

The high oxygen requirement of neurons makes them among the most delicate cells in the body. They begin to suffer permanent damage if deprived of blood supply for more than a few minutes. This is why cardiopulmonary resuscitation must begin within just a few minutes after cardiac arrest if there is to be any chance of complete recovery. The main divisions of the nervous system are the central nervous system, the peripheral nervous system, and the autonomic nervous system.

The central nervous system consists of accumulations of nerve cell bodies, nerve fibers (axons), and supporting cells in the brain and spinal cord. The brain, consisting of the cerebrum, cerebellum, and brain stem, is housed in the skull. The spinal cord is housed in the vertebral canal formed by the vertebrae. Together they form the main control systems for the rest of the body.

The cerebrum is the largest, most rostral part of the brain. The functions of the cerebrum are very complex and poorly understood. It is the center of higher learning and intelligence, and it functions in perception, maintenance of consciousness, thinking and reasoning, and initiating responses to sensory stimuli.

The cerebellum is located just caudal to the cerebrum. The cerebellum does not initiate movements but serves to coordinate, adjust, and generally fine-tune movements directed by the cerebrum.

The brain stem is the most primitive part of the brain. It forms the stem to which the cerebrum, cerebellum, and spinal cord are attached. Functionally, the brain stem maintains the vital functions of the body. Centers in the brain stem control respiration, body temperature, heart rate, gastrointestinal tract function, blood pressure, appetite, thirst, and sleep/wake cycles. Severe damage to vital centers in the brain stem usually results in immediate death.

The spinal cord is the caudal continuation of the brain stem. Spinal nerves exit and enter the spinal cord between each set of adjacent vertebrae. They carry information to and from the peripheral portion of the nervous system.

The peripheral nervous system consists of cordlike nerves that run throughout the body. The nerves are actually bundles of axons that carry impulses between the central nervous system and the rest of the body. Nerves that carry only information toward the central nervous system are called **sensory nerves.** Those that carry only instructions from the central nervous system out to the body are called **motor nerves.** Most nerves are mixed nerves, a combination of both sensory and motor nerves. The peripheral nervous system includes cranial nerves and **spinal nerves.**

The autonomic nervous system is the self-governing portion of the nervous system. It operates independent of conscious thought to maintain **homeostasis,** a constant internal environment in the body. Primarily a motor system, the autonomic nervous system consists of two parts, the sympathetic system and the parasympathetic system, which have opposite effects and are in constant balance with each other.

The sympathetic system produces the "fight or flight" reaction in response to real or perceived threats. In a time of crisis or physical threat, the heart rate and blood pressure increase, the air passageways in the lungs and the pupils of the eyes dilate, digestive tract activity decreases, and the hairs stand on end, producing raised hackles. The net effect is to prepare the body for intense physical exertion and to make the animal look larger and more threatening.

The parasympathetic system has the opposite effect. It is the "rest and restore" system. It predominates during relaxed, routine, business-as-usual states. The heart rate and blood pressure decrease, the air passageways in the lung and the pupils of the eyes constrict, and digestive tract activity increases. The net effect is to allow the body to relax and rejuvenate itself.

Neurologic evaluation can localize and determine the progression of the injury. Pupillary size and response to light are noted (Table 22-5). Normal, responsive pupils or equally constricted (miotic) pupils are associated with damage to the cerebral cortex or subcortical structures. Dilated or midrange fixed pupils are most commonly related to midbrain injury and are a grave sign. Eye position is noted, with ventral or lateral **strabismus** (crossed eyes) indicating a midbrain lesion. **Nystagmus** (repeated sweeping movement) is caused by a vestibular problem, either in the inner ear or within the brain stem. In an unconscious patient, changes in posture, with the forelimbs and neck in extensor rigidity (decerebrate rigidity), are a grave neurologic sign, indicating a midbrain lesion.

TABLE 22-5 Terminology to Describe Ocular Abnormalities

TERM	DESCRIPTION
Enophthalmos	Recession of the eyeball within the orbit
Miosis	Pupil constriction
Mydriasis	Excessive dilation of the pupil
Nystagmus	Rapid, rhythmic involuntary eye movement
Ptosis	Abnormally low position (drooping) of the upper eyelid
Strabismus	One eye is misaligned with the other when focusing

Respiratory Rate and Effort

Respiratory changes imply serious central nervous system damage. A rhythmic waxing and waning of respiration (Cheyne-Stokes respiration) is caused by severe, diffuse cortical injury. Apneustic breathing (holding the breath) and uncontrolled hyperventilation indicate a brain stem lesion.

The lungs, airways, larynx, pharynx, and nasal passages make up the respiratory tract. The rate, pattern, and effort of breathing are controlled by the brain and respiratory muscles (intercostal muscles and diaphragm). The diaphragm is a dome-shaped sheetlike muscle that completely separates the thoracic cavity from the abdominal cavity. The contraction of the diaphragm pushes the abdominal organs down and increases the volume of the thoracic cavity. The lungs expand passively as the thoracic cavity enlarges, and air is drawn into them through the upper respiratory passages.

Two systems control the process of respiration: a mechanical control system and a chemical control system. The mechanical control system sets normal limits on inspiration and expiration to allow rhythmic, resting respiration. The inspiratory center in the brain initiates impulses at regular intervals. These impulses travel to the diaphragm, allowing it to contract and the lungs to inflate. Stretch receptors in the lungs sense when the preset limit of inflation has been reached. They initiate impulses that travel to the respiratory centers in the brain, stopping inspiration and starting passive expiration. The chemical control system monitors the chemical composition of the blood. If it senses fluctuations in O_2 and CO_2 levels or pH, it initiates adjustments in respiration necessary to restore normal values.

Respiratory rate and effort can be affected by disease of the respiratory tract, respiratory center of the brain, or respiratory muscles. Thoracic trauma (e.g., diaphragm rupture, pressure on the diaphragm, rib fractures, intercostal muscle damage) can hinder respiration from pain and also by disrupting the mechanics of breathing. Metabolic changes leading to acid-base imbalances and pain can cause abnormal breathing. Auscultation can help distinguish pleural disease from lung disease. Moist lung sounds suggest fluid in lung tissues. Dry, coarse sounds on inspiration and expiration suggest fibrosis of the lung. Absence of lung sounds indicates interruption of sound transmission by air or fluid in the pleural space.

The first subtle sign of respiratory distress is increased respiratory rate (Table 22-6). In general, respiratory rates below 8 or above 30 per minute are considered abnormal. This is followed by a change in respiratory pattern, which is determined by the site of the injury or disease. Difficult or labored breathing is called **dyspnea.** As distress progresses, the patient assumes various postures in attempts to bring relief, followed by open-mouth and labored breathing. With increasing respiratory distress, the patient assumes a posture that aids the respiratory effort. Cats often crouch, with the sternum elevated. Dogs extend their necks, abduct their elbows, and arch their backs. **Cyanosis** (bluish mucosae) is a late sign of respiratory distress and is often followed quickly by death. Respiratory patterns can suggest the anatomic site of disease and guide lifesaving intervention (Table 22-7).

Heart Rate

An increase in heart rate (**tachycardia**) and contractility increases the force and volume of blood flow to tissues. Tachycardia can be normal or may be associated with shock, stress, excitement, fever, or hyperthyroidism. However, when the heart rate increases above a critical level, the heart muscle becomes exhausted and coronary perfusion decreases, causing myocardial hypoxia. Cardiac arrhythmias and myocardial failure can result, leading to systemic hypoxia and organ failure.

A decreased heart rate (**bradycardia**) can decrease cardiac output. Causes of bradycardia include hypothermia, metabolic disorders (e.g., hyperkalemia, hypoglycemia, hypothyroidism), and parasympathetic (vagal) stimulation. Parasympathetic stimulation can occur with brain, pulmonary, and gastrointestinal diseases, or a diseased sinoatrial node. Heart rates below a critical level can lead to tissue hypoxia, organ failure, and death.

TABLE 22-6 Possible Causes of Respiratory Rate Abnormalities

RESPIRATORY RATE	POTENTIAL CAUSES
Decreased rates	Trauma to the brain or spinal cord Diseases affecting respiratory drive (e.g., chronic obstructive pulmonary disease, low blood carbon dioxide level) Drugs (e.g., sedatives)
Increased rates	Fever Pain Anxiety Trauma to the brain or chest Metabolic alterations (e.g., alkalosis) Pulmonary disease (e.g., pneumonia or edema of the lungs) Drugs (e.g., oxymorphone)

TABLE 22-7 Relationship of Respiratory Pattern and Anatomic Site of Disease

RESPIRATORY PATTERN	ANATOMIC SITE OF DISEASE
Stridor (loud breathing heard without stethoscope)	Upper airway (nasal passages, larynx/pharynx, trachea)
Inspiratory stridor	Extrathoracic airways, especially the larynx
Expiratory stridor	Intrathoracic tracheal changes
Rapid, shallow breathing	Infringement of the pleural space (e.g., by air or fluid)
Labored breathing on both inspiration and expiration	Lung parenchymal
Distress on expiration, with a short inspiration	Small airways

Heart Rhythm

An **arrhythmia** is an irregular heartbeat. Arrhythmias can be detected by auscultating the heart or by electrocardiography. An abnormal conduction system or diseased heart muscle causes an arrhythmia. When ventricular contraction does not forcefully propel blood to the periphery, a **pulse deficit** is detected.

Not all arrhythmias are pathologic. When the ECG has a P wave associated with most QRS complexes and the QRS complexes are of normal width, the rhythm is termed supraventricular. **Sinus arrhythmia** is fluctuation of heart rate with respiration, decreasing with expiration and increasing with inspiration; this is normal in dogs. Ventricular rhythm is characterized by QRS complexes that are wide and bizarre and not associated with P waves. Supraventricular and ventricular arrhythmias can be subdivided into bradyarrhythmias or tachyarrhythmias. Additional information regarding the ECG is located in Chapter 24.

Listen to the heart by placing the stethoscope over the left and right side of the patient's thorax at the fourth to sixth intercostal space, while palpating the pulse (Fig. 22-8).

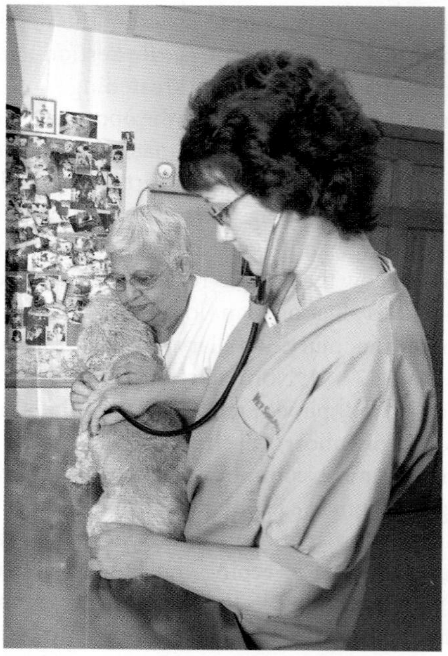

FIGURE 22-8 The pulse can be evaluated while the thorax is auscultated. Any difference between heart and pulse is termed a pulse deficit.

Any difference between heart and pulse rate is termed a pulse deficit. Pericardial fluid, pleural air or fluid, severe hypovolemia, or herniated abdominal organs cause muffled heart sounds. Tachycardia, bradycardia, muffled heart sounds, and pulse deficits require immediate attention by the veterinary team.

Indications of Perfusion

Mucous membrane color, capillary refill time, pulse strength and quality, and body temperature reflect perfusion of (blood flow to) peripheral tissues. Blood pumped into the aorta during ventricular contraction creates a fluid wave that travels from the heart to the peripheral arteries. This wave is called a pulse. Evaluation of pulse strength is based on the difference between the systolic (heart contracting) and diastolic (heart filling) pressure, called the pulse pressure. With normal pulse pressure, the pulse is easily palpated and strong. When the difference is great, the pulse is bounding. Causes of a bounding pulse include fever, hyperthyroidism, patent ductus arteriosus, and early shock. When the difference is small or the time to maximum systolic pressure is prolonged, the pulse feels weak. Any condition that decreases cardiac output (e.g., late shock, heart failure, arrhythmia) causes a weak pulse.

> *TECHNICIAN NOTE* Evaluation of perfusion involves assessment of mucous membrane color, capillary refill time, pulse strength and quality, and body temperature.

The pulse is palpated by lightly placing the tips of the index and middle fingers at a site where an artery crosses over bone or firm tissue. The most common pulse points assessed are the femoral and dorsal pedal arteries. In cats both femoral pulses should be assessed simultaneously to detect caudal aortic obstruction, as seen with a saddle thrombus. In large animals the pulse can be assessed where the facial artery crosses the ventral border of the mandible.

A bounding pulse may reflect pain, fever, or early shock, and it indicates the need for intervention with analgesics (pain relievers) and fluid replacement. A weak pulse is cause for immediate concern and warrants aggressive measures to improve cardiac output (e.g., IV fluids for shock, appropriate cardiac medications for heart failure).

Capillary refill time is the time required for blood to refill capillaries after displacement by finger pressure. Prompt refilling of capillaries depends on cardiac output and vascular tone.

To measure the capillary refill time, apply pressure with the index finger to an unpigmented area of mucous membrane and then release (Fig. 22-9). The time for the color to return to the blanched area is the capillary refill time. Normal values are 1 to 2 seconds. A prolonged capillary refill time (more than 2 seconds) suggests poor peripheral perfusion (e.g., late shock, severe vasodilation or vasoconstriction, pericardial effusion, heart failure). A short capillary refill time (less than 1 second) can be related to anxiety, compensatory shock, fever, and pain.

Although mucous membrane color is most commonly assessed by examining the gums, one can also use the conjunctiva of the eye and the membranes of the vulva and penis. The normal pink color of unpigmented mucous membranes requires adequate blood hemoglobin concentration, tissue oxygen tension, and peripheral capillary blood flow (Table 22-8). Pale gums with prolonged capillary refill time warrant oxygen administration and a rapid search for the underlying cause. Patients with these signs may require aggressive fluid therapy.

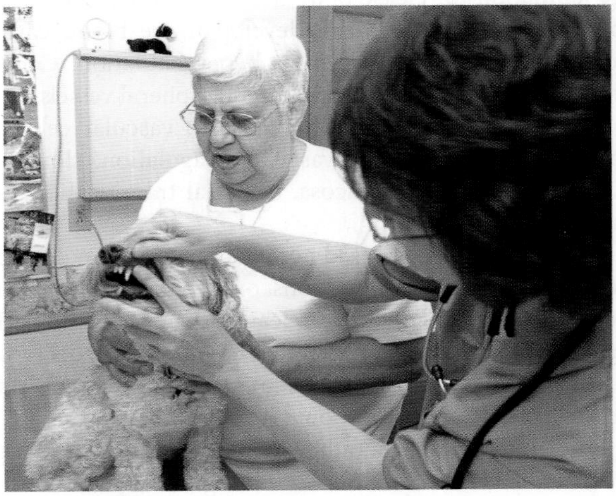

FIGURE 22-9 To measure the capillary refill time, apply pressure with the index finger to an unpigmented area of mucous membrane and then release.

TABLE 22-8 Interpretation of Mucous Membrane Color

MEMBRANE COLOR	INTERPRETATION	CAUSES
Pink	Normal	Adequate perfusion and oxygenation of peripheral tissues
Pale	Anemia, poor perfusion vasoconstriction	Blood loss, shock vasopressors
Blue	Cyanosis, inadequate oxygenation	Hypoxemia
Brick red	Hyperdynamic perfusion vasodilation	Early shock sepsis, fever, systemic inflammatory response syndrome
Icteric	Bilirubin accumulation	Hepatic/biliary disorder, hemolysis
Brown	Methemoglobinemia	Acetaminophen toxicity in cats
Petechiae or ecchymoses	Coagulation disorder	Platelet disorder, disseminated intravascular coagulation, coagulation factor deficiencies

Evaluating Body Temperature

The body maintains its normal temperature by balancing heat production with heat loss through a thermostatic feedback mechanism in the hypothalamus. This mechanism can be altered by disease of the central nervous system or other illness. Chemical substances released in disease can affect the thermoregulatory center and increase the metabolic rate body temperature. These chemicals may be pyrogens secreted by bacteria or cytokines associated with inflammation. Brain disease (e.g., cerebral edema, neurosurgery, trauma, tumors) can reset the thermostat to a higher level.

Hyperthermia (increased body temperature) increases tissue oxygen requirements. The body responds by increasing ventilation to release body heat. Cerebral vasoconstriction and brain hypoxia can develop if the blood carbon dioxide levels fall too low from hyperventilation. Cardiac work and oxygen demands increase. Peripheral vessels dilate in an effort to release heat. Damage to vascular cells can lead to disseminated intravascular coagulation, sloughing of the gastrointestinal mucosa, bacterial translocation, and hypovolemia.

Hypothermia (decreased body temperature) reduces the metabolic rate, enzyme functions, oxygen consumption, and the ability of hemoglobin to release oxygen to tissues. Hypothermia can cause peripheral vasoconstriction, decreased heart rate, and hypotension. Gastrointestinal motility is decreased, and **ileus** (lack of bowel motility) may occur.

Body temperature should be monitored from a single site, usually the rectum. Serial readings are more informative than a single reading. Other sites include the axillary and inguinal regions. Readings in these areas generally are 1 to 2 degrees lower than the rectal temperature. Body temperatures can also be measured with an ear probe inserted carefully into the external ear canal.

SYSTEMATIC APPROACH TO PHYSICAL EXAMINATION

After the vital signs are recorded, proceed to the physical examination, beginning at the tip of the nose and concluding at the tip of the tail. The examination can be divided into several areas: head and neck; trunk and forelimbs; thorax; abdomen; hind limbs; and external genitalia and perineum.

EXAMINATION OF THE HEAD AND NECK

Observing the patient at arm's length allows comparison of the two sides of the face and head for symmetry. Look for unilateral (one-sided) facial paralysis and unilateral or bilateral (two-sided) nasal/ocular discharge, and note any irregularities in head shape or size.

Assess the eyes for size, position, and any discharge. Observe for **ectropion** (everted eyelids) or **entropion** (inverted eyelids). Assess pupil size and the response to light. Check the cornea for clarity and contour, looking for scars, ulcers, infiltrates, and pigmentation. Assess the color and condition of the sclera and conjunctiva. Note any signs of jaundice, hemorrhage, or increased vascularization.

Evaluate the nose and nares for symmetry and conformation, as well as evidence of nasal discharge. If there is swelling evident or a history of chronic nasal discharge, determine patency of the nares. If the patient allows it, close the mouth, cover one nostril first and then the other, and assess nasal airflow. Note any areas with increased malleability of facial bones.

Check the lips for areas of inflammation, swelling, masses, or lip-fold pyoderma. Retract the lips and assess the oral mucosa and gingival tissues for color, capillary refill time, inflammation, jaundice, and ulcers. Check for fractured, missing, or loose teeth and periodontal disease. Assess the soft and hard palates for tumors, ulcerations, and foreign bodies.

Evaluate the carriage and position of the ears, thickness and malleability of the pinnae, and cleanliness of the ear canals. Check for odors, fluid, or exudate in the ear canal. Patients exhibiting pain or discomfort during examination of the ear canal should have a more detailed otoscopic examination.

After examining the ears, palpate the peripheral lymph nodes, salivary glands, larynx, and thyroid gland (Fig. 22-10). Palpate the trachea to determine if it is on the midline. In patients with inspiratory dyspnea, gently palpate the trachea to detect tracheal ring abnormalities. A sustained cough, retching, or gagging after gentle compression of the larynx and trachea is abnormal.

EXAMINATION OF THE TRUNK AND FORELIMBS

Palpate each forelimb, feeling for abnormalities in angulation, deformities, swelling, bleeding, bony protrusions, obvious fractures, or joint luxations. Assess both limbs in weight-bearing and non-weight-bearing positions. Assess for masses or lymph node abnormalities. Palpate for points of tenderness, stiffness, or crepitus at the joints. Note the condition of the feet, nails, or hooves; nail bed or hoof color may give an indication of perfusion. Palpate both brachial pulses for quality and strength.

Examine the haircoat for **alopecia** (hair loss), eruptions, parasites, dryness, or excessive oil. Palpate for any skin masses or lacerations. Assess the elasticity of the skin.

EXAMINATION OF THE THORAX

Observe the patient's respiratory rate, effort, and depth. Look for evidence of dyspnea, such as rapid open-mouth breathing, increased effort, an increased abdominal component, abnormal posture to assist in breathing, and cyanosis.

Observe and palpate the thorax for conformation, symmetry, and movement of the ribs, sternum, or vertebral column. Palpate for masses. Palpate the area between the fourth and sixth intercostal spaces on both sides of the thorax for the point of maximum intensity of the heartbeat and cardiac thrills.

Assess the respiratory tract. Listen for noisy breathing at the mouth and nares without the use of a stethoscope. Use a stethoscope to auscultate the lungs. Divide each side of the thorax (left and right) into four quadrants: craniodorsal,

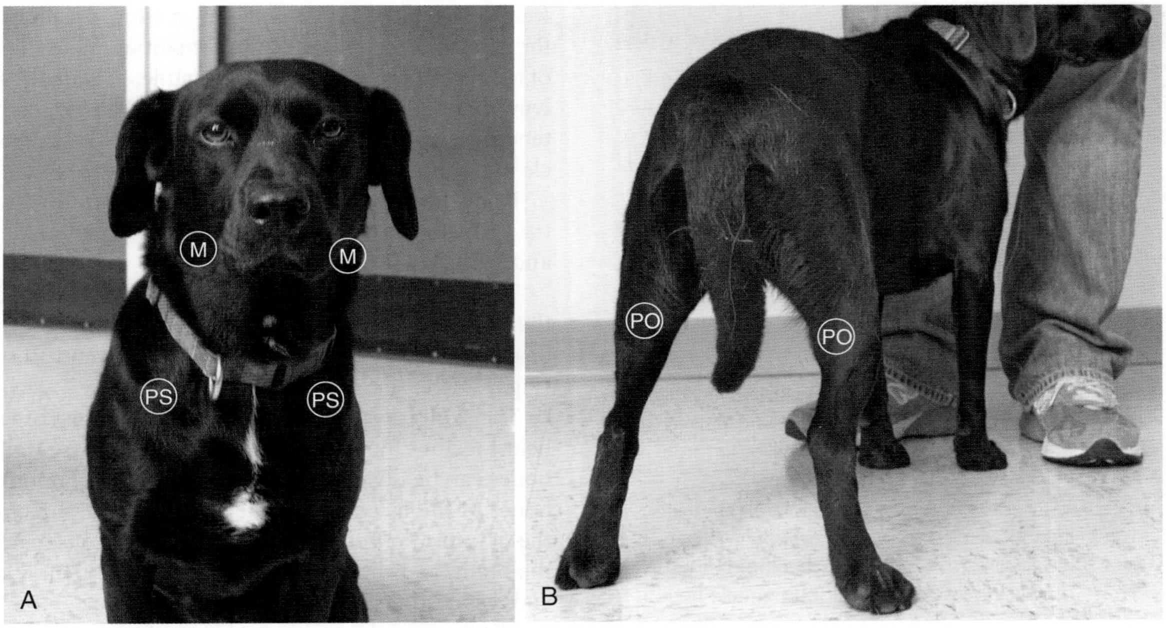

FIGURE 22-10 A, Dog showing the location of mandibular and prescapular lymph nodes. B, Dog showing the location of popliteal lymph nodes. (From Figure 7-18 in Bassert J, Thomas J: *McCurnin's clinical textbook for veterinary technicians,* ed 8, St Louis, 2014, Saunders.)

caudodorsal, cranioventral, and caudoventral. Begin by auscultating the right side at the craniodorsal quadrant, and continue in a clockwise fashion. Then do the same on the left side.

The upper respiratory tract starts at the tip of the nose. Inhaled air enters the nostrils and passes back through the nasal passages. From the nasal passages, inhaled air passes through the pharynx, or throat. This is a common passageway for both the digestive and respiratory systems. Through a series of intricate reflexes, the pharynx and larynx help prevent swallowed material from entering the lower respiratory tract.

The larynx, commonly called the voice box, is a short, irregular tube of cartilage and muscle that connects the pharynx with the trachea. In addition to its voice-producing function, it also acts as a valve to control airflow to and from the lungs. At the junction of the pharynx and the larynx is the epiglottis, a flap of cartilage that acts as a "trap door" to cover the opening of the larynx during swallowing.

Carrying air from the larynx to the lungs is the trachea, or windpipe. The trachea is composed of several C-shaped incomplete rings of hyaline cartilage, which prevent it from collapsing during inhalation. At its caudal end, the trachea divides into the left and right bronchi, which enter the lungs.

Lower Respiratory Tract

Beginning at the lower respiratory tract, the bronchi enter the lungs and branch into smaller and smaller air passageways that eventually lead to tiny grapelike clusters of thin cells called alveoli. The alveolus is the actual site of gas exchange in the lungs. Normal respiratory sounds are described as vesicular or bronchial, depending on where they are auscultated.

Vesicular sounds are heard over normal lung parenchyma and are produced by movement of air through small bronchi, bronchioles, and alveoli. Vesicular sounds are best heard on inspiration. They have been described as resembling the sound made by wind blowing through trees or the sound of rustling leaves.

Bronchial sounds are produced by movement of air through the trachea and large bronchi. They are usually heard over the area of the trachea and carina, most noticeably during expiration. Abnormal lung sounds include crackles (sometimes referred to as rales), wheezes, dull lung sounds, or muffled lung sounds. The type and location of the sound can aid in identifying the source of a problem (Table 22-9).

Cardiac auscultation can detect murmurs, arrhythmias, and muffled heart sounds. When assessing murmurs, it is important to determine in which quadrant the murmur is the loudest; this helps identify the valvular area involved. Arrhythmias most commonly detected are sinus arrhythmia (normal), atrial fibrillation, heart block, premature ventricular contractions, and gallop rhythm. Muffled heart sounds can be caused by obesity, pericardial effusion, pleural effusion, an intrathoracic mass, or diaphragmatic hernia.

EXAMINATION OF THE ABDOMEN

The abdomen should be inspected for distention, deformity, displacement, symmetry, and bruising. In trauma patients examine the umbilicus for red discoloration, suggestive of intra-abdominal bleeding. If the abdomen is distended, use percussion to determine if the distention is caused by peritoneal effusion, gastric dilatation or volvulus, an intra-abdominal mass, or obesity. Percussion that produces tympanic sounds suggests gastric or small intestinal obstruction and gas entrapment.

TABLE 22-9 Causes of Abnormal Lung Sounds

ABNORMAL LUNG SOUND	CAUSES
Crackles	Caused by air movement through small airways within the lumen reduced by fluid, mucus, or thickened walls. Mostly heard in conditions such as pulmonary edema, bronchopneumonia, and pulmonary fibrosis
Dry crackles	Associated with passage of air through relatively solid material in the bronchi or trachea
Moist crackles	Caused by passage of air through fluid material
Wheezes	High-pitched, musical sounds heard mostly on expiration Associated with infectious or allergic bronchitis (e.g., asthma in cats)
Dull or muffled lung sounds	Caused by collapse or consolidation of a lung lobe, tension pneumothorax, pneumomediastinum, hydrothorax, pyothorax, a mass displacing the lung, or diaphragmatic hernia

Auscultate the abdomen to detect intestinal hypermotility (increased frequency or intensity of intestinal sounds) or hypomotility (decreased frequency or intensity of intestinal sounds). Absence of bowel sounds suggests ileus (lack of intestinal motility) or a fluid-filled abdomen.

The abdomen of most small animals can be readily palpated, but this may not be feasible in patients with tense abdominal muscles. Abdominal palpation in large animals is more in the form of **ballottement,** in which the fist is rhythmically pressed into an area of the abdomen in an attempt to bump any large underlying masses or organs.

> *TECHNICIAN NOTE* Palpate the abdomen starting at the cranial area, proceeding systematically to the caudal area so all abdominal organs are palpated.

Palpate the abdomen in an orderly fashion. Divide the abdomen into three areas: cranial, middle, and caudal. Start the procedure at the cranial portion, and conclude at the caudal portion. Palpate the cranial abdomen to assess the stomach, duodenum, biliary structures, liver, and the area of the pancreas (seeking pain on palpation). In the midabdominal area, assess the spleen, kidneys, adrenal glands, mesenteric lymph nodes, and intestines. Organs assessed upon caudal abdominal palpation are the urinary bladder, prostate, uterus (in the intact female if enlarged), and colon. A normal uterus is not ordinarily palpable. Also note any indications of pain or tenderness or any evidence of swelling or masses during palpation.

EXAMINATION OF THE HIND LIMBS

Palpate each hind limb, feeling for abnormalities in angulation, deformities, swelling, bleeding, bony protrusions, obvious fractures, or joint luxations. Assess both limbs in weight-bearing and non-weight-bearing positions. Assess for masses or lymph node abnormalities. Note the position of the patellas when assessing the stifle. Palpate the popliteal lymph nodes for size and consistency. Palpate for points of tenderness, stiffness, or crepitus at joints. Also evaluate muscle mass and tone.

Palpate the pelvic region for conformation and symmetry. Palpate the vertebral column to assess for deviations and pain.

The axial skeleton is composed of the bones located on the axis or midline of the body. It is composed of the bones of the skull, the spinal column, the ribs, and the sternum (Fig. 22-11).

The skull is composed of many bones, most of which are held together by immovable joints called sutures. The skull bones can be divided into the bones of the cranium and the bones of the face (which extend in a rostral direction from the cranium). The bones of the cranium house and protect the brain, and the bones of the face house mainly digestive and respiratory structures.

The spinal column is composed of a series of individual bones called vertebrae. The vertebrae form a long, flexible tube called the vertebral canal. The vertebral canal houses and protects the spinal cord. The vertebrae are divided into five groups, and each vertebra is numbered within each group from cranial to caudal. The cervical vertebrae (C) are in the neck region. The first cervical vertebra (C1) is the atlas that forms a joint with the skull. The thoracic vertebrae (T) are dorsal to the chest region and form joints with the dorsal ends of the ribs. The lumbar vertebrae (L), which are dorsal to the abdominal region, are fairly large and heavy, because they serve as the site of attachment for the large sling muscles that support the abdomen. The sacral vertebrae (S) in the pelvic region are fused together into a solid structure called the sacrum, which forms a joint with the pelvis. The caudalmost vertebrae, the coccygeal vertebrae (Cy), form the tail. The number of vertebrae in each region varies with species. Following is the vertebral formula of different species.

Dog: C 7, T 13, L 7, S 3, Cy 20-23
Cow: C 7, T 13, L 6, S 5, Cy 18-20
Horse: C 7, T 18, L 6, S 5, Cy 15-20

EXAMINATION OF EXTERNAL GENITALIA AND PERINEUM

The male reproductive system is organized to produce male reproductive cells and transmit them to the female. Its main components are the testes, the epididymis, the vas deferens, the accessory sex glands, and the penis.

In males, inspect the prepuce and penis, noting any discharge. In dogs, expose the penis by retracting the preputial sheath. Look for masses and evidence of trauma, and note any color abnormalities (such as jaundice or bruising). If the patient is intact (not castrated), inspect both testicles for symmetry, size, location (within the scrotum), and conformation. If you detect only one testicle (cryptorchidism), palpate the inguinal area and caudal abdominal region for

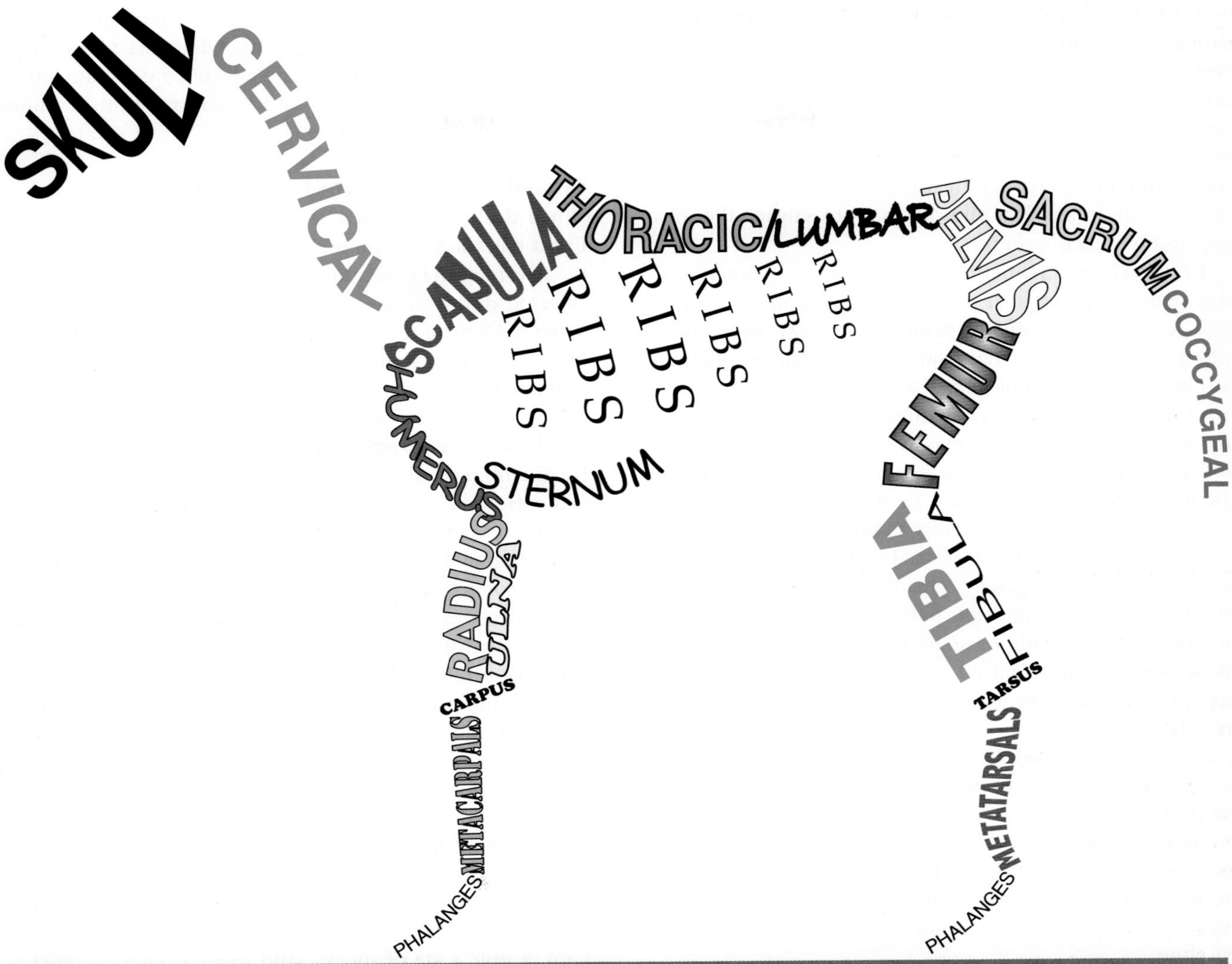

FIGURE 22-11 Word skeleton. The main bones of axial and appendicular portions of the skeleton. (From Colville TP, Bassert JM: *Clinical anatomy and physiology for veterinary technicians*, ed 2, St Louis, 2008, Mosby.)

a retained testicle. A rectal examination to determine texture, size, and conformation of the prostate is done by the veterinarian.

The female reproductive system is organized to produce female reproductive cells, accept male reproductive cells (spermatozoa), allow one sperm cell to unite with each female reproductive cell, and then shelter and nourish the resulting developing fetuses until birth. The organs of the female reproductive system are ovaries, oviducts, uterus, cervix, vagina, and vulva.

Female genital examination includes inspection and palpation of the mammary glands for tumors or cysts. In the lactating bitch or female dogs in pseudopregnancy, determine if there is evidence of mastitis or milk. In lactating cows, palpate for excessive heat and areas of firmness (induration). A California mastitis test can quickly assess the milk of lactating cows. Inspect the vulva for any discharge (blood, pus), polyps, tumors, or structural defects.

Rectal examination is done with a finger in small animals and with the hand and arm in large animals. Assess the sublumbar lymph nodes in the dorsal aspect of the pelvic canal. Feel for evidence of pelvic fracture and note anal tone and fecal consistency. Check for masses in the pelvic canal and caudal abdomen. In large animals, feel for displaced or distended loops of bowel, and assess the kidneys, if within reach.

Inspect the perianal area for hair mats, hernias, feces, masses, and evidence of discharge. In dogs, palpate for impacted or abscessed anal sacs.

PHYSICAL EXAMINATION IN EMERGENCIES

TRIAGE, PRIMARY SURVEY, AND SECONDARY SURVEY

The procedure called triage (French for "to sort") is used to classify patients according to the severity of illness or injury to determine their relative priority for treatment. In its original application in combat, triage was used by French military medical personnel to sort wounded soldiers into three categories: those that would survive without immediate treatment; those that would die despite immediate treatment; and those that would survive only if given immediate treatment. Emergency treatment of only the last group (those likely to survive) allowed them to salvage the most lives using limited resources.

In veterinary medicine, triage is used primarily in emergency situations. It can also be used in the critical care setting as a means of prioritization and assessment, and it guides the veterinary care team in efficient delivery of medical and patient care. Using triage, the treatment team focuses initially on life-threatening conditions (e.g., an obstructed airway or massive external hemorrhage) and institutes immediate measures to correct them with the most efficient use of available manpower and skills. A primary survey is used to detect any life-threatening problems. A secondary survey is used to broaden the evaluation to include all organ systems in a progressive, detailed manner. In triage of multiple patients (e.g., after a barn fire or horse trailer accident, or in a busy emergency clinic), those with a compromised airway, breathing difficulties, and/or circulatory problems (ABCs) should be assessed and treated first.

Vital signs assessed during triage include level of consciousness, respiratory rate and effort, heart rate and rhythm, and indications of perfusion (pulse, mucous membrane color, capillary refill time, temperature). These vital signs can indicate trends of deterioration, warning the team of complications. Vital signs should be assessed at frequent, regular intervals to detect trends, using initial values as the baseline.

In the emergency setting, no disease, injury, or physiologic abnormality should be considered as an isolated entity. The team should consider the current status, physiologic reserve, and potential for deterioration of each organ system or problem, rather than just the primary problem (e.g., fractured femur), and develop a plan of action.

During the primary survey and initial management, life-threatening conditions are addressed in the following order of priority:

1. Airway patency (open airway)
2. Breathing
3. Circulation
4. Neurologic deficit assessment

During the primary survey, neurologic status can be evaluated with the aid of the acronym AVPU: Is the patient **A**lert and aware of its surroundings? Is it **V**oice responsive? Is it **P**ain responsive? Is it **U**nresponsive?

After the ABC areas have been addressed and resuscitation measures have been initiated, the secondary survey is performed. Vital signs are reassessed, and the patient is rapidly and thoroughly examined from head to tail. The thorax, abdomen, pelvis, and extremities are visually inspected, palpated, and auscultated where appropriate. Neurologic status is repeatedly assessed. Appropriate radiographic and laboratory studies are obtained. Other diagnostic procedures that may be done at this time include, but are not limited to, an ECG, measurement of blood pressure and central venous pressure, and pulse oximetry.

Classification System for Triage

When dealing with more than one emergency or critically ill patient, the team can use a classification system based on the nature of the presenting complaint, as well as vital signs assessed during triage. There are a variety of classification systems Many of these are based on the Emergency Severity Index (ESI) used in human medicine. The ESI is designed to evaluate the patient as well as identify any resources to address the patient's condition.

Class I—Life Threatening. Patients in class I must receive treatment immediately and are usually those suffering from acute trauma, respiratory or cardiorespiratory arrest or failure, or airway obstruction, or are unconscious. Class I patients may be dying before your eyes. They are usually in a decompensatory stage of shock. The decompensatory stage of shock is characterized by cyanosis, ashen white mucous membranes, prolonged capillary refill time or no capillary refill, cold skin, a decreased rectal temperature, weak or undetectable femoral pulses, and oliguria (reduced urine production). They may be unconscious, stuporous, or losing consciousness. The bleeding patient may have seizures as a result of low blood pressure if the hemorrhage is substantial.

Class II—Emergent. Patients in class II are critically ill. These patients are suffering from multiple injuries, shock, or severe bleeding but have adequate respiratory function. They require treatment within minutes to an hour. They may be in a mild state of shock. Mild shock is characterized by pale or ashen mucous membranes, prolonged refill time, cool skin, a decreased rectal temperature, and weak femoral pulses. Class II patients may show tachycardia, oliguria, and altered mentation (e.g., depression, seizures, excitation). Hemorrhage may be profuse or a slow trickle.

Class III—Urgent. Patients in class III are seriously ill but not critically ill. These patients usually have severe open wounds or fractures, burns, penetrating wounds to the abdomen without active bleeding, or blunt trauma. They are not in shock or exhibiting an altered level of consciousness. They require treatment within a few hours.

Class IV—Non-urgent. Patients in class IV are less seriously ill but are still of concern. This classification does not apply to most trauma patients. The mucous membranes may be red or pale pink and capillary refill time under 1 second. The skin and rectal temperatures are normal, and femoral pulses are normal or bounding. These patients often have normal respiration, tachycardia or a normal heart rate, normal urine output, and normal mentation, evidenced by alertness and awareness of their surroundings. Usually these patients are mildly depressed to slightly excited and generally are not actively hemorrhaging. Class IV patients require treatment within 24 hours.

REVIEW QUESTIONS

Fill in Blank

Provide the best answers to complete the following statements.

1. The interview is most successfully conducted when the technician is ____________________ but cheerful, friendly, and genuinely concerned about the patient.
2. When conducting a patient history, it is generally more effective to ask ________, ____________, and ____________ than "why."
3. Tapping the body's surface to produce a vibration and sound is called ________________.
4. Percussion ventral to the fluid line in the thorax will produce a ______ ____________ sound.
5. Percussion dorsal to the fluid line produces a ______________ or __________________ sound.
6. Listening to sounds produced by the body is termed ____________________________.
7. Relaxation of heart chambers is referred to as ________________, and contraction of heart chambers is referred to as ______________.
8. The body is normally ____________________, meaning both sides are complementary or balanced.
9. Vital signs include the __________ rate and effort, ____________ rate and rhythm, and indications of ______________________.
10. A prolonged capillary refill time is more than ________ seconds.
11. Body temperature is maintained by a thermostatic feedback mechanism in the __________________.
12. The autonomic nervous system consists of two parts, the ______________ ________ and the ______________ ____________.
13. Cerebral vasoconstriction and brain hypoxia can develop from ____________________________.
14. Body temperature is monitored in animals via the ________________.
15. The common passageway for both the digestive and respiratory systems is the __________.
16. The ____________ is a flap of cartilage that acts as a "trap door" to cover the opening of the larynx during swallowing.
17. Obesity, pericardial effusion, pleural effusion, an intrathoracic mass, or diaphragmatic hernia can muffle ______________ sounds.
18. Increased frequency or intensity of intestinal sounds is called ______________; decreased frequency or intensity of intestinal sounds is called ________________.
19. The term ________________ is used to classify patients according to the severity of illness or injury to determine their relative priority for treatment.
20. In an emergency clinic, those patients with ______________________ or ____________________ issues are treated first.

Fill in the Chart

Animal	Heart Rate (beats/min)	Respiration Rate (breaths/min)	Temperature (°C)
Dog			
Cat			
Horse			
Cow			
Sheep			
Pig			
Rabbit			
Hamster			
Guinea Pig			

RECOMMENDED READING

Battaglia AM, Steele A: *Small animal emergency and critical care*, ed 3, St Louis, 2015, Saunders.

Crow SE, et al.: *Manual of clinical procedures in dogs, cats, rabbits, and rodents*, ed 3, Indianapolis, IN, 2009, Wiley-Blackwell.

Ford RB, Mazzaferro E: *Kirk and Bistner's handbook of veterinary procedures and emergency treatment*, ed 9, St Louis, 2011, Saunders.

The Merck veterinary manual: clinical values and procedures, ed 10, Rahway, NJ, 2010, Merck.

Nelson RW, Couto GC, editors: *Small animal internal medicine*, ed 4, St Louis, 2013, Mosby.

Rijnberk A, van Sluijs FJ: *Medical history and physical examination in companion animals*, ed 2, Oxford, UK, 2008, Saunders.

Silverstein D, Hopper K: *Veterinary emergency and critical care medicine*, St Louis, 2008, Saunders.

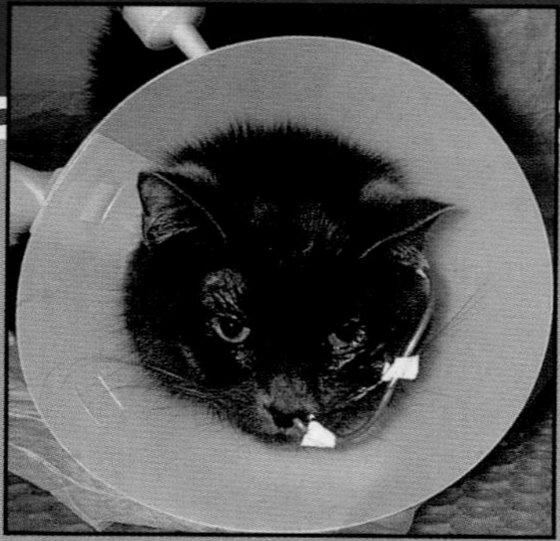

23 Nutrition

OUTLINE

LEARNING OBJECTIVES

After reviewing this chapter, the reader will be able to:

1. List basic energy-producing and non–energy-producing nutrients.
2. Describe considerations for feeding young and adult dogs.
3. Describe considerations for feeding young and adult cats.
4. Discuss the fundamentals of exotic pet diet considerations.
5. Explain nutritional peculiarities of livestock.
6. Give examples of methods used in feeding livestock.
7. Discuss basic differences in the digestive tracts of ruminants and monogastric animals.

KEY TERMS

Ad libitum
Agammaglobulinemic
Body condition scoring
Byproduct feeds
Colostrometer
Concentrates
Energy-producing nutrient
Ensiling
Essential amino acids
Fat-soluble vitamins
Feed analysis
Feedstuff
Forages
Hay
Lignin
Microbial fermentation
Nitrogen-free extract (NFE)
Non–energy-producing nutrient
Nonessential amino acids
Nonnutritive feed additives
Nutrient
Proximate analysis
Silage
Spoilage
Water-soluble vitamins

DIGESTIVE SYSTEM

The digestive or alimentary system converts food eaten by an animal into nutrient compounds that body cells can use for metabolic fuel. The digestive system consists of a tube running from the mouth to the anus, with accessory digestive organs attached to it. Food moving through the tube is broken down into smaller, simpler compounds through the process of digestion. These simple compounds then pass through the wall of the digestive tract into the bloodstream through the process of absorption for distribution of nutrients to body cells.

The structure of a species' digestive system is largely dependent on its diet. Nutrients in the plant-matter diet of herbivores, such as horses and cattle, are incorporated within hard-to-digest cellulose. Herbivores depend on the help of microorganisms, such as protozoa and bacteria, to help break down cellulose through a process called **microbial fermentation.** At some point in their digestive tract, herbivores have a large "fermentation vat," where cellulose can be broken down into usable nutrients. In cattle this is the rumen, and in horses it is the much-enlarged cecum, part of the large intestine. The digestive system of carnivores (meat eaters), such as dogs and cats, is much simpler. Carnivores depend on enzymes to break down easy-to-digest animal-source nutrients through the process of enzymatic digestion. Therefore, no large fermentation vat is needed. Omnivores (species eating a mixed diet), such as pigs, are somewhat intermediate. They depend primarily on enzymatic digestion, with a minor amount of microbial fermentation occurring in their large intestine.

ENERGY-PRODUCING NUTRIENTS

The most common question in veterinary practices today is, "What should I feed my pet?" This common inquiry compels all members of the veterinary health care team to maintain a high level of current knowledge about the best feeding recommendations for pets. Veterinary clinical practice continues to successfully integrate the application of nutrition to include both the healthy and the ill patient. The quality of a pet's life can be dramatically influenced by the intake of nutrients balanced to its lifestyle and state of health.

A **nutrient** is any constituent of food that is ingested to support life. The six basic nutrients are proteins, fats, carbohydrates, water, vitamins, and minerals. **Energy-producing nutrients** have a hydrocarbon structure that produces energy through digestion, metabolism, or transformation. Energy is used for all metabolism, cell rejuvenation, maintenance of homeostasis, and production of new cells. **Non–energy-producing nutrients** play an important role throughout the body system and are often called the "gatekeepers of metabolism" (Box 23-1).

PROTEINS

Dietary protein is used to build body tissues. Amino acids, the building blocks of protein, are categorized into essential and nonessential types. **Essential amino acids** cannot be synthesized in the body and so must be supplied by the diet (Box 23-2). **Nonessential amino acids** are synthesized in the body. The proportion of essential and nonessential amino acids largely determines the quality, or biologic value, of a particular protein source. A protein's biologic value represents the amount that is retained by the body after ingestion. A protein with a 100% biologic value is entirely retained by the body after ingestion. A protein of very low biologic value, such as 5%, is almost entirely excreted by the body after ingestion.

BOX 23-1 Nutrients

Energy-Producing
- Fats
- Carbohydrates
- Proteins

Non–Energy-Producing
- Water
- Vitamins
- Minerals

BOX 23-2 Essential Amino Acids

- Arginine
- Histidine
- Isoleucine
- Leucine
- Lysine
- Methionine
- Phenylalanine
- Threonine
- Tryptophan
- Valine
- Taurine (cats; conditionally essential)

FATS

Vegetable and animal fats, oils, and lipids are composed of fatty acids and contain more energy per unit of weight than any other nutrient. There is a direct correlation between fat content and caloric density in a diet; the more fat there is in a diet, the more calories it contains. Cats require three essential fatty acids in their diet, whereas only two are essential in dogs (Box 23-3).

TECHNICIAN NOTE Fat has more energy per gram than all other nutrients.

CARBOHYDRATES

Carbohydrates are classified as soluble or insoluble, based on their digestibility. Mammals cannot digest insoluble carbohydrates, such as fiber, although bacteria can degrade fiber in the stomach of herbivores. Fiber decreases a diet's digestibility and caloric density. Soluble carbohydrates,

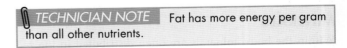

BOX 23-3 Essential Fatty Acids

Dogs
- Linolenic
- Linoleic

Cats
- Linolenic
- Linoleic
- Arachidonic

such as sugar and starches, can be readily digested and are metabolized for energy needs.

> **TECHNICIAN NOTE** Fiber is added to a diet for treatment of obesity or management of GI disorders.

NON–ENERGY-PRODUCING NUTRIENTS

WATER

Water provides the foundation for metabolism of all nutrients in the body. Minor alterations in the body's water content and distribution can result in dramatic alterations in nutritional requirements. Water balance in the system affects the ability to excrete waste into the urine by the kidneys. Water is also essential for absorption and metabolism of water-soluble vitamins B and C. Access to fresh, clean water is imperative for all animals. An animal's water needs may not be met if the water source freezes during inclement weather or if the water container is tipped over. It is important to educate clients on providing access to fresh, clean water in all seasons.

VITAMINS

Vitamins play a very important role in maintaining normal physiologic functions. These organic molecules are required only in minute amounts to exert their function as coenzymes, enzymes, or precursors in metabolism. **Water-soluble vitamins** are passively absorbed from the small intestine, and excess amounts are excreted in the urine. **Fat-soluble vitamins** are metabolized in a manner similar to fats and stored in the liver. Because of this storage mechanism, toxicity from excessive intake of fat-soluble vitamins can occur. A deficiency of fat-soluble vitamins is not as common as with water-soluble vitamins (Box 23-4).

MINERALS

Within the body, minerals are often distributed in ionized form as a cation or anion electrolyte. In this form they are involved with acid/base balance, clotting factors, osmolality, nerve conduction, muscle contraction, and a variety of other cellular activities.

Deficiencies or excesses in mineral intake can lead to problems through imbalances. Minerals are closely interrelated, and an imbalance in one mineral can affect several others. Dietary minerals include calcium, phosphorus, potassium, sodium, chloride, magnesium, iron, zinc, copper, manganese, selenium, iodine, and boron (Box 23-5).

BOX 23-4 Vitamins

Water-Soluble
- Thiamin
- Riboflavin
- Niacin
- Pyridoxine
- Pantothenic acid
- Folic acid
- Cobalamin
- Vitamin C
- Choline
- L-carnitine

Fat-Soluble
- A
- D
- E
- K

BOX 23-5 Minerals

- Calcium
- Phosphorus
- Potassium
- Sodium
- Chloride
- Magnesium
- Iron
- Zinc
- Copper
- Manganese
- Selenium
- Iodine
- Boron

FEEDING CONSIDERATIONS FOR DOGS

Contrary to popular belief, domestic dogs do not need variety in their diet. Frequent changes in diet have few positive effects, encourage finicky eating, and precipitate digestive disorders. It is best to consistently feed a diet formulated to meet the animal's needs at each stage of life. Regular assessment of weight can help determine the amount to feed. Weight loss or gain indicates a need to reevaluate the amount being fed or diet selection. **Body condition scoring** is a valuable way to assess the appropriate amount of food; a review of the body condition scoring system used for small animals can be found in Figure 23-1. Similar systems exist for evaluation of nutritional status of horses and production animals (Figs. 23-2 and 23-3).

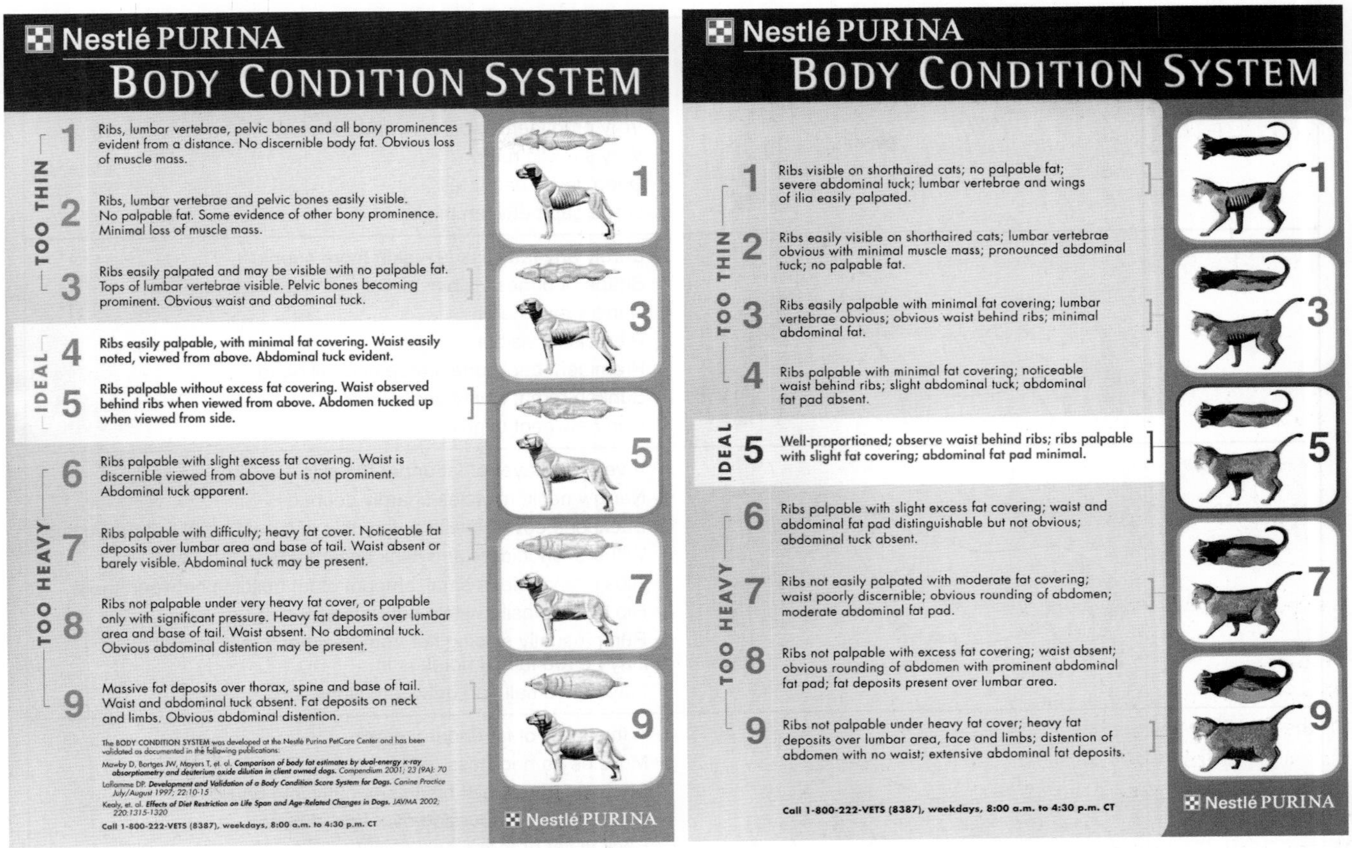

FIGURE 23-1 Body conditioning scoring system for small animals.

FEEDING METHODS

Portion Control

Portion control is currently the most popular way to feed dogs. After determining the animal's nutritional requirements, the daily portion is offered to the animal, either in a single feeding or divided into several portions offered several times per day. The animal is then allowed to consume the food throughout the day or during 5 to 10 minutes for each divided portion.

Free Choice

In free-choice feeding, the animal is allowed access to food 24 hours per day. The food supply is replenished as needed. It may be difficult to detect subtle changes in food intake with this method. Free-choice feeding is not recommended for puppies and obese dogs, but it works well for cats.

Time Control

In time-controlled feeding, a portion of food is offered and the animal is allowed access for only 5 or 10 minutes. Any remaining food is taken away after that time. Puppies are commonly fed in this manner.

FEEDING THE GESTATING OR LACTATING DOG

The daily energy requirement during gestation in the bitch increases during the length of the pregnancy. Although clients may have the impulse to dramatically increase food consumption, it is important to educate them on how to feed an appropriate amount. Excessive weight gain in the gestating bitch can make parturition more difficult and affect the overall health of the dog. The goal is to increase food intake gradually assessing weight gain carefully during the pregnancy. In the lactation phase, many dogs will require free feeding as they will need to eat smaller meals more frequently to reduce their absence from the puppies during this critical growth phase. Figure 23-4 shows the relationship between body weight and food intake during lactation and gestation in the dog.

FEEDING PUPPIES

With puppies born by cesarean section or if the bitch has no milk, the veterinary technician must intervene and provide nutritional support to neonatal puppies. Fortunately, they can be raised successfully on canine milk replacer. Cow's milk is not an acceptable substitute because it contains inappropriate levels of protein and lactose. Initially it may be necessary to use orogastric intubation or a feeding syringe and then gradually adopt a regular small-animal feeding bottle as the puppies begin to thrive.

Daily or twice-daily weighing and physical examination of the puppies helps identify problems early enough to adjust feeding protocols or begin other therapeutic measures to avoid mortality. Puppies typically gain 2 to 4 g/kg of anticipated adult weight each day.

0 – Emaciated	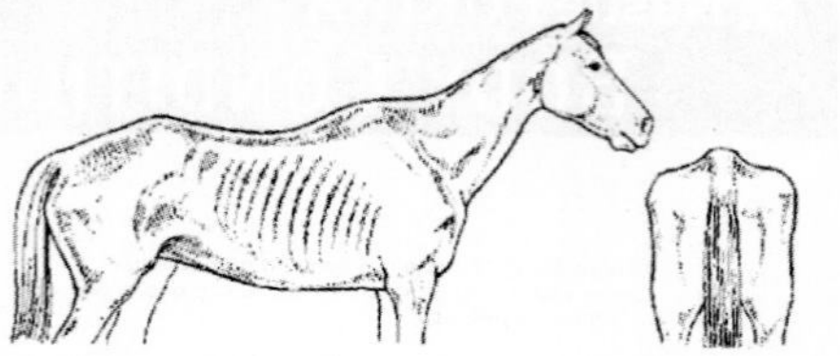	• No fatty tissue can be felt – skin tight over bones • Shape of individual bones visible • Marked ewe-neck • Very prominent backbone and pelvis • Very sunken rump • Deep cavity under tail • Large gap between thighs
1 – Very thin	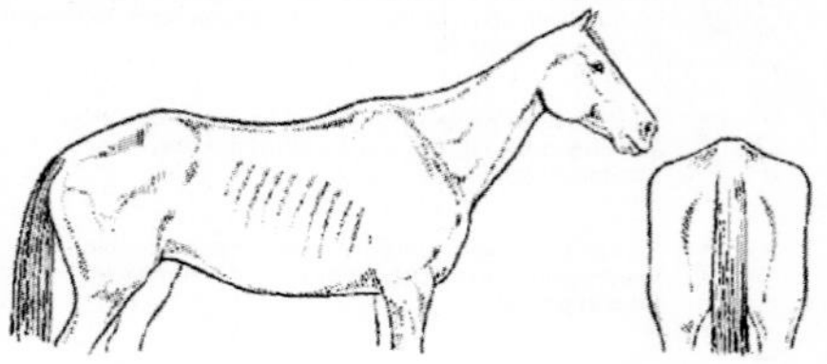	• Barely any fatty tissue – skin more supple • Shape of bones visible • Narrow ewe-neck • Ribs easily visible • Prominent backbone, croup and tail head • Sunken rump; cavity under tail • Gap betweent thighs
2 – Very lean	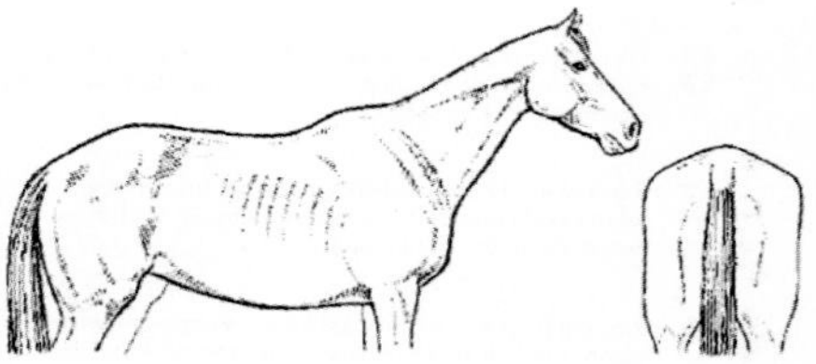	• A very thin layer of fat under the skin • Narrow neck; muscles sharply defined • Backbone covered with a very thin layer of fat but still protruding • Withers, shoulders and neck accentuated • Ribs just visible, a small amount of fat building between them • Hip bones easily visible but rounded • Rump usually sloping flat from backbone to point of hips, may be rounded if horse is fit • May be a small gap between thighs
3 – Healthy weight	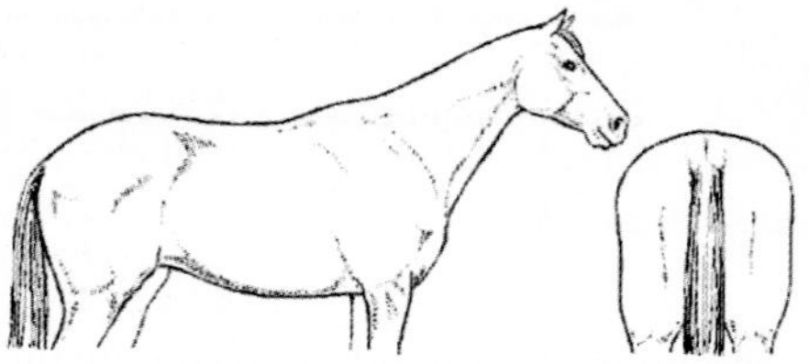	• A thin layer of fat under the skin • Muscles on neck less defined • Shoulders and neck blend smoothly into body • Withers appear rounded over tips of bones • Back is flat or forms only a slight ridge • Ribs not visible but easily felt • A thin layer of fat building around tail head • Rump beginning to appear rounded • Hip bones just visible
4 – Fat	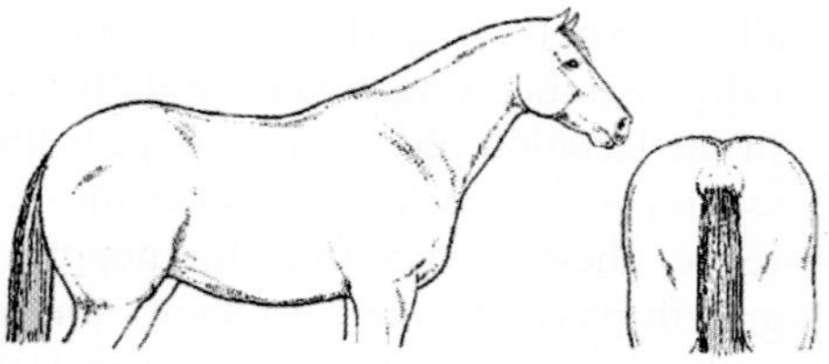	• Muscles hard to determine beneath fat layer • Spongy fat developing on crest • Fat deposits along withers, behind shoulders, and along neck • Ribs covered by spongy fat • Spongy fat around tail head • Gutter along back • Rump well rounded • From behind rump looks apple shaped • Hip bones difficult to feel
5 – Obese	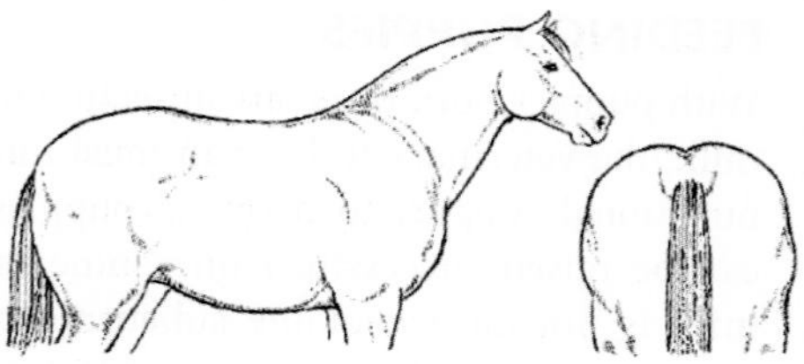	• Horse takes on a bloated or blocky appearance • Muscles not visible – covered by a layer of fat • Pronounced crest with hard fat • Pads of fat along withers, behind shoulders, along neck and on ribs, ribs cannot be felt • Extremely obvious gutter along back and rump • Flank filled in flush • Lumps of fat around tail head • Very bulging apple shaped rump, bony points buried • Inner thighs pressing together

FIGURE 23-2 Body conditioning scoring system for horses. (From Holtgrew-Bohling K: *Large animal clinical procedures for veterinary technicians,* ed 2, St Louis, 2012, Mosby.)

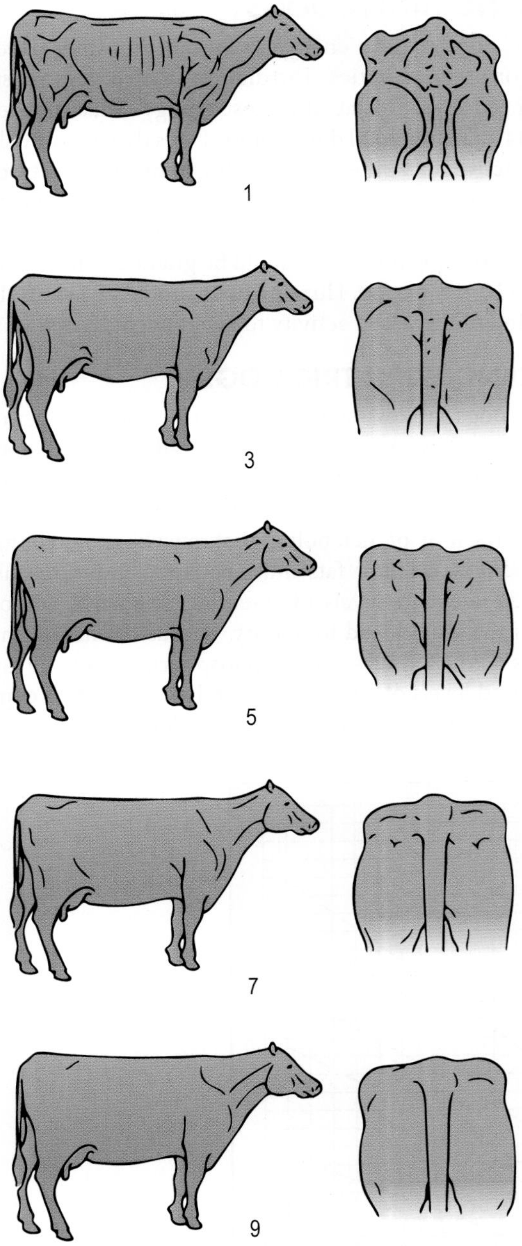

FIGURE 23-3 Body conditioning scoring system for beef production animals. (From Holtgrew-Bohling K: *Large animal clinical procedures for veterinary technicians,* ed 2, St Louis, 2012, Mosby.)

> **TECHNICIAN NOTE** Any variance in a puppy's normal daily weight gain of 2 to 4 g/kg of anticipated adult weight demands closer investigation.

Some neonatal puppies fail to gain weight when nursing the bitch because they cannot compete with siblings for a nipple. Puppies in this situation tend to be restless and whimper inordinately. Normal weight can be restored by allowing such puppies to nurse the bitch without competition three to four times daily.

Weaning begins around 3 to 4 weeks of age in large-breed puppies and at 4 to 5 weeks of age in smaller breeds.

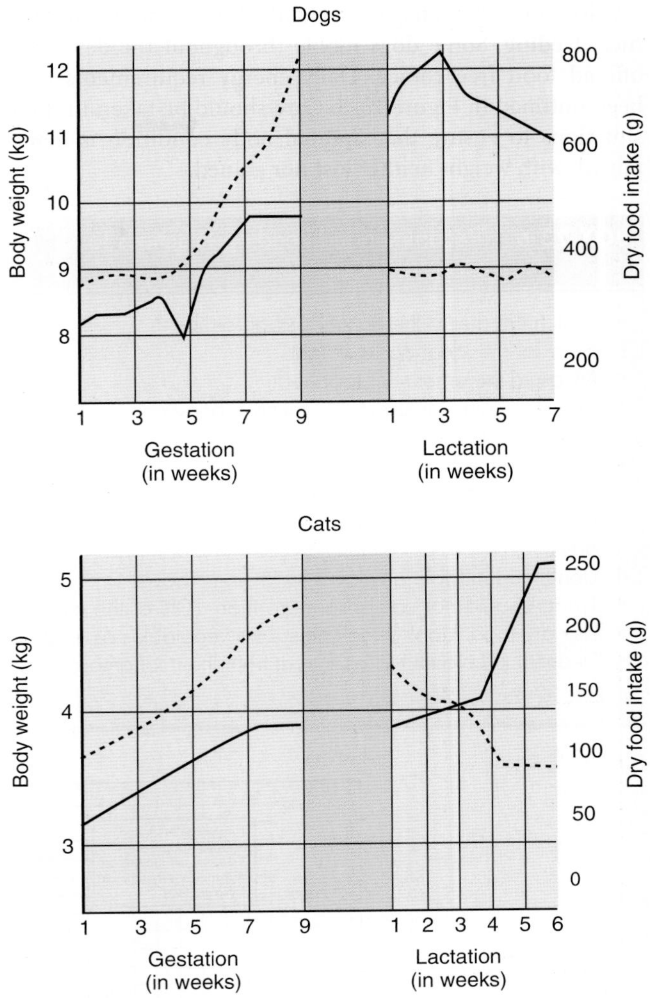

FIGURE 23-4 The pattern of normal weight gain during gestation and loss in the postpartum and lactation periods differs between cats and dogs. Solid line indicates food intake. Dashed line indicates body weight. (Courtesy Hill's Pet Nutrition, Inc., Topeka, KS.)

To facilitate the transition to solid foods, begin by making a gruel or slurry of a growth type of diet. Gruel is created by mixing equal parts of food and water together to form a homogeneous consistency. The mixture should have the texture of cooked oatmeal. Puppies initially may play with or walk through the slurry, but eventually they consume it in increasing volumes. Gruel should be offered three to four times daily during the weaning process. Feed the puppy increasing amounts until the puppy can be maintained without nursing, at 5 to 7 weeks in large-breed puppies and at 6 to 7 weeks in smaller breeds. Once weaning is complete, decrease the volume of water added to the mixture until the puppy is eating the desired diet and voluntarily drinking water.

FEEDING ADULT DOGS

As a dog matures, be sure to monitor activity level and predisposition to obesity to preserve a neutral energy equilibrium. Reassess feeding methods, because inappropriate techniques commonly result in excessive nutrient intake and obesity. Review feeding habits with clients to preclude future problems (Box 23-6).

Most dogs are managed efficiently through time-restricted meal feeding. Some dogs nibble throughout the day when offered food free choice. Daily energy requirements have been outlined in Figure 23-5. Care should be taken in these situations to ensure that optimal body condition is maintained, with weight neither lost nor gained.

BOX 23-6 Recommended Feeding Practices for Dogs and Cats

- Match the diet to the animal's stage of life.
- Feed for the ideal body weight.
- Measure the amount of food fed.
- Adjust the amount fed to the animal's body condition.
- Don't feed table scraps.
- Don't overfeed.
- Don't change the diet frequently.
- If the diet is to be changed, do so gradually, over 3 to 5 days.
- Don't feed multiple animals from a single bowl.
- Treats should not comprise more than 10% of the diet.
- Use dry food (kibble), ice chips, and vegetables as treats.
- Deduct the amount fed as a treat from the total amount fed daily.

FEEDING ACTIVE DOGS

Active dogs require energy to sustain hunting, obedience trial, or other activities. The diets for active dogs must have enhanced levels of fat, the most energy-dense nutrient, as well as increased total digestibility. Dogs that are only slightly more active than others need slightly more food, but working dogs with significant energy demands require a substantial increase in food portions. Any increase in food portions, to condition a dog for work, should be gradually instituted over a 7- to 10-day period. Hunting dogs should be fed just before a period of increased activity to avoid hypoglycemia.

FEEDING GERIATRIC DOGS

Older dogs are less able to adjust to prolonged periods of poor nutrition. Any changes in an older dog's diet should be based on careful patient assessment and not solely on the dog's age. Dietary protein should be of high biologic value to reduce the level of metabolites that must be excreted through the kidneys. Dietary fats must be sufficiently digestible to provide adequate levels of essential fatty acids without an excess that could lead to obesity. Because of its detrimental effects on the kidneys, dietary phosphorus should be limited. Increased levels of zinc, copper, and vitamins A, B complex, and E may be required in the diet of older dogs.

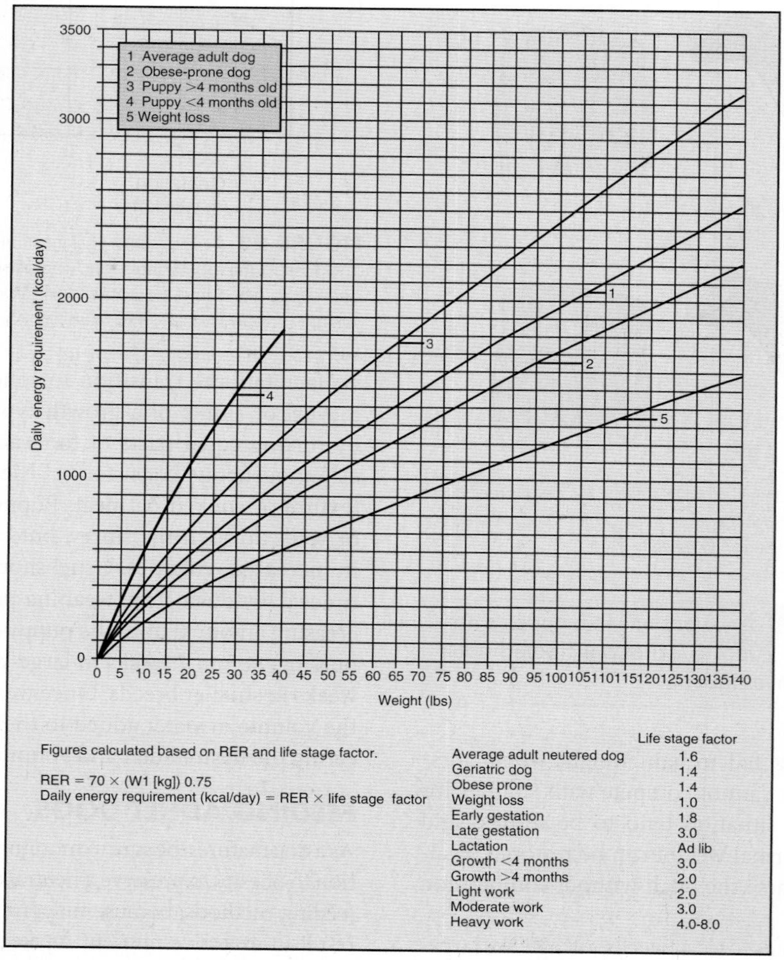

FIGURE 23-5 Canine daily energy requirements. (Courtesy Hill's Pet Nutrition, Inc., Topeka, KS.)

FEEDING OVERWEIGHT DOGS

Obesity is the most common nutritional disorder of pets. Obesity places significant stress on the body system and may predispose to diabetes mellitus, cardiovascular disease, and skeletal problems. Early counseling of owners can alert them to weight gain. Educate clients on the potential adverse effects of weight gain. Additional considerations for feeding overweight pets can be found in Box 23-6.

A review of nutritional considerations for different life stages in the cat and dog can be found in Table 23-1.

FEEDING CONSIDERATIONS FOR CATS

FEEDING KITTENS

Kittens that are orphaned or born to queens unable to nurse must be hand-fed. Weaning should not commence until 7 weeks of age. Kittens can be gradually introduced to a diet by first offering a slurry of canned food mixed with kitten milk replacer. As with puppies, the amount of liquid is gradually reduced. Later they can be offered a dry diet if preferred.

FEEDING ADULT CATS

Adult cats typically eat several small meals throughout a 24-hour period. Unfortunately, many clients provide food to their cats in unlimited amounts, filling the food dish each time their cat empties it. Such free-choice feeding predisposes to obesity. Overfeeding can be prevented by offering limited amounts of food throughout the day. This gives the cat the opportunity to nibble throughout the day while avoiding excessive caloric intake.

Caution owners against offering a constantly changing diet, such as various brands and types of commercial diets, because this can result in undesirable eating behavior.

FEEDING CATS WITH LOWER URINARY TRACT DISEASE

Feline urinary tract disease is a complex disease characterized by bouts of frequent painful urination, bloody urine, and, in males, possible urethral obstruction. It tends to occur more often in obese, sedentary cats. Factors other than diet are involved in lower urinary tract disease, but careful attention to the diet of affected cats can help prevent future episodes.

Depending on the type of uroliths (small stones composed of cellular debris and mineral crystals) present in the urinary tract (struvite or calcium oxalate), prevention involves manipulation of dietary mineral, fiber, and water intake. Special commercial diets are available for dietary management of feline urologic syndrome.

FEEDING GERIATRIC CATS

Because aging can diminish the senses of smell and taste, it is sometimes necessary to enhance the aroma and taste of foods to improve their palatability for aged cats. Successful techniques include warming canned food to body temperature in the microwave to improve the aroma, applying garlic powder to canned food before it is warmed, and addition of aromatic foodstuffs, such as clam juice or bits of canned fish.

FEEDING THE GESTATING AND LACTATING CAT

Food intake for the gestating queen is not as dramatic as that found in the canine. Allow the queen to have free access to food during the last 30 days of gestation. Assess weight gain and body condition on a weekly basis to reduce the occurrence of excess weight gain. Free food should be available to the queen throughout lactation to assure ample milk availability to the kittens. Figure 23-4 shows the relationship between food intake and body weight during lactation and gestation in the cat. Feline daily energy requirements have been calculated in Figure 23-6.

PET FOOD CONSIDERATIONS

When a nutritional assessment is made for a pet, the need of fulfilling dietary requirements is only partially met by the veterinary health care team. To fully gratify all the dietary needs, it is also necessary to understand the broad assortment of types, classifications, and varieties of diets available commercially today. Often questions arise regarding effective techniques in comparing diets. The effective veterinary technician must be able to answer these questions with insight and full understanding of the pet's nutritional need. To accurately evaluate commercial diets for dogs and cats, it is necessary to obtain accurate information about the common pet foods that clients consider feeding and that are recommended by the veterinary practice.

> **TECHNICIAN NOTE** Attention by the veterinary technician should be made to build a comprehensive collection of information to have available when clients have questions.

Occasionally, clients inquire regarding their potential to produce a homemade diet. This presents a multifaceted dilemma because of the difficulty in maintaining balance from batch to batch. Most homemade diet recipes have not been analyzed for adequacy, possess ingredients often hard to come by, and are hard to reproduce consistently. Clients should be alerted to these concerns and be reminded of the reliability and convenience of many commercial pet foods available today.

Assessing pet food begins with making an overview of general considerations then progresses to more specific evaluations as the diet continues to meet nutritional expectations. The following section is a review of common questions to assist in effective comparisons and determinations of pet foods. It is essential to review the information available on a pet food label to assess its ability to meet the needs of pets during different stages of life. A review of information available on a pet food label is shown in Figure 23-7.

TABLE 23-1 Nutrient Considerations for Different Life Stages in Cats and Dogs

LIFE STAGE	FOOD CHARACTERISTICS	COMMENTS
Cats		
Kittens 8 weeks to 1 year Gestation/lactation	Metabolizable energy 4.5 kcal/g dry matter Digestibility >80% Protein 35%-50% Fat 17%-30% Fiber ≥5% Calcium/phosphorus ratio 1.0-1.8 to 0.8-1.5 Magnesium ≤20 mg/100 kcal	Transition the queen to a growth diet at 3 weeks of gestation.
Adult cat	Metabolizable energy 3.75 kcal/g dry matter Digestibility >78% Protein 0%-45% Fat 9%-25% Magnesium <20 mg/100 kcal	Ad lib feeding is acceptable to kittens and queens. Free feeding adults may result in overnutrition.
Obese-prone cat	Metabolizable energy 3.50-3.75 kcal/g dry matter Digestibility >75% Protein 30%-45% Fiber 7%-12% Fat 9%-25% Magnesium <20 mg/100 kcal	Feed multiple times (3-4) daily. Fiber provides satiety and decreased caloric density
Geriatric cat	Metabolizable energy 3.75 kcal/g dry matter Digestibility >80% Protein 35%-45% Fiber 7%-12% Fat 9%-25% Magnesium <20 mg/100 kcal	Watch excess sodium and energy intake. Increased palatability may be needed.
Dogs		
Puppies Gestation/lactation	Metabolizable energy >3.9 kcal/g of diet Digestibility >80% Protein 27%-30% Fiber <4% Fat 8%-20% Calcium/phosphorus 1.0-1.8 to 0.8-1.6	Avoid excessive weight during pregnancy. Puppies reach skeletal maturity at approximately 12 months of age.
Adult dog	Metabolizable energy >3.5 kcal/g of diet Digestibility >75% Protein 15%-25% Fiber ≥5% Fat 7%-15%	Food and feeding consistency encouraged.
Obese-prone dog	Metabolizable energy <3.5 kcal/g of diet Digestibility >80% Protein 15%-25% Fiber >5% Fat 6%-10%	Free feeding can contribute to obesity.
Increased activity or stressed dog	Metabolizable energy >4.2 kcal/g of diet Digestibility >82% Protein 25%-32% Fiber <4% Fat 23%-27%	
Geriatric dog	Metabolizable energy = 3.75 kcal/g of diet Digestibility >80% Protein 14%-21% Fiber >4% Fat 10%-12% Control sodium	The average small-medium breed dog is considered geriatric after 7 years. Giant and large breeds are geriatric at 5 years of age.

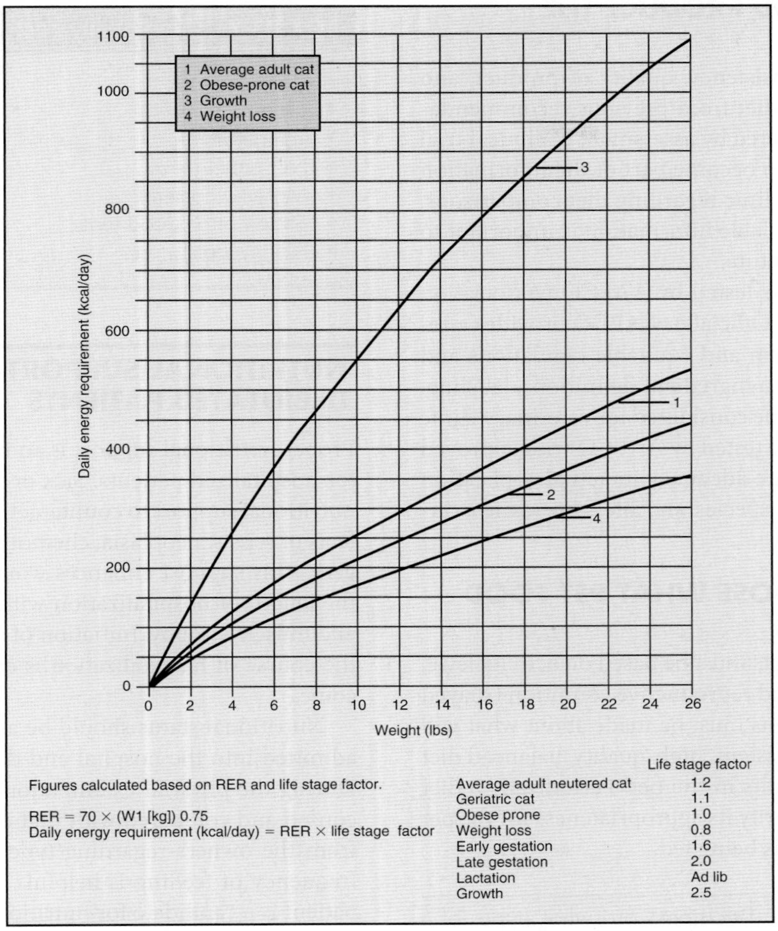

FIGURE 23-6 Feline daily energy requirements. (Courtesy Hill's Pet Nutrition, Inc., Topeka, KS.)

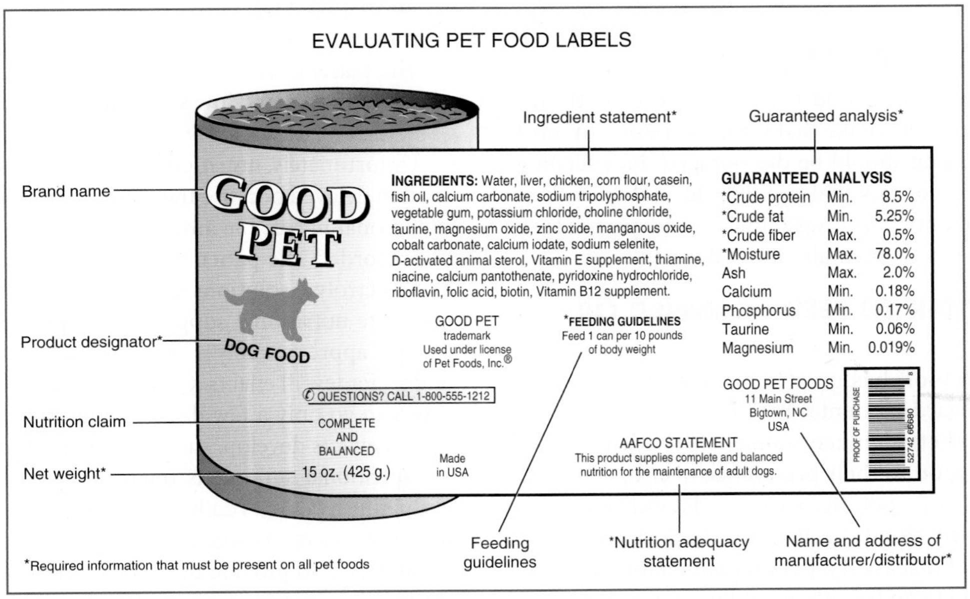

FIGURE 23-7 A pet food label is the contract between the manufacturer and the consumer. A label provides information required by law and may have optional information, such as a statement of calorie content, the Universal Product Code, batch information, or a freshness date. (Courtesy Hill's Pet Nutrition, Inc., Topeka, KS.)

DOES THIS PET FOOD PRODUCE THE DESIRED RESULTS?

Questions about fecal consistency, quality of product, and physiologic response to a diet from previous recommendations, which must be answered by assessment of clinical trial and experience, should also become part of the information retained at the veterinary clinic regarding diet comparisons. Keeping records of this valuable information is important to be able to draw on in the future.

Pet foods should also be tested by AAFCO (Association of American Feed Control Officials). AAFCO provides a resource to formulate uniform and equitable regulations and policies. These laws apply to ingredient definitions, labeling, and feeding trials. Diets to be considered for veterinary clinic recommendation should be tested by AAFCO with approved feeding trials to substantiate adequacy in actual application of the diet to a particular species and life stage as it is intended to be fed.

HOW DO YOU CHOOSE WHAT PET FOOD TO FEED?

Decisions on feeding for pets must be based on activity level, breed, age, health status, and reproductive condition (spayed or neutered). Considerations must be made about what will provide the pet with a consistent, high-quality, balanced diet that produces the best results in the pet. Periodically a diet should be reevaluated to verify its appropriateness for the pet and that the right amount is being fed.

> **TECHNICIAN NOTE** Decisions on what type of food and how often to feed a pet are based on activity level, breed, age, health status, and reproductive condition.

CAN I FREE FEED MY PET?

Allowing pets free access to food at any time increases the incidence of excess caloric intake that leads to obesity. In most situations, free feeding should be discouraged. Free feeding may be acceptable for cats that are able to maintain their weight without obesity, lactating females, and particularly fussy pets. The goal is to maintain optimal weight.

WHICH IS BETTER TO FEED—CANNED OR DRY?

Although canned food has greater palatability, there are some concerns regarding dental health. For that purpose, dry food may be a better choice. Some pets that are finicky may find canned food to their preference over dry food. If caloric intake falls in a pet, increasing palatability can assist in rectifying the situation. It is also important to rule out the presence of disease if a pet's feeding habits change. Palatability of a diet can be enhanced by warming canned food to body temperature or by adding warm water to dry food as well as using a small amount of fat/oil as a top dressing for dogs. Additional palatability factors can be found in Box 23-7.

BOX 23-7 Palatability Factors

- Texture
- Odor
- Temperature
- Fat/protein levels
- Moisture content
- Shape of dry food (cats)
- Acidity (cats)

NUTRITIONAL SUPPORT FOR ILL OR DEBILITATED PATIENTS

Proper nutritional support is an important aspect of therapy for hospitalized patients. Sick or injured patients need good nutritional support to counteract the immunosuppressive effects of sepsis, neoplasia, chemotherapy, anesthesia, and surgery. This support enhances wound healing and minimizes the length of hospitalization without significant weight loss and muscle atrophy. Initiation of nutritional support early in the course of hospitalization is crucial for a successful outcome.

Nutritional status should be assessed when the patient is admitted into the hospital and daily during hospitalization. During the physical examination, the patient's weight is recorded and compared with that of previous visits. A history from the owners regarding type of food, quantity fed, and frequency of feeding is helpful. During hospitalization, the patient is a candidate for nutritional support if the following occurs:

- The patient loses more than 10% of body weight.
- The patient has a decreased appetite or anorexia.
- The patient loses body condition from vomiting, diarrhea, trauma, or wounds.
- The patient has increased needs because of fever, sepsis, wounds, surgery, low serum albumin, organ dysfunction, or chronic disease.

Unfortunately, nutritional support in hospitalized patients is often delayed because the patient is not reassessed daily for nutritional needs, the amount of food a patient consumes is not recorded, the patient is not weighed daily, and dextrose and electrolyte solutions are erroneously thought to provide adequate nutritional support. Most previously healthy dogs can go approximately 1 week without nutritional support and suffer few ill effects. Cats, however, especially overweight cats, can go only a few days without nutritional support before ill effects develop, such as hepatic lipidosis.

Nutritional support is often the last consideration when evaluating a patient's daily treatment regimen, until the patient does not recover as quickly as expected. The goal of nutritional support is to provide the patient's nutritional requirements while it is recovering from its disease process and/or anorexia, trauma, or surgery, until the patient is able to eat enough on a regular basis to accommodate any ongoing losses. With nutritional support, patients can gain weight and have an improved response to medical or surgical therapy.

> **TECHNICIAN NOTE** Parenteral nutritional support is used with patients that are unable to digest or absorb nutrients via the GI tract or have uncontrolled vomiting.

The route of nutritional support administration can be enteral, parenteral, or a combination of both. Enteral feeding may be accomplished with orogastric, nasogastric, nasoesophageal, pharyngostomy, gastrostomy, and jejunostomy tubes. Parenteral nutrition is administered via a catheter placed in the cranial or caudal vena cava.

The route selected depends on such factors as function of the gastrointestinal (GI) tract, the disease process, duration of support, equipment and personnel available to provide the necessary support, and cost of the chosen method. Enteral support is chosen most often because it is physiologically sound, easy, relatively free of complications, and inexpensive. If the gastrointestinal tract is functional and the patient can swallow, use as much as possible. Parenteral support should be used if the patient has a medical or surgical condition that prevents ingestion or digestion of nutrients (e.g., vomiting, diarrhea, ileus, pancreatitis, malabsorption, reconstructive surgery, coma), and as adjunctive therapy for patients with organ failure or when malnutrition is severe.

ENTERAL NUTRITIONAL SUPPORT

Hand feeding favorite foods and tempting with warm, odoriferous foods in multiple, small meals can be used in conjunction with other methods of nutritional support. Forced feeding can be stressful to the patient and may deliver only a portion of the nutrition required for recovery.

Orogastric intubation is excellent for rapid administration but can cause aspiration and trauma and is very stressful for patients other than neonates. This method is for short-term use only.

Placement of a nasoesophageal or nasogastric tube is an easy, simple, and relatively inexpensive procedure that allows liquid nutritional support for an extended time and can be easily administered by the owner at home for continued convalescence (Box 23-8).

BOX 23-8 Methods of Enteral Feeding

- Oral feeding (increased palatability)
- Oral feeding (forced feeding)
- Orogastric tube feeding
- Nasogastric tube feeding
- Pharyngostomy tube feeding
- Esophagostomy tube feeding
- Gastrostomy tube feeding
- Jejunostomy tube feeding

A nasoesophageal or nasogastric tube is placed through the nasal cavity into the distal esophagus or stomach to bypass the oral cavity (Procedure 23-1). Placement is contraindicated in patients with nasal masses, esophageal disorders (e.g., megaesophagus), or no gag reflex. A nasoesophageal or nasogastric tube can usually be placed without chemical restraint (ideal for animals unable to tolerate general anesthesia). It is tolerated by most patients and used when the animal is anorexic, too stressed for forced feeding, and not receiving enough nutrition through hand feeding. The tube can remain in place for a week or longer, until the patient's appetite increases or the oral cavity can be used again. Feedings through the tube can start immediately after placement, unlike pharyngostomy or gastrostomy tubes. Have the patient in a sitting position when tube feeding. Common problems with nasoesophageal or nasogastric tubes include epistaxis (nosebleed) when the tube is first placed, accidental placement in the trachea, patient intolerance of the tube, and tube obstruction by medications or diet.

Soft, flexible pediatric feeding tubes, red rubber tubes, and seamless, polyurethane tubes (in a variety of lengths and diameters) are used for cats and dogs. Animals weighing less than 5 kg require a 5-French feeding tube, whereas some cats and all dogs weighing 5 to 15 kg can accept an 8-French tube. In larger dogs, the larger-diameter feeding tubes require a guidewire for placement in the esophagus or stomach.

For nasoesophageal placement with the tube tip at the level of the midthoracic esophagus, measure from the tip of the nose to the eighth or ninth rib. For nasogastric placement, measure from the tip of the nose to the thirteenth rib to assure safety in its position. Occasionally tubes placed in the stomach may cause gastroesophageal reflux and irritation, but this is usually not a problem with a small-diameter tube. Mark the premeasured length on the tube with a permanent marker.

For nasoesophageal tube feeding, aspirate the tube before each feeding. If air is aspirated, do not feed. During aspiration, there should be negative pressure on the syringe if the tube is correctly placed. Accidental tracheal intubation can cause aspiration pneumonia. Before each feeding, also assess tube location by injecting 3 ml of sterile water through the tube and listening for coughing or gagging. If this occurs, do not administer the feeding; remove the tube.

A pharyngostomy tube is placed through the wall of the pharynx into the esophagus or stomach, bypassing the oral cavity. Placement requires general anesthesia and surgery. The many possible complications (e.g., esophagitis, pharyngitis, laryngitis, vomiting, regurgitation, aspiration pneumonia) and the difficulty of pharyngostomy tube placement outweigh the benefits.

A jejunostomy tube is a feeding tube surgically placed in the mid- to distal duodenum or proximal jejunum, bypassing the stomach. Continuous feeding of easily digestible diets through the jejunostomy tube requires prolonged hospitalization, without the benefits of home care. This procedure is rarely used because of the cost of placement and maintenance and possible complications.

A gastrostomy or PEG tube is placed through the body wall into the lumen of the stomach, bypassing the mouth and esophagus. A gastrostomy tube is used for patients requiring long-term nutritional supplementation because of orofacial neoplasia, surgery or trauma, esophageal disor-

PROCEDURE 23-1 Nasoesophageal Tube Placement

1. Restrain the animal in sternal recumbency or sitting, with the head held level or slightly elevated. Anesthetize the nostril with a few drops of topical ophthalmic anesthetic. While waiting for the topical anesthetic to take effect, lubricate the tip of the feeding tube with a water-soluble lubricant or 5% lidocaine jelly.
2. Place the tip of the tube in the nares and direct the tube dorsomedial to the alar fold. After the tip has been inserted 1 or 2 cm into the nostril, direct the tube caudoventrally into the esophagus.
3. When the tube is inserted to the premeasured line, infuse a small amount of sterile saline into the tube. If coughing occurs, the tube is probably in the trachea. Remove and reinsert the tube. If no coughing occurs, aspirate the syringe. If air is removed from the tube, the tube could be in the trachea. If negative pressure is evident, the tube is in the esophagus. If fluid is aspirated, the tube is in the stomach. If there is any question of tube location, make a lateral radiograph to determine placement.
4. Move the proximal end of the tube laterally alongside the nares, place a small strip of elastic tape around the tube, and either suture or glue it alongside the nares. The tube may be sutured without tape using a series of hand ties around the tube. Move the tube caudally between the eyes (alongside the dorsal nasal midline) and suture or glue. Cap the end of the tube to prevent air from entering.
5. Apply an Elizabethan collar to prevent the patient from removing the feeding tube (Figure 1). Evaluate the sutures or glue at each feeding to ensure that the tube is stable and not malpositioned.
6. To remove the tube, flush the tube with air to clear fluid out of the tube. Remove the sutures or gently pull the glued tube away from the skin, and pull the tube out of the nose.

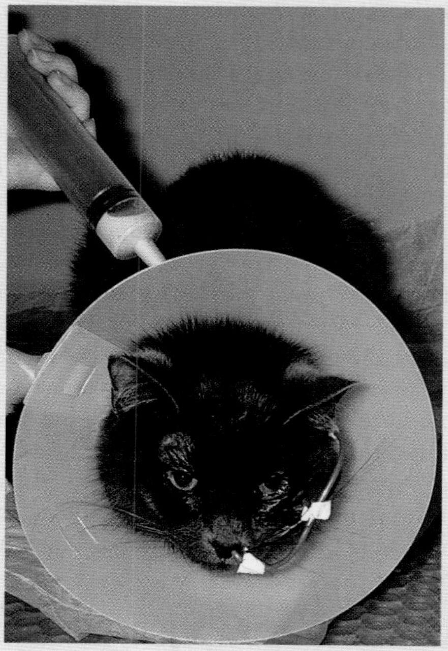

FIGURE 1 Nasoesophageal tube in place in a cat being fed a liquid enteral diet. (From Nelson RW, Couto G: *Small animal internal medicine*, ed 4, St Louis, 2009, Mosby.)

ders, or liver disease. The diet can be easily prepared and administered by the owner, increasing owner compliance. The tube's bulb or mushroom tip helps retain the tube in the desired location (Fig. 23-8). Gastrostomy tubes can be placed with use of endoscopic equipment (i.e., percutaneous endoscopic gastrostomy) or without endoscopic equipment (i.e., blind percutaneous gastrostomy). Placement requires general anesthesia and trained personnel. Additional details on placement of feeding tubes are located in Chapter 24.

ENTERAL NUTRITION DAILY CALORIC REQUIREMENTS

Diet selection is based on caloric density, diameter of the feeding tube, and daily caloric needs of the patient. Each illness is assigned a factor to increase the calculated estimate of the patient's basal energy requirements by 25% to 75%. The volume and consistency of the diet are limited by the size of the animal's stomach and diameter of the feeding tube, but total caloric requirements can usually be delivered when using a calorically dense diet. Stomach volume is approximately 20 ml/kg body weight. Daily water requirement is 12 ml/kg.

Patients with a nasoesophageal or nasogastric tube require a liquid diet (because of small tube diameter). Human enteral feeding products are easily administered through these tubes but are not developed for veterinary patients and may need supplementation with additional nutrients. Hyperosmolar diets can cause diarrhea. Liquid veterinary products are available. Also, canned diets, such as Hill's a/d and Eukanuba Nutritional Recovery Formula, can be delivered through a feeding tube as small as 8-French.

Select the appropriate diet of canned food, and calculate the caloric density (kcal/ml) of the diet based on information on the label or supplied by the manufacturer. The total volume (ml) to be delivered per day is calculated by using the maintenance energy requirement (MER) and caloric density (Box 23-9).

For anorexic patients, after placement of the tube, the volume fed is gradually increased over 3 days, with 5 ml of water administered through the tube every 2 hours for 12 hours. Change to the selected diet, and double the volume to 10 ml every 2 hours for 12 to 24 hours. Gradually increase the volume to achieve full caloric intake, divided into four to six feedings per day, by the third day. For patients with delayed or inadequate gastric emptying, a meal may need to be skipped, or smaller, more frequent feedings administered if too much food remains in the stomach. If the patient vomits, skip the next scheduled feeding and adjust the amount, rate, and frequency of the feeding.

To prepare the diet using canned food, place one can of food in a blender and add enough water to achieve a consis-

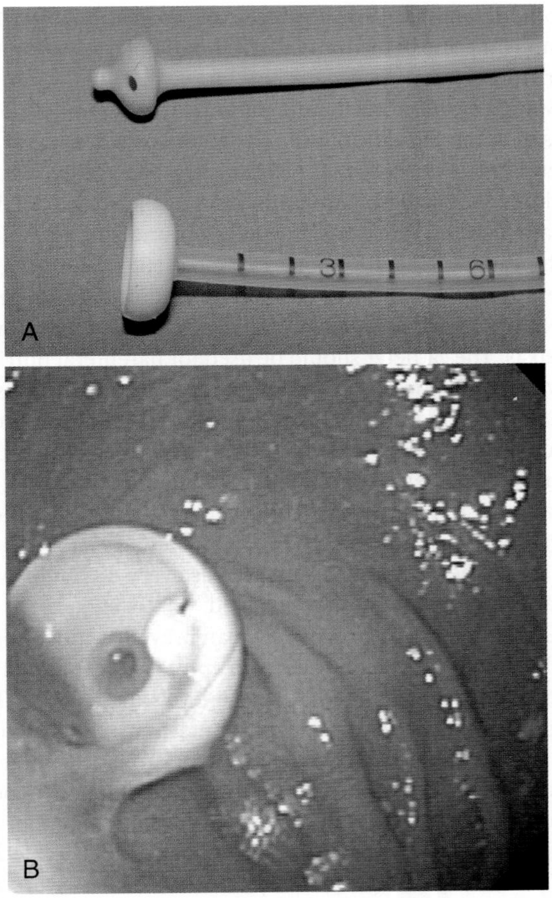

FIGURE 23-8 **A,** Illustration of a typical gastrostomy tube available commercially. **B,** Endoscopic view of the PEG tube in place in the stomach wall. (From August J: *Consultations in feline internal medicine,* vol 5, St Louis, 2006, Saunders.)

BOX 23-9 Enteral Feeding Calculation

- Calculate Resting Energy Requirement (RER):

  RER = 70 × bw (body weight in kg)

- Calculate Illness/Infection/Injury Energy Requirements (IER):

  Factor = 1.2 – 1.5

- Multiply chosen factor by RER to equal IER.
- Choose a veterinary-specific critical care formula.
- Calculate the volume of diet required, and identify amount of kcals per ml:

  IER/Kcals per ml = ml of diet per day

- Calculate the number and volume of feedings:

  ml of diet per day/number of feedings per day = ml diet/feeding

tency that will pass through a large-bore nasogastric tube or a gastrostomy tube. You can also use dry food by allowing the food to soak thoroughly in water before blending. The mixture must be blended well and then strained twice to remove any large chunks that would occlude the feeding tube. All food should be able to pass through a syringe without occluding the tip. For example, one can of Hill's Feline p/d mixed with 340 ml of warm water is of the consistency to pass through the feeding tube; it has a caloric density of 0.8 kcal/ml.

The volume of water added to the canned food when blended is usually adequate for the patient's water requirement. All feedings should be administered slowly, at room temperature. Hill's a/d and Iams Eukanuba Nutritional Recovery Formula can be given straight out of the can through an 8-French feeding tube, at room temperature or slightly warmed, with no premixing with water. The a/d provides 1.2 kcal/ml, and Nutritional Recovery Formula provides 2.1 kcal/ml. If a smaller-diameter tube is used, mixing two 5.5-oz. cans of a/d with 50 ml of water provides a caloric density of 1.0 kcal/ml. Flush the tube with 5 or 10 ml of water after each feeding to prevent tube occlusion.

Animals with feeding tubes in place should be offered fresh food before each feeding once the oral cavity and esophagus can be used. Most animals begin to eat with the feeding tube still in place. When the animal begins to voluntarily eat at least half of its maintenance energy requirement daily, the amount of food given through the feeding tube can be decreased until the patient is consuming its full caloric intake per os. The change from enteral feedings to the normal diet should be gradual over 3 to 5 days if the patient's normal diet is not used for enteral feedings.

Clients can be instructed on how to feed their animal through the tube at home, if necessary. Ease of administration, minimal maintenance, and owner compliance makes this method of nutritional support a viable alternative for patient care in a nonhospital situation.

PARENTERAL NUTRITIONAL SUPPORT

Patients that cannot receive enteral nutrients must be supported by total parenteral nutrition (TPN), which involves intravenous infusion of nutrient solutions. This is a practical alternative for patients that cannot absorb nutrients through the GI tract (e.g., malabsorption), require rest of the GI tract (e.g., vomiting due to severe pancreatitis), cannot swallow (e.g., comatose patients), or are so debilitated that additional nutrition must be administered by another route.

Carbohydrates are administered in the form of dextrose. The most common concentration used is 50% dextrose, which provides 1.7 kcal/ml. Dextrose and lipids each provide 50% of the canine patient's daily MER. Dextrose and lipids are used in a 1:1 ratio to meet the MER.

Gradual introduction of dextrose is necessary to avoid hyperglycemia. On the first day of TPN, only half of the calculated amount of dextrose is administered. If the patient's urine glucose remains negative and the blood glucose level is below 200 mg/dl, the entire calculated dose of dextrose can be administered on day two. Occasionally a patient requires addition of insulin to the TPN solution. This should be added immediately before administration of the parenteral nutrition.

Lipids (including essential fatty acids) provide the fat required by the patient. These are available in 10% and 20%

solutions, with 20% more commonly used. Made of soybean or safflower oil, egg yolk phospholipids, and glycerol, they provide a concentrated energy source that supplies 50% of the patient's energy requirements. Visually checking the patient's plasma for lipemia on a daily basis can help decrease hyperlipidemia. Patients with hepatic, pancreatic, or endocrine disease may develop hyperlipidemia. For patients with severe hyperlipidemia, decrease the rate of infusion or the concentration of the lipids, or discontinue use of lipids altogether.

Proteins are supplied in the form of crystalline amino acids, made of essential and nonessential amino acids, available in a variety of concentrations, with or without electrolytes. The most common concentration used is 8.5% with electrolytes. The basic solutions of amino acids contain all of the essential amino acids required by dogs and cats, except taurine. If TPN is to be continued for longer than 1 week, supplementation of taurine is essential in cats. For patients with renal or hepatic insufficiency, reduced amounts of amino acids or specially formulated amino acid products should be administered.

Electrolytes can be included in the amino acid solutions. This is usually sufficient to maintain a normal electrolyte balance. Hypokalemia is the most common electrolyte abnormality. For patients with ongoing potassium losses (e.g., vomiting), additional supplementation may be necessary. If the patient is in renal failure, amino acids are administered without electrolytes.

Vitamins are administered as a multivitamin supplement. B complex vitamins should be added daily to the feeding solution. Vitamin K is incompatible with parenteral solutions and should be administered by subcutaneous or intramuscular injection only if parenteral nutrition is continued longer than 1 week.

Trace elements only need to be supplemented if long-term (more than 1 week) parenteral nutritional support is needed. Zinc may need to be supplemented after 1 week in patients with GI disease. Phosphorus may be added for diabetics.

The total daily fluid volume for maintenance TPN is 30 ml/lb of body weight. If the total volume of TPN is less than the calculated required amount, add an additional amount of balanced electrolyte solution or sterile water to equal the calculated fluid requirements. If the patient is experiencing ongoing fluid losses, a second catheter or an additional lumen on a central catheter can be used to deliver the fluids.

When mixing the appropriate solutions, strict asepsis is essential. Using a laminar flow hood, an automatic mixing pump, or an "all-in-one" bag will help keep contamination to a minimum. Add the dextrose and amino acids before the lipids to prevent lipid destabilization. Add the water or electrolyte solutions next, and any vitamins last.

Parenteral nutrition is administered via a catheter in the cranial or caudal vena cava. A double-lumen catheter is of benefit if additional medication, fluids, blood products, or blood sampling are needed. Administration by a fluid pump is the most accurate method of delivering parenteral nutrition.

Many complications of parenteral nutrition involve problems with the catheter. Sepsis is another complication of parenteral nutrition. Nutrient solutions are an excellent growth medium for bacteria. Contamination of the solutions, lines, or catheters can cause fever, depression, and pain or swelling at the catheter insertion site. Daily patient monitoring can help eliminate or minimize this complication. Administering TPN through a dedicated IV line can decrease the likelihood of sepsis. The catheter should be used for parenteral nutrition only, and not for blood sampling, medication administration, or CVP monitoring. New bags of TPN solution should be made daily for the patient and hung for a maximum of 24 hours at room temperature before changing to another bag. All administration lines should be changed every 48 hours when the bag is changed. The catheter bandage should be replaced whenever it is soiled, as well as every 48 hours, when the administration lines are changed.

Gradually tapering off of TPN can prevent hypoglycemia. If TPN must be discontinued abruptly, use a 5% dextrose solution to maintain blood glucose levels. Patients on TPN longer than 1 week may develop intestinal villus atrophy. Partial parenteral nutrition in conjunction with enteral nutrition may be advised when parenteral nutrition is being withdrawn. Care must be taken when changing from one diet to another; the transition should be gradual. Table 23-2 summarizes the nutritional requirements of pets with various diseases.

FEEDING CONSIDERATIONS FOR SMALL MAMMALS

Pet rodents can be fed commercial rodent chows or pellets. "Party mix" diets containing seeds and nuts are not recommended. These are high in fat, and many rodents prefer these to the formulated pellets. Seeds and nuts can be offered as an occasional treat (less than 10% of the daily diet). Fresh, well-cleaned vegetables and occasionally a small amount of fruit can be offered as well. Leafy green vegetables (not lettuce or celery) can be offered, as well as yellow and orange vegetables. The total daily amount of these "people foods" should not make up more than 10% of the diet. The diet should consist of 90% commercial pellets, 5% to 10% vegetables and fruits, and a few seeds or nuts as occasional treats. Hay (alfalfa or clover) may be offered free-choice as a source of fiber.

Unlike most other pets, guinea pigs require a dietary source of vitamin C. They should be fed guinea pig chow (pellets), which is supplemented with vitamin C. However, the shelf-life of vitamin C is about 90 days from the time of milling, not from the time of purchase. Therefore, vitamin C should also be supplied in the drinking water. A simple way to do this is to crush a 200-mg vitamin C tablet into powder. Mix the powder in 1 liter of water. This solution should be made fresh daily and used as the pet's drinking water. Fresh

TABLE 23-2 Summary of Small Animal Clinical Nutrition*

OBJECTIVES	CONSIDERATIONS	PRODUCT†	COMMENTS
Allergy, Food			
Dogs			
Reduce antigen ingestion	Novel highly digestible protein source or protein hydrolysate Reduce total protein content Simplify food Distilled H_2O	Prescription Diet Canine d/d or Canine z/d	8- to 10-week trial period Avoid treats, snacks, access to other food sources, chewable medications, supplements
Cats			
Reduce antigen ingestion	Same as dog except Control Mg^{2+} intake Provide taurine Control urine pH	Prescription Diet Feline d/d or Feline z/d	
Anemia			
Support RBC production	↑ Iron, cobalt, and copper ↑ B-complex vitamins ↑ Protein	Prescription Diet Canine p/d Feline p/d	
Anorexia			
Prevent protein/caloric malnutrition Stimulate appetite	Establish fluid/electrolyte balance Acid-base balance ↑ Protein and fat ↑ Micronutrients	Prescription Diet Feline/Canine a/d Canine p/d Feline p/d	Cat foods are suitable for dogs in acute care settings
Ascites			
Reduce fluid retention	Restrict sodium chloride Maintain hydration	Prescription Diet Canine h/d, k/d Feline h/d, k/d	h/d = marked salt restriction k/d = moderate salt restriction
Bone Loss and Fracture Healing			
Correct deficiency of energy and protein	↑ Protein ↑ Energy Avoid supplementation	Prescription Diet Canine p/d Feline p/d	Extra dietary calcium does not increase rate of fracture healing
Cancer			
Increase longevity and quality of life	↓ Soluble carbohydrate ↑ Fat and n-3 fatty acids ↑ Arginine	Prescription Diet Canine n/d Canine/Feline a/d	Use in conjunction with chemotherapy or other forms of cancer therapy
Colitis			
Normalize gastrointestinal motility Rebalance microflora Provide local healing factors	Feed small meals 3-6 times/day Control dietary antigens Vary levels of dietary fiber	Prescription Diet Canine w/d, i/d, d/d Feline w/d, d/d	
Constipation			
Normalize gastrointestinal motility Maintain stool water Maintain stool bulk	>10% fiber	Prescription Diet Canine w/d Feline w/d	No table scraps or bones Increase exercise Encourage water intake Cats: keep litter box clean
Copper Storage Disease			
Restrict copper intake	<1.2 mg copper/100 g dry diet	Prescription Diet Canine i/d	No table scraps or treats
Debilitation			
Restore tissue, plasma, and nutrients	↑ Protein ↑ Fat ↑ Macronutrients and micronutrients	Prescription Diet Canine/Feline a/d	Assist feed if needed

Continued

TABLE 23-2 Summary of Small Animal Clinical Nutrition*—cont'd

OBJECTIVES	CONSIDERATIONS	PRODUCT†	COMMENTS
Developmental Orthopedic Disease			
Reduce rapid growth	↓ Fat and energy density ↓ Calcium	Prescription Diet Canine p/d Large breed	Avoid calcium-phosphorus supplements
Diabetes Mellitus			
Even rate of glucose absorption Consistent caloric intake	>10% fiber ↓ Soluble carbohydrates	Prescription Diet Canine w/d Feline w/d	Weigh animal frequently and note in medical record
Diarrhea, Acute			
Normalize gastrointestinal tract motility and secretion	Withhold food for 1-2 days Feed small amounts 3-6 times/day ↓ Fiber ↓ Sugar ↑ Digestibility	Prescription Diet Canine i/d Feline i/d	Electrolyte disturbances and dehydration are common
Eclampsia			
Provide Ca/P in correct quantity and ratio prepartum	High digestibility of diet Balanced minerals/vitamins	Prescription Diet Canine p/d Feline p/d	Avoid supplementation
Flatulence			
Decrease aerophagia Avoid food fermentation	Avoid milk or milk products Feed small meals 3-6 times/day ↑ Caloric density	Prescription Diet Canine i/d Feline i/d	Feed in a flat, open dish Avoid vitamin or fatty acid supplementation Separate competitive eaters
Gastric Dilatation/Bloat (Postoperative)			
Prevent gastric distension	Avoid exercise before and after feeding ↑ Digestibility of diet Small frequent feedings	Prescription Diet Canine i/d	Diet form or type is *NOT* related to risk of occurrence or recurrence
Heart Failure			
Dogs			
Control Na+ retention	↓ Na^+ intake Maintain energy and protein intake ↑ B-complex vitamins ↓ Na^+ intake	Prescription Diet Canine h/d Canine k/d	Prescription Diet k/d has moderate Na^+ restriction
Cats			
Control Na^+ retention	↑ Taurine Control Mg^{2+} levels	Prescription Diet Feline h/d Feline k/d	Avoid high Na^+ treats and water
Hyperlipidemia			
Control fat intake	↑ Fiber intake ↓ Fat intake	Prescription Diet Canine w/d Feline w/d	Common in Schnauzers Consider fat in treats, table foods, and supplements
Hyperthyroidism (Cats)			
Support increased energy need	↑ Energy intake ↑ Vitamins and minerals ↑ Protein	Prescription Diet Feline a/d	Monitor for evidence of concurrent renal disease
Liver Disease (Fat-Tolerant)			
Reduce protein metabolism Maintain liver glycogen Prevent ammonia toxicity	↑ Digestible energy Protein restriction High biologic value proteins Control Na^+ intake	Prescription Diet Canine l/d Feline l/d	May feed small meals (4-6 times/day)

TABLE 23-2 Summary of Small Animal Clinical Nutrition*—cont'd

OBJECTIVES	CONSIDERATIONS	PRODUCT†	COMMENTS
Lymphangiectasia			
Decrease dietary fat	↓ Intake of long-chain triglycerides Control protein levels Consider medium-chain triglycerides	Prescription Diet Canine w/d or r/d	Medium-chain triglyceride oils and powder can increase caloric density
Obesity			
Maintain intake of all nutrients except energy	↓ Energy digestibility Replace digestible calories with indigestible fiber Increase bulk to control hunger Added carnitine	Prescription Diet Canine r/d Feline r/d	Requires professional advice and teamwork with veterinary technician and client
Oral Disease: Gingivitis (Gum Inflammation), Periodontitis (Loss of Tooth Attachment)			
Control accumulation of plaque, stains, and calculus Maintain gingival health	Food that promotes chewing and mechanical cleansing of teeth	Prescription Diet Canine t/d Feline t/d	Many treats make dental claims but are not effective
Pancreatitis, Acute (Recovery Phase)			
Control pancreas secretions	↓ Fat ↑ Digestibility Feed small meals 3-6 times/day	Prescription Diet Canine i/d Feline i/d	Frequent, small meals
Pancreatic Exocrine Insufficiency			
Reduce requirements for digestive enzymes	↓ Fiber ↓ Fat Highly digestible carbohydrates ↑ Caloric density	Prescription Diet Canine i/d Feline i/d	Pancreatic enzymes complement highly digestible food
Renal Failure			
Reduce signs of uremia Slow progression of disease	↓ Protein (↑ biologic value of protein) ↑ Nonprotein calories ↓ Phosphorus and sodium ↑ B-complex vitamins	Prescription Diet Canine k/d Canine g/d Canine u/d Prescription Diet Feline k/d Feline g/d	Small meals 4-6 times/day Conversion to a protein-restricted diet may take 7-10 days Water available at all times
Canine Urolithiasis (Struvite)			
Treatment			
Urine volume Urine pH Restrict Mg^{2+}, PO_4	↓ Protein ↓ PO_4, Mg^{2+} ↑ Na^+ ↓ Urine pH (5.9-6.1)	Prescription Diet Canine s/d	Evaluate and treat urinary tract infection Average duration of stone dissolution is 36 days; follow up via radiography
Prevention			
Maintain physiologic level of urinary solutes and urine pH	Control protein excess ↓ Ca^{2+}, P, Ma^{2+} ↓ Sodium mildly ↓ Urine pH (6.2-6.4)	Prescription Diet Canine c/d	Monitor urine sediment for crystalluria and infection
Canine Urolithiasis (Ammonium Urate)			
Prevention			
	↓ Protein ↑ Nonprotein calories ↓ Nucleic acids ↓ Ca^{2+}, P, Mg^{2+}, Na^+ Urine pH (6.7-7.0)	Prescription Diet Canine u/d	Drugs plus diet may be successful treatment Monitor urinary crystalluria Prevention may require long-term drug treatment

Continued

TABLE 23-2 Summary of Small Animal Clinical Nutrition*—cont'd

OBJECTIVES	CONSIDERATIONS	PRODUCT†	COMMENTS
Canine Urolithiasis (Calcium Oxalate and Cystine)			
Prevention			
↓ Urinary concentration of calcium oxalate or cystine	↓ Protein ↑ Nonprotein calories ↓ Ca^{2+}, P, Na^{+}, Mg^{2+} ↑ Urine pH (6.1-7.0)	Prescription Diet Canine u/d	Treatment by surgical removal Prevention by dietary management ± drugs
Feline Urolithiasis (Struvite)			
Treatment			
↑ Urine volume ↓ Urine pH (5.9-6.1) Restrict Mg^{2+}, Ca^{2+}, PO_4	↑ Caloric density ↓ P and Ca^{2+} Mg^{2+} >20 mg/100 kcal ↑ Na^{+} Urine pH (6.2-6.4)	Prescription Diet Feline s/d	Dissolution is complete 1 month after negative radiographs Recurrence is high if prevention is not implemented
Prevention			
Maintain physiologic levels of urinary solutes and urine pH	Mg^{2+} >20 mg/100 kcal (0.1% DMB) ↓ P ↑ Caloric density Urine pH (6.2-6.4)	Prescription Diet Feline c/d-s	In obesity, use calorie-restricted diets that maintain urine pH 6.2-6.4 (Prescription Diet w/d is suggested)
Feline Urolithiasis (Calcium Oxalate)			
Prevention			
↑ Urine volume ↓ Urinary Ca^{2+}, oxalate ↑ Urine pH	↓ Protein ↑ Nonprotein calories ↓ P, Ca^{2+}, Na^{+} Mg^{2+} <20 mg/100 kcal	Prescription Diet Feline c/d-oxl	Monitor urinary crystalluria
Vomiting			
Minimize gastric secretion Gastrointestinal rest	↑ Digestibility ↑ Caloric density	Prescription Diet Canine i/d Feline i/d	Frequent, small meals

*Nutrients in table are expressed on a dry weight basis.
†Other North American therapeutic brands with wide distribution include CNM (Purina), VMD, Medi-Cal, and IVD Select Care (Heinz), Eukanuba Veterinary Diets (Iams), and Waltham Veterinary Diets (Mars).
Ca, Calcium; DMB, dry matter basis; Mg, magnesium; Na, sodium; P, phosphorus; PO, phosphate; RBC, red blood cells.

green vegetables (broccoli, cabbage, bok choy) can also be used to supply vitamin C.

> **TECHNICIAN NOTE** Guinea pigs require a dietary source of vitamin C.

Rabbits should be fed mainly free-choice hay. Alfalfa hay can be offered in small amounts, but it is too rich to be the sole source of fiber. Timothy grass or clover hay are better choices. Commercial pelleted feed should be offered each day at no more than ¼ cup per 5 pounds of body weight. The increased fiber helps prevent diarrhea and formation of trichobezoars (hairballs).

Ferrets can be fed commercial kitten food or cat food, or specially formulated ferret diets. As with dogs and cats, periodontal disease is common in ferrets. A dry diet can help reduce tartar accumulation.

FEEDING CONSIDERATIONS FOR REPTILES AND AMPHIBIANS

The subject of feeding reptiles and amphibians is vast and beyond the scope of this chapter. However, it is important to understand the dietary needs of reptiles, especially because improper diet is a common cause of many diseases in pet reptiles. This section discusses the general dietary needs of common pet reptiles and amphibians.

IGUANAS

Regardless of what pet store clerks tell clients, iguanas are herbivorous. This means that a major portion of the diet must be plant material. There is some controversy among veterinarians as to whether it is acceptable to feed iguanas small amounts of animal protein, such as crickets, moths, or worms. Most veterinarians would probably agree that limiting these animal protein sources to no more than 10% of the diet is safe, although the iguana may not even require these foods (and some iguanas will not eat them).

Most of an iguana's diet should consist of flowers (and leaves), such as roses, hibiscus, carnations, and mums, and green leafy vegetables (not celery and iceberg lettuce, which are low in nutritional value). A small amount of fruits can also be offered. Commercial dog and cat foods are too high in protein and vitamin D and are not recommended. Vegetable and flower "salad" should be chopped into pieces suitable for the iguana's size and offered fresh daily or every other day. A light dusting of calcium powder (daily) and vitamin powder (weekly) is often recommended. Fresh water should be available at all times. Metabolic bone disease is common in green iguanas and results from a deficiency of dietary calcium, such as when only lettuce and fruit or lettuce and crickets are fed.

SNAKES

Most species of snakes are carnivorous and eat whole prey. Suitable prey items include rats, mice, hamsters, and gerbils. Some species prefer one type of rodent, so it is wise to check reference texts regarding the snake species in question. To prevent injury or death of the snake, it is best to feed killed prey, either freshly killed (or stunned) or thawed frozen prey. If the snake will eat only live prey, the owner must observe the snake after feeding it the prey. If the snake has not killed and eaten the prey within 15 minutes, the prey should be removed and the snake fed at a later time.

BOX TURTLES

Like iguanas, box turtles eat a large amount of plant material; like snakes, they also eat animal protein. As a rule, the diet should consist of about 50% plant material (similar to that for the iguana; hay can also be offered) and 50% animal protein. This can include commercial turtle pellets, tofu, sardines, crickets, or worms. Vitamin A deficiency commonly results when turtles are offered only lettuce and fruit or lettuce and crickets. A proper diet helps prevent this common disorder. As with iguanas, a light daily sprinkling of calcium and weekly sprinkling of vitamins can help supplement the diet of box turtles.

AMPHIBIANS

Most amphibians are carnivorous as adults. Improper diet, such as a diet consisting of only crickets, can cause nutritional problems, such as metabolic bone disease. An improper diet, such as one consisting entirely of dog or cat food, may cause the opposite problem and lead to hypervitaminosis D or gout. Reference texts should be consulted regarding the proper diet for the species of amphibian in question.

FEEDING CONSIDERATIONS FOR LABORATORY ANIMALS

Animals should be fed a clean, wholesome, and nutritious diet **ad libitum.** It is important to feed a balanced diet, freshly milled, formulated for that particular species. In most instances the food should be placed in a feeder hung in the animal's cage. This prevents soiling of the food with urine and feces, keeping it dry and clean. If vegetables or fruit are offered to supplement the diet, they should be fresh and washed before feeding them. Any uneaten vegetables or fruits should be removed daily. Animals should have access to fresh water via an automatic watering system or water bottles with sipper tubes.

NUTRITION OF LIVESTOCK

Livestock species (cattle, horses, pigs, sheep, goats) require certain essential nutrients to meet metabolic and physiologic needs. Essential nutrients include water, energy, amino acids (proteins), fatty acids, minerals, and vitamins; these are discussed in the first part of this chapter.

There is a unique feature to protein nutrition in ruminants (cattle, sheep, goats). As a result of their pregastric fermentation system, nonprotein nitrogen (e.g., urea), in addition to rumen-degradable dietary protein, can be used by the resident microbes as a nitrogen source of synthesis of microbial proteins. Microbial protein then passes into the abomasum (true stomach) and is digested like any other dietary protein. Microbial protein can account for a significant amount of dietary protein in ruminants.

Dietary fiber is required to maintain adequate gastrointestinal function in herbivores (plant-eating animals) with active microbial fermentation chambers. These include ruminants and hind gut fermenting animals (horses). Therefore, gastrointestinal anatomy has a very critical role in the animal's ability to derive essential nutrients from the feedstuffs available. Domestic livestock extract essential nutrients from plant materials. The plant material consumed by livestock species contains cellulose, hemicellulose, pectin, and lignin compounds that are indigestible by people and carnivorous predators. Microbes within the gut use these plant compounds, and the animal uses the end products of microbial fermentation. Animals have evolved in many ways to take advantage of microbial fermentation in their digestive process.

The alimentary tract includes the mouth and associated structures, esophagus, stomach, small intestine, cecum, and colon (large intestine). The rumen of cattle, sheep, and goats functions as a pregastric fermentation vat (Fig. 23-9). This allows ruminants to efficiently derive nutrients from plant material. In hind gut fermenters, such as horses, a greatly enlarged colon serves as a fermentation vat. These animals can also digest plant material, but not to the same extent as ruminants. As a result of differences in their anatomy, ruminants digest prefermented feed material, whereas hind gut herbivores ferment predigested feed material. Pigs are considered omnivores, which means that they can digest materials of both plant and animal origin, although they are primarily fed less bulky plant materials. Pigs have some microbial fermentation capacity in their enlarged, sacculated colon, but not to the extent of hind gut fermenters or ruminants.

FEEDSTUFFS

A **feedstuff** is any dietary component that provides some essential nutrient or serves some other function. Nonnutritive feedstuffs may provide bulk, flavor, odor, or color, or act as an antioxidant to protect other dietary components. More than 2000 different feedstuffs have been fed to domestic livestock throughout the world. The variety of feedstuffs available for use in a given geographic area depends on the crops grown locally. Potential feedstuffs must be matched with the appropriate livestock species, based on nutrient requirements and gastrointestinal tract capabilities. Feedstuffs may be divided into a number of categories, based on their source and nutrient concentration. General categories include forages (roughages), concentrates, byproducts, mineral and vitamin supplements, and nonnutritive additives.

Forages are feeds made up of most or all of the plant. Forages generally have large amounts of fiber, low energy density, and high bulk (low weight per unit volume). This is a direct result of the amount of plant cell wall material present. Plant cell walls are composed of cellulose, hemicelluose, lignin, and other compounds. A forager's protein content depends on the type of plant and stage at harvesting. For example, alfalfa hay has much higher protein levels than grass hays at a comparable stage of plant growth. Within plant species, there is an increase in fiber content and a decrease in protein content, energy content, and overall digestibility with advancing maturity of the plant. The decrease in digestibility with maturity is because of increasing **lignin** content of the plant. Lignin is an inert compound that increases rigidity of the plant cell wall. Straw represents the most mature and indigestible form of forages.

Forages fed to livestock belong to either the legume or grass plant families. Legumes commonly used for forage production include alfalfa, red and white clover, bird's foot trefoil, and vetch. Grasses offer more variety for forage production and include Bahia grass, Bermuda grass, bluegrass, bromegrass, fescue, timothy, orchard grass, reed canary grass, ryegrass, and Sudan grass. Other grass forages that can be used for cereal grain production include corn, wheat, rye, oats, and sorghum. Of these, corn is the most important forage and cereal grain product grown for livestock.

Forage products are harvested and stored for livestock feeding purposes in a number of ways. Livestock may graze grasses, legumes, and other broadleaf vegetation (forbs and browse). Allowing livestock to harvest forage avoids costs incurred in mechanical harvesting and storage. However, forage quality and quantity can be extremely variable, depending on plant maturity and environmental conditions. A more controlled method of grazing called intensive rotational grazing is being adopted. In this method, animals are allowed to graze restricted areas of forage for limited periods and are then moved to another area; the forage in the grazed area is allowed to regrow until the animals are returned for grazing. With highly managed rotational grazing, forage quality can be maintained at a very high level.

Forage crops can also be mechanically harvested, stored, and fed using various methods. Green chop or **spoilage** represents forage harvested at a given stage of development and fed directly. Green chop contains a high water content (75% to 85%) and available nutrients; however, it must be harvested daily to avoid rapid deterioration with storage.

Ensiling is a harvesting process by which forage is chopped and placed into a storage unit (e.g., silo), which excludes oxygen. As the forage ferments, lactic acid is produced and the pH decreases. This effectively "pickles" the forage to a partially fermented state called **silage.** Good-quality silage can be stored indefinitely in upright silos, bunker silos, or

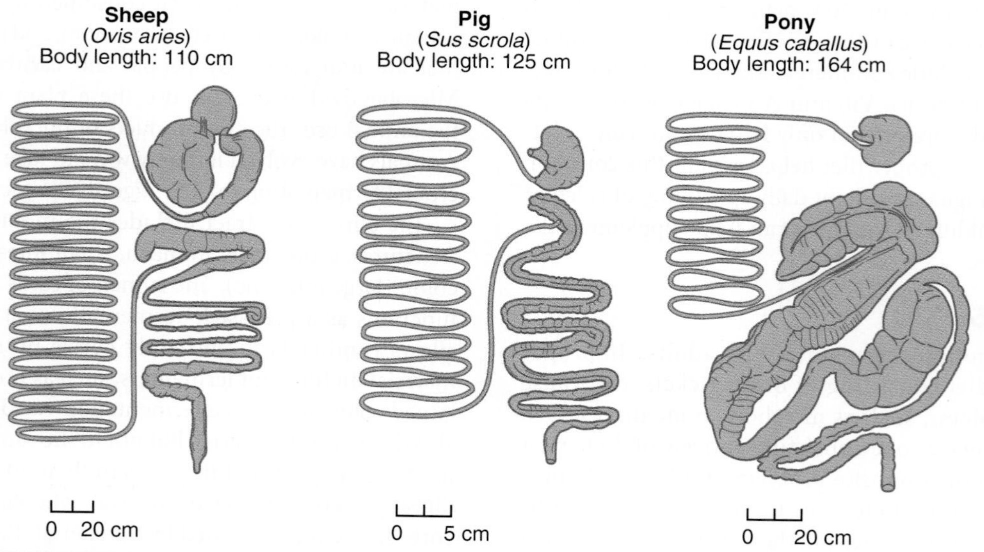

FIGURE 23-9 Schematic diagrams comparing the gastrointestinal tract of ruminants (sheep), pigs, and horses.

plastic bags, the important feature being exclusion of oxygen. Silage has an intermediate water content (55% to 75%) and has the least loss of nutrients from harvesting and storage. Grass, legume, and corn silages are the most common ensiled forages fed to livestock.

Hay is forage that is cut and allowed to dry before being collected into bales for storage. Hay should have less than 15% water to be stable in storage. Harvesting losses are high in hay making, but storage losses are usually minimal if it is properly dried.

> **TECHNICIAN NOTE** Feedstuff types include forages (roughages), concentrates, byproducts, mineral and vitamin supplements, and nonnutritive additives.

Concentrates are generally low in fiber and high in energy and/or protein. Cereal grains, such as barley, corn, millet, oats, rye, sorghum, and wheat, are the seeds of many of the grass species. Corn is the most common grain fed to livestock and the standard with which others are compared. Cereal grains contain large amounts of energy in the form of starch and are added to diets to increase energy density. Other feed products used as energy concentrates include molasses, root crops (e.g., turnips, beets, carrots), and potatoes. Fats and oils of plant or animal origin contain 2.25 times the energy density of carbohydrates and are also used as energy concentrates.

Concentrate feeds that contain more than 20% crude protein are subclassified as protein supplements. Protein supplements may be of plant or animal origin, including marine fish. Plant-based protein products are derived from oilseed crops, such as soybean, canola, cottonseed, sunflower, and peanut seed meals. Of these, soybean meal is by far the most common oilseed meal fed to livestock. Oil from the seeds is harvested for a variety of industrial and nutritional uses; the remaining seed contains more than 40% crude protein. Animal-based protein supplements are derived from rendered animal or fish tissues or from dried-milk products. Animal proteins generally range from more than 50% crude protein to 90% crude protein. As compared with plant-based protein sources, animal protein sources have a better amino acid composition relative to requirements. However, there is much variability in the quality of animal-based products and the way in which they are manufactured.

Byproduct feeds are residues of the feed-processing industry and span a wide array of feedstuffs. Examples of byproduct feeds include sugar beet pulp, bakery waste, blood, bone meal, brewer's grains, tallow, and whey. Many byproduct feeds contain substantial amounts of fermentable fiber, energy, and protein.

Mineral and vitamin supplements are sources of individual or combination of minerals, with or without vitamins. Fat-soluble vitamins are supplemented primarily in the form of premixes. Fat-soluble vitamins are sensitive to oxidation, sunlight, heat, and fungal growth. Certain water-soluble vitamins may be supplemented in swine and horse diets; they are not routinely supplemented in ruminant diets. Yeast cultures are good sources of B complex vitamins and are commonly added to livestock diets.

Nonnutritive feed additives can include buffers, hormones, binders, and medications. Feed medications may include antibiotics, antifungals, anthelmintics, antiparasitics, and ionophores (antibiotics with growth-promoting effects). Their use is regulated by the Food and Drug Administration in an effort to prevent tissue residues (see Chapter 11). Nonnutritive additives are used to stimulate animal performance, improve feed efficiency, and improve animal health or metabolic status.

FEED ANALYSIS

Different classes of feedstuffs contribute variable amounts of the essential nutrients (Table 23-3). Even within cer-

TABLE 23-3 Relative Nutrient Content of Various Feedstuffs for Livestock

	RELATIVE NUTRIENT CONTENT						
FEEDSTUFF GROUP	PROTEIN	ENERGY	MINERALS		VITAMINS		FIBER
			MACRO	MICRO	FAT-SOL	B-COMPLEX	
High-quality roughage	+++	++	++	++	+++	+	+++
Low-quality roughage	+	+	+	+	—	—	++++
Cereal grains	++	+++	+	+	+	+	+
Grain mill feeds	++	++	++	++	+	++	++
Fats and oils	—	++++	—	—	—	—	—
Molasses	+	+++	++	++	—	+	—
Fermentation products	+++	++	+	++	—	++++	±
Oil seed proteins	++++	+++	++	++	+	++	+
Animal proteins	++++	+++	+++	+++	++	+++	+

+ to ++++: low to very high content.
±: may or may not be present in significant amounts.
—: not present.

tain feed groups, such as forages, nutrient composition can vary tremendously. **Feed analysis** is a procedure by which chemical analysis determines the proportion of specific components of a feedstuff. The **proximate analysis** includes determinations of dry matter (DM), crude protein (CP), ether extract (EE, crude fat), crude fiber (CF), and ash. The nonfiber carbohydrate portion of the feed, termed **nitrogen-free extract (NFE),** is determined using the equation 100 minus (CP% + CF% + moisture% + ash%). More recently crude fiber analysis has been replaced with neutral and acid detergent fiber analysis, improving our estimate of cell wall components and their availability. Feed analysis should be routinely completed in any nutritional diagnostic problem.

FEEDING MANAGEMENT OF LIVESTOCK

The goal of any livestock feeding management program is to provide sufficient daily amounts of the essential nutrients for optimal (cost-effective) productivity. Because feed costs account for the greatest amount of total production costs in the livestock industry, we must minimize feed costs to ensure profitability. Byproduct feeds are so widely used when available, because they usually are of lower cost.

DAIRY CATTLE

Dairy cattle are segregated and housed by production stages and fed according to specific nutrient requirements. Typical feeding groups on a dairy farm include milk-fed calves, growing replacement heifers, nonlactating pregnant cows (dry cows), and lactation groups. Lactation groups are usually based on level of milk production, parity (first lactation vs. older cows), days in milk, or a combination of these factors.

Feeding systems and housing facilities vary among dairy farms, depending on prevailing environmental conditions. Smaller family dairies with fewer than 100 cows generally have individual tie stalls, and cows are fed individually. The amount of forage and concentrates are fed according to production level and body condition score (Table 23-4). These farms are predominantly found in the northeastern and midwestern United States as a result of the cold winters. In larger dairies cows are generally housed in free-stall barns or in open drylots, depending on environmental conditions. Drylots are found primarily in the southern and western United States, whereas free-stall barns are found anywhere in the United States. In larger dairy management systems, cattle are fed in groups at a common feedbunk, rather than individually. Feedbunks may be located within the free-stall facility or along one side of the drylot.

Although feeding management of dairy cattle depends on the type of facility available, there are some options as to how feed is delivered to the animals. Forage (hay, silage) may be fed separately from concentrates in any of the feeding management systems described. Concentrates may be fed separately in the milking parlor or from computerized feeders. Parlor grain feeding and computerized feeding are becoming more common with current interest in pasture-grazing management systems. In large dairies, the most common method of feed delivery is by total mixed ration (TMR). In this system, all individual feed ingredients are mechanically mixed in a feed wagon and presented as a single mixture to the cows. This allows cows to consume the same blend of nutrients in each bite and minimizes selectivity. Some dairies feed what might be termed a partial TMR in that dry hay is fed separate from the rest of the diet.

BEEF CATTLE

Beef cattle management can be divided into cow-calf and cattle feeding (feedlot) operations. Cow-calf enterprises produce calves that enter the breeding herd or are sent to cattle-feeding operations (feedlots). Forage use is the basis of cow-calf enterprises. Feed costs account for more than 60% of production costs and therefore must be minimized.

TABLE 23-4 Body Condition Scoring Classifications for Livestock

BODY CONDITION SCORING SCALE*		GENERALIZED ANIMAL DESCRIPTION†
1.0	1	*Emaciated.* All bones obviously protruding; no subcutaneous fat evident
1.5	2	*Very thin.* Bones visible and easily palpated; minimal subcutaneous fat
2.0	3	*Thin.* Thin, flat musculature; prominent ribs, pelvic bones, and spinal processes
2.5	4	*Moderately thin.* Minimal subcutaneous fat; individual ribs not obvious
3.0	5	*Moderate.* Smooth musculature; bones not visible but palpable
3.5	6	*Moderately fleshy.* Fat palpable; soft fat over ribs and covering pelvis
4.0	7	*Fleshy.* Fat visible; ribs barely visible; spinal processes buried in fat
4.5	8	*Fat.* Thick neck; ribs difficult to palpate; rounded appearance to pelvis
5.0	9	*Grossly obese.* Bulging fat all over; patchy fat pads around tailhead

*The body condition scoring scale used depends on the species. Dairy cattle, sheep, pigs, and goats are typically scored on a scale of 1 to 5, whereas beef cattle and horses are scored on a scale of 1 to 9.

†When determining body condition score, evaluate for the presence or absence of fatty tissue over the neck, ribs, spine, and pelvis, independent of animal body weight and frame size.

Cows are allowed to graze pasture or range land, depending on availability, and then are supplemented with energy, protein, and vitamin-mineral supplements as necessary to meet specific nutritional requirements. Depending on geographic location and season, pasture grazing may be replaced with feeding of dry hay or silage. Supplementation programs depend on prevailing forage quality relative to nutrient requirements of the various production units. Cow-calf operations may have feeding groups for bulls, replacement heifers, growing calves, maintenance, and pregnant or lactating cattle.

Cattle-feeding enterprises involve feeding calves from weaning to slaughter and include backgrounding, stocker, and feedlot systems. In backgrounding and stocker feeding systems, weanling calves are placed on low-cost pasture and supplementation feeding programs to gain weight at a moderate rate and then sold to feedlot operations. The goal of a feedlot enterprise is to maximize rate of gain and feed conversion efficiency for the lowest cost. New arrivals at the feedlot are initially fed a high-forage, low-concentrate diet to acclimate the animal to the operation. The proportion of forage is gradually reduced and concentrate increased to facilitate the desired rate of gain. To minimize feeding costs, a wide variety of byproduct feeds and grain products is fed. To ensure animal health with high-grain feeding, ionophores, buffers, and antimicrobial agents are incorporated into the feedlot diet. Generally, the feedlot diet is fed as a TMR similar to the method for dairy cattle.

NUTRITION IN THE DEBILITATED CALF

Feeding Colostrum

Because calves are born essentially **agammaglobulinemic** (without immunoglobulins), provision of colostrum shortly after birth is critically important for the calf to obtain passive maternal antibodies. As a rule of thumb, beef calves should be fed all of the dam's first-milking colostrum as soon as they develop a suckle reflex. If dairy cow colostrum is used, be sure that the colostrum is of sufficient quality. The quality of colostrum is a rough measure of the concentration of immunoglobulin. This is most easily determined by use of a **colostrometer,** a simple tool that measures the specific gravity of the colostrum.

Dairy cows produce much more colostrum than beef cows do, but generally the quality and the concentration of immunoglobulin is lower. As a rule of thumb, if calves are provided with dairy cow colostrum, it can be administered orally at 10% of body weight over the first 24 hours of life. Absorption of maternal colostral immunoglobulin by the calf's intestine usually begins to decrease after the first feeding of colostrum or at about 8 hours of age. Therefore it is important that the first feeding of colostrum is usually of fairly large magnitude. If the calf has a vigorous suckle reflex, allow the calf to nurse all of the dam's colostrum that it will consume. If more colostrum is available, continue to feed it throughout the first 24 hours, offering it at 2-hour intervals and allowing the calf to suckle. If the calf does not have a suckle reflex, continue to offer the colostrum frequently, looking for development of a suckle reflex up to about 6 hours of age. If the calf has not developed a suckle response at that time, intubate the calf and give all of the colostrum from a beef cow or 5% of the calf's body weight in colostrum from a dairy cow.

For administration of colostrum or milk, allowing the calf to suckle versus intubating is an important question. If the calf has already been nursing the dam and is presented for treatment beyond the first several days of age, it is common for the calf to refuse a rubber nipple feeder. It may be worthwhile to reintroduce the calf to the dam because it may then suckle the dam quite readily. On the other hand, if it is a newborn calf that has not yet suckled the dam, it will usually suckle from a nipple feeder as readily as from the dam's teats.

Development of a suckle reflex is a very important indicator of the calf's status. Calves with a variety of problems, including hypoxemia, hypoglycemia, hypothermia, or acidosis resulting from dystocia, frequently do not develop the reflex until these problems are corrected. Therefore lack of a suckle reflex is a good indicator of one or more of these problems. In some cases if these problems are present, the calf may not absorb immunoglobulin, even if colostrum is provided via intubation.

Development of a suckle reflex usually suggests improvement in an underlying condition. Further, when other problems are present, the calf's gastrointestinal tract may not be fully functional. Therefore repeated intubation of newborn calves or calves of older ages suffering from similar problems may result in large accumulations of fluid in the forestomachs or abomasum. If you resort to intubation to supply the calf with oral fluids or milk, carefully monitor the calf for fecal production and palpate its abdomen, looking for evidence that the fluid administered is sequestering in the gastrointestinal tract, rather than proceeding on through and being absorbed. If the calf will not suckle and there is evidence that fluid has accumulated in the gastrointestinal tract, continue to offer fluids frequently via nipple feeder but discontinue orogastric intubation.

Stimulation of the calf to develop a suckle reflex is another important function of the dam. Most calves are very responsive to stroking or rubbing along the back, especially near the tailhead. If the calf is not suckling well, such rubbing stimulation can often provide very rewarding results. If the calf has been sleeping or is compromised by one of the aforementioned problems, it may require several minutes before the calf begins to suckle. Therefore it is worthwhile to repeatedly introduce the nipple into the calf's mouth and try to deliver a small amount of milk before giving up and assuming the calf does not have a suckle reflex.

Newborn ruminants, such as calves and lambs, essentially function as monogastric animals while they are nursing. Fermentation of the swallowed milk in the rumen and reticulum would likely result in digestive upsets. Closure of a structure called the esophageal groove enables the swallowed milk to bypass the rumen and reticulum, and pass directly into the omasum and abomasum. Closure of the groove is stimulated by the act of nursing, and by the presence of milk. When the maturing animal begins eating solid foods, the groove does not close, and the swallowed food enters the rumen and reticulum for microbial fermentation, as in adult animals.

Feeding Milk

Beyond colostral feeding, provision of milk as nutrition is obviously of critical importance. Although dairy calves are often raised with the provision of only 10% of body weight per day as fluid milk, this practice should not be mistakenly construed as providing optimal nutrition. The strategy of providing 10% of body weight per day is geared to enhancing intake of solid feeds so that dairy calves can be weaned at an early age. Most calves, if given the opportunity, freely consume between 20% and 30% of their body weight in milk per day. Although sick calves may not have a very hearty appetite, a recovering calf or premature calf commonly has an exaggerated appetite. For these reasons provide a calf with up to 3% of its body weight per feeding and offer milk feedings at approximately 2-hour intervals. With this regimen some calves consume more than 30% of their body weight in milk per day.

Feeding Electrolytes

For calves with fluid loss because of neonatal enteritis, oral electrolyte solutions are commonly offered as a means to provide additional fluid therapy. Calves with mild to moderate dehydration may respond adequately with only oral fluid supplementation, whereas calves with severe dehydration require intravenous fluid support. It has been a common practice to withhold milk from calves with enteritis. You do not have to hold to that practice, but rather offer milk via nipple feeder if the calf will accept it. Because milk alone will not provide the electrolytes that have been lost through the gastrointestinal tract, provide oral electrolyte solutions at alternate feedings with the milk. The electrolyte fluids and milk or milk replacer should not be mixed, because this adversely influences normal milk digestion. Offer milk at 2% to 3% of body weight maximum, alternating with oral fluid feedings offered at 5% of body weight per feeding, with the alternate feedings at 2-hour intervals. Many calves refuse the milk feedings but eagerly suckle the electrolyte. With this regimen even when calves do refuse the milk, they can be provided as much as 30% of body weight per day in additional oral electrolyte fluids.

HORSES

Horse feeding management is primarily designed to meet the nutritional requirements of individual horses. Although horses are not ruminants, they require a substantial amount of dietary fiber, in the form of forage, to maintain a healthy digestive tract. Forages fed to horses are primarily hay and pasture. Silage is not commonly fed to horses because of their sensitivity to the molds and mycotoxins potentially found in silage. Many varieties of grasses and legumes can be suitable forages for horses. The need for energy, protein, and mineral-vitamin supplementation depends on forage quality and nutrient requirements of the horse. Corn, barley, and oats are common grain supplements fed to horses for added energy. Recently, fat supplementation has been advocated to provide energy for growing, lactating, and working horses. Protein sources such as linseed, canola, and soybean meal are commonly used. Byproducts containing fermentable fiber, such as rice bran and beet pulp, are becoming more popular.

Many commercial horse feeds are available to horse owners. These range from complete feeds (no supplementation required) to specific vitamin-mineral supplements. Various grain supplements containing energy, protein, minerals, and vitamins are available. These commercial grain supplements may be formulated specifically for growing foals, lactating mares, or geriatric horses, or they may be more generic in purpose. Horse owners should match the concentrate to their forage relative to energy, protein, mineral, and vitamin requirements. A proper horse-feeding program would provide adequate amounts of water and provide sufficient energy to achieve and maintain proper body condition. The diet must then be balanced for protein, minerals, and vitamins according to the National Research Council recommendations. Appropriate dental care and parasite management programs should accompany all horse-feeding systems.

Feeding and Watering Hospitalized Horses

Hospitalized horses often have special dietary needs. Their diseases can often create a catabolic state. The horse may require extra calories to maintain its weight. Horses that can chew and swallow normally should be fed their usual diet if their disease permits. Good-quality alfalfa or grass hay, such as timothy hay, can be fed. Good-quality oat hay is also a suitable feed. Horses with gastrointestinal disturbances, such as colic or diarrhea, need special consideration. Horses recovering from impactions may need more laxative feeds, such as alfalfa hay, grass pasture, and even bran mashes. Horses with diarrhea or those that have been operated on for colic may benefit from a diet that is not so rich, such as timothy or oat hay. Hay pellets or cubes that contain alfalfa or a mixture of alfalfa and Bermuda or oat hay can also be used. If added carbohydrate is needed, a pelleted feed that also contains grains may be fed.

Pelleted feed produces less dust and may be better for horses recovering from respiratory allergies or pneumonia. Horses recovering from gastrointestinal ulceration may also need to be fed a pelleted ration, because the increased fiber and stem in hay may irritate and exacerbate certain kinds of ulcers. Pellets soaked to make gruel can be fed to horses with oral lesions, facial fractures, dental problems, or recurrent episodes of choke. Feed softened in this manner is easier for the animal to chew and swallow. Horses with neuromuscular disorders, such as botulism, may be unable to chew and swallow normally. A pelleted ration that has been soaked may be the only feed the animal can eat.

Fresh water should always be available. Some horses may not know how to use an automatic waterer if it requires the horse to push on a lever to fill the water cup. Water buckets or tubs should always be provided in these cases. Salt may need to be provided topically on the feed or in the form of a salt lick during hot weather, or for horses that have diseases that create a sodium deficiency, such as colitis.

PIGS

Pig feeding management is similar to beef cattle management in that there are breeding-farrowing (reproductive) and growing enterprises. The farrowing unit produces baby pigs as reproductive replacements or to enter the growing unit for feeding to slaughter weight. The pig industry is one of the most intensively managed agricultural enterprises. Current pig production units are moving to total confinement farrow-to-finish operations containing many animals. Within these operations, feeding groups are segregated according to nutrient requirements, with diets for lactating and gestating sows and gilts, boars, nursery pigs, and growing pigs. For the most part, animals in the farrowing unit are housed and fed as individuals to better control body weight and condition. Within the feeding operation, starting with the nursery pigs, all animals are group-housed and fed according to age and moved between groups as an entire unit.

As omnivores, pigs have a digestive tract that can accommodate a certain level of dietary fiber. Given the economics of rate of gain from forages versus grains, pig diets consist primarily of concentrates, along with energy, protein, mineral, and vitamin supplements. All feed ingredients are thoroughly mixed and provided as a single diet, like the TMR for cattle. Dietary ingredients depend on the nutritional requirements of the specific group of animals being fed. The classic pig diet consists of corn grain and soybean meal, with a vitamin-mineral premix. Learning more about the specific nutrient requirements of pigs has resulted in more sophisticated diets for pigs. Crystalline amino acids, high-quality animal byproduct protein meals, fiber sources, and vitamin-mineral supplements have been incorporated into specific pig diets to improve growth efficiency.

> *TECHNICIAN NOTE* Pig diets consist primarily of concentrates, along with energy, protein, mineral, and vitamin supplements.

SHEEP

Sheep are managed similarly to beef cattle in that there are reproductive and lamb-growing enterprises. Sheep are raised under a wide variety of conditions, ranging from large flocks on western rangelands to small flocks in confinement. The basis of any sheep production system is forage. The advantage of feeding sheep is their ability to selectively graze. This allows sheep to consume a diet of higher nutritional value than the quality of the total forage. A variety of forage types including harvested and stored forages can be used for feeding sheep. As ruminants, sheep can also use a wide variety of byproduct feeds efficiently.

For the most part, sheep diets consist of vitamin-mineral supplements added to the base forage. The composition of the vitamin-mineral supplement depends on the forage. Grazing sheep are provided with minerals as a block (salt lick) or loose from a feeder. Additional energy and protein supplementation may be used for late gestation, lactation, and growing diets. A wide variety of feed sources may be used, with cost being of primary concern. These supplements may be top-dressed on (spread on top of) the forage or fed by themselves in a feed bunk. Commercial concentrate pellets are also available for ewes and growing lamb diets. Growing lambs may be sent to slaughter directly from grazing high-quality forage or after feeding in a feedlot. Lamb feedlots are similar in organization and feeding practices to beef feedlots. Lambs are acclimated from a high-forage to high-concentrate TMR diet to increase grain and feed efficiency.

GOATS

Goats are managed similarly to dairy cattle because of their milk production. However, some breeds of goats are primarily used for mohair (wool) or meat production. Forage is the primary component of goat-feeding programs. Like sheep, goats can selectively graze the more nutritious parts of plants. Goats raised for mohair and meat are managed with grazing or browsing rangeland or pasture and appropriate energy and protein supplementation when necessary. Dairy goats are managed more intensively because of their higher nutritional requirements for milk production.

Dairy goats are usually housed in smaller areas and fed stored forages, such as dry hay. Pasture grazing alone cannot support milk production, so supplements are necessary. The energy and protein feed supplements for goats are similar to those of dairy cattle. Many commercial concentrate products used for horses, sheep, and dairy cattle can also be fed to goats. The amount and nutrient composition of the supplement depend on the nutrient requirements of the animal being fed and on forage quality. Lactating goats require substantial energy supplementation and should be fed the highest-quality forages. Supplements may be top-dressed on forage in a feedbunk or provided in the milking parlor.

LIVESTOCK CLINICAL NUTRITION

A basic understanding of nutrition can be applied to medical management of livestock. The most important part of clinical nutrition is obtaining an appropriate nutritional history. This is used to determine the potential role of nutrition in a medical problem. Questions one should ask in obtaining a nutritional history are outlined in Table 23-5.

Following the history taking, assess the nutritional status of the animal through physical assessment and via blood chemistry determinations. Physical assessment of the animal involves obtaining an accurate body weight, height measure-

TABLE 23-5 Nutritional History in Livestock (Specific Information Depends on the Species of Livestock)

GENERAL CATEGORIES OF INFORMATION	SPECIFIC INFORMATION
Identify the people involved	Names and telephone numbers of the owner, herdsman, veterinarian, nutritionist, others
Owner's primary concern	Pertaining to the presenting problem
Historical information about the agribusiness.	Ask questions relating to years of ownership, number of hired hands, new animal purchases, acreage, other farms, etc.
Herd information	Function, breeds, average weights, and age distribution of animals on the farm
Production information	Level of performance (milk production, weaning weights, litter size, etc.) in the herd over time; use production record systems if available
Housing facilities	Type of housing, stall surfaces, and bedding used for each group of animals; adequacy of ventilation
Feeding system	Feed storage facilities, feeding system used, feed and water availability, bunk space per animal, number of times fed per day, etc.
Dietary information	Feed ingredients and their nutrient analyses, specific feeds for each feeding group; obtain feed samples if feed analysis or feed tag information is unavailable
Herd disease information	Disease prevalence for pertinent disease problems, animal culling and mortality rates over the past month, 6 months, and year
Reproductive information	Measures of fertility, pregnancy losses, etc.
Preventive medicine practices	Vaccinations, treatments, and dewormings administered and when; ask if routine herd health visits are made by the veterinarian

ment, and body condition score. Body height at the shoulders (withers) can be used to assess frame size and growth. Body weight and height measurements can be compared with those in standardized growth charts to assess growth performance.

Body condition scoring is a method of subjectively quantifying subcutaneous body fat reserves. Animals are scored on a scale of 1 to 5 or 1 to 9, with the low and high scores representing emaciated and obese animals, respectively. Changes in body condition score represent either a positive (increased) or negative (decreased) energy balance. A negative energy balance suggests that the diet contains insufficient energy to meet needs and that body fat reserves are being mobilized.

Beyond this quantitative measure, physical assessment of the animal may include observations of hair coat, hoof quality, hydration status, manure consistency, and attitude. Assess these factors and record them in the animal's records daily for hospitalized patients. Indirect measures of nutritional status may be evaluated through metabolite concentrations in blood.

REVIEW QUESTIONS

True or False

Indicate whether each of the following statements is True or False.

____ **1.** Allowing livestock to harvest forage avoids costs incurred in mechanical harvesting.

____ **2.** Concentrates are generally low in fiber and high in energy and protein.

____ **3.** During aspiration of a feeding tube, there should never be negative pressure on the syringe if the feeding tube is placed correctly.

____ **4.** It is acceptable for clients to constantly change their cat's diet with various brands and types of commercial diets.

____ **5.** Weaning of kittens should begin at 5 weeks of age.

____ **6.** Feline urinary tract disease tends to occur more often in obese sedentary cats.

____ **7.** Domestic dogs do not need variety in their diets.

____ **8.** Puppies should begin weaning at 3 to 4 weeks.

____ **9.** Many complications of parenteral nutrition involve the catheter.

____ **10.** It is acceptable to feed iguanas commercially prepared food.

____ **11.** Domestic livestock extract essential nutrients from plant material.

____ **12.** Grass hay has a much higher level of protein than alfalfa.

____ **13.** Aging diminishes the sense of taste and smell.

____ **14.** Force feeding is preferred because it is a stress-free way to get nutrients into the pet.

____ **15.** Iguanas are herbivores.

Matching

Match each term with its description.

___ 1. body conditioning score
___ 2. forage
___ 3. byproduct feeds
___ 4. herbivore
___ 5. obesity
___ 6. portion-control feeding
___ 7. free-choice feeding
___ 8. time-controlled feeding
___ 9. water
___10. essential amino acids
___11. nonessential amino acids
___12. nutrient
___13. carnivore
___14. water-soluble vitamins
___15. fat-soluble vitamins

A. amino acid that is synthesized in the body
B. meat eater
C. vitamins absorbed from the small intestines—excess amount excreted in urine
D. vitamins metabolized and stored in the liver
E. plant eater
F. method of subjectively qualifying body fat reserves
G. residues of food-processing industry
H. daily portion offered either in single feeding or divided into several portions
I. foundation for metabolism of all nutrients in the body
J. most common nutritional disorder of pets
K. feeds made up of most or all plant material
L. access to food 24 hours a day
M. amino acid that can't be synthesized in the body
N. any constituent of food that can be ingested to support life
O. portion fed with access for only 10-15 minutes

RECOMMENDED READING

Case LP, et al.: *Canine and feline nutrition*, ed 3, St Louis, 2011, Mosby.

Cheeke PR: *Applied animal nutrition: feeds and feeding*, ed 3, New York, 2004, Macmillan.

Church DC: *Livestock feeds and feeding*, ed 6, Englewood Cliffs, NJ, 2009, Prentice-Hall.

Ensminger ME, Olentine CG, Heinemann WW: *Feeds and nutrition*, ed 2, Clovis, CA, 1990, Ensminger.

Morris ML, et al.: *Small animal clinical nutrition*, ed 5, Topeka, KS, 2010, Mark Morris Institute.

National Research Council: *Nutrient requirements of beef cattle*, ed 7, Washington, DC, 2000, National Academies Press.

National Research Council: *Nutrient requirements of dairy cattle*, ed 7, Washington, DC, 2001, National Academies Press.

National Research Council: *Nutrient requirements of goats: angora, dairy, and meat goats in temperate and tropical countries*, Washington, DC, 1981, National Academies Press.

National Research Council: *Nutrient requirements of horses*, ed 6, Washington, DC, 2007, National Academies Press.

National Research Council: *Nutrient requirements of small ruminants*, Washington, DC, 1985, National Academies Press.

National Research Council: *Nutrient requirements of swine*, ed 11, Washington, DC, 1988, National Academies Press.

Wortinger A, Burns K: *Nutrition and disease management for veterinary technicians and nurses*, ed 2, Ames, Iowa, 2015, Wiley Blackwell.

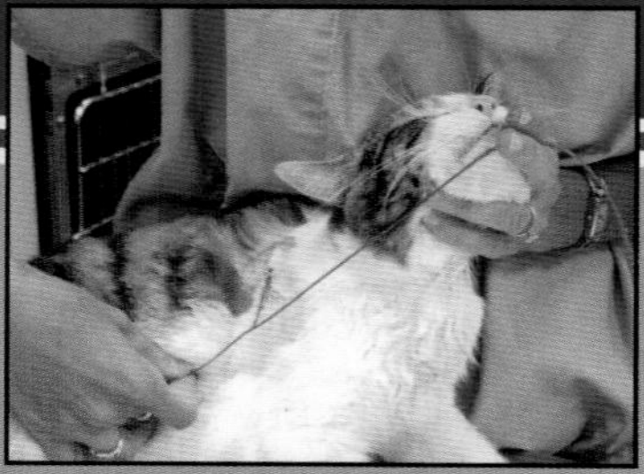

24 Nursing Care of Dogs and Cats

OUTLINE

LEARNING OBJECTIVES

After reviewing this chapter, the reader will be able to:

1. Describe techniques used in the general nursing care of dogs and cats.
2. Discuss techniques used in the recording of patient care.
3. Describe procedures used in grooming, skin, nail, and ear care.
4. List common routes of administration of medication and describe procedure used in administration of medications.
5. List and describe methods of parenteral administration.
6. List and describe methods of intravenous catheterization.
7. List and describe methods of urethral catheterization.
8. List and describe methods of orogastric and nasogastric intubation.
9. Discuss procedures used in nursing in special circumstances.
10. Describe methods of respiratory support.
11. Discuss procedures used in caring for recumbent patients.
12. Discuss issues related to techniques used in the care of neonatal puppies and kittens.
13. Discuss issues related to techniques used in the care of geriatric patients.

KEY TERMS

- Analgesia
- Anaphylaxis
- Apnea
- Arrhythmia
- Atelectasis
- Auscultation
- Bradycardia
- Buccal
- Central catheter
- Central venous pressure
- Cyanosis
- Decubital ulcer
- Diastolic blood pressure
- Dyspnea
- Euthanasia
- Intraosseous
- Nebulization
- Normothermia
- Nystagmus
- Percussion
- Petechia
- Phlebitis
- Strabismus
- Systolic blood pressure
- Tachycardia
- Tenesmus

GENERAL NURSING CARE

ATTENDING TO THE PHYSICAL NEEDS OF DOGS AND CATS

Companion animals should be kept in clean, dry, comfortable, and secure housing. Every effort should be made to eliminate environmental stress. Each animal should be adequately identified with cage cards and paper ID neck bands (Fig. 24-1). Soiled cages should be cleaned promptly with approved disinfectants and the bedding replaced. When medically permitted, exercise should be scheduled and carried out. Clean water and food are supplied if medically permitted. The veterinary technician is instrumental in providing physical comfort and safety to hospitalized pets.

ATTENDING TO THE PSYCHOLOGICAL NEEDS OF DOGS AND CATS

An often overlooked aspect of nursing care includes petting and simple touch or verbal praise to the patient. The hospitalized pet can be afraid and uncomfortable in a new environment, which can have a negative effect on appetite, temperature, and mentation. Make friends with the patients by always talking gently and quietly. When interacting with the patient, place yourself on the patient's level by sitting on the cage edge or squatting down to pet and stroke the chest or chin. Repeat this at every opportunity. Establish a rapport with the patient. At treatment times, double the amount of positive interaction, especially when the procedure or treatment involves pain or discomfort. Patients respond positively to gentle reassurance and support. If the patient's condition permits, provide special snacks or food. Each patient has individual needs and it requires observation and often owner input to help make the patient's hospitalization as positive as possible.

MONITORING VITALS AND ELIMINATION

Level of Consciousness

Recording vital signs should always begin with level of consciousness (LOC). It is important to note that problems associated with the central nervous system (CNS) may be the first clue of forthcoming complications. CNS signs may reflect a systemic disorder or a disorder secondary to either anesthesia or a surgical procedure. Such disorders include lethargy, aggression, coma, blindness, or hyperexcitability. If any abnormalities in the LOC exist, an extensive physical examination, including appropriate laboratory diagnostic testing, should be completed.

Assessment of patients' LOC can give important information on the direction of their care and treatment. Note whether the patient is alert, depressed, sedated (recovering from anesthesia), agitated, quiet, or comatose. Pain may be assessed depending on the patient's attitude. Signs of pain may include anorexia and depression. Other signs include whimpering or crying, sharp yipping when moved or touched, growling when approached, anxiety, avoidance behavior, restlessness, frequent repositioning in the cage, reluctance to lie down, arching of the spine, abdominal tucking, head pressing, limping or non–weight-bearing on a limb, and chewing at a specific area.

Owner					Name									
Date in:			Ph #1											
Est. date out:			Ph #2											
	Sunday		Monday		Tuesday		Wednesday		Thursday		Friday		Saturday	
	AM	PM	AM	PM	AM	PM	AM	PM	AM	PM	AM	PM	AM	PM
Fed														
Ate														
Water														
Urine														
Stool														
Meds														
Walked														

FIGURE 24-1 Stable, hospitalized patients require minimally a daily weight and record of eating, drinking, and elimination. This example of a cage card is conveniently graphed for recording this information. This type is also a sticker that can be applied to the permanent medical record after use.

Monitoring Weight

Weigh each patient daily, at the same time and on the same scale, to help monitor hydration and nutrition status. Daily weighing is of particular importance in patients on high intravenous fluid rates (e.g., renal failure). All animals seen as office appointments should also have a body weight recorded, regardless of the reason for the visit.

Monitoring Body Temperature

Get a baseline temperature on every patient immediately on admittance to the hospital, and during every routine appointment. Body temperature can be monitored rectally with a standard mercury thermometer, a digital thermometer (battery operated), or an electronic probe for continuous monitoring rectally. Leave the thermometer in the rectum for 2 or 3 minutes (count the pulse and respiratory rates while waiting) and record the temperature. Disposable thermometer covers should be used to prevent nosocomial infection (Fig. 24-2).

Temperature change can be an early sign of a metabolic derangement; for example, temperature can decrease in renal failure and increase in bacterial infection. Monitoring temperature can be an important indicator and early sign of a patient's condition improving or deteriorating. Monitoring temperature is critical in any patient undergoing surgery or anesthesia.

Maintenance of normal body temperature (**normothermia**) involves regulating the external environment as well as the internal environment of the patient. Hypothermia (subnormal body temperature) can occur with shock, severe sepsis, severe cardiac insufficiency, multiple organ failure, poor perfusion secondary to anesthesia or surgery, or with low environmental temperatures. Hypothermia can be combatted with circulating warm-water blankets (not electric heating pads), forced-air warming devices, warm-water bottles, warmed towels or blankets, a warm bath, blow dryer, heat lamp, or incubator. For patients with severely low temperatures, intravenous fluids can help increase perfusion and subsequently increase core body temperature. Fluids may be warmed to 37° C (98.6° F) with a fluid warmer, or the IV line can be run through a bowl of warm water.

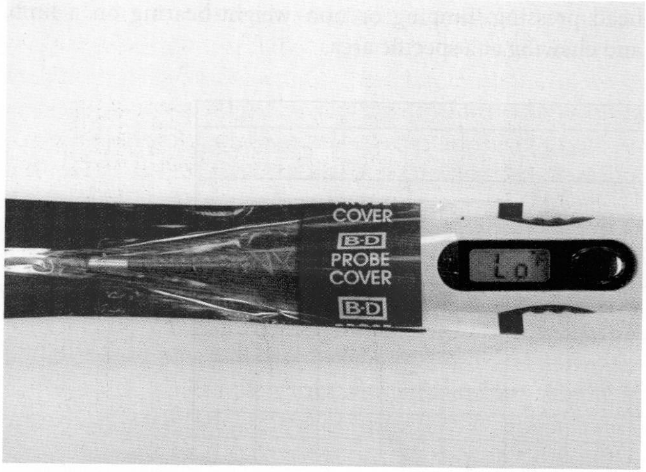

FIGURE 24-2 When taking a patient's temperature, disposable thermometer covers should be used to prevent nosocomial infection.

Monitor the rectal temperature at least every 30 minutes in patients with marked hypothermia (<97° F). Discontinue warming when the rectal temperature approaches the normal range (99° F). Do not overheat the patient. Most water blankets can be adjusted (lowered) to normal body temperature to maintain normothermia and not overheat patients. Always have a towel or pad between the water blanket and the patient. Electric heating pads are not recommended because of the possibility of electric shock, overheating, and burns. If a heat lamp is used, the patient must be able to move away from the heat source. When using an incubator or oxygen cage, extreme care must be taken to avoid overheating the patient; temperatures should be monitored and recorded frequently.

Hyperthermia (abnormally high body temperature) may occur with infection, sepsis, toxicity, inflammation, brain lesions or tumors (loss of thermoregulation), heat stroke, seizures, stress, and excitation. Patients with extreme and persistent hyperthermia (>104.5° F) require constant monitoring. Hyperthermia can be controlled with ice wrapped in towels in front of fans, alcohol application, and tepid drinking water. Lukewarm water applied to the jugular and femoral arteries will cool the patient more quickly. Cold water and ice will cause extreme peripheral vasoconstriction, inhibiting the patient's ability to dissipate heat through conductive and convective cooling mechanisms. As a result, core body temperature will continue to rise. Discontinue cooling when the rectal temperature reaches 103° F (39.5° C). Do not overcool the patient; vasoconstriction may occur which may impair perfusion.

> **TECHNICIAN NOTE** For severe hyperthermia, apply isopropyl alcohol to the foot pads, in addition to spraying tepid water on the patient and placing a fan nearby for convection.

Monitoring Pulse

Determination of the heart rate is the first diagnostic clue as to the cardiovascular status of the patient. Normal heart rate for the dog ranges from 70 beats per minute in larger dogs to as high as 220 beats per minute in puppies. Normal heart rates for cats and kittens range from 120 to 240 beats per minute. A slower than normal heart rate is termed **bradycardia,** and a faster than normal rate is termed **tachycardia.** Abnormalities in heart rate or rhythm must be identified and characterized by performing electrocardiography to determine the precise nature of the rate and/or rhythm abnormality. Assessment of the pulse quality, heart rate, and heart rhythm can also help determine the patient's hemodynamic status and help guide the course of treatment.

Auscultate the heart while palpating the pulse. A pulse deficit (a difference in the number of heartbeats and pulse beats) may indicate an **arrhythmia** (Fig. 24-3). Pulses can be described as absent, weak and thready, normal, bounding, or irregular. Pulse quality should be assessed in both the dorsal pedal and femoral regions of the dog and cat; differences in pulse strength may indicate a perfusion abnormality.

There are two normal rhythm variations in the dog. Normal sinus rhythm has regular beat with a normal rate. A normal respiratory sinus arrhythmia has a normal to slow heart rate and is characterized by an increase in heart rate during inspiration and a decrease in heart rate during expiration. Respiratory sinus arrhythmia is common in dogs, but very uncommon in the cat. Other common rhythm abnormalities include beats that occur prematurely, and may be associated with pulse deficits, such as atrial and ventricular premature complexes. Arrhythmias that are characterized by intermittent prolonged periods of asystole are termed bradyarrhythmias (e.g., with severe second-degree AV block).

Presence of a cardiac murmur should also be noted during cardiac **auscultation.** In general, the patient should be in sternal or standing position during auscultation, because a murmur can be positional. Murmurs are caused by turbulence disturbing the normal laminar flow of blood. They are most often caused by dysfunctional valves or septal defects. Characterization of murmurs is based on several criteria, of which timing in the cycle, location or point of maximal intensity (PMI) of the murmur, and intensity (loudness) are the most important (Table 24-1).

If the murmur occurs between the first heart sounds (S1) and second heart sound (S2), it is systolic (common in small animals). If it occurs between S2 of one beat, and S1 of the following beat, it is diastolic (extremely uncommon in small animals). Continuous murmurs (e.g., such as heard with left-to-right shunting patent ductus arteriosus) are heard throughout the cardiac cycle and peak in intensity at about the position of S2. Correct recognition of the PMI can be very helpful in identifying the specific cardiac abnormality.

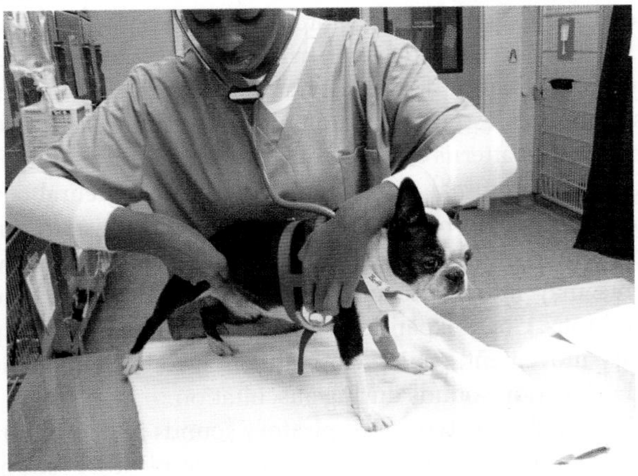

FIGURE 24-3 Auscultation of heart rate and rhythm in conjunction with the palpation of an arterial pulse will detect presence of "dropped beats" or arrhythmias.

TABLE 24-1 Classifying a Heart Murmur

GRADE	DESCRIPTION
1/6	Softest murmur audible
2/6	Soft, readily heard, but focal over one valve only
3/6	Prominent, easily heard, radiates to other areas
4/6	Loud, radiates widely, but not accompanied by a palpable thrill
5/6	Loud and accompanied by a palpable thrill
6/6	Very loud and auscultated with the stethoscope held off the thorax

Note that murmurs can often be heard in young puppies and kittens. Such murmurs are generally soft systolic murmurs heard best at the mitral or aortic valves. Termed "innocent murmurs," they are often transient and disappear by 3 to 4 months of age. Their cause is not known. It is speculated that the murmur may be related to the lower packed cell volume of young animals. Physiologic murmurs are categorized as murmurs that occur in animals that are anemic and occur as a result of changes in blood viscosity (which results in disruption of normal blood flow). These are soft murmurs that resolve with resolution of the underlying disease.

Examination of the jugular vein is an important evaluation of the cardiac system. It is often necessary to clip the area over the jugular veins to visualize jugular pulsations or jugular distention, although persistent jugular distention can frequently be palpated. Persistent jugular distention is an important indicator of right heart failure. It is typically seen with a pericardial effusion, but can also occur with other causes of right-sided congestive heart failure (e.g., dilated cardiomyopathy). A jugular pulse that extends more than about one third of the way up the neck frequently indicates tricuspid regurgitation. Blood pressure should be evaluated in the presence of jugular distension or pulsation.

If there are unusual findings related to the heart rate, heart rhythm, or pulse quality, the patient should be monitored with an electrocardiogram (ECG). The ECG is an indicator of the electrical activity of the heart muscle. Atrial depolarization is indicated by the P wave. Following the P wave there is a short delay represented by the P-R segment, after which the ventricles depolarize and produce the QRS complex. The S-T segment and the T wave represent ventricular repolarization. (Fig. 24-4). Common abnormal ECG waveforms are summarized in Box 24-1.

Place the patient in right lateral recumbency and attach the alligator clips to the skin caudal to the elbows and on

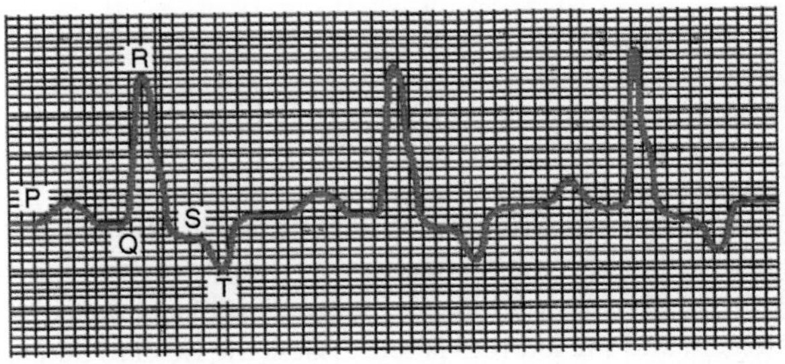

FIGURE 24-4 Normal canine P-QRS-T complex. Normal lead II electrocardiographic complex. Atrial depolarization is indicated by the P wave. Following the P wave there is a short delay in the A-V node (P-R segment), after which the ventricles depolarize and produce the QRS complex. This S-T segment and the T wave represent ventricular repolarization. (From Edwards NJ: *ECG manual for the veterinary technician*, St Louis, 1993, Elsevier.)

BOX 24-1 Common Abnormalities Seen on ECG

Atrial Fibrillation
No P waves or QRS complexes

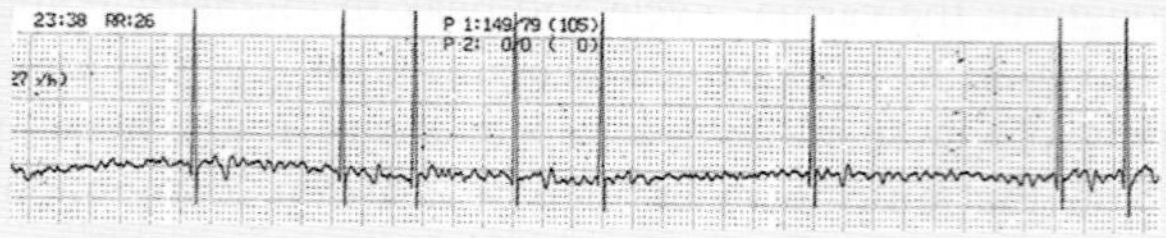

Atrial Standstill
Absent P waves
Widened QRS complexes
Tall T waves

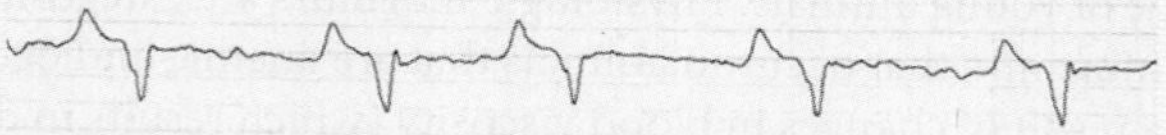

Premature Supraventricular (Atrial) Contraction
Premature negative P wave

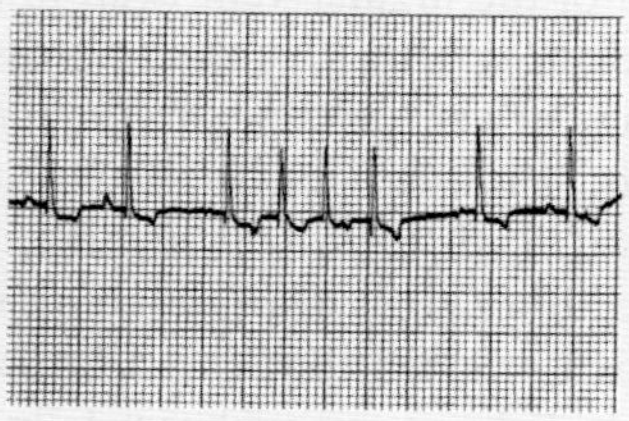

Third-Degree AVBlock
Nonconducter P waves

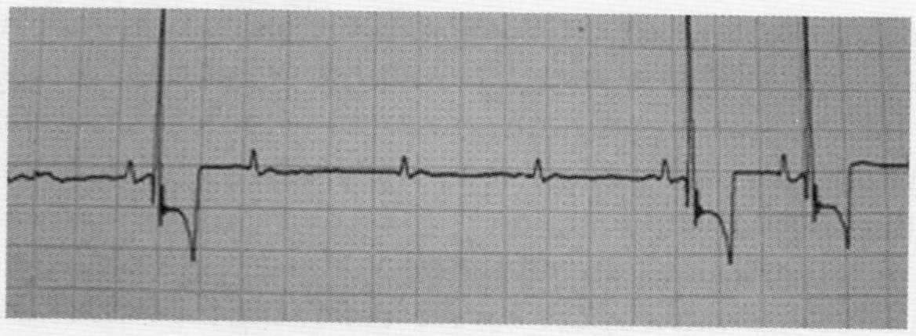

Premature Ventricular Contraction
Widened QRS comlex
Nonrelated T waves

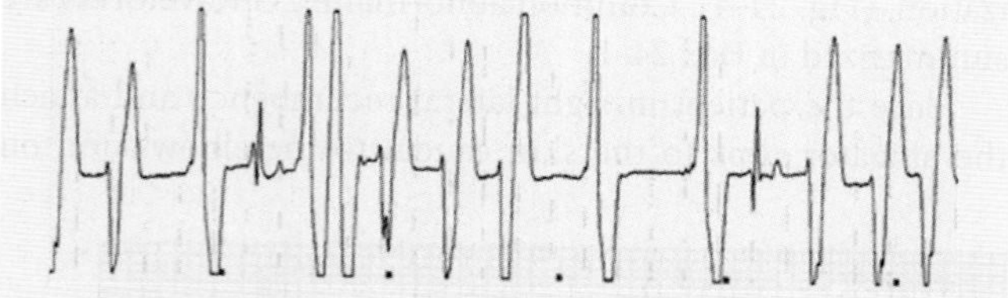

From Sirois, M: *Mosby's veterinary PDQ*, St Louis, 2009, Mosby.

the stifles (Fig. 24-5). Alcohol or ultrasonic gel on the contact points will help with transmission. If the clips are color coded, the right front is white, the left front is black, the right rear is green, and the left rear is red. Assess the ECG to determine if continuous monitoring is advisable.

Monitoring Respiration

Auscultation is an important nursing tool in assessing the respiratory system. Proper technique for accuracy and expediency is paramount. Observe the patient's respiratory effort

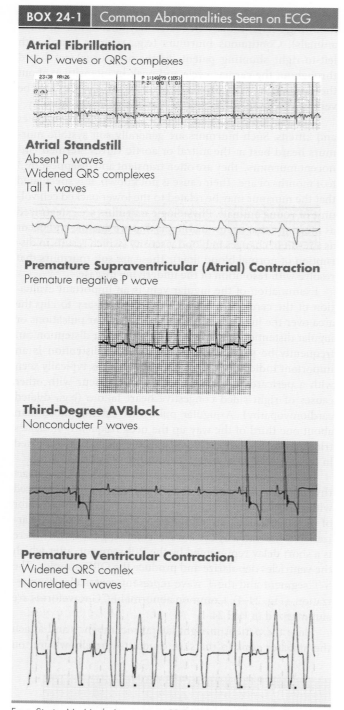

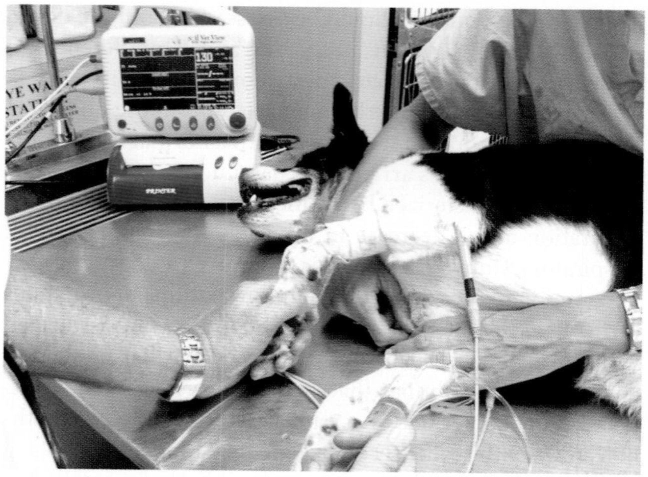

FIGURE 24-5 Attaching "alligator" or pinch clips onto leads of an ECG will ensure a quick and steady contact.

when it is relaxed and breathing normally if possible. Check the rate and depth of respiration. Normal respiratory rates in small animals are approximately 18 to 30 breaths/minute. The patient should be in sternal recumbency and allowed to inhale oxygen during the exam if stressed, to facilitate lung expansion and accurate auscultation. It is recommended that the pediatric head of the stethoscope be used in smaller patients to avoid referred sounds. The auscultation should include both sides of the chest, ventrally and dorsally, while paying close attention to the respiratory pattern. Respiratory effort should be noted in conjunction with the respiratory component.

In general, respiratory patterns and lung sounds are subtler in cats than in dogs. Respiratory patterns should be assessed before restraint or manipulation when possible. Note that certain patterns can provide diagnostic information. For example, abdominal components can indicate pleural complications (fluid or air), neurological compromise, trauma (cervical lesions), or chest wall trauma. Paradoxical movements may indicate diaphragmatic hernia or neurological conditions. Chest expansion should be assessed in any respiratory movement, paying close attention to both inhalation and exhalation sounds during auscultation.

Identifying the type of respiratory sounds in ill or injured patients can be difficult. Common respiratory sounds (Box 24-2) include harsh or static sounding lungs (indicative of trauma, parenchymal disease, early signs of fluid overload), crackles or popping sounds (indicative of parenchymal disease, severe fluid overload, asthma), wheezes or musical sounds (asthma or chronic bronchitis), or upper airway (referred) sounds (indicative of stenosis, elongated soft palate, tracheal collapse, or constriction). It is important to combine lung sounds with other physical exam findings such as patient mentation, respiratory rate, respiratory effort, respiratory pattern, heart rate, pulse quality, temperature, and mucus membrane color. Monitoring the trends of such exam findings is critical in providing good nursing care. Note that pediatric patients may fluctuate more easily than adults because of a more fragile, immature immune system.

Other respiratory sounds include inspiratory dyspnea, characterized by a prolonged, labored inspiratory effort, and

BOX 24-2 Significance of Common Respiratory Sounds

Harsh or Static Sounds
Trauma
Lung parenchymal disease
Early fluid overload
Asthma
Crackles or popping sounds
Lung parenchymal disease
Severe fluid overload
Asthma

Wheezes or Musical Sounds
Asthma
Chronic bronchitis

Upper Airway (Referred) Sounds
Stenosis
Elongated soft palate
Tracheal collapse
Tracheal constriction

Muffled or Absent Lung Sounds
Pneumothorax
Hemothorax
Chylothorax
Diaphragmatic hernia

Noisy Breathing (Inspiratory Stridor)
Upper airway obstruction
Laryngeal paralysis

a quicker, easier expiratory phase. Inspiratory dyspnea usually indicates an upper airway disorder (e.g., laryngeal paralysis). Stertors and/or stridors frequently accompany inspiratory dyspnea. Stertor is defined as a low-pitched snoring noise, whereas stridor is a high-pitched harsh, wheezy noise. Expiratory dyspnea is often characterized by a prolonged, labored expiratory effort and may indicate an intrathoracic airway disorder (e.g., chronic bronchitis, pulmonary edema caused by congestive heart failure) and/or a restrictive disorder (e.g., pleural effusion). Intrathoracic disease will frequently cause both inspiratory and expiratory dyspnea.

Patient posture is noted as a part of respiratory evaluation. Dyspnea may be manifested as a refusal to lie down. Note the quality of the animal's breathing. Note the presence of any difficulty on inspiration or expiration. Difficult respirations may be characterized by abdominal breathing. Orthopnea is a term applied to respiratory distress that is exacerbated by recumbency. Animals showing orthopnea assume a standing or sitting position with elbows abducted and head and neck extended. Movement of the abdominal muscles that assist ventilation is often exaggerated. Such animals vigorously resist being placed in lateral recumbency. Finally, note any coughing, muscle wasting, or abdominal distention. Presence of a cough may indicate bronchial diseases in cats, causing abnormal airway sounds.

The mucous membrane color can also supply a wealth of information in assessing the respiratory system. Keep in mind that pink membranes may not necessarily indicate a stable, well-perfused patient. Combine pulse quality with the mucous membrane analysis to better determine hemodynamic stability. Note differences between pedal and femoral pulse quality; femoral pulses may be difficult to find in the cat versus the dog, particularly if the patient is overweight. Pale or white mucous membranes may not indicate respiratory dysfunction, but rather hypothermia, pain, decreased cardiac output, anemia, or peripheral vasoconstriction. In addition, brick red membranes may indicate a hyperemic, hypercapnic state, indicating poor ventilation. Cyanotic mucous membranes (blue-colored) may indicate an increase in the concentration of deoxygenated hemoglobin. **Cyanosis** is seen with right-to-left shunting defects (such as Tetralogy of Fallot), severe respiratory disease, or marked hypothermia (Fig. 24-6).

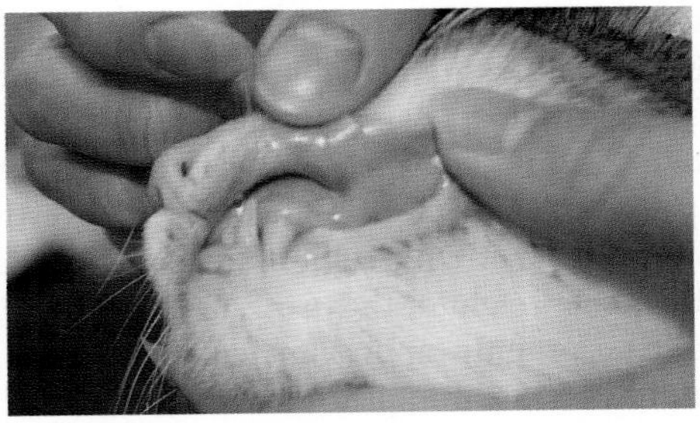

FIGURE 24-6 Cyanosis. (From Studdert V: *Saunders comprehensive veterinary dictionary*, ed 4, St Louis, 2012, Saunders.)

> **TECHNICIAN NOTE** Careful examination of the respiratory rate, effort, body posture, and respiratory pattern can help locate the source of respiratory distress. Pay close attention to each inspiratory and expiratory phase of respiration.

Monitoring Urine Production

Urination frequency should be recorded on all patients, particularly critical pets. Walk dogs regularly and record any urination. Evaluate frequency of urination on cats by cleaning out the litter box often, making sure to also check bedding and underneath cage mats for possible eliminations. Patients on IV fluids may have an increased amount of urine production and may need to be walked more frequently.

The veterinary technician is required to record frequency of urination, strength of urine stream, and gross visual analysis of the urine. Further laboratory analysis and methods of collection are explained in detail in Chapter 9. The urinalysis can aid diagnosis and monitor response to treatment. Urine production and composition reflect perfusion, renal function, hydration status, bladder function, and endocrine function.

Measuring Urine Production

Dogs can be taken outside to urinate if no urinary catheter is in place to collect and measure urine. Walk ambulatory canine patients outside every 4 hours during the day to eliminate. A bedpan works well for catching the urine; then pour the urine into a graduated container to measure. Disposable pads or diapers can be used in recumbent patients to facilitate cleaning and measure urine output by weight. After a patient urinates on the diapers, remove them and weigh. Subtract the initial weight of the paper or diaper; the remainder is the weight of the urine. Convert that into milliliters to determine the approximate urine output. Normal urine output is 1 to 2 ml/kg/hr. Recumbent animals can be placed on "trampolines" or cots; urine can be measured by placing paper, diapers, or even a bowl underneath the cot (Fig. 24-7).

Urinary catheterization permits accurate measurement of urine output, facilitates collection of urine for analysis, promotes cleanliness of recumbent patients, and reduces exposure of other patients or personnel to contaminated urine (e.g., leptospirosis, chemotherapy). A urinary catheter and collection system also keeps the bladder empty in patients with bladder dysfunction or patients on high fluid administration rates. Indwelling urinary catheters should be placed and handled with sterile technique. Urine collection bags can either be made by using an intravenous administration set and a fluid bag, or by using a specialized collection bag designed to prevent urine backflow (Fig. 24-8).

TECHNICIAN NOTE Always wear gloves when handling animal urine. This is of particular importance in dogs that may have leptospirosis.

In cats with lower urinary tract disease, urinary catheters prevent reobstruction. Cats without urinary catheters can have their urine output quantitated by using an empty litter pan, paper litter, plastic beads, or diapers. The paper litter and the litter pan should be weighed before placing in the cage. Plastic beads can be used as litter; urine can be collected by use of a strainer and bowl.

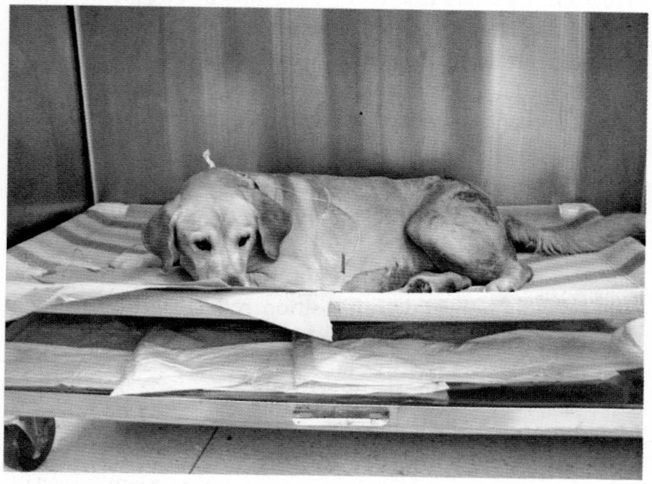

FIGURE 24-7 Trampolines will prevent decubital ulcers and urine scalding in the recumbent patient.

Patients that cannot completely empty the bladder may need to have the bladder manually expressed. Bladder expression is necessary to prevent bladder atony and to decrease the chance of a urinary tract infection. Nonambulatory patients may be carefully taken outside on a gurney, assisted to stand, and, if necessary, have the bladder expressed to stimulate urination. Bladder expression keeps the patient much cleaner and reduces the chance of urine scalding. Patients with neurologic abnormalities (e.g., intervertebral disc disease) should have bladders palpated and expressed at least three times daily. Veterinary technicians should differentiate between bladder overflow and conscious urination.

The urinary system can also be evaluated by noting the hydration status of the animal. Assessing dehydration from physical examination can be determined as indicated in Table 24-2, Assessing Dehydration.

GASTROINTESTINAL MONITORING

Monitor all excretions (urine, feces, vomit, saliva) from the patient and record a description (including estimated quantity) on the patient's chart. Characterizing the color and content of the vomitus (e.g., yellow or bile-looking, green, coffee-ground, partially or undigested food, watery, or foul-smelling) and the feces (e.g., black, red with frank blood, mucoid, watery) can help aid the diagnosis. Regurgitation must

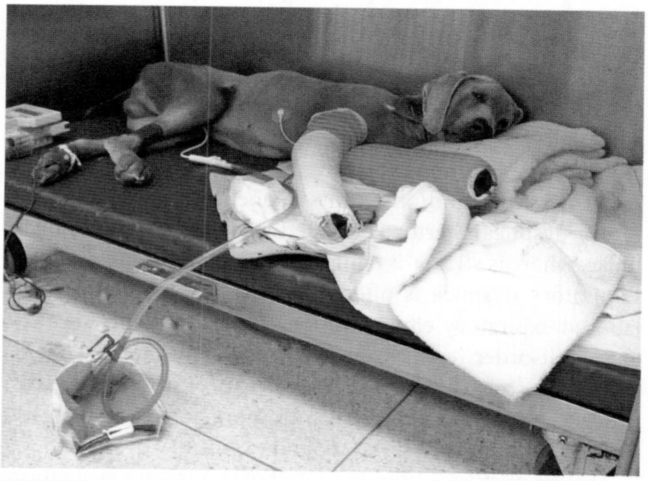

FIGURE 24-8 Specialized collection bags are designed to prevent urine backflow, thus helping prevent a urinary tract infection.

TABLE 24-2 Assessing Dehydration

PERCENTAGE OF DEHYDRATION	PHYSICAL EXAMINATION FINDINGS
<5 %	No detectable abnormalities
5 %	Slightly "doughy" inelasticity of skin
7%	Definite inelasticity of skin. Capillary refill time 2-3 seconds; slight depression of eyes into orbits. Dry mucous membranes
10%-12%	Severe skin inelasticity; capillary refill time >3 seconds; markedly sunken eyeballs; shock in debilitated animals; involuntary muscle twitching

be differentiated from vomiting. Vomiting is typically active and projectile; regurgitation is typically passive, quiet, and is often associated with movement. In patients that do not or cannot drink water, calculated fluid losses should be replaced with IV fluids.

The patient's body must be kept clean and free of body waste and excretions. Cleaning and flushing the oral cavity with saline, water, or a weak tea solution can help prevent or heal oral ulcers. Flushing or suctioning any vomitus out of the mouth also makes the patient feel better. The mouth of patients that cannot take food or water per os may be moistened with a gauze sponge and water. The skin around the mouth should be kept clean of vomitus and saliva to prevent scalding and secondary bacterial infections. In comatose patients, or patients intubated for extended periods, the tongue should be kept moist by either frequent water application or kept wrapped with moist gauze.

Patients with diarrhea must be kept as clean and dry as possible. Clean the cage or run thoroughly and replace any soiled bedding. Frequent walks outside to eliminate help the patient feel better and reduce cage cleanup. Any abnormal stool should be characterized in the medical record; include the color, amount, and general composition. Large, watery stools are more typical of small bowel diarrhea, whereas bloody or tarry stools can indicate a potentially life-threatening condition such as GI bleeding or ulceration. The veterinary technician should help question the owner concerning diet history. The dietary history is paramount because in small animals, diarrhea is often dietary induced. Recent diet changes to a moist, high-fat, or meat-based diet; more frequent feeding of table scraps; or access to garbage or dead animals can be responsible.

Patients that have not had a bowel movement in the past 2 days but are still eating should be closely monitored and encouraged to eliminate (e.g., take outside on a long leash, place in an outdoor run, provide a larger litterbox or different litter). Diet changes may be necessary (e.g., canned food, addition of fiber). Enemas may be indicated if constipation is diagnosed. Patients with certain neurologic abnormalities or patients in a drug-induced coma should have their colon manually evacuated. Any **tenesmus** (straining to defecate) should be reported to the veterinarian. Gut sounds should be monitored at least twice daily by placing a stethoscope ventral to the last rib and monitoring for gaseous, gurgling stomach sounds.

> *TECHNICIAN NOTE* Gut sounds are important to monitor in any patient with a history of vomiting, diarrhea, inappetence, or recumbency. Place a stethoscope ventral to the last rib and monitor for gaseous, gurgling stomach sounds.

NEUROLOGIC SYSTEM MONITORING

Assessment of the neurologic system should begin with attitude or level of consciousness. Patients that are demented or semicomatose are often diagnosed with intracranial diseases or injury. Note body posture for presence of a head tilt or any other abnormal head posture, indicating a possible lesion in the area of the brain corresponding with the same side as the head tilt. Evaluate gait by noting coordinated movement of all four limbs, as well as postural reactions or conscious proprioception. Tests such as hopping, hemiwalking, wheelbarrowing, and extensor postural thrust evaluate the ability of the animal to recognize that its limb is in an abnormal position to bear weight and the ability of it to place it in a more normal position. Cranial nerve examination is also performed to test for neurologic insufficiency and is numbered sequentially from cranial to caudal. A comprehensive neurology reference should be consulted for information on proper performance of evaluation of postural reactions and cranial and spinal nerve examination.

Ocular inspection is also important in the neurologic examination. Pupils should be symmetrical and responsive to light (both direct and consensual). Abnormal movement (**nystagmus**) or position (**strabismus**) of the eye should be duly noted. Vision should be evaluated by observing movement and ability to follow objects. Menace response should be performed by making a menacing gesture toward the eye and looking for a blink response.

INTEGUMENTARY SYSTEM MONITORING

Vascular and skin integrity should also be noted on the physical exam. Any abnormal areas of alopecia, presence of ticks or fleas, pitting edema, icterus, ecchymosis, **petechia** (Fig. 24-9), or abnormal bleeding during phlebotomy should be duly noted to the veterinarian.

> *TECHNICIAN NOTE* Petechia and/or ecchymosis usually indicate a coagulopathy. Common sites of eruption are the ear pinnae, ventral abdomen, and mucous membranes. Avoid jugular venipuncture and/or jugular catheterization unless directed by the veterinarian when signs of coagulopathy are present.

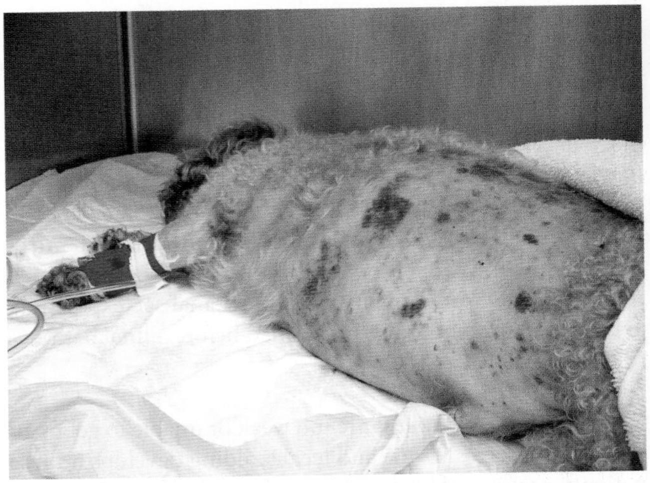

FIGURE 24-9 Petechia may signify a coagulation abnormality. It often appears as small red dots on the ventral abdomen, mucous membranes, or the ear pinnae.

NUTRITIONAL SUPPORT

The primary goal of nutritional assessment is to identify whether a patient is at risk for malnutrition. Because altered nutritional status is associated with adverse clinical outcomes, it is important to address the nutritional needs early in the critically ill patient. Although clinical status alone may dictate the need for nutritional intervention, a thorough nutritional assessment consists of evaluating both clinical and biochemical data, including patient history, and a thorough physical exam including body weight and body condition scoring. A baseline nutritional assessment should be followed by serial assessments throughout the course of hospitalization. The veterinary technician is in a crucial position to identify baseline data and ongoing changes in nutritional status, because the technician spends the most time with the patient. Nutritional intervention is crucial to recovery and survival, particularly with the critical patient, and appropriate consideration as to the type and route of nutrition should be given based on the underlying disease process or diagnosis.

In summary, sick or injured patients need good nutritional support to counteract the immunosuppressive effects of sepsis, neoplasia, chemotherapy, anesthesia, and surgery. This support enhances wound healing and minimizes the length of hospitalization without significant weight loss and muscle atrophy. Initiation of nutritional support early in the course of hospitalization is crucial for a successful outcome. Refer to Chapter 23 for detailed information on nutritional support for hospitalized patients.

GROOMING AND SKIN CARE

Some hospitalized patients develop skin problems (e.g., decubital ulcers, pyoderma, urine scald, dry scaly skin) because of recumbency, urinary or fecal incontinence, stress, electrolyte imbalances, poor hydration, and general lack of appropriate care. Others have been healthy until admitted for trauma. Regardless of the reason for admittance to the hospital, all patients require routine grooming and skin care. Patients also feel better when kept clean and dry.

When a patient is admitted and its condition has been stabilized, any vomit, diarrhea, urine, or blood should be removed from the skin to prevent secondary infections. Skin care of the hospitalized patient involves bathing to remove body fluids, skin oil, or exudates; brushing to prevent mat formation; padding to prevent decubital ulcer formation; and medicating affected areas of skin. Surgical patients with diarrhea should be cleaned frequently to prevent incisional infections. Before the patient is discharged from the hospital, such routine procedures as toenail trimming, anal sac expression, and ear cleaning should be performed before a final bath.

Skin Care

Many critically ill patients are too weak or unable to get up to relieve themselves. Urine and fecal scalding develops if these patients are not cleaned after each occurrence. However, use good judgment before partially or completely bathing a critically ill patient. For example, if a dyspneic animal in an oxygen cage urinates on itself, remove the soiled bedding and spot clean the patient. Do not jeopardize the patient's overall health to completely bathe the animal. Also, do not let the patient continue to lie in body waste without attempting to clean it. Sick pediatric patients should be dried thoroughly and kept warm if bathing is necessary, because thermoregulation may be impaired.

Any long hair should be trimmed to prevent moisture from being trapped and causing a secondary infection. Carefully shave the hair around the perianal and inguinal areas for ease of cleaning. Avoid nicking or cutting the patient with the clippers. Apply a light tail wrap on long-haired patients with diarrhea to help keep the tail clean and prevent scalding. Wrap the tail loosely and incorporate some of the hair to keep the wrap in place. Change the wrap after each episode of diarrhea.

Patients with minor soiling can be spot cleaned with mild solutions (e.g., Peri-Wash, Sween). Continuous diarrhea can cause perineal irritation and ulceration and may cause ascending urinary tract infection. A complete bath is recommended when large areas are soiled. Clean contaminated incision areas gently with water and a washcloth. Soak off any dried organic material. Pat the incision dry. Remove as much organic material from the patient as possible before placing in a bathtub and bathing. Apply a light layer of triple antibiotic ointment to the incision to prevent contact with water and shampoo.

Recumbent patients can be kept cleaner and drier if a urinary catheter is placed to prevent urine scald. If the patient is large, transfer the patient on a gurney to a tub with a grate placed over it, or slide the patient out of the cage onto a rack elevated above a floor drain. Have shampoo, several buckets of warm water, and towels ready before starting. If the patient does not have a urinary catheter, encourage urination before bathing. Express the bladder if necessary. If the patient has not defecated in days, enemas or digital removal of feces may be necessary. Use this opportunity to make the patient more comfortable before bathing. Cover any clean and dry bandages with plastic to reduce the need for bandaging after the bath. Change any contaminated bandages. Patients with indwelling urinary catheters should have preputial or vaginal areas free of any fecal material to prevent ascending urinary tract infections.

Wet the patient on the exposed side, apply shampoo, and scrub gently with the hands. Rinse thoroughly and turn the patient to the other side. Repeat the shampooing. Remove all wet and soiled bandages at this time. Clean and completely dry the areas under the bandages before replacing. Squeeze excess water from the hair and towel dry. Use a blow dryer to dry the exposed side; then turn the patient over and repeat on the other side. Completely dry the patient with a handheld dryer. Patients can become overheated quickly if left unattended with in a cage dryer with the dryer on a high setting. Monitor patients frequently during drying, particularly obese or brachycephalic breeds.

Insecticidal spot-ons, sprays, powders, or mousses may be applied after drying. It is contraindicated to use dryers after some therapeutic dips. Read the instructions on the dip for these recommendations. Numerous products on the market are available in spot-on treatments. Their efficacy can be affected by improper application. Read and follow all instructions and be able to educate the client about their proper use as well.

Medicated shampoos may be prescribed by the veterinarian. Medicated shampoos can be antiseptic, moisturizing, degreasing, antipruritic, antifungal, or insecticidal. Massaging the shampoo into the coat disperses the medication while loosening any scales and crusts. Contact time for therapeutic shampoos is important; review product instructions before application. Patients with bacterial dermatitis may need to be carefully shaved before shampooing. Avoid clipper burns and irritating the skin when shaving.

If insecticidal dips are used, pay strict attention to the package insert. Insecticides may cause toxicities in cats and certain dog breeds, such as Collies, Shelties, and Old English Sheepdogs. Signs of toxicity include vomiting, diarrhea, excessive salivation, bradycardia, miosis, ataxia, and seizures; these need immediate medical attention. Mildly affected animals can be treated by rebathing with a nonmedicated shampoo to remove any insecticide remaining on the hair.

A comb or brush may be used while drying the patient to decrease drying time. Use care when brushing thin-skinned patients with a slicker brush. The wire bristles can scratch the skin easily. Remove mats with scissors or electric clippers while the hair is dry, preferably before bathing. Before replacing the patient back in the cage, make sure the patient is completely dry and all irritated areas on the skin are examined, shaved if necessary, cleaned, and treated appropriately. Ointments, creams, lotions, drying solutions, or powders can be reapplied at this time. For recumbent patients, place clean towels or padding placed between the patient's legs to aerate the skin, make the patient more comfortable, and prevent scrotal edema. Roll stockinette into a donut-shape to pad any decubital ulcers, which typically form on bony prominences such as the scapula or femur.

Nail Care

The nails of cats and dogs are regularly trimmed to prevent ingrown nails, injury from traumatic nail fractures, and impaired walking from overlong nails that impinge on the footpads. Trimming also minimizes damage to the environment (e.g., bedding and padding) and injury to handlers and other animals. The nail should not extend beyond the level of the foot-pad and should be trimmed accordingly (Fig. 24-10). However, animals that do not have their nails trimmed routinely can have an overlong "quick" or ungual blood vessel that bleeds with trimming; this vessel will gradually regress with frequent nail trimming. To avoid injury of veterinary staff, cats should have their nails trimmed before starting any procedure.

> **TECHNICIAN NOTE** A Dremel tool may be used to ensure the nail bed is trimmed down to the shortest possible length without eliciting trauma or bleeding.

Purposely "quicking" the nails (cutting the nail short, causing bleeding) is unnecessarily cruel and painful. "Quicking" is viewed unfavorably by clients and causes the animal to resist subsequent nail trimming. Unless the patient has a history of painful nail trims, most animals do not resent nail trimming.

The patient should be in lateral or sternal recumbency or sitting. An assistant may be necessary to help restrain the animal. Hold the toe between thumb and forefinger, with the foot grasped firmly in that hand. Push the toe distally to extend the nail and allow the trimmer to slide over the tip of the nail (Fig. 24-11).

The nail should be cut cleanly, with no frayed edges; smooth off any rough edges with nail file or Dremel (Fig. 24-12). After trimming, examine each nail for bleeding before going on to the next nail. Examine each foot to ensure that all nails, including the dewclaws, have been trimmed cleanly and are not frayed.

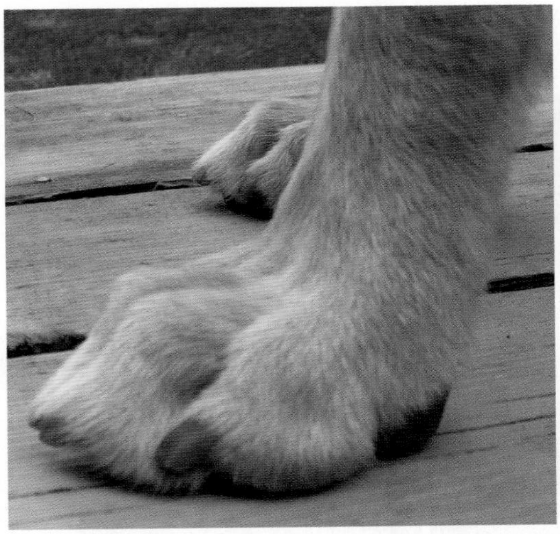

FIGURE 24-10 Example of a dog's foot with toenails of proper length. Note that nails do not contact the ground. (From Bassert J, Thomas J: *McCurnin's clinical textbook for veterinary technicians*, ed 8, St Louis, 2014, Saunders.)

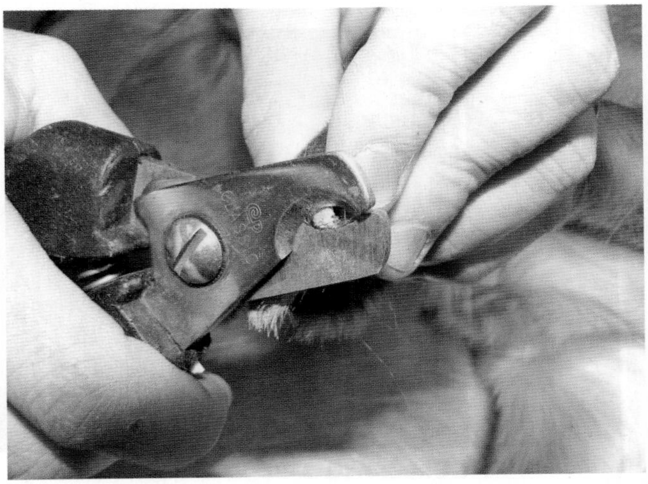

FIGURE 24-11 Nail trimmer placed over the edge of the nail that extends beyond the foot pad.

If the quick is accidentally cut, apply a cauterizing agent, such as hemostatic powder. If no cauterizing agent is available, apply pressure with a cotton ball or gauze sponge directly on the quick to gradually stop the bleeding. Cauterizing a nail with silver nitrate application may cause some discomfort in patients, so be prepared for the patient to attempt to withdraw the foot.

> **TECHNICIAN NOTE** Silver nitrate may permanently stain countertops or exam tables; place a towel under the patient before application.

Anal Sac Care

The anal sacs are paired sacs located beneath the skin on either side of the anus at the 5 o'clock and 7 o'clock positions, each with a duct opening directly into the terminal rectum (Fig. 24-13A). The anal sacs normally empty their malodorous secretions during defecation. Occasionally animals (rarely cats) may not be able to empty the anal sacs naturally and develop painful distention or impaction of the anal sacs. Signs include "scooting" on the hindquarters and licking of the anal area. The anal sacs of dogs can be expressed (emptied manually) as a routine part of grooming, as part of the physical examination, and before bathing. The anal sacs are emptied with the dog restrained in the standing position. Anal sac expression may cause discomfort and a muzzle may be necessary.

For internal anal sac expression, wear exam gloves, well-lubricated with a water-soluble lubricant or 2% lidocaine jelly. With the handler holding the tail dorsally or laterally, insert the first joint of the index finger into the rectum and gently palpate the anal sac between thumb (externally) and forefinger (Fig. 24-13B). Gently massage with light to moderate pressure, milking the secretions medially into the anal opening; repeat on the other side. Notify the veterinarian of any unusual secretions, such as thick, yellow mucopurulent liquid or if the discharge contains blood. Clean the perineum with a deodorizer or spot cleaner if not bathing immediately after expression.

For external anal sac expression, place a gauze sponge or paper towel over the anus while applying gentle, firm pressure craniomedially against the perineum. Examine the secretions and repeat on the opposite side. External expression does not completely empty the anal sacs but may cause less discomfort than internal expression.

Anal sac abscesses may need to be treated with hot packs to the perineum, instilling medication into the anal sacs, drains, or surgical intervention. Patients with recent rectal surgery should not have the anal sacs expressed.

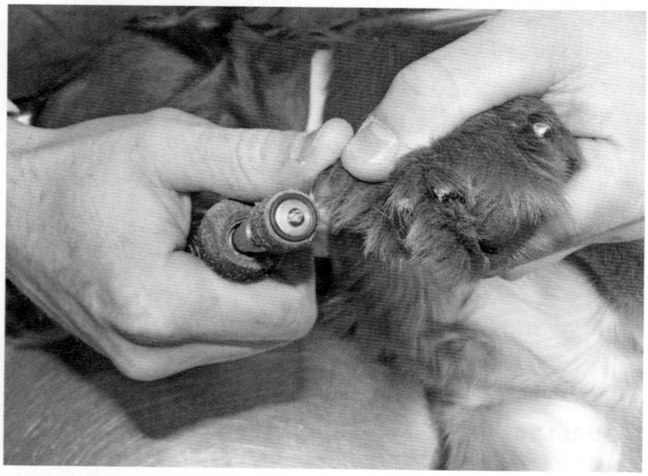

FIGURE 24-12 A Dremel tool may be used to smooth off any rough nail edges.

Ear Care

Before cleaning ears, visually examine the external ear canal and tympanic membrane for any irregularity (Fig. 24-14). Cleaning the ears and instilling medication without examination may cause further damage to the tympanic membrane and result in loss of hearing, temporary loss of vestibular function, or facial nerve paralysis. The tympanic membrane must be intact before any products other than saline or water

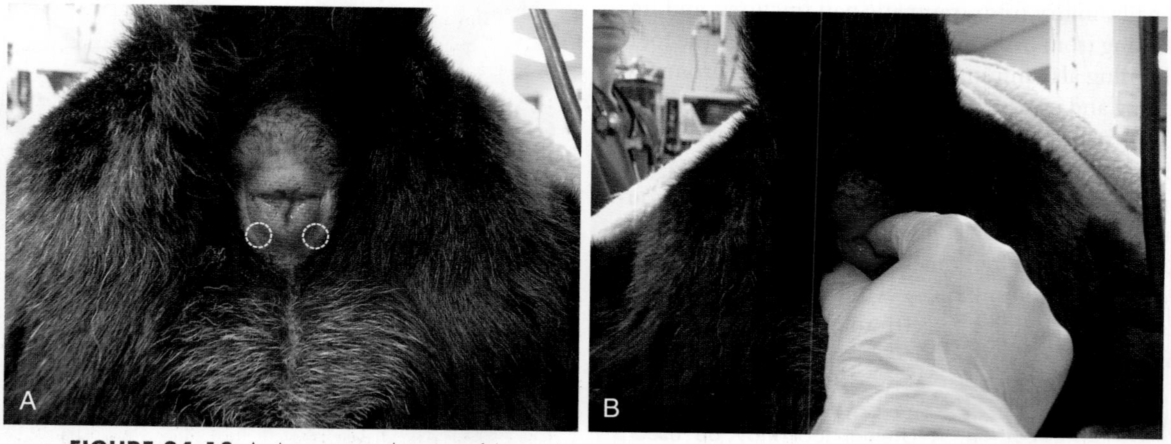

FIGURE 24-13 A, Approximate location of the anal sacs in a dog *(dotted circles)*. B, Technique for expression of the left anal sac in a dog. (From Bassert J, Thomas J: *McCurnin's clinical textbook for veterinary technicians*, ed 8, St Louis, 2014, Saunders.)

are instilled into the ear. Look for any redness, discharge, ulceration, excessive tissue formation, narrowing (stenosis) of the canal, abnormal odor, or debris in the outer ear and on the pinna. Evaluate the patient for signs of pain during the aural exam. These could indicate a bacterial or yeast infection, ear mite infestation, or tumors. Thickening of the pinna could indicate an aural hematoma. Signs of ear disease include excessive shaking of the head, scratching at the ears, head tilt, nystagmus, and ataxia.

If the animal has an ear problem, examine the less affected ear first. Most patients tolerate ear examination with minimal restraint while sitting or in sternal recumbency. Patients with painful ears or chronic ear disease typically require general anesthesia or chemical restraint for ear examination and cleaning. Use a separate clean otoscope cone for each ear to avoid contaminating a normal ear with organisms from an infected ear. Cytology is recommended on both ears for diagnosis.

Gently grasp the pinna and carefully insert the otoscope cone into the ear canal. Straighten the ear canal by gently pulling the pinna laterally while advancing the otoscope cone into the canal to visualize the tympanic membrane. Occasionally, the ear canal is occluded with debris and must be cleaned and flushed with saline to visualize the tympanic membrane. If cultures or cytologic samples are required, obtain the samples before cleaning the ears.

Some dog breeds, such as Poodles, have hair growth in the ear canal. This hair traps moisture and debris and increases the likelihood of infection. Hair in the ear canal should be plucked out with hemostats or the fingertips, a few strands at a time. This procedure may be painful, so appropriate restraint of the head is necessary. Sedation or tranquilization may be necessary. Grasp a few hairs at a time with the hemostats and quickly pluck the hair out. Grasping too much hair in the hemostats is painful and may cause more inflammation.

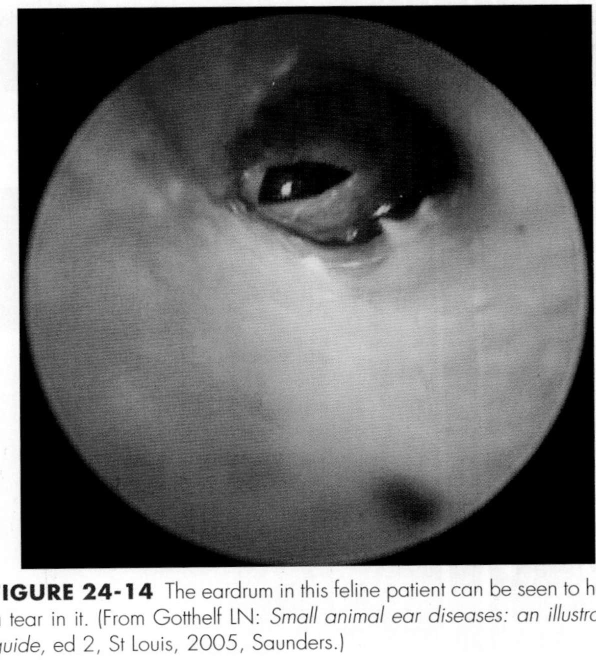

FIGURE 24-14 The eardrum in this feline patient can be seen to have a tear in it. (From Gotthelf LN: *Small animal ear diseases: an illustrated guide*, ed 2, St Louis, 2005, Saunders.)

Ensure the tympanic membrane is intact before any cleaning. Most cleaning solutions are ototoxic if the tympanic membrane is not intact. If the membrane is not intact, use a saline solution to clean the ears. Antimicrobial agents may be used if the membrane is intact. Various ceruminolytics are available for breaking up debris and cleansing. Cleansing products with a drying agent are good for cleaning the ears of dogs with long, droopy ears, such as Poodles and Cocker Spaniels (Procedure 24-1).

It is good public relations to have the patient looking better (as well as feeling better) upon discharge than when it was admitted. Examine every patient before discharge to ensure that all extraneous bandages are removed. Ensure that the patient is bathed, groomed, dematted, and smelling good and that the nails are trimmed, ears cleaned, and anal sacs expressed. Brush one last time and spray with a lightly scented spray. Educating clients on proper skin care and grooming can prevent many problems and will keep the animal in better health.

ADMINISTERING MEDICATIONS

TOPICAL ADMINISTRATION

Medication applied to the skin provides a local effect and is also absorbed through the skin. Shaving and cleaning the area or parting the hair before application facilitates absorption of the medication. Wear exam gloves and/or plastic aprons when giving a medicated bath or applying topical

PROCEDURE 24-1 Cleaning Dogs' Ears

Materials

- Basin
- Bulb syringe
- Cotton balls or cotton swabs
- Hemostats
- Ceruminolytic agents, saline solution, cleansing solution, or dilute vinegar

Procedure

1. Obtain cytology samples (if needed) from both ears by using cotton swabs and a glass slide.
2. To clean, tip the head and ear slightly ventrally, grasp the pinna, and place the solution into the ear canal, with the bulb syringe directed ventromedially into the canal. Have the basin ready below the ear to catch the excess.
3. Massage the base of the ear to distribute the cleansing solution and loosen any debris. Flush the ear again. Use cotton balls on a hemostat to clean the debris in the ear canal, or 4×4 gauze squares. Never insert cotton-tipped swabs into the canal of an inadequately restrained patient. These cotton swabs should be used for the external ear canal and interior of the pinna only. Allow the patient to shake its head occasionally to loosen more debris.
4. Flush and clean the ears until debris is no longer visible. Dry the ear canal with cotton balls or 4×4 gauze squares.
5. Examine the ears with an otoscope and apply any medications necessary. Massage the ear canal to distribute the medication evenly and thoroughly.

medication. Topical medications include medicated shampoos for skin diseases, fentanyl transdermal patches for analgesia, spot-on flea and tick control, topical anesthetics, nitroglycerin ointment for cardiac disease, and other various antibiotic and cortisone creams/ointments.

ORAL ADMINISTRATION

Oral administration is the route most commonly used to administer medications. Medications given orally are metabolized slowly. A different route of administration is necessary if more rapid absorption of medication is required. The patient must be able to swallow and have normal digestive function if medication is given per os (PO, by mouth).

Oral medications are available in tablet, capsule, and liquid form. If necessary, tablets can be crushed or capsule contents dissolved in water and given with a syringe or feeding tube. Always check the product insert before doing this as some medications should not be modified in this way. If multiple medications are prescribed, ensure no contraindications exist if given simultaneously. Compounding pharmacies are now available to make medicine solutions with tasty flavorings. If the patient has a good appetite, the medication may be placed in a meatball of canned food (this does not work well with sick cats). If the oral cavity is damaged, the medication can be given directly into the gastrointestinal tract via nasogastric or gastrostomy tube after mixing with water for easy tube passage.

A pilling device can be used to avoid being bitten. This is a plastic rod with a rubber-tipped plunger to hold the medication (Fig. 24-15). Hemostats should not be used to administer medication, because they can damage the teeth or soft palate. Teach animal owners how to correctly administer oral medication and how to check the animal's mouth to ensure that all medications have been swallowed.

Place small patients at waist level and large dogs on the floor. Medicate cats by grasping the upper jaw over the top of the head and tipping the head back. The lower jaw will drop open, or it may need to be pried open slightly with the middle finger of the dominant hand, with the pill held between the thumb and forefinger of that hand. Place the pill in the center groove of the tongue, at the back of the throat. After swallowing, reopen the mouth to ensure pill passage. Follow this procedure with a small amount of water via a syringe for large pills. Do not scratch the soft palate with your fingers. With aggressive cats, wrapping the cat in a towel or using a cat bag may be necessary.

In dogs, grasp the muzzle using the fingers and thumb to press the skin against the teeth (Fig. 24-16). Slip the thumb of the left hand into the mouth and press up on the hard palate, keeping the lips against the teeth. Place the pill on the base of the tongue at the back of the throat. Keep the head slightly elevated, close the mouth, and hold it shut, while rubbing the throat until the patient swallows. Swallowing can be facilitated by blowing into its nose. After administering medication, always examine the patient's mouth for complete swallowing of the medication. Follow medication with a small amount of water via syringe for large pills.

To administer liquid medication in a syringe, tilt the head back slightly and pull the lips outward slightly to form a pocket (Fig. 24-17). Place the syringe between the lips and back teeth so that the liquid flows between the molars and

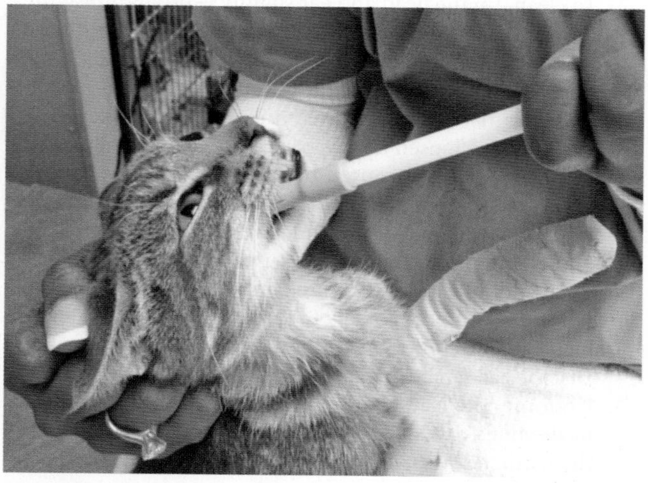

FIGURE 24-15 A pill gun is useful in administering medications to the difficult patient.

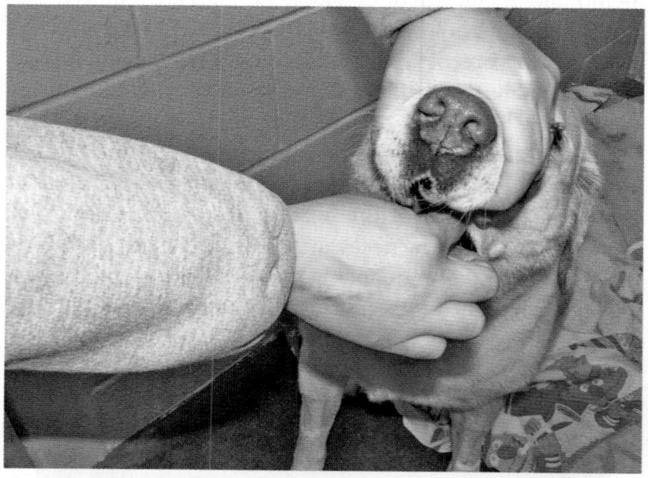

FIGURE 24-16 Oral administration of a tablet or pill.

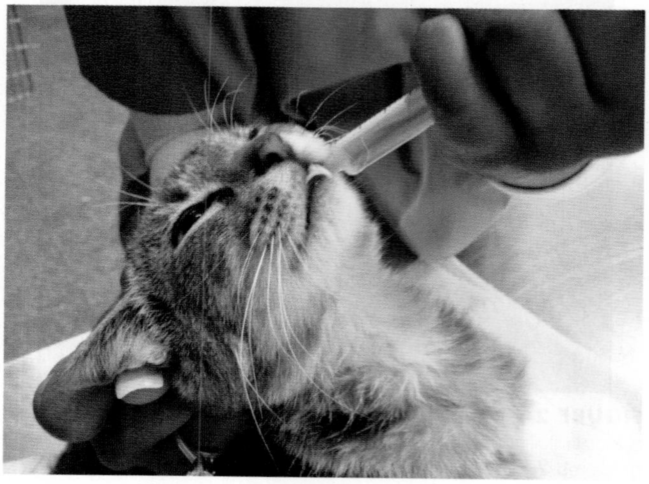

FIGURE 24-17 Liquid administration.

into the throat. Administer slowly in small boluses to allow the patient to swallow and not aspirate. Buccal or transmucosal administration of medications can also be effectively achieved in the feline patient. Specifically, use of the buccal route to deliver analgesia such as buprenorphine is more effective than the intravenous route because of the alkaline (pH 8 to 9) environment of the cat's mouth. Ease of administration of buccal medication is also an advantage to the owner, who can safely provide pain control to the pet.

RECTAL ADMINISTRATION

An enema introduces fluids into the rectum and colon to stimulate bowel activity, evacuate the large intestine for diagnostic procedures, and irrigate the colon (Procedure 24-2). Enemas soften feces and stimulate colonic motility. Tap water or saline adds bulk, whereas petrolatum oils soften, lubricate, and promote evacuation of hardened feces. Glycerin and water, mild soap and water, or commercial enema preparations can also be used for enema solutions. However, phosphate enemas (e.g., Fleet) should not be administered to cats or small dogs. Large volumes of warm water are administered with a bucket elevated above the patient and attached to soft red rubber tubing. Smaller volumes can be administered with a 60-ml syringe attached to the tubing. The solution should be at room temperature or tepid.

Enemas are contraindicated if the bowel is perforated or recent colon surgery has been performed. Complications of enema administration include perforating the colon and leakage of fluid into the peritoneal cavity, vomiting if fluid is administered too quickly, and hemorrhage if the colon is irritated. Hydration status is important to evaluate in the constipated patient. Intravenous or subcutaneous fluids, in addition to the enema, may be indicated for colonic emptying and to prevent or correct dehydration or poor perfusion.

NASAL ADMINISTRATION

Some medications may be administered into the nasal cavity to be absorbed through the nasal mucosa. Occasionally, nasal cannulas are inserted through the nares to administer oxygen and humidified air to the lungs; nasoesophageal and nasogastric tubes are inserted to provide nutrition. Respiratory vaccines and local anesthetics also may be placed into the nasal passages. Nasal administration, via syringe or dropper, is usually not stressful and most dogs and cats tolerate it very well.

Have all medications and materials ready and within reach before starting. With the patient in sternal recumbency or sitting, tip the animal's head back so that the nose is slightly elevated, and instill the medication into the nares (Fig. 24-18). It may be helpful to cover the eyes during the procedure with the hand that is holding the head back. Once the medication is administered, keep the nose elevated until the medication is absorbed through the mucosa.

OPHTHALMIC APPLICATION

Medication can be applied topically onto the eye to treat the cornea, conjunctiva, and anterior chamber. Ophthalmic medications are available in liquid and ointment forms. Most eye conditions are very painful and may require firm restraint for application. Before applying the medication, the eye must be cleaned of any exudates, including any excess hair that may deter application. An ophthalmic irrigating solution and cotton balls are used to clean the surrounding area. A clean comb can be invaluable when removing exudate from hair surrounding the eye. Have all materials and medications ready and within reach before restraining the patient.

Restrain the patient in a sternal position or sitting, with the head tipped back and the nose pointed toward the ceiling. Grasp the muzzle to prevent the patient from moving its head. Gently clean the eye area with wet cotton balls. Flush the cornea and conjunctival sac by everting the eyelids and applying a gentle stream of irrigating solution from medial to lateral. If excessive ocular discharge has caused irritation of surrounding skin, apply a thin layer of petrolatum-based ointment onto the skin.

PROCEDURE 24-2 Giving an Enema

1. For an evacuation enema, place the animal in a tub, run, or large cage. Lubricate the tubing with water-soluble lubricating jelly.
2. Wearing gloves and with the animal restrained in a standing position, insert the lubricated tube into the rectum, at least 5 cm cranial to the anal sphincter, and administer the solution slowly. Warm water enemas to evacuate the bowel are safely given at 10 to 20 ml/kg of body weight. Rapid administration may cause the patient to vomit. A small amount of liquid soap (½ tsp) and 1 to 2 tsp of sterile lubricating jelly may be safely added to the warm water solution.
3. Remove the tubing from the rectum and allow the animal to evacuate in a large area. This may take minutes to hours.

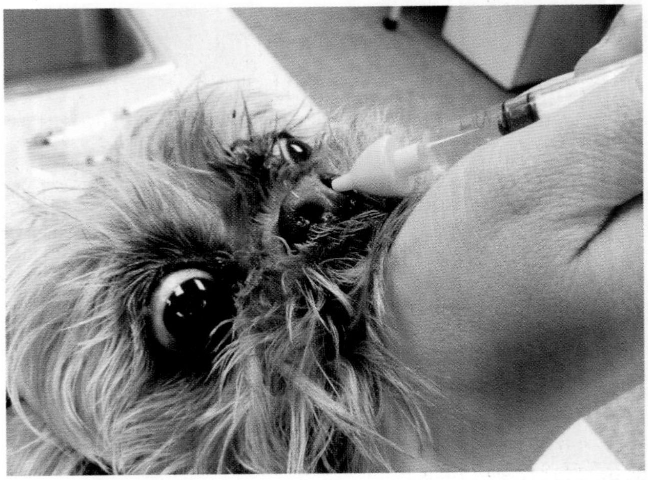

FIGURE 24-18 Intranasal administration of medication or vaccines. Note that the head is elevated to allow flow of the medication into the nasal passages.

Ophthalmic solutions are easier to administer but may need to be administered more frequently than ointments. Most solutions are applied every few hours to maintain their effect. With the dropper or bottle held 1 or 2 inches above the eye and the upper eyelid pulled up, apply the solution directly onto the sclera; then release the eyelid (Fig. 24-19). To avoid contaminating the dropper bottle or tube, do not touch the eye or eyelid with it. If more than one solution is to be applied, wait about 5 minutes between applications. If both a solution and an ointment are to be used, apply the solution several minutes before the ointment. Autologous serum is sometimes used as a treatment for certain ophthalmic conditions. Serum has anticollagenase properties and is used to counteract the destructive effects of collagenase produced by certain bacteria. If administration of autologous serum is prescribed by the veterinarian, place the blood into a serum-separating blood collection tube and centrifuge the sample. Using sterile technique, remove the serum and store in a sterile tube in the refrigerator for up to one week. An insulin or tuberculin syringe may be used to draw serum out of the tube for ocular administration. The technician should always wipe the top of the tube with alcohol to keep contents sterile. Because the patient may paw or scratch its eye after medications, an Elizabethan collar is generally recommended.

Ointment is slightly more difficult to apply. Ointments are usually applied every 4 to 6 hours; they do not wash out but may soil the skin around the eye. The ointment tube must be held close to, but not in contact with, the eye. Evert the eyelid and place a ⅛- or ¼-inch strip of ointment medial to lateral onto the cornea or lower border of the eyelid, making sure not to touch the tube to the eye or eyelid. Gently pinch together the upper and lower eyelids to disperse the ointment.

> **TECHNICIAN NOTE** If multiple eye medications are prescribed, wait several minutes between administrations. Ophthalmic solutions should be applied first, followed by ointments.

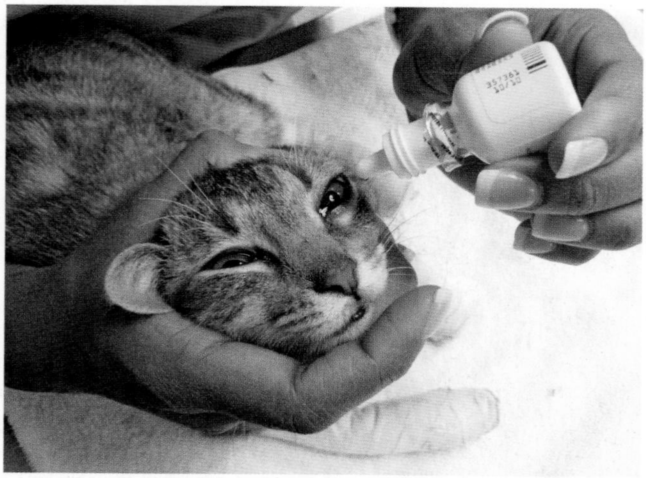

FIGURE 24-19 Instillation of ophthalmic drops to the eye. Note that the container does not touch the eye.

OTIC APPLICATION

Liquids can be instilled into the ear canal to medicate or clean the ear. The ear should be cleaned before instilling medication to ensure that the medication is absorbed and fully dispersed. Otoscopic examination is necessary to ensure that the tympanic membrane is intact before ear cleaning or applying medication. Obtain culture or cytologic samples, if necessary, before the ears are cleaned.

The simplest technique to clean ears is to rinse with a cleanser. The ears are first filled with a cleanser followed by gentle massage of the ear cartilage. After the pet shakes the material out or after tilting the head, swab the external orifice with either gauze sponges or cotton balls. Never put cotton tipped applicators down the vertical canal!

The ear can also be cleaned by using a bulb syringe. This is more effective than an ear rinse with the cleanser. Fill the bulb syringe with lukewarm cleanser or ceruminolytic agent; a mixture of white vinegar and water solution mixed in equal parts can also be used as a disinfectant. Place a bulb syringe loosely into the external orifice of the ear canal (Fig. 24-20). Squeeze the bulb gently to administer the cleanser, followed by gentle massage of the ear cartilage. Remove fluid and debris by gauze sponges and/or cotton tip applicators.

Most patients tolerate medication of the ear with minimal restraint. Start with the less affected ear first, to avoid contaminating the other ear. To straighten the ear canal, apply lateral tension on the pinna (ear flap).

PARENTERAL ADMINISTRATION

Fluids and medications administered parenterally are injected via sterile syringe and needle or through a catheter. Parenteral routes include intradermal (ID), subcutaneous (SC), intramuscular (IM), intravenous (IV), intraosseous (IO),

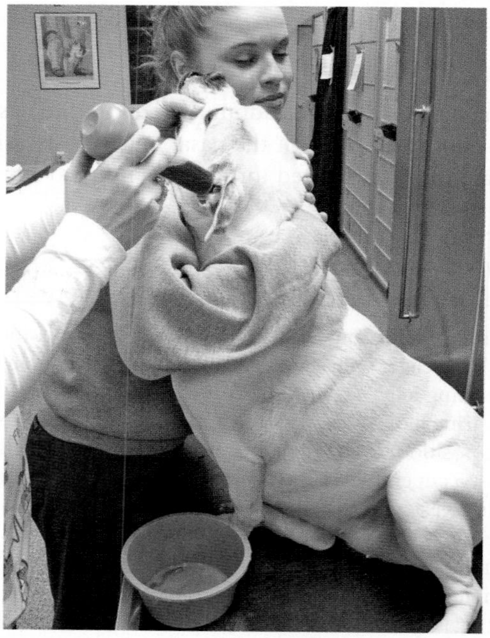

FIGURE 24-20 Ear lavage with bulb syringe; ensure syringe is directed ventromedially into the canal. A basin should be ready below the ear to catch the irrigant solution.

epidural, and intraperitoneal (IP). Local inflammation, pain, infection, nerve damage, anaphylactic or allergic reactions, and necrosis at the injection site are possible complications of parenteral administration.

Before aspirating medications into a syringe, swab the rubber stopper of the medication vial with alcohol. Select the appropriate syringe and needle size for the dose and route chosen (Table 24-3). The angle at which the needle enters the patient differs with different injection routes (Fig. 24-21). Aspirate the medication into the syringe, hold the syringe vertically, and tap it to expel any air bubbles. Change the needle before patient administration. The technician and animal handler must wear latex or chemotherapy gloves when administering chemotherapeutic agents by any route. Protective eyewear, gowns, and masks may also be indicated.

Intradermal Administration

Intradermal (ID) injections are used primarily for skin testing and local anesthesia. Skin testing may require sedating the patient before placing in lateral recumbency. Local anesthesia may or may not require sedation.

Prepare the skin for skin testing by shaving a large area over the lateral thorax or abdomen, being careful to prevent "clipper burn." Do not use antiseptics to clean the area. For local anesthesia of wounds, skin biopsies, and excision of small lesions, shave and prepare the area as for surgery.

Hold the skin taut between the thumb and forefinger of the left hand and insert the needle (bevel up) into the skin at an angle of approximately 10 degrees (see Fig. 24-21). The bevel of the needle should be within the dermis and not visible. Inject a small amount of allergen or local anesthetic intradermally to form a bleb at the site. If no bleb forms, the injection may have been subcutaneous and not intradermal.

TABLE 24-3 Syringe and Needle Sizes for Injection Route

ROUTE	NEEDLE SIZE
Intradermal	22- to 27-gauge
Subcutaneous	18- to 22-gauge
Intramuscular	22-gauge
Intravenous	20- to 25-gauge
Intraperitoneal	20- to 22-gauge
Epidural	22- to 25-gauge

Subcutaneous Administration

Subcutaneous (SC) injections are used for sustained absorption of fluids and medications and administration of some vaccines. Medication and fluids are absorbed slowly over 20 or 30 minutes or longer for larger volumes of fluids (6 to 8 hours). Clients can easily be taught to give SC injections of medication (e.g., insulin) and fluids to patients at home.

Fluids are not readily absorbed when injected SC in severely dehydrated, debilitated, or patients with poor perfusion or shock. The IV route should be used in such cases. Hypertonic, caustic, or irritating solutions administered SC can cause damage and sloughing of the skin and can not be administered by this route. Fluids given SC should not contain any additives such as dextrose or potassium chloride exceeding 20 mEq/L. Read the drug's package insert before administering medications subcutaneously.

Large volumes of room-temperature fluids may be administered by gravity flow via fluid bag and administration set with a needle attached (Fig. 24-22). This allows for patient comfort during the long process of administering larger volumes of fluid. The needle should be changed with each injection site change to prevent abscessation. 18-gauge needles are recommended for the average size cat or dog, and 16-gauge for large dogs. The patient should be restrained in a comfortable sitting, standing, or sternal position. Most cats and dogs tolerate SC administration well. Carefully part the hair, clean the skin if excessively dirty, and apply a skin antiseptic, such as 70% alcohol. Between 50 and 100 ml of fluid may be safely administered at each site without discomfort. Common sites of SC fluid administration include the dorsal scapula (between the shoulder blades) as well as the dorsal spine (T-L region). The skin is "tented" and the needle inserted gently. As the fluids are administered, the needle should be held in place and fluid should not leak out during initial administration. Remove the needle after administration, gently pinch the injection site, and massage the area. This prevents leakage and facilitates dispersal and absorption of

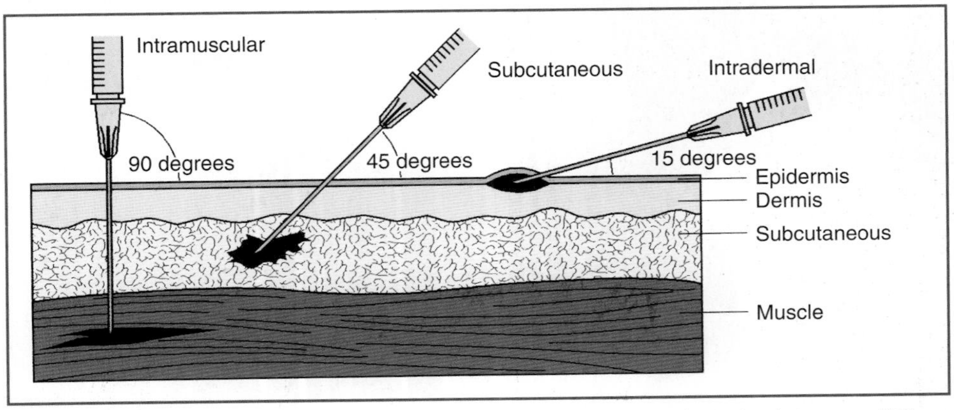

FIGURE 24-21 Comparison of angle of injection and location of medication deposit for intramuscular (IM), subcutaneous (SC), and intradermal (ID) injections. (From Bassert JM, McCurnin DM: *McCurnin's clinical textbook for veterinary technicians*, ed 7, Philadelphia, 2009, WB Saunders.)

fluid or medication. Large volumes of fluid may gradually migrate ventrally before being absorbed completely.

To give a single SC injection, grasp the skin between thumb and forefinger along the dorsal aspect of the neck or back and lift gently to form a tent (Fig. 24-23). Insert the needle into the skin fold and aspirate. If blood is aspirated, withdraw the needle and use another injection site. If no blood is aspirated, inject the medication or fluids slowly. Multiple injection sites can be used along the dorsum and lateral to the spine. Patient restraint may be necessary, because some substances can be painful on injection.

Vaccines

In all subcutaneous vaccinations, sites of the SC injection should be discussed with the veterinarian before administration.

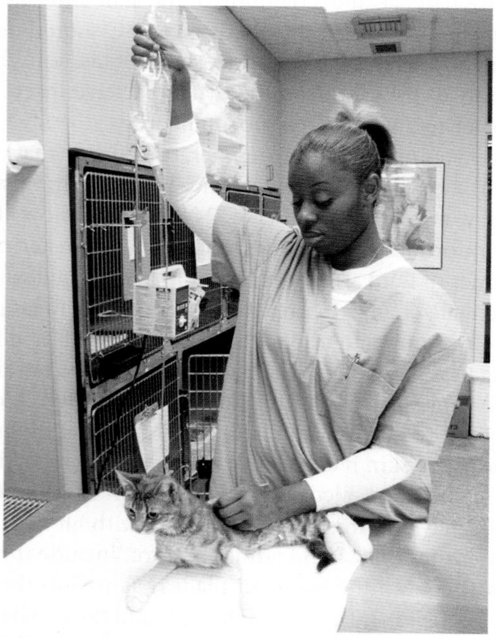

FIGURE 24-22 Administration of SC fluids. Hang fluid bag above patient; use a large gauge needle for faster administration.

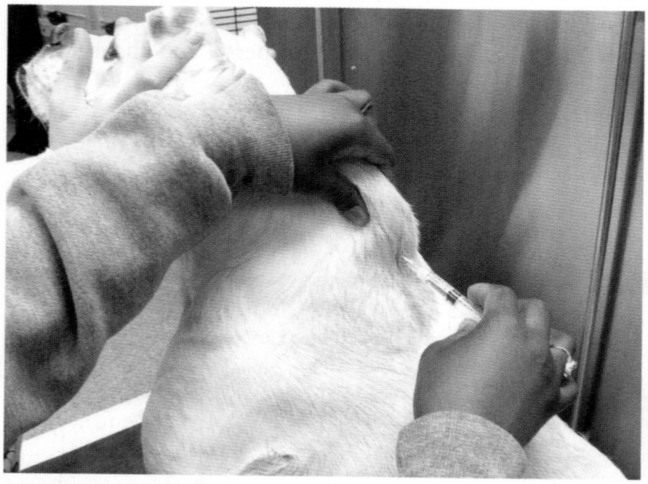

FIGURE 24-23 To give a single SC injection, grasp the skin between thumb and forefinger along the dorsal aspect of the neck or back and lift gently to form a tent.

Injections of the feline leukemia vaccine have been linked to feline injection site-associated sarcoma (FISAS) or vaccination-associated sarcoma. Sarcomas are malignant tumors; FISASs are reported to have an incidence of 1 to 10 per 10,000 cats. Many studies investigating FISAS are ongoing because of their reported linkage to certain types of vaccine.

All pets should be monitored for vaccine reactions several hours post vaccine administration. Typical clinical signs of vaccine reactions include facial swelling, urticaria, hypersalivation, and vomiting. **Anaphylaxis,** an acute and severe multi-systemic hypersensitivity reaction, may occur although it is rare. Epinephrine is the drug of choice for life-threatening anaphylaxis, whereas corticosteroids and antihistamines are used for non–life-threatening reactions. Epinephrine can be given intramuscularly in the early stages of anaphylaxis, whereas intravenous administration is preferred in poorly perfused patients.

Insulin Therapy

Insulin is typically administered SC, although in the unstable, ketotic diabetic patient insulin may be given intravenously as a single injection or as a CRI. SC administration of insulin is preferred at sites along the lateral abdomen and thorax. There are two types of insulin syringes: U-40 (for insulin of the 40 units per cc concentration) and U-100 syringes (for insulin of the 100 units per cc concentration) (Fig. 24-24). Insulin syringes come in 0.5 cc and 0.3 cc volumes and are graded in units. The smaller the syringe volume, the easier it is to read the unit gradations. It is critical that the type of syringes used match the insulin used! One (1) unit on a U-40 syringe is 0.025 ml; one (1) unit on a U100 is 0.01 ml. Consequently, two (2) units on a U-40 syringe are 0.05 ml, which is 5 units on a U100 syringe.

> *TECHNICIAN NOTE* Clipping or shaving a 1-x 1-inch square of haired skin on the lateral thorax or abdomen will assist the owner in accurate insulin administration

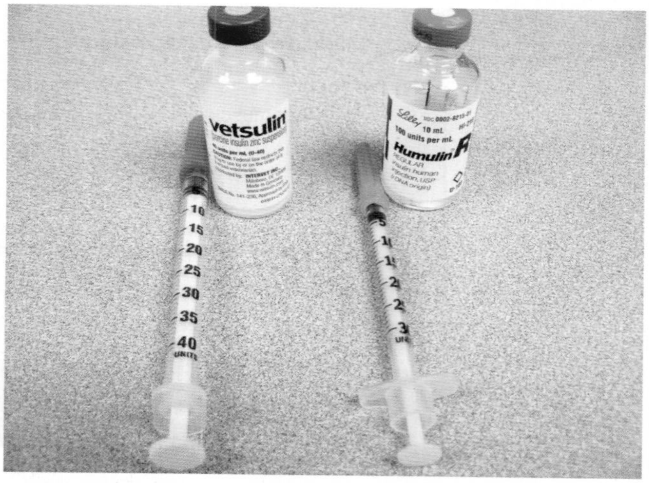

FIGURE 24-24 Insulin syringes come in 0.5 cc and 0.3 cc volumes and are graded in units.

For patients requiring small amounts of insulin, it is generally recommended to use the 0.3-cc syringes. Insulin syringes are made extra fine; patients should not object to injections. Most human insulins (e.g., Lantus and Humulin) are 100 units per cc, whereas most veterinary insulin (e.g., PZI) are more dilute at 40 units per cc. When drawing up the insulin, always hold the bottle vertically to avoid unnecessary bubbles in the syringe. Never shake an insulin bottle; roll the bottle between your hands to mix the solution.

Insulin syringes can also be used to administer small doses of other types of medications. Keep in mind that the needle is very flimsy and will dull after penetrating a vial or bend when penetrating the skin.

> **TECHNICIAN NOTE** Always match the insulin type to the correct syringe. All insulins have the proper syringe size indicated on the bottle. Warning! Life-threatening situations can arise by administering insulin in the wrong syringe.

Intramuscular Administration

Muscles are more vascular than subcutaneous tissue and medication is more readily absorbed after intramuscular (IM) administration than if given SC. However, muscle tissue cannot accommodate more than 2 to 5 ml of medication at any one site, and IM injections can be painful. Slow to moderate rates of administration with small-gauge (22- to 25-gauge) needles may be less painful than rapid injections. Intramuscular administration is never used for fluid therapy. Some medications that are poorly soluble and mildly irritating can be administered IM but not SC or IV.

Large muscle groups are used for IM injections, such as the epaxial muscles lateral to the dorsal spinous process of lumbar vertebrae 3 to 5, quadriceps muscles of the cranial thigh, and triceps muscles caudal to the humerus (Fig. 24-25). The epaxial muscles are the best site for IM injections in small patients. The semimembranosus/semitendinosus muscles on the caudal thigh should be avoided because of possible sciatic nerve damage from incorrect IM injection. If that muscle group must be used, insert the needle at a 45-degree angle directed caudally to avoid the sciatic nerve. Repeated IM injections should be alternated between muscle groups and given on different sides of the body.

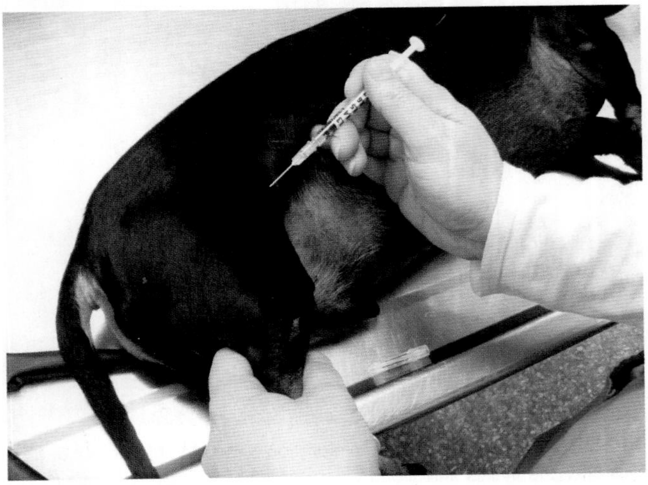

FIGURE 24-25 Large muscle groups are used for IM injections.

Proper patient restraint is necessary to avoid painful injections. Restrain the patient's head and body during IM administration. After locating the muscle group by palpation, swab the injection site with a disinfectant. With the needle attached to the syringe, quickly insert the needle 1 to 2 cm at a 90-degree angle (see Fig. 24-21). Aspirate the syringe to ensure the needle is not placed in a blood vessel. If blood is aspirated, withdraw the needle and insert into a different site. This step is crucial when injecting potent medications, oil-based drugs, or microcrystalline suspensions. If no blood is aspirated, inject the medication at a slow to moderate rate. Remove the needle and massage the muscle to disperse the medication.

Intravenous Administration

Medications and fluids administered intravenously (IV) are rapidly absorbed and reach a higher blood level faster than by other routes. Large volumes of solutions may be given in a short time. Caustic, irritating, or hypertonic medications can be given IV with fewer problems than with other routes. IV injections typically do not produce a lasting effect unless a continual infusion is given. A general rule is that if the solution is opaque, it cannot be safely given IV, except for parenteral nutrient solutions and propofol. Vaccines are never administered IV. All intravenous injections should be performed using sterile technique.

Drugs can be given IV with a syringe and needle, winged infusion set, or catheter (Procedure 24-3). The most commonly used veins for IV administration using a syringe and needle are the cephalic vein and the saphenous vein. The patient should be restrained sitting or in sternal recumbency if the cephalic vessel is being used and in lateral recumbency if the saphenous vessel is used. The use of rubbing alcohol onto the targeted area may facilitate vessel identification and provide a cleaner surface for injection.

Patient restraint is very important if using a syringe and needle for administration of medication. The limb being used must remain immobile during administration. Any movement of the patient may lacerate the vessel with the needle and/or result in extravascular administration of medication. When injecting a caustic or irritating solution, an IV catheter or winged butterfly set should be placed to prevent extravascular injection.

Always attempt venipuncture initially at a distal point on the limb. If the needle lacerates the vessel, moving more proximally or using another vein may be indicated. Light pressure should be applied at all venipuncture sites after injection to prevent hematoma formation. To place a needle into small, rolling vessels or vessels surrounded by fat (i.e., in obese patients), insert the needle into the skin lateral to the vessel. To prevent the vessel from rolling or moving, place a finger alongside of the vessel and then puncture the vessel.

Intraosseous Administration

Intraosseous (IO) administration is used to inject medication and fluids in pediatric patients in which an IV cannot be placed. The intraosseous space is always available regardless of the degree of hypovolemia or dehydration; catheters can be placed to provide short-term access quickly as opposed to struggling with a small peripheral catheter. The intraosseous space rapidly absorbs crystalloid fluids, colloids, and drugs. Catheterization can be performed by using an 18-gauge bone marrow needle or a 20- to 22-gauge 1-inch spinal needle. The needle or catheter can be inserted into the trochanteric fossa of the femur, the tibial tuberosity, or the greater tubercle of the humerus after quick clipping of hair and a surgical prep. It is helpful to use a stylet so as to avoid clogging up the needle with bone. Fluids should be warmed before delivery through an IO catheter. Intraosseous catheters can be painful and should be replaced every 72 hours.

Intraperitoneal Administration

Medication or fluids may be administered into the peritoneal space in neonates with vessels too small for IV catheterization, or in patients needing peritoneal lavage (e.g., with pancreatitis). Debilitated or hypovolemic patients do not absorb IP fluids or medication readily. Intraperitoneal administration is the least desirable route of administration because of the serious potential complications. The only routine uses of intraperitoneal procedures in small animal practice are diagnostic peritoneal lavage or IP administration of chemotherapy. More information on diagnostic peritoneal lavage is located in Chapter 17.

PROCEDURE 24-3 Intravenous Injection

1. The assistant restrains the patient, immobilizes the limb, and occludes the vessel proximal to the administration site to distend the vein. The venipuncture site may be shaved to visualize the vessel easier. The site can be prepared using 70% alcohol swabs to moisten the hair, clean the skin, and aid visualization of the vein. Surgical preparation of the site is not necessary for IV administration with a syringe and needle, unlike catheter placement.
2. Grasp the metacarpal/metatarsal area and straighten the leg. Palpate by using forefinger; the vein will feel elastic or spring-like with gentle touch.
3. Using a 20- to 22-gauge needle attached to a syringe full of medication, direct the bevel of the needle up, and insert the needle at a 30-degree angle through the skin and into the vessel lumen. Aspirate blood into the syringe to ensure venipuncture. Redirect the needle into the vessel if necessary, but do not "see-saw" back and forth. Keep in mind that wherever the needle enters the leg isn't necessarily where the vein will be accessed. Aim for the most visible, distal aspect of the vessel. The syringe and needle size should correlate with vessel size and amount of medication to be injected. Ensure that there are few, if any, air bubbles in the syringe.
4. Once the needle is in the vessel, have the veterinary technician's assistant release pressure on the vein while still holding the limb immobile.
5. Inject the medication slowly or rapidly, depending on the drug (e.g., thiopental is injected fairly rapidly, chemotherapeutic agents are given slowly and through a winged infusion set or catheter).
6. After the medication is administered, withdraw the needle and apply pressure at the venipuncture site. A light compression bandage can minimize hematoma formation.

Epidural Administration

Epidural administration is used for injection of analgesics and anesthetics. Injection of local anesthetics or analgesics into the lumbosacral junction (L7-S1) provides complete analgesia and muscle relaxation caudal to the block (Fig. 24-26).

Epidural analgesia is a useful technique for providing pain relief during painful rear limb procedures. The technique can be performed as either a single injection through a spinal needle placed into the epidural space at the lumbosacral junction or through an epidural catheter. Sterile technique is critical. Contraindications to epidural injections include patients with coagulation disorders, septicemia, or spinal trauma.

Epidural catheters can also be placed to provide a continuous infusion of analgesia. Skin preparation is similar to that for an epidural. Once the site is cleansed, a Tuohy needle is used to facilitate catheter placement. Once the positioning of the Tuohy needle is confirmed by standard methods used for epidurals, the catheter may be placed through the needle. The catheter is then secured to the skin by suturing. Before each injection into the catheter, gentle aspiration should be performed to guard against inadvertent intravenous or spinal injection. A filter should always be used before any injections.

INTRAVENOUS CATHETERIZATION

Intravenous catheters provide access to circulating blood for administration of medication, fluids, nutrients, and blood products, as well as monitoring blood pressure and collecting

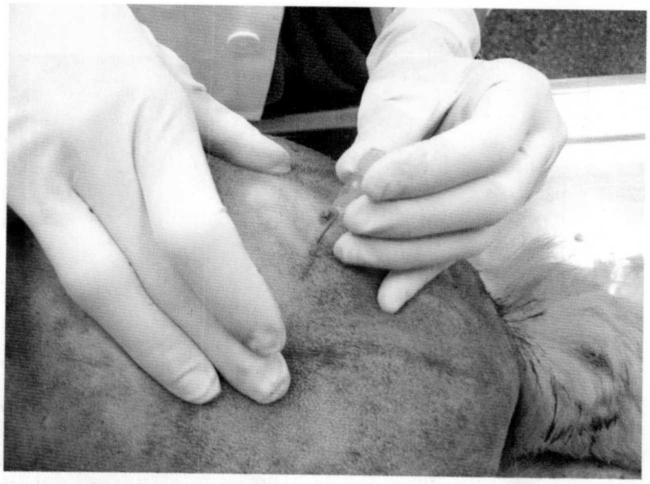

FIGURE 24-26 Epidural administration is used for injection of analgesics and anesthetics. Injection of local anesthetics or analgesics typically occurs at the lumbosacral junction (L7-S1).

blood samples. Catheters are available in a wide variety of lengths and diameters (Fig. 24-27). Types of catheters include winged infusion needles (butterfly catheters), over-the-needle catheters, and through-the-needle catheters. Common insertion sites are the cephalic vein, the saphenous vein, and the jugular vein. The medial or lateral auricular (ear) vein can be accessed in some patients where peripheral catheterization is difficult, such as in the Bassett Hound or Dachshund breeds.

The longer the catheter, the more stable it is in the vessel and the less likely it is to cause mechanical irritation with resulting phlebitis. A short, peripheral over-the-needle catheter may be inserted distal to an area of flexion, such as in a cephalic vein distal to the elbow. A **central catheter** placed in a large vessel, such as the jugular vein, is less likely to cause mechanical or chemical irritation. Hypertonic or hyperosmolar solutions such as partial parental nutrition (PPN) can be delivered through the central catheter with less incidence of phlebitis or extravasation.

The diameter (gauge) of the catheter chosen depends on the diameter of the vessel. In general, although smaller diameter catheters may be easier to place and can be less traumatic to a vessel, rapid fluid administration of fluids can become problematic. Larger, more rigid catheters are typically easier to advance through the skin but have the potential to cause more damage to vessel walls compared with the smaller diameter catheters. The general recommendation is to place the largest bore catheter possible without causing significant vascular trauma or stress in any patient requiring intravenous access A fluid pump can facilitate delivery of fluids through a small catheter. Small-diameter catheters are easily occluded with fibrin clots and blood sample collection through the catheter is not recommended. See Chapter 16 for more details on fluid therapy.

Winged Infusion (Butterfly) Catheters

Winged infusion (butterfly) catheters are for patients that need multiple intravenous medications (e.g., chemotherapeutic agents) but not long-term fluid therapy. Several medications can be given if the catheter is flushed with 0.9% saline between infusions of each medication. These catheters are simple to insert and cause the fewest local infections. However, they can cause irritation and may perforate the vessel. Winged infusion catheters require constant monitoring while in place and stabilization of the catheter can be difficult. Once the blood starts flowing into the catheter tubing, attach the heparinized saline-filled syringe, aspirate the air out of the tubing, and flush to ensure catheter patency before administering medications. The catheter can be taped in place for a short period of time by placing tape behind the catheter wings. Administer the medication while holding the leg and the catheter steady (Fig. 24-28). Occasionally aspirate to check catheter patency while administering medications. Once the medication has been administered, flush the tubing and the catheter with heparinized saline before removing the catheter. If multiple drugs are to be administered, flush between medications with heparinized saline.

> **TECHNICIAN NOTE** The cap should be removed before insertion of the butterfly catheter or there will be no "flash" of blood flow indicating correct placement into the vessel.

Over-the-Needle Peripheral Catheters

Over-the-needle peripheral catheters are quick and relatively atraumatic to place, inexpensive, and easily stabilized with a light bandage (Procedure 24-4). They are used for infusion of fluids, medication, anesthetics, and blood products. They can be left in place for 72 hours before changing to another vessel. Unless sterile technique is practiced during placement, the catheter can easily be contaminated (Fig. 24-29). These catheters usually cannot be used for blood sampling. Easy removal by patients, subcutaneous infusion of fluids, phlebitis, or thrombosis are potential complications of short over-the-needle catheters.

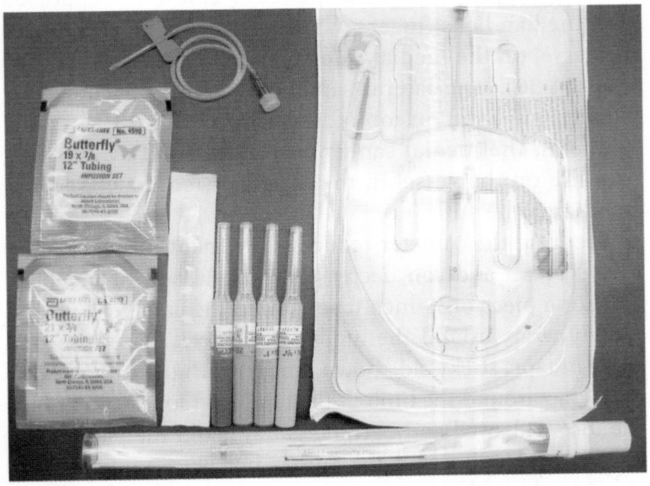

FIGURE 24-27 Catheters are available in a wide variety of lengths and diameters.

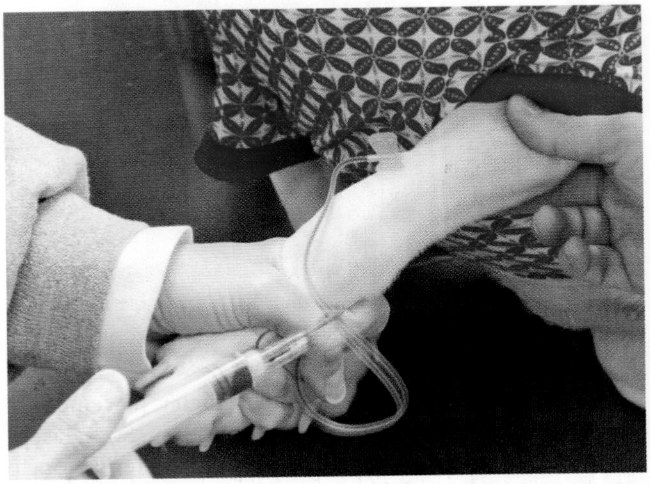

FIGURE 24-28 Winged infusion (butterfly) catheters are convenient for quick, multiple intravenous medications.

PROCEDURE 24-4 Peripheral Intravenous Catheter Insertion

Materials

- Catheter of appropriate type, length, and diameter
- Clippers with a #40 blade
- Cotton balls or gauze sponges soaked in povidone-iodine or chlorhexidine gluconate
- Cotton balls or gauze sponges soaked in 70% isopropyl alcohol
- Dry, sterile gauze sponges
- Two pieces of ½-inch-wide porous adhesive tape long enough to go around patient's limb two times or a ½-inch-wide roll of tape that has been unrolled and then loosely rerolled
- Two pieces of 1-inch porous adhesive tape long enough to go around patient's limb two times or a 1-inch-wide roll of tape that has been unrolled and then loosely rerolled
- Povidone-iodine ointment
- 2- or 3-inch roll of Kling (Johnson & Johnson, New Brunswick, NJ)
- 2- or 4-inch roll of Vetrap (3M, St. Paul, MN)
- Extension set primed with heparinized saline (2 I.U. of heparin/1 ml of 0.9% saline) or the fluids to be administered
- Injection cap

Procedure

1. Shave approximately 1 clipper blade width on each side of the vessel, with the shaved length (proximal to distal) approximately twice that of the width. This allows a second attempt at catheterization more proximal than the first, as well as providing a sterile field.
2. Prepare the insertion site using a surgical soap and antiseptic; alternate between surgical scrub or soap with alcohol to ensure a sterile field. Prepping should start at the center of the targeted vessel and cleaned in circular motions directed away from the sterile center. After prep, wash hands and apply sterile examination gloves.
3. While the handler occludes the vessel, grasp the limb with the left hand while the right hand holds the catheter with the bevel directed up.
4. With over-the-needle catheters, direct venipuncture is performed by holding the catheter at a 15- to 30-degree angle over the vein, puncturing the skin, and advancing the catheter needle into the vessel in a single, quick, smooth motion. Indirect venipuncture is performed by holding the catheter needle at a 45-degree angle slightly distal and to one side of the desired site of catheter entry into the vessel (e.g., arterial catheterization).
5. Once the catheter needle is inserted into the skin, decrease the angle of the needle, advance the catheter needle into the vein, and slide the catheter into the vessel. If the catheter does not advance into the vessel, replace the catheter and attempt catheterization more proximal than the first attempt. With a winged infusion catheter, grasp the wings between thumb and forefinger and advance directly into the vessel, keeping the vessel steady until the catheter is stabilized. Tape the catheter in place using ½-inch tape attached behind the wings and wrapped around the limb.
6. Once the catheter is advanced to the hub, remove the catheter needle and hold the catheter in place while attaching the injection cap or primed extension set. Flush a small amount of fluid or heparinized saline into the vessel to ensure catheter patency. For very small, pediatric patients, monitor the amount of fluid used to flush the catheter.

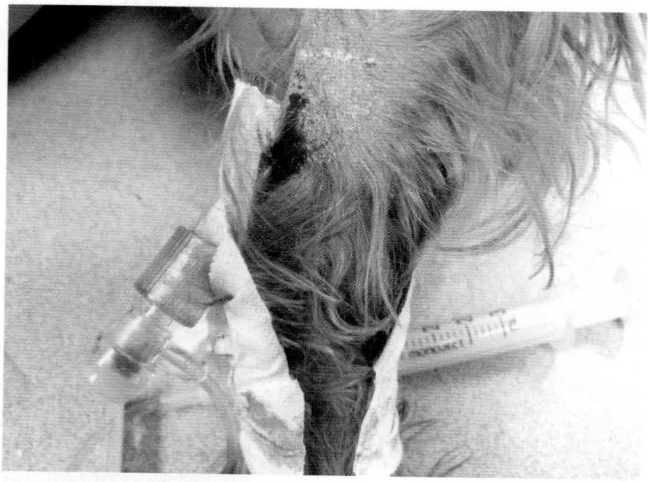

FIGURE 24-29 Intravenous catheter contamination; note areas of redness and swelling.

Proper skin preparation before catheter placement is essential to prevent phlebitis and infection. Strict aseptic technique must be followed during catheterization to avoid sepsis. Proper hand washing is done after clipping and before catheter placement. Sterile surgical gloves are indicated. The catheter must be secured with tape or sutures and covered with a light bandage to protect the insertion site. Daily bandage changes should be performed and the site inspected for signs of irritation or infection.

The selected vessel is occluded to raise the pressure in the vessel and allow for easier visualization and palpation. For the cephalic vein, the patient's elbow is supported with the handler's fingers, while the thumb is placed over the vessel on the medial side and slightly rotated laterally (Fig. 24-30). The lateral saphenous vein is occluded by placing one hand on top of and around the stifle, medial to lateral; the medial saphenous is occluded by applying pressure on the vessel in the inguinal (femoral) area and stabilizing the stifle.

Securing the catheter reduces movement of the catheter in the vessel and can decrease the likelihood of phlebitis. Anchor a piece of ½-inch tape around the catheter hub and loosely wrap around the limb (Fig. 24-31). Place a second piece of tape, sticky side down, underneath the catheter hub and wrap around the limb. If the tape is wrapped too tightly, the foot will swell and become painful, and the patient will chew at the catheter. If the tape is not placed immediately distal to the catheter insertion point and stuck to the hair, the catheter may back out of the vessel. Place a light bandage

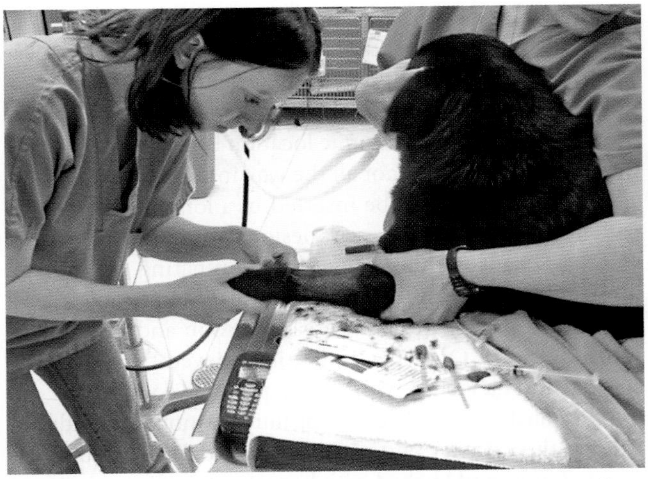

FIGURE 24-30 For easy cephalic vessel access, the patient's elbow is supported with the handler's fingers, while the thumb is placed over the vessel on the medial side and slightly rotated laterally.

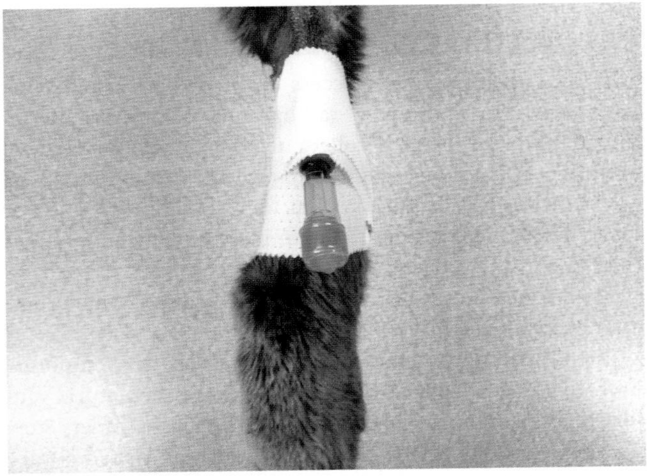

FIGURE 24-31 Securing the catheter with tape reduces movement of the catheter in the vessel and can decrease the likelihood of phlebitis.

over tape using rolled gauze and Vetrap to prevent catheter migration and gross contamination.

For an over-the-needle jugular catheter in a pediatric patient, wrap the rerolled ½-inch tape around the catheter hub and secure loosely around the neck. A light, protective bandage may be necessary to prevent catheter migration.

IV Catheter Care

Conscientious nursing care of the catheter is necessary to maintain a catheter and prevent complications from catheterization. Catheter management can prevent sepsis, the most serious complication associated with catheters. **Phlebitis,** or local venous inflammation, can be caused by contamination of the catheter during placement, or chemical or mechanical irritation. Signs of phlebitis include swelling at the catheter site, redness, pain, thickening, pitting edema, or general irritation of the vessel (Fig. 24-32). Septicemia, thrombosis, or bacterial endocarditis can be caused by indwelling catheters.

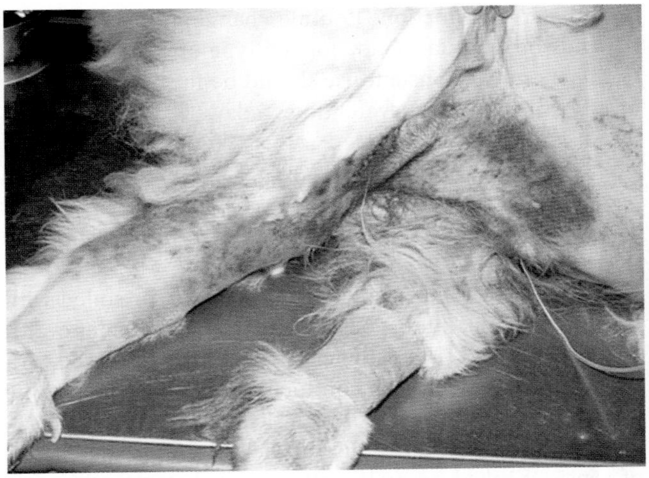

FIGURE 24-32 Signs of phlebitis include swelling at the catheter site, redness, pain, thickening, pitting edema, or general irritation of the vessel.

BOX 24-3 Signs of Catheter Phlebitis or Thrombosis

Phlebitis
- Erythema
- Pitting edema
- Pain on palpation
- Thickened appearance of the limb
- Limb feels hot on palpation

Thrombosis
- Rope-like vessel on palpation
- Pain on palpation
- Limb feels cool on palpation
- Vessel stands up without being held-off

Signs of septicemia and bacterial endocarditis include cardiac arrhythmias or murmurs, injected mucous membranes, fever, and leukocytosis. Signs of thrombosis include a vein that stands up without being held off and a thick cordlike feeling to the vein; the limb may feel cold and painful to the patient (Box 24-3). When signs of phlebitis or thrombosis are apparent, the catheter should be removed and a new one placed at a different site

TECHNICIAN NOTE If thrombosis is suspected in a limb, use a Doppler blood pressure machine to assess perfusion by monitoring presence of an audible arterial pulse. Toe pads can also be inspected for evidence of a bluish-tint, indicating poor blood flow.

The catheter bandage must be kept clean and dry, the catheter and extension set clear of any blood clots, and a closed administration system established to prevent contamination. The patient's body temperature should be measured at least once daily, the site proximal to the catheter monitored for any signs of phlebitis or subcutaneous fluid accumulation, and the toes checked for swelling. The catheter should be removed at the first sign of phlebitis, thrombosis, sepsis, or catheter malfunction. Routine changing of the catheter depends on hospital policy for the type of catheter placed. Catheters not in constant use should be flushed with saline or heparinized saline several times a day.

> **TECHNICIAN NOTE** Any unexplained fever in the patient should warrant IV catheter replacement.

When the catheter bandage becomes wet or soiled with organic material, it must be changed and the catheter evaluated for problems. The catheter may need to be covered with plastic to keep clean in incontinent patients. Swabbing the injection port with alcohol or a disinfectant before flushing or injecting medications can help decrease the chance of sepsis. Kinked or malfunctioning catheters and extension tubing with blood clots occluding the ports must be replaced.

The amount of time a catheter can be safely left in place is controversial. Depending on the established hospital policy, a short peripheral catheter is usually moved to another vessel (new catheter inserted) every 72 hours. Leaving it in place longer can contribute to instances of phlebitis. If the catheter is properly maintained and patent, it can remain in place as long as needed. Continuous rotation of the veins used allows indefinite IV catheterization for therapy. Central catheters may be left in place for an extended period, with routine catheter bandage changes, provided the catheter is still functional.

Patients receiving hyperalimentation require a central catheter for nutritional support and an additional peripheral catheter for medication and fluid therapy. Another central catheter is also necessary if central venous pressure (CVP) monitoring or blood sampling is required. Placement of one multilumen central catheter for CVP monitoring, blood sampling, nutritional support, fluid therapy, and medication administration reduces the need for a second catheter and can be maintained for long periods.

Central catheters are long catheters made of an inert material that causes little tissue reaction and can be left in for extended periods. Placement in the cranial or caudal vena cava does not compromise venous return and decreases the possibility of phlebitis from mechanical irritation. Two types of central catheters are the over-the-guidewire (Seldinger) catheters and the through-the-needle catheters. Placement in large vessels allows greater dilution of hypertonic fluids, rapid infusion rates, administration of blood products, blood sampling, and central venous pressure monitoring. However, the cost of these catheters may be prohibitive for short-term (less than 3 days) fluid therapy. The length of central catheters needed to reach the cranial or caudal vena cava for measuring central venous pressure depends on the size of the patient. For jugular catheterization, the handler immobilizes and hyperextends the patient's head and neck while placing one finger in the thoracic inlet and applying pressure on the vessel. (Refer to Chapter 16 and 17 for placement techniques and central venous pressure monitoring technique.)

For jugular insertion, measure from the insertion point to the third intercostal space; for a saphenous insertion, measure from the insertion point to the seventh lumbar vertebra. If central venous pressures are indicated, radiographic confirmation for correct anatomic location is necessary—within the thoracic cavity but not all the way in the left atrium.

The catheter should be inserted in a long, straight vessel with no nearby infection, scars, lesions, wounds, or fractures, and little chance of the patient's contaminating the catheter insertion site. The catheter should be placed in the distal part of the vessel, away from any area of flexion and inserted toward the heart. Once placement is achieved the catheter is sutured and bandaged with a light, protective wrap.

If a constant rate infusion of fluids is not being administered, the catheter end must be capped with an injection cap or T-port and flushed with heparinized saline solution at least four times daily to prevent clot formation. Daily catheter inspection and bandage changes should be performed to assess the catheter for migration, extravasation, patient discomfort, or signs of infection.

URINARY TRACT CATHETERIZATION

Urinary catheters provide access to the urinary bladder via the urethra to administer radiographic contrast material directly into the bladder, collect urine for urinalysis, relieve urethral obstruction, maintain urine flow, and provide a closed urinary collection system for precise monitoring of urine output, collection of contaminated urine, and patient cleanliness.

Urinary catheters are available in a variety of materials, diameters, and lengths (Fig. 24-33).

Metal urethral catheters can be used to temporarily catheterize a female dog but can cause hematuria and potentially serious injury to the urethra and bladder. Sterile polypropylene urinary catheters are ideal for temporary female catheterization in lieu of a metal urethral catheter; short, "olive-tipped" metal catheters can be used to relieve an obstruction at the tip of a male cat's penis. Softer, red-rubber

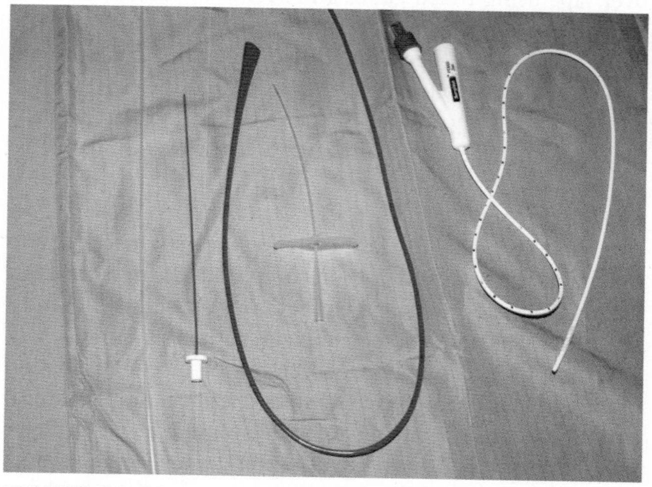

FIGURE 24-33 Urinary catheters are available in a variety of materials, diameters, and lengths.

catheters should be used for male urinary catheterization or for continuous urine collection in male cats or small dogs.

> **TECHNICIAN NOTE** 3.5 to 5.0 Fr red-rubber urinary catheters can be kept in a freezer so that they remain stiff for ease of placement in a blocked cat or small dog.

Careful placement of the most flexible, smallest-diameter catheter minimizes trauma to the urethra and bladder. However, an overly small catheter diameter may allow leakage of urine around the catheter unless a Foley catheter (containing a balloon) is used. Always examine the catheter for defects and test the bulb of Foley catheters before use by gently inflating with sterile water or saline before placement. Overinflation of the Foley balloon may cause urethral trauma or rupture; use the smallest amount of saline required. Most Foley catheters will indicate the amount of saline needed for balloon dilation on the inflation port (Fig. 24-34).

Measure the distance from the tip of the penis or vulva to the neck of the bladder before placing the catheter. Catheters that are too rigid or long can traumatize the wall of the bladder. Flexible catheters that are too long or advanced too far into the bladder can become kinked, knotted, or folded within the bladder and may require surgical removal. Foley catheters that are too short or inflated in the urethra and not in the bladder can damage the urethra.

In patients with a possible ruptured bladder, urethral stricture, or urolithiasis (bladder stones), air or radiographic contrast material may be administered through a urethral catheter to evaluate the bladder and urethra. When percutaneous cystocentesis is difficult or impossible, a urinary catheter may be passed aseptically to collect urine. Once the catheter is placed, a syringe is attached to the catheter, the sample is aspirated, and the urinary catheter is removed. Patients with lower urinary tract disease, urolithiasis, or urethral stricture require a more rigid urinary catheter placed initially to pass the problem area in the urethra, followed by a softer, more flexible urinary catheter placed for continuous urine collection. Patients with bladder atony need a urinary catheter to keep the bladder small and to prevent urine retention. Large, nonambulatory patients with leg, pelvic, or spinal fractures or recent spinal surgery require a urinary catheter collection system to avoid moving the patient excessively for nursing care.

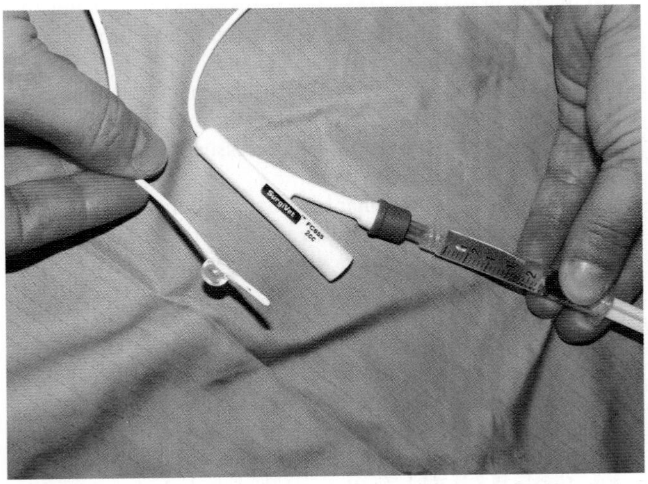

FIGURE 24-34 The bulb of a Foley catheter is gently inflated with sterile water or saline to prevent leakage around a urinary catheter. Overinflation of the balloon may cause urethral trauma or rupture.

Complications of urethral catheterization include iatrogenic ascending urinary tract infections, catheter breakage, and trauma to the urethra or bladder. Urinary catheters must be placed aseptically. Indwelling urinary catheters that are left open and exposed can lead to infection. A closed urinary system can decrease infection rates. Changing the collection system (and only if possible to replace easily, the urinary catheter) every 72 hours also helps prevent infection. Daily nursing duties include inspecting the system for kinks and blood clots, cleansing the vulva or prepuce with an antiseptic, and emptying the urine bag at scheduled times. Urinary collection bags that prevent retrograde flow are also beneficial in preventing urinary tract infections.

Most healthy cats require sedation or general anesthesia to place a urinary catheter, but very sick cats may not require chemical restraint. Most dogs do not require any chemical restraint and can be physically restrained. All patients should be placed in lateral recumbency for urinary catheterization. However, female dogs may also remain standing or be placed in sternal recumbency. Male cats may also be placed in dorsal or lateral recumbency.

> **TECHNICIAN NOTE** A laryngoscope blade can be used to visualize the urethral orifice or papilla. Hyperextend the vaginal fold ventrally and insert the blade slightly.

In female dogs, urinary catheters can be placed by visualization of the urethral orifice or by palpation. Palpation is usually better tolerated in canine patients and allows the catheter to be placed as quickly and easily as the visual method. The vagina of cats and small dogs may be too small for palpation, but a small, sterile, slit otoscope or a small laryngoscope blade can be used with a light source to visualize the papilla for placement of a flexible urinary catheter with or without a stylet. A semirigid urinary catheter may be placed with the "blind" technique but can cause trauma to the tissues. Usually a Foley catheter is placed in females to prevent leakage of urine around the catheter. The smallest Foley (5 Fr) can be placed in female cats.

Before placing a urinary catheter, gather all of the materials needed (Procedure 24-5). Clip any long hair around the prepuce or vulva and clean the immediate area with chlorhexidine or Betadine solution. Wear sterile gloves when handling the catheter and use sterile water-soluble lubricant to prevent contamination and for ease of catheter placement. Use of sterile 2% lidocaine jelly on the gloves, speculum, and urinary catheter minimizes patient discomfort.

PROCEDURE 24-5 Urinary Catheterization

Materials

- Clippers with a #40 blade
- Gauze sponges for cleaning skin
- Cleaning solution
- Sterile water-soluble lubricating jelly
- Sterile gloves
- Urinary catheter of appropriate type and size
- Flexible wire stylet, or plastic stylet for very flexible catheters
- Light source and sterile speculum for female patients
- Urinary collection system and connecting tubes
- Material to stabilize the urinary catheter in place (e.g., 1-inch tape, suture material, gauze sponges, Kling, 3-inch elastic tape)

Procedure: Catheter Placement in Male Dogs

1. Shave the hair around the prepuce and apply thumb pressure caudally where the prepuce attaches to the abdomen.
2. Retract the prepuce to expose the distal glans penis.
3. Clean away exudates with the gauze sponges and cleaning solution such as chlorhexidine or Betadine. The veterinary technician's assistant continues to hold the penis in this manner during catheterization.
4. With gloves on, place lubricating jelly onto the tip of the urinary catheter and insert the catheter into the distal urethral orifice.
5. Advance the catheter into the bladder until urine flows out continuously, then advance 1 to 2 cm farther to place all catheter fenestrations in the bladder. If resistance is met early during catheter advancement, the assistant may loosen their grip slightly on the prepuce to facilitate passage past the os penis.
6. For Foley catheters, advance the catheter 4 or 5 cm farther to ensure the balloon is in the bladder. Inflate the balloon slowly with saline so that it does not burst (see Figure 24-33). To minimize the length of catheter in the bladder, gently withdraw the Foley catheter until the balloon halts withdrawal.
7. To place urinary catheters aseptically, without gloves, keep the catheter in its sterile package while advancing the lubricated tip of the catheter into the urethra (Figure 1). A paper tab can be made with the package and used to advance the catheter without directly touching the catheter. Avoid touching the penis with the paper tab. Advance the catheter as directed above.

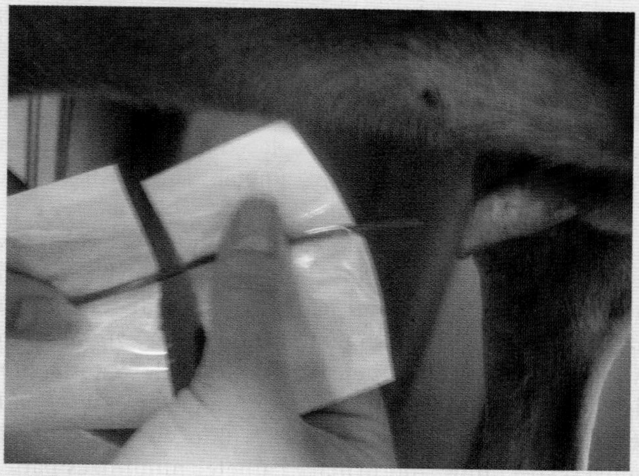

FIGURE 1 Urinary catheters can be aseptically placed in the male patient by keeping the catheter in its sterile package while advancing the lubricated tip of the catheter into the urethra.

8. Once the catheter is placed and urine is flowing freely, release the os penis and allow the prepuce to retract over the glans penis. Secure the catheter as described in the text.

Procedure: Catheter Placement in Male Cats

1. Clean the perineal area without saturating the fur.
2. The assistant extrudes the penis from the prepuce by placing the thumb and index finger on each side of the prepuce and applying gentle pressure toward the ischium. The penis may be easier to extract if the patient is sedated and in a ventral, dorsal position.
3. With gloves on, place lubricating jelly on the catheter tip and insert it into the penis (Figure 2). The catheter will not be able to advance beyond 1 or 2 cm because of the curve of the penile urethra.

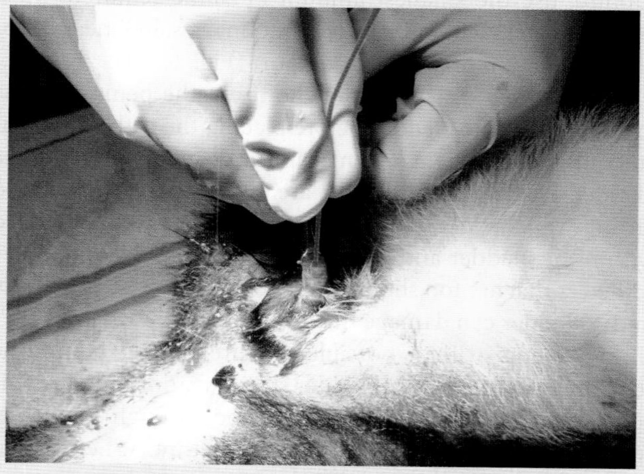

FIGURE 2 Insertion of an open-ended tomcat catheter; the catheter will not be able to advance beyond 1 or 2 cm because of the curve of the penile urethra.

4. To straighten the penile urethra, allow the penis to retract into the prepuce, then gently pull the prepuce distally while advancing the catheter through the urethra into the bladder. Continue to advance the catheter until urine flows freely.
5. Allow the prepuce to cover the penis with the catheter in place. Attach elastic tape to the catheter if no suture wings are available on the catheter.
6. Suture the urinary catheter to the prepuce and then attach the collection system. Always have a security loop attached to the patient to avoid excessive pressure on the catheter.
7. Apply an Elizabethan collar before the patient awakens. For patient comfort, it is generally recommended to replace the short, stiff tomcat catheters with longer, more flexible, red rubber catheters after the urethra is unobstructed.

Procedure: Catheter Placement in Female Dogs

1. Shave the excess hair away from the vulva and clean the perineal area.
2. For placement of the urinary catheter by visualization, lubricate a sterile speculum, the catheter tip, and the stylet tip. Insert the stylet into the catheter. A slight bend in the stylet approximately 1 cm from the tip may help direct the catheter ventrally into the urethral orifice. Ensure patency of the Foley by adding saline to the balloon.

PROCEDURE 24-5 Urinary Catheterization—cont'd

3. Gently place the speculum into the vagina and direct it dorsally and then cranially until the angle becomes more horizontal. The speculum is not inserted very far in female cats. Look through the speculum while slowly backing out of the vagina. The urethral orifice is on the ventral aspect of the vagina, cranial to the vulva.
4. Holding the speculum and light source steady, guide the urinary catheter and stylet gently through the speculum into the urethral orifice. Gently advance the catheter through the urethral orifice into the bladder. Once the catheter is placed into the bladder, and urine is freely flowing through the catheter, advance the catheter 1 or 2 cm farther to ensure that the fenestrations or the entire balloon is in the bladder and inflate the balloon if using a Foley catheter.
5. Remove the speculum from the vagina and back the Foley catheter out until the balloon stops at the neck of the bladder. If using the sterile slit otoscope cone, remove the cone from the catheter by sliding the catheter through the slit. If using a red rubber or non-Foley catheter in a cat, the catheter will need butterfly wings attached to the catheter before suturing to the perineal area. Attach the extension of the collection system to the leg of the patient (see Figure 24-35). Place an Elizabethan collar if necessary.
6. For placement of a urinary catheter in a female by palpation, apply sterile lubricating jelly to the gloved finger tip, catheter tip, and, if using a stylet, the tip of the stylet. If the patient is small, using the smallest digit to palpate is least painful for the patient.
7. Bending the stylet tip, once it is inserted into the catheter, may facilitate placement of the catheter but is not necessary, because the catheter is directed into the orifice with the tip of the finger. A stylet may or may not be used, depending on the preference of the person placing the catheter.
8. Identify the urethral papilla; it is a firm, round mass on the ventral aspect of the vagina 3 to 5 cm cranial to the vulva in dogs. Bend the tip of the finger just cranial to the papilla to guide the catheter into the urethral orifice. Insert the catheter into the vagina and ventrally into the urethra and on into the bladder.
9. Once the catheter is advanced into the bladder, remove the finger and inflate the balloon of the Foley catheter. Back the urinary catheter out gently until the balloon stops at the neck of the bladder. Attach the urinary system to the catheter and tape to the patient.

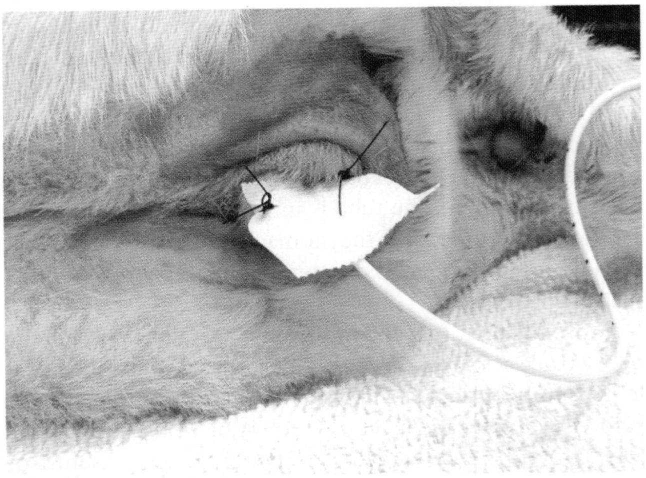

FIGURE 24-35 For urinary catheters without suture wings or balloons, make a butterfly wing with elastic tape around the catheter and suture each wing onto prepuce.

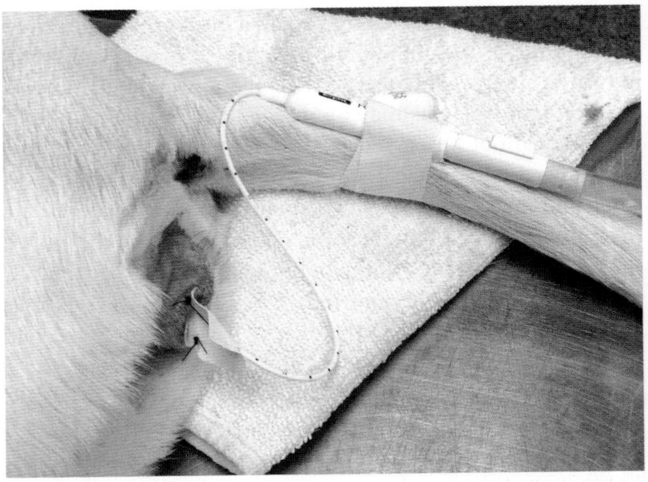

FIGURE 24-36 Female dogs may have the urinary catheter extension attached to the rear leg or tail base. Ensure enough slack to prevent tension on the catheter during tail movement.

For urinary catheters without suture wings or balloons, make a butterfly wing with elastic tape around the catheter approximately 0.5 cm from the tip of the prepuce. Suture the tape wings on each side of the prepuce (Fig. 24-35). Attach the urinary catheter collection system aseptically. Depending on the patient and the type of catheter placed, a light abdominal wrap may be necessary. For male dogs, place an abdominal bandage (not necessary for Foley catheters) to keep the urinary catheter straight and clean, or secure 1-inch tape around the catheter and wrap loosely around the abdomen. For male dogs with Foley catheters, attach 1-inch porous tape around the distal end of the catheter and loosely wrap around the abdomen.

Female dogs may have the extension attached to the rear leg or tail base, with enough slack to prevent tension on the catheter during movement (Fig. 24-36). Cats have the extension tubing looped and attached to the tail or rear leg. Place the collection bag below the level of the patient to prevent backflow of urine into the bladder. Urinary bags should be emptied and urine production quantified every 4 hours.

OROGASTRIC INTUBATION

Orogastric tubes are inserted through the mouth to the stomach and used for administering liquid medication, barium, short-term feeding of gruel type diets and flushing the stomach (gastric lavage). The animal must have a swallowing reflex to prevent aspiration if the patient regurgitates. Another cause of aspiration is passing the orogastric tube into the trachea, instead of the esophagus, and administering the medication.

A soft, flexible feeding tube is used, of appropriate diameter and length and with a slightly rounded tip. Premeasure the distance from the tip of the nose to just caudal to the last rib. Mark the tube with a piece of tape or permanent marker. Lubricate the tube with water-soluble lubricating jelly.

Place the patient in sternal recumbency or in a sitting position. Placing the dog in a sitting position or an upright position by supporting the elbows may help the distended stomach to fall away from the diaphragm and facilitates passage of a lubricated large diameter tube. Two people may need to restrain the patient if chemical restraint is not used. Elevate the head slightly and extend the neck, while passing the tube slowly and gently into the esophagus. Palpate the neck to ensure esophageal placement. Inadvertent passage of the tube and subsequent administration of medication into the trachea may result in severe lung damage and possibly death. Once the tube reaches the line marked, inject air through the tube followed by a small amount of sterile saline and auscultate for air bubbling in the stomach. Coughing may indicate tracheal tube placement and warrants immediate tube removal. Gas may be smelled as it exits the tube. If the tube cannot be passed to the line marked on the tube, withdraw it and try again. Administer the fluid with a syringe and flush the tube with a small amount of water or air to empty the tube of medication. Occlude or kink the end of the tubing to prevent spilling of liquid into mouth or trachea while the tube is being removed.

TECHNICIAN NOTE Placing the animal in different positions may facilitate the passing of the gastric tube. To ensure the tube is not in the trachea, place an end-tidal CO_2 monitor at the end of the tube; CO_2 levels should be zero (nonexistent).

NASOESOPHAGEAL AND NASOGASTRIC INTUBATION

Restrain the animal in sternal recumbency or sitting, with the head held level or slightly elevated. Anesthetize the nostril with 1 to 2 drops of topical ophthalmic anesthetic or 1 to 2 drops of 2% lidocaine. While waiting for the topical anesthetic to take effect, lubricate the tip of the feeding tube with a water-soluble lubricant or 5% lidocaine jelly.

Premeasure the tube from the tip of the nose to mid thorax and mark with a permanent marker (Fig. 24-37). Place the tip of the tube in the nares and direct the tube medially and ventrally. After the tip has been inserted 1 or 2 cm into the nostril, direct the tube caudoventrally into the esophagus (Procedure 24-6).

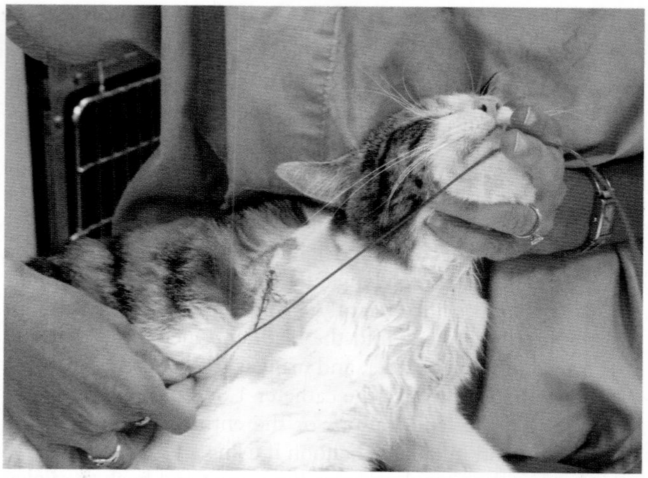

FIGURE 24-37 For nasogastric tube placement, premeasure the tube from the tip of the nose to mid thorax and mark with a permanent marker.

TECHNICIAN NOTE Pushing nares upward in a "pig-nose" position may facilitate nasogastric tube passage.

When the tube is inserted to the premeasured line, aspirate the tube first to ensure negative pressure. If excessive air is obtained, pull tube and reinsert. Infuse a small amount of sterile saline into the tube. If coughing occurs, the tube is probably in the trachea. Remove and reinsert the tube. If no coughing occurs, aspirate the syringe. If air is removed from the tube, the tube could be in the trachea. If negative pressure is evident, the tube is in the esophagus. If fluid is aspirated, the tube is in the stomach. If there is any question of tube location, make a lateral radiograph to determine placement.

Move the proximal end of the tube laterally alongside the nares, place a small strip of elastic tape around the tube, and either suture or staple it alongside the nares. The tube may be sutured without tape using a series of hand ties around the tube. Move the tube caudally between the eyes and suture or staple. Cap the end of the tube to prevent air from entering. The tube should be aspirated before every feeding to ensure patency. Any excessive amounts of air should warrant immediate tube removal.

Apply an Elizabethan collar to prevent the patient from removing the feeding tube. Evaluate the sutures or glue at each feeding to ensure that the tube is stable and not malpositioned. To remove the tube, flush the tube with air to clear fluid out of the tube. Remove the suture or staples and pull the tube out of the nose.

ENDOTRACHEAL ADMINISTRATION

Oxygen, inhalant anesthetics, medication, and small volumes of fluid can be administered through the trachea for direct absorption through the mucosa or for diagnostic

PROCEDURE 24-6 Nasoesophageal/Nasogastric Tube Placement

Indications

- Short-term feeding of liquid diet
- Decompression of esophagus or stomach

Materials Needed

- 3.5 to 12 Fr tube
- Sterile KY jelly
- Sterile saline
- 1-inch white tape
- Suture or staple gun
- Lidocaine
- Stethoscope
- Elizabethan collar

Method

1. Use 3.5 to 12 Fr tube; lube distal end with sterile lube.
2. Place 1 to 3 drops of proparacaine or lidocaine into nostril while elevating the animal's head to allow for gravity to disperse anesthetic.
3. For nasoesophageal tube, premeasure to level of xiphoid and mark tube with tape or permanent marker.
4. For nasogastric tube, premeasure to last rib and mark tube with tape or permanent marker.
5. Hold head in neutral or flexed position to allow passage into esophagus; *do not* hyperextend head and neck, as this may predispose passage into the trachea.
6. Push upward on nasal planum ("pig nose") and insert tube in ventromedial direction, introducing tube in short insertions, similar to throwing a dart.
7. If resistance is met, the tube may have passed into the dorsal nasal cavity; withdraw tube and reinsert in a more ventral direction.
8. Slide tube to designated mark; aspirate tube with syringe.
9. If a significant amount of air is aspirated, the catheter tip is either in the trachea or coiled in the pharynx; withdraw and reinsert.
10. Monitor patient response; if patient coughs or the tube exits mouth or other nares, withdraw and reinsert.
11. Using a stethoscope placed dorsally at the last rib, instill a small of amount of sterile saline into tube, followed by a small amount of air. Clearly audible gurgling sounds while rapidly injecting into the tube usually verifies correct tube placement.
12. Suture or staple tube to the skin as it courses along the side of the face.
13. Place an Elizabethan collar to keep the patient from removing the catheter.
14. If unsure of location of tip of tube, always radiograph prior to using.
15. Cap tube to prevent air influx.

evaluation of tracheal/bronchial secretions (tracheal wash). Placement of an endotracheal tube allows direct administration of oxygen or anesthetics. Humidification and nebulization for respiratory therapy can be administered through an oxygen mask, nasal insufflation tube, tracheostomy tube, endotracheal tube, or a hand-held nebulizer. Medications may be placed into the humidifier/nebulizer for direct administration, by aerosolization, to the bronchioles (refer to Chapter 17). For diagnostic evaluations of bronchial secretions, a sterile polypropylene catheter can be inserted through the skin and tracheal rings (transtracheal wash). To avoid respiratory distress, fluid volumes injected depend on the animal's size.

NURSING CARE IN SPECIAL CIRCUMSTANCES

Table 24-4 contains more details regarding nursing management of patients with specific diseases.

BLOOD PRESSURE MONITORING

Blood pressure monitoring is also used in assessment of critically ill patients. Blood pressure (BP) is the pressure exerted by the blood on the luminal wall of the vessel. The **systolic blood pressure** is the maximum force caused by contraction of the left ventricle of the heart. **Diastolic blood pressure** is the minimum force during the relaxation phase, when the aortic and pulmonic valves are closed.

Blood pressure monitoring can be accomplished by using either indirect or direct methods. The most common method, the indirect blood pressure method, uses oscillometric devices with veterinary software to compile patient data. Oscillometric indirect blood pressure measurement senses amplitude of oscillations in a pressurized cuff. These oscillations are produced by changes in arterial diameter caused by changes in pulse pressure. Measuring indirect blood pressure via oscillometry is noninvasive and does not require anesthesia or a specialty catheter. Oscillometric devices have the advantage of giving systolic, diastolic, and the mean arterial pressure. Requiring only the proper size cuff, measurements can be taken on the dorsal pedal artery or the tail base on feline patients. Disadvantages to oscillometric devices include inconsistencies in relation to patient movement, limb edema, and improper positioning or cuff size.

Another method of measuring indirect blood pressure includes using ultrasonic techniques. Devices such as the Doppler and ultrasonic pulse detectors use ultrasound kinetoarteriography to detect arterial wall motion using ultrasonic waves to amplify the sound of pulsating blood. Gradual deflation of cuff pressure allows blood flow as pressures drop below systolic blood pressure. The Doppler technique often provides more consistent and accurate results than oscillometric devices, although the Doppler only yields a systolic blood pressure and may be more difficult to obtain. Measured by a crystal probe on the ventral digital artery, an audible signal is detected as a cuff is placed above

TABLE 24-4 Nursing Management of Specific Diseases

DISEASE	CLINICAL SIGNS	NURSING MANAGEMENT
Heart Disease	Nocturnal cough (dogs) Abnormal heart rate Abnormal CRT Heart murmur ± arrhythmias Abnormal BP Poor mentation Abnormal temperature Poor MM color Dyspnea Cachexia	Blood pressure ECG Heart rate Pulse quality MM color Body temperature LOC Pulse oximetry Lung sounds Nutritional intake
Renal Insufficiency	Oliguria, polyuria, polydipsia Chronic weight loss Lethargy Halitosis Hypertension Anorexia Pale mucuos membranes Cachexia Oral ulcerations	Urine production Blood pressure Lung sounds in response to fluids Heart rate Body weight in response to fluids CVP Body temperature Nutritional intake Packed cell volume
Respiratory Distress	Tachypnea Dyspnea Cyanotic mucous membranes Abnormal lung sounds Abnormal body temperature Abnormal pulse quality Lethargy Coughing	Oxygen therapy Pulse oximetry Arterial blood gas Blood pressure Heart rate Body temperature Mentation Mucous membrane color Lung sounds Ecchymosis (with fluid therapy) Nasal discharge Body position (keep sternal)
Diabetes Mellitus	Polyuria, polydipsia Chronic weight loss Polyphagia Halitosis	Hydration status Body temperature Mentation Blood glucose Urinalysis (ketones) Blood pH Nutritional intake
Hepatic Lipidosis	Chronic anorexia Icterus Weight loss Abnormal body temperature Poor mentation Vomiting/diarrhea	Body weight Nutritional intake Electrolytes Hydration status Mentation Body temperature
Viral Enteritis	Diarrhea ± melena Dehydration Vomiting Poor mentation Abnormal body temperature	Hydration status Electrolytes Packed cell volume Body weight Gut sounds Body temperature Nutritional intake (once vomiting subsides) Mentation
Anemia	Dull mentation Anorexia Lethargy Pale mucous membranes Increased CRT Tachycardia Abnormal cardiac rhythm Tachypnea ± dyspnea	Packed cell volume Body temperature Blood pressure MM color, CRT Oxygen therapy Pulse oximetry Heart rate and rhythm Nutritional intake Hydration status
Pancreatitis	Tachypnea Mid-abdominal pain Absence of gut sounds Vomiting Diarrhea Fever Abnormal heart rate Anorexia	Hydration status Mentation Gut sounds Blood pressure Body temperature Heart rate Analgesia administration Stool production Nutritional intake once vomiting subsides
Tick-Borne Rickettsial	Fever Anorexia Vomiting Diarrhea Poor vascular integrity (edema) Petechia Lymphadenopathy Joint pain or lameness Lethargy	Body temperature Nutritional intake Hydration status Packed cell volume and total protein Colloid oncotic pressure Coagulation profile Mentation Joint stiffness or gait abnormalities
Geriatric Vestibular Syndrome	Head tilt Nystagmus Strabismus Disorientation Recumbency or ataxia Anorexia Seizures (rare)	Hydration status Nutritional intake Bladder management Physical therapy ± massage Seizure management

TABLE 24-4 Nursing Management of Specific Diseases—cont'd

DISEASE	CLINICAL SIGNS	NURSING MANAGEMENT
Sepsis	Lethargy Abnormal temperature Abnormal blood pressure Brick red mucous membranes Increased CRT Abnormal heart rate Seizures (hypoglycemia) Tachypnea	Blood pressure Hydration MM color Heart rate Body temperature Blood glucose Oxygen therapy Pulse oximetry
Dystocia	Active, prolonged straining without fetus produced Green, purulent, or hemorrhagic vaginal discharge Pain Tachycardia Restlessness Abnormal body temperature Tachypnea Vomiting (occasional)	Body temperature Hydration status Heart rate Analgesia Nutritional intake (after delivery or C-section)
Heartworm Disease	Exercise intolerance (dogs) Tachypnea ±dyspnea Coughing Ascites (dogs) Vomiting (cats) Abnormal heart rate Arrhythmia (occasional)	Oxygen therapy if dyspneic Pulse oximetry Strict cage confinement Heart rate and rhythm Hydration status Nutritional delivery
Addison's Disease	Polyuria and polydipsia Extreme lethargy or collapse in acute cases Seizures (hypoglycemia) Hemorrhagic gastroenteritis	Intravenous fluid therapy Blood pressure Heart rate Blood glucose Serial electrolyte analysis Body temperature Nutritional intake
Cushing's Disease	Polyuria, polydipsia Pendulous, "pot-belly" Bilaterally symmetric alopecia Thin skin Muscle weakness Muscle atrophy Panting Dyspnea (rare) Inappetence Lethargy Hypertension	Blood pressure Heart rate Hydration status Nutritional intake Serial electrolytes Oxygen therapy if dyspneic Body temperature
Collapsing Trachea	Honking cough Exercise intolerance Tachypnea ± dyspnea Fever Tachycardia	Antitussive administration Oxygen therapy Pulse oximetry Exercise restriction
	Increased lung sounds Wheezes	Hydration Nutritional intake Body temperature
Head Trauma	Coma or stupor Seizures Anisocoria Head tilt Hyphema Abnormal heart rate Abnormal blood pressure Tachypnea or Dyspnea	Oxygen administration Intubation if comatose Pulse oximetry Blood pressure Heart rate Body temperature Elevation of head/neck to 30 degrees Judicious intravenous fluid therapy Analgesia Packed cell volume Nutritional intake
Seizures	Facial twitching Hypersalivation Exaggerated chewing motions Whole body tremors Acute extensor rigidity Paddling Acute vocalization Involuntary urination, defecation Acute hyperthermia Tachycardia	Place sternal immediately Obtain IV access Monitor blood glucose Anticonvulsant administration Oxygen administration Body temperature Heart rate Clear airway of vomitus or hypersecretions
Spinal Trauma	Schiff-Sherrington phenomenon Flaccid paralysis to rear limbs Tachypnea Tachycardia Pain Abnormal BP Abnormal body temperature Inability to urinate Absence of anal tone	Secure to rigid surface if transported Monitor deep pain sensation Monitor presence of anal tone Hydration status Analgesia Blood pressure Body temperature Bladder management Stool production/evacuation
Hit-by-car	Pulmonary contusions Pneumothorax Fractures Hemorrhage Hypotension Head trauma Ruptured bladder Soft tissue damage	Auscultation Oxygen therapy Pulse oximetry Serial PCV/TS Blood pressure Radiographs Serial PLR Monitor urination Monitor deep pain sensation Intravenous fluids Analgesia

the probe and inflated by using a hand-held sphygmomanometer to a point where the signal can no longer be heard (Fig. 24-38). The cuff is then deflated and the pressure gauge monitored. The reading at which the pulse is first heard is the systolic blood pressure. It is important to measure the systolic pressure several times and take the average of the reading, because patients may be anxious because of both restraint and the sound emitted from the machine. Combine other data with mechanical findings, such as the pulse quality, mucous membrane color, and heart rate, as opposed to relying solely on equipment to assess perfusion. Trends should be mapped out and parameters established for proper nursing care regimens.

Proper and consistent technique is important to ensure accurate and consistent blood pressure readings (Procedure 24-7). The patient should be calm because excitement and struggling before taking a reading will falsely elevate the actual BP. For indirect blood pressure monitoring, the patient should be in lateral recumbency. The cuff should be placed on the "down" rear limb, or the limb at heart level. Elevating a limb above heart level will result in a lower reading, whereas placing the limb below heart level will falsely elevate BP readings. The cuff should be placed as close to the dorsal pedal artery as possible. The tail can be used as an alternate site; locate a pulse and place a cuff proximal to it for obtaining a BP measurement.

Cuff size is important in obtaining reliable readings. A cuff that is too large (wide) will result in a BP reading that will be falsely lowered, whereas a cuff that is too small (narrow) will result in a falsely elevated reading. Cuff width should be about one-third the limb circumference at the site the cuff is to be applied.

TECHNICIAN NOTE Avoid use of blue electrode gel, because it contains sodium chloride and will corrode the crystal BP probe. Wash the probe after each use.

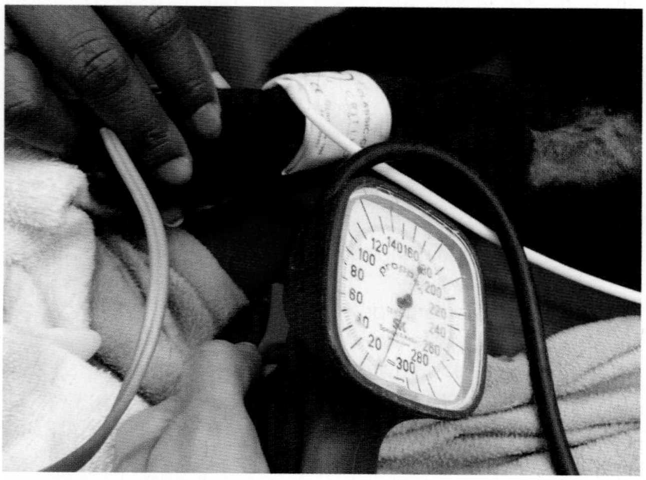

FIGURE 24-38 A hand-held sphygmomanometer is used to obtain blood pressure by cuff inflation to a point where the signal can no longer be heard.

Direct blood pressure monitoring is the most accurate method in assessing blood pressure. Designed for continuous assessment of arterial perfusion to the major organ systems of the body, direct measurements are accomplished through an arterial catheter and a transducer. Special arterial catheters are available that use the Seldinger technique or guidewire system, or regular over-the-needle peripheral catheters may be used. The transducers necessary to monitor direct blood pressure vary. Most commercial transducers come in kits with multiple administration sets and specialty tubing with

PROCEDURE 24-7 Indirect Systolic Blood Pressure Measurement

Materials Needed

- Doppler unit
- Clippers
- Sphygmomanometer
- Blood pressure cuff (single tube)
- Ultrasound gel or KY jelly
- White tape

Procedure

1. Clip hair from over pulse point (dorsal plantar surface of the digital artery) of selected limb; other common sites include the anterior tibial artery on the anterior-medial aspect of the hock/proximal metatarsus, or the caudal tail base.
2. Select proper sized cuff based on limb circumference.
3. Apply cuff to the limb at heart level, proximal to hock or carpus. The tail may be used if an audible pulse is detected.
4. Wrap the cuff snugly around the limb, securing it with the Velcro fastener and a small piece of white tape. Do not wrap it tightly or place tape around the entire circumference of the cuff.
5. Attach the sphygmomanometer to the cuff.
6. Place the patient in lateral recumbency.
7. Apply gel to *concave* surface of Doppler probe.
8. Gently place probe in the indentation over the pulse. Turn on the Doppler unit with the volume turned down to the lowest audible level. Be careful not to press the probe down over the artery with too much pressure.
9. Slightly move the probe to find the pulse if not initially detected.
10. Once you can you hear the pulse flow, hold the probe in place or tape probe in place.
11. Inflate the cuff until you can no longer hear blood flow by pushing the red exhaust lever on the sphygmomanometer *up* (i.e., closed).
12. Allow the cuff to deflate slowly or gradually release air by using the red exhaust lever while watching the pressure dial.
13. The pressure at which you can *first* hear blood flow return is the systolic pressure.
14. Take five readings and discard the highest and the lowest readings, then average the middle three for the average BP.
15. Rinse the probe and store properly.

three-way stopcocks. It is important to know particular equipment specifications in order to purchase the correct transducer at the lowest cost, because large numbers of tubing and administration sets may not be needed.

The transducer is hooked directly into a monitor that gives a readout of the systolic, diastolic, and the mean pressure through a series of waveforms. The waveform is a valuable tool in assessing cardiac function, or specifically, left ventricular ejection. As the veterinary technician palpates a pulse, it is the pressure wave or the ventricular ejection that is perceived. Direct blood pressure monitoring is useful in any critical patient or for hemodynamic monitoring during invasive surgical procedures.

> TECHNICIAN NOTE A mean arterial pressure needs to be greater than 60 mm Hg to perfuse vital organs such as the brain and kidneys.

CENTRAL VENOUS PRESSURE

Central venous pressure (CVP) is the pressure within the cranial vena cava. It reflects the condition of the cardiovascular system and is influenced by many factors, including blood volume and cardiac function. The CVP is monitored in patients receiving large volumes of IV fluids, patients with poor cardiac or renal function, critical patients, or patients with encephalopathies. It is monitored by catheterization of the cranial vena cava via the jugular vein. The catheter is connected to a fluid-filled column (manometer) and a source of fluid (syringe or bag). Normal central venous pressure is less than 5 cm water; however, the trend of CVP changes is more important than a single reading. (Refer to Chapters 16 and 17 for additional information.)

> TECHNICIAN NOTE CVP readings should be performed with the patient in right lateral recumbency for consistent results.

PAIN CONTROL

Analgesia (pain relief) can speed recovery and improve the patient's mental status. Pain can cause cardiovascular and respiratory irregularities, illicit poor wound healing, aggression, and hysteria. The ability to recognize a patient in pain and provide pain relief can prevent the patient from harming itself or the handler, improve patient health, and shorten the length of hospitalization.

Individual animals react differently to pain. If the patient is resting quietly in the cage, signs of pain may not be detected unless a physical examination is performed. Signs may include anorexia, depression, mydriasis (dilated pupils), partially closed eyes, third eyelid protrusion, tachypnea (increased respiratory rate), tachycardia (increased heart rate), pale mucous membranes, and ptyalism (excessive salivation). Other signs include whimpering or crying, sharp yipping when moved or touched, growling when approached, anxiety, avoidance behavior, restlessness, frequent repositioning in the cage, reluctance to lie down, abdominal splinting, arching of the spine, limping or non–weight-bearing on a limb, and chewing at a specific area.

Attempt to determine the location and severity of the pain, and, if possible, eliminate the cause or factors contributing to the pain. Application of heat or cold to the affected area, additional padding or bedding, massage, quietly speaking to the patient while stroking, and handfeeding highly palatable food may be of some comfort to the patient. Monitor the patient at regular intervals for change in the degree of pain.

When using medication to control pain, consult the package insert for the onset of analgesic effect. The route used may alter the onset and duration of action. For example, pain may be relieved immediately with IV analgesia, but the duration of action is short.

The common practice of waiting until a specified time has elapsed between doses of analgesic medication is not humane. Preemptive application of pain management is more effective than giving the drug after the pain is present. At the conclusion of surgery, systemic, regional, epidural, or local analgesia can be administered before the animal is removed from inhalation anesthesia. A fentanyl citrate skin patch can be applied for pain relief, but will not provide immediate relief. Fentanyl patches typically take 8 to 12 hours before being effective. Refer to Chapter 14 for more information on analgesia.

> TECHNICIAN NOTE Acepromazine is a sedative, and should not be used for analgesic effect.

RESPIRATORY SUPPORT

Respiration supplies body cells with oxygen and eliminates carbon dioxide from the body. **Dyspnea** is difficult or labored breathing, resulting from airway obstruction (e.g., infection, trauma, neoplasia, laryngeal paralysis, asthma), changes in the lungs or thorax (i.e., metastasis, pulmonary contusions, pneumothorax, diaphragmatic hernia, pneumonia, pleural effusion), or cardiovascular or hematologic abnormalities (e.g., anemia, heart failure, heartworm disease). Tachypnea refers to increased respiratory rate, but not necessarily respiratory effort.

Respiratory therapy can improve or maintain pulmonary function and tissue oxygenation. The therapeutic objective is to maintain alveolar ventilation (with oxygen, ventilator therapy, or chest tube placement), control secretions (by decreasing production and increasing clearance), and normalize pulmonary reflexes.

Respiratory support may involve placement of an oxygen mask, nasal insufflation tube, tracheostomy tube, or endotracheal tube, or placing the patient in an oxygen cage or on a ventilator to provide oxygen to the lungs and prevent hypoxia. It may also involve placement of a chest tube to remove fluid or air surrounding the lungs and allow expansion of the lungs. Refer to Chapter 17 for oxygen therapy methods.

TECHNICIAN NOTE Any patient having respiratory difficulty should be placed in sternal recumbency to facilitate chest expansion and oxygen administered by the least stressful route.

Respiratory Physiotherapy-Nebulization

Ultrasonic **nebulization** provides humidification of inspired gases and promotes mobilization of the mucous layer to aid removal of secretions in patients with respiratory disease. In conjunction with percussion and vibration (coupage), postural drainage (using gravity) moves secretions from small airways into the bronchi, where they can be coughed up. Exercise and stimulation of the cough reflex (e.g., by tracheal manipulation) also improves clearance of secretions.

Ultrasonic nebulizers produce a dense mist of microdroplets. They are used to administer medication (e.g., bronchodilators, antibiotics, detergents, mucolytics) directly to the lungs, humidify air inhaled by the patient, hydrate and loosen dried bronchial secretions, restore the epithelium in the lungs, and promote coughing (Fig. 24-39). Effective nebulization must also be accompanied by other physical therapy techniques (e.g., coupage, postural drainage, exercise, cough stimulation) to be effective in clearing the lungs. Nebulization for 15 to 30 minutes every 4 to 6 hours, with additional respiratory therapy, is more effective than continuous ultrasonic aerosolization.

The nebulizer equipment should be cleaned and all removable parts sterilized before use on each patient. Each patient should have its own sterile fluid reservoir and hoses leading from the nebulizer. Sterile fluids should be used whenever possible. Complications can also occur if the dried secretions are not suctioned immediately after nebulization therapy. The patient can become more dyspneic from swelling of the rehydrated secretions. The patient should never be left unattended once ultrasonic nebulization therapy has begun, and should always be placed in sternal recumbency to avoid aspiration.

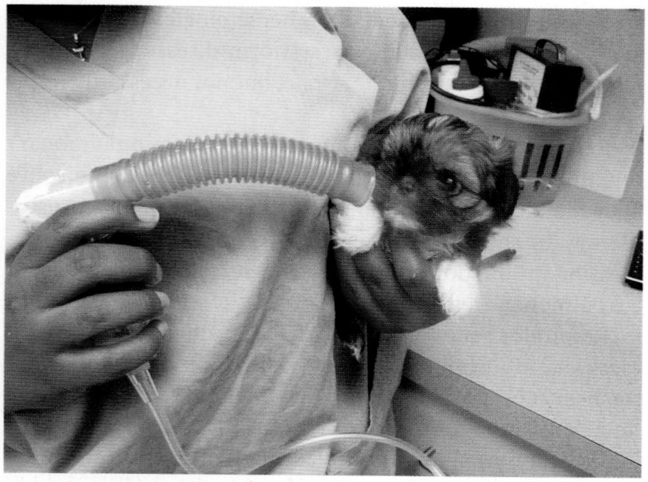

FIGURE 24-39 A nebulizer provides humidity directly to the lungs, to hydrate and loosen dried bronchial secretions, restore the epithelium in the lungs, and promote coughing.

The nebulizer hose may be attached to an oxygen mask for direct administration to the patient. Patients that do not tolerate a face mask may allow an Elizabethan collar to be placed and covered with plastic to form a tent over the head. The nebulizer hose can be attached to the tent to permit aerosolization of the patient. Another method of administration is by covering the cage door with plastic and nebulizing the cage, although this method is not as effective as direct nebulization. A cage specifically for nebulization may be used, but this can cause cross-contamination between patients if the unit is not thoroughly cleaned between uses.

Percussion is the creation of waves of air to loosen secretions in the lungs. Vibration is high-frequency compression of the chest wall. For manual percussion (or coupage), the cupped hands are clapped against each side of the chest, trapping air between the hands and the chest wall, starting with the caudal lung lobes and working cranially to move the secretions out of the tract. Care must be taken to strike the chest wall without causing discomfort or bruising. Rhythmic percussion loosens and mobilizes secretions; postural drainage, exercise, and coughing help expel the secretions. Contraindications for nebulization and coupage therapy include the patient with flail chest, pneumothorax, severe soft tissue trauma to thoracic area, bleeding disorders, or patients with chest tubes. If the patient is oxygen dependant, nasal oxygen can be used during therapy, if not already in use.

Recumbent patients may be turned to the other side or placed sternally, with the head lower than the chest to augment gravitational drainage of secretions. After nebulization and coupage, dogs may be walked outside to help increase drainage of secretions. Cats may be placed in a large cage to encourage physical activity, which increases clearance of secretions.

NURSING CARE FOR RECUMBENT PATIENTS

A number of conditions can cause recumbency in patients, including pelvic fractures, head trauma, and herniated intervertebral discs. A major concern in recumbent patients is formation of **decubital ulcers** (e.g., bed sores, pressure sores). Increased skin moisture and irritation contribute to the development of decubital ulcers; therefore, patients should be kept clean and dry, and should be bathed frequently. Because decubital ulcers are primarily caused by pressure, they can be avoided or minimized by using bedding such as sheepskin, foam or air mattresses, trampolines, or bandaging techniques. The best treatment is prevention; animals must be kept clean. Urine and feces should not be allowed to remain on the skin and hair coat. Poor sanitation promotes skin breakdown and formation of decubital ulcers. Shaving the hair around the perineal region on animals that are incontinent or have diarrhea can save time in baths and drying. Sponge baths can be done instead.

Decubital ulcers (Fig. 24-40) develop rapidly (within 2 or 3 days) but heal slowly. The extent of tissue damage is often graded from least severe (Grade I—darkened area of thickened skin, no exposure of subcutaneous tissue) to most severe (Grade IV—deep tissue loss with exposure of bone). Grade II decubital ulcers involve exposure of subcutaneous fat, and Grade III ulcers involve tissue defects to the level of deep fascial layers. Once the underlying muscle and/or bone is exposed, it can become infected. Small, superficial ulcers can be managed conservatively with doughnut bandages and topical astringents and antibiotics. Ointments with a petroleum base are not recommended, because these can trap moisture and harbor bacteria. If bone is exposed, proper care is to be taken to prevent the periosteum from drying. Prevention and treatment of infection are essential. Areas affected most are the sternum, shoulders, sides of the fifth digits, stifles, and hips. Surgical intervention may be required for decubital ulcers, especially if they are Grade III or IV in severity. Such intervention may include debridement and primary closure, delayed wound closure, or use of cutaneous or myocutaneous flaps.

TECHNICIAN NOTE Preparation-H is believed to stimulate wound healing when applied to decubital ulcers.

TURNING

Turning the patients every 2 to 4 hours helps prevent formation of ulcers and dependent pulmonary **atelectasis.** After turning, the pressure points should be checked. Redness should be only temporary. If redness persists 30 minutes or longer, decrease the time on that side. After a position change, stimulate areas over pressure points by massage and flexion/extension exercises, which will increase circulation to affected areas.

PADDING

Padding the recumbent patient is essential in preventing the formation of decubital ulcers and is also used when treating decubital ulcers. Paralyzed animals frequently thrash about; padding helps prevent animals from harming themselves. Any animal with paralysis or paresis, seizures, vestibular problems, encephalopathy resulting from neoplasia of the brain, orthopedic disease, or metabolic disease should have padding placed in the cage. Animals with vestibular disease, neoplasia of the brain, or frequent seizures should be placed in cages with padded doors and walls. Types of padding include fleece pads, sponge rubber egg crates, diapers, and waterbeds. Household items, such as blankets, sheets, and foam rubber placed in plastic bags, can be used as padding. Fleece pads are synthetic sheep skins. They are washable, absorbent, very soft, and airy. These can be combined with other forms of padding. If used alone, they are best for patients under 25 pounds.

Foam rubber egg crates are especially good for larger patients. A big disadvantage, however, is that they act like a sponge, absorbing urine and water. Place them in plastic bags to keep them clean and dry. Owners can purchase these crates at medical supply stores or in the bedding department of retail stores. Veterinary "trampolines" or cots can also facilitate patient cleanliness and may help prevent the formation of pressure sores.

Waterbeds are especially good in preventing decubital ulcers. Animal waterbeds are made in various sizes so that most standard veterinary cages will accommodate them. The bed should be placed in a cage of nearly the same area so that the patient will not fall off and become stuck between the bed and the cage wall. Animal waterbeds are thermostatically heated and provide warmth and comfort to animals placed on them. If they become unplugged, they require about 12 hours to heat up before they can be used. Temperature can be adjusted easily on the waterbeds to prevent the animal from becoming overheated or too cold. Heat eases muscle soreness, stimulates circulation, and helps animals relax. Waterbeds should never be used without turning on the heat. A cold waterbed draws heat from the animal and produces hypothermia.

Disposable diapers or bed pads are placed on top of all padding to help keep the padding clean. Use of diapers saves valuable nursing time. Soiled diapers are simply thrown away, leaving the underlying padding reasonably clean and dry. In pet stores, they are called puppy training pads.

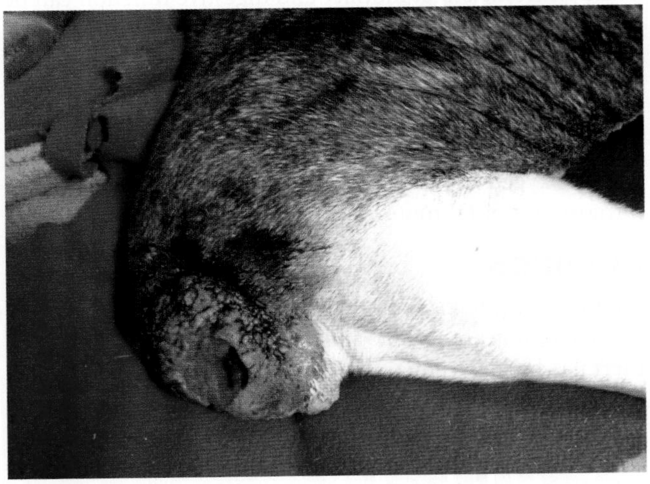

FIGURE 24-40 A major concern in recumbent patients is formation of decubital ulcers, commonly referred to as bed sores or pressure sores.

BLADDER MAINTENANCE

Every effort should be made to promote voluntary urination so that expressing the bladder and catheterization are kept to a minimum. Taking the animal outside may stimulate or promote voluntary urination. Before expressing, allow the patient to urinate. Attention should be given to bladder size, the act of urination, and the amount, color, and odor of the urine. When motor function starts to return, some bladder function usually returns, also. Time should be allowed for the patient to totally evacuate its bladder.

Palpate the bladder with even, steady pressure. Sudden movement may cause the patient to tense the abdominal muscles. In toy breeds and cats, it is easiest to use one hand. Use both hands for larger breeds. Placing patients on their side is easier than trying to hold them up while expressing the bladder, especially if the patient starts to struggle. Once the bladder is palpated, apply pressure. Several seconds may be required to override the sphincter tone, especially in animals with neurologic injury.

A urinary catheter and collection set may be used in a paralyzed animal for better nursing care. The urinary catheter should be left in place only 3 to 4 days because of the risk of infection. If hematuria or some other change in urine color develops, removal of the catheter should be considered. The risk of infection can be decreased if the animal is catheterized only when necessary. The major disadvantage is the time required to catheterize the animal.

BOWEL MAINTENANCE

Keep a record of the patient's bowel movements on the medical record or treatment sheet. An enema or digital removal of feces may be required if the patient becomes constipated. If the patient has a flaccid anal sphincter, nursing care and adequate sanitation can be especially difficult. The hindquarters of long-haired dogs and cats should be clipped closely so that feces do not smear or entangle in the hair coat. Clipping also facilitates bathing and drying if the animal becomes soiled.

CARE OF NEONATAL PUPPIES AND KITTENS

PHYSICAL EXAMINATION AND TRIAGE PROTOCOLS

The normal neonate is warm to the touch and is vigorous and vocal in its objection to handling. Body temperature ranges from 35.5 to 36.5° C. The mucous membranes should be pink to red and moist. Normal capillary refill time is less than 2 seconds. Respiration is regular (15 to 35 breaths per minute), and no fluid is auscultated over the lung fields. Minimal clear nasal discharge may be evident. The heart rate is rapid, usually 180 to 250 beats per minute. Normal hydration is evidenced by normal skin turgor. Urination and defecation are easily elicited by gentle stimulation of the anogenital area with a moistened cotton ball.

Clinical signs of sick neonates typically begin with excessive crying. Excessive crying is generally considered greater than a 20-minute period. Other signs of abnormal mentation include listlessness and the inability to nurse or remain with the bitch/queen or other littermates. A sick neonate will be limp and relaxed. Owners may report weight loss or the inability to gain weight. Physical exam findings include poor muscle tone, pale or gray mucous membranes (healthy neonates will have hyperemic mucous membranes until day 4 to 7), increased respiratory rate and effort, increased lung sounds, diarrhea, and the absence of guttural sounds. Diarrhea is present in approximately 60% of sick neonates. A sick neonate should be immediately isolated from the mother and the rest of litter.

There are particular aspects that must be addressed quickly in the pediatric patient. These include respiratory care, environmental temperature and humidity, nutrition, and fluid requirements.

RESPIRATORY CARE

Weak neonates unable to nurse following parturition may have atelectatic lungs, aspiration of amniotic fluid, or anoxia from premature placental separation. Puppies can also develop pulmonary contusions following trauma from the birth canal. Oxygen may be administered by mask or intranasal catheter if the patient is cyanotic, or if experiencing increased respiratory effort. Small portable fish tanks can also be used for an oxygenated environment. If intranasal catheters are used, fenestration is not recommended. If the patient is recumbent, place in sternal recumbency to facilitate chest expansion, or turn hourly. Although arterial blood gases are nearly impossible to collect on the neonate, a pulse oximeter can be placed on the hairless skin of the ventral abdomen. Normal oxygen saturation is >92%. Keep in mind that hypothermic patients are vasoconstricted; consequently, the pulse oximeter may read falsely low.

ENVIRONMENTAL TEMPERATURE

External warming should be provided if the neonate is separated from its mother. Hypothermia of neonates predisposes to hypoglycemia, hypoxemia, and poor digestive function. Nest box surfaces should be lined with smooth, nonporous materials to facilitate cleaning and avoid abrading the neonates. Warming protocols should include the use of circulating hot water blankets only; electric heating pads are not recommended. Other alternatives include warmed rice bags, hot water bottles, heat lamps, or Bair Hugger units. A pan of water can increase the humidity in the environment. Neonatal incubators can be used to provide a temperature of 85 to 90° F and a humidity of 55% to 65%.

Whichever heat source is used, the neonate should be able to crawl away from the heat source, and the temperature monitored at least every 20 to 30 minutes on the recumbent patient. A thermometer should be placed near the neonate to check ambient temperature. Hypothermia is common in neonates and is associated with shallow respirations, bradycardia, gastrointestinal paralysis, and coma. Feeding is contraindicated if the patient is hypothermic (<94° F), because gastrointestinal motility and digestive function can be impaired.

Neonatal body temperature should be increased slowly. The most effective method is the use of warm inspired air because it warms the core as well as the external shell (such as provided by the Bair Hugger units), or by an incubator or heated oxygen cage. Warm fluids can also be given by the intraosseous or IV route, or as an enema.

NUTRITION

Enteral food intake should always be encouraged once the animal is normothermic and adequately hydrated. Hypothermia, hypoglycemia, and poor perfusion must be corrected before orogastric nutrition is attempted. If the animal is dehydrated or too weak for oral intake, administer warm fluids slowly by intravenous or intraosseous route. Percent dehydration can be difficult to assess, but dehydration can safely be assumed if the mucous membranes are dry and of an abnormal pallor. The animal should be weighed before fluid therapy and then weighed three to four times a day. Regular assessment of the cardiopulmonary status should be performed, as it is extremely easy to overhydrate an ill puppy or kitten. Respiratory patterns should also be monitored to aide in avoiding overhydration.

Neonatal malnutrition can result from poor milk production or quality, crowding, and ineffectual nursing. Malnutrition is evidenced by failure to gain weight steadily. The birth weight should double by 12 days of age. Rotating neonates in the whelping box gives smaller, weaker individuals first access to the teats. Supplemental feeding with commercially available artificial bitch and queen milk is often indicated. Approximately 22 to 26 kcal per 100 g of body weight should be fed daily. Commercial milk replacers generally provide 1 to 1.24 kcal/ml of formula. The neonate should receive 13 to 22 ml of formula per 100 g of body weight, divided into four meals daily, over the first 4 weeks of life.

> **TECHNICIAN NOTE** Do not feed neonatal or pediatric pets if hypothermic, because digestive function may be impaired.

After dehydration and hypoglycemia are corrected, oral feeding can be initiated if bowel sounds are present. Bitch milk replacer (Esbilac, Pet Ag, Inc., Elgin, IL) or kitten milk replacer (KMR, Pet Ag, Inc.) can be used. If the animal has a strong suckling reflex, a small animal nursing bottle or doll's baby bottle may be used. Pierce the nipple with a hot needle so that a drop forms over 1 to 2 seconds when the full bottle is tipped upside-down. A syringe or eyedropper is not recommended, but can be used in an urgent situation where a bottle is not available. It is essential to deliver the liquid into the mouth slowly to prevent aspiration.

If a feeding tube is used, care must be taken not to place it in the trachea. The stomach capacity of the neonate is approximately 50 ml/kg. Although feeding frequencies vary, generally the first 3 days of life are the most critical.

> **TECHNICIAN NOTE** Improper tube placement is more likely in neonates because the gag reflex does not develop until 10 days of age.

Typically, the stomach is full from feeding when the belly is distended or the animal turns its head away from the nursing bottle and squirms. New formula should be made at each feeding and not stored reconstituted to avoid bacterial contamination. Food substances should be room temperature before administration. All equipment should be meticulously clean or sterile.

A 5-Fr or 8-Fr infant feeding tube is typically used for gavage (Fig. 24-41). Placement techniques include measuring from the tip of the nose to the last rib, marking the tube, and passing it down the left side of the mouth. A gag reflex is not present until 10 days, but easy passage to the premeasured distance usually indicates correct placement. The passage of larger tubes can be felt in the esophagus. After delivery of the fluid, kink the tube before withdrawal and withdraw it quickly to prevent aspiration. The animal should be burped after feeding by holding it at a 45-degree angle, massaging the stomach, and patting it gently on the back with fingertips only. Residual stomach volume should be measured by gentle aspiration of stomach contents (which are then returned to the stomach) before each treatment/feeding to document that fluids are being absorbed and gastric motility is adequate.

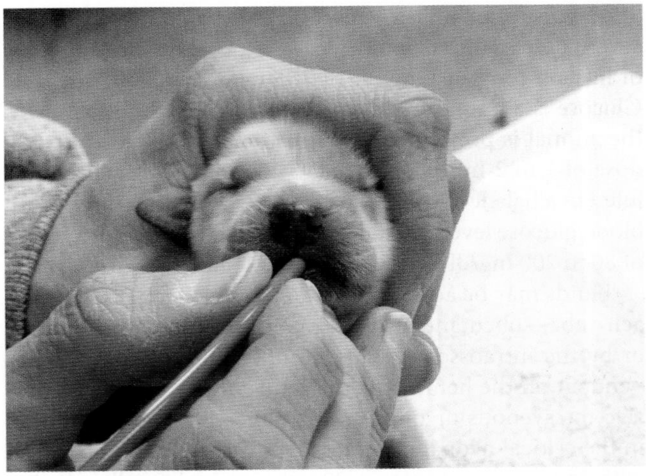

FIGURE 24-41 Gavage is sometimes necessary for nutritional delivery in the neonate. A gag reflex is not present until 10 days, but easy passage to the pre-measured distance usually indicates correct placement.

> **TECHNICIAN NOTE** Healthy puppies are expected to gain 1 to 1.5 g daily for each pound of anticipated adult weight.

Constipation or diarrhea may occur with formula feeding. If diarrhea occurs, the formula should be diluted 1:2 with balanced electrolyte solution until diarrhea resolves. A baseline birth weight should be recorded; healthy puppies are expected to gain 1 to 1.5 g daily for each pound of anticipated adult weight. Assist elimination every 2 to 4 hours (or after each feeding) for up to 4 weeks using cotton balls soaked in warm water to wipe the caudal abdomen and anogenital region. Wipe down the entire animal with a slightly damp, warm face cloth or soft nail brush 1 to 2 times/day.

FLUID REQUIREMENTS

Pediatric patients have increased fluid requirements and reduced ability to maintain glucose homeostasis compared with adult animals. Most sick neonates are hypoglycemic because of depletion of glycogen stores and immature hepatic function. Glucose can be provided orally (initially, 1 to 2 ml of 5% to 15% dextrose) to neonates which are not dehydrated or hypothermic. If mild dehydration is present, fluids containing 2.5% dextrose and 0.45% NaCl can be given subcutaneously. Hypertonic dextrose solutions must never be given

SC. Neonates exhibiting neurologic dysfunction, shock, or severe dehydration should receive glucose parenterally (IV or intraosseous) at a dosage of 0.25 ml/25 g of 20% dextrose. Glucose is administered before resuscitative fluid therapy if the animal is profoundly depressed or having seizures, at a dose of 1 to 2 ml/kg of a 10% to 20% dextrose solution diluted in a balanced electrolyte solution at a 1:10 ratio. Serum blood glucose levels should be maintained at a concentration of 80 to 200 mg/dl for normal physiologic processes.

Fluids may be administered to the sick neonate by stomach tube, subcutaneously, intraperitoneally, intravenously, or by the intraosseous route. Route of fluid therapy is dependent on the hemodynamic status of the animal; aggressive intravenous or intraosseous fluid therapy is indicated in the critical neonate. Intraosseous catheters can be placed with ease in the neonate; a 22-gauge spinal needle or standard 18- to 25-gauge hypodermic needle is an effective route for fluid administration. The most commonly used sites are the tibial tuberosity, medial surface of the proximal tibia, trochanteric fossa and greater tubercle of the proximal humerus. The wing of the ilium may also be used, but the structure is quite thin and the tip of the needle may exit the thin part of the wing. The site should be clipped and aseptically prepared, and a minimal amount of local anesthetic (such as diluted lidocaine) can be injected into the skin before placing the needle. A well-placed needle should feel firmly seated.

Dehydration occurs rapidly in neonates because of rapid water turnover. Hydration status can also be difficult to assess in neonates. Skin turgor is not reliable because of the increased water and decreased fat content of the skin. Mucous membranes should be moist and not tacky, with normal membrane color a deep red (hyperemic) for the first 4 to 7 days of life. Pale mucous membranes and slow capillary refill time (in the absence of anemia) may indicate circulatory collapse and 12% to 15% dehydration. Warmed IV fluids can be given at an initial rate of 1 ml/30 g over 5 to 10 minutes. Fluid loading is continued until color, CRT, heart rate, and body temperature have improved. The patient is reassessed every 30 minutes until stable, and then fluids are administered at a maintenance level of 60 to 90 ml/lb/day. Vitamin K should be administered to any sick neonate less than 48 hours old or exhibiting signs of hemorrhage (.01 to 0.1 mg SC or IM); note that puppies can have decreased thrombin levels at birth and are more prone to hemorrhage than adult animals.

Blood transfusions may be given IV, IO, or IP (absorption takes several days). Fluids should be warmed to 95 to 98.6° F. Maintenance fluid requirements in neonates are about 120 to 220 ml/kg/24h. Fluid requirements are significantly increased with dehydration, fever, or sepsis.

PEDIATRIC HYGIENE

Poor sanitation can lead to infections of the skin, eyes, and umbilicus (Fig. 24-42). External parasites, such as fleas and ticks, can cause severe debilitation. Flea and tick products should not be used in nursing animals, although newer products containing pyrethrins contain appropriate label directions for nursing mothers. The mother should be treated but nipples should be avoided or rinsed. Bedding should be washed or discarded. Young puppies and kittens can be treated topically by spraying a towel with pyrethrin insecticide and wrapping the animal's body in the towel, leaving the head out. A flea comb can then be used to remove dead and dying fleas. If the infant is bathed, extreme care must be taken to avoid hypothermia.

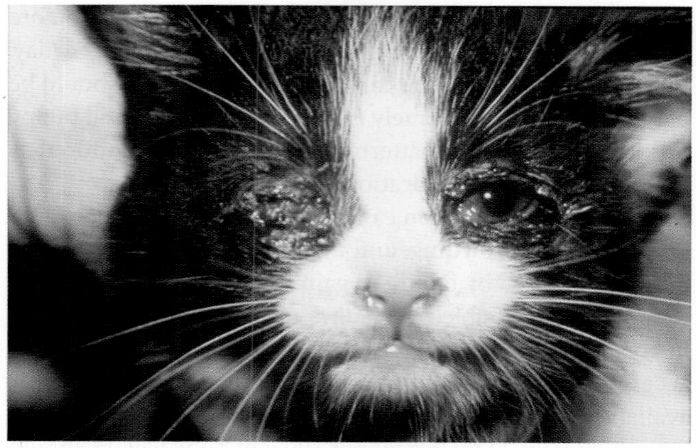

FIGURE 24-42 Poor sanitation can lead to infections of the skin, eyes, and umbilicus.

The bedding of the nest box should not show evidence of diarrhea. Disinfectants used on nest box surfaces must not leave caustic or toxic residues. Bedding material should not impair respiration or obscure neonates from the dam's view, but it should provide good footing and absorb wastes. Shredded, unprinted newspaper and washable terry cloth toweling are superior.

TECHNICIAN NOTE It is abnormal for a neonate to cry for longer than 20 minutes. A sick neonate is limp and relaxed, and often has poor muscle tone.

RESUSCITATION

Resuscitation of the neonate is necessary when the bitch or queen fails or is unable to perform this (such as after cesarean section or with maternal behavioral problems), or when a puppy or kitten does not respond to typical maternal manipulation (licking and nuzzling by the bitch or queen). An airway free of amniotic fluid, placental membranes, and meconium (first neonatal feces) should be established within 3 to 5 minutes after birth. The placental membranes, if present, are removed first, by tearing from the neonate's face. The oral cavity and trachea are cleared by swabbing with cotton-tipped applicators or gentle suction with a bulb syringe. Clearing the airway prevents aspiration of potentially damaging meconium-containing fluids.

Respiration can be stimulated by thoracic and facial massage with a dry, warm towel. Oxygen can be supplied by a small face mask if cyanosis persists.

The neonate should be completely dried and warmed. Immediate suckling is encouraged, because it provides colostrum (first milk), calories, and glucose, sparing the neonate's limited glycogen stores. If nursing is not immediately available, glucose should be provided via oral administration of one or two drops of Karo (corn) syrup. Subcutaneous administration of 5% dextrose (2 to 4 ml/kg) is possible, but this runs the risk of abscessation. Fluids administered by any route should be first warmed to body temperature.

Poorly responsive neonates can benefit from drug therapy. For the purposes of drug dosing, normal puppies weigh 100 to 700 g (0.1 to 0.7 kg) at birth, whereas normal kittens weigh approximately 100 g (0.1 kg). Reversal of the effects of any narcotic or barbiturate anesthetic agent used during anesthesia of the dam can improve the status of neonates born by cesarean section. Naloxone, a narcotic antagonist, and doxapram, a respiratory stimulant, can be administered (0.1 to 0.2 ml) into the tongue (or other muscle) or umbilical vein of the neonate.

Apnea (lack of breathing) lasting longer than 5 minutes can warrant therapeutic intervention to correct acidemia and provide substrate for myocardial metabolism. Sodium bicarbonate, diluted 1:1 with 5% dextrose (0.5 mEq/ml), can be administered at 0.5 to 1 mEq/kg via the umbilical vein, over 2 to 4 minutes. Prolonged bradycardia or cardiac standstill can be treated with epinephrine (1:10,000 solution given IV at 0.1 ml/kg) and atropine (0.03 mg/kg IM or IV).

Acquired disorders of the postpartum period include immunodeficiencies, malnutrition, and infectious disease. Orphaned neonates are at increased risk. Neonatal congenital immunodeficiencies associated with thymus dysfunction have been proposed. Acquired immunodeficiencies result from failure of passive transfer of maternally derived antibodies, acquired primarily by ingestion of colostrum during the first 24 hours of life. Acquired immunodeficiencies also occur secondary to distemper and parvoviral infections and dietary zinc deficiencies.

CARE OF GERIATRIC PATIENTS

THE EFFECTS OF AGING

Old age brings about numerous gradual degenerative changes. Body weight changes, the skin loses elasticity and becomes dry and scaly, and the hair coat becomes dull and sparse. The footpads become hyperkeratinized and the nails become brittle. In carnivores dental calculus increases. Digestion is less efficient and reduced colonic motility leads to constipation.

Cardiac output decreases with age, usually as a result of mitral valve insufficiency. The lungs lose elasticity, and increased susceptibility to respiratory infection can lead to chronic obstructive pulmonary disease, chronic bronchitis, bronchiectasis, and emphysema. Diminished kidney function leads to polydipsia, polyuria, urinary incontinence, anemia, and wasting.

In addition, muscle and bone atrophy is imminent. Degenerative joint disease and vertebral spondylosis are common in older animals. Changes in the nervous system lead to loss of short-term memory, changes in sleep patterns, and incontinence. Hearing, vision, and taste decrease; the sense of smell is preserved to some extent in most aged companion animals. Altered immune function may lead to reduced antibody response to antigens, autoimmune diseases, and a higher incidence of neoplasia.

Geriatric pets are less able to adjust to stressful conditions and some react with stereotypic, destructive, or aggressive behaviors or depression and anorexia. Separation anxiety or excessive vocalization is certainly a consideration whenever the geriatric patient is hospitalized. An animal with failing vision or hearing is more apt to be startled and overreact aggressively. House soiling is another common geriatric problem. Musculoskeletal disease may make movement to the appropriate place for elimination difficult or painful. Inappropriate elimination caused by medical problems must be differentiated from that related to behavior.

Aging pets often suffer a decline in cognitive function such as memory, learning, perception, or awareness. The geriatric pet may become disorientated, forget learned behaviors such as housetraining, or develop new fears or anxiety. Not all such changes in the aging pet are caused by cognitive dysfunction, because a variety of medical problems, including other forms of brain pathology, can contribute to these behavioral signs.

GERIATRIC CRITERIA

When the changes described above have taken a toll on the animal's well-being, that animal can be considered geriatric. The age at which this occurs depends on the expected life span of the species, as well as various individual factors. In general, species that grow to large size live longer than smaller mammals. If there is wide variation in size within a species, such as with the many dog breeds, the smaller breeds tend to live longer than the largest breeds. See Tables 12-9 and 12-10 for more information on age equivalents in dogs and cats.

NURSING CONSIDERATIONS FOR GERIATRIC PATIENTS

Handling

When providing nursing care for a geriatric companion animal, assume that the effects of aging are affecting the health and behavior of that animal. Old pets brought to the veterinary hospital may be overly anxious and have any number of problems, such as impaired vision and hearing; poor appetite; painful joints; thin bones; weak muscles; poor kidney function; congestive heart failure; chronic bronchitis; decreased liver, pancreatic, and gastrointestinal function; periodontal disease; malodorous breath; flaky skin; and a sparse hair coat.

Schedule office visits for geriatric patients during less busy times of the day and week. Never rush examinations or sample collection. Take time for discussion with the owner. Handle the geriatric animal gently and deliberately. Avoid sudden movements. Let the animal know where you are at all times. Keep your hands on the animal and gently stroke it. Be careful moving or manipulating the limbs. If the animal is to be left at the hospital, expect separation anxiety. Placing the pet's blanket or food dish or a piece of the owners' clothing in the cage or run may help reduce stress. Polydipsia and polyuria necessitate attention to the water supply and may require more frequent cleaning of the enclosure. Provide adequate bedding for patients with osteoarthritis. If possible, do not leave a geriatric patient overnight unattended in the hospital.

Drug Therapy

Drug absorption, disposition, and excretion are affected by age-related organ and metabolic changes. These alterations should be considered to ensure efficacy and avoid toxicity during drug therapy. Absorption of orally administered drugs is affected by an increase in gastric pH, loss of intestinal absorptive surface area, prolonged intestinal transit time, and decreased blood flow to the liver and gastrointestinal tract. Absorption of parenterally administered drugs is affected by increased fat deposits and decreased vascular integrity.

Although body fat increases, muscle and body fluid decrease in many older patients. Lipophilic drugs, such as some anesthetics, will be distributed more to body fat and less to the plasma, altering their effects and rate of elimination. Hydrophilic drugs, such as aminoglycosides, accumulate less in fat-containing tissues and more in plasma. Renal excretion of drugs may be reduced; the likelihood of nephrotoxicity can be reduced by reducing the frequency of dosing or reducing the drug dose.

Anesthesia

Any geriatric pet requiring anesthesia should be thoroughly examined and have a panel of laboratory tests performed (e.g., CBC, blood chemistry panel) to obtain baseline blood values. Auscultation of a heart murmur should warrant a blood pressure, an ECG reading, and/or an echocardiogram or thoracic radiographs before anesthesia. The doses of preanesthetics and anesthetics may need to be altered and usually reduced. Drugs with profound effects on the cardiovascular system should be avoided. Of the inhalant anesthetics, sevoflurane is preferred. It has minimal effects on cardiac, renal, and hepatic function, and it provides rapid induction and recovery. Chapter 14 contains detailed information on anesthetic agents available for geriatric patients. Special care must be taken when handling anesthetized geriatric patients. The animal's airway should never be compromised. The animal should be supported and handled with extreme care especially when unconscious. Intravenous fluid therapy should be monitored closely to avoid overload in the geriatric patient with a history of cardiac or respiratory insufficiency.

Client Education

Many owners fail to discuss geriatric behavior changes with the veterinarian because they incorrectly assume that these problems are untreatable aspects of aging. Educate the owners about the need for regular comprehensive geriatric evaluations, or use questionnaires to identify problems that owners might not otherwise mention during an office visit.

Aging affects all animals, but the effects of aging on each individual vary. Serious problems can be prevented by knowing the history of the geriatric patient and scheduling regular physical examinations, with appropriate laboratory tests. Veterinary technicians should educate the client on the effects of aging and the special requirements of geriatric animals. Discussions should include diet, body condition, grooming, dental problems, vaccinations, internal parasites, and the value of regular examinations. Solicit questions from the client during office visits and periodically contact the client to inquire about the patient's well-being. A healthcare program for the geriatric patient is more apt to be implemented by animal owners if they are convinced of the benefits.

EUTHANASIA METHODS

The term **euthanasia** is derived from the Greek *eu-*, meaning good, and *thanatos-*, meaning death. The goal is to provide the animal with a quick and painless death, while minimizing stress and anxiety. Considerations that help determine the method of euthanasia include safety of the individual performing the task and of the animal; ability of the agent to produce rapid loss of consciousness and death without pain, distress, or anxiety; reliability and availability of the agent; and age and species limitations. Depending on the technique used, death is produced by hypoxia, depression of neurons vital for life's function, or disruption of brain activity.

Animals can be euthanized by inhalation or injection methods. An enclosed chamber or induction mask is used to deliver inhalant anesthetics such as isoflurane. Inhalant anesthetics can also be used to render an animal unconscious while a second method is used to cause death.

Intravenous injection of an anesthetic (barbiturates) is the most rapid, the most reliable, and a very desirable method for performing euthanasia. An animal that is anxious, wild, or aggressive should be sedated before intravenous administration of any euthanasia agent. Once the animal is sufficiently sedated an IV or butterfly catheter will provide a controlled means for administration of the barbiturate. In small animals such as neonates (less than 2 kg), intraperitoneal injection is acceptable, provided the euthanasia agent is nonirritating. Intracardiac injection is acceptable in an animal that is heavily sedated, anesthetized, or comatose.

When it becomes necessary to euthanize any animal, death should be induced as quickly and painlessly as possible. It should be carried out by individuals trained and qualified to do so. When a necropsy is to be performed immediately after euthanasia, the method of euthanasia should be one that causes the least amount of artifactual changes in the tissues and leaves the animal as intact as possible.

REVIEW QUESTIONS

Matching

Match the disease or injury with the proper nursing response. Choose only one answer per situation.

_____1. diabetes mellitus	A. monitor for deep pain sensation
_____2. hepatic lipidosis	B. nutritional intake
_____3. renal failure	C. aggressive fluid therapy
_____4. respiratory distress	D. establish IV access
_____5. seizures	E. blood glucose
_____6. head trauma	F. electrolyte analysis
_____7. spinal trauma	G. serial PCV/TS
_____8. Addison's disease	H. avoid excessive IV fluid resuscitation
_____9. heartworm disease	I. strict exercise restriction post treatment
_____10. hit-by-car	J. oxygen therapy

True or False

Indicate whether each of the following statements is True or False.

_____1. Lung sounds are more subtle in the dog than the cat.
_____2. Pulmonary crackles found on auscultation usually indicates severe dehydration.
_____3. A patient's posture can help assess ventilation efficiency.
_____4. Presence of a cough usually always indicates heart disease in the cat.
_____5. Buccal or transmucosal administration of medications can be effectively achieved in both the canine and the feline patient.
_____6. A pulse deficit may indicate an arrhythmia.
_____7. Respiratory sinus arrhythmia is common in dogs, but very uncommon in cats.
_____8. Persistent jugular distention is an important indicator of right heart failure.
_____9. Mild soapy water can be an effective enema solution in the constipated patient.
_____10. Paradoxical ventilatory movements may indicate diaphragmatic hernia or some neurological condition.

Short Answer

Answer the following questions related to specific clinical scenarios.

1. A French Bulldog presents with labored breathing. Auscultation is difficult due to referred airway sounds. What are some other means to assess ventilation?
2. What is the difference between vomiting and regurgitation? Why is this clinically important?
3. During a physical exam of a dog with a history of lethargy, you note small pin-point red dots on the ventral abdomen. The mucous membranes are pale. What could this be indicative of?
4. a. List some common signs of pain in the small animal.
   b. What are some physiologic consequences of pain?
5. A Great Dane is recovering from spinal surgery for a ruptured cervical disc. His vitals are as follows: T = 97.0, HR = 200, R = 79, MM are pale, and pulse quality is poor. Auscultation is difficult over shivering and growling.
   a. What are some possible explanations for the elevated heart rate?
   b. The dog will not be able to walk for several days. What is standard protocol for any recumbent patient?

RECOMMENDED READING

Aspinall V: *Clinical procedures in veterinary nursing*, ed 3, Burlington, MA, 2014, Butterworth Heinemann.

Aspinall V: *The complete textbook of veterinary nursing*, ed 2, St Louis, 2011, Saunders.

Ford R, Mazzaferro E: *Kirk & Bistner's handbook of veterinary procedures and emergency treatment*, ed 9, St Louis, 2012, Saunders.

Lane DR: *Veterinary nursing*, Burlington, MA, 2003, Butterworth Heinemann.

Macintire DK: *Manual of small animal emergency and critical care medicine*, New York, 2005, Wiley-Blackwell.

Schaer M: *Clinical medicine of the dog and cat*, ed 2, London, 2010, Manson Publishing.

Taylor S: *Small animal clinical techniques*, St Louis, 2009, Elsevier.

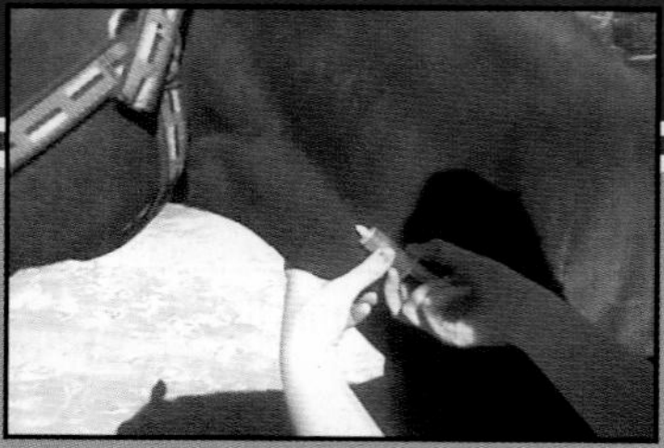

25 Nursing Care of Horses

OUTLINE

LEARNING OBJECTIVES

After reviewing this chapter, the reader should be able to do the following:

1. Discuss the principles of feeding, watering, exercising, and bedding of horses.
2. Explain and demonstrate routine procedures used in grooming and foot care.
3. Discuss the techniques used in general nursing care of horses.
4. Identify specific nursing procedures used in caring for recumbent horses.
5. Discuss the methods of sample collection for laboratory analysis.
6. State the pros and cons of using various routes of administration of medication.
7. List the steps necessary for the proper intravenous catheterization of horses.

KEY TERMS

Catabolic	Dyspnea	Hypovolemia	Pneumonia
Colic	Ethmoturbinates	Isoerythrolysis	Tachypnea
Decubital ulcers	Gastroenteropathies	Laminitis	Thrombophlebitis
Diastema	Hyperechoic	Nasogastric	Thrush
Dysphagia	Hypothermic	Perivascular	Urticaria

GENERAL CARE FOR HORSES

FEEDING AND WATERING

Proper feeding and watering of horses is a critical component of good nursing care. In addition to providing the usual maintenance requirements, the food and water given to sick or injured animals must meet their added nutritional requirements for healing. Additional information on general feeding of horses is located in Chapter 23.

Hospitalized horses often have special dietary needs. Their diseases can often create a **catabolic** state. The horse may require extra calories to maintain its weight. Horses that can chew and swallow normally should be fed their usual diet if their disease permits. Good quality alfalfa or grass hay, such as timothy hay, can be fed. Good quality oat hay is also a suitable feed. Horses with gastrointestinal disturbances, such as **colic** or diarrhea, need special consideration. Horses recovering from impactions may need more laxative feeds, such as alfalfa hay, grass pasture, and even bran mashes. Horses with diarrhea or ones that have had an operation because of colic may benefit from a diet that is not quite so rich, such as timothy or oat hay. Hay pellets or cubes that contain alfalfa or a mixture of alfalfa and Bermuda or oat hay can also be used. If added carbohydrate is needed, a pelleted feed that also contains grains may be fed.

Pelleted feed produces less dust and may be better for horses with heaves or for those suffering from respiratory allergies or **pneumonia.** Horses recovering from gastrointestinal ulceration may also need to be fed a pelleted ration, because the increased fiber and stem in hay may irritate and exacerbate certain kinds of ulcers. Pellets soaked to make a gruel can be fed to horses with oral lesions, facial fractures, dental problems, or recurrent episodes of choke. Feed softened in this manner is easier for the animal to chew and swallow. Horses with neuromuscular disorders, such as botulism, may be unable to chew and swallow normally. For these animals, a pelleted ration that has been soaked in water may be the only type of feed they can eat.

Fresh, clean water should be available at all times. Many horses will require 10 to 15 gallons of water daily; therefore, providing a continuous supply of water becomes critical in meeting this requirement. Some horses can learn to use an automatic watering cup which refills as the horse drinks the water; however, water buckets or tubs are usually used. When supplying water to buckets or tubs, the water level must be checked at least twice a day to ensure a continuous supply is available.

BEDDING

Horses can be bedded on a variety of materials. It is important that the bedding be clean, as dust free as possible, and relatively deep. Another important consideration when choosing bedding is its usefulness as a fertilizer after composting. Pine shavings are adequate for most patients, but they tend to be very dusty. This may not be acceptable for horses with open wounds or respiratory disorders. Pine shavings with minimal dust or shredded paper bedding is preferable for horses with severe respiratory problems. It is best to obtain wood shavings from a known source to prevent accidental exposure to black walnut shavings, which can cause **laminitis** when the horse stands in the shavings. Black walnut wood is darker than pine but can be difficult to recognize if the bedding is soiled or if multiple types of wood chips have been mixed. Straw bedding is often used for mares with newborn foals. Bedding should always be deep unless the horse has a problem that necessitates a firmer surface for standing. Regardless of the type of bedding used, it should be kept very clean by removing soiled bedding at least once daily. The use of rubber stall mats has also reduced the amount of bedding that has to be used.

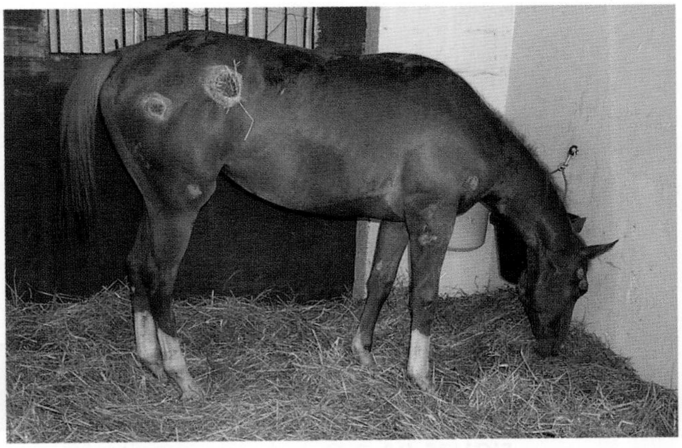

FIGURE 25-1 Patient with decubital ulcers. (From Bassert J, McCurnin D: *McCurnin's clinical textbook for veterinary technicians*, ed 7, St Louis, 2010, Saunders.)

Recumbent adult horses must have very deep bedding to help prevent formation of **decubital ulcers** (pressure sores) (Fig. 25-1). Alternatively, large mattresses or specially designed water beds can be used. Critically ill foals can be kept on mattresses with waterproof covers and fleece pads to keep them clean and dry. It may be necessary to clean the stall or change the bedding each time the horse or foal urinates or defecates if the animal is recumbent. Strategically placed diapers or absorbent mats may help reduce the number of bedding changes needed with a recumbent foal.

FLY CONTROL

The best method of fly control is to maintain a clean barn with frequent manure removal. Various topical fly sprays are available. Those containing permethrins, pyrethrins, or citronella sprays are the safest for sick horses. Overhead fly systems that release fly repellents at regular intervals can also minimize the fly population. A soft cloth can be used to apply fly repellent to the horse's face, taking care to apply the repellent around the eyes without getting any into the eyes. Fly masks are available for the face and the ears of sensitive patients and a fly sheet can also be used to cover most of the body, except the distal parts of the legs.

> *TECHNICIAN NOTE* Fly repellents containing organophosphates should not be applied to debilitated horses or foals.

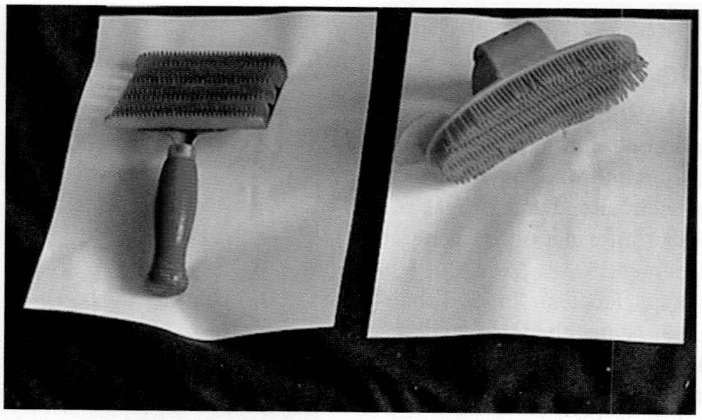

FIGURE 25-2 Grooming equipment. Metal curry comb and plastic curry comb. (From Aspinall V: *The complete textbook of veterinary nursing*, ed 2, St Louis, 2011, Elsevier.)

EXERCISE

Adult horses and foals should have some form of exercise daily unless their medical problem requires stall rest. Walking on soft dirt or grass surfaces is preferable to walking on concrete or asphalt. Foals may be allowed to run freely alongside the mare if they do not have a condition that warrants more restricted activity, and if the area is properly fenced with no hazards, such as drains or moving vehicles. If the foal's activity must be controlled, the foal can be walked using a halter and a rope around the foal's hindquarters in the area of the semimembranosus and semitendinosus muscles. Good judgment and caution are needed to prevent the foal from rearing and flipping over backward. Neonates whose exercise must be limited can be walked by placing one arm in front of the foal's chest and one arm behind the foal to cradle it while walking. Alternatively, an adult horse halter can be used over the foal's body like a harness, with the nose piece around the foal's neck, the buckle strapped around the ventral thorax, and the rope clip located on the caudodorsal portion of the foal's back. The hind end of the foal may still need to be supported.

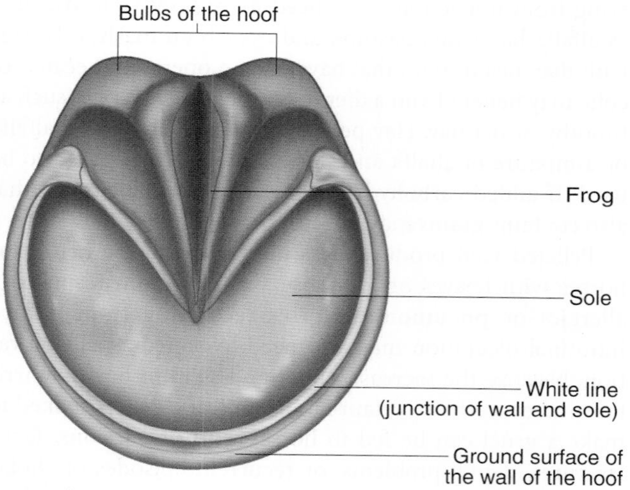

FIGURE 25-3 Ground surface of the right fore hoof. (From Aspinall V: *The complete textbook of veterinary nursing*, ed 2, St Louis, 2011, Elsevier.)

GROOMING

Equine patients should be groomed daily, unless the horse has a condition whereby vigorous grooming would be painful or damaging (e.g., severe skin infections, cutaneous burns). A rubber curry comb (Fig. 25-2) should be used in a circular motion to remove dried sweat or mud. Next a stiff-bristled brush can be used to remove dirt and loose hair. If stiff brushes and rubber curry combs are used on the horse's face and distal limbs, they should be used gently, because overly vigorous grooming may be uncomfortable for the animal. Metal curry combs should not be used on the horse's head or distal limbs. A soft brush can be used to finish removing loose hair and dirt. If needed, a damp or dry cloth can be used to remove the remaining dust from the horse's coat. A stiff brush, hair brush, or metal mane comb should be used on the tail and mane.

HOOF PICKING

A horse's hooves should be picked clean daily. Most adult horses raise the foot when a hand is run down the caudal aspect of the distal limb and gentle pressure is exerted over the caudal aspect of the limb at the level of the distal splint bones. The hoof is then cleaned with a hoof pick by removing debris from the lateral and central sulci, starting at the heel and working toward the toe, and then from the rest of the hoof (Fig. 25-3). A degenerative condition called **thrush** is common in feet that are infrequently cleaned, or if the horse stands for long periods in damp bedding or muddy soil. Thrush may occur secondary to a bacterial infection and appears as black, malodorous material in the region of the frog. A 10% sodium hypochlorite (bleach) solution or 2% iodine solution can be applied to the lateral and central sulci to dry the foot and kill the bacteria. Commercial formulations containing formaldehyde or copper sulfate can also be used. Care must always be used to avoid spilling caustic solutions on the coronary band or other parts of the horse's leg. The technician should wear gloves to protect herself/himself from the solutions. Some animals with severe thrush require foot trimming to remove diseased hoof tissue and wraps to help keep the foot clean and dry during the length of the treatment program.

MONITORING PATIENTS

Hospitalized patients must be monitored regularly for changes in their condition. Horses only slightly ill can develop more severe and even life-threatening illness while receiving treatment. For instance, a horse receiving antibiotic therapy for a mild respiratory infection can develop life-threatening diarrhea from changes in bowel microflora. A horse receiving nonsteroidal anti-inflammatory drugs for an orthopedic problem can develop gastrointestinal ulceration or renal dysfunction secondary to the anti-inflammatory medication, particularly if the animal is not eating and drinking normally.

The heart rate, respiratory rate, rectal temperature, mucous membrane color (Fig. 25-4), capillary refill time, attitude, digital pulses, urine and fecal output, gastrointestinal motility, and appetite should all be monitored at least once or twice daily. Critically ill neonates require more frequent monitoring, sometimes as often as every 2 hours, as their condition can deteriorate rapidly. Adult horses should be weighed at admission with a walk-on scale, if available, or a weight tape can be used to estimate the horse's weight. Neonates should be weighed at admission and then daily. Most newborn foals can be weighed by picking them up and weighing the handler and foal together on a conventional scale and then subtracting the handler's weight. This may not be feasible with larger foals.

CARE OF RECUMBENT HORSES

Nursing care for recumbent animals must be meticulous. Caring for a horse that is unable to rise is tedious and often unrewarding. Horses that remain recumbent for prolonged periods eventually develop various complications, regardless of the primary disease. Because of the weight of the animal, several people are needed to frequently turn the animal from one side to the other. This is usually done with long ropes looped, not tied, around the pasterns so that the handlers can stand farther from the limbs of the horse, or by using a winch and harness, when available. If the size of the horse permits, it would be preferable to flex the legs up next to the body then roll the horse's torso over the flexed legs rather than roll the horse over on its back. Rolling the horse on its back may cause a twisted intestine and add another unneeded complication to an already sick or injured animal. When a horse is turned from one side to another, the animal often kicks, which can be very dangerous for anyone standing in the vicinity. The animal must be turned as frequently as possible to prevent development of decubital ulcers on the skin and edema and congestion in the dependent portion of the lung. Helmets can be applied to horses that tend to flail about and hit their head against the wall or ground. The technician should also pay particular attention to the eyes of a recumbent animal because the corneas can become ulcerated if the animal rubs its eyes on the ground.

> *TECHNICIAN NOTE* No one should stand within striking distance of the limbs of a recumbent horse.

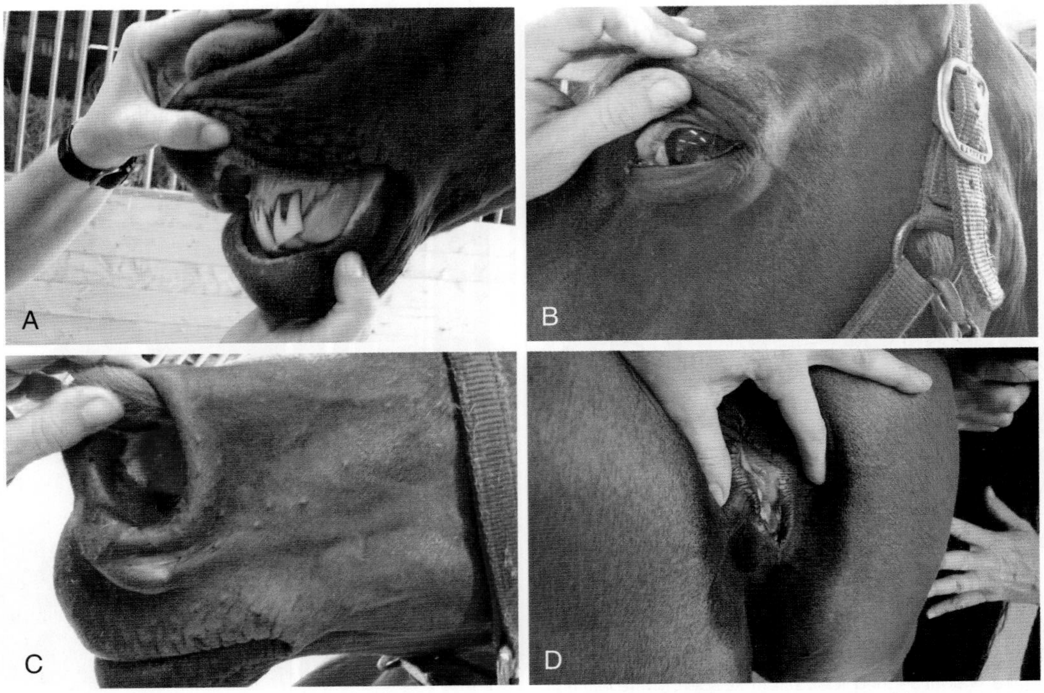

FIGURE 25-4 Examination of mucous membranes. **A,** Examination of the gums. **B,** Examination of the conjunctiva. **C,** Examination of the mucosa of the nares. **D,** Examination of the vulva in the female. (From Hanie EA: *Large animal clinical procedures for veterinary technicians,* St Louis, 2006, Mosby.)

The primary disease must be resolved as quickly as possible so that the animal may once again stand. If the horse can stand but only with assistance, the hind limbs can be supported by suspending a rope attached to the tail from a ceiling beam. The head may also need to be supported. Commercial slings are available that provide support for horses that have some ability to support themselves but require additional help. A sling cannot be used for horses with flaccid paralysis or other conditions that make them unable to support themselves at all, because they can only slump down in the sling. Slings must be well padded to prevent development of pressure sores (Fig. 25-5).

Regardless of how meticulous the nursing care, decubital ulcers may develop over bony prominences, such as the tuber coxae, carpus, hock, shoulder joint, or elbow. These must be cleaned with a mild antibacterial soap. Topical antibacterial powders or sprays can also be used. A spray that creates a "breathable" bandage may provide the best protection. Any bony protuberance that can be protected by wraps should be wrapped. It is important to keep the animal clean and dry. Frequent cleaning can help to prevent urine scalding and reduce the severity of decubital ulcers. Additional bedding may also help minimize the formation of decubital sores.

The recumbent animal may not eat or drink well. Soft, highly palatable feeds should be offered. If mashes are offered but not eaten, they must be replaced frequently to ensure palatability. Fresh, clean water should be offered to the recumbent animal every 2 hours, if possible. The food and water may have to be given by nasogastric tube because the animal may aspirate feed or water into the lungs when trying to eat or drink in lateral recumbency. If possible, it is preferable to feed the horse while it is in a more sternal position. Infusion of IV fluids may be required in more debilitated or dehydrated animals.

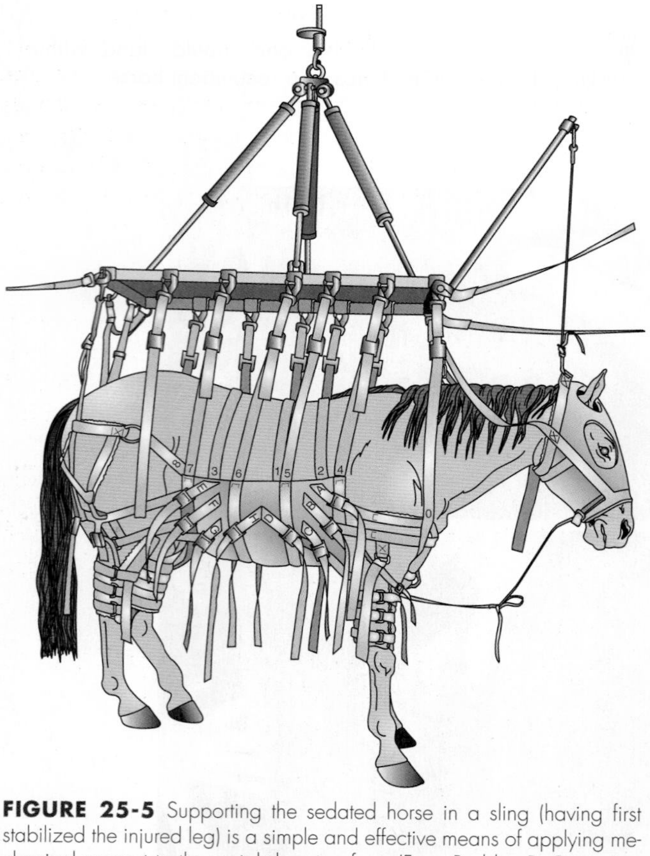

FIGURE 25-5 Supporting the sedated horse in a sling (having first stabilized the injured leg) is a simple and effective means of applying mechanical support to the weight-bearing foot. (From Redden R: *Preventing laminitis in the contralateral limb of Horses with nonweight-bearing lameness, Clinical Techniques in Equine Practice,* St Louis, 2004, Elsevier.)

BANDAGING

Materials needed to bandage the distal limbs include cotton quilts or sheet cotton (three sheets), and track wraps, brown roll gauze, or some type of conforming bandage material. Leg wraps can be used to protect a wound, to give additional support, or to cover a medicated area. The wrap should be applied with even pressure so that the tendons running along the caudal aspect of the leg (superficial and deep digital flexor tendons) are protected and pressure is evenly applied over the entire length of the tendons.

To start, a quilt or some other thick padding is wrapped around the leg. Sheet cotton can be used; at least three sheets are needed for sufficient padding. Start the wrap at the front portion of the leg and then bring the quilt across the outside of the leg, around the back and then inside of the leg, maintaining even tension at all times (Fig. 25-6). Once the quilt is in place, a track wrap brown gauze roll or other type of outer wrap is used. The same principle is followed, with the wrap being placed from lateral toward medial across the back of the leg. It is best to start this part of the wrap near the bottom of the leg (distally) and work up (proximally).

The outer wrap is secured with Velcro attachments, ties or adhesive tape. If adhesive tape is used, the ends should not overlap, because the tape is relatively inelastic and may produce uneven pressure across the tendons. If roll gauze is used, this can be secured with adhesive tape; alternatively, an additional layer can be applied using a conforming bandage

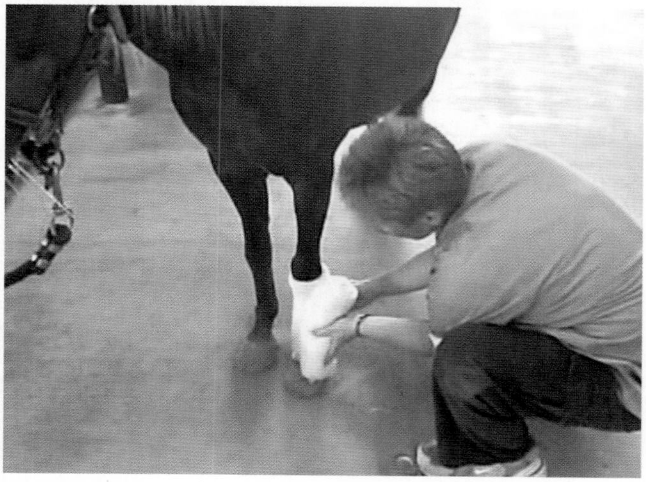

FIGURE 25-6 Application of sheet cotton for placement of a wrap to the distal limb of a standing horse.

wrap. When the wrap is finished, a small strip of padding should be visible in the innermost layer of the wrap both proximally and distally (Fig. 25-7). Care must be taken to make sure that the wrap is snug but not too tight. Two fingers should be able to fit snugly between the leg and the wrap, but the wrap should feel firm and should not slip down the leg. If the wrap is applied to protect a wound, antibacterial ointment and a nonstick dressing must first be applied to the area and held in place with a layer of stretch gauze.

If the full length of the leg must be wrapped, an additional wrap can be applied so that it overlaps the lower limb wrap to some extent. This additional wrap is applied in a similar manner. The proximal wrap should overlap the distal wrap and extend to the mid-radius area. Often a piece of the wrap is cut out over the accessory carpal bone to prevent development of pressure sores over this bone. This is more difficult to do on the hind leg, because special consideration must be given to the highly movable hock joint. Often the conforming bandage material is applied in a figure-of-eight around the hock so that only the sheet cotton contacts the point of the hock.

FOOT WRAPS

There are many different ways to wrap feet. The foot is first picked clean and then washed and dried if needed. If the foot requires medication, this can be applied and then covered with a gauze sponge secured with a layer of rolled gauze. If padding is needed for protection, roll cotton or two to three sheets of cotton are used to wrap around the foot. Next, rolled brown gauze or stretch gauze can be used to secure the sheet cotton. This is applied in figure-of-eight fashion to make the sheet cottons lie flat across the bottom of the foot. Finally, elastic tape or duct tape is applied to provide additional support and protection, and secure the bandage in place. It is very important to have the ground surface of the foot wrap flat, rather than convex and bulging, so that even pressure is applied to the bottom of the foot. If no padding is needed and the foot wrap is being used to apply medication to an area of the foot, the duct tape or a conforming bandage material can be applied directly to the foot after a nonsticking dressing or gauze sponge is placed over the medication.

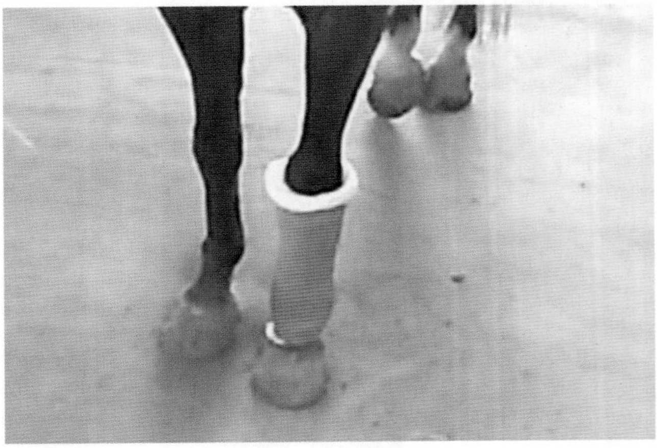

FIGURE 25-7 Leg wrap with outer covering of elastic wrap over sheet cotton.

Be careful not to wrap up over the coronary band if no protective padding is in place. Excessive pressure directly on the coronary band can reduce circulation to hoof tissues and cause damage or sloughing of the hoof. If there is any question about the amount of pressure on the coronary band, one or more vertical slits can be cut in the bandage where it covers the coronary band to relieve pressure.

TAIL BANDAGES

Tail wraps can consist of stall bandages, rolled brown gauze, or even commercial tail bags. If the tail wrap is intended to be left on the horse for many days, it is important that the wrap not extend proximally to include the tail bones (coccygeal vertebrae), because the tail has little muscular padding and a tight wrap can occlude blood circulation to the tail and create a tissue slough or even loss of the entire tail. If it is necessary to wrap more proximally on the tail, a nonconstricting wrap should be loosely applied and changed daily.

At times it is necessary to wrap the tail of a horse with severe diarrhea to keep the tail clean. This can be done using a plastic rectal sleeve. Holes can be cut in the sleeve to help keep the tail from "sweating." The tail hair should first be braided and the sleeve slid over the tail and tied at the most proximal part of the braid. The sleeve can also be anchored to the most proximal part of the tail with a strip of adhesive tape or duct tape placed lengthwise from the sleeve cranially along the midline of the back.

The tail may also need to be wrapped when a mare is about to foal or for a reproductive examination. Rolled brown gauze is applied, starting at the tail head (proximal area) and working distally, being sure to incorporate all of the tail hairs within the wrap. When the wrap reaches just distal to the last tail bone, the remaining tail hairs can be folded and incorporated within this section of the wrap (Fig. 25-8). The brown gauze is then tied to itself to end and secure the wrap.

ABDOMINAL BANDAGES

It may be necessary to wrap a horse's abdomen to protect a wound or an abdominal incision following colic surgery. A sterile nonstick pad is placed over the wound. Next, a dressing made from large folded sheet cotton can

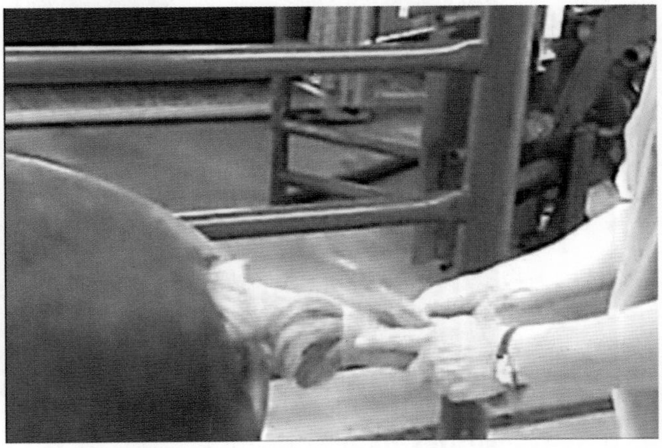

FIGURE 25-8 Tail hairs should all be incorporated into the wrap.

be placed against the sterile dressing. A conforming bandage material is wrapped around the abdomen and over the back to hold the bandage in place. It may be necessary to use four to six rolls of this material when applying a full abdominal bandage.

Padding in the form of leg rolls or quilts should be used across the horse's back to protect the skin if the backbone is prominent. Because pressure is applied with the wrap, skin necrosis can occur in this area if there is little muscle or fat across the back. The same application principles are used as for leg wraps. The material is applied evenly, starting at the cranial part of the abdomen and working caudally. It is applied snugly to provide support, but not too tight. Each layer of the material should overlap the last pass until the wrap is completed. This type of wrap is very expensive and usually does not need changing unless there is excessive drainage, or if the wound or incision must be evaluated. Thoracic wraps can be applied in a similar manner to cover a thoracic wound or protect a thoracic drain.

Chapter 13 contains detailed information on wound management and bandaging.

DIAGNOSTIC SAMPLE COLLECTION

Body fluids that can be collected include venous and arterial blood, abdominal fluid, pleural fluid, airway fluid, joint fluid, cerebrospinal fluid (CSF), feces, and urine. Tissue samples include skin and mucosal scrapings/swabs, fine needle aspirates, and biopsy tissue sections. Additional information on collection of samples by centesis and skin and mucosal scrapings is located in Chapter 9.

Collecting Blood Samples

To obtain a blood sample from a horse, the animal must be properly restrained. The jugular vein is most commonly used to obtain blood samples and lies directly under the skin in the jugular furrow. The vein should be entered at the most cranial one third of the neck, where the vein is more superficial and somewhat better separated from the carotid artery. The jugular vein and carotid artery exit the thoracic inlet closely together but become more separated as the vessels course cranially toward the head (Fig. 25-9).

The vein is distended by occluding it with a thumb placed proximal (ventral) to the venipuncture site. Once the vein fills, a 20-gauge or larger needle, attached to a syringe, is quickly and smoothly inserted (Fig. 25-10). The entire length of the needle's shaft should be well seated in the vein. The syringe is then aspirated to withdraw the sample. Alternatively, a double-ended Vacutainer blood collection needle can be used by inserting the unsheathed longer portion into the vein and attaching the collection vials to the shorter, sheathed end. The vacuum within the collection vials allows the blood to flow freely into the vial (Fig. 25-11). For either method, the needle is removed after the pressure on the vein has been released. By releasing the pressure before removing the needle, the chance of developing a hematoma at the collection site is reduced.

In a seriously ill horse, the jugular veins may need to be preserved to allow continued venous access for delivery of medications and fluids. In this case another site should be used for routine blood collection. A venous sinus ventral to the facial crest can be used for obtaining blood samples. It

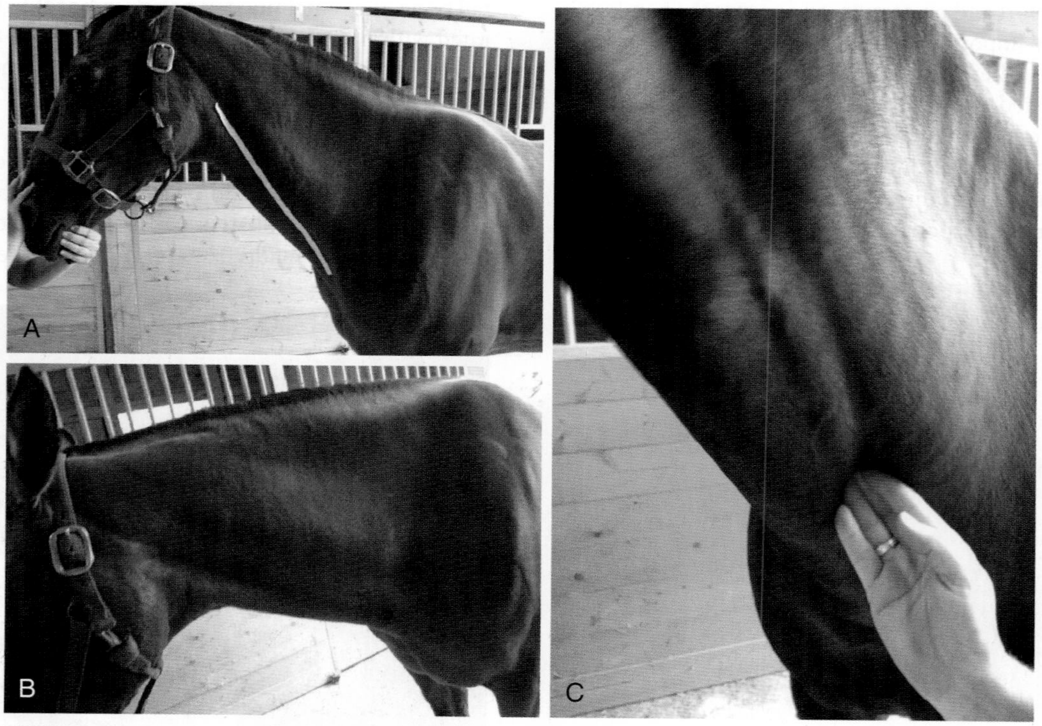

FIGURE 25-9 Anatomy of the jugular vein area. **A,** Location of the jugular groove. **B,** The jugular groove. **C,** Distension of the jugular vein. (From Hanie EA: *Large animal clinical procedures for veterinary technicians,* St Louis, 2006, Mosby.)

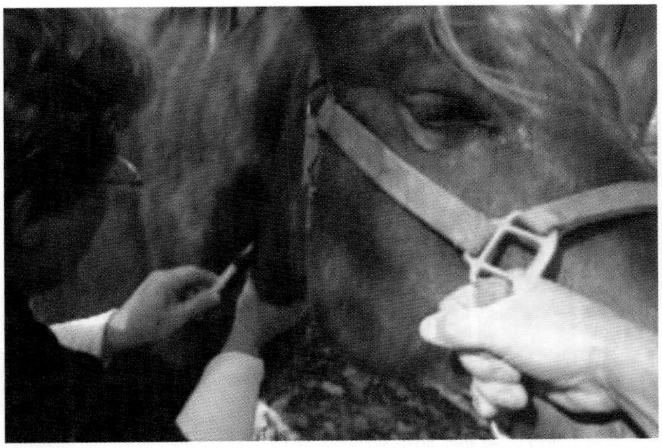

FIGURE 25-10 Collecting blood from the jugular vein with needle and syringe.

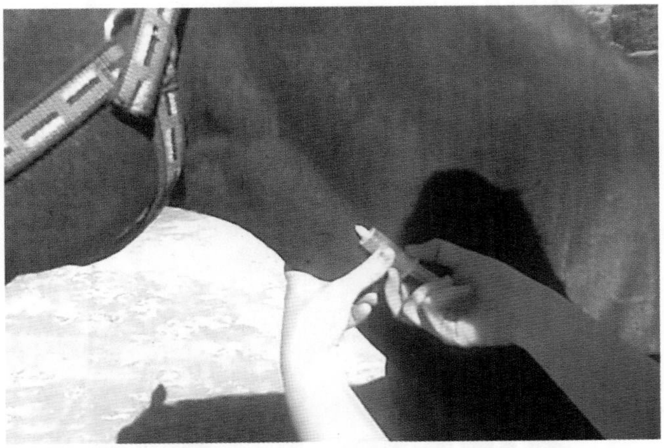

FIGURE 25-11 Collecting blood from the jugular vein with the Vacutainer system.

should be entered just caudal to its midpoint between the medial canthus of the eye and the rostral end of the facial crest, just ventral to the facial crest. This should only be attempted by experienced technicians or veterinarians because of the proximity to the horse's eye. Care must be taken to avoid inadvertently puncturing the eyeball if the horse turns its head suddenly.

ADMINISTRATION OF MEDICATION

ORAL ADMINISTRATION

Medications that are in liquid form and required in only small doses may be administered with a dose syringe or a syringe with the locking tip removed. The syringe is placed through the side of the mouth in the area of the **diastema,** or interdental space (space between the incisors and premolars) (Fig. 25-12). The medication is deposited on the caudal portion of the tongue if possible. Medications in pill form can be crushed with a mortar and pestle and then mixed with something sweet, such as molasses, and given in a similar manner. It is best not to mix medication with the feed, because horses often eat around the medication and do not consume the full dose. Medication that must be given in large volumes requires use of a nasogastric tube for delivery into the stomach.

NASOGASTRIC INTUBATION

A horse that cannot chew or swallow normally, but with a functional gastrointestinal tract, can be fed and hydrated through a nasogastric tube. Nasogastric intubation should be done in the presence of a veterinarian until the technician has become proficient in the technique. Feeding through a

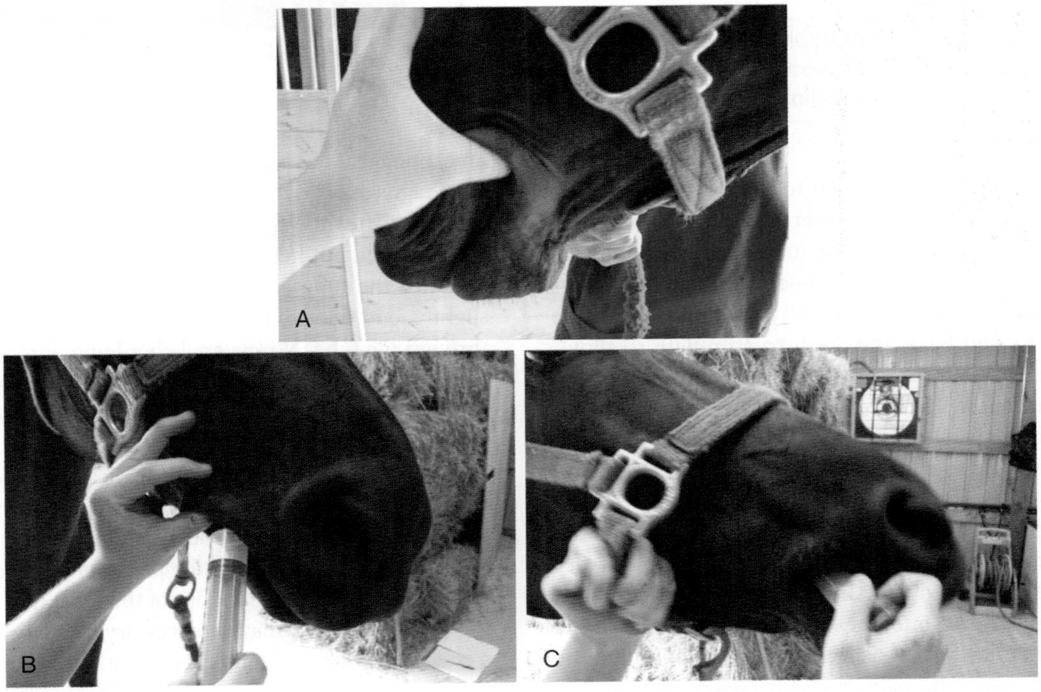

FIGURE 25-12 **A,** Opening the lips before placing the oral syringe in the mouth. **B,** Placement of the dose syringe near the commissure of the lips. **C,** Proper positioning of the oral syringe. (From Hanie EA: *Large animal clinical procedures for veterinary technicians,* St Louis, 2006, Mosby.)

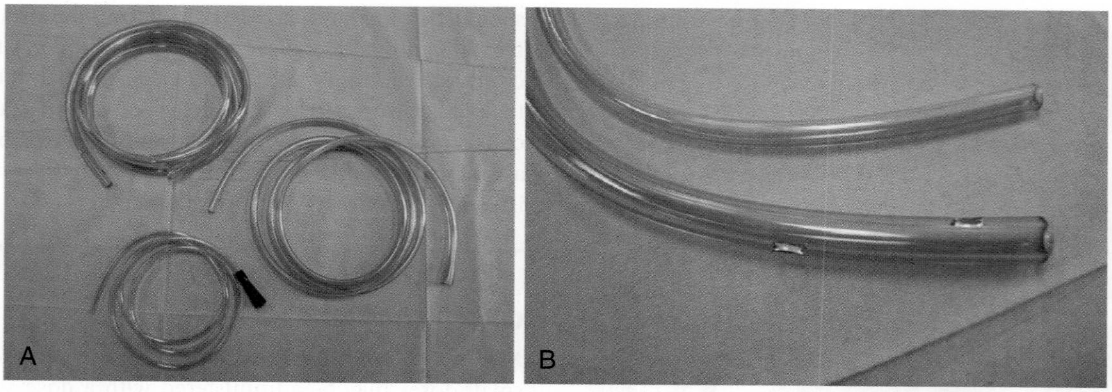

FIGURE 25-13 A, Nasogastric tubes are available in different diameters. B, Single opening (*top*) and multiple side ports (*bottom*). (From Hanie EA: *Large animal clinical procedures for veterinary technicians*, St Louis, 2006, Mosby.)

nasogastric tube requires a larger-bore stomach tube than does water administration (Fig. 25-13). The length of tube necessary to reach the horse's stomach should be determined before the procedure.

The tube is first lubricated with a water-soluble lubricant jelly (e.g., K-Y Jelly) or even plain water. The tube is then inserted into the nostril with one hand. The other hand is used to guide the tube through the most ventral portion of the nasal passage, the ventral meatus (Fig. 25-14). Care must be taken to ensure that the tube is directed caudoventrally, because it will not easily pass into the pharynx if it is inserted into the middle or dorsal meatus. The tube should never be forced if it will not pass easily. If the tube strikes the **ethmoturbinates** as it is being passed through the ventral meatus to the pharynx, the nasal membranes may bleed profusely. This may happen if the horse moves at the wrong moment, or if the technician or veterinarian is not careful.

> TECHNICIAN NOTE CAUTION: Improper nasogastric tube placement is one of the most frequent malpractice claims against veterinarians or technicians.

Once the tube has been inserted to the level of the pharynx, the horse's head should be lowered and the neck flexed slightly to facilitate entrance of the tube into the esophagus and not the trachea. The tube is passed into the esophagus as the horse swallows. If the horse will not swallow, the tube can be gently moved back and forth to stimulate swallowing. If the tube passes into the trachea by mistake, the horse may cough and resist. However, sedated or severely debilitated horses may not resist or cough if the tube is erroneously placed into the trachea. If the trachea is grasped in one hand and moved back and forth, the tube can be felt rattling within the cartilaginous structure. The tube will not rattle if it is in the esophagus, because this is a collapsible structure composed of striated and smooth muscle. If the tube is in the esophagus, it can often be seen on the left side of the neck near the jugular furrow as it is being passed. If the tube cannot be seen, it can be palpated as it passes through the esophagus. The tube may be difficult to pass if the horse has an esophageal obstruction. Care should be used because the esophagus may be ruptured by overaggressive nasogastric intubation. The tube should be passed caudally, all the way into the stomach, but never forced.

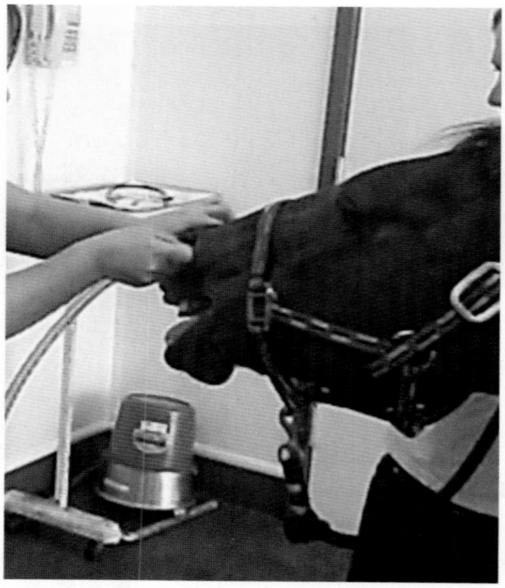

FIGURE 25-14 When placing the nasogastric tube, one hand is used to guide the tube through the ventral meatus.

Once the tube enters the stomach, the typical sweet and slightly fetid odor of the stomach contents may be discernible through the tube. No material should be pumped through the stomach tube unless you are absolutely certain that the tube is in the stomach and not in the trachea. Horses cannot vomit, so always check for excessive gastric contents (gastric reflux) before administration of fluid, feed, or medication. Checking for gastric reflux is done by creating a siphon effect by injecting a small amount of water into the tube with a stomach pump or dose syringes and disconnecting the pump or syringe to see if fluid or ingesta flows freely back out of the tube. If excessive fluid or ingesta is present, it may be necessary to medicate the horse at a later time, when no reflux is present. Overfilling the stomach can result in gastric rupture and death. The adult horse's stomach can hold 8 to 15 liters, but this varies between horses.

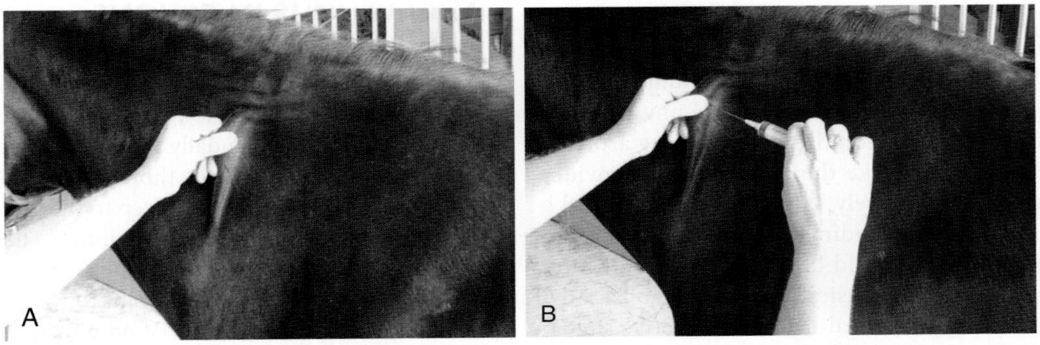

FIGURE 25-15 A, Elevating the skin for subcutaneous injection. B, Injection technique for subcutaneous injection. (From Hanie EA: *Large animal clinical procedures for veterinary technicians*, St Louis, 2006, Mosby.)

Medication or fluid should be given by gravity flow through a funnel, when possible, to prevent overfilling of the stomach. If a stomach pump must be used to administer water or mineral oil, it should be periodically disconnected to check for increased pressure and backflow of fluid out of the stomach tube. Before the nasogastric tube is withdrawn, all of the fluid should be removed from the tube. This can be done by pumping or blowing a small amount of air through the tube while it is still in the stomach and then kinking the end of the tube or placing a finger over the end while it is being removed. This prevents the horse from aspirating fluid into the lungs as the tube is being removed.

Horses can be rehydrated by administering water through the nasogastric tube. If IV administration of fluids is not possible or practical, the stomach tube can be taped or sutured where it exits the nostril and then taped to the horse's halter. The tube is then wrapped around and taped in one additional site on the halter to minimize movement of the tube. A syringe or cork can be placed in the end of the tube to prevent air from filling the stomach. Water can be given every 2 hours or as needed in this manner. Horses must not be allowed to eat or drink with a large-bore stomach tube in place, because they cannot adequately protect their airway when they swallow.

PARENTERAL INJECTIONS

Drugs and other liquids can be injected into a muscle (IM) or vein (IV), under the skin (SC), or into a layer of the skin (ID). Some medications can be given by multiple routes, either intravenously or intramuscularly. It is very important to know which routes of administration are acceptable for each drug administered, because injection by an inappropriate route can have harmful or even lethal effects on the horse. For example, procaine penicillin should be given only in the muscle (IM). If this medication is given in the vein (IV), the procaine component may cause excitation, seizures, and death. Some medications, such as phenylbutazone, should be administered intravenously only. These medications can be very caustic and cause tissue sloughing if administered outside the vein (**perivascular**) or in the muscle.

INTRADERMAL INJECTIONS

Rarely an injection must be given into the upper layers of the skin. Some forms of allergy testing use intradermal injections of allergens. A very small amount of test material, usually 0.1 to 1 ml, is injected using a 25-gauge, ⅝-inch needle. The skin is cleaned with alcohol if needed, and the needle is inserted into the skin (not underneath it). The plunger is withdrawn slightly to make sure a blood vessel has not been entered. If no blood is aspirated, the medication is injected. Because the medication is being injected into the skin, a small bleb, called a wheal, becomes visible in the skin.

SUBCUTANEOUS INJECTIONS

Occasionally medications are injected subcutaneously. These medications are usually given in smaller doses, such as for allergy desensitization. A 20- or 21-gauge, 1-inch needle should be used. Any area where the skin can easily be lifted from the underlying muscle and fascia may be used; the lateral aspect of the neck where IM injections are also given is a suitable site. The skin is first cleaned with alcohol if necessary and then pulled laterally to form a "tent." The needle is then inserted under the skin (Fig. 25-15). Always aspirate to make sure no blood enters the syringe and then inject.

INTRAMUSCULAR INJECTIONS

Various sites can be used for IM injections. The safest muscle for technicians to use is in the lateral surfaces of the neck area. The neck muscles of the horse can be used only for administering small volumes of medication. The area to be used is a triangular portion on the side of the neck formed by the ligamentum nuchae dorsally, the spine ventrally, and the scapula caudally (Fig. 25-16). Another common area for IM injection is in the semitendinosus and semimembranosus muscles of the hind leg. This is the preferred site for IM injections in neonates because they are usually the largest muscle masses available in young and minimally developed foals. However, this is a very vulnerable position for the technician and horses that are known to kick should not be injected at this site. Yet another available site would be the pectoral muscles found on the cranial chest wall between the front legs. Care must be taken to avoid inserting the needle directly on the midline between the muscle masses as the sternum (breastbone) is located there and is unprotected by any muscle. Standing laterally to either front leg and reaching around the front of the horse to make the injection will provide the technician with a relatively safe place to stand. Additionally, if either the semitendinosus/semimembranosus area or the pectoral area should develop an injection site abscess, these would be the easiest areas to establish adequate drainage to allow for healing. An alternative site is in the gluteal (hip) muscles. This allows the person giving the injection to stand in a somewhat safer position, but if the horse develops an abscess subsequent to a gluteal injection, it can be very difficult to establish adequate drainage. For this reason, many veterinarians will avoid giving any IM injections there. In any case, there should always be an experienced handler available to properly restrain the horse when administering any IM injections in the horse.

A 16- or 18-gauge, 1.5-inch needle should be used for IM injections in adults. A 20-gauge, 1-inch needle should be used for small equines and neonates. The site is cleaned with alcohol if necessary, and the needle, without an attached syringe, is inserted with a quick jab. Some people prefer to tap on the area to be injected a few times with their fist before injecting in an attempt to desensitize the area. When injecting the neck muscles, a fold of skin can be grasped and pulled slightly away from the neck to act as a skin twitch and distract the horse before inserting the needle. Always disconnect the needle from the syringe before inserting it so that if the horse kicks or jumps, the needle will remain in place and not be pulled out by the weight of the syringe. Then the syringe is attached and the plunger aspirated to make sure a blood vessel has not been entered. If no blood is visible in the syringe, the medication can be injected safely. The needle and syringe are then removed. No more than 20 ml of solution should be given to mature horses in one IM site.

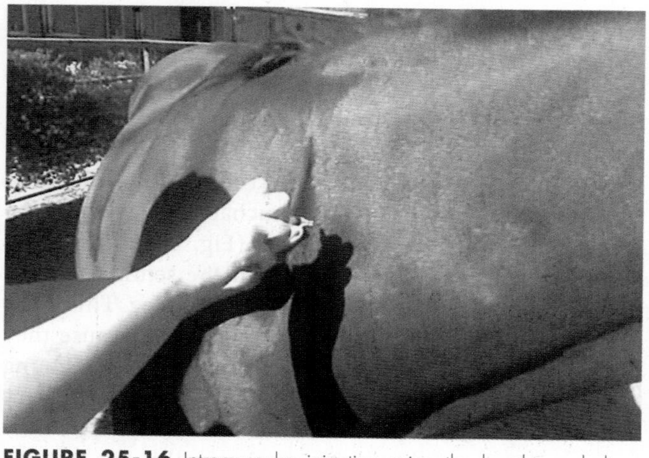

FIGURE 25-16 Intramuscular injection using the brachiocephalicus muscle.

INTRAVENOUS INJECTIONS

When administering medication IV, the blood dilutes the medication causing it to become less caustic. The jugular vein is the only appropriate vein for IV injections in horses. The jugular vein runs caudally along the jugular furrow from the head and then enters the thoracic inlet on its way to the heart. The carotid artery runs deep to the jugular vein in the same vicinity, but it courses deeper into the neck and is separated from the jugular vein in the more cranial portion of the neck. This is a very important point to remember. It is safer to attempt venipuncture and IV administration of medications in the cranial one third of the neck, because you are less likely to inadvertently enter the carotid artery when aiming for the jugular vein. If a large-bore needle (18-gauge) is used and the syringe is removed before venipuncture, it should be apparent which blood vessel has been entered. Blood drips out of the hub of an 18-gauge needle if it has been placed in the jugular vein but spurts out of the needle if it is within the high-pressure carotid artery. Smaller-bore needles (20-gauge or smaller) are suitable for obtaining blood samples; however, they do not allow differentiation between arterial or venous puncture, because in both cases blood drips from the needle. Medications inadvertently injected into the carotid artery pass directly to the brain and can cause severe seizures, collapse, and even death.

When drugs are administered IV, the needle may be inserted in the direction of the flow of blood in the jugular vein, pointed caudally. Some people prefer to insert the needle pointed cranially. Regardless of which direction the needle is placed, it should be well seated into the vein so that there is little chance for perivascular or intra-arterial injection. The vein is distended by occluding it with the thumb of one hand and then the needle is inserted into the vein with the other hand. Blood should drip from the hub of the needle while the vein remains occluded. The syringe is then attached to the needle and the plunger is gently withdrawn to produce a back flow of blood which confirms that the needle is still in the vein. The medication is then injected slowly.

> **TECHNICIAN NOTE** CAUTION: Never give any medications by the IV route without checking, THEN RECHECKING, to be sure it is the correct medicine for this patient.

Medication should not be quickly injected as a bolus, because this could cause an adverse reaction. If the medication is given slowly, administration can be halted if a reaction occurs. Even with good technique, movement of the horse during injection can drive the needle through the jugular vein and into the carotid artery. If the horse moves after connection of the syringe to the needle, the syringe should once again be removed from the needle to check the needle's position. If all is well, the injection can be continued. Remember that it is not reliable to try to distinguish arterial blood from venous blood by color when withdrawn into a syringe filled with a drug. If multiple IV injections are required daily or if large volumes of fluid must be administered, placement of an indwelling catheter is advisable.

ADVERSE REACTIONS

Adverse reactions may occur to medications given by any route. In general, however, these reactions occur more rapidly with intravascular injections. Reactions can range from mild sweating, **urticaria** (hives), and colic, to respiratory distress, collapse, and death. With any reaction, administration of the medication should be stopped immediately and, if time allows, the veterinarian should be contacted. Epinephrine 1:1000 given SC or IM at 3 to 5 ml/450 kg of body weight, as well as dexamethasone given IV at 0.02 to 2 mg/kg, may be needed to stop an anaphylactic reaction and save the horse's life. It is always wise to know the appropriate dosage for these drugs and to have them within reach when medication is to be given. The horse's medical record should always be tagged to indicate medications to which the animal has previously reacted.

INTRAVENOUS CATHETERIZATION

Procedure 25-1 details the procedure for intravenous catheterization.

PROCEDURE 25-1 Procedure for Intravenous Catheterization

Materials

- Gauze sponges, povidone-iodine scrub, povidone-iodine solution, alcohol, water, hair clipper, 2% lidocaine
- For adults, 14- to 16-gauge, 140-mm Teflon catheter or 150-mm polyurethane catheter for the jugular vein
- 2-0 or 0 nonabsorbable suture, such as polypropylene
- Injection plug
- Sterile latex gloves
- Heparinized saline (2500 units in 250 ml saline for adults; 1000 units in 250 ml saline for neonates)
- T-port (optional)
- For foals, elastic tape, sterile gauze sponges and antibacterial ointment. For adults, similar to foal or stent bandage using stretch gauze roll bandage and umbilical tape

Procedure

1. Shave and aseptically prepare the site to be catheterized.
2. Inject 1 ml of lidocaine subcutaneously to block the skin if desired.
3. Wearing sterile gloves, take the catheter from the package and place the end of the stylet at the appropriate site. Always insert the catheter in the direction of blood flow.
4. With a sharp and quick jab, insert the catheter through the skin and into the vein. Hold the catheter at about a 45-degree angle to the skin until the vein is penetrated (Figure 1). Blood should flow freely into the hub if the vein is occluded (jugular) or flows freely without holding the vein off for the other sites. If the horse is severely dehydrated or hypovolemic, backflow of blood may not occur. For the compromised patient, it may be helpful to have the catheter filled with heparinized saline so that once the vein is penetrated, the heparinized saline starts to flow retrograde out the hub of the catheter.
5. Once the vein has been entered, orient the catheter and stylet parallel to the vein and advance the catheter ½ inch for adults and ¼ inch for foals. This ensures that both the catheter and stylet are within the lumen of the vein.
6. Hold the stylet in place and slide the catheter down the stylet and into the vein (Figure 2). This should be a smooth action; the catheter should easily slide down the stylet and not feel like it is sticking. Never advance the stylet into the catheter or pull the catheter onto the stylet once the catheter has been advanced, because this could sever the tip of the catheter off within the vein. If the catheter is not correctly placed with the lumen of the vein, simply remove the entire unit and try again. Advance the catheter until only the hub protrudes from the skin (Figure 3).
7. Once the catheter is in place, remove the stylet and place a T-port with injection plug or just an injection plug over the end of the catheter.
8. The catheter should be sutured in place using the grooves in the hub to mark the site for the first suture, then around the narrow portion of the injection plug or T-port. If a T-port is used, another suture should be placed over the "T" to secure it. In adults, it may be advantageous to also suture the arm of the T-port loosely to add stability without creating tension at the catheter insertion site. The arm of the T-port should slide easily through the loose loop of suture as the horse changes its neck position.
9. Flush the catheter with 3 ml of saline or heparinized saline.

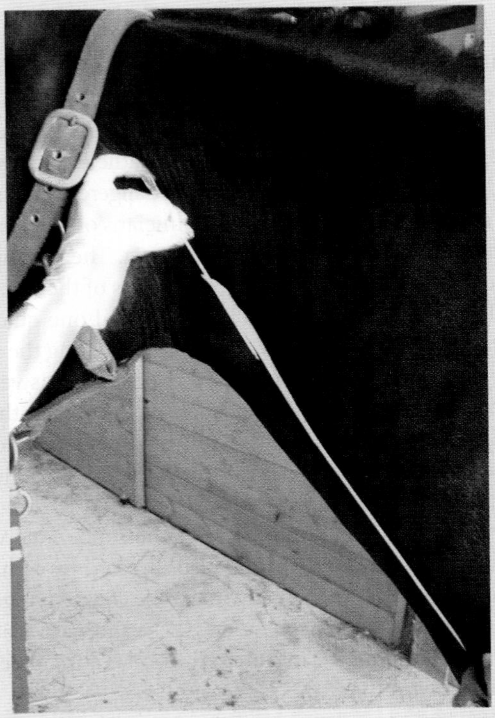

FIGURE 1 Proper insertion angle for an intravenous (IV) catheter. (From Hanie EA: *Large animal clinical procedures for veterinary technicians*, St Louis, 2006, Mosby.)

Continued

PROCEDURE 25-1 Procedure for Intravenous Catheterization—Cont'd

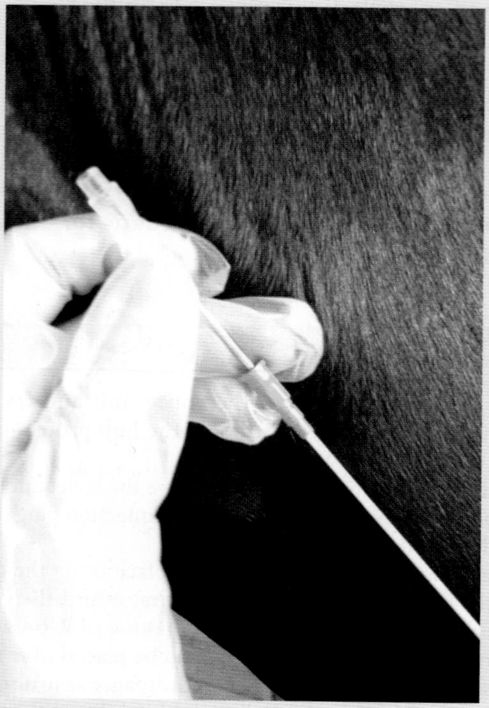

FIGURE 2 Partial withdrawal of the stylet. (From Hanie EA: *Large animal clinical procedures for veterinary technicians,* St Louis, 2006, Mosby.)

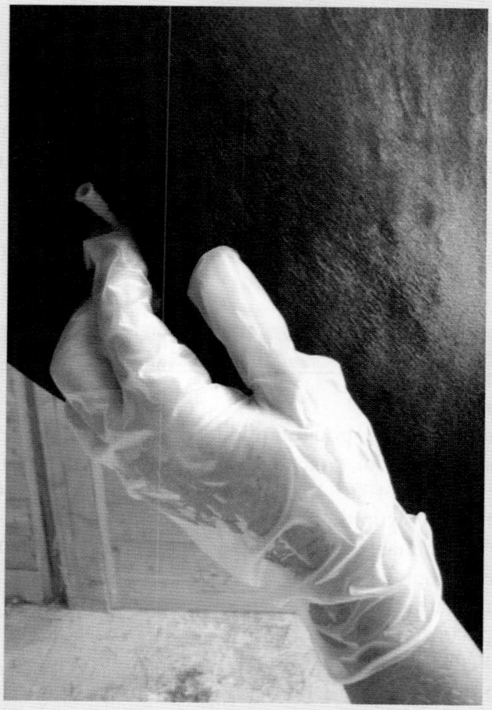

FIGURE 3 The catheter is advanced until the hub reaches the skin. (From Hanie EA: *Large animal clinical procedures for veterinary technicians,* St Louis, 2006, Mosby.)

Sites

In adult horses, the jugular vein is preferred for catheter placement. Alternative sites include the lateral thoracic vein, cephalic vein, and, in extreme cases when there are no remaining accessible veins, the saphenous vein. Catheterizing veins in the hind legs of adult horses can be very dangerous and should only be attempted by experienced technicians or veterinarians when the horse is under general anesthesia. The principles of venous catheterization are similar, regardless of the site.

The lateral thoracic vein lies in the ventral one quarter of the thorax on either side. It is visible coursing along the side of the thorax and runs cranially toward the axilla. This vein can be catheterized from its mid to caudal section. The catheter is directed cranially so that it runs with the flow of the blood. It can be secured by suturing in the same manner as for a jugular catheter. The cephalic vein is entered proximal to the carpus and the catheter directed proximally. The saphenous vein is entered proximal to the hock and also directed proximally. It is advisable to wrap the catheter with sterile gauze sponges and an elastic bandage when using one of these alternative sites for catheterization. If long-term catheterization is anticipated, it is best to use polyurethane or silastic catheters.

Catheter Care

If the insertion site has not been bandaged, clean the insertion site gently with povidone-iodine solution and then apply an antibacterial ointment over the insertion site at least once daily or more often if needed. Catheters that have been bandaged should have the dressing changed as needed. Foals that spend much time lying down should always have the catheter site bandaged. Bandages covering cephalic catheters usually do not need changing until it is time for the catheter to be removed. Bandages over jugular vein catheters frequently need changing because the wrap becomes loose and allows bedding material to accumulate under it.

Stent bandages can be used instead of elastic bandages to protect the catheter site. Four sutures are placed around the insertion site to form a rectangle that is smaller than the size of a gauze roll. These sutures are placed loosely so that a loop remains, through which a piece of umbilical tape can be placed. The umbilical tape is threaded through the sutures and then tied to keep a gauze roll in place over the catheter at its insertion site. The insertion site can be cleaned daily and a new gauze roll placed over the insertion site.

Teflon catheters can be left in the vein for 3 to 5 days if the insertion site is kept clean and there is no sign of swelling or **thrombophlebitis.** Silastic or polyurethane catheters can be left in the vein for up to 2 weeks if adequate care is used in preserving the catheter. This type of catheter is much less likely to cause clot formation than the Teflon type and causes less irritation to the vein. The injection plug and IV tubing should be changed every 24 hours because bacteria may proliferate within the lines. The injection plug should be cleaned with an alcohol swab before administration of medication or fluids through the port. Sterile technique must always be used when handling IV catheters or giving IV infusions because thrombophlebitis can result from bacterial contamination.

Catheter Complications

Teflon catheters can kink, obstructing the flow of IV solutions. The smaller-gauge catheters used in foals (18-gauge) have been known to break off if the catheter is placed in an area where there is much mobility, such as the jugular vein. The catheter first bends and then develops a crease. As the foal continues to move its head, the catheter may become weaker at the kinked site and can eventually break. For this reason, the cephalic vein may be a better site for IV catheter placement in newborn foals.

Catheter sites should be checked frequently to avoid major complications. Local reactions at the insertion site can occur at any time. The swelling may not involve the vein itself but only the skin and subcutaneous tissues. This type of swelling may resolve with careful, gentle cleaning of the insertion site. If the swelling persists or progresses, the catheter should be removed and a new catheter inserted at a different site.

Thrombosis can develop secondary to irritation of the vessel walls, with subsequent release of thrombogenic factors that initiate the clotting cascade and platelet adherence. This occurs more frequently with severely compromised patients that may already be prone to coagulation disorders. Horses with endotoxemia, any type of gastrointestinal disorder, or gram-negative infections are at highest risk. A thrombosed vein appears corded and feels firm to the touch; however, it may not be painful if it is not infected. It is best to avoid use of the remaining patent jugular vein, because if the remaining jugular vein also develops thrombosis, venous return from the head is impaired, and the horse may develop severe swelling of the face and head. This may cause **dyspnea** (difficult breathing) and **dysphagia** (difficulty in eating). If jugular thrombosis develops, the horse should be fed from an elevated position to prevent dependent edema in the head. Softer feed is sometimes beneficial, such as water-soaked hay pellets and mashes. Thrombosed veins can be treated with application of warm compresses two or three times daily and application of dimethyl sulfoxide gel.

Thrombophlebitis can occur after administration of irritating substances, such as tetracycline, phenylbutazone, or dimethyl sulfoxide solution at concentrations greater than 10%. Thrombophlebitis can also result from bacterial colonization (infection) of the vein. This can lead to disastrous effects for the horse. The infected vein may be larger than normal size, corded, painful, and warm to the touch. The horse may resent having the vein manipulated. Ultrasound examination may show the vein to be **hyperechoic,** with or without fluid (blood) centrally. A hyperechoic core may also be present. If the vein is infected, an aspirate can be taken aseptically and cultured for bacterial growth. Alternatively, the catheter tip can be cultured immediately after catheter removal. Affected horses will require appropriate systemic antibiotics, as well as local therapy consisting of hot compresses.

INTRAVENOUS INFUSIONS

Various intravenous infusions can be used to treat sick horses. Crystalloid fluids, such as lactated Ringer's solution or sodium chloride (saline), can be used to combat dehydration and **hypovolemia.** Colloid solutions, such as plasma or serum, can also be administered to animals requiring protein or antibody supplementation. Large volumes of fluids may be rapidly infused as a bolus in adult horses, but various fluid delivery systems are available to provide continuous fluid drip administration when needed. Care must be taken to change or remove the IV fluid bag when the fluids run out so that blood does not back up from the catheter into the IV line. If blood is allowed to fill the catheter, it may become clotted.

Fluid bags can be hung from a swivel hook and line fixed at the top of the stall. Alternatively, IV fluid administration lines and extension tubes can be attached to rubber tubing that extends from the hook holding the IV fluids and is attached to the horse's halter on the same side as the catheter. The IV line is secured to the rubber tubing so that it forms loops as it travels down the rubber tubing. This allows the horse to move freely in the stall without pulling out the IV line. If continuous fluid therapy is not necessary, the horse can be restrained in stocks and fluids given as a bolus infusion using a pressure bulb.

> *TECHNICIAN NOTE* Fill the IV tubing with medicine to displace all trapped air before attaching the tubing to the needle hub or catheter port.

Foals require special consideration. Care must be taken not to overhydrate neonates. Special IV delivery pumps can be used to continuously deliver fluids at the desired rate. Administration systems with an in-line reservoir that holds up to 150 ml of fluid can prevent accidental delivery of excessive fluid volumes. Critically ill neonates are often **hypothermic,** so IV fluids should be warmed to body temperature before infusion. This can be done by heating the fluids in a bucket of warm water, or by microwaving the fluids (only if they are in plastic bags!). It is important to check the fluids to make sure they have not become too hot. Seriously compromised adult horses may also benefit from warm fluids, although this may not be practical.

Medication may be given through an injection port of the IV line if no other drugs have been added to the fluid bag. Various fluid additives are incompatible with certain medications and form a precipitate in the IV line. If there is any doubt about the compatibility of the medication with the fluids, administration of the fluids should be stopped. The catheter is then flushed with sterile saline and the medication is delivered through the injection port. The catheter is flushed again with saline to clear the medication and then fluid administration can be resumed.

The volume of saline needed to flush the catheter depends on the catheter used. In general, 3 ml are sufficient to flush a catheter and T-port. If extension tubing is used, more flush solution may be required. If more than one type of medication is to be given, the catheter must be flushed with saline between injections of each medication. If fluids are not being infused, the final flush should be with heparinized saline to prevent clotting within the lumen of the catheter. Catheters must be flushed with heparinized saline every 4 to 6 hours when fluids are not being given. As a general rule-of-thumb, most medications should not be given in IV lines delivering plasma, blood products, or parenteral nutrition.

Horses with protein-losing **gastroenteropathies,** such as gastric ulcers, colitis, or right dorsal colon ulcers, may require IV plasma therapy. Plasma provides for volume expansion and much-needed protein. Foals with failure of passive transfer of maternal antibodies may also require IV plasma administration to obtain protective antibodies that were not absorbed from the mare's colostrum. Plasma can be harvested directly from an appropriate donor previously screened for compatibility, or more conveniently obtained from commercial sources. Plasma is also available from donors hyperimmunized against *Rhodococcus equi, Salmonella, Clostridium botulinum,* and the J-5 endotoxin. This plasma contains antibodies directed against specific bacteria or the toxins produced by the bacteria.

Plasma is stored frozen and requires thawing in warm water, not in the microwave. This should be done as quickly as possible without overheating the plasma and denaturing the protein. Water that is warm to the touch, but not hot, should be added frequently to facilitate thawing. Special IV administration sets that contain a filter to catch any fibrin clots are necessary when administering plasma or blood products. Some serum products that can be stored in the refrigerator instead of the freezer are also available in concentrated form. These also require warming to body temperature.

Whole-blood transfusions may be needed in cases of severe blood loss or with such conditions as neonatal **isoerythrolysis.** Blood transfusions should be considered when the hematocrit falls below 12% to 15%. Horses that become anemic or lose blood gradually over a longer period can tolerate relatively lower hematocrits. If a neonate or adult rapidly loses blood to a hematocrit of 15% or less, arrangements should be made to obtain fresh, whole blood. This should be harvested from a donor that has previously been screened for compatibility or, in an emergency, from a gelding that has not received any blood or plasma transfusions. Foals with neonatal isoerythrolysis may be transfused with the dam's red blood cells after they have been separated from the plasma and washed with saline to remove the mare's antibodies that are responsible for lysis of the foal's red blood cells. The mare's washed red blood cells must then be resuspended in saline to a packed cell volume of 50% before administration.

Plasma, serum, and blood should be infused slowly, giving 1 L/hr, if possible, to reduce the chance of an adverse reaction. Plasma or blood is administered very slowly at first to observe for reactions. The speed of the drip can be increased to the desired rate if the horse or foal tolerates it well, however, rapid administration may be necessary if the horse is hemorrhaging. Adverse reactions range from mild **tachypnea** (rapid breathing), shivering, hives, or fever, to severe respiratory distress, colic, hypotension, collapse, and death.

EYE MEDICATION

Topical ointments or solutions can be applied directly to the eye. Once the horse is adequately restrained, the eye is gently pried open with clean fingers, being careful to touch only the outer lids (Fig. 25-17). Ointments can be applied by placing a small bead of ointment into the lower conjunctival sac. Care must be taken not to scratch the surface of the cornea. Ophthalmic drops can be placed in the lower conjunctival sac using the plastic dispenser vial provided or using a sterile tuberculin syringe without an attached needle if the solution is to be used on multiple horses.

Severe corneal ulcers may require topical treatments as often as every 1 to 2 hours. For horses that become head shy and resentful with this frequent treatment schedule, alternative medication delivery systems can be used. Lavage systems can be placed in the upper eyelid (subpalpebral) or inserted into the tear duct (nasolacrimal duct) and liquid medications can then be delivered easily through either of these systems. Severe corneal ulcers and some other abnormalities may require extra protection for the eye. A protective eye cup can be used to protect the eye and keep the horse from dislodging the lavage system. The black plastic cup also protects the eye from direct sunlight that could cause pain. This may be very important, because many corneal ulcers require treatment with atropine to inhibit ciliary spasm. This makes the horse unable to constrict the pupil when exposed to direct sunlight. Netted fly masks can also be used to provide some protection for the eyes. Horses that spend a lot of time lying down may accumulate shavings or bedding in the eyes. Eye cups or netted fly masks can also be used to help keep the shavings out.

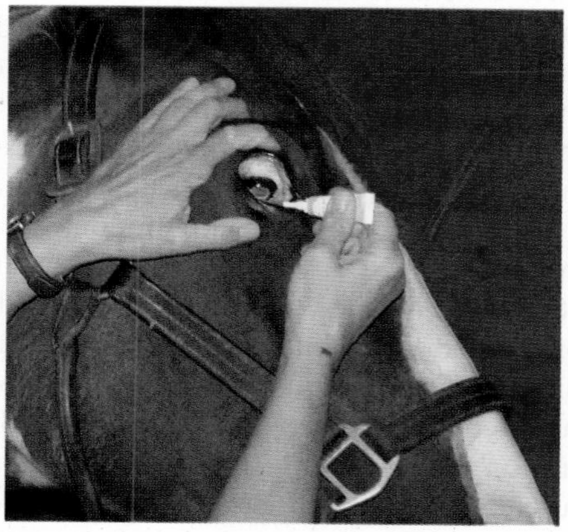

FIGURE 25-17 Proper technique for medicating the eye. (From Gilger B: *Equine opthalmology,* ed 2, St Louis, 2010, Saunders.)

DIAGNOSTIC IMAGING

The common principles of radiography and radiation safety that apply to dogs and cats also apply to horses, with the major differences being size and positioning. Review Chapter 6 for more details on radiation principles and safety. Special consideration is needed for areas of patient restraint, equipment, preparation, radiation safety, and positioning devices. The extensive use of portable machines in equine facilities can be particularly dangerous with regard to radiation exposure. These machines can be aimed in any direction, and because of their limited power, they must use longer exposure times to produce diagnostic images. Caution must be taken to ensure no one is in the path of the primary beam and that all personnel have donned appropriate protective equipment and dosimeters. Never hold image receptors by hand. Use cassette holders and stand back as far from the primary x-ray beam as possible (Fig. 25-18). Make sure that the primary beam is collimated to include only the area of interest.

Proper patient preparation is essential to obtain high-quality radiographs and to minimize radiation exposure. Horses can easily become startled when confronted with unfamiliar objects, so it is important to minimize sudden movements and loud noises. Sedation can help calm the animal and curtail startling it to help diminish movement blur. Movement artifacts, poor positioning of the patient or the x-ray beam, and inadequate exposure are the most common reasons that radiographs must be repeated. Among other inconveniences, any repetition means further radiation dose for the restrainer or the patient.

To help minimize repeat radiographs, take the time to make sure that the patient is properly positioned, the image receptor is properly placed, and the central ray is properly directed. The hair coat should be dry, brushed, and cleared of dirt or other debris. If the foot is being radiographed, it is important to prevent overlying shadows superimposed on the field of view. This is especially true of dorsopalmar/dorsoplantar and oblique views. Remove the shoe and trim back any overgrown portions of the foot. Pick and thoroughly clean the sole and clefts, and then pack the sulci adjacent to and in the center of the frog with a substance of similar radiographic opacity, such as Play-Doh, methylcellulose, or softened soap, to eliminate gas shadows caused by the grooves of the frog (Fig. 25-19).

Because the construction of x-ray machines does not allow the primary beam to be centered less than about 10 cm from the ground, a positioning block may need to be used to raise the affected foot. This is especially true for the lateromedial view of the foot. A cassette tunnel is also useful for radiographs of the digits to protect the image receptors for dorsopalmar or dorsoplantar and oblique views of the foot. A cassette tunnel can be purchased or can be manufactured out of radiolucent wood (avoid use of nails) or

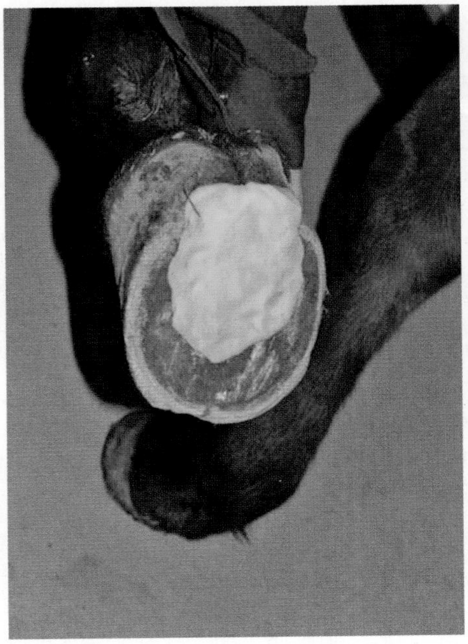

FIGURE 25-18 For diagnostic radiographs of the distal foot the shoe should be removed, the sole cleaned, and then packed with a radiolucent material. (From Brown M, Brown L: *Lavin's radiography for veterinary technicians,* ed 5, St Louis, 2014, Saunders.)

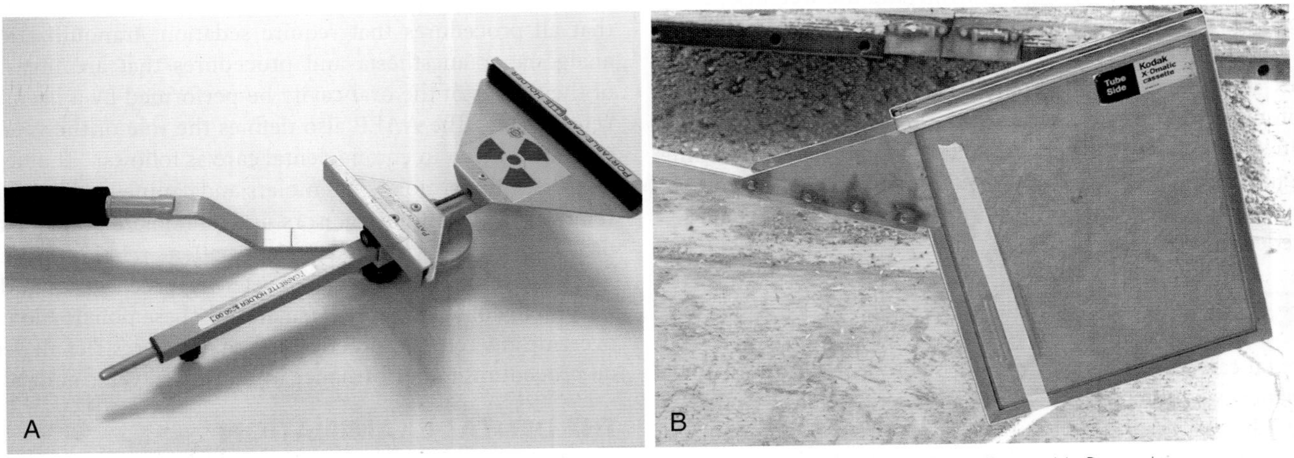

FIGURE 25-19 A and B, Commercial cassette holders used for equine positioning. (From Brown M, Brown L: *Lavin's radiography for veterinary technicians,* ed 5, St Louis, 2014, Saunders.)

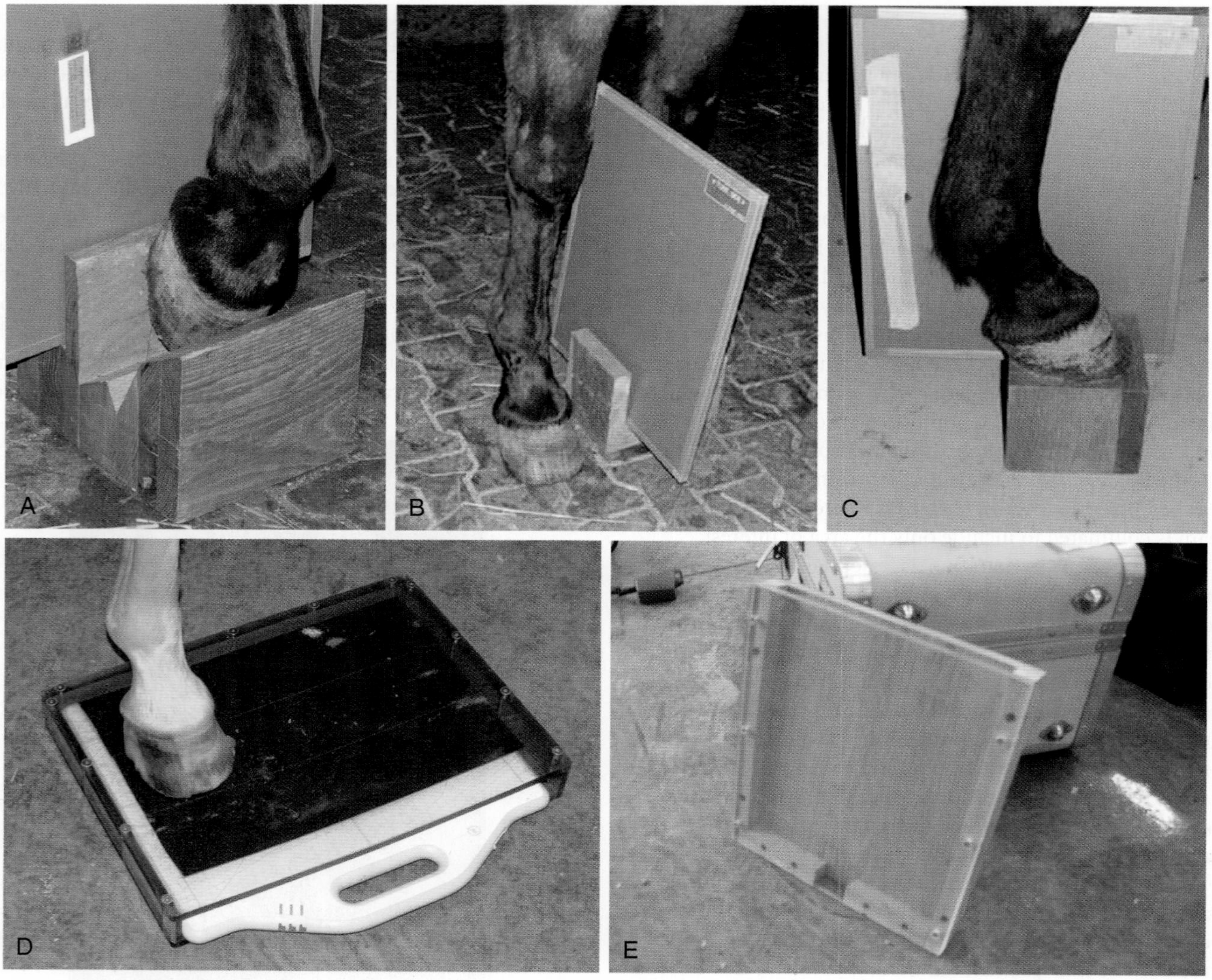

FIGURE 25-20 An example of positioning devices used to hold the cassette. **A,** Used for the upright pedal route DP positions. **B,** Ideal for lateral views of the metacarpus. **C,** Used for the lateral phalanx and sesamoids. The block can be rotated for a DP weight-bearing view so the beam is parallel to the ground. **D,** Use of a radiolucent cassette tunnel for the digital plate. **E,** Homemade cassette tunnel for film cassette. (From Brown M, Brown L: *Lavin's radiography for veterinary technicians,* ed 5, St Louis, 2014, Saunders.)

hard plastic durable enough to withstand the weight of the horse (Fig. 25-20).

Because equine skeletal structures are large and complex, multiple views are required. Horses generally require a minimum of four views for most positions, and six for many joints. A review of the views used for the proximal limb is in Figure 25-21. A comprehensive equine imaging text should be consulted for detailed information on imaging views needed in the equine patient.

EQUINE DENTISTRY

Dental care should be part of a horse's routine health maintenance program. The oral cavity and teeth should be examined at least once per year by a veterinarian. Some dental procedures do not require sedation of the horse and can be completed by the veterinary technician. The American Association of Equine Practitioners (AAEP) recommends that all procedures that require sedation, tranquilization, analgesia or anesthesia and procedures that are invasive of the tissues of the oral cavity be performed by a licensed veterinarian. The AAEP also defines the role of the veterinary technician in equine dental care as follows: "The rasping (floating) of molars, premolars and canine teeth and the removal of deciduous incisors and premolars (caps) may, provided a valid veterinary-client patient relationship exists, be performed by a certified veterinary technician under the employ of a licensed veterinarian." These policies do not override any relevant practice acts that may restrict all dental procedures to performance by a licensed veterinarian.

THE DENTAL EXAMINATION

The dental examination requires minimal equipment; a light source such as a penlight or flashlight and a dental speculum

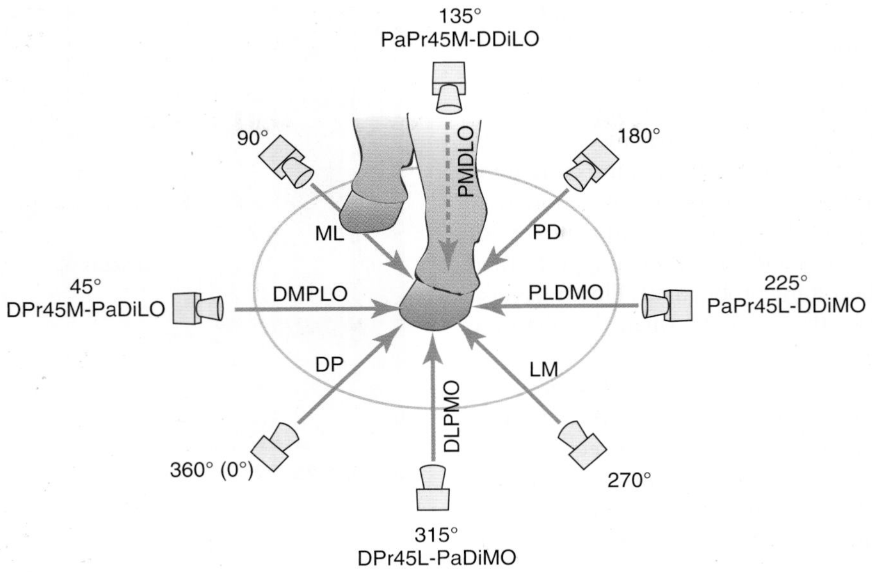

FIGURE 25-21 Terminology of the equine proximal limb views. *Inner circle:* Common terminology and angles. *Outer circle:* Proper directional terms for the oblique views taken at the level of the metacarpus. P and Pa, palmar; D, dorsal; Pr, proximal; Di, distal; M, medial; L, lateral; O, oblique. (From Brown M, Brown L: *Lavin's radiography for veterinary technicians*, ed 5, St Louis, 2014, Saunders.)

are all that are needed for many patients. A dose syringe to flush out the mouth is helpful. Physical restraint and the need for sedation depends on the individual horse. The dental examination begins with an evaluation of the incisors. The lips are separated with the hands to reveal the incisors and gums. The incisors are checked for number and proper occlusion and the occlusal surfaces checked for wear. The examiner then places the thumb into the interdental space and presses on the hard palate to encourage the horse to open the mouth. The canines (if present) and rostral cheek teeth can be visually and manually examined and the presence of wolf teeth (premolar 1) determined.

Full examination of the rest of the cheek teeth and oral cavity requires use of a speculum. In cooperative individuals, the tongue can be pulled laterally out of the mouth and held caudally against the commissure of the lips. In this position, the horse tends to hold the mouth open to avoid biting its own tongue. Most individuals, however, require a mechanical mouth speculum to hold the mouth open for a thorough examination. The cheek teeth are examined for number, sharp points, and occlusion.

Radiographs are sometimes required as part of the dental examination, especially when involvement of tooth roots and accompanying sinus disease is suspected. Sedation is almost always necessary. Common views include straight lateral and lateral oblique projections for the cheek teeth.

REMOVAL OF CAPS

The deciduous premolars, commonly referred to as "caps," are normally shed when the underlying permanent premolar teeth erupt. Occasionally, the caps are not shed and are referred to as "retained." Retained caps are often loose and may cause pain and reluctance to chew, swallow, or accept a bit. Retained caps should be removed. If the area is painful or the patient is uncooperative, sedation may be required.

Removal is usually accomplished with an elevator to pry the cap loose and a grasping instrument such as cap-extracting forceps or wolf tooth forceps to remove the cap. The elevator is used to loosen any remaining tissue or tissue tags between the cap and the underlying permanent tooth. Once the cap is grasped with the forceps, the cap is gently rocked from side to side until it is removed. Bleeding is usually minimal, and no special aftercare is required.

DENTAL FLOATING

Filing or rasping of the teeth is known as floating. It is the most common dental procedure in horses and is part of the routine healthcare program. Several factors contribute to the need for floating. The cheek teeth (premolars and molars) advance slowly from their alveoli into the mouth continuously for most of the horse's life. The occlusal surfaces are continually worn down by a natural side-to-side chewing motion, combined with sand and grit in the horse's diet. However, the maxilla is approximately 30% wider than the mandible so that the upper and lower cheek teeth do not meet squarely. The buccal margin of the upper cheek teeth and the lingual margin of the lower cheek teeth are left without contact with an opposing surface. These surfaces tend to become more prominent as the central portions are worn down. This results in formation of sharp edges, known as points, over time. Additionally, the upper and lower cheek teeth usually do not meet perfectly in the rostral–caudal plane. The upper cheek teeth are usually shifted slightly more rostrally, leaving the rostral margin of the upper 2nd premolar and the caudal margin of the lower 3rd molar without direct occlusion.

Sharp points, referred to as hooks (upper arcade) and ramps (lower arcade), tend to form along these surfaces.

Points, hooks, and sharp edges can cause pain and discomfort to the horse, resulting in ulcerations and lacerations of the tongue and oral tissues, poor performance, and problems with mastication. Severe cases often require cutting the teeth with special instruments to remove points before they can be filed smooth. Horses should be checked regularly for developing points and hooks and dental floating performed to prevent them from becoming problematic. Floating is also used to prevent overgrowth of a tooth when the opposing tooth has been lost.

Most horses' teeth need floating by age 3 to 4 years, but it is not uncommon for horses as young as 2 years to have sharp points requiring treatment. Most horses require floating at least once per year, but many need it twice yearly. Some horses, especially geriatric horses and horses with missing cheek teeth, may need floating three to four times per year.

The procedure is performed with the horse standing, except in intractable patients that may require general anesthesia. If horses become accustomed to the procedure at a young age and the procedure is performed by a patient operator, minimal physical restraint may be necessary. However, many horses dislike the noise and vibration associated with floating, and more aggressive physical restraint and/or chemical restraint must be used. The safety of personnel must be of primary concern, especially given the vulnerable position of the operator.

A minimum amount of equipment is required for floating. A good light source is mandatory; a mouth speculum usually is necessary. A stainless steel bucket with water and disinfectant is useful for cleaning the instruments during and after use. A dose syringe for flushing the mouth before and after the procedure also is useful.

A wide array of dental floats is available. Float handles and float blades are usually purchased separately, allowing replacement of the blade when it becomes worn or when a different blade texture (fine, medium, or coarse) is desired. Carbide blades are usually preferred over steel for their durability.

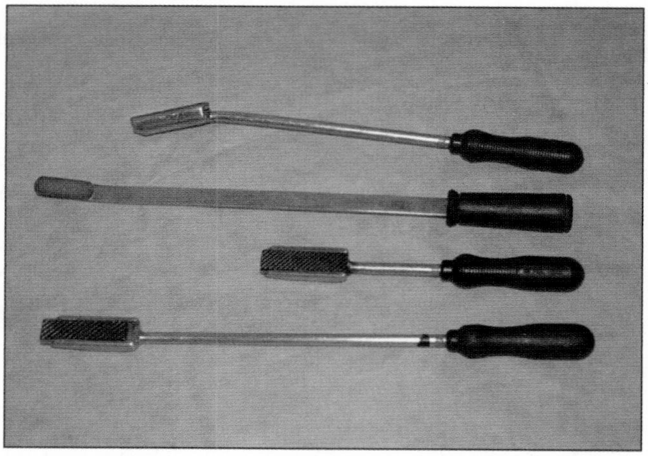

FIGURE 25-22 Typical handheld dental floats. (From Easley J, Dixon P, Schumacher J: *Equine dentistry*, ed 3, St Louis, 2011, Saunders.)

The basic float set includes a long, straight float handle/shaft and blade for the lower cheek teeth and a shorter, angled float handle/shaft and blade for the upper cheek teeth. Additional handles and blades with specialized shapes can be added to the basic set (Fig. 25-22). Motor-driven power floats are also available and may be more effective for individuals who lack the physical strength and stamina needed to manually float the teeth. However, power floats are expensive, and horses may resent the noise they create.

COMMON DISEASES

Horses are prone to many of the same types of bacterial, viral, fungal, and parasitic diseases as small animals. A thorough review of equine diseases and disorders is beyond the scope of this chapter. A comprehensive medicine textbook should be consulted for more details.

Common parasites of equines are summarized in Table 25-1. Many common diseases of horses can be prevented with proper vaccination. A summary of AAEP guidelines for vaccination of horses is located in Table 25-2.

TABLE 25-1 Equine Parasites

COMMON NAME/ILLUSTRATION*	SCIENTIFIC NAME	IMPORTANCE	DIAGNOSIS	COMMON TREATMENTS
Large Strongyle				
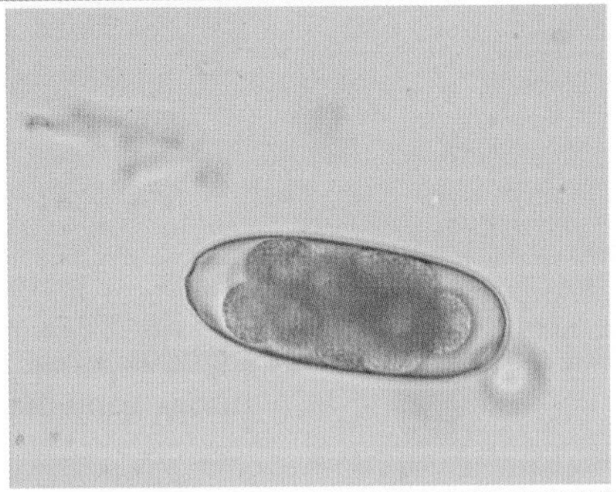	*Strongylus vulgaris*	Larval migration can result in blockage of intestinal circulation leading to deathAdults can cause anemia	Eggs in fecal flotation or identification using Baermann apparatus	Ivermectin, moxidectin, fenbendazole
Small Strongyle				
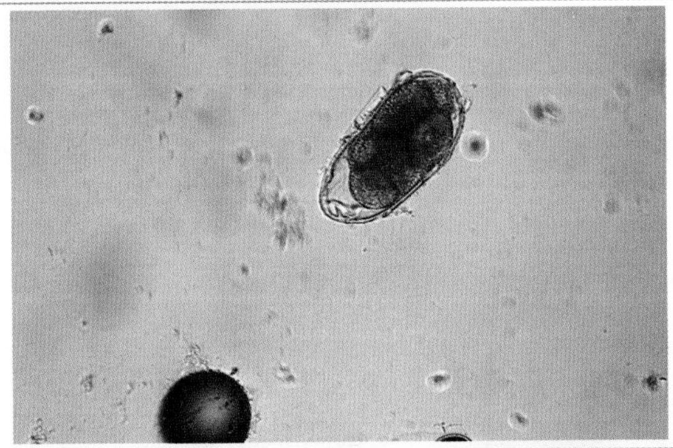	*Cylicocephalus, Cyathostomum, Gyalocephalus*	Inflammation of the intestine	Eggs in fecal flotation or identification using Baermann apparatus	Ivermectin, moxidectin, piperazine, pyrantel pamoate
Pinworm				
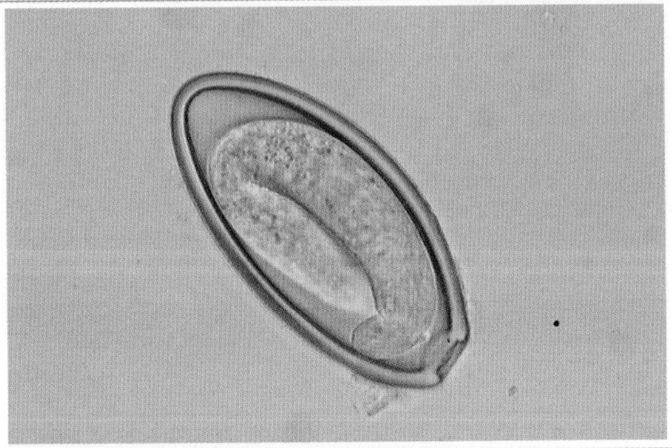	*Oxyuris equi*	Rubbing the tail or hair loss at the tail head	Cellophane tape test or eggs identified in fecal flotation	Moxidectin, piperazine, pyrantel

Continued

TABLE 25-1 Equine Parasites—cont'd

COMMON NAME/ILLUSTRATION*	SCIENTIFIC NAME	IMPORTANCE	DIAGNOSIS	COMMON TREATMENTS
Bot Fly				
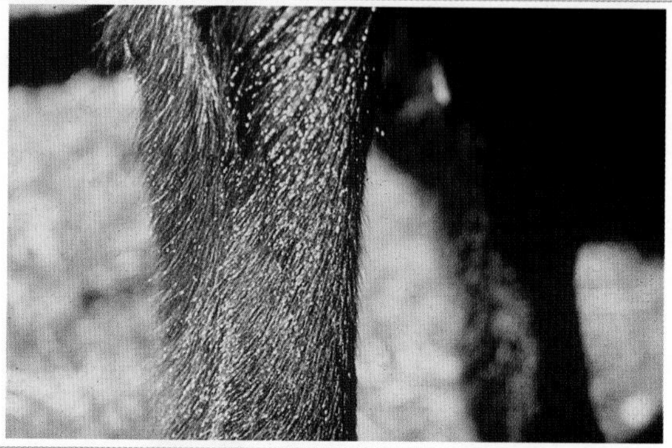	*Gastrophilus* spp.	Rare; can cause gastric ulcers	Yellow eggs on hair of legs and face Larvae in stomach at necropsy	Dichlorvos, ivermectin, moxidectin, trichlorfan
Ascarid or Roundworm				
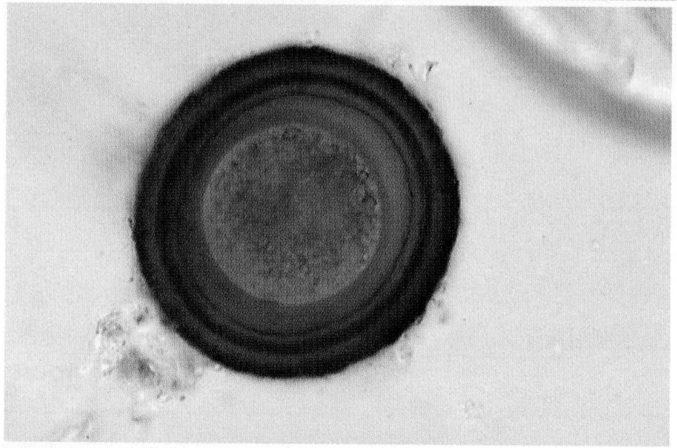	*Parascaris equorum*	Foals can get colic Migrating larvae can cause liver and lung damage	Eggs in fecal flotation	Piperazine, pyrantel pamoate, mebendazole, ivermectin, moxidectin
Stomach Worm				
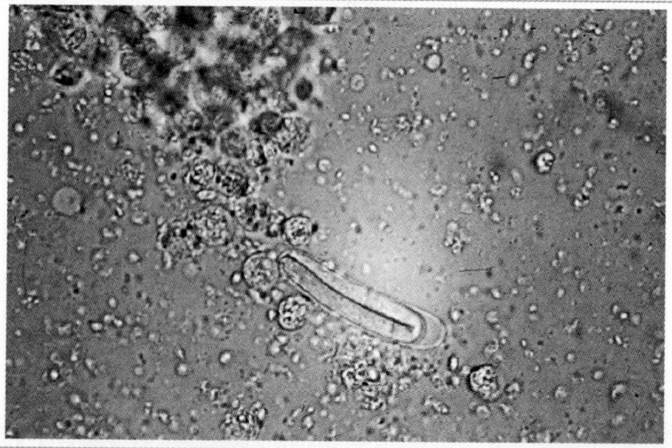	*Habronema* spp.	Migrating larvae can cause "summer sores." Adults can cause gastric inflammation or gastric tumors	Eggs in fecal flotation Larvae upon skin scraping of "summer sore"	Ivermectin, moxidectin

Threadworm				
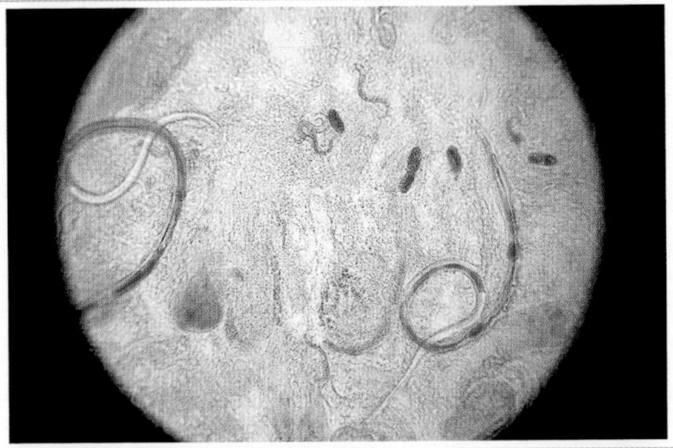	*Strongyloides westeri*	Can be cause of acute diarrhea and coughing	Eggs in fecal flotation	Ivermectin, oxibendazole
Tapeworm				
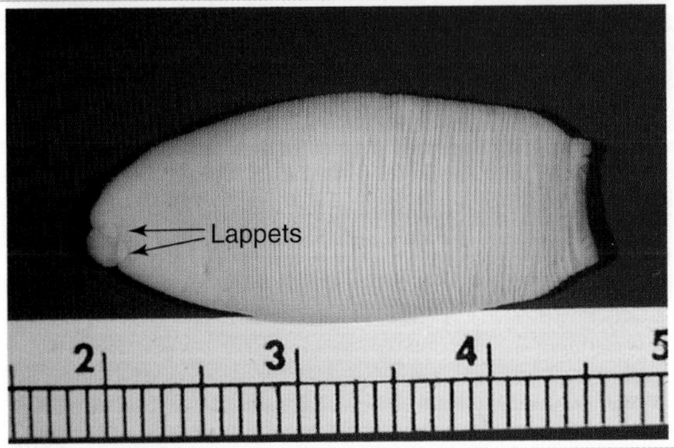	*Anoplocephala* spp.	Ileocecalitis	Tapeworm segments found in feces Eggs in fecal flotation	Albendazole, mebendazole, pyrantel pamoate, praziquantel
Apicomplexa				
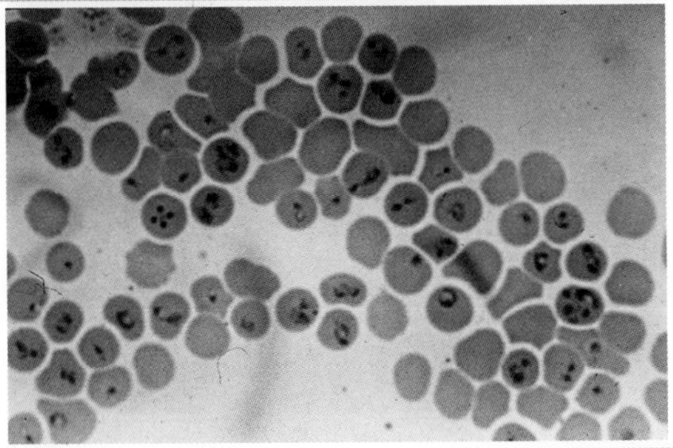	*Babesia* spp.	Fever, anemia, splenomegaly, icterus	Blood smear evaluation	Phenamidine

Continued

TABLE 25-1 Equine Parasites—cont'd

COMMON NAME/ILLUSTRATION*	SCIENTIFIC NAME	IMPORTANCE	DIAGNOSIS	COMMON TREATMENTS
Lice				
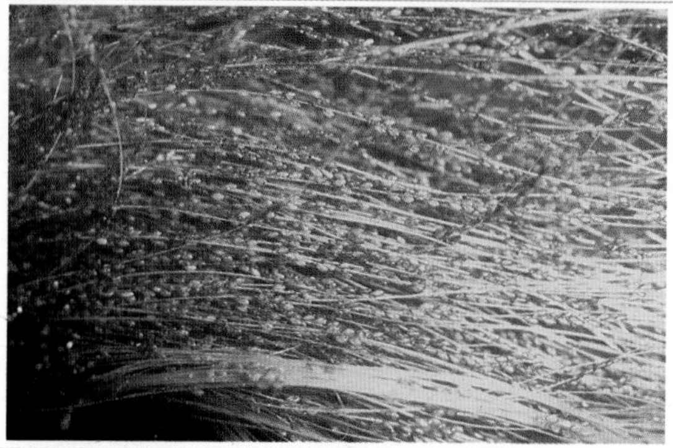	*Bovicola* spp. (biting louse) *Haematopinus asini* (sucking louse) *Microthoracius* spp. (sucking louse)			Sprays, dusts, oral, injectable, pour-on
Flies				
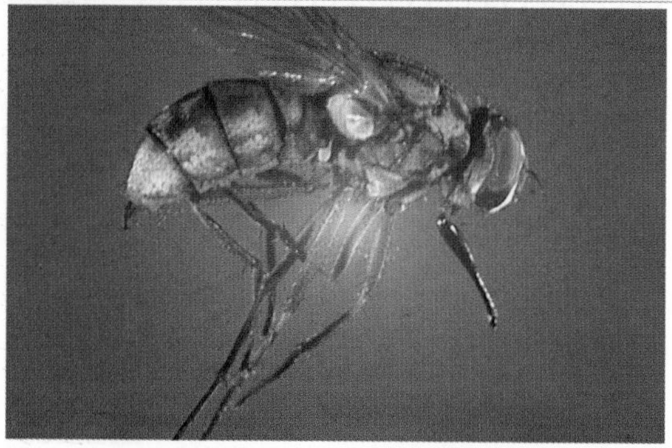 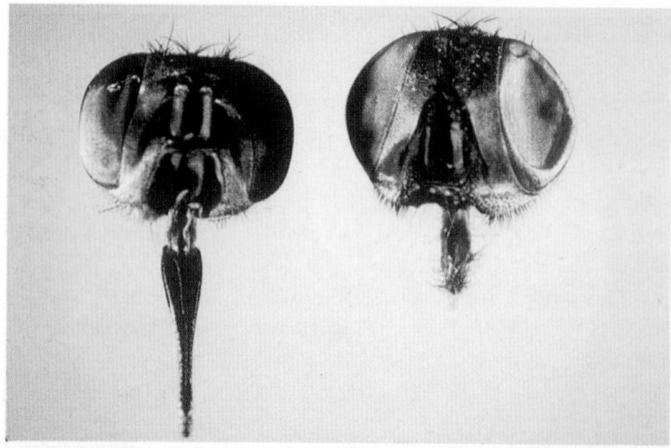	*Musca domestica* (house fly) *Musca autumnalis* (face fly) *Siphona (Haematobia)* (horn fly) *Stomoxys calcitrans* (stable fly) *Tabanus* and *Chrysops* spp. (horse fly/deer fly) Mosquitoes *Hypoderma* spp. (cattle grubs)			Sprays, dusts, oral, injectable, pour-on

Mites		
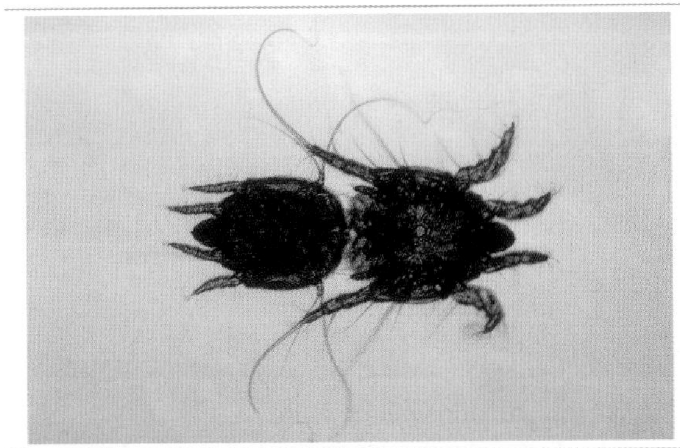	*Sarcoptes scabiei* (dry mange) *Psoroptes equi* (scale and wet mange) *Chorioptes bovis* (tail and hock mange) *Demodex* spp. (nodular mange)	Sprays, dusts, oral, injectable, pour-on
Ticks		
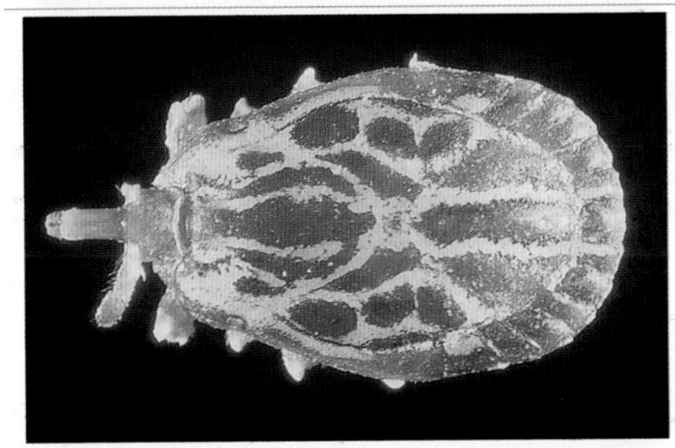		Sprays, dusts, oral, injectable, pour-on

*Illustrations from Hendrix CM, Robinson E: *Diagnostic parasitology for veterinary technicians,* ed 4, St Louis, 2012, Mosby.
From Holtgrew-Bohling K: *Large animal clinical procedures for veterinary technicians,* ed 2, St Louis, 2012, Mosby.

TABLE 25-2 AAEP Guidelines for Vaccination of Horses

The schedule below is a suggested vaccination schedule provided by the AAEP and is based on generally accepted veterinary practices. These guidelines are neither regulations nor directives for all situations and should not be interpreted as such. It is the responsibility of attending veterinarians, through an appropriate veterinarian–client–patient relationship, to utilize this information coupled with available products to determine the best professional care for their patients. For complete discussion of vaccination guidelines, please see the AAEP resource guide "Guidelines for Vaccination of Horses."

DISEASE/VACCINE	FOALS/WEANLINGS	YEARLINGS	PERFORMANCE HORSES	PLEASURE HORSES	BROODMARES	COMMENTS
West Nile virus	First dose: 3-4 months Second dose: 1 month later (plus third dose at 6 months in endemic areas)	Annual booster, before expected risk. Vaccinate semi-annually or more frequently (every 4 months), depending on risk.	Annual booster, before expected risk. Vaccinate semi-annually or more frequently (every 4 months), depending on the risk.	Annual booster, before expected risk. Vaccinate semi-annually or more frequently (every 4 months), depending on the risk.	Annual, 4-6 weeks prepartum	Annual booster is after primary series. In endemic areas, booster as required or warranted due to local conditions conductive to disease risk. Vaccinate semiannually or more frequently (every 4 months), depending on risk.
Tetanus toxoid	**From nonvaccinated mare:** First dose: 3-4 months Second dose: 4-5 months **From vaccinated mare:** First dose: 6 months Second dose: 7 months Third dose: 8-9 months	Annual	Annual	Annual	Annual, 4-6 weeks prepartum	Booster at time of penetrating injury or surgery if last dose not administered within 6 months.
Encephalomyelitis (EEE, WEE, VEE)	**EEE (in high-risk areas):** First dose: 3-4 months Second dose: 4-5 months Third dose: 5-6 months	Annual, spring	Annual, spring	Annual, spring	Annual, 4-6 weeks prepartum	In endemic areas, booster EEE and WEE every 6 months; VEE only needed when threat of exposure; VEE may only be available as a combination vaccine with EEE and WEE
	WEE, EEE (in low-risk areas) and VEE: From nonvaccinated mare: First dose: 3-4 months Second dose: 4-5 months Third dose: 5-6 months **From vaccinated mare:** First dose: 6 months Second dose: 7 months Third dose: 8 months	Annual, spring	Annual, spring	Annual, spring	Annual, 4-6 weeks prepartum	

Influenza	**Inactivated injectable: From nonvaccinated mare:** First dose: 6 months Second dose: 7 months Third dose: 8 months, then at 3-month intervals **From vaccinated mare:** First dose: 9 months Second dose: 10 months Third dose: 11-12 months, then at 3-month intervals	Every 3-4 months	Every 3-4 months	Annual, with added boosters before likely exposure	At least semi-annual, with one booster 4-6 weeks prepartum	Series of at least three doses is recommended for primary immunization of foals. Not recommended for pregnant mares until data are available. Use inactivated vaccine for prepartum booster. If first dose is administered to foals <11 months of age, administer second dose at or after 11 months.
	Intranasal modified live virus: First dose: 11 months (has been safely administered to foals <11 months)	Every 6 months	Every 6 months	Every 6 months	Annual before breeding (see comments)	
Rhinopneumonitis (EHV-1 and EHV-4)	First dose: 4-6 months Second dose: 5-7 months Third dose: 6-8 months, then at 3-month intervals	Booster every 3–4 months up to annually	Booster every 3-4 months up to annually	Optional: Semi-annual if elected	Fifth, seventh, and ninth months of gestation (inactivated EHV-1 vaccine); optional dose at third month of gestation	Vaccination of mares before breeding and 4-6 weeks prepartum is suggested. Breeding stallions should be vaccinated before the breeding season and semi-annually.
Strangles	**Injectable:** First dose: 4-6 months Second dose: 5-7 months Third dose: 7-8 months (depending on product used) Fourth dose: 12 months **Intranasal:** First dose: 6-9 months Second dose: 3 weeks later	Semi-annual	Optional: Semi-annual if risk is high	Optional: Semi-annual if risk is high	Semi-annual, with one dose of inactivated M-protein vaccine 4-6 weeks prepartum	Vaccines containing M-protein extract may be less reactive than whole-cell vaccines. Use when endemic conditions exist or risk is high. Foals as young as 6 weeks of age may safely receive the intranasal product. Third dose should be administered 2-4 weeks before weaning.
Rabies	**Foal born to nonvaccinated mare:** First dose: 3-4 months Second dose: 12 months **Foal born to vaccinated mare:** First dose: 6 months Second dose: 7 months Third dose: 12 months	Annual	Annual	Annual	Annual, before breeding	Vaccination recommended in endemic areas. Do not use modified live virus vaccines in horses.
Potomac horse fever	First dose: 5-6 months Second dose: 6-7 months	Semi-annual	Semi-annual	Semi-annual	Semi-annual, with one dose 4-6 weeks prepartum	Booster during May to June in endemic areas.

Continued

TABLE 25-2 AAEP Guidelines for Vaccination of Horses—cont'd

DISEASE/VACCINE	FOALS/WEANLINGS	YEARLINGS	PERFORMANCE HORSES	PLEASURE HORSES	BROODMARES	COMMENTS
Botulism	**Foal from vaccinated mare:** Three-dose series of toxoid at 30-day intervals starting at age 2-3 months **Foal from nonvaccinated mare:** See comments	Consult your veterinarian	Consult your veterinarian	Consult your veterinarian	Initial three-dose series at 30-day intervals, with last dose 4-6 weeks prepartum. Annually thereafter, 4-6 weeks prepartum	Only in endemic areas. Third dose administered 4-6 weeks after second dose may improve response of foal to primary immunization. Foal from nonvaccinated mare may benefit from (1) toxoid at age 2, 4, and 8 weeks; (2) transfusion of plasma from vaccinated horse; or (3) antitoxin. Efficiency requires further study.
Equine viral arteritis	**Intact colt intended to be breeding stallion:** One dose at age 6-12 months	Annual for colt intended to be breeding stallion	Annual for colt intended to be breeding stallion	Annual for colt intended to be breeding stallion	Annual for sero-negative open mares before breeding to carrier stallion; isolate mare for 21 days after breeding to carrier stallion	Annual for breeding stallions and teasers, 28 days before start of breeding season. Virus may be shed in semen for up to 21 days. Vaccinated mares do not develop clinical signs even though they become transiently infected and may shed virus for a short time.
Rotavirus A	Little value in vaccinating foal because of insufficient time to develop antibodies to protect during susceptible age	Not applicable	Not applicable	Not applicable	Vaccinate mare at 8, 9, and 10 months of gestation, each pregnancy. Passive transfer of colostral antibodies aids in preventing rotaviral diarrhea in foal	Check concentrations of immunoglobulins in foal to ensure no failure of passive transfer.

Adapted from http://www.anslab.iastate.edu/Class/AnS216/Health%20Hints.htm.

As with administration of all medications, the label and product insert should be read before administration of all vaccines. Schedules for stallions should be consistent with the vaccination program of the adult horse population on the farm and modified according to risk.

AAEP, American Association of Equine Practitioners; *EEE*, Eastern equine encephalomyelitis; *EHV-1*, equine herpesvirus type 1; *EHV-4*, equine herpesvirus type 4; *VEE*, Venezuelan equine encephalomyelitis; *WEE*, western equine encephalomyelitis.

REVIEW QUESTIONS

Fill in the Chart

1. Complete the left column of the following chart with the type of feed most appropriate for a horse with the disease or condition listed in the right column.
2. In the left column, list the four sites on a horse where an intramuscular (IM) injection can be given. In the right column, list an appropriate safety precaution for the site being used.

Feed	Disease or Condition
	Chews and swallows normally
	Impactions
	Diarrhea
	Allergies or pneumonia
	GI ulcerations
	Oral lesions or choking
	Neuromuscular—botulism

Muscle / Site	Safety Precaution

Fill in the Blank

Provide the best answers to complete the following statements.

1. Horses require __________ gallons of water daily.
2. ________ shavings are not acceptable bedding for horses with open wounds or respiratory disorders.
3. Black walnut shavings can cause __________ when the horse stands in the shavings.
4. Recumbent adult horses must have very deep bedding to help prevent formation of ____________ __________.
5. Fly sprays containing ______________, ______________ or __________________ are the safest for sick horses.
6. _________ currycombs should not be used on the horse's head or distal limbs.
7. ___________ appears as black, malodorous material in the region of the frog.
8. Antibiotic therapy can develop into life-threatening diarrhea from changes in bowel ______________.
9. Nonsteroidal anti-inflammatory drugs for an orthopedic problem can cause __________ __________ or ______________ ______________.
10. Critically ill neonates require frequent monitoring, as often as every ____ hours.
11. In seriously ill horses an alternative to the use of the jugular vein for blood collection is the ________ _________, which is ventral to the facial crest.
12. If the nasogastric tube strikes the ethmoturbinates as it passes through the pharynx, the ___________ ___________ may bleed profusely.
13. No more than _____ ml of solution should be given to mature horses in one IM injection site.
14. The _______________ is the only appropriate vein for IV injections in horses.
15. Medications inadvertently injected into the carotid artery pass directly to the brain and can cause severe ______________, ____________, and even ______________.

RECOMMENDED READING

Holtgrew-Bohling K: *Large animal clinical procedures for veterinary technicians*, ed 2, St Louis, 2012, Mosby.

McAuliffe S: *Knottenbelt and Pascoe's color atlas of diseases and disorders of the horse*, ed 2, St Louis, 2013, Mosby.

Orsini JA, Divers TJ: *Equine emergencies: treatments and procedures*, ed 4, St Louis, 2013, Saunders.

Reed S, Bailey W, Sellon D, editors: *Equine internal medicine*, ed 3, St Louis, 2010, Saunders.

Smith BP, editor: *Large animal internal medicine*, ed 4, St Louis, 2014, Mosby.

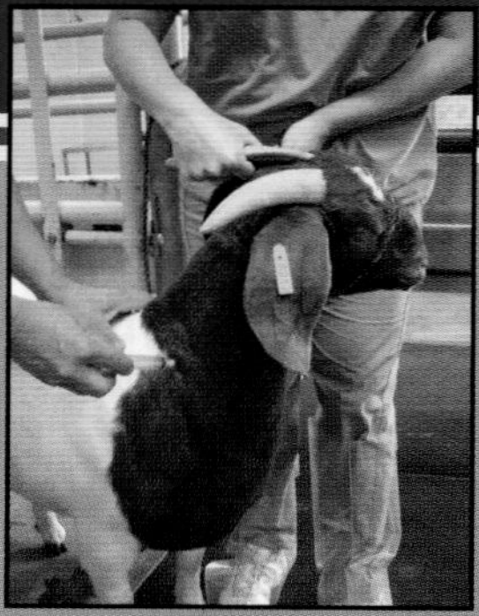

26 Nursing Care of Production Animals, Camelids, and Ratites

OUTLINE

LEARNING OBJECTIVES

After reviewing this chapter, the reader will be able to:

1. Explain general husbandry terms and techniques used with food animals and ratites.
2. Compare and contrast various routes of administration of medication in food animals and ratites.
3. Explain the techniques used in general nursing care of food animals and ratites.
4. Identify and describe various methods of sample collection for laboratory analysis.
5. State the steps necessary for the proper procedure for intravenous catheterization.
6. Demonstrate proper procedures used in grooming and foot care.

KEY TERMS

Bolus
Bronchoalveolar lavage
Cervix
Coccygeal vertebrae
Colostrum
Commissure
Crutched
Cut-down
Dental pad
Drenching
Gestation
Interdental space
Orogastric administration
Parturition
Perianal
Perivascular
Simplex system
Wheal
Withdrawal time

INTRODUCTION

This chapter focuses on the general care of cattle, sheep, goats, and the routine techniques performed in the veterinary clinic on those species. These techniques include administration of oral, parenteral, intrauterine, and intramammary medications; venipunctures; urine collection; milk sampling; and foot care. Camelids and ratites have their own sections to conclude the chapter. The importance of the correct method of application of medications and correct dosage for the species cannot be overemphasized. The veterinary technician must be familiar with several basic principles of pharmacology and behavior to choose the best route of administration of medications or sample collection.

CARE OF CATTLE (BOVINE)

The cattle industry can be divided into two distinctly different areas, each with its own set of production goals and management techniques. The beef industry uses heavily muscled breeds of cattle that are capable of efficient conversion of hay and grain into skeletal muscle mass for maximum meat production. Common breeds of beef cattle include American Salers, Angus, Beefmaster, Brahman, Charolais, Hereford, Shorthorn, and Texas Longhorn (Fig. 26-1). The dairy industry uses other breeds of cattle that are more efficient in converting cattle food into the production of large volumes of saleable milk as the main production goal. Common breeds of dairy cattle include Ayrshire, Guernsey, Holstein, and Jersey (Fig. 26-2). Labor expenses in the beef industry are mainly centered on processing and moving the cattle with additional demands around calving time. The labor involved with milking cows in the dairy industry is essentially an all-day, 365-days-a-year requirement.

Breeding in the beef industry still occurs by allowing bulls (intact males) to roam the pastures with cows (adult females) seeking those who are "in heat" (estrus); however, many operations are now using artificial insemination (AI) with frozen bull semen as a common method of breeding. The dairy industry uses AI almost exclusively as the preferred method of breeding. The **gestation** period (pregnancy length) for cattle ranges from 276 to 295 days. The female calf is called a heifer (until she has had a calf) and the male calf is called a bull calf until he is castrated (at which time he is called a steer).

All cattle require various vaccinations and/or blood tests before being sold or transported between states. Some of the vaccinations and tests must be done by an accredited veterinarian on behalf of state or federal regulatory departments that require the procedure. Private-practice veterinarians can become accredited by learning the required laws and rules and by passing a test to demonstrate that knowledge.

Veterinary personnel who deliver or prescribe any medications to any food-producing animal must inform the farm manager about the proper **withdrawal time** for that medication. The

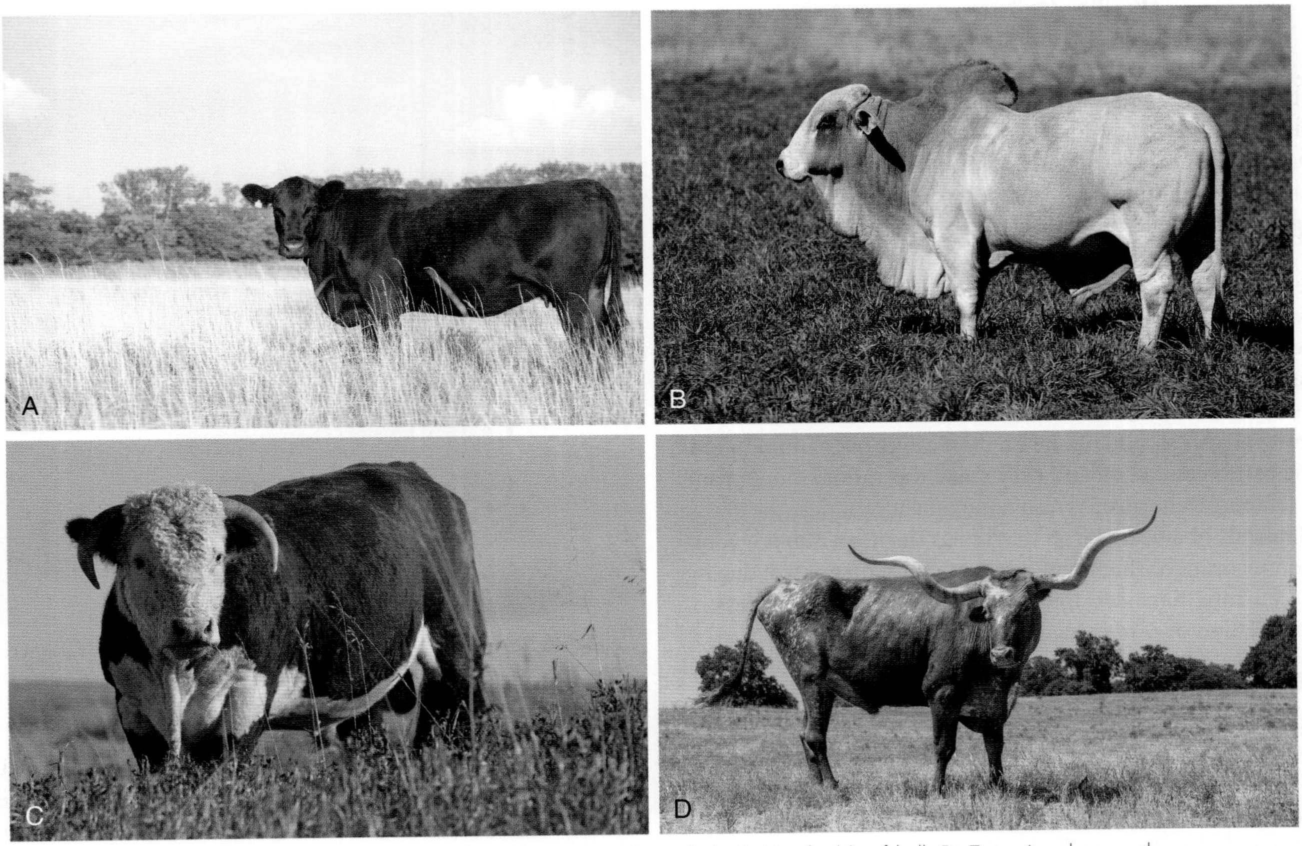

FIGURE 26-1 Beef cattle breeds. **A,** Angus. **B,** Brahman bull. **C,** Hereford beef bull. **D,** Texas Longhorn cattle. (From Holtgrew-Bohling K: *Large animal clinical procedures for veterinary technicians*, ed 2, St Louis, 2012, Mosby.)

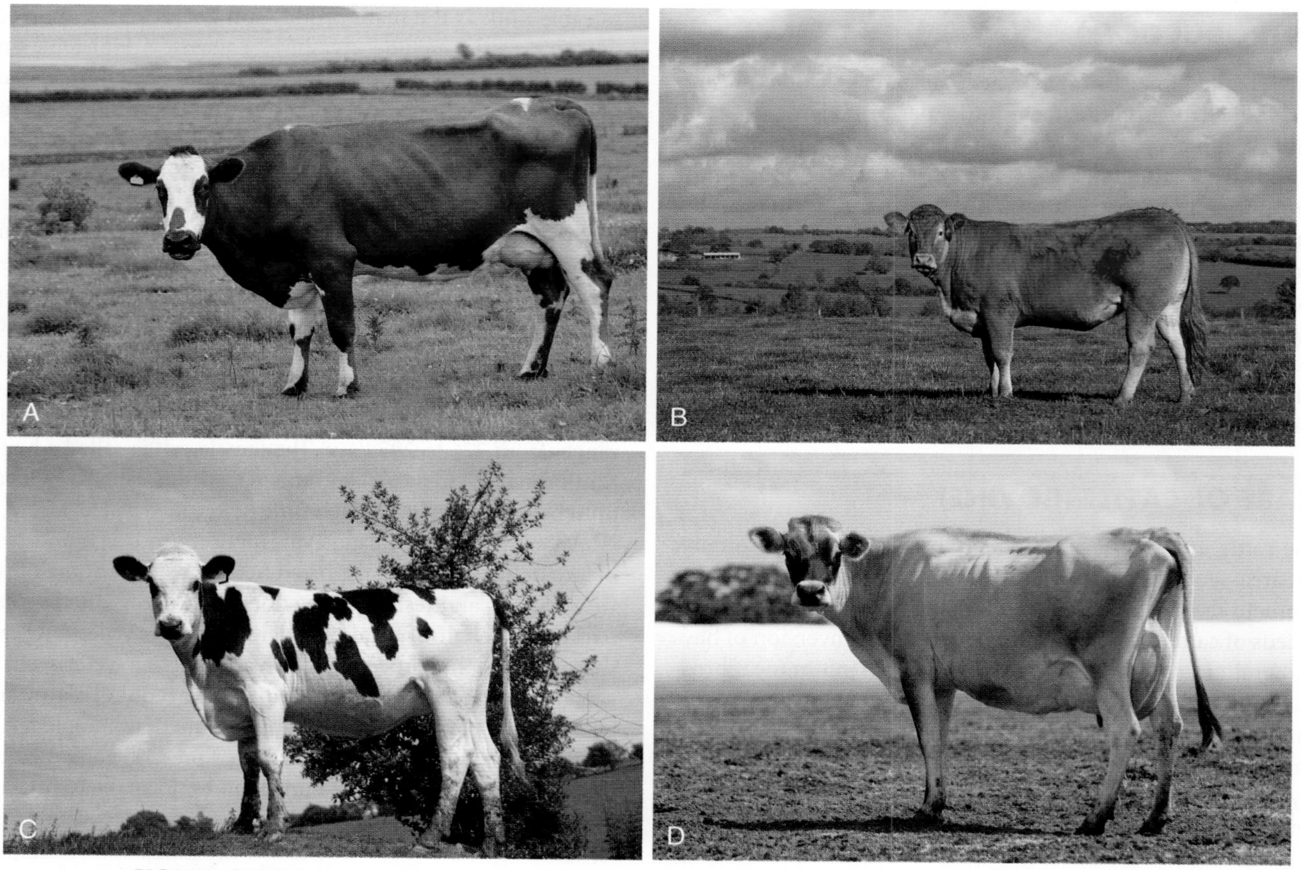

FIGURE 26-2 Dairy cattle breeds. **A,** Ayrshire. **B,** Guernsey. **C,** Holstein. **D,** Jersey. (From Holtgrew-Bohling K: *Large animal clinical procedures for veterinary technicians*, ed 2, St Louis, 2012, Mosby.)

withdrawal time refers to the minimum length of time that must pass from the last administration of the medicine until the time that the animal is slaughtered for food or the milk is collected for human consumption. Failure to do so can lead to serious legal repercussions for the prescribing veterinarian.

Male calves are usually castrated at a fairly young age depending on the owner's preferences. They can be castrated using an emasculator which will surgically remove the testicle from the body. Some producers will use the elastrator, an elastic band that goes around the testicle causing circulation loss, which will make the testicles fall off in about a week; however, this should not be used on calves over 1 month old. The bands can fall off and they make the animal more prone to tetanus. Dehorning is also done on young stock; the use of chemicals or a heated iron that burns the horn nub is a common technique. The use of lidocaine for pain control during the burning has been found to greatly reduce the stress of this method of dehorning.

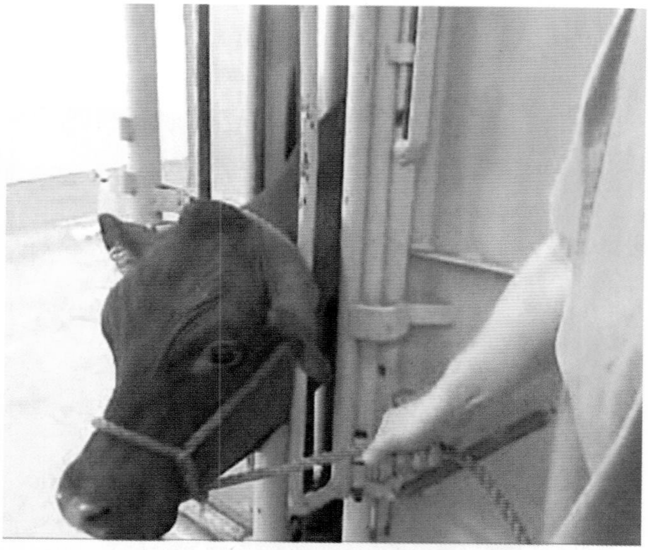

FIGURE 26-3 Cattle restrained in a squeeze chute. A rope halter has also been placed to allow further control of the head. (From Hanie, EA: *Large animal clinical procedures for veterinary technicians*, St Louis, 2006, Mosby.)

RESTRAINT

Dairy cattle are usually used to human handling and can be vaccinated or medicated while haltered and in a stanchion or head gate. However, care should be taken at all times to protect the handler from harm. Beef cattle are not used to being handled and so should be placed in a chute and haltered for most procedures (Fig. 26-3). If available, vaccinations or medications can be given intramuscularly (IM) or subcutaneously (SC) to cattle that are in an alley, as long as they are crowded in fairly tightly so they cannot move forward or backward. Serious injuries can occur by being kicked. While working on the back end, place a bar or bale of hay behind their rear legs. Dairy cattle will tolerate antikicking chains being placed just above the hocks, or you can tie a foot up with a long rope (Fig. 26-4).

CARE OF SHEEP (OVINE)

Sheep are raised for meat and wool. There are particular breeds that are selected to do one or the other specifically. However, all sheep have wool of some type; it just may not be very much or of as good quality as from sheep raised specifically for wool. Fine wool breeds include the Merino and Rambouillet (Fig. 26-5). Breeds commonly raised for meat include the Dorset and Suffolk (Fig. 26-6).

Some husbandry terms related to the sheep industry include the following: The ewe (adult female) gives birth to one to three lambs (lambing) that are called ram lambs (male) or ewe lambs (female). The gestation for sheep is about 148 days, and breeding usually occurs in the fall of the year resulting in spring lambs. The buck or ram is the name of an intact adult male, and a castrated male is called a wether.

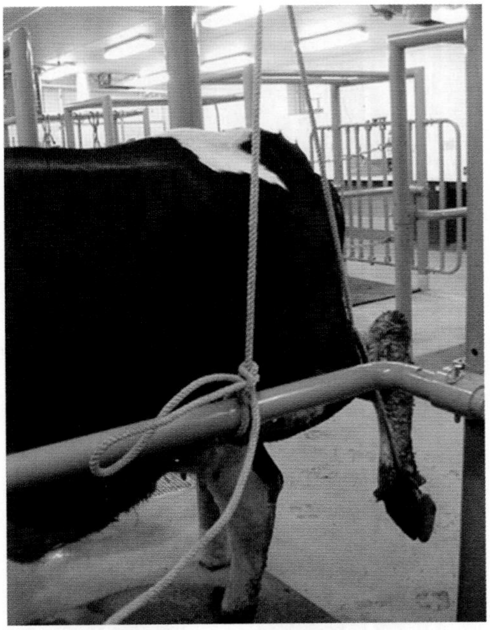

FIGURE 26-4 Cow with back leg tied up. (From Sheldon CC, Sonsthagen T, Topel JA: *Animal restraint for veterinary professionals*, St Louis, 2006, Mosby.)

RESTRAINT

Remember that sheep have a strong flocking instinct and can be moved easily as a group. A singled out sheep may panic and hurt itself or the handler while trying to get back to the flock. Using small pens that can crowd the sheep together or moving a single sheep out of the pen in view of the rest of the flock are good ways to handle these sensitive animals. Setting a sheep up on its rump is often used for venipuncture, intradermal (ID) injections, and foot trimming (Fig. 26-7). Backing the sheep into a corner and pinning its body up against a wall with a hand under the chin will usually suffice for most procedures.

CRUTCHING (OR TAGGING)

Ewes close to **parturition** should be **crutched** or tagged. This procedure removes the wool from around the vulva and the udder. A clean vulva area facilitates passage of the lamb and allows the birthing process to proceed easily. Removing the wool from around the udder assists the lambs in finding and suckling the teats. Lambs suck on anything on the ewe's body, including wool and fecal tags. Trimming this debris from around the vulva and udder areas prevents the lambs from sucking inappropriately.

TAIL DOCKING AND CASTRATING

The tail of lambs is commonly docked to reduce the incidence of fecal material collecting on and around the anus. This in turn causes scalding. Flies will lay eggs in the skin which hatch into maggots. This can cause serious injury to the lamb and even death. The tail is docked or banded below the webbing on the tail using a clean, tail docking instrument, or an elastrator with an elastic band is placed around the tail, which impairs the circulation and causes the tail to fall off in about 1 week. If the tail is docked too short it can cause prolapse of the rectum. Castration can also be done with the elastrator at the same time as the tail docking. The

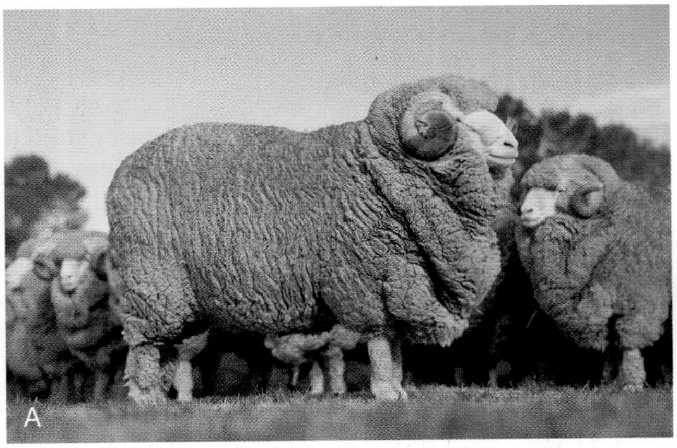

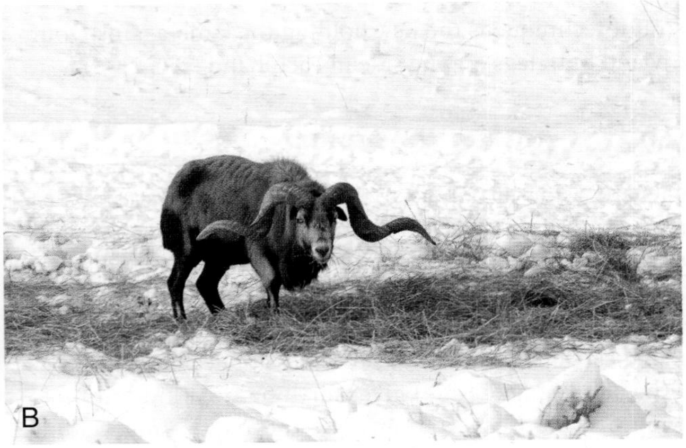

FIGURE 26-5 Fine wool breeds include the Merino (**A**) and Rambouillet (**B**). (From Holtgrew-Bohling K: *Large animal clinical procedures for veterinary technicians*, ed 2, St Louis, 2012, Mosby.)

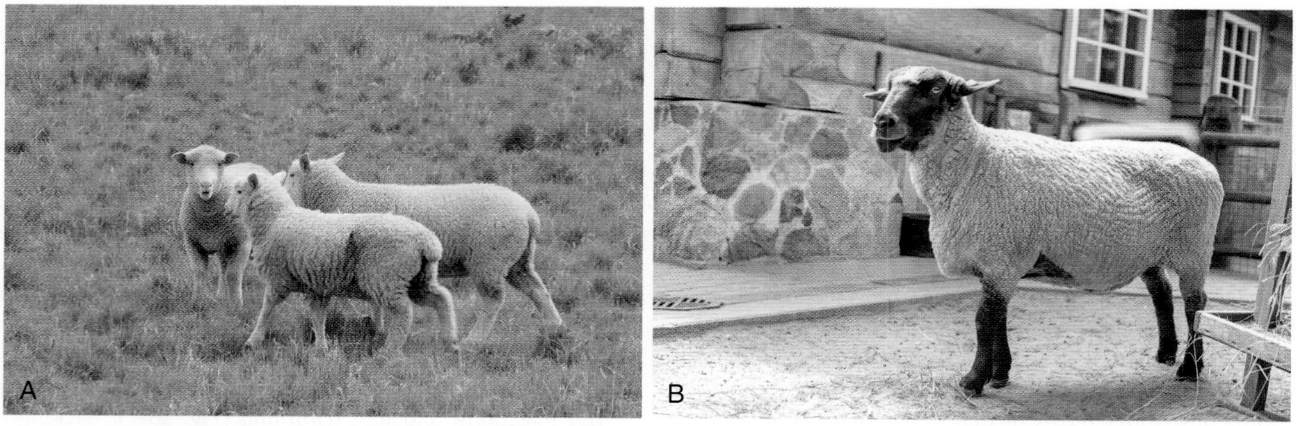

FIGURE 26-6 Sheep breeds commonly raised for meat include the Dorset (**A**) and Suffolk (**B**). (From Holtgrew-Bohling K: *Large animal clinical procedures for veterinary technicians*, ed 2, St Louis, 2012, Mosby.)

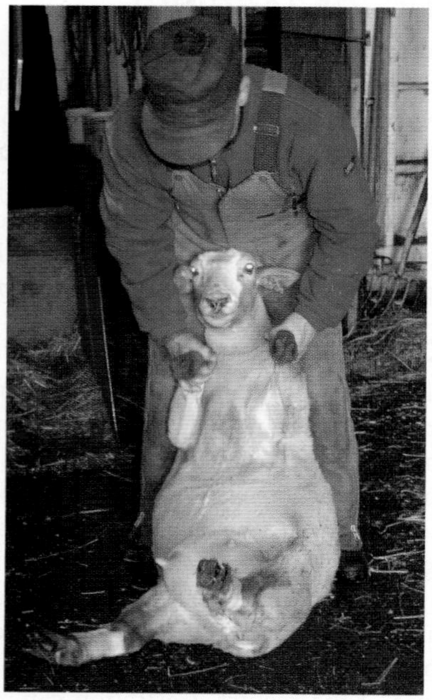

FIGURE 26-7 Setting a sheep up on its rump. (From Sheldon CC, Sonsthagen T, Topel JA: *Animal restraint for veterinary professionals*, St Louis, 2006, Mosby.)

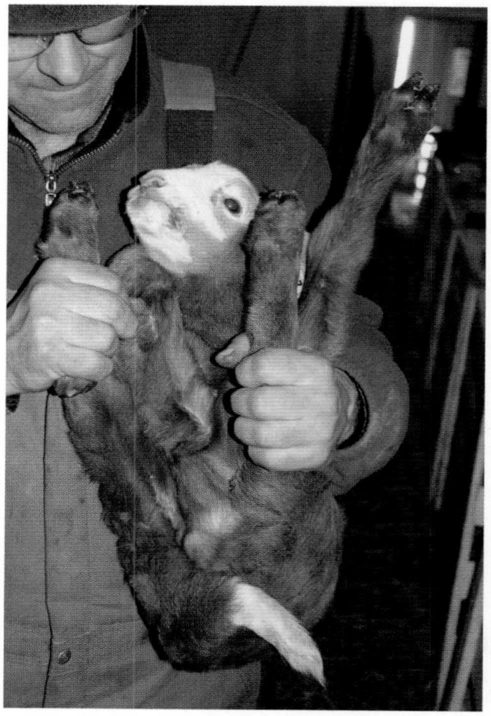

FIGURE 26-8 Holding a lamb for tail docking and castration. (From Sheldon CC, Sonsthagen T, Topel JA: *Animal restraint for veterinary professionals*, St Louis, 2006, Mosby.)

restraint technique is the key, holding the lamb against your body and both legs on one side in each hand (Fig. 26-8).

CARE OF GOATS (CAPRINE)

Goats are rising in popularity as an alternative farming enterprise and as pets. They are also used in many teaching and research institutions as models for animal or human diseases. The rise in popularity of goats has increased the need for veterinary team members to familiarize themselves with the nursing care and treatment techniques applicable to goats.

The adult female (doe) gives birth to kids (kidding) following a 5-month gestation (140-160 days). Intact adult males are called a billy or ram, and castrated males are called wethers. The kids are castrated at a young age with an elastrator. The billy goats have a strong musky smell that is attractive to the females; however, it permeates through the entire farm as well. Although there is some demand for goat meat and fleece, the major use of goats today is milk production for milk or cheese. Dairy goat breeds include the Alpine and LaMancha. Angora goats are commonly raised for fleece while Spanish goats are commonly raised for meat (Fig. 26-9).

RESTRAINT

Goats can often be handled like sheep; however, many milking goats are halter broken and can be led to a small

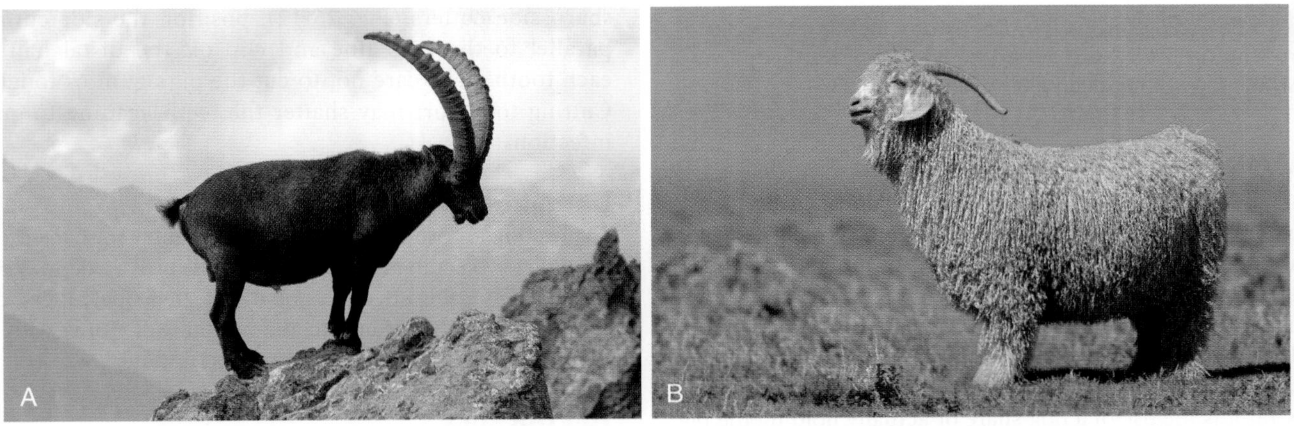

FIGURE 26-9 Common goat breeds. **A,** French Alpine. **B,** Angora. (From Holtgrew-Bohling K: *Large animal clinical procedures for veterinary technicians*, ed 2, St Louis, 2012, Mosby.)

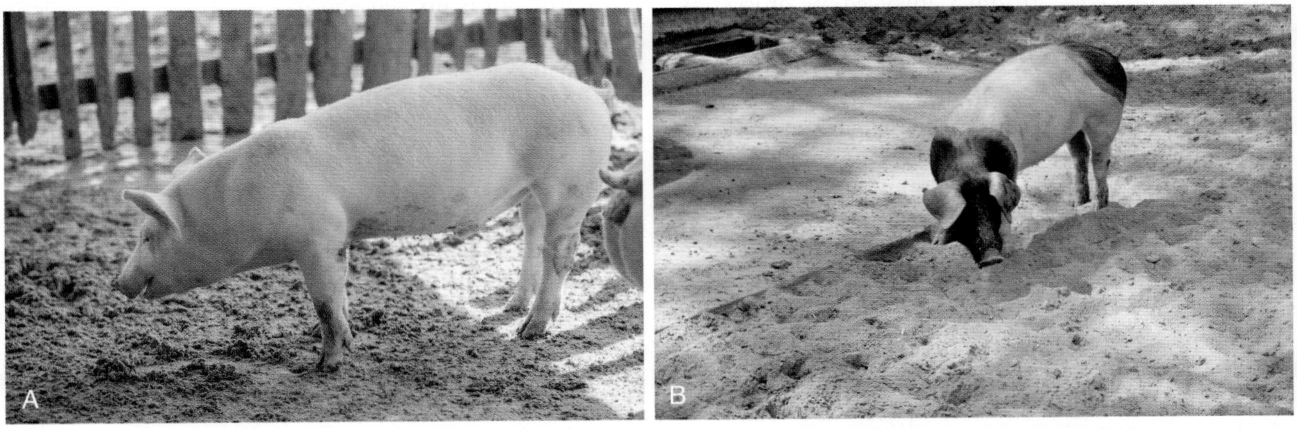

FIGURE 26-10 Common breeds of swine include the Landrace (**A**), Hampshire (**B**), Duroc. (From Holtgrew-Bohling K: *Large animal clinical procedures for veterinary technicians*, ed 2, St Louis, 2012, Mosby.)

stanchion or tied to a post for procedures. They do not like to be set up like sheep; therefore lateral recumbency, like a big dog, is often used if they need to be off their feet. Otherwise, they can be treated by backing them into a corner and placing your hands on either side of their chin. This prevents backward and forward motion.

CARE OF SWINE (PORCINE)

The present trend in swine production is the use of confinement rearing facilities. However, total confinement operations have received some criticism from organizations concerned with the lack of natural environments being available for the swine under these conditions. Confinement housing facilities allow producers to raise more pigs per farm and to market pigs in 5 to 6 months. The increase in pig density raises concerns in regard to prevention of disease. If a disease occurs, the entire herd can be affected and the economic loss can be devastating. Pigs become unhealthy because of disease transmission from adjacent pigs or infections from outside sources (e.g., trucking, feed personnel, wind, or other species of animals). Therefore it is imperative when visiting a confinement swine unit that you follow their rules for dress and foot coverings. Never enter a unit without their personnel present. Disease is best prevented by ensuring good health status, nutrition, housing, management, and husbandry.

Common breeds of swine include the Landrace, Hampshire, Duroc, and Yorkshire (Fig. 26-10). The adult female (sow) gives birth to piglets (an act called farrowing) after a gestation of about 114 days (3 months, 3 weeks, and 3 days). The intact adult male is a boar, and the castrated male is called a barrow. Young females are called gilts until they farrow.

Sows enter the farrowing room a few days before expected parturition. The use of traditional farrowing crates limits the movement of the sows and provides an area for the piglets to avoid being lain on and stay warm and dry. Litter sizes range from 7 to 12, and the average birth weight is approximately 1.5 kg. Hypothermia is a problem in newborn piglets. The piglet's body temperature at birth is 39° C but decreases to 37° C within a few hours. Over the next 24 hours the piglet's body temperature returns to 39° C. An environmental temperature of 30° to 35° C should be maintained with heat lamps and heat mats during this time of relative hypothermia.

TECHNICIAN NOTE Be aware that some postfarrowing sows can become very aggressive toward handlers when you are handling their newborn piglets.

HANDLING AND RESTRAINT

A significant animal welfare and production concern is the potential for stress from improper handling of pigs. Proper handling reduces stress during routine production practices, such as moving of swine, blood sampling, vaccinating, clipping tails and teeth, ear notching, detusking, castration, and administration of therapeutics. Chapter 21 presents information on handling of pigs. The most common method of restraint is the use of a hog snare or actually holding the pig up by the back legs.

SURGICAL AND PROCESSING PROCEDURES

Veterinary technicians are often involved in processing procedures as part of the herd health program. Although most producers are quite skilled in performing these procedures, technicians familiar with these procedures can assist new producers or help train farm employees. Processing includes clipping teeth, umbilical cord clipping, tail docking, ear notching, and castration. Supplies and equipment needed for these practices are a disinfectant (chlorhexidine), tincture of iodine, side cutters, ear notching tool, and a castration knife or scalpel. Place the instruments in the disinfectant between uses.

Clipping Teeth

The newborn piglet has eight very sharp canine (wolf) teeth (Fig. 26-11). In large litters, if the needle teeth are left intact, the piglets scratch each other, causing infection and cause significant irritation to the sow's teats. Cutting the teeth in smaller litters may be unnecessary, but many producers clip teeth as a precaution. Using clean, sharp side cutters (Fig. 26-12), position the side cutters parallel to the gum line and clip off the distal half of each tooth. Take care not to cut the pig's gum or tongue. Cutting too short may shatter the teeth, leading to gum infection.

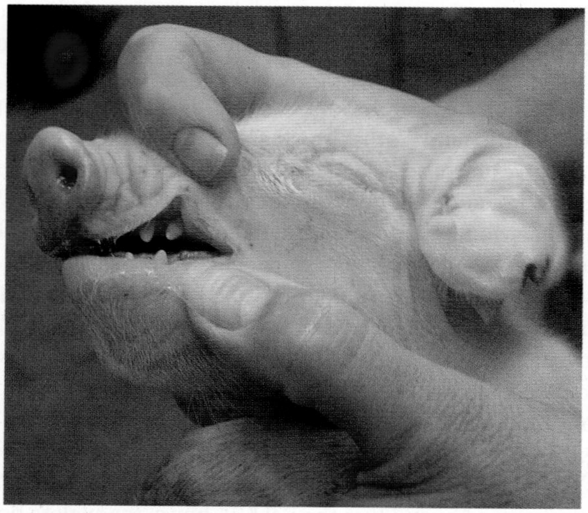

FIGURE 26-11 Needle teeth in neonatal pigs should be clipped to prevent bite injuries to the dam and littermates. (From Bassert JM, McCurnin DM: *McCurnin's clinical textbook for veterinary technicians*, ed 7, St Louis, 2010, Saunders.)

Umbilical Cord Clipping

The umbilical cord can act as a portal of entry for bacteria. If the piglet is bleeding from the umbilical cord, tie off the cord immediately using string. Using disinfected side cutters, cut the cord 4 to 5 cm from the abdominal wall. Spray with or dip the end of the cord in 2% povidone-iodine.

Tail Docking

The tail of piglets is commonly clipped to reduce the incidence of tail biting later in the grower-finisher stage. This behavioral vice may result in stress, lameness, and paralysis. The tail is docked approximately 2 cm from the base of the tail using clean, slightly dull side cutters to crush the tail. Cauterizing clippers tend to reduce the amount of bleeding. Cutting the tail too short may result in anal prolapse.

Castration and Inguinal Hernia Repair

After puberty male pigs may have an offensive odor or "boar taint" that is evident in pork during cooking. There are various techniques of castration, each determined by the age and size of the pig. The best time to castrate is before 3 weeks of age. However, one disadvantage to early castration is reduced detection of inguinal hernias. A knife blade can be used in boars of any size. A hooked blade (No. 12) works well with pigs weighing less than 15 kg.

Pigs castrated between 2 weeks and 16 weeks of age can be held by the back legs, with the abdomen toward the operator and the back of the pig cradled between the restrainer's legs.

TECHNICIAN NOTE Before attempting to deliver medication by any method, be sure the animal is adequately restrained for the method used.

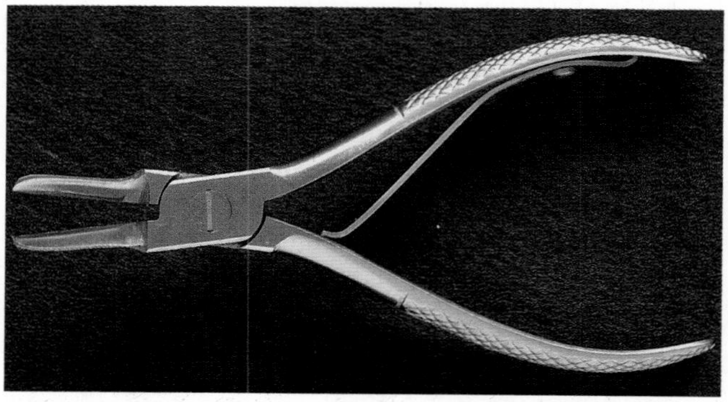

FIGURE 26-12 Pig tooth nipper. (From Sonsthagen TF: *Veterinary instruments and equipment: a pocket guide*, ed 2, St Louis, 2011, Mosby.)

DIAGNOSTIC AND THERAPEUTIC TECHNIQUES

ORAL ADMINISTRATION OF MEDICATION

Balling Gun

Boluses (large tablets), capsules, or magnets may be given per os (PO) with a balling gun. This instrument is available in various sizes for use in different species. Cattle require a balling gun with a large head and long handle, with a metal or flexible plastic head. The plastic head produces less trauma to the pharyngeal tissue than a metal head but is easily damaged by teeth. Small balling guns are manufactured for use in calves, sheep/lambs, and goats/kids.

The methods of introducing a balling gun, dose syringe, drench bottle, or Frick's speculum are similar in all species. For cattle, sheep, and goats: stand cranial to the animal's shoulder and, facing the same direction as the animal, reach across the bridge of the nose with the animal's head positioned on your hip (Fig. 26-13). Insert the fingers of this hand into the mouth at the **interdental space** and apply pressure to the hard palate, which causes the animal to open its mouth. Lubricate the bolus and balling gun before inserting it into the animal's mouth. Insert the balling gun or similar instrument straight in over the incisors on the bottom jaw; the fingers inside the mouth can guide it as it moves to the center of the tongue. Once it reaches the tongue you'll feel it bump over the esophageal groove; advance the balling gun until the rings of the handle touch the lips (Fig. 26-14). This ensures that the balling gun is back far enough in the mouth to deposit the bolus, forcing the animal to swallow and preventing expulsion of the medication. Depress the plunger a couple of times to eject the bolus then remove the instrument. Observe the animal to be sure the medication was swallowed. It is not necessary to elevate the head until the bolus is swallowed if the bolus was deposited correctly.

If working on sheep that are short enough, straddle them to insert the balling gun (Fig. 26-15).

Frick's Speculum

A Frick's speculum may be used to give two or more boluses to cattle. Insert the speculum in the same manner as the balling gun. Once the speculum is placed over the base of the tongue, the boluses are inserted into the speculum. Allow the boluses to travel down the speculum and into the esophagus. Remove the speculum and observe for swallowing. This method is used to save time but has the added danger of aspiration of medication.

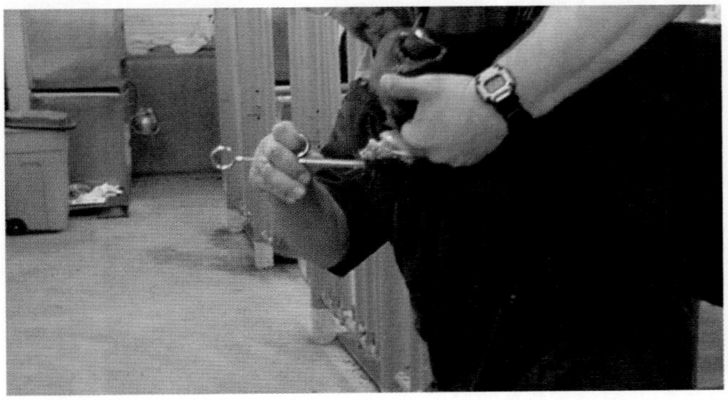

FIGURE 26-13 Correct positioning of a cow's head and insertion of the balling gun. (From Sheldon CC, Sonsthagen T, Topel JA: *Animal restraint for veterinary professionals*, St Louis, 2006, Mosby.)

Drenching

Giving small volumes of liquids PO is often referred to as **drenching.** Drenching is done with a dose syringe with various sized nozzles to fit the animal or a drench bottle (Fig. 26-16). A 60-ml catheter-tipped syringe or a bulb syringe may be used as a dose syringe in calves, lambs, and kids. The drench bottle should be made of strong glass and have a long, tapered neck and smooth mouth.

The technique for drenching is similar to that described for the balling gun except you insert the bottle at the **commissure** of the lips in the interdental space. The animal's head should be held slightly elevated so that the nose is level with the animal's eye. If the head is raised excessively, the

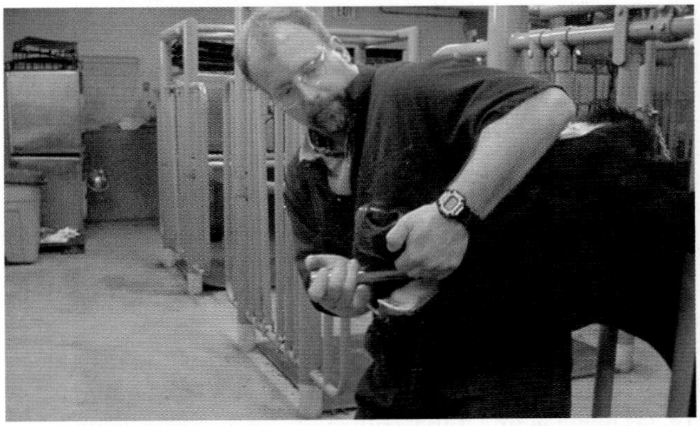

FIGURE 26-14 Balling gun at the right point to engage the plunger. (From Sheldon CC, Sonsthagen T, Topel JA: *Animal restraint for veterinary professionals*, St Louis, 2006, Mosby.)

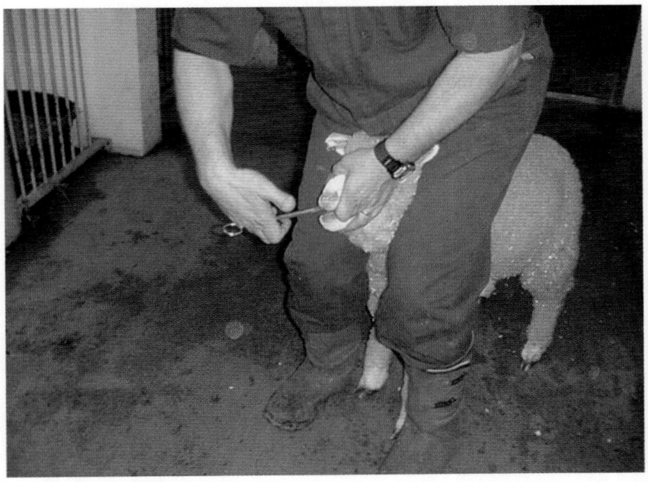

FIGURE 26-15 Oral administration using a balling gun in a sheep. (From Sheldon CC, Sonsthagen T, Topel JA: *Animal restraint for veterinary professionals*, St Louis, 2006, Mosby.)

animal could aspirate some of the medication. Give the medication slowly, allowing the animal to swallow at its own pace. There is a Drench-Matic dose syringe that can be used to medicate a herd of animals. When the handles are squeezed, a set amount of medication is delivered to each animal. It is attached to a hose that is inserted into a gallon container that holds the medication. If administering medications in a crowd pen, make sure to mark each animal as it is done so you don't double-dose or miss one.

Pastes

Commercially prepared paste syringes containing medication are inserted the same as for the balling gun. The paste is usually deposited on the tongue and not down the esophagus.

Orogastric Intubation

Orogastric administration, also called "stomach tubing," is a quick and relatively painless method to deliver large quantities of liquid medication or fluids. A stomach tube may be passed through the nasal cavity (nasogastric administration), as in horses, but this method is not commonly used in food animals. In food animals, the stomach tube is usually passed through the oral cavity with the aid of a mouth speculum (Fig. 26-17).

An oral speculum is required to prevent damage to the soft stomach tube from the animal's teeth or be closed off by the animal biting down on the tube. The Frick's, Drinkwater, or Bayer speculum is inserted into the mouth and held in place by an assistant or the person inserting the tube.

Stomach tubes are available in different lengths and diameters. Choose an appropriately sized tube for the individual animal. A tube with an outside diameter of ⅝ to 1 inch is the average size used for adult cattle. A foal stomach tube is often used for "tubing" calves, sheep, and goats. A 14-French feeding tube will work on neonate lambs and kids. A stomach pump, syringe, or funnel can be used to facilitate administration.

Measure the distance externally from the mouth to the rumen and insert the tube approximately this distance. The first 3 feet of the tube should be lubricated with water or water-soluble lubricating jelly before intubation. With an assistant holding an oral speculum in place, insert the tube into the speculum and advance it with gentle pressure. Some resistance may be felt when the tube reaches the esophagus. Observe for swallowing, then advance the tube into the esophagus. If passage is difficult, rotate the tube slightly and apply gentle pressure to advance the tube. Blowing air into the tube as it passes through the esophagus will inflate the esophagus and makes the passage of the tube easier.

After inserting the tube the measured distance, check for correct placement in the rumen. If the stomach tube was inadvertently placed in the trachea, the animal may cough, although this should not be used alone to determine correct placement. If the tube has been inadvertently passed down the trachea, air may be felt exiting the tube on exhalation. Remove the tube and reinsert. Another test used to check if the tube has been passed into the rumen is to have one person blow air into the end of the tube while another listens with a stethoscope at the rumen. Gurgling should be heard as air is blown into the tube. The smell of rumen gas may sometimes be detected exiting the tube. In some lightly muscled animals, the tube can be observed progressing caudally down the esophagus. In these animals one may also palpate the neck for two tubular structures, i.e., the trachea and the stomach tube within the esophagus.

Once the stomach tube is correctly positioned, the medication can be given. After the medication has been infused, rinse the tube with water to flush out remaining medication. Kink the tube or occlude its end and withdraw it quickly. This prevents any fluid remaining in the tube from entering the trachea on tube removal.

PARENTERAL ADMINISTRATION OF MEDICATION

Parenteral administration routes routinely used in food animals are subcutaneous, intramuscular, and intravenous. Whenever the efficacy of treatment is not compromised,

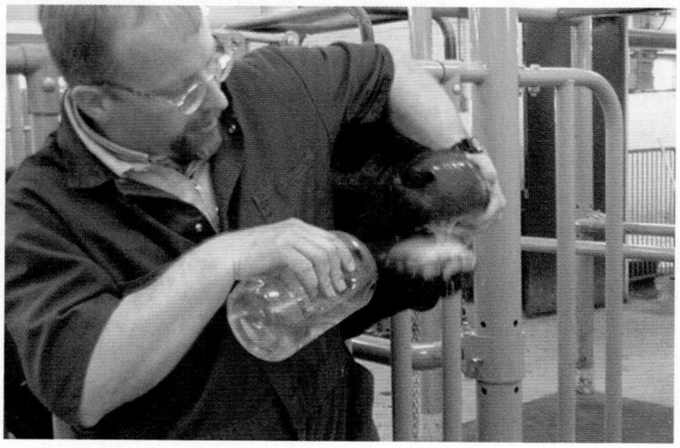

FIGURE 26-16 Drenching a cow with the animal restrained in a stanchion. (From Sheldon CC, Sonsthagen T, Topel JA: *Animal restraint for veterinary professionals,* St Louis, 2006, Mosby.)

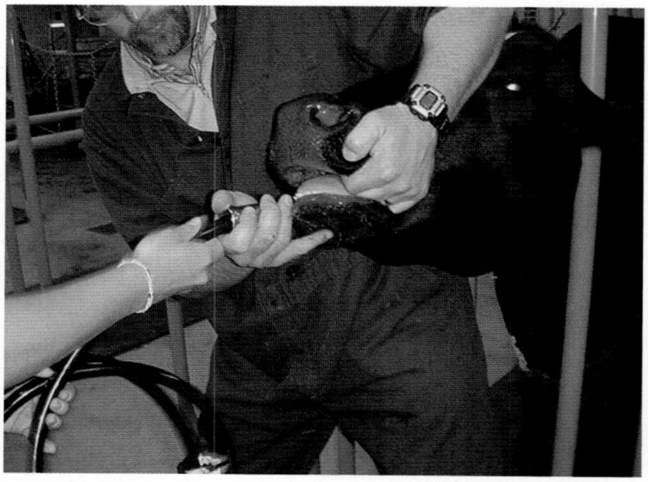

FIGURE 26-17 A Frick's speculum has been placed to allow passage of a stomach (ororumen) tube. (From Hanie, EA: *Large animal clinical procedures for veterinary technicians,* St Louis, 2006, Mosby.)

drugs and vaccines should be given subcutaneously rather than intramuscularly to minimize damage to muscle tissue and decrease the incidence of abscesses.

Intramuscular Injections

Intramuscular (IM) injections are not as commonly used in food animals now as in previous years. The movement to reduce injection abscesses and scarring in the muscles used for prime cuts of meat has prompted the medical community to limit IM injections to the lateral cervical muscles. These muscles are cranial to the scapula, dorsal to the cervical vertebrae, and ventral to the ligamentum nuchae. Care must be taken to place the needle in the center of the muscle area; too high and it will be inserted into the ligamentum nuchae. The volume of injection should not be more than 5 ml per site in calves, goats, and sheep and no more than 10 ml in adult cattle per site. With pigs, use the area of the neck muscle caudal to the ear. Do not inject more than 2 ml of medication into one site. Try to use the same injection site for each product. If a particular site shows signs of irritation, you can determine which product is causing the reaction.

Materials. The needle selected for IM injection depends on the viscosity (thickness) of the medication to be administered and the size of the muscle mass selected. A 16-, 18- or 20-gauge, 1.5-inch needle is commonly used for adults. A smaller-gauge needle, 18-, 20-, or 22-gauge, 1- to 1.5-inch, is used for calves, sheep/lambs, goats/kids, and piglets.

Restraint. Dairy cattle can be given IM injections in a stanchion or head gate; a halter is usually not necessary. Beef cattle should be placed in a chute and, if running a large group of cattle at one time, the injection can be given in the alley way as they are waiting to go through the chute. Calves, sheep, and goats are backed into a corner and the head is restrained by placing an arm around their necks. Pigs will require a hog snare if they are adults; if under 40 to 50 pounds they can be picked up by their back legs or crowded into a small pen with a marker crayon to mark each pig after an injection.

Technique. Select the appropriate needle for the animal and syringe size to fit your medication dose. If medicating a single animal, wipe the area of the neck described above with alcohol-soaked cotton. On sheep and goats, make sure to part the wool/hair to expose the skin. Remove the needle from the syringe and cap, holding the hub by index finger and thumb in your dominant hand. Using the side of that hand, "thump" the area you wiped with alcohol twice, then in the next swing turn your hand so the needle can be directed into the muscle. The thumping distracts the animal from what you are doing, and the force of the thump pushes the needle in so fast they don't even react. Attach the syringe to the needle, aspirate, and if there is no blood, inject the medication (Fig. 26-18). If you get blood on aspiration, remove the needle and place it using the same technique in a different spot on the neck. An alternate technique would be to hold the syringe with needle attached between your thumb and index finger. Quickly thrust the needle into the muscle, aspirate to check for blood, and inject if there is no blood. Remove the needle and try a different spot if blood is aspirated. This works fine on the thinner skinned animals.

If administering medication to a herd of animals, an automatic dose syringe is more efficient to use. Most syringes will hold 50 ml of medication or vaccine, and there is a dial that can be set to deliver 1 to 5 ml at a time when the handles are squeezed. The injection sites are not wiped with alcohol so the chance of an injection abscess increases. The animals are usually put into an alley or crowded into a pen.

Subcutaneous Injections

Some vaccines and anthelmintics are given subcutaneously. The lower vascularity of the subcutaneous layer allows for slower release of product into the system. Subcutaneous (SC) injections are given in the lateral aspect of the neck, over the ribs or in front of the shoulder for every animal except the pig. Subcutaneous injections in pigs less than 25 kg are given primarily in the loose skin of the flank or caudal to the elbow. If injecting into the flank, inject into the folds of the skin and not into the peritoneal cavity. In larger pigs the preferred injection site is the loose skin caudal to the ear. It is not necessary to tent the skin as we do in small animals if you use a short enough needle. This technique is used if vaccinating numerous animals in an alley or crowd pen, otherwise pinching the skin to make a tent works well. For sheep, limit the volume of medication to 5 ml per site. If a large volume is to be injected, divide the dose into several portions injected at different sites. If done correctly, subcutaneous injection should leave a bleb under the skin.

Materials. An 18-, or 20-gauge, ¾- to 1-inch needle is used for SC injections in calves, sheep/lambs, and goats/kids. A 16, or 18-gauge, ¾- to 1-inch needle is used for cattle and pigs. The needle size selected depends on the viscosity of the drug and thickness of the skin. A syringe is used to inject

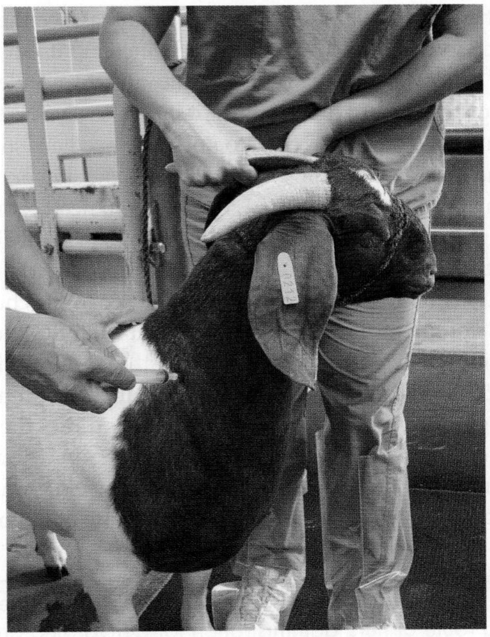

FIGURE 26-18 Site for IM injection in neck of goat. (From Bassert JM, McCurnin DM: *McCurnin's clinical textbook for veterinary technicians*, ed 7, St Louis, 2010, Saunders.)

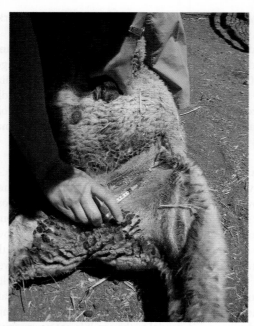

FIGURE 26-19 Administration of SC injection in inguinal area of sheep. (From Bassert JM, McCurnin DM: *McCurnin's clinical textbook for veterinary technicians*, ed 7, St Louis, 2010, Saunders.)

small quantities. A **simplex system** may be used to administer larger quantities of SC fluids. If using the tent technique, use of a 1.5-inch needle is appropriate.

Technique. The site should be cleaned with an antiseptic, such as 70% alcohol. Pinch the skin and raise it to form a tent, taking care not to penetrate the other side with the needle (Fig. 26-19). After the needle is positioned, aspirate. If blood is not observed on aspiration, inject the medication. If there is blood present in the needle, withdraw the needle and attempt the injection at a new site. When the injection is completed, withdraw the needle, release the skin fold, and massage the area to enhance spread of the medication and increase its absorption rate. If processing a herd of beef cattle, a short needle can be inserted straight into the animal; if it injects easily, it is through the skin. If the plunger is hard to push, the needle is still in the skin and must be either pushed further into the skin or changed to a longer length. If using the 1.5-inch length needle, the insertion angle must be very shallow so it isn't inadvertently injected into the muscle (Fig. 26-20). This technique is used when working a large number of cattle in an alley way or in the chute.

The volume of medication injected at each SC site varies according to personal preference and the animal's size. For cattle, 50 to 250 ml per site is the recommended maximum. When giving large volumes, intermittently direct the needle to prevent depositing large quantities in one site. The amount that can be injected at each SC site for the other animals varies from 2 to 30 ml, with a maximum volume of 50 ml.

> *TECHNICIAN NOTE* SC injection is not the preferred route of fluid administration for dehydrated animals or animals in shock because poor tissue perfusion to the area may delay the uptake of the medication.

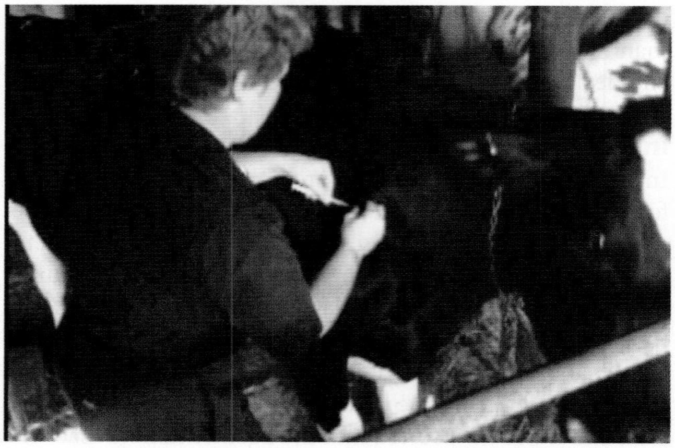

FIGURE 26-20 Subcutaneous injection in cattle.

Intradermal Injections

Intradermal (ID) injection is directed into the dermis, the skin layer underlying the most superficial epidermis. ID injections are used mainly to aid in diagnosis of certain diseases. Animals are tested for tuberculosis using ID injection of tuberculin. ID injections are also used for allergy testing, a procedure usually limited to companion animals. Local anesthetics are injected ID to anesthetize sites for surgery or other invasive procedures.

The caudal tail fold is the site used most often for ID injections of tuberculin. They may also be given on the lateral aspect of the neck, the axillary or inguinal regions, and abdomen.

Materials

Food animals require a 22- to 23-gauge, 1-inch needle because of their thick skin. A tuberculin or 3-ml syringe is adequate for injecting small volumes ID. A 25-gauge, ⅝-inch or 26-gauge, ⅜-inch needle is used for sheep and goats.

Restraint. The restraint required depends on the site chosen, the number of injections to be given, and the animal's temperament. A chute for beef cattle and a stanchion for dairy cattle is appropriate restraint. If giving the injection into the caudal fold of the tail, a bar or bale of hay can be used to prevent the animal from kicking. Sheep can be set up to use the wool-free areas of the axillary and inguinal regions to prevent damage to the pelts. Goats are usually allowed to stand with a halter tied to a post. Pigs may need to be turned on their backs.

Technique. The sites must be free of hair before ID injection is attempted. If a diagnostic test is to be performed, the site should not be cleaned with antiseptics, because they might create a skin reaction and interfere with test results. Usually removal of dirt and feces is all that is required for preparation. Antiseptics can be applied to the site if local anesthetics are being deposited before surgery.

The needle, with the syringe attached, is placed parallel to the skin. The free hand is used to pinch the skin firmly which helps stabilize it. With the bevel directed up, insert the needle into the dermis of the skin. Aspirate if the injection is for local anesthesia over a vessel. A bleb (**wheal**) should be visualized as the drug is deposited. If a bleb does not form, the needle is too deep; retract it a small distance and inject the drug. It is not appropriate to massage the site, because the goal is to keep the drug localized in the dermis.

Intravenous Injections

The veins most often used for IV injections are the jugular veins; in cattle, the coccygeal (tail) vein and subcutaneous abdominal (milk) veins also can be used. The jugular veins are most often used for large-volume IV injections. In addition to their accessibility, there is less chance of being kicked when using these veins. The jugular vein is always used for IV injections in calves, sheep, and goats because it is the largest accessible vessel. The auricular vein is used in pigs.

The coccygeal (tail) vein is used for IV injection of small volumes (0.3 to 0.5 ml) of drugs that are noncaustic to the surrounding tissues in case it goes **perivascular.** Most dairy cattle are tolerant of tail injections; however, there is a chance of being kicked. This can be minimized with proper restraint, which can be a bar or bale of hay placed behind the back legs.

The subcutaneous abdominal vein, also called the mammary or milk vein, is used mainly when the jugular veins are thrombosed (occluded) or cannot be located. There are several disadvantages to milk vein injections. The technician has an increased risk of being kicked. A second person may be required to provide additional restraint. The milk vein rolls easily under the skin, making it hard to puncture the vein and thread the needle. Finally, hematomas are easily formed and may result in thrombosis of the vein.

The auricular vein in pigs is often used to deliver IV medications. A winged (butterfly) infusion set can be used to access the vein and secured with Tegaderm, a transparent dressing that adheres well to bare skin. The injection should be fairly slow because the vein will often balloon out if it is given too fast.

Preparation for IV injection is similar for all four veins. Cotton soaked in 70% alcohol should be applied to the injection site to remove gross contamination and increase visibility of the vein. IV injections should not be made through dirt or fecal material because phlebitis, septicemia, and/or contamination of medication and samples may result. Clipping the hair over the injection site may be necessary if it cannot be readily visualized.

Restraint. Beef cattle are placed into a chute and their heads are haltered for the jugular vein injection. For tail injections, a bar should be placed behind their back legs to prevent kicking. The subcutaneous abdominal vein is rarely used on beef cattle but can be accessed by lowering the side panels on the chute. Tying the back legs may be necessary because they can kick forward with their rear legs. Dairy cattle can be given IV injections in a stanchion. Using the other restraint devices and techniques as previously discussed is also a good idea to ensure your safety.

The veins can be easily accessed on sheep if the animal is set up on its rump. Goats, adult sheep, and small calves can be backed into a corner and pinned up against the wall with the restrainer's body. Reach both hands around the head and grasp the jaws with each hand. The cephalic and femoral veins may be used also, with the sheep and goats in a standing or lateral recumbency position.

The needle selected for IV injection of large volumes of fluids varies according to personal preference and the flow rate desired. It also depends on the viscosity of the drug to be administered. Use the smallest needle possible, because this reduces discomfort to the patient and minimizes trauma. A 14-, 16-, or 18-gauge, 1.5- to 2-inch needle is best for giving large volumes to adult cattle. A correctly threaded needle is not likely to slip from the vein if the cow thrashes around, decreasing the chances of perivascular infiltration of irritants and hypertonic solutions. For injections of small volumes into the jugular vein, use of a 16-, 18-, or 20-gauge, 1.5-inch needle is recommended for cows and calves. Depending on the size of the sheep or goat, an 18- or 20-gauge, 1- to 1.5-inch needle and syringe can be used.

A rubber IV line, referred to as a simplex, is used for IV infusions. A syringe may also be used to inject medication. Its size depends on the volume of medication to be injected.

Cotton and 70% alcohol are also needed to clean the injection site of manure and dirt.

Jugular Vein Technique. For jugular vein injections, have your medication ready with the correct needle size attached to the syringe before approaching the animal. Occlude the jugular vein by pushing the fingers of your nondominant hand into the jugular furrow, about two thirds of the way caudad on the neck. Wipe the area over the injection site with alcohol-soaked cotton. This will make the vein fill and become more visible. The needle may be directed toward the head for administration of small volumes, but larger volumes should be given with the needle directed toward the heart. Center the syringe and needle over the vein and insert at a 30- to 40-degree angle through the skin and into the vein in an upward motion. Aspirate and, if blood flows into the syringe, inject. Occasionally the needle only penetrates the skin. When this occurs, relocate the vein, withdraw the needle about half way and angle it deeper to hit the vein. Redirection of the needle from side to side may also be necessary to find the vein. Thread the needle to its hub into the vein; this allows for movement of the animal and keeps the needle from being dislodged. If the needle has been inserted too deeply and has penetrated entirely through the vessel, pull the syringe and needle back slowly until the blood flows freely at aspiration; at this point the needle can be threaded. Apposition of the bevel of the needle against the vessel wall may also occlude it. This may be corrected by slightly rotating the needle along its long axis. Do not inject the medication unless you are sure you are in the vein; redirect the needle if necessary. Care must be taken when redirecting the needle to prevent laceration of the vein and consequent hematoma formation. If giving a caustic medication, aspirate after every few milliliters injected to check that you are still in the vein. Withdraw the needle while attached to the syringe and apply pressure over the injection site to prevent formation of a hematoma.

With sheep, you start by parting the wool along the jugular furrow and wiping the area with cotton soaked in alcohol in a stroking motion; this will help define the borders of the vessel. Occlude the vessel at or slightly cranial to the thoracic inlet. Insert the needle at a 30- to 45-degree angle, threading the needle into the vessel. Aspirate to check for blood. If the needle is positioned in the vessel, inject the medication slowly. The jugular vein appears deeper in an unshorn sheep because the wool prevents the technician from resting the syringe against the animal's skin. The jugular vein also sits fairly close to the trachea and is very superficial compared with a cow.

Tail Vein Technique. To access the tail vein, the tail is lifted straight (tail jacked) up to expose the area just above the anus. The needle is inserted perpendicular to the tail, centered on the midline. The needle may hit bone; if it does, back it out while aspirating. As soon as you see blood, stop backing the needle out and inject slowly. The medication injected into this area should NOT be caustic to the tissues if it goes perivascularly. Use 20- to 22-gauge needles at 1-inch in length.

Subcutaneous Abdominal Vein Technique. The subcutaneous abdominal vein (milk vein) is used when the jugular veins cannot be raised or are inaccessible for other reasons. These veins should be used for administration of large volumes of medication only. It is too dangerous to obtain routine blood samples from them.

The animal should be tied securely or restrained in a stanchion or chute. Stand close to the cow's flank, facing the same direction as the cow. One should not face the cow's rear, as cows can kick forward with their back legs.

A 16-gauge, 2- to 3-inch needle and syringe may be used to inject medication; however, a simplex system is frequently used. Because blood flows slowly in this vein, administration through a simplex may require more time than anticipated.

It is not necessary to occlude the milk vein before puncturing it, because it is normally distended. The preferred site is immediately caudal to the point where the vessel enters the abdomen; this section of the vein is the most stable. As with jugular injections, it takes some force to introduce the needle through the skin. If blood is not aspirated, check the position of the needle and redirect it. Exercise caution when redirecting the needle, because it is easy to create hematomas in this area. Observe the area for perivascular infiltration during administration. When the injection has been completed, remove the needle and apply digital pressure for several minutes. Even with digital pressure, hematomas form easily.

Auricular Vein Technique. Intravenous injections are commonly given in the auricular vein (Table 26-1) on pigs and some large cattle. Pigs less than 15 kg can be held, whereas larger pigs should be restrained using a snare. The auricular vein, near the lateral border of the ear, is prominent when held off using thumb pressure or a rubber band as a tourniquet at the base of the ear. After a minute the ear veins become engorged. A 20- to 22-gauge, ¾- to 1-inch infusion set (butterfly catheter) works very well for administration of solutions. If you need to leave the catheter in, a Tegaderm bandage is a clear bandage that works well on the bare skin of the ear.

INTRAPERITONEAL INJECTION

The intraperitoneal (IP) route is usually used in neonates for fluid therapy. The fold between the ventral midline and flank is the best site for IP injections. The site is prepared by clipping the area and prepping with a surgical scrub. The animal is restrained in dorsal recumbency, with the

TABLE 26-1 Recommended Needle Sizes, Injection Volumes, and Blood Sample Volumes, Based on Pig Size

	INJECTIONS					BLOOD SAMPLING		
IM	SC	IV	CRANIAL VENA CAVA	JUGULAR VEIN	EAR VEIN	MEDIAL CANTHUS	TAIL VEIN	CEPHALIC VEIN
Piglet								
Needle	18-20 gauge, 11 mm	21 gauge, 11 mm	20 gauge, 38 mm	20 gauge, 38 mm		20 gauge, 25 mm		
Quantity	1-2 ml/site		Unlimited			5-10 ml		
Weaner								
Needle	18-20 gauge, 18 mm	21 gauge, 25 mm	20 gauge, 38 mm			20 gauge, 25 mm		20 gauge, 38 mm
Quantity	1-2 ml/site		Unlimited			5-10 ml		5-10 ml
Grower-Finisher								
Needle	16 gauge, 18-25 mm	18 gauge, 25 mm	18 gauge, 65 mm	20 gauge, 38 mm	20 gauge, 25 mm	16 gauge, 38 mm		
Quantity	1-3 ml/site		Unlimited		1-2 ml	5-10 ml		
Breeding Stock								
Needle	14-16 gauge, 38 mm	18 gauge, 38 mm	16 gauge, 90 mm	20 gauge, 38 mm	20 gauge, 25 mm	14 gauge, 38 mm	20 gauge, 25 mm	
Quantity	1-3 ml/site		Unlimited		1-2 ml	5-10 ml	5-10 ml	

hindquarters elevated or, if it is a piglet, held by the back legs. To avoid puncturing the bladder or injuring the penis in males, insert the needle slightly off midline. Gently insert a 16- to 18-gauge, ¾- to 1-inch needle, just deep enough to enter the abdominal cavity. Hold onto the needle to prevent it from moving around as it can damage the internal organs. The fluids should flow easily if the needle is in the abdominal cavity. Many problems, such as peritonitis from improper site preparation or puncturing of abdominal organs, can result if improper technique is used in this procedure. In larger pigs, the injection is performed through the paralumbar fossa with the animal in the standing position. A 16- to 18-gauge × 3-inch needle is usually used.

INTRANASAL INSUFFLATION

The intranasal route is used to administer vaccines and local anesthetics. Only vaccines designed for intranasal use should be given by in this manner. Other vaccines are not effective when given by this route. Intranasal anesthetics may be given before potentially painful procedures on the nasal cavity, such as nasogastric intubation, **bronchoalveolar lavage,** and endoscopy. Restraint of the head is a necessity. Calves may be manually restrained, whereas adults should be secured with a halter and in a chute or stanchion. Pigs less than 15 kg can be held, whereas larger pigs should be snared and the head elevated.

Technique

Nasal secretions should be wiped from the nostril with moist cotton before medication administration. A 3- to 5-ml syringe is filled with the vaccine or local anesthetic, with a disposable, blunt tip attached to inject the drug, although the syringe alone may be used. For all animals except the pig, start by facing the same direction as the animal. Place one hand over the bridge of the nose, grasping the jaw bone to elevate it and pull it close to your body. The head must be slightly elevated to prevent the medication from running out of the nostril. The free hand is used to quickly insert the syringe into the nostril and quickly inject the solution. When the injection is completed, elevate the head for 10 to 15 seconds before releasing it. Another technique to prevent the animal from ejecting the solution by sneezing is to time the injection with inspiration.

INTRAMAMMARY INFUSION

Veterinarians and dairy farmers often use intramammary infusions to treat mastitis or to infuse udder quarters when cows and goats are dry (not lactating). It may be necessary to check or treat sheep for mastitis. A physical examination is best performed with the sheep in a set-up position. Treatments or milk testing in the ewe are usually done with the ewe in a standing position.

The best time to infuse the udder is after the last milking of the day, which allows the medication to remain in the udder overnight. The udder should not be infused immediately before milking because the beneficial effect of the medication would be lost. Because intramammary antibiotic therapy affects the results of milk culture, milk samples from mastitic quarters must be obtained before treatment (Fig. 26-21). If you need to, collect a sample for bacteriologic examination and somatic cell count and California Mastitis Test (CMT). Each teat end should be cleaned with an alcohol-soaked cotton swab. The teat on the far side of the udder is disinfected first, sampled, and then the one on the near side is disinfected and sampled. Before a sample is collected, a small squirt of milk is discarded from each teat to flush out any bacteria present in the teat canal. The sterile sample tubes are labeled as to the particular side of the udder, the stopper is removed, and milk is directed into the tube held at a 45-degree angle, rather than vertically. This prevents any debris from falling into the sample and contaminating it. As previously mentioned, samples are usually collected first from the far side teats then from the near side teats. Look for flakes or blood in the milk and perform a test to confirm mastitis. This should be done after the udder is thoroughly cleaned.

Restraint

Minimal restraint is required for intramammary infusion with dairy cattle and goats. Rear leg and tail restraint may be necessary for fractious cows. Care must be taken with beef cows, especially if they have been separated from their calves, because they are protective of their calves as well as unused to being touched by a human in that area. Placing them into a chute and tying a foot back may be necessary to ensure safety. Goats will usually tolerate being touched, so being haltered and tied to a post should work just fine.

Technique

Crouching down beside the udder to work makes it easier to avoid injury from kicking, but never sit down or kneel.

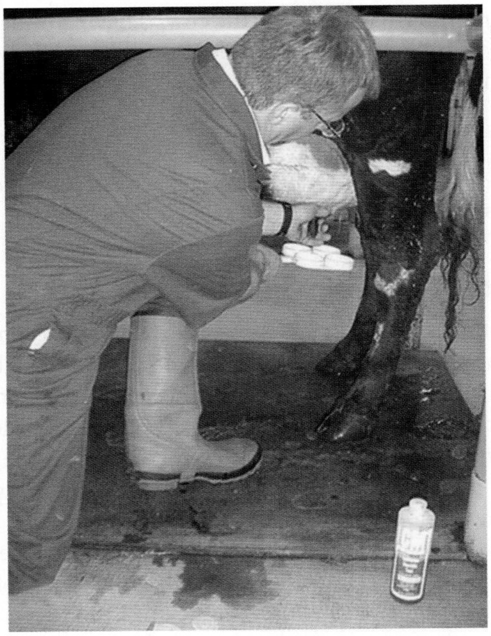

FIGURE 26-21 Collection of milk sample for mastitis testing. (From Sheldon CC, Sonsthagen T, Topel JA: *Animal restraint for veterinary professionals*, St Louis, 2006, Mosby.)

Thoroughly clean the udder before treatment, using warm water and antiseptic soap. Use a separate cloth or paper towel to wash each teat to decrease the spread of microorganisms among the quarters. Use a liquid germicidal teat dip, allowing 30 seconds of contact time before drying with a paper towel. Dry each teat with a separate towel to remove contaminated water droplets. Wipe the teat orifice with an alcohol swab and allow to air dry. If all four quarters are to be infused, swab the far teats before swabbing the near ones, to prevent contamination when reaching past the near teats.

Empty the quarter by manually "stripping out" the milk before infusing medication, because residual milk mixes with the medication and dilutes it. Collect the discarded milk in a bucket to prevent contamination of the environment by the bacteria in the milk. After the teat is prepared, grasp it near the base and insert a teat cannula or sterile, disposable mammary infusion cannula into the teat orifice. More commonly, commercially prepared, disposable syringes with an attached cannula are used. Advance the cannula just through the teat sphincter a short distance and inject the medication slowly; pinch the teat orifice gently to prevent the medication from leaking around the cannula. Do not insert the cannula to the hub, because this stretches the teat sphincter and predisposes the quarter to mastitis. The typical commercial intramammary preparation is 10 to 20 ml, all of which may be infused into a quarter. Any volume over that is most likely an extra-label use and should be evaluated carefully by a veterinarian. Remove the cannula, continue to pinch the teat orifice closed, and gently massage the teat and quarter to disseminate the medication. When the procedure is completed, dip the teat in germicidal teat dip to prevent invasion of microbes. If the weather is extremely cold (0° C or less), do not allow the cow to go outside until the udder is dry, to prevent chapping and frostbite. Mark the cow as having been treated so that its milk can be discarded. This is often accomplished with ankle bands.

> **TECHNICIAN NOTE** Medication withdrawal times must be observed with lactating goats in the same manner as they are with lactating cattle.

INTRAUTERINE MEDICATION

Medication is placed in the uterus to locally treat retained placenta or metritis. Although this technique still may be performed, most uterine infections are now treated systemically.

Uterine medication is available as boluses, capsules, and solutions. The form of the drug used depends on the condition of the uterus, stage of the reproductive cycle, types of drugs available, and personal preference.

Usually done on cows, they should be restrained in a chute or stanchion for this procedure. A bar or bale of hay is placed behind the legs to prevent kicking. The tail should be secured away from the **perianal** region by tying it to the animal's neck. Feces should be raked (manually removed) from the rectum before the vulva is cleaned, to aid in palpation and prevent contamination of the area and equipment. An antiseptic soap, warm water, and cotton are used to wash the vulva and surrounding area. Wipe the vulva, starting at the dorsal commissure of the labia and progressing down to the ventral commissure. The soap should be rinsed off before treatment.

Intrauterine Infusion Technique

A uterine pipette is used to infuse solutions into the uterus, using a syringe to inject the medication through the pipette. A hazard associated with this technique is that the vaginal and rectal walls may be penetrated if excessive force is used. This could result in such complications as peritonitis, metritis, abscesses, and reproductive disorders.

Intrauterine infusion is done in goats to treat retained placenta or metritis. The vulva should be scrubbed and rinsed thoroughly to remove contaminants. A sterile vaginal speculum and a light source are needed. The vaginal speculum, lubricated with sterile, water-soluble jelly, is inserted into the vagina. The light source is inserted inside the speculum, and the speculum is rotated cranially until the **cervix** is located. A sterile bovine insemination pipette is then inserted into the cervix by applying moderate pressure to penetrate the cervix and enter the uterus. A syringe is attached to the end of the pipette, and the appropriate amount of medicated fluid is infused into the uterus.

Intrauterine Boluses

A sterile sleeve should be worn to insert boluses or capsules into the uterus. There are fewer complications with this method of intrauterine medication than with infusion. The primary complication is introduction of bacteria into the uterus by using poor sanitary techniques. Rough handling can damage vaginal and cervical tissue.

The owners need to be informed of drug withdrawal times so that meat or milk from treated animals is not immediately sold.

URINE COLLECTION

A female generally urinates just after standing. However, urine samples for bacteriologic, chemical, and microscopic testing can be collected directly from the bladder by inserting a catheter using aseptic technique.

The animal should be suitably restrained and the vulva cleaned. For goats a double-bladed small animal vaginal speculum is inserted into the vagina. Under visual control with illumination from a light, a sterile curved metal urinary catheter is inserted into the urethra. For cattle a catheter is guided in with one hand in the rectum, so the feces needs to be raked out and the vulva cleaned thoroughly before placing the catheter.

Urethral catheterization of males cannot be performed. The presence of a urethral diverticulum at the level of the ischial arch makes it impossible to introduce a catheter into the urinary bladder.

Collecting urine from sheep is easier than with many other animals. Have a specimen cup ready before starting.

Hold the sheep in a standing position and pinch the nostrils closed until urination occurs. Generally the sheep will urinate within 30 seconds. The nostrils may be held closed for up to 1 minute. If the sheep does not urinate in that minute, allow the animal to rest for 1 or 2 minutes. Repeat the procedure as necessary to obtain a sample.

BLOOD SAMPLING

Jugular Venipuncture

Materials. All required materials should be assembled before attempting a venipuncture. An evacuated tube with holder and needle system (see Fig. 7-4) can be used as well as a needle and syringe. The evacuated tube system reduces materials as the blood flows directly into the tube with just a new needle being used on each animal. The appropriate-sized needle for adult cattle is 16- to 18-gauge, 1.5 inch in length. Cotton with 70% alcohol is needed to cleanse the insertion site.

Restraint. Good restraint is necessary when attempting any venipuncture. Cattle should be haltered and restrained in a chute or stanchion. Drawing blood from the jugular vein of an animal that is not properly restrained is difficult and dangerous. Therefore never attempt venipuncture on a free-moving large animal. Once haltered the head is raised and pulled to one side, tying the halter rope with a quick-release knot. Tying the head to one side secures it, making the vein accessible, but it may also make it more difficult to distend the vein if tied too tightly. A nose lead also may be used if the animal is very wild and aggressive. Care must be taken with nose leads because they can damage the nasal septum if used improperly. If the animal should fall during the procedure, the head can be released immediately to prevent injury to the animal. If blood must be collected from a recumbent cow, its head can be secured by tying the free end of the halter back above the hock with a quick-release knot.

A calf or goat may be restrained by backing it into a corner and pinning its body against a wall, then immobilizing its head by grasping its chin with both hands. Older calves can be restrained like adult cattle. A recumbent calf or goat should have its head firmly held with the neck extended. If the calf moves excessively, a second person should aid in restraint. Tying the legs together will prevent any inadvertent kicking.

Swine from 40 lbs and up are restrained by a hog snare. A sheep can be handled like a goat or set up on its rump.

> TECHNICIAN NOTE Bovine skin is difficult to puncture. Expect the animal to react during jugular venipuncture when it feels the needle poke the skin of the neck.

Technique. One should never kneel or stand directly in front of the animal during jugular venipuncture; moving to the side is a safer place to stand or squat down. Distend the jugular vein by applying pressure at the jugular furrow, about two thirds of the way caudad on the neck. Wipe the jugular in a downward motion to allow time for the vein to fill. Briskly stroking the vein with the cotton soaked with alcohol helps raise it for easy visualization. Unless the animal is in shock or is severely dehydrated, jugular venipuncture should not be attempted without sufficiently raising the vein.

Bovine skin is thick and may be difficult to penetrate, therefore the needle must be inserted with considerable force. Grasp the holder or syringe by the barrel using the thumb and index finger, thrusting it through the skin at a 35- to 45-degree angle to the vessel, with the needle directed toward the head. Engage the evacuated tube or aspirate the plunger on the syringe. If blood flows into the tube or syringe, don't move the needle any further; allow the tube to fill or continue aspirating until the syringe is full. If blood does not appear, redirect the needle as described in IV Injection section, again stopping the motion when blood starts to fill the tube or syringe. If using the evacuated tube system, do not pull the needle all the way out of the skin because this will cause the vacuum in the tube to be released, rendering it useless. Keep the jugular vein occluded until the tube or syringe has filled. If using the evacuated tube system, slide the tube off of the short needle inside the holder before sliding the insertion needle out of the vein. This avoids sucking contaminates into the tube if the entire vacuum was not used.

To collect blood from the jugular vein in pigs, the collector identifies the deepest hollow in the jugular furrow approximately 5 to 8 cm cranial to and to the right of the manubrium. The needle, usually seated on a Vacutainer, is positioned perpendicular to the skin. The needle and Vacutainer are then directed toward the same shoulder blade of the pig. The advantage of jugular venipuncture is the high degree of safety for the pig. The needle length (3.8 cm) is unlikely to penetrate the vagus nerve and lymphatics. The jugular vein is not as large as the cranial vena cava, however, and the shorter needle makes the jugular vein more difficult to penetrate in older and overweight pigs.

The jugular vein (as well as cranial vena cava) is most commonly used to retrieve 5 to 20 ml of blood from a large number of pigs. These techniques are cost effective and expedient; however, some skill is required by the handler and the blood collector. The methods used and anatomy of the area have been described elsewhere. The handler, restraining the pig with a snare, should ensure that the pig is aligned with the shaft of the snare, with the head raised, and neck extended to expose the jugular fossa.

Cranial Vena Cava

To access the cranial vena cava, the collector should identify the right jugular furrow to the point just cranial to and to the right of the manubrium. The approach is made from the pig's right side because the right vagus nerve provides less innervation to the heart and diaphragm than the left vagus (accidental puncture of the vagus nerve can cause cyanosis, dyspnea, and convulsive struggling). The needle is directed toward the top of the opposite shoulder blade while a slight vacuum is maintained in the syringe (Fig. 26-22). When the vena cava is entered, blood fills the test tube or syringe.

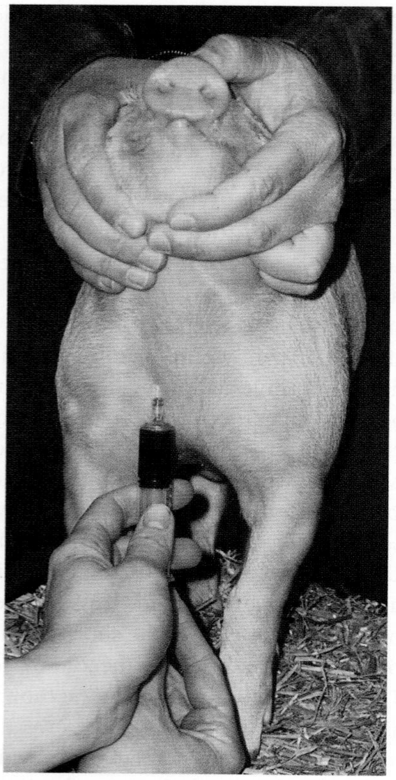

FIGURE 26-22 Collecting blood from the cranial vena cava in a standing pig. The needle is inserted at the caudal extent of the right jugular furrow, lateral to the manubrium. (From Hanie, EA: *Large animal clinical procedures for veterinary technicians*, St Louis, 2006, Mosby.)

Auricular Vein

This vein is generally used for collecting small samples of only 2 to 5 ml and is most commonly used on pigs and sometimes large cattle breeds. The procedure is the same as for intravenous injection. A 20- to 22-gauge winged (butterfly catheter) infusion set can be used for collection of blood.

Coccygeal Venipuncture

The coccygeal (tail) vein is often used rather than the jugular vein. Cattle are usually less agitated when the tail is used for venipuncture. This method also usually requires less restraint than when the jugular vein is used.

> TECHNICIAN NOTE CAUTION: Standing directly behind the animal to perform coccygeal venipuncture puts you in a very vulnerable position to get kicked.

Materials. A 20-gauge, 1-inch needle attached to a 3- to 10-ml syringe or a 20-gauge, 1-inch vacuum system needle, holder, and tube are appropriate for coccygeal venipuncture. Tube size can vary depending on the amount needed for the tests being performed.

Restraint. Limited restraint is needed for coccygeal venipuncture. Dairy cattle require a halter or stanchion and a "tail jack." Beef cattle generally are more fractious and require restraint in a chute. A bar across the back legs or a bale of hay can prevent being kicked. A tail jack can be used for coccygeal venipuncture, as it allows for good visualization and simultaneously serves as restraint. However, it is possible to lift the tail slightly and get the blood sample. It does take an experienced venipuncturist to use this "low tail" technique. The coccygeal artery lies very close to the vein and may inadvertently be punctured instead of the vein. This is usually not a huge problem; just apply digital pressure for 30 to 60 seconds to help ensure hemostasis.

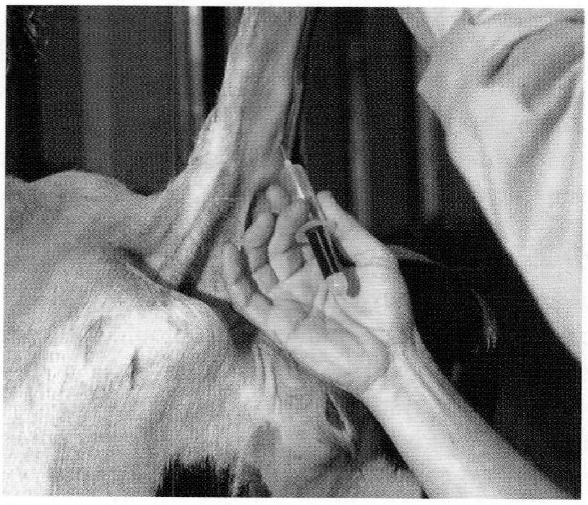

FIGURE 26-23 Blood collection from the tail vein. (From Hanie, EA: *Large animal clinical procedures for veterinary technicians*, St Louis, 2006, Mosby.)

Technique. The first three coccygeal vertebrae (near the tail base) are the best sites for the coccygeal venipuncture. To locate the correct site, apply a tail jack and clean the ventral surface of the tail with cotton soaked with alcohol to remove gross contamination. Palpate the tail for the bony protrusions (hemal arches) of the vertebrae. Insert the needle directly on the midline perpendicular to the tail (Fig. 26-23). If the blood does not flow into the tube, advance or retreat the needle to locate the vein. Avoid moving the needle excessively because that can cause a hematoma to develop and decreases the chances of getting a blood sample from the tail. As soon as the blood starts to flow into the tube, stop moving the needle. Once the tube is full, remove the needle, lower the tail, and apply digital pressure for 30 to 60 seconds. Hematoma formation is usually not a problem, although digital pressure should be applied if the artery was punctured.

Blood collection from the tail vein is limited to adult pigs without docked tails. The tail vein is found on the ventral midline of the tail at the junction of the tail with the body. The volume of blood typically obtained is approximately 2 to 5 ml.

> TECHNICIAN NOTE All blood samples must be marked with the animal's ID, species, sex, and owner's name. This is extremely important when drawing blood for regulatory tests.

INTRAVENOUS CATHETERIZATION

Intravenous catheterization is used primarily for prolonged fluid therapy, but it is also used for administration of injectable anesthetics, administration of irritating medications, or repeated IV injections.

Technique

The technique for all food animals is basically the same with just a few minor adjustments needed for each species; that information will follow this description.

The site should be clipped and a local anesthesia is administered if a **cut-down** is required. A surgical scrub with antiseptic is applied and wiped off with 70% alcohol to complete skin preparation. Because many of the food animals have thick skin, attempts to introduce a catheter through it may bend or damage the tip of the catheter. To help introduce a catheter, a disposable needle of the same gauge or one size larger is used to create a pilot hole or a small cut is made through the skin over the jugular vein with a surgical blade. Care must be taken to not poke or cut into the vein. This enables the catheter to pass into the vein with ease. An IV catheter should be placed in a sterile manner, which includes wearing sterile gloves. Occlude the jugular vein by pushing the fingers of your nondominant hand into the jugular furrow, about two thirds of the way caudad on the neck. Hold on to the indwelling catheter by the hub; insert the catheter at a 15- to 30-degree angle, aiming it toward the heart. When blood starts to flow freely from the catheter, stop advancing the needle portion of the catheter and advance the catheter off of the needle until its entire length is in the vein; discard the needle portion of the catheter. Cap the catheter with an injection port and flush with 10 to 15 ml of heparinized saline.

> TECHNICIAN NOTE A #10 or #20 surgical blade or the bevel edge of a 14- or 16-gauge needle can also be used to do a cut-down over the vein or create a pilot hole in the skin for easier insertion through thick skin.

The catheter must be secured to the neck because bandaging alone is not sufficient to keep the catheter from slipping out of place. Wings can be fashioned on the hub of the catheter with adhesive tape. The wings are then sutured to the skin with a simple interrupted stitch using 1/0 or 1 nonabsorbable suture. Catheters can also be secured by placing the first suture caudal to the hub and a second suture cranial to the hub on the extension or IV line. At least two sutures should be placed to secure the catheter. Suturing the catheter increases the likelihood that the catheter will stay in place. Cyanoacrylate glue can also be used to bond the hub of the catheter to the skin.

A simplex (Fig. 26-24) or IV drip set is attached to the catheter directly or a needle is placed on the end of the tube and inserted through the injection port. The fluids should be held in an inverted position higher than the heart. This allows gravity to do its thing. If using a simplex system, a steady stream of bubbles in the bottle indicates that the medication is flowing into the vein and is being replaced by air. If the bubbling becomes irregular or if the drops on an IV drip set stop, it can indicate that the catheter is occluded or out of the vein. In such cases lower the bottle below the heart; blood should fill the hub of the catheter indicating the catheter is still in place. If no blood shows, check the catheter for correct positioning and make the appropriate adjustments, which could mean putting in another catheter.

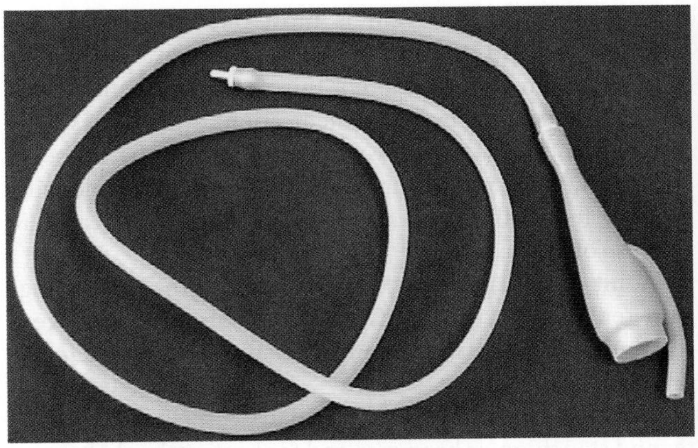

FIGURE 26-24 Simplex IV Bell Set. (From Sonsthagen TF: *Veterinary instruments and equipment: a pocket guide*, ed 2, St Louis, 2011, Mosby.)

After the fluids have been administered, disconnect the drip set. Check the jugular furrow for swelling around the insertion point. If there is swelling, it can mean the fluid has gone perivascular and the catheter will have to be placed in a different vein. If all looks well, apply an antibiotic ointment over the catheter insertion point with a sterile tongue depressor. Place a sterile gauze pad over the ointment and secure the catheter with elastic tape around the animal's neck.

If long-term catheterization is necessary, a longer, flexible, 5.5-inch catheter is used. The catheter must be flushed every 4 hours to help keep the catheter patent. An extension set is attached to the catheter and wrapped such that the injection port is accessible. Swab the port with alcohol before flushing or attaching the drip set. The catheter insertion point should be observed daily for redness, swelling, or discharge. If any of those signs are observed, the catheter will need to be removed.

Indwelling catheters and IV lines should be changed every 3 days to prevent thrombophlebitis and infection. The longer central line type catheters can be left in place as long as there are no signs of infection.

The efficacy of fluid support is evaluated by frequent weight determination, urine production, and signs of overhydration.

After the IV fluids are no longer needed remove the catheter by applying digital pressure for 30 to 45 seconds over the insertion site with a cotton ball to prevent a hematoma.

Cattle. The jugular vein is most often chosen for IV catheterization in cattle. The caudal auricular vein can be catheterized in cattle, although this vein is used mainly for injection of small volumes of medication. A local anesthetic is used to decrease ear movement and to give the ear some stability. Insert a roll of gauze into the ear before bandaging the ear. It is difficult to secure a catheter in the ear vein because of its location.

Adult cattle can be catheterized with a 16- to 18-gauge catheter, either a 2-inch indwelling or a longer 5.5-inch central line. Newborn calves require a smaller-gauge catheter, 18 or 20 gauge.

Restraint for catheterization in dairy cattle involves a halter and stanchion or head gate and for beef cattle a halter and chute. Some of the larger bulls may also need a nose lead to keep their heads still.

Sheep and Goats. The jugular vein is most often used; however, the cephalic or femoral veins may be used if the jugular vein is not patent. Both can be restrained by backing them into a corner and placing hands on either side of the head grasping the chin. The wool and hair should be sheared from the jugular furrow and occluded at the thoracic inlet. Elevate and slightly turn the head to the side.

Catheter dimensions vary, depending on the size of the sheep. In adults use 18- or 20-gauge, 2- to 3½-inch catheters. In lambs use a 20- or 22-gauge, 1½- to 2-inch catheter.

Swine. The auricular vein is the preferred site for IV catheterization in swine. A 20- to 22-gauge, 1-inch infusion set (butterfly catheter) is inserted in the lateral vein on the ear. The technique is exactly as described for venipuncture in the ear. Tegaderm bandage is also very useful as its clear window allows you to see if the insertion point is in good condition or if it is infected. A small indwelling catheter may also be used to run fluids into the ear vein. An extension set, not unlike the tube on the infusion set, allows a drip set to be attached without fear of dislodging the catheter.

HOOF TRIMMING

Periodic trimming of the hooves is required for the comfort and humane treatment of the animals. Damaged or overgrown hooves can be trimmed and shaped by using various types of knives, shears, and electric grinders.

Restraint

Cattle must be properly restrained by using, at least, a squeeze chute. Hydraulically operated tilt tables made specifically for trimming cattle feet make the task safe and efficient. The cattle are secured to the table then laid over on their side (tilted) so the operator has the legs safely restrained and the hooves at a comfortable working height (Fig. 26-25).

Sheep and goats that are not allowed to graze or that are raised in confinement tend to develop overgrown feet. Typically the sidewalls and the toes overgrow. Sheep can be set up on their rumps, and goats can be done standing. The sidewalls should be trimmed to keep the sole flat and the toes pointing forward. Toes are normally squared off. Trimming is done with heavy scissors, hoof rot shears, or a sharp knife (Fig. 26-26). If bleeding occurs, apply hemostatic powder or copper naphthenate solution. Severe bleeding may require bandaging.

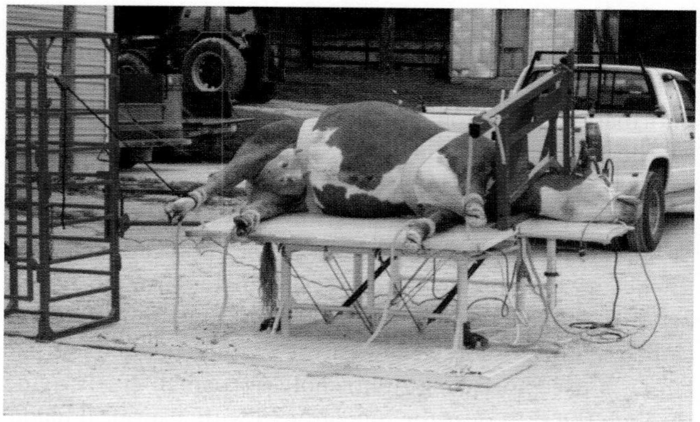

FIGURE 26-25 Hoof-trimming table and chute. (From Sonsthagen TF: *Veterinary instruments and equipment: a pocket guide*, ed 2, St Louis, 2011, Mosby.)

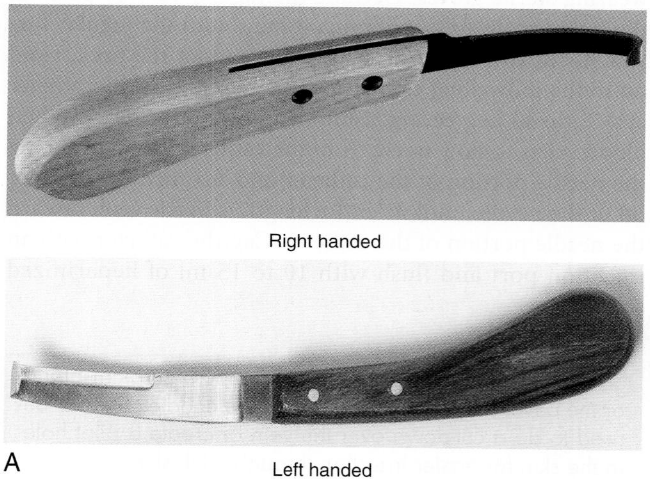

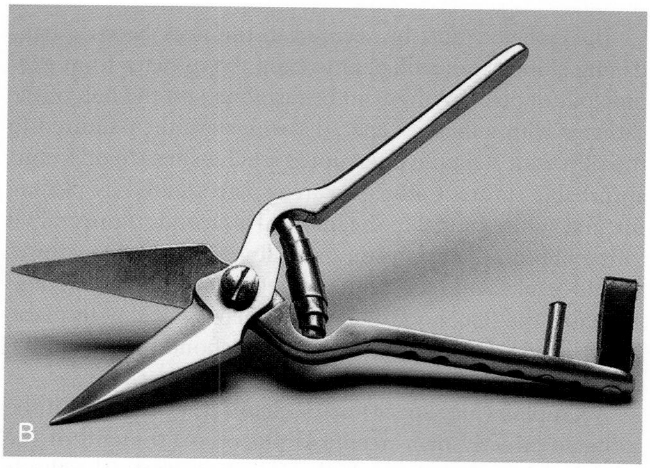

FIGURE 26-26 **A**, Hoof knife. **B**, Hoof trimmer. (From Sonsthagen TF: *Veterinary instruments and equipment: a pocket guide*, ed 2, St Louis, 2011, Mosby.)

CARE OF CAMELIDS

Llamas and alpacas are part of a larger group of South American camelids or New World camelids. In recent years South American camelids have gained popularity and increasing numbers are now being raised in the United States. Four species of the Lamini tribe are found in South America (Fig. 26-27). The llama *(Lama glama)* and the alpaca *(Lama pacos)* were domesticated about 5000 years ago, whereas the guanaco *(Lama guanicoe)* and the vicuña *(Vicugna vicugna)* are undomesticated.

ANATOMIC AND PHYSIOLOGIC CHARACTERISTICS

The llama is the largest of the four species. The face is usually free of wool, with a long, straight to slightly rounded nose. The ears are also long and erect. The wool covers much of the neck and the body. The back is flat, ending in a tail that curls up and back. The colors are solid black, white, brown, or shaded, but they can also be spotted (Appaloosa), patched, or multicolored.

The alpaca is smaller than the llama. It has short ears, a wooly face, a rounded rump, and a straight tail. In the United States, 22 colors are recognized. The guanaco is slightly smaller than the llama but of similar conformation. The ears and nose are smaller than those of the llama. All guanacos have the same color pattern: soft brown to rust on the upper body and a white underbelly. Guanacos can be unpredictable and are undomesticated. The vicuña is the smallest and the rarest of the four species. They have a small head and a long, thin neck. Their color pattern is consistently golden brown, with a white chest. The vicuña is also undomesticated and in South America is protected from hunting.

A unique feature of camelids is that they have a stomach with three compartments, rather than four like other ruminants. For this reason they are not considered true ruminants, although they do ruminate, chew their cud, and digest cellulose. The first compartment represents more than 80% of the total stomach in volume and is equivalent to the rumen and reticulum of true ruminants.

A split upper lip facilitates food prehension. Only three pairs of incisors are found in the lower jaw. Together with the upper **dental pad,** these teeth facilitate browsing and nipping. Eruption of the adult incisors starts at 2 years for the central incisors, 3 years for the middle incisors, and 4 years for the corner incisors. The upper corner incisors and upper and lower canines develop into sharp scimitar-shaped teeth that are used by males in fighting. These teeth erupt in males around 2 to 3 years and are usually removed surgically.

Llamas have two digits on each foot. The second and third phalanges are positioned horizontally and do not bear weight, whereas the first phalanx is in an upright position. The end of the foot is protected by a nail (not a hoof), and the remainder of the foot is supported by a digital cushion and a soft pad on the palmar surface. The nail may need periodic trimming.

The skin in the cranial cervical region is very thick (up to 1 cm in adult males) and the ventral projection of the transverse processes of the caudal cervical vertebrae forms an inverted U, covering the vessel of the neck. The jugular vein is deep in the neck and close to the carotid artery. The location of the jugular vein makes blood sampling and intravenous injection difficult.

The uterus of the female llama is bicornuate, with a small uterine body. Most pregnancies occur in the left horn. Although pregnancies have been observed in female llamas as young as 6 months, it is recommended to delay breeding until 12 months of age. Breeding usually takes place while the female assumes a sternal recumbent position with the male straddling her. Copulation usually lasts about 20 minutes. Ovulation is induced during copulation. Pregnancy is confirmed by rectal palpation at 35 to

FIGURE 26-27 Four South American camelids: top left, vicuña; top right, guanaco; bottom left, alpaca; bottom right, llama. (From Fowler ME Miller RE: *Zoo and wild animal medicine current therapy*, vol 6, St Louis, 2008, Saunders.)

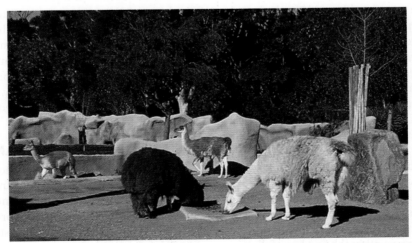

TABLE 26-2 Physical and Physiologic Characteristics of South American Camelids

	LLAMA	ALPACA	GUANACO	VICUNA
Height (CM)				
At the withers	115-130	75-95	—	90
At the poll	150-180			
Weight (KG)				
Male	132-244	60-80	100-150	40-65
Female	108-200	55	100-120	30-40
Rectal temperature (° Celsius)	37.2-38.7	37.2-38.7	37.2-38.7	37.2-38.7
Heart rate (beats/min)	60-90	60-90	60-90	60-90
Respiratory rate (resp./min.)	10-30	10-30	10-30	10-30

40 days, ultrasound findings, or serum progesterone levels above 1 ng/ml at 21 days. The normal gestation period is 335 to 350 days. Most births occur rapidly and typically during daylight hours. Teat enlargement can start 1 to 3 weeks prepartum, with milk letdown 48 to 72 hours before parturition, although the teats can also enlarge after parturition.

Table 26-2 lists physical and physiologic characteristics of camelids.

NEONATAL CARE

At birth, crias (baby camelids) are covered by a semitransparent epidermal membrane attached to all mucocutaneous junctions. Within an hour after birth, normal crias can stand and nurse. Average birth weight ranges from 8 to 18 kg. Llama crias weighing less than 8 kg are considered premature or dysmature and may require some special attention. Alpaca crias are somewhat smaller; crias weighing less than 5 kg are considered premature.

The first consideration is to make sure the cria can breathe by clearing the membranes and mucus away from the mouth and nostrils. A bulb syringe can be used to carefully suction mucus from the nostril. In addition, lifting and supporting the cria can help clear amniotic fluid from the respiratory tract. Respiration can be stimulated by rubbing the back or tickling the nose with a piece of straw. Artificial respiration can be done by mouth to nose resuscitation or more effectively by placing a small rubber tube (6 to 7 mm in diameter) in the cria's nostril and gently blowing intermittently at about 10 times/minute. Choanal atresia is a frequent congenital abnormality of llamas of which to be aware. Because llamas and alpacas are obligate nasal breathers, crias with these congenital abnormalities show difficulty in breathing, even when fluids have been cleared.

Postpartum care of the cria should include dipping the umbilical cord in 7% tincture of iodine or chlorhexidine diluted to a 0.5% solution. This should be done three times within the first 24 hours. Additional care includes drying and weighing the cria and watching for nursing of the **colostrum.** Normal crias nurse within the first hour following delivery. Crias nurse three or four times per hour, usually for less than 30 seconds each time. If the cria has not been observed nursing for 6 hours, supportive care should be given and llama colostrum should be given in feedings of about 100 to 200 ml every 2 to 3 hours. Goat or cow colostrum can be used as a substitute. Passage of meconium (first bowel movement) should occur within the first 18 to 20 hours.

For compromised crias, oxygen support is provided with a small tube inserted in one nostril and taped to the bridge of the nose. The tube is connected to humidified oxygen and is advanced to the premeasured level of the eye. Initially, the oxygen flow rate is set at 5 L/minute and adjusted to the patient's needs, based on serial evaluations of arterial blood gases.

If the cria does not or is not able to nurse, nutritional support can be provided by bottle feeding (soft plastic bottle with a lamb nipple) or orogastric tubing. Tube feeding a cria is easy. A stallion catheter or soft rubber feeding tube is convenient for this use. Before insertion, the tube is held against the cria's side and the distance from the mouth to the base of the neck is measured. Water-soluble lubricant (e.g., K-Y jelly) is applied to the tube, which is then slowly passed into the mouth. As the tube is swallowed and advanced to the premeasured length, it should be seen and felt on the side of the neck next to the trachea. To ensure the tube is in the esophagus and not in the trachea, blow on the end of the tube and watch for the stomach to expand, or listen for gurgling sounds. Inject 10 to 15 ml of water into the tube before feeding. If the animal gags and/or coughs, the tube is probably in the lungs and should be withdrawn. If a substitute for the dam's milk is necessary, straight goat's milk or a 3:1 volume to volume mixture of goat milk and goat yogurt is recommended.

BEHAVIOR, HANDLING, AND RESTRAINT

Llamas and alpacas are shy but curious animals that are usually easy to handle. They are social animals with a strong herd instinct. In a comfortable environment the ears of the llama are erect and directed rostrally (forward). When a llama is upset, the ears are flattened against the head and the nose is elevated and they begin to vocalize (orgle) (Fig. 26-28). If it remains agitated, the llama may spit (actually regurgitate stomach contents) and continue to vocalize. Although llamas

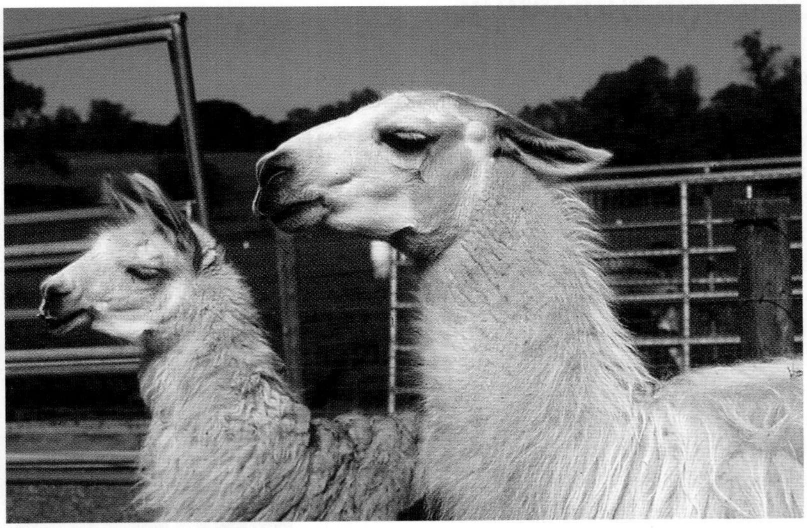

FIGURE 26-28 Ear position: alert in back, mild aggression in front. (From Fowler ME Miller RE: *Zoo and wild animal medicine current therapy*, vol 6, St Louis, 2008, Saunders.)

frequently spit at each other when competing for food or to assess territoriality, they rarely spit at humans. To handle a spitting animal, a towel or other type of cloth can be placed over the muzzle.

Male llamas may bite, charge, and butt with their chest. They can also kick with their rear legs and inflict injury. Llamas rarely charge or bite humans, except for the so-called berserk male syndrome or aberrant male syndrome displayed by some bottle-raised male llamas.

In most cases a satisfactory approach to working with llamas is to have the owner catch and halter the animal before the animal is seen by the veterinarian. If it has not been caught, it is easier to move the whole herd to a smaller enclosure before trying to isolate one animal for examination. Once cornered, the animal can be approached to place a lead rope or an arm around the neck or apply a halter. The person placing the halter should avoid direct eye contact; touching the head of the llama should be minimized. Adult llamas can be easily restrained with a halter and lead rope. Juvenile llamas can be handled by placing a hand around the front of the neck and grasping around the rump or at the base of the tail. A restraining chute can be very useful for veterinary procedures. Temporary restraint can be achieved using an ear twitch. The base of the ear is encircled with the palm of the hand and squeezed. The ear should not be twisted. The owner should be consulted before using this method.

HERD HEALTH

Immunization

A minimal vaccination program should include *Clostridium perfringens* C/D and tetanus. Recommendations include annual C/D and tetanus administration for all juveniles (starting at 3 months) and adults. Pregnant females should receive a C/D and tetanus booster 1 month before the anticipated parturition date. Recent information indicates that vaccination of the cria within the first week of age, followed by two monthly boosters, is effective irrespective of colostral immunity. Immunization with 7- or 8-way clostridial vaccine may cause significant injection site reactions. Other vaccinations to consider vary with the area of the country. If leptospirosis is a problem in the region, biannual vaccination of brood females should be considered. No rabies vaccine efficacy testing has been conducted in the llama, yet no adverse reaction following administration of the killed vaccine has been reported.

Parasite Control

New World camelids are susceptible to all the nematode parasites that affect ruminants. *Parelaphostrongylus tenuis* is a major concern in areas inhabited by white tail deer. In enzootic liver fluke areas, llamas should be checked periodically for flukes. Coccidiosis may be a significant cause of diarrhea in young animals. Establishment of a parasite-control program depends on the geographic area, climatic conditions, number of animals, and stocking rate. Fenbendazole and ivermectin have been used successfully to control most nematodes. A minimum of two dewormings (spring and fall) is recommended. In areas with meningeal worms, monthly deworming with ivermectin or daily administration of Strongid C can be used.

Lice are the most common external parasites of llama herds. Topical treatment with organophosphate or carbamate powder is effective. Mange mite infestation is not very common, probably because of extensive use of ivermectin.

Common Procedures

Male llamas generally need to have their fighting teeth (incisors and canines) cut by 2 to 2.5 years of age. This procedure can be rapidly done in a restraining chute or under general anesthesia using a surgical wire. Castration is usually performed after 2 years of age but can be done earlier if necessary.

COMMON DIAGNOSTIC AND THERAPEUTIC TECHNIQUES

Orogastric Intubation

Medication, fluids, or food can be administered with a stomach tube. The technique is fairly similar to the procedure for sheep and cattle. Adult llamas usually resist and may regurgitate, increasing the likelihood of aspiration pneumonia. Restraint is important and use of a chute with cross-ties is helpful. A speculum is necessary to protect the tube. The Frick's speculum used in cattle is usually too big, except for the largest llamas. A 20-cm-long segment of PVC pipe, slightly wider than the stomach tube, can be used. The edges must be smoothed or wrapped with adhesive tape. Once the head is secured and slightly flexed, the lubricated tip of the stomach tube is advanced caudally through the speculum to the throat. Gentle pressure and rotation of the tube encourages swallowing. A little resistance should be felt as the tube is advanced into the esophagus. The most reliable sign of correct tube placement is palpating it in the left cervical region.

Intravenous Injections

The landmarks and the technique are similar to those used for blood collection. The tip of the needle is directed caudally so that the operator is warned of inadvertent carotid artery penetration by high-pressure, bright red blood exiting the hub of the needle.

Intramuscular Injections

The general rules for giving injections are similar to those for other species, including the need for proper restraint, swabbing of the injection site, and checking for the presence of blood by pulling back on the syringe plunger before injecting the product. Intramuscular injections can be done in any large muscle mass using a 4-cm, 22- to 16-gauge needle, depending on the viscosity of the drug. The neck region should be avoided. On most llamas restrained in a chute, the hind legs are most accessible. The semimembranosus and semitendinosus muscles are the sites of choice. If frequent injections are needed, the injection sites should be rotated to avoid soreness. The area of the triceps in the angle formed by the scapula and the humerus may also be used.

Subcutaneous Injections

The technique is similar to that used in other species. The preferred sites include the skin of the thorax and caudal to the elbow, where wool is usually absent.

Blood Collection

Superficial veins are not readily accessible. There is no jugular groove and visualization of the jugular vein is impossible. Jugular venipuncture can be done at a cranial or caudal location on the neck (Fig. 26-29). The landmark in the cranial location is ventral to a line extending from the ventral border of the mandible to the lateral surface of the neck. The tendon of the sternocephalicus muscle should be located on the neck, and the vein should be penetrated just caudal to the tendon. The site on the caudal neck is identified by palpation of the vertebral process of the fifth or sixth cervical vertebra. The needle is inserted slightly medial to the tip of the process and directed toward the center of the neck. This must be done carefully because the carotid artery is close to the jugular vein. Blood can also be collected from an ear vein near the caudal edge of the pinna. The ear is bent and a needle is inserted into the vein. Blood is collected while dripping from the hub. This method is less desirable because llamas are usually head shy. The midventral vein of the tail is located in a similar location as in cattle. The saphenous artery and vein can be used for blood collection in recumbent llamas. The artery and vein can be located on the medial aspect of the stifle. In crias, the cephalic vein can also be used. The location is similar to the position of the cephalic vein in dogs.

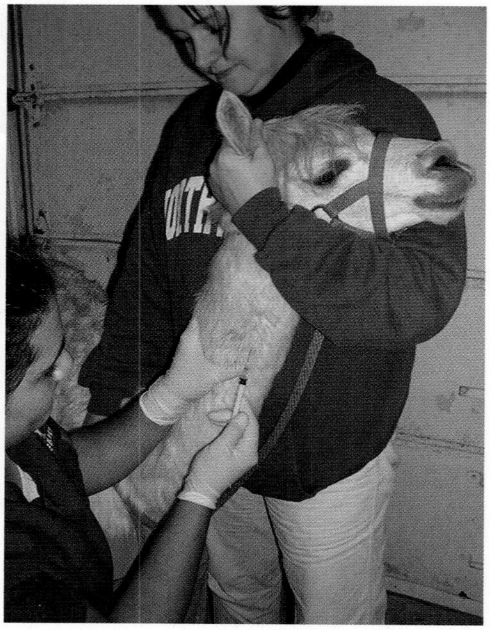

FIGURE 26-29 Jugular venipuncture may be achieved high on the neck near the ramus of the mandible. (From Bassert JM, McCurnin DM: *McCurnin's clinical textbook for veterinary technicians*, ed 7, St Louis, 2010, Saunders.)

Urine Collection

If urine cannot be collected by free catch, bladder catheterization can be performed in female llamas. Free-catch collection of urine is better done in the morning, when llamas go to the dung pile. Bladder catheterization is virtually impossible in the male. In the female llama, catheterization is fairly easy. The external urethral orifice is easily palpated on the floor of the vulva. The ventral suburethral diverticulum complicates catheterization. After the vulva has been thoroughly cleaned, a sterile gloved finger is advanced in the vulva to palpate the meatus. The finger is withdrawn slightly and the catheter (No. 5 French) is advanced into the urethra above the finger to avoid the diverticulum. If the meatus is difficult to palpate, a sterile bitch speculum can be used to visualize it.

CARE OF RATITES

Ratites are a group of nonflying birds that include the ostrich *(Struthio casmelus),* the emu *(Dromaius novaehollandiae),* and the rhea *(Rhea americana).* The cassowary *(Casuarius casuarius)* is also included in this group; they are primarily concentrated on the west coast of the United States.

VISUAL EVALUATION

Visual assessment of the entire flock may provide pertinent information about individual health. The birds' activity level should be noted. The initial response when a stranger approaches and enters a pen is for the birds to run from the intruder. Most will then return out of curiosity. When possible, the birds should be observed while they are eating. A food bolus can normally be observed as it passes down the cervical esophagus. Unhealthy or sick birds may go through the motions as if they are eating, pecking and throwing their head upward as if to swallow, but no food bolus is seen passing down the neck. Closer examination should be performed on birds that are inactive, that lag behind, or that are not actively eating.

Note asymmetry of the neck and dorsal spine, and deviations of the appendages. During the visual examination note the condition of the integumentary system. Unthrifty plumage may indicate trauma, ectoparasites, nutritional deficiency, or feather plucking by other birds, suggesting overcrowding or boredom.

PHYSICAL EXAMINATION

The heart rate (60 to 120 beats/min) is most easily determined by auscultation laterally, between the ribs. The respiratory rate (10 to 40 breaths/min) is best determined visually in the unrestrained patient. Temperature (100° to 104° F) can be measured with a rectal or tympanic membrane thermometer. The external ear canal is a large opening caudal to the mandible at the base of the skull. Cloacal temperatures may be 1 or 2 degrees lower than tympanic membrane temperature.

The eye can be superficially examined with a good penlight. The ear canal is easily explored with an otoscope for parasites, hemorrhage, or masses. When the mouth is opened, the mucous membranes are evaluated for color (pink) and capillary refill time (≤2.5 sec). Symmetry of the choana (nasopharynx), glottis, and rostral trachea should be noted. Choanal or tracheal swabs can be made for bacterial culture and cytology when a discharge is noted. The neck is palpated for asymmetry of the trachea, right jugular vein, and vertebrae.

The thorax is auscultated and palpated. Auscultation is performed, noting abnormal respiratory sounds associated with the lungs or air sacs. Heart murmurs can also be detected by auscultation of the thorax. There is very little muscle over the thorax, making palpation easy for any signs of asymmetry associated with rib fractures or masses.

The abdomen is easily palpated in the chick. Structures that should be noted include the proventriculus and yolk sac. The proventriculus lies just to the left of the midline, caudal to the rib cage. The structure is firm to the touch and should have feed material within it that is easily compressed with gentle pressure. An empty proventriculus is firm. The yolk sac has the feel of a large bladder, decreasing in size over a 2-week period, when it should be absorbed. As the yolk sac is absorbed, the intestines become more palpable in the young chick.

These structures are not as evident in the adult bird. However, impaction associated with the proventriculus or egg retention can be recognized during careful evaluation of the adult bird's abdomen.

The cloaca should be examined for accumulation of fecal matter and urates on the feathers surrounding the opening. This commonly indicates illness or depression. Mucosal prolapse may be indicative of intestinal obstruction or local trauma. The genitalia can also be evaluated within the cloacal sphincter.

The skin and feathers are evaluated for parasites and trauma. These birds groom themselves, so the feathers should be relatively clean and well separated, unless they have recently given themselves a dust bath. Feather regrowth is a good indicator of adequate nutrition.

The wings and limbs of the birds should be examined closely, both visually and by palpation. Ostriches and rheas have well-developed wings, whereas the wing of the emu is vestigial and difficult to see when it is held close to the body. Asymmetry is noted and the structures are palpated for fractures and dislocations.

The thigh and calf regions are well muscled, making direct palpation of the femur and tibiotarsus difficult. The tarsometatarsus and phalanges are easily palpated, because there is very little tissue covering these areas. Swollen joints should be noted and the cause explored. The tendons and their sheaths should be examined for pain and swelling. Tendon luxation over the tibiotarsus and the metatarsophalangeal joint are common injuries. The foot should always be examined closely for heat, pain, and swelling. Asymmetry surrounding a phalangeal joint should be carefully explored because of the common incidence of puncture wounds involving these joints. Traumatic avulsion of the toenails may lead to localized infection.

RESTRAINT

Restraining is one of the most important skills to master when working with ratites. Many owners are unable to restrain their own birds, and frequently their facilities are less than ideal. The birds have very powerful legs that can inflict severe trauma from kicking. The emu, rhea, and cassowary have sharp claws that can easily lacerate the handler. The danger zone when working on ratites is directly in front of the birds, because they strike forward when they kick. The emu and rhea can also kick to the side, but the most powerful segment of the kick is in front.

Chicks can easily be handled by placing a hand between their legs while cupping the sternum and picking them up, much like holding a football. While in a sitting position, the handler can treat small juvenile birds by placing the bird in the lap, with the bird's legs squeezed between the handler's knees. Larger juveniles can be held standing from the back or from the side, keeping the bird close to the handler's body. When restraining from the back, your feet should be spread apart to help maintain balance, but your knees should be held close together to prevent the bird from backing under you.

Adult birds are more difficult and risky to handle. It is frequently necessary to capture large juveniles or adult ostriches in an open pen. Applying a loose, tubular cloth hood over the head and covering the eyes commonly calms the bird so that evaluation and treatment can be carried out. These birds are generally curious and will approach strangers. The hood is placed over the handler's forearm. When the bird is within reach, the neck is grasped and pulled down parallel to the ground with the opposite hand. Simultaneously the beak is grasped and the hood is everted over the head, leaving the nares exposed. If the bird does not approach the handler, a shepherd's hook can be used to capture the head (Fig. 26-30). The hood is then applied as described. To move the bird, a second handler grasps the tail from behind, pushing forward as gentle traction on the neck steers in the desired direction. Ostriches can also be restrained in stocks or in chutes designed for the birds. When this type of facility is not available, the birds can be restrained by squeezing the bird between a solid gate and a wall. Caution should be used when working around adult birds, especially males during the breeding season, as these birds can be aggressive.

Emus in general are not aggressive and males frequently become more docile during the breeding season. Adult emus present more difficulty in handling, because they commonly become very fractious when restrained. Their sharp claws and rough, scaly tarsometatarsus can tear clothing and severely abrade the handler's skin. Many emus do not resist mild restraint. To catch and restrain them, pass an arm around the neck near the sternum and pull the bird firmly into your upper legs and trunk, tilting the bird into an upright position. Low placement of the arm minimizes the chance of injury from kicking. The bird can be moved from this position, being careful to keep the animal in contact with your body. Sometimes moving the bird backward is easier than moving forward, and it is occasionally necessary to simply pick the birds up to move them.

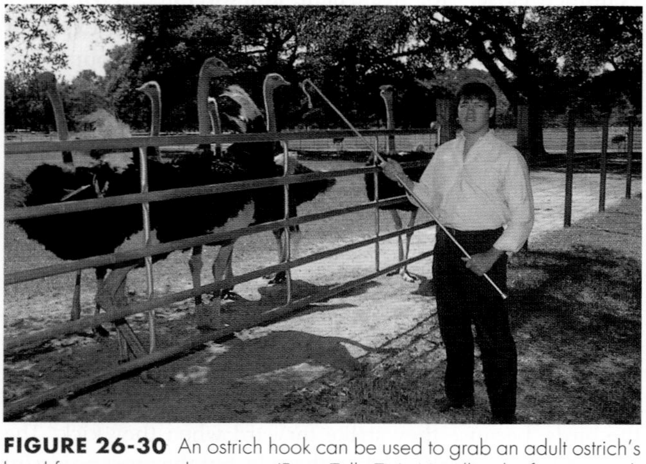

FIGURE 26-30 An ostrich hook can be used to grab an adult ostrich's head for capture and restraint. (From Tully TN: *Handbook of avian medicine*, ed 2, St Louis, 2009, Saunders.)

Male rheas are the most aggressive of the three common species. Restraint is most easily accomplished by two handlers. The first handler catches the bird as described for emus. The second handler then grasps the bird's legs and pulls the bird to the ground between the first handler's legs. With the bird's legs held, one individual straddles the recumbent bird on his or her knees, placing gentle pressure on the dorsum of the bird.

A hood can be applied to rheas, but the results are much less predictable than with ostriches. Another option that should be considered, when possible, is working on the birds in a darkened enclosure. This environment has a calming effect on the birds.

COMMON DIAGNOSTIC AND THERAPEUTIC TECHNIQUES

Orogastric Tube Placement

Gastric intubation is used to administer fluids, nutrients, and medication. The mouth is opened by grasping the upper beak and the tube is then directed over the glottis. Once past the glottis, the tube is easily visualized externally, passing down the cervical esophagus. Care is taken to prevent regurgitation while administering substances through the tube. Esophagostomy tube placement should be considered when long-term enteral nutrition is indicated.

Pill Administration

Pills or boluses can be given by grasping the upper beak and gently prying the mouth open. Occasionally a finger must be inserted into the commissure to assist in opening the mouth. The pill is then placed over the glottis and a finger is used to push it into the cervical esophagus.

Injections

Subcutaneous injections can be given over the lateral thorax caudal to the leg. The skin is lifted and the needle is inserted with care to prevent inadvertent penetration into the chest cavity. Intramuscular injections are usually given in the abaxial muscles over the rump and in the proximal thigh. Intravenous injections are administered in the same locations as described for blood sampling, although the metatarsal vein is seldom used for this purpose.

Blood Sampling and Catheterization

Blood sampling and catheterization can be performed on the right jugular, cutaneous ulnar, and medial metatarsal veins. The jugular vein is easily distended and visualized in the ostrich and rhea. Watching for feather motion along the course of the distending vein, on the neck, helps to visualize and locate it on the emu. Feathers can be plucked to help visualize the vessel. When this vessel is catheterized, placement is in the upper (cranial) one third of the neck, to prevent the bird from pulling it out. Care is taken not to penetrate the trachea or esophagus.

In the ostrich and rhea, the cutaneous ulnar vein is located on the ventral aspect of the wing, coursing over the distal antebrachium. The vestigial wing in the emu makes this vein impractical for blood sampling and catheterization. Catheters placed in the wing vein should be protected to prevent the bird from pulling them out.

The medial metatarsal vein is located on the medial aspect of the leg, paralleling the metatarsus. Care is taken when collecting blood from this area, because the vessel is easily lacerated if the bird kicks during sampling.

Needles and catheters of 20- to 22-gauge are commonly used in these birds. Larger catheters can be placed in the jugular vein when rapid fluid volume replacement is indicated.

Blood should be collected into tubes containing heparin anticoagulant. This sample can be used for both hematologic and serum chemistry evaluations. EDTA and serum separator or plain sterile tubes are suitable for blood collection in emus and rheas.

Fluid Therapy

Fluids can be administered parenterally or enterally. Parenteral administration is performed subcutaneously or intravenously. Maintenance fluids are administered at 13 ml/kg/hr (range 5 to 28 ml/kg/hr). Enteral fluid administration is performed via an orogastric tube.

COMMON DISEASES

A complete review of all diseases of cattle, sheep, goats, swine, camelids, and ratites is beyond the scope of this chapter. A comprehensive large animal medicine reference should be consulted. Commonly encountered parasites of production animals are summarized in Table 26-3. Many diseases of production animals are preventable through vaccination. A review of vaccination protocols recommended for these species is presented in Tables 26-4 through 26-8.

TABLE 26-3 Common Parasites of Production Animals

BOVINE PARASITES				
COMMON NAME/PHOTOGRAPH	**SCIENTIFIC NAME**	**IMPORTANCE**	**DIAGNOSIS**	**TREATMENT**
Brown Stomach Worm*				
Table 26-3, 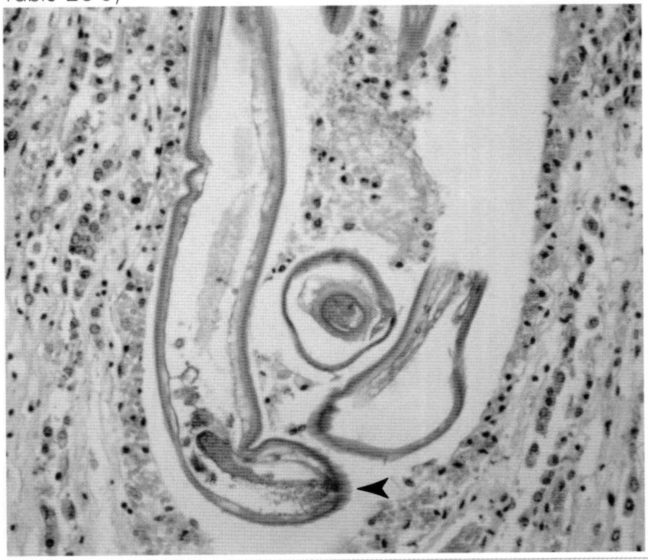	*Ostertagia ostertagi*	Larval destruction of gastric glands causes severe diarrhea and weight loss Type I: Produce eggs Pre-type II: Not clinically apparent, fourth-stage larvae inhibited in gastric glands Type II: Eggs often not found in feces	Fecal flotation and identification at necropsy	Fenbendazole, doramectin, eprinomectin, ivermectin, morantel tartrate, moxidectin

Continued

TABLE 26-3 Common Parasites of Production Animals—cont'd

BOVINE PARASITES				
COMMON NAME/PHOTOGRAPH	SCIENTIFIC NAME	IMPORTANCE	DIAGNOSIS	TREATMENT
Bankrupt Worm or Small Stomach Worm*				
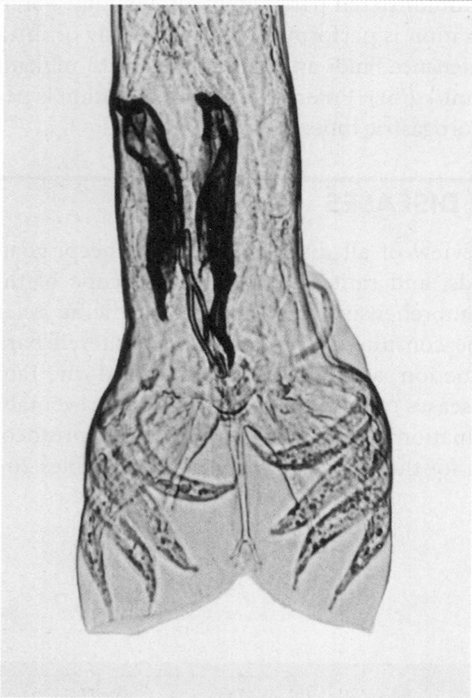	*Trichostrongylus axei*	Loss of weight, dehydration, diarrhea, bottle jaw Prepatent period is 3 weeks	Eggs in fecal flotation and identification at necropsy	Ivermectin, doramectin, eprinomectin, fenbendazole, moxidectin, morantel tartrate
Nodular Worm*				
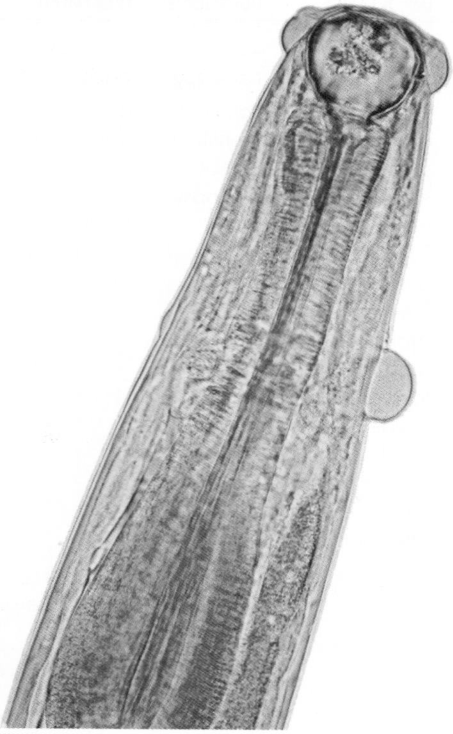	*Oesophagostomum radiatum*	Possible diarrhea Prepatent period is 40 days	Eggs in fecal flotation and identification at necropsy	Moxidectin, morantel tartrate, levamisole, eprinomectin, doramectin

TABLE 26-3 Common Parasites of Production Animals—cont'd

BOVINE PARASITES

COMMON NAME/PHOTOGRAPH	SCIENTIFIC NAME	IMPORTANCE	DIAGNOSIS	TREATMENT
Cattle Bankrupt Worm* 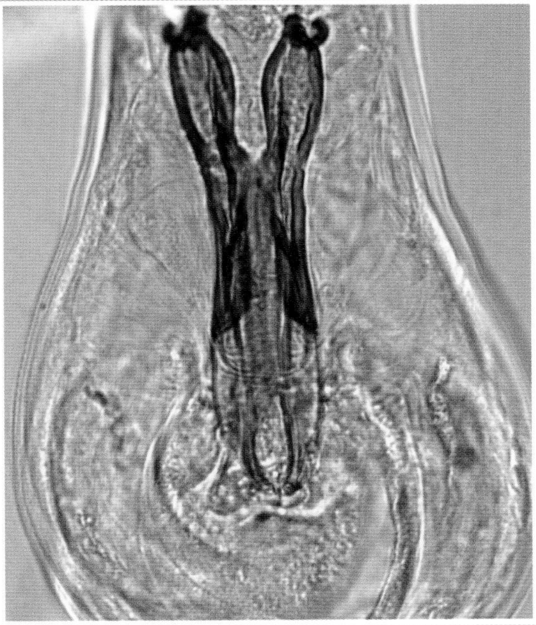	*Cooperia pectinata* *Cooperia punctata* *Cooperia spatulata* *Cooperia mcmasteri (surnabada)*	Decreased growth, anorexia	Eggs in fecal flotation and identification at necropsy	Doramectin, ivermectin, moxidectin, eprinomectin, albendazole, fenbendazole, levamisole, morantel tartrate
Hookworm* 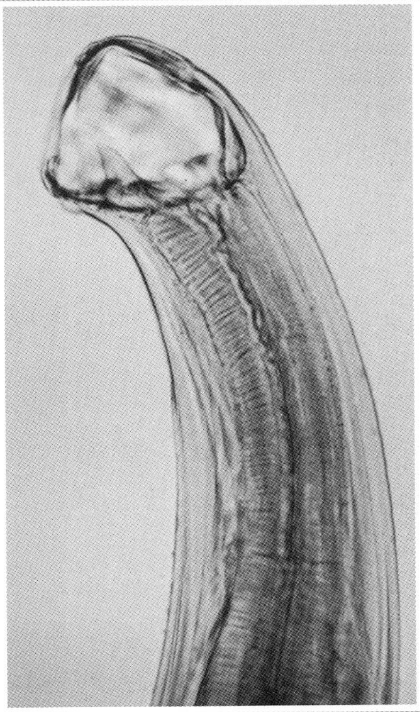	*Bunostomum phlebotomum*	Loss of weight, diarrhea, anemia, death in young animals	Eggs in fecal flotation and identification at necropsy	Ivermectin, moxidectin, doramectin, eprinomectin, fenbendazole

Continued

TABLE 26-3 Common Parasites of Production Animals—cont'd

BOVINE PARASITES				
COMMON NAME/PHOTOGRAPH	**SCIENTIFIC NAME**	**IMPORTANCE**	**DIAGNOSIS**	**TREATMENT**
Whipworm*				
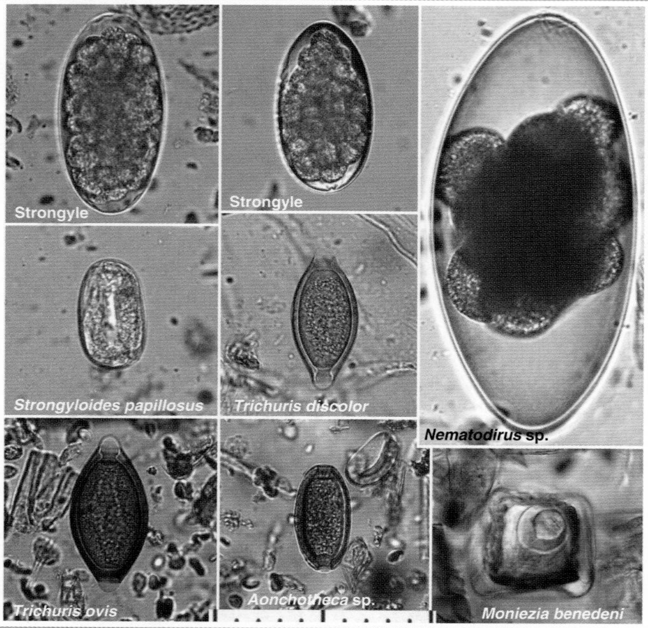	*Trichuris ovis*	Extreme infections can cause fatal hemorrhage into cecum Prepatent period is 2 months	Eggs in fecal flotation Adults in cecum and large intestine at necropsy	Ivermectin, fenbendazole, eprinomectin
Capillary Worm†				
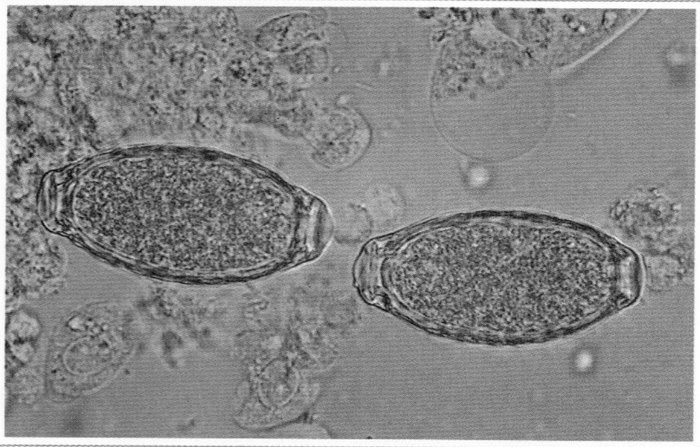	*Capillaria* spp.	Egg may be confused with *Trichuris* spp. Prepatent period is 6 weeks	Eggs in fecal flotation	Ivermectin, doramectin, eprinomectin, fenbendazole
Threadworm*				
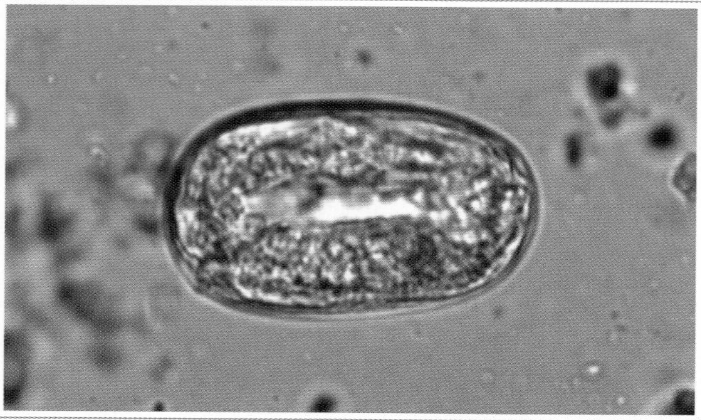	*Strongyloides papillosus*	Prepatent period is 1–2 weeks	Larvated eggs or larvae in fecal flotation	Eprinomectin

TABLE 26-3 Common Parasites of Production Animals—cont'd

BOVINE PARASITES				
COMMON NAME/PHOTOGRAPH	**SCIENTIFIC NAME**	**IMPORTANCE**	**DIAGNOSIS**	**TREATMENT**
Hair Worm, Black Scour Worm[†]				
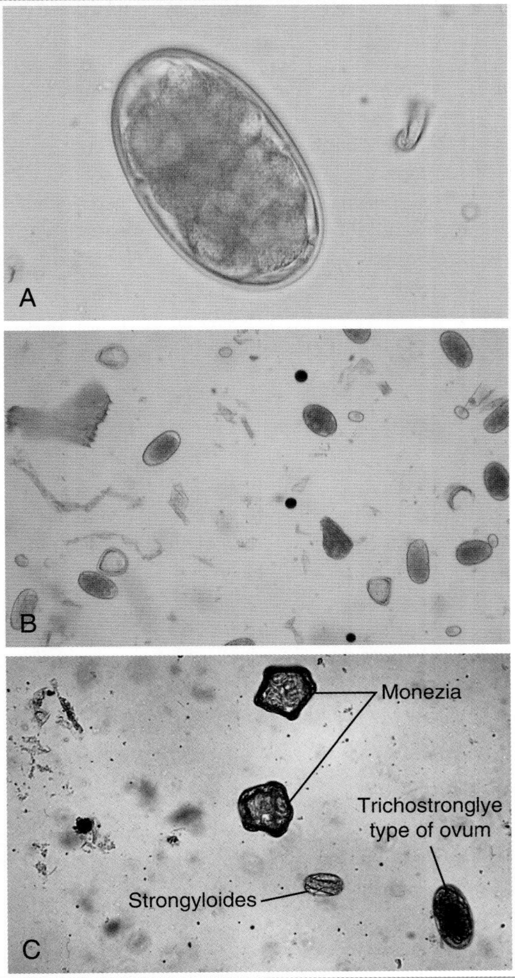	*Trichostrongylus colubriformis*		Eggs in fecal flotation Adults in small intestine at necropsy	Levamisole, morantel tartrate, doramectin, eprinomectin, fenbendazole, moxidectin
Barber's Pole or Wire Worm*				
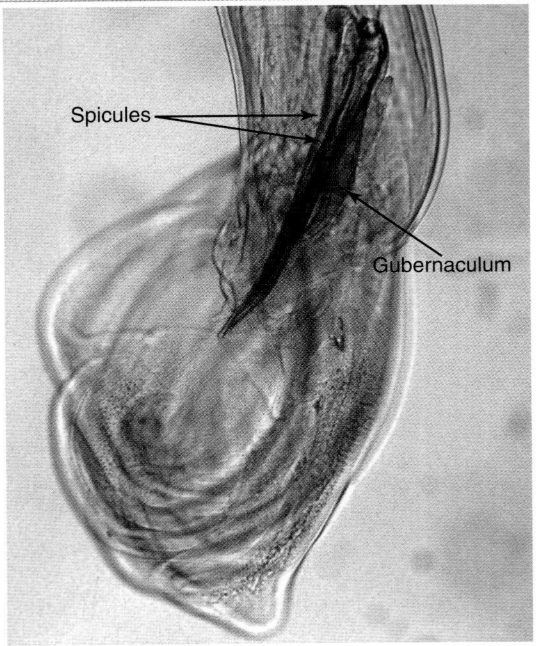	*Haemonchus placei*	Prepatent period is 17–21 days Eggs will not larvate after 4–5 days of refrigeration	Fecal flotation Adults in abomasum at necropsy	Levamisole, ivermectin, albendazole, doramectin, morantel tartrate, moxidectin, eprinomectin, tetramisole

Continued

TABLE 26-3 Common Parasites of Production Animals—cont'd

BOVINE PARASITES				
COMMON NAME/PHOTOGRAPH	**SCIENTIFIC NAME**	**IMPORTANCE**	**DIAGNOSIS**	**TREATMENT**
Lungworm† 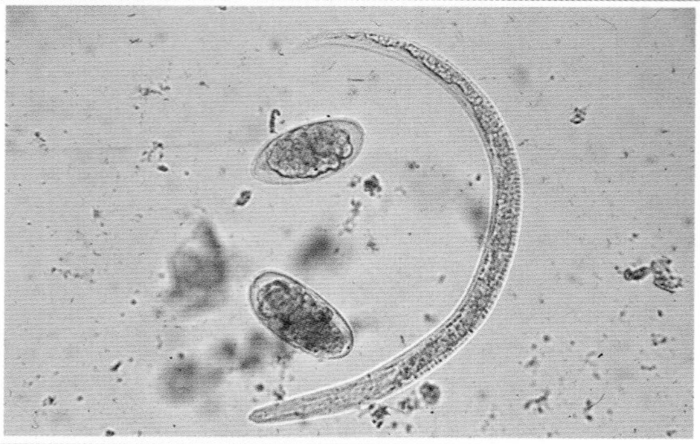	*Dictyocaulus viviparous*	Respiratory symptoms (e.g., cough, cyanosis, dyspnea) Prepatent period is 4 weeks	Baermann technique for larvae from feces Fecal flotation Adults in lung at necropsy	Ivermectin, doramectin, eprinomectin, moxidectin, levamisole, fenbendazole
Common Liver Fluke 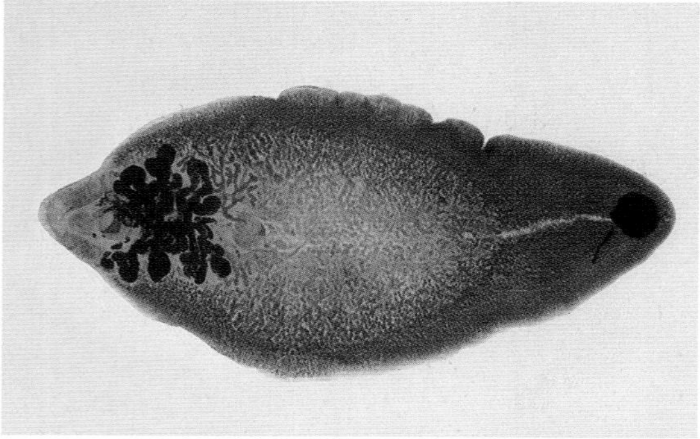	*Fasciola hepatica*	Anemia, weight loss, decreased performance, hepatitis, death Prepatent period is 10–12 weeks	Eggs in fecal sedimentation Flukes in liver and bile ducts at necropsy Enzyme-linked immunosorbent assay	Clorsulon, nitroxynil, rafoxanide
Tapeworm† 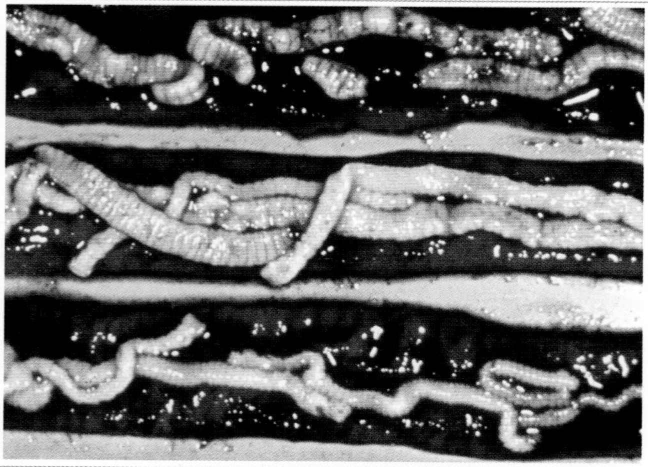	*Moniezia benedeni*	Prepatent period is 40 days	Proglottids in feces Fecal flotation Adults in small intestine at necropsy	Fenbendazole, albendazole, dichlorophen, lead arsenate, niclosamide

TABLE 26-3 Common Parasites of Production Animals—cont'd

BOVINE PARASITES

COMMON NAME/PHOTOGRAPH	SCIENTIFIC NAME	IMPORTANCE	DIAGNOSIS	TREATMENT
Beef Cysticercosis, Measles† 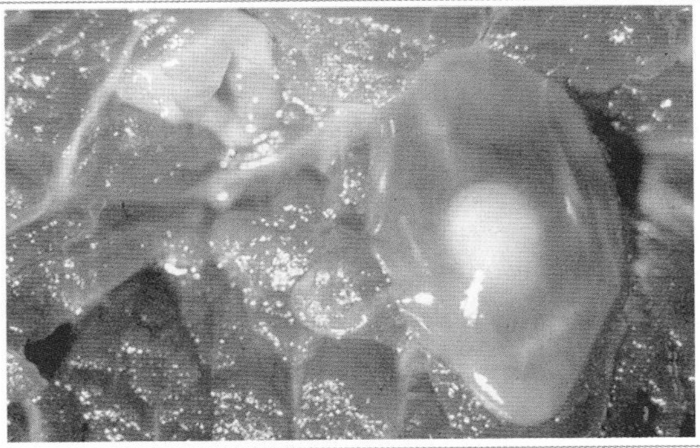	*Taenia saginata*	Carcass condemnation or trimming Transmission is from eggs in human feces orally consumed by cattle	Serologic tests and confirmation upon necropsy	None that are economically justified
Rumen Fluke† 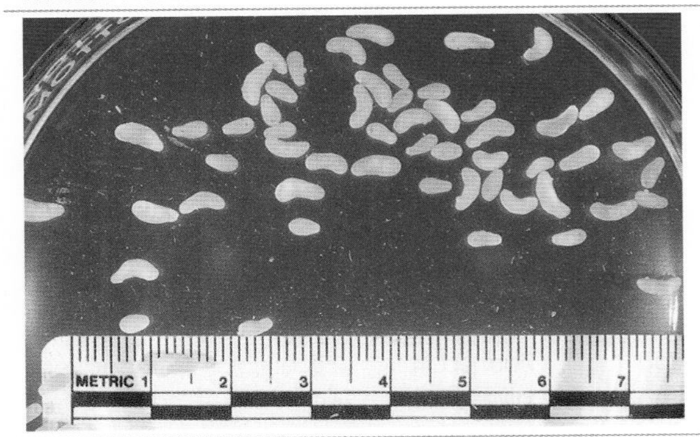	*Paramphistomum* spp.	Diarrhea	Fecal sedimentation	Oxyclozanide, niclosamide
Babesia or Pyroplasma† 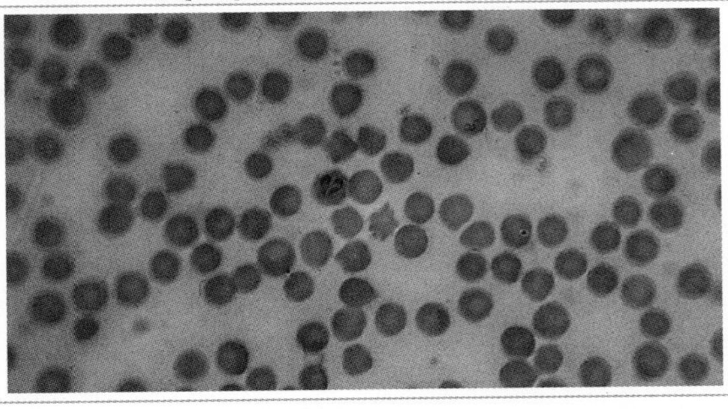	*Babesia bigemina*	Texas cattle fever, anemia, splenomegaly, fever Incubation period is variable (14–70 days)	Stained blood smear	Berenil, phenamide, acriflavine
Thin Necked Intestinal Worm: Sheep and Cattle† 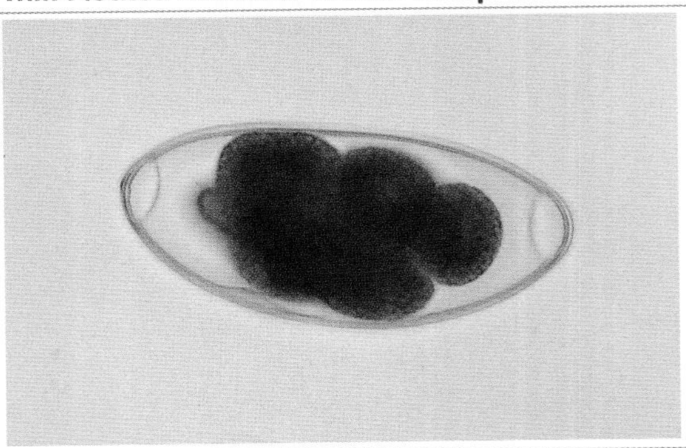	*Nematodirus filicollis, Nematodirus battus, Nematodirus spathiger*	*N. battus* is especially dangerous Prepatent period is 14–21 days	Fecal flotation Adults in small intestine at necropsy	Eprinomectin, ivermectin, moxidectin, albendazole, fenbendazole, levamisole, morantel tartrate

Continued

TABLE 26-3 Common Parasites of Production Animals—cont'd

BOVINE PARASITES				
COMMON NAME/PHOTOGRAPH	**SCIENTIFIC NAME**	**IMPORTANCE**	**DIAGNOSIS**	**TREATMENT**
Coccidia[†]				
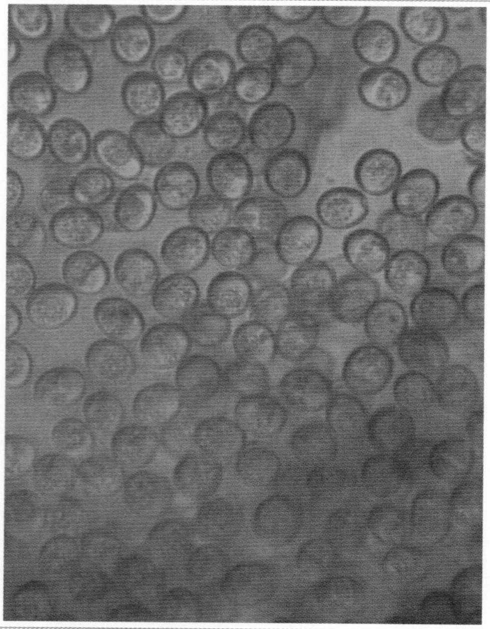	*Eimeria bukidnonensis, Eimeria aubemensis, Eimeria bovis, Eimeria cylindrical, Eimeria alabamensis, Eimeria zurnii, Eimeria ellipsoidalis*	Coccidiosis, bloody diarrhea, decreased performance, death Prepatent period is 12–18 days	Fecal flotation Hemorrhagic intestines with white raised lesions on necropsy	Sulfaguanidine, monensin, lasalocid
Crypto[†]				
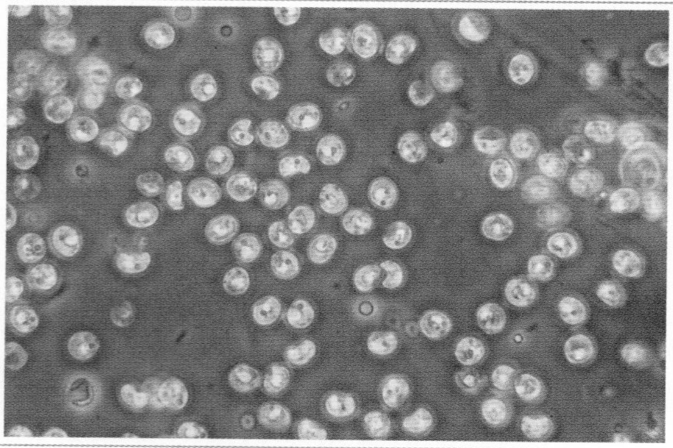	*Cryptosporidium* spp.	Diarrhea in calves 2–4 weeks of age Zoonotic to humans	Fecal flotation	Supportive care
Esophageal Worm[†]				
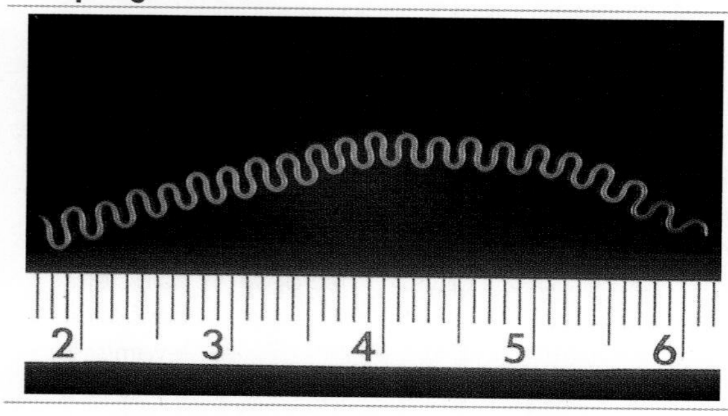	*Gongylonema pulchrum*		Eggs in fecal flotation	None available

TABLE 26-3 Common Parasites of Production Animals—cont'd

BOVINE PARASITES				
COMMON NAME/PHOTOGRAPH	SCIENTIFIC NAME	IMPORTANCE	DIAGNOSIS	TREATMENT
Brisket Worm†				
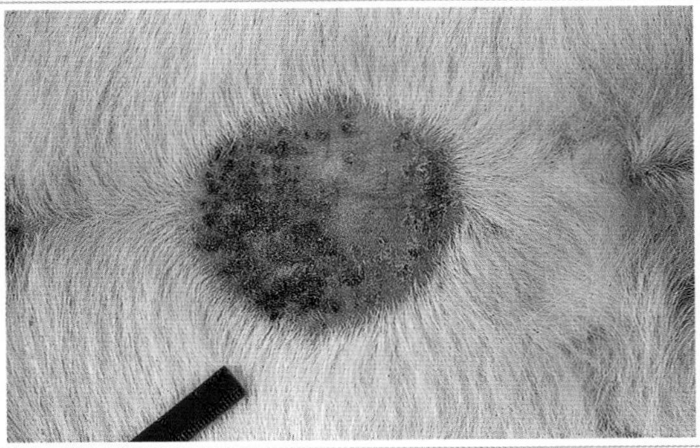	*Stephanofilaria stilesi*	Lesions on ventral abdomen Prepatent period is 6–8 weeks	Deep skin scrapings	Control horn flies
Skin Nodular Worm†				
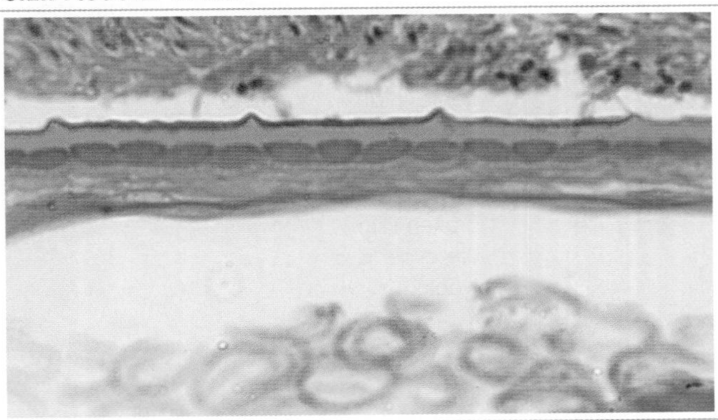	*Onchocerca* spp.	Keratitis or iritis Possibility of condemned carcass Prepatent period is 6–12 months	Microfilaria identification in skin sample from near skin nodule	None
Abdominal Worm†				
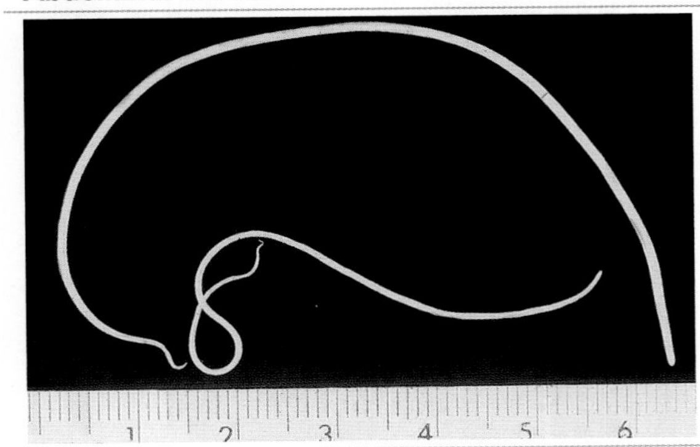	*Setaria cervi*	May cause cerebral nematodiasis Prepatent period is variable	Microfilaria in the blood	None

Continued

TABLE 26-3 Common Parasites of Production Animals—cont'd

BOVINE PARASITES				
COMMON NAME/PHOTOGRAPH	**SCIENTIFIC NAME**	**IMPORTANCE**	**DIAGNOSIS**	**TREATMENT**
Common Cattle Bot Fly and Northern Cattle Bot Fly*				
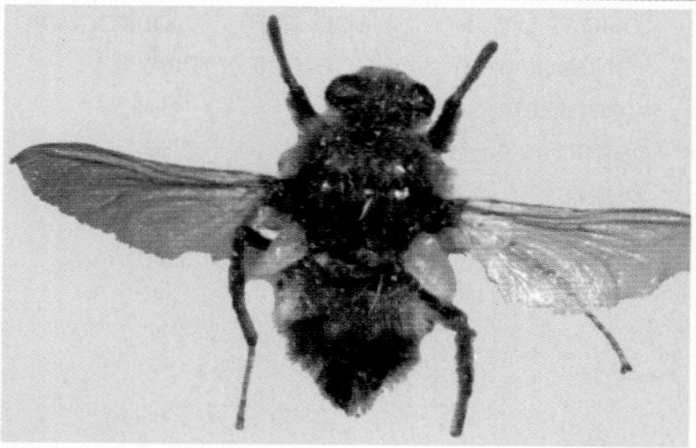 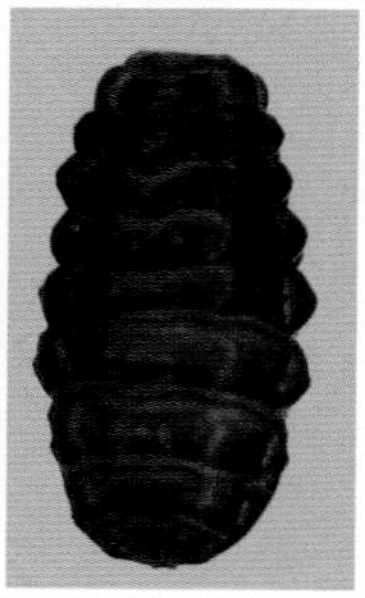	*Hypoderma lineatum* *Hypoderma bovis*	Reduction in weight gain, decreased hide value Migration to esophagus or spinal column causes warbles Life cycle is 10–12 months	Warbles	Pour-on ivermectin, trichlorfon, famphur, organophosphates, coumaphos, fenthion, moxidectin
Screwworm†				
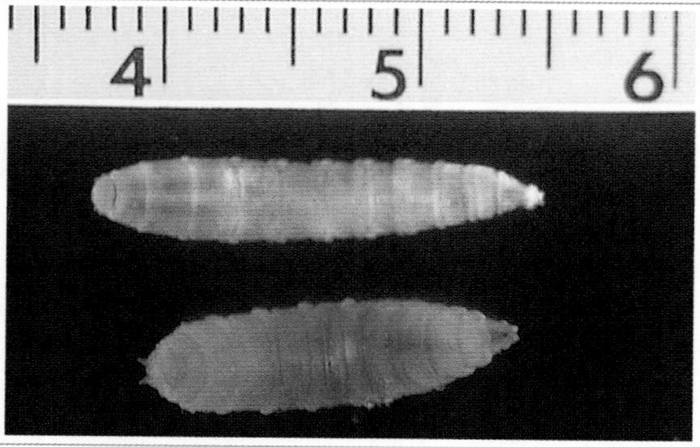	*Cochliomyia hominivorax*	Reportable disease in United States Highly pathogenic, high mortality Maggots penetrate through broken skin Life cycle is 3 weeks	Larvae from wounds should be sent to the state diagnostic laboratory	Ivermectin, organophosphates
Face Fly†				
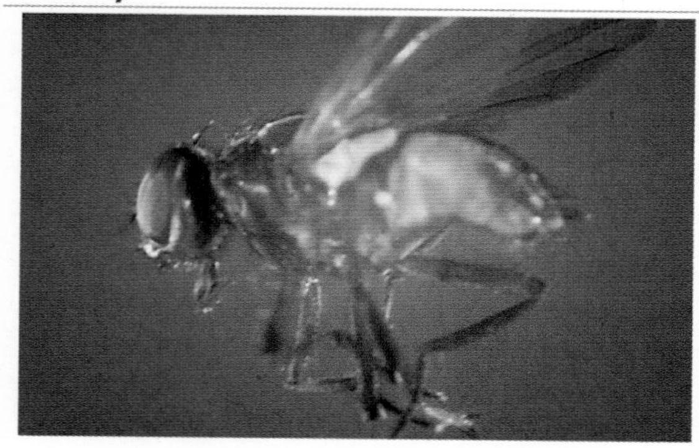	*Musca autumnalis*	May predispose to bacterial keratoconjunctivitis (pink eye) Can transmit eyeworms (*Thelazia* spp.), infectious bovine rhinotracheitis Life cycle is variable, ~10–14 days	Identification of flies	Pour-ons, dips, sprays, dusts, back rubbers, orals, injectables, feed additives

TABLE 26-3 Common Parasites of Production Animals—cont'd

BOVINE PARASITES				
COMMON NAME/PHOTOGRAPH	SCIENTIFIC NAME	IMPORTANCE	DIAGNOSIS	TREATMENT
House Fly* 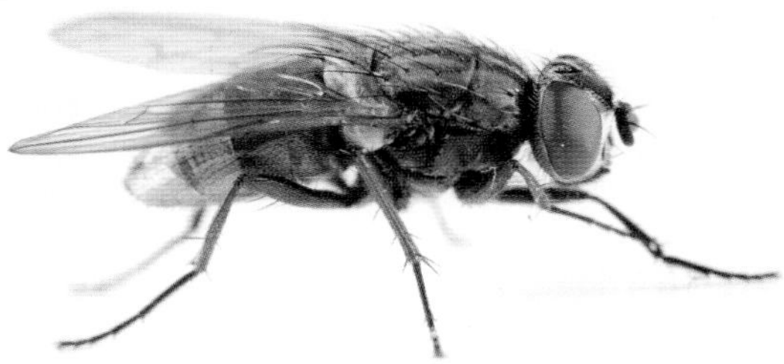	*Musca domestica*	Production loss Life cycle is 10–14 days	Identification of flies	Pour-ons, dips, sprays, dusts, back rubbers, orals, injectables, feed additives
Horn Fly* 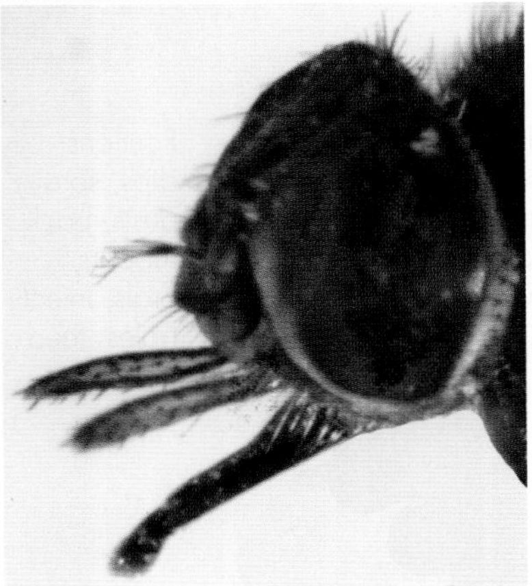	*Siphona (Haematobia) irritans*	Production loss Life cycle is ≥3 weeks	Identification of adult fly Smaller than house fly and usually feeds with head down	Pour-ons, dips, sprays, dusts, back rubbers, orals, injectables, feed additives
Stable Fly† 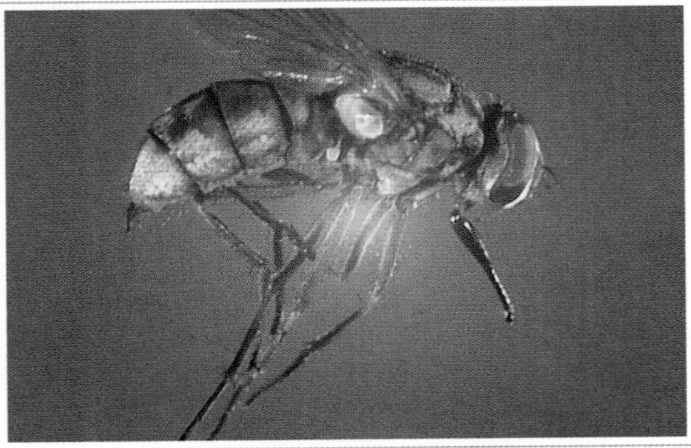	*Stomoxys calcitrans*	Production loss Life cycle is ≥4 weeks	Identification of adult fly Size of house fly	Pour-ons, dips, sprays, dusts, back rubbers, orals, injectables, feed additives
Horse Fly† 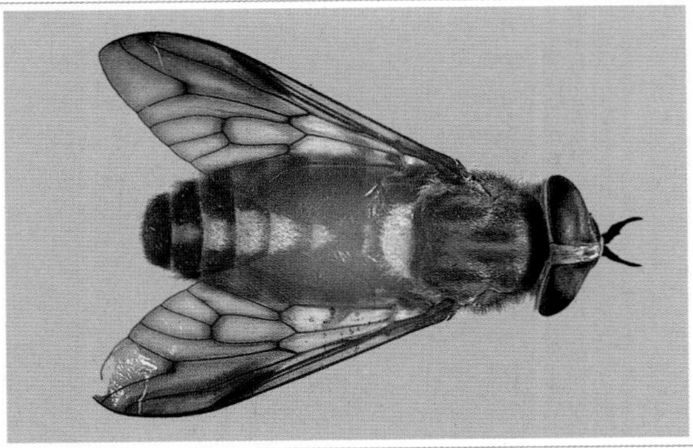	*Tabanus* spp.	Transmit anaplasmosis Production loss Bites may cause stampedes; very painful	Identification of adult fly	Pour-ons, dips, sprays, dusts, back rubbers, orals, injectables, feed additives

Continued

TABLE 26-3 Common Parasites of Production Animals—cont'd

BOVINE PARASITES				
COMMON NAME/PHOTOGRAPH	**SCIENTIFIC NAME**	**IMPORTANCE**	**DIAGNOSIS**	**TREATMENT**
Biting Louse†				
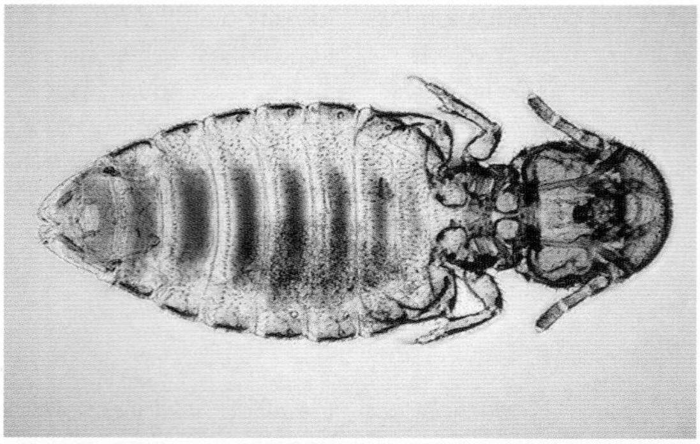	*Bovicola (Damalinia) bovis*	Production loss Most common in fall and winter Usually on neck, brisket, head, and between legs in cattle Life cycle is about 4 weeks	Identification of eggs, nymphs, adult lice	Pour-ons, dips, sprays, dusts, back rubbers, orals, injectables, feed additives
Sucking Louse*				
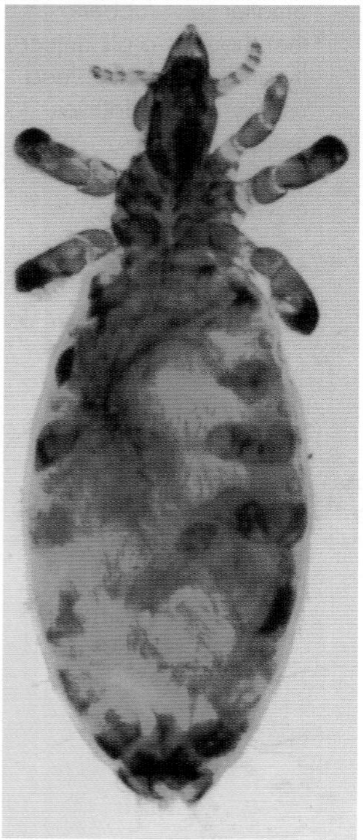	*Linognathus vituli* (long-nosed or blue cattle louse) *Haematopinus eurysternus* (short-nosed cattle louse)	Production loss may cause anemia Life cycle is about 4 weeks	Identification of eggs, nymphs, adults	Pour-ons, dips, sprays, dusts, back rubbers, orals, injectables, feed additives
Mange Mite or Scab Mite†				
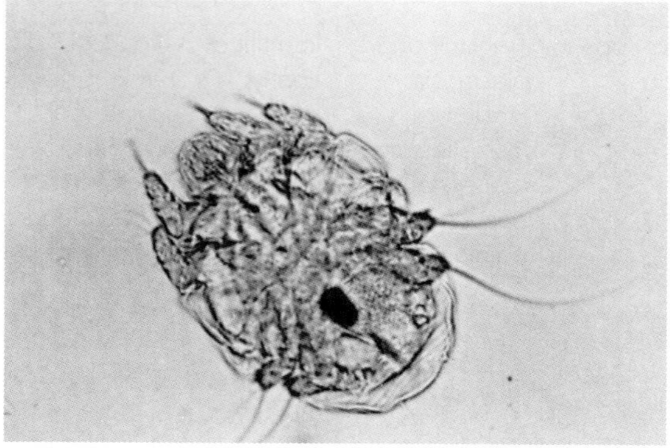	Psoroptes spp.	Reportable disease in some states Dramatic weight loss Life cycle is about 3 weeks	Skin scrapings	Pour-ons, dips, sprays, dusts, back rubbers, orals, injectables, feed additives

TABLE 26-3 Common Parasites of Production Animals—cont'd

BOVINE PARASITES				
COMMON NAME/PHOTOGRAPH	**SCIENTIFIC NAME**	**IMPORTANCE**	**DIAGNOSIS**	**TREATMENT**
Mange Mite†				
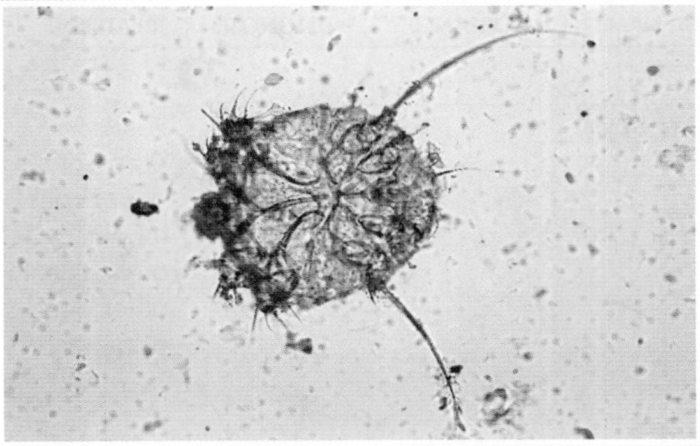	*Sarcoptes scabiei*	Reportable disease in some states Life cycle is about 3 weeks	Skin scrapings	Pour-ons, dips, sprays, dusts, back rubbers, orals, injectables, feed additives
Mange Mite†				
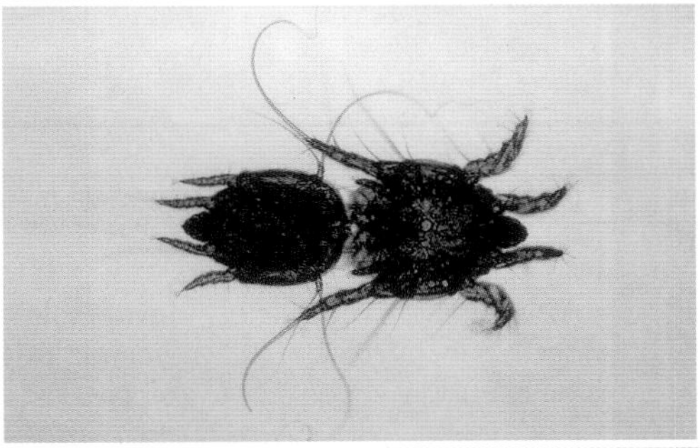	*Chorioptes* spp.	Reportable disease of cattle in some states Causes tail or foot mange Life cycle is about 3 weeks	Skin scrapings	Pour-ons, dips, sprays, dusts, back rubbers, orals, injectables, feed additives
Ticks†				
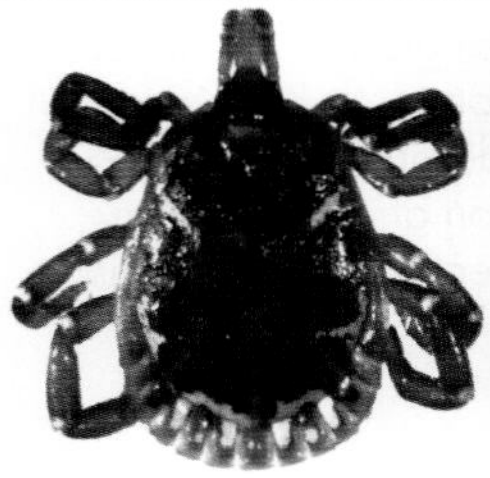 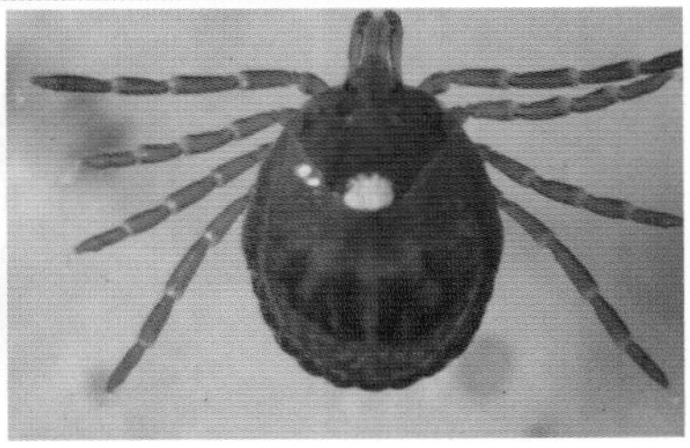	*Dermacentor variabilis* (American dog tick), *Dermacentor andersoni* (Rocky Mountain wood tick), *Dermacentor albipictus* (winter tick), *Dermacentor occidentalis* (Pacific Coast tick), *Ixodes scapularis* (black-legged tick), *Amblyomma americanum* (Lone Star tick), *Amblyomma maculatum* (Gulf Coast tick), *Boophilus annulatus* (cattle tick), *Boophilus microplus* (southern cattle tick), *Otobius megninii* (spinose ear tick), *Ornithodoros coriaceus* (Pajaroello tick)	Possible transmission of anaplasmosis		Pour-ons, dips, sprays, dusts, back rubbers, orals, injectables, feed additives

Continued

TABLE 26-3 Common Parasites of Production Animals—cont'd

BOVINE PARASITES

COMMON NAME/PHOTOGRAPH	SCIENTIFIC NAME	IMPORTANCE	DIAGNOSIS	TREATMENT
Mange Mite†				
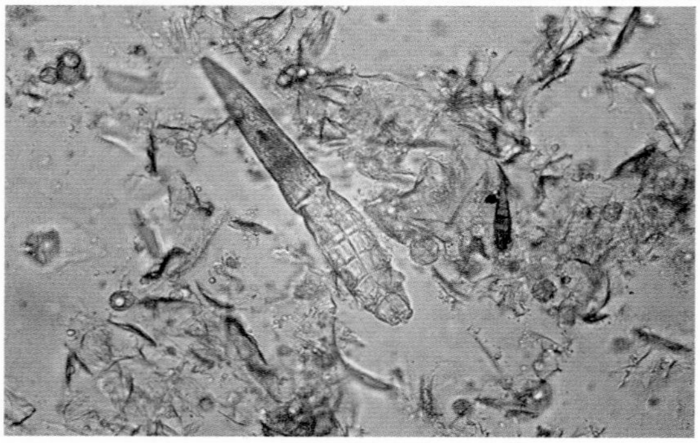	*Demodex bovis*			Pour-ons, dips, sprays, dusts, back rubbers, orals, injectables, feed additives

SHEEP AND GOATS

COMMON NAME/PHOTOGRAPH	SCIENTIFIC NAME	IMPORTANCE	DIAGNOSIS	TREATMENT
Barber's Pole or Wire Worm*: Sheep				
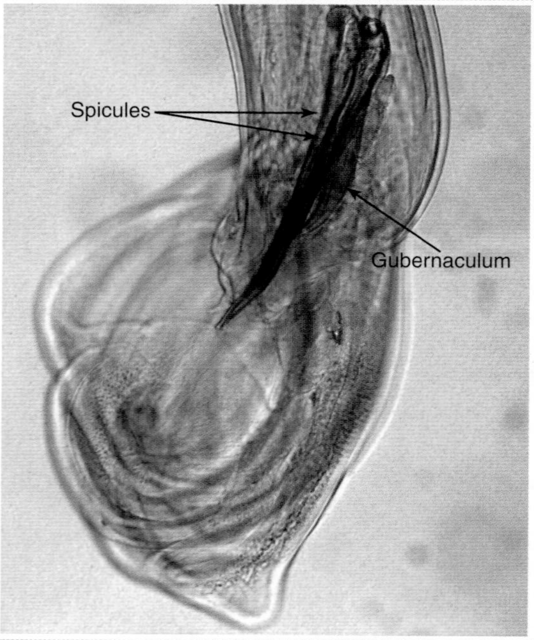	*Haemonchus contortus*	Acute anemia in lambs; bottle jaw, death, chronic weight loss in adults Prepatent period is 17–21 days	Fecal flotation. Eggs do not larvate after 4–5 days of refrigeration Identification at necropsy	Levamisole, ivermectin, albendazole, doramectin, morantel tartrate, moxidectin, eprinomectin, tetramisole

TABLE 26-3 Common Parasites of Production Animals—cont'd

SHEEP AND GOATS				
COMMON NAME/PHOTOGRAPH	SCIENTIFIC NAME	IMPORTANCE	DIAGNOSIS	TREATMENT
Brown Stomach Worm*: Sheep				
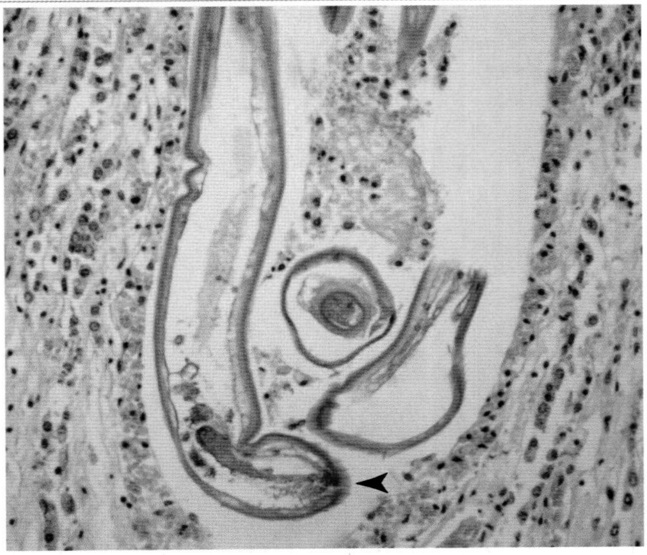	*Ostertagia ostertagi*	Larval destruction of gastric glands causes severe diarrhea and weight loss. Type I: Produce eggs Pre-type II: Not clinically apparent, and fourth-stage larvae are inhibited in gastric glands Type II: Eggs often not found in feces	Fecal flotation and identification at necropsy	Fenbendazole, doramectin, eprinomectin, ivermectin, morantel tartrate, moxidectin
Bankrupt Worm or Small Stomach Worm*: Sheep and Goats				
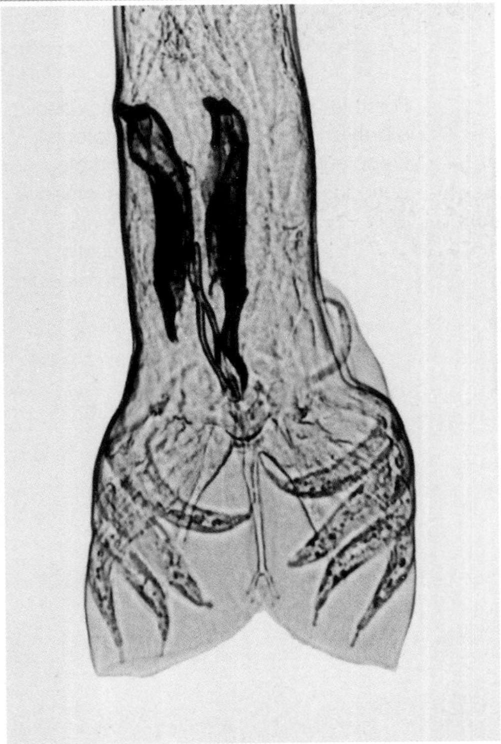	*Trichostrongylus axei*	Diarrhea, dehydration, bottle jaw, emaciation in stressed animals Prepatent period is 3 weeks	Eggs in fecal flotation and identification at necropsy	Ivermectin, doramectin, eprinomectin, fenbendazole, moxidectin, morantel tartrate

Continued

TABLE 26-3 Common Parasites of Production Animals—cont'd

SHEEP AND GOATS				
COMMON NAME/PHOTOGRAPH	**SCIENTIFIC NAME**	**IMPORTANCE**	**DIAGNOSIS**	**TREATMENT**
Thin Necked Intestinal Worm†: Sheep and Cattle				
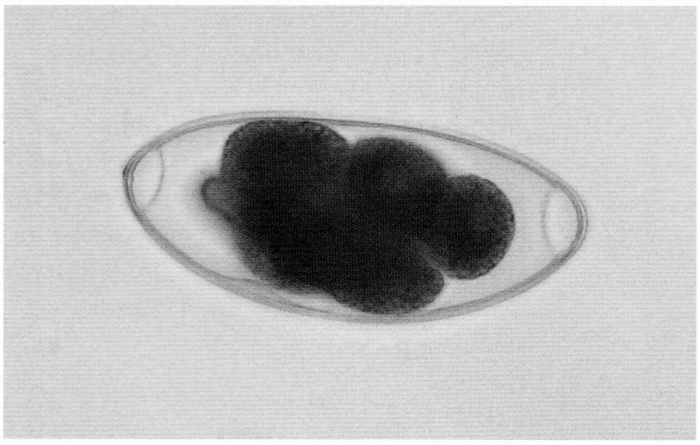	*Nematodirus filicollis, Nematodirus battus, Nematodirus spathiger*	*N. battus* is especially dangerous Prepatent period is 14–21 days	Fecal flotation and identification at necropsy	Eprinomectin, ivermectin, moxidectin, albendazole, fenbendazole, levamisole, morantel tartrate
Threadworm*: Sheep and Cattle				
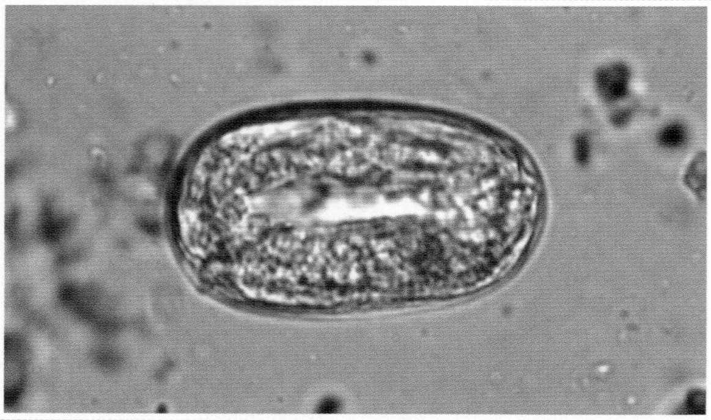	*Strongyloides papillosus*	Foot rot, diarrhea Prepatent period is 1–2 weeks	Eggs in fecal flotation and identification at necropsy	Ivermectin, eprinomectin
Nodular Worm*: Sheep and Goats				
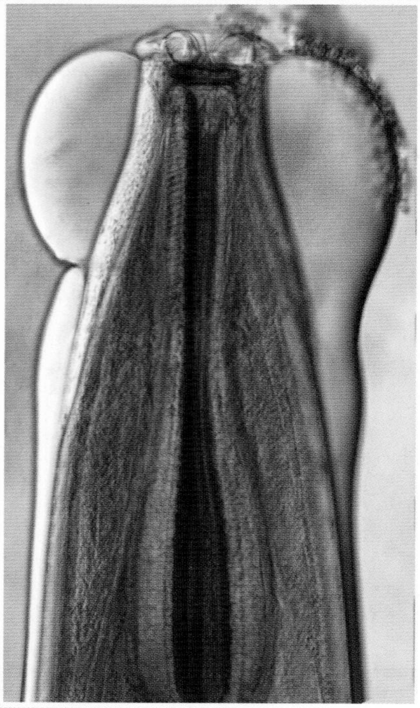	*Oesophagostomum columbianum, Oesophagostomum venulosum*	Possible diarrhea Prepatent period is 40 days	Eggs in fecal flotation and identification at necropsy	Moxidectin, morantel tartrate, levamisole, eprinomectin, doramectin

TABLE 26-3 Common Parasites of Production Animals—cont'd

COMMON NAME/PHOTOGRAPH	SCIENTIFIC NAME	IMPORTANCE	DIAGNOSIS	TREATMENT
SHEEP AND GOATS				
Hair Worm, Black Scour Worm†: Sheep and Goats				
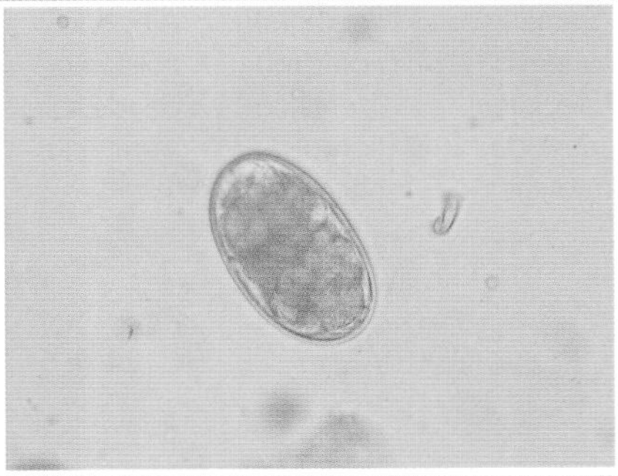	*Trichostrongylus colubriformis*	Diarrhea May cause bottle jaw, decreased weight gain Prepatent period is 3 weeks	Eggs in fecal flotation. Adults in small intestine at necropsy	Levamisole, morantel tartrate, doramectin, eprinomectin, fenbendazole, moxidectin
Cattle Bankrupt Worm*: Sheep and Goats				
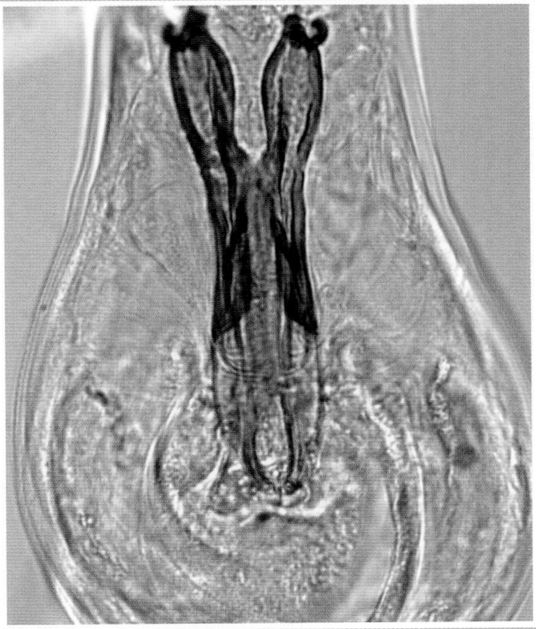	*Cooperia punctata, Cooperia pectinata*	Decreased growth, anorexia	Eggs in fecal flotation and identification at necropsy	Doramectin, ivermectin, moxidectin, eprinomectin, albendazole, fenbendazole, levamisole, morantel tartrate
Hookworm*: Sheep				
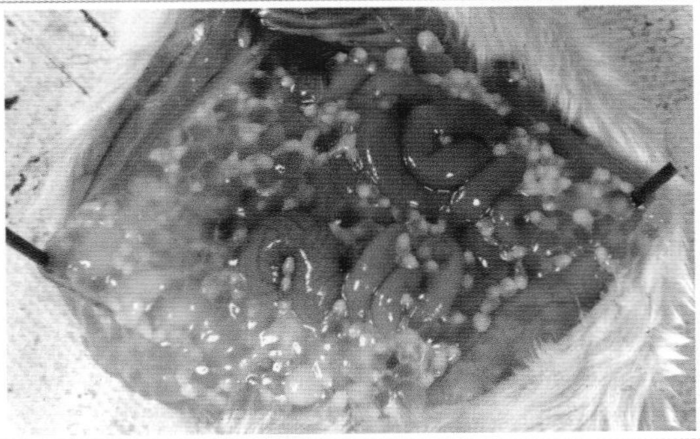	*Bunostomum trigonocephalum*	Weight loss, diarrhea, anemia, death in young animals	Eggs in fecal flotation and identification at necropsy	Ivermectin, moxidectin, doramectin, eprinomectin, fenbendazole

Continued

TABLE 26-3 Common Parasites of Production Animals—cont'd

SHEEP AND GOATS				
COMMON NAME/PHOTOGRAPH	**SCIENTIFIC NAME**	**IMPORTANCE**	**DIAGNOSIS**	**TREATMENT**
Large-Mouthed Bowel Worm*: Sheep 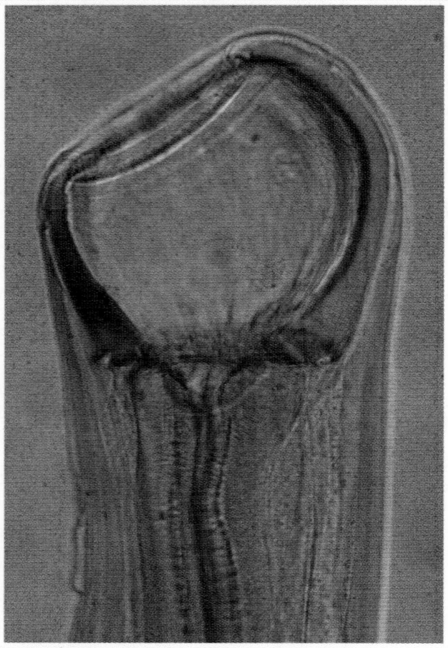	*Chabertia ovina*	Sometimes anemia Prepatent period is 2 months	Fecal flotation and identification at necropsy	Albendazole, fenbendazole, ivermectin
Whipworm*: Sheep 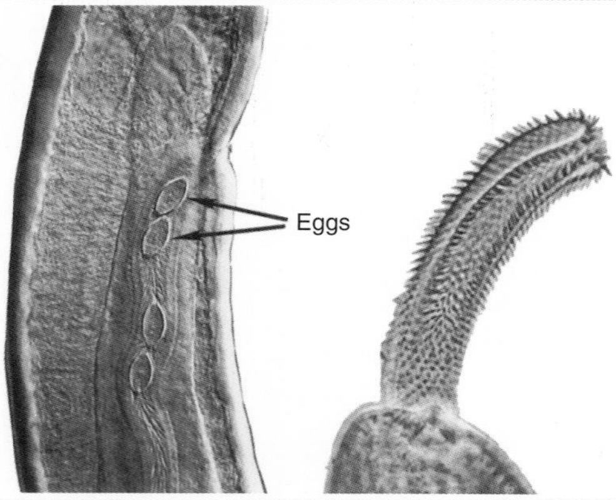	*Trichuris ovis*	Extreme infections can cause fatal hemorrhage into cecum Prepatent period is 2 months	Eggs in fecal flotation and identification upon necropsy	Ivermectin, fenbendazole, eprinomectin
Capillary Worm†: Sheep 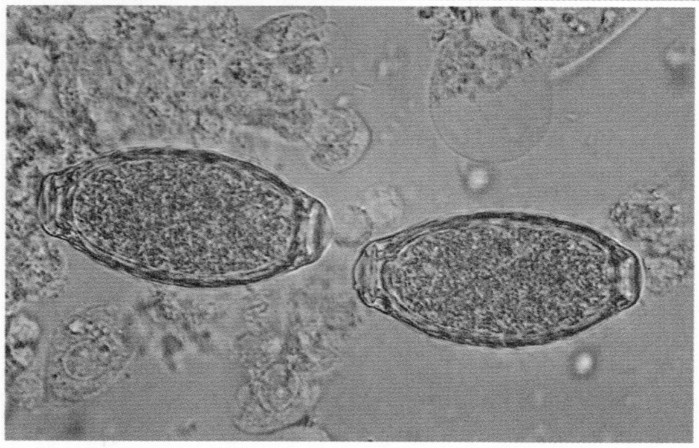	*Capillaria* spp.	Prepatent period is 6 weeks	Eggs in fecal flotation	Ivermectin, doramectin, eprinomectin, fenbendazole

TABLE 26-3 Common Parasites of Production Animals—cont'd

SHEEP AND GOATS				
COMMON NAME/PHOTOGRAPH	**SCIENTIFIC NAME**	**IMPORTANCE**	**DIAGNOSIS**	**TREATMENT**
Lungworm*: Sheep				
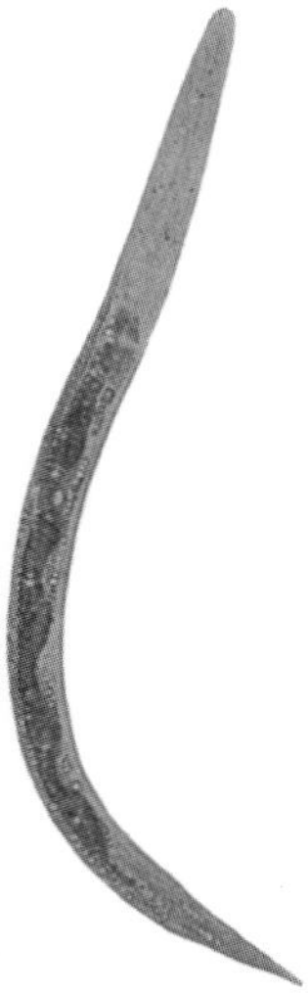 *Dictyocaulus viviparus* (×250) 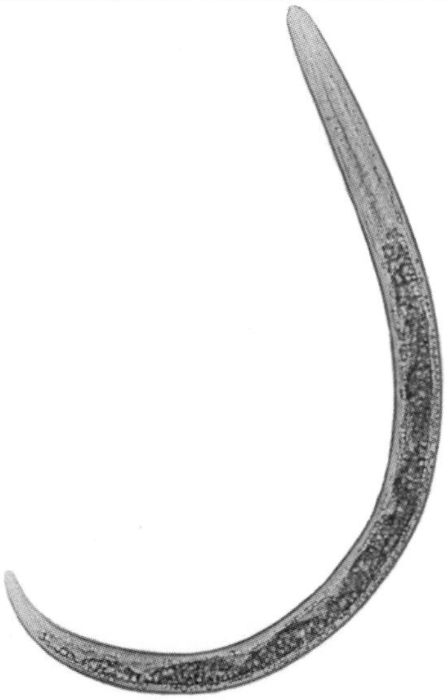 *Dictyocaulus filaria* (×250) 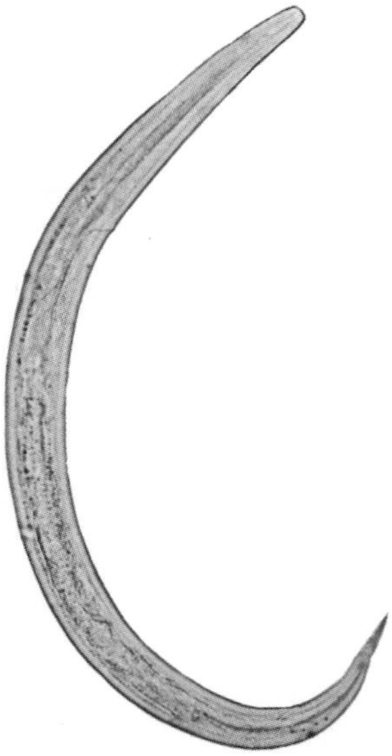 *Protostrongylus* sp. (×425) 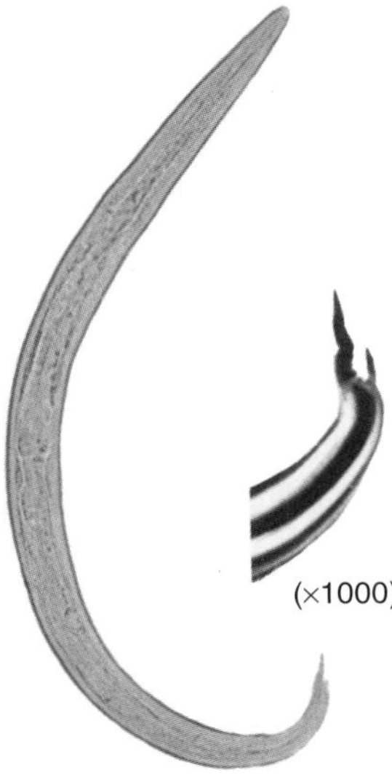 (×1000) *Muellerius* sp. (×425)	*Dictyocaulus filaria*	Respiratory symptoms (e.g., cough, cyanosis, dyspnea) Prepatent period is 4 weeks	Baermann technique for larvae from feces Fecal flotation Adults in lung at necropsy	Ivermectin, doramectin, eprinomectin, moxidectin, levamisole, fenbendazole

Continued

TABLE 26-3 Common Parasites of Production Animals—cont'd

SHEEP AND GOATS				
COMMON NAME/PHOTOGRAPH	**SCIENTIFIC NAME**	**IMPORTANCE**	**DIAGNOSIS**	**TREATMENT**
Bighorn Sheep Lungworm*: Sheep				
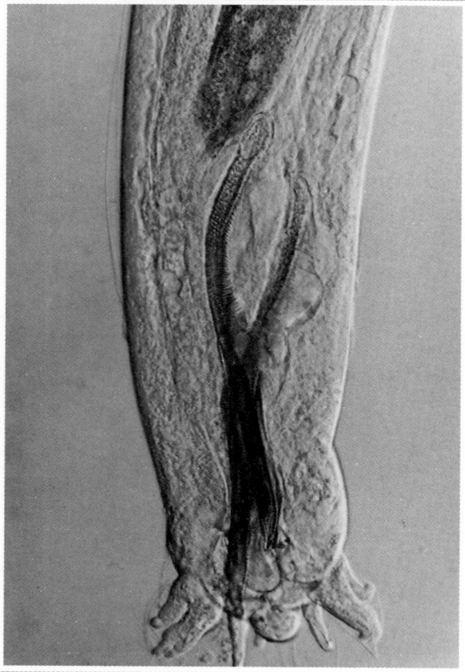	*Protostrongylus rufescens, P. rushi, P. stilesi* (bighorn sheep)	Predisposes sheep to pneumonia Transplacental transmission in bighorn sheep Prepatent period is 5 weeks Uncommon in domestic sheep	Eggs in fecal sedimentation Flukes found in liver and bile ducts at necropsy ELISA	Ivermectin, albendazole, fenbendazole
Goat Lungworm†: Goats				
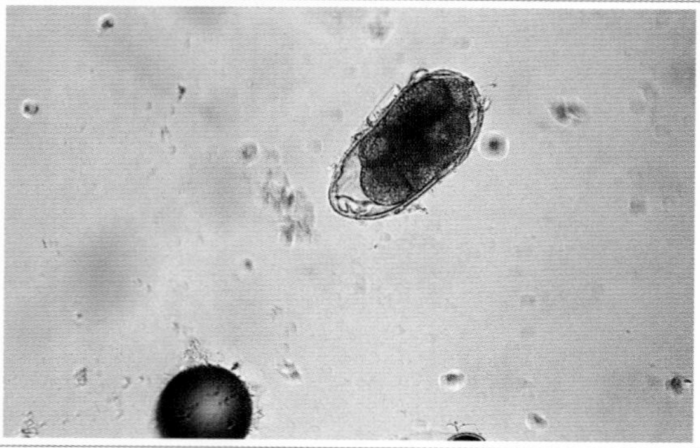	*Muellerius capillaris*	Predisposes goats to pneumonia	Baermann technique	Ivermectin, fenbendazole, albendazole
Common Liver Fluke (Fasciolidae)†				
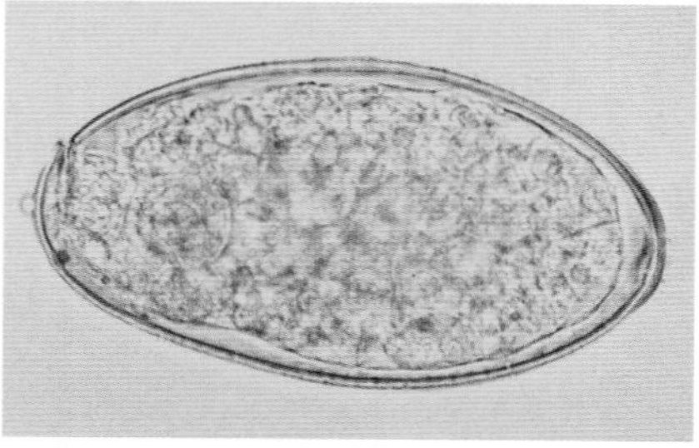	*Fasciola hepatica*	Anemia, weight loss, decreased performance, hepatitis, death Prepatent period is 10–12 weeks	Eggs in fecal sedimentation Flukes in liver and bile ducts at necropsy ELISA	Clorsulon, nitroxynil, rafoxanide

TABLE 26-3 Common Parasites of Production Animals—cont'd

COMMON NAME/PHOTOGRAPH	SCIENTIFIC NAME	IMPORTANCE	DIAGNOSIS	TREATMENT
SHEEP AND GOATS				
Tapeworm†: Sheep 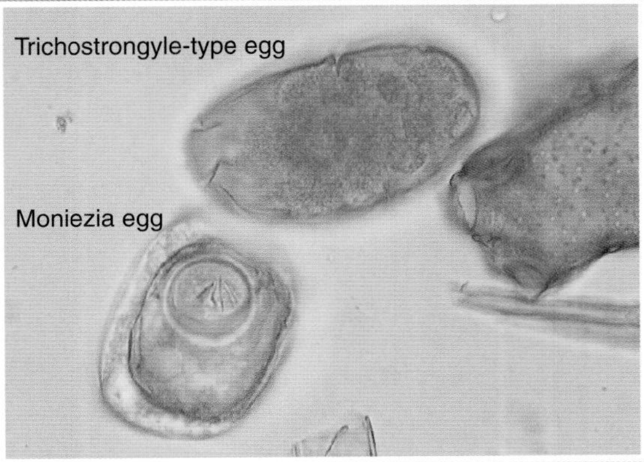	*Moniezia expansa*	Prepatent period is 40 days	Proglottids in feces Fecal flotation Adults in small intestine at necropsy	Fenbendazole, albendazole, dichlorophen, lead arsenate, niclosamide
Abdominal Worm†: Sheep and Goats 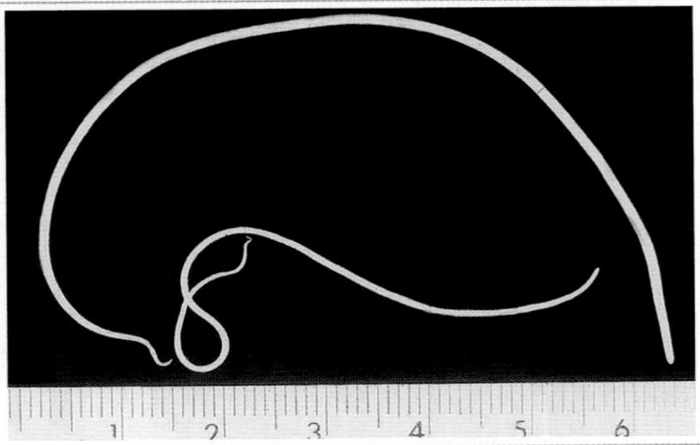	*Setaria cervi*	May cause cerebral nematodiasis Prepatent period is variable	Microfilaria in blood	None
Fringed Tapeworm†: Sheep 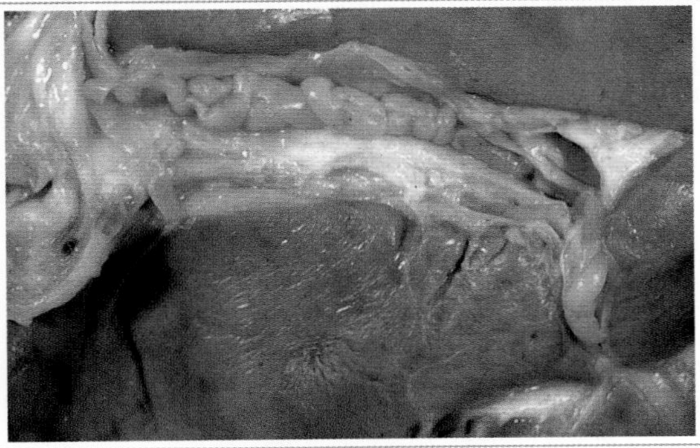	*Thysanosoma actinoides*	Liver condemnation, weight loss Prepatent period is 1 month	Proglottids in feces	Fenbendazole, albendazole

Continued

TABLE 26-3 Common Parasites of Production Animals—cont'd

SHEEP AND GOATS				
COMMON NAME/PHOTOGRAPH	**SCIENTIFIC NAME**	**IMPORTANCE**	**DIAGNOSIS**	**TREATMENT**
Cysticercus Tenuicollis†: Sheep				
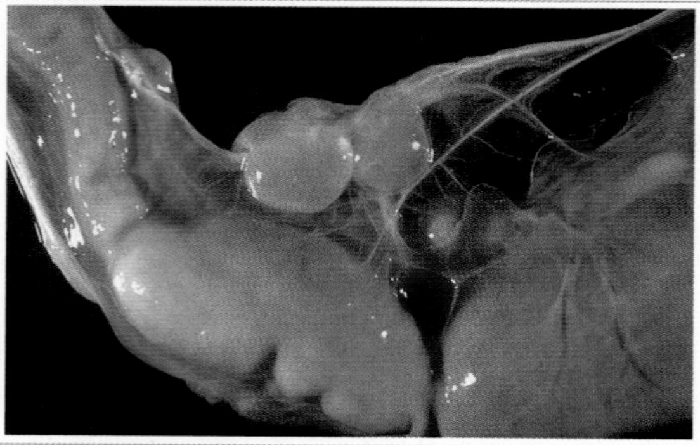	*Taenia hydatigena*	Prepatent period in dogs is 51 days	Identification upon necropsy	None
Hydatid Cyst*: Sheep				
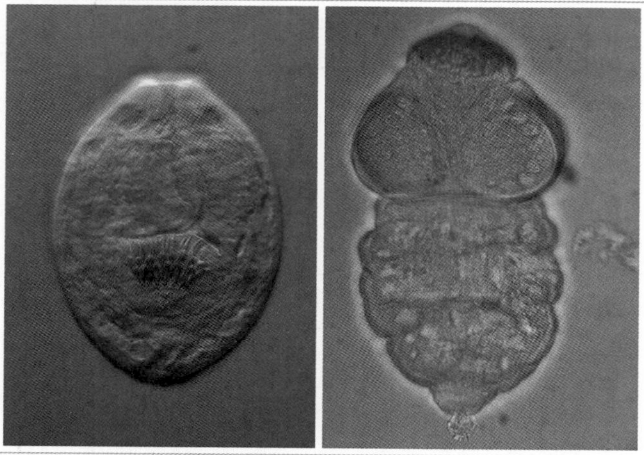	*Echinococcus granulosus*	Intermediate host and source of infection for carnivores Prepatent period in dogs is 7–9 weeks	Identification upon necropsy	None
Sheep Cysticercosis*: Sheep				
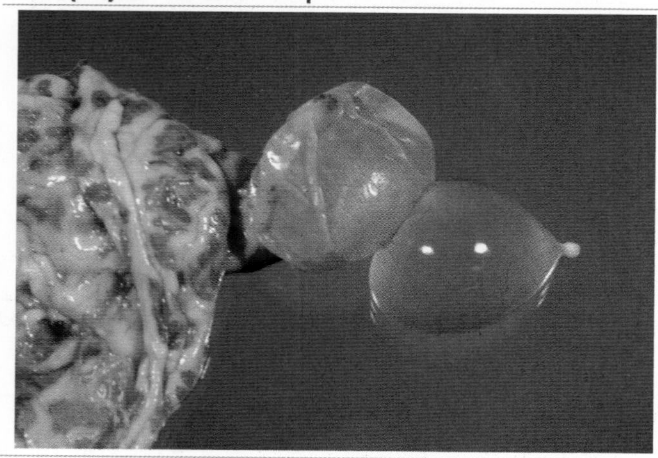	*Taenia ovis*	Responsible for condemnation, trimming Prepatent period in dogs is 60 days	Identification upon necropsy	None

TABLE 26-3 Common Parasites of Production Animals—cont'd

SHEEP AND GOATS				
COMMON NAME/PHOTOGRAPH	**SCIENTIFIC NAME**	**IMPORTANCE**	**DIAGNOSIS**	**TREATMENT**
Gid†: Sheep				
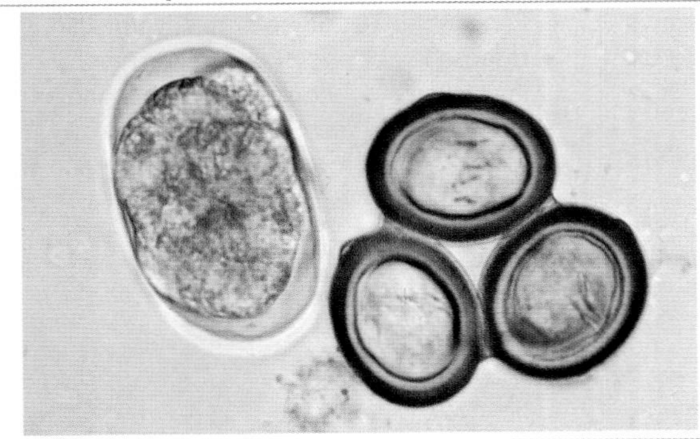	*Taenia multiceps*	Causes central nervous system disorder but is rare in the United States Prepatent period in dogs is 2–3 months	Identification upon necropsy	None
Sorehead, Filarial Dermatitis: Sheep				
	Elaeophora schneideri	Commonly found in mule deer in the western United States Causes filarial dermatitis "sorehead," most often in older sheep Prepatent period is 4–5 months	Identification of microfilariae in skin	None
Sheep Blowflies or Bottle Flies*: Sheep				
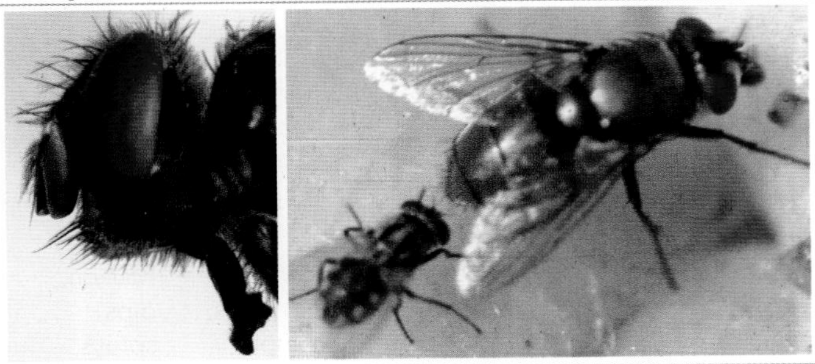	*Lucilia, Phormia, Calliphora*	Responsible for strike Life cycle is 10 days	Identification of larvae in rotting wool	Wound treatment, organophosphates

Continued

TABLE 26-3 Common Parasites of Production Animals—cont'd

SHEEP AND GOATS				
COMMON NAME/PHOTOGRAPH	**SCIENTIFIC NAME**	**IMPORTANCE**	**DIAGNOSIS**	**TREATMENT**
Screwworm†: Sheep and Goats				
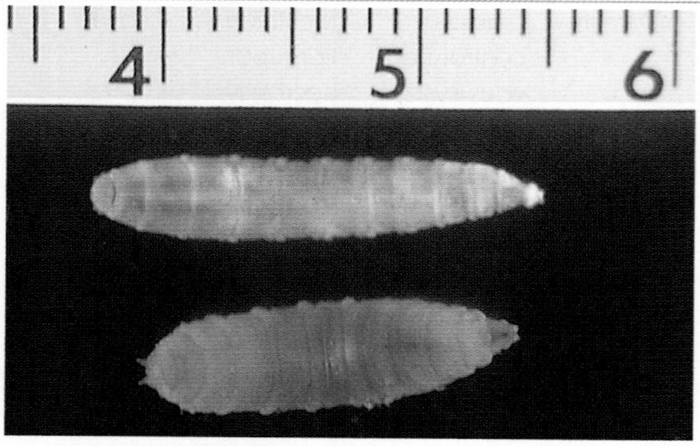	*Cochliomyia hominivorax*	Reportable disease in the United States Highly pathogenic, high mortality Maggots penetrate through broken skin Life cycle is 3 weeks	Larvae from wounds should be sent to state diagnostic laboratory	Ivermectin, organophosphates
Sheep Nasal Bot Fly*: Sheep				
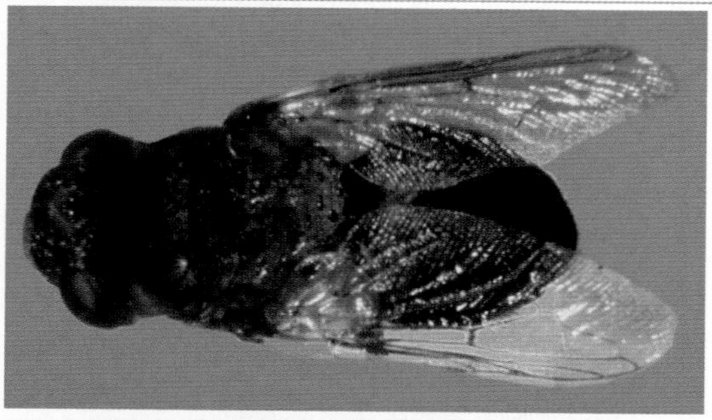 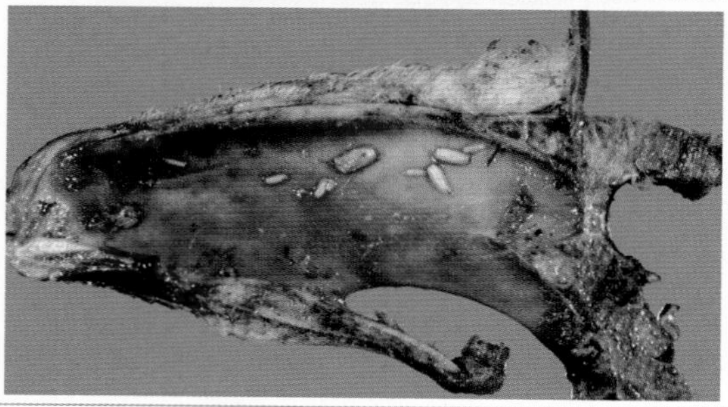	*Oestrus ovis*	Dyspnea, nasal discharge	Identification upon necropsy	Ivermectin, *Bacillus thuringiensis* aerosol
Biting Louse†: Sheep and Goats				
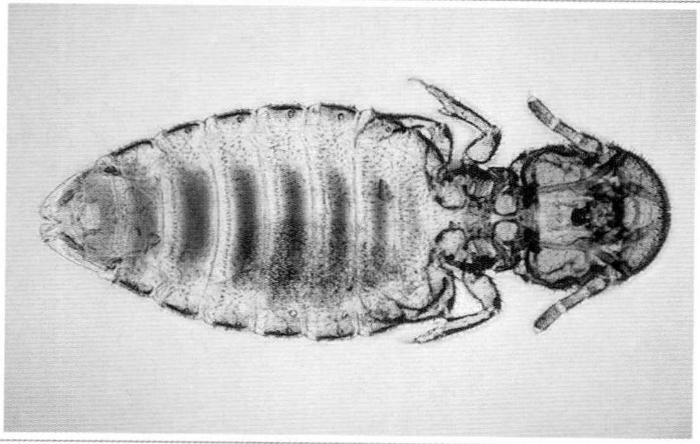	*Bovicola (Damalinia) bovis*	Production losses Most common in fall and winter Usually on neck, brisket, head, and between legs in cattle	Identification eggs, nymphs, adult lice	Pour-on, dips, sprays, dusts, back rubbers, orals, injectables, feed additives

TABLE 26-3 Common Parasites of Production Animals—cont'd

COMMON NAME/PHOTOGRAPH	SCIENTIFIC NAME	IMPORTANCE	DIAGNOSIS	TREATMENT
SHEEP AND GOATS				
Sucking Lice*: Sheep and Goats				
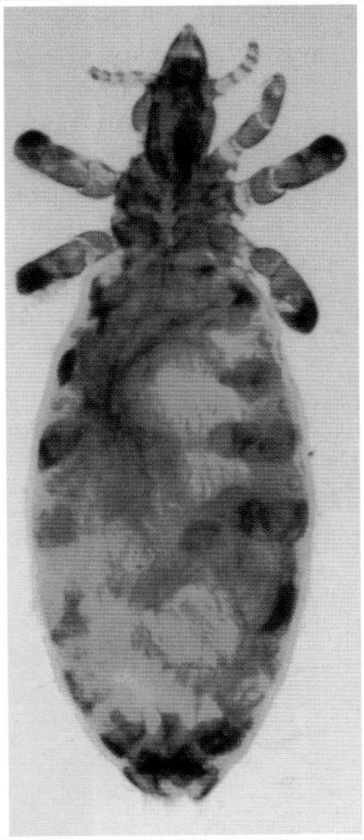	*Linognathus pedalis* (sheep foot louse), *Linognathus ovillus* (sheep face and body louse)	Production losses, may cause anemia Life cycle is about 4 weeks	Identification of eggs, nymphs, adults	Pour-ons, dips, sprays, dusts, back rubbers, orals, injectables, feed additives
Mange Mite or Scab Mite†: Sheep and Goats				
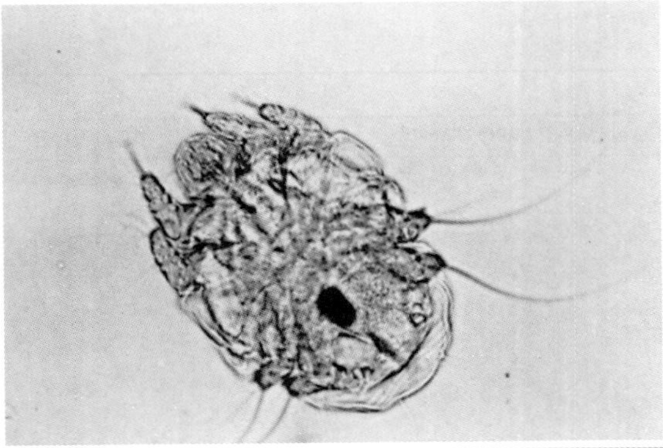	*Psoroptes* spp.	Reportable disease in some states Dramatic weight loss Life cycle is about 3 weeks	Skin scrapings	Pour-ons, dips, sprays, dusts, back rubbers, orals, injectables, feed additives
Mange Mite†: Sheep				
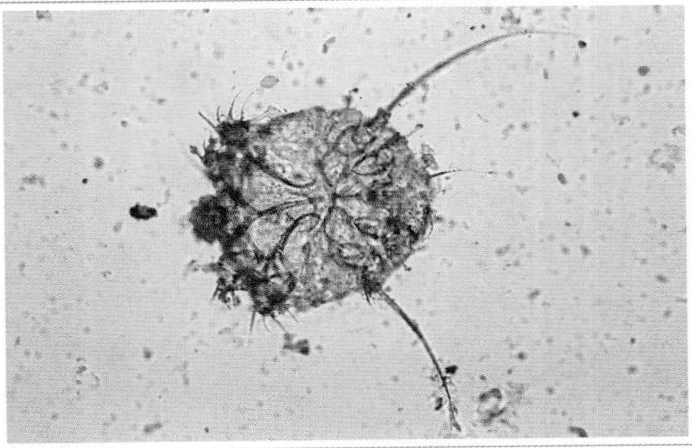	*Sarcoptes scabiei*	Reportable disease in some states Life cycle is about 3 weeks	Skin scrapings	Pour-ons, dips, sprays, dusts, back rubbers, orals, injectables, feed additives

Continued

TABLE 26-3 Common Parasites of Production Animals—cont'd

SHEEP AND GOATS

COMMON NAME/PHOTOGRAPH	SCIENTIFIC NAME	IMPORTANCE	DIAGNOSIS	TREATMENT
Mange Mite[†]: Sheep and Goats				
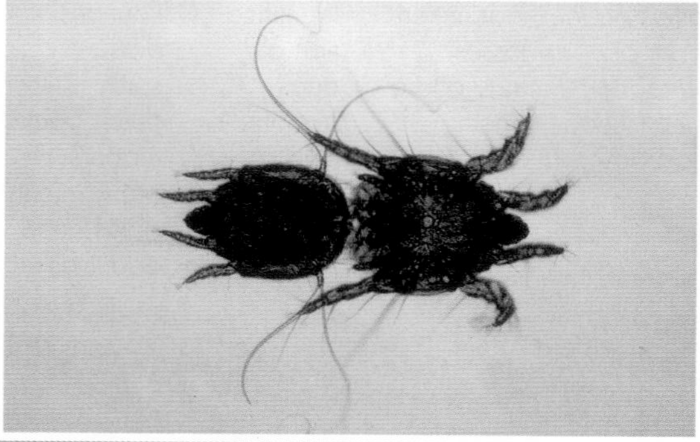	*Chorioptes* spp.	Reportable disease in cattle in some states Causes tail or foot mange	Skin scrapings	Pour-ons, dips, sprays, dusts, back rubbers, orals, injectables, feed additives
Sheep Ked, Erroneously Called a Sheep Tick[†]: Sheep				
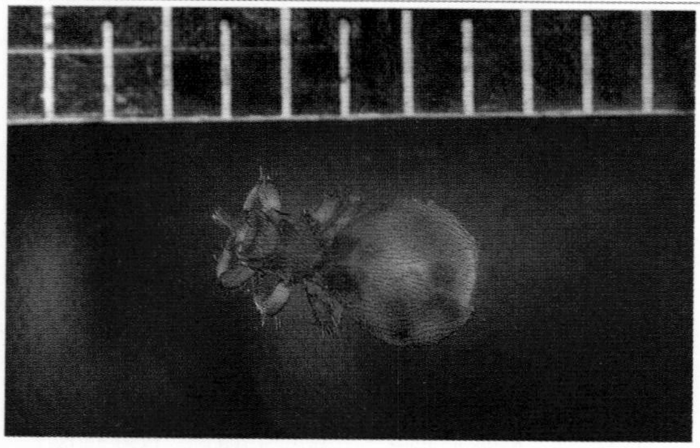	*Melophagus ovinus*	Skin irritation, anemia, weight loss, wool loss Life cycle is about 3 months Adults live about 3 months	Visual observation	Trichlorphon, fenchlorphos, coumaphos, crotoxyphos, tetrachlorvinphos, phosmet

SWINE

COMMON NAME/PHOTOGRAPH	SCIENTIFIC NAME	IMPORTANCE	DIAGNOSIS	TREATMENT
Mange Mite[*]				
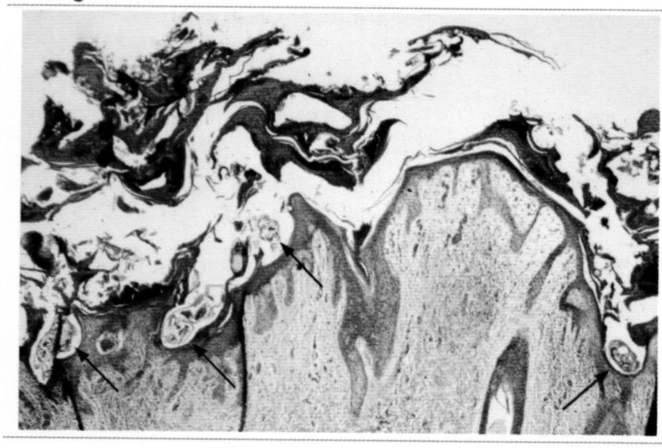	*Sarcoptes scabiei*	Most common clinical indication is pruritus Life cycle is 3 weeks	Skin scrapings	Ivermectin

TABLE 26-3 Common Parasites of Production Animals—cont'd

SWINE				
COMMON NAME/PHOTOGRAPH	SCIENTIFIC NAME	IMPORTANCE	DIAGNOSIS	TREATMENT
Hog Louse*				
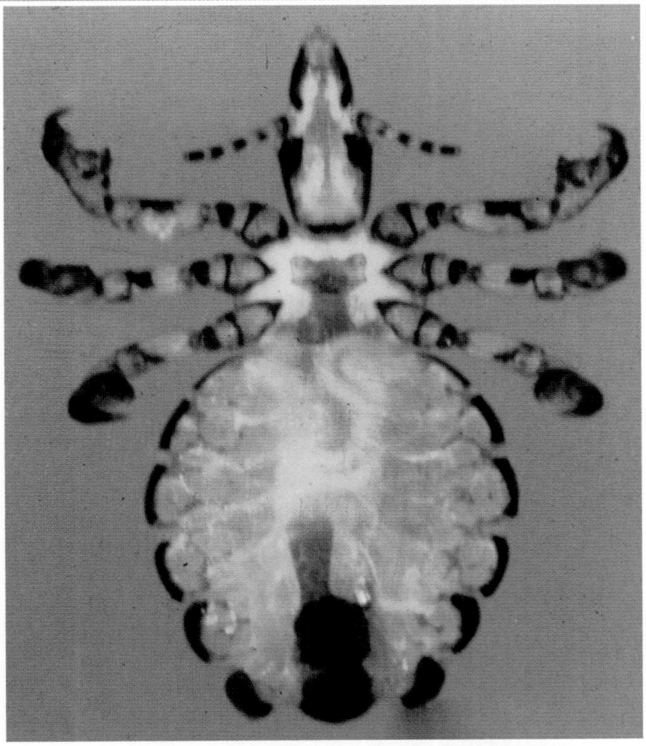 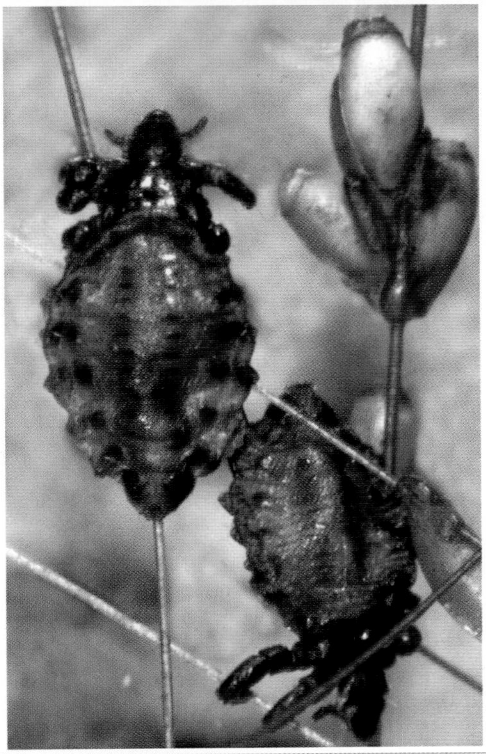	*Haematopinus suis*	Most common clinical indication is pruritus Life cycle is 3–4 weeks	Examination of skin for lice	Amitraz, ivermectin

Continued

TABLE 26-3 Common Parasites of Production Animals—cont'd

SWINE				
COMMON NAME/PHOTOGRAPH	**SCIENTIFIC NAME**	**IMPORTANCE**	**DIAGNOSIS**	**TREATMENT**
Roundworm*				
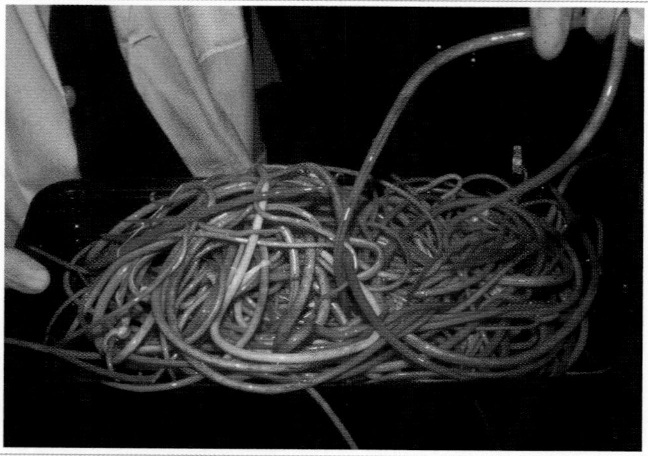	*Ascaris suum*	Reduced weight gain, stunted growth, abdominal breathing, referred to as "thumps" Prepatent period is 8 weeks *Zoonotic:* Contracted through ingestion of larvated eggs	Eggs in fecal flotation Presence of worms in intestine or "milk spots" in liver at necropsy	Ivermectin, fenbendazole, dichlorvos, doramectin, hygromycin, levamisole, piperazine
Whipworm*				
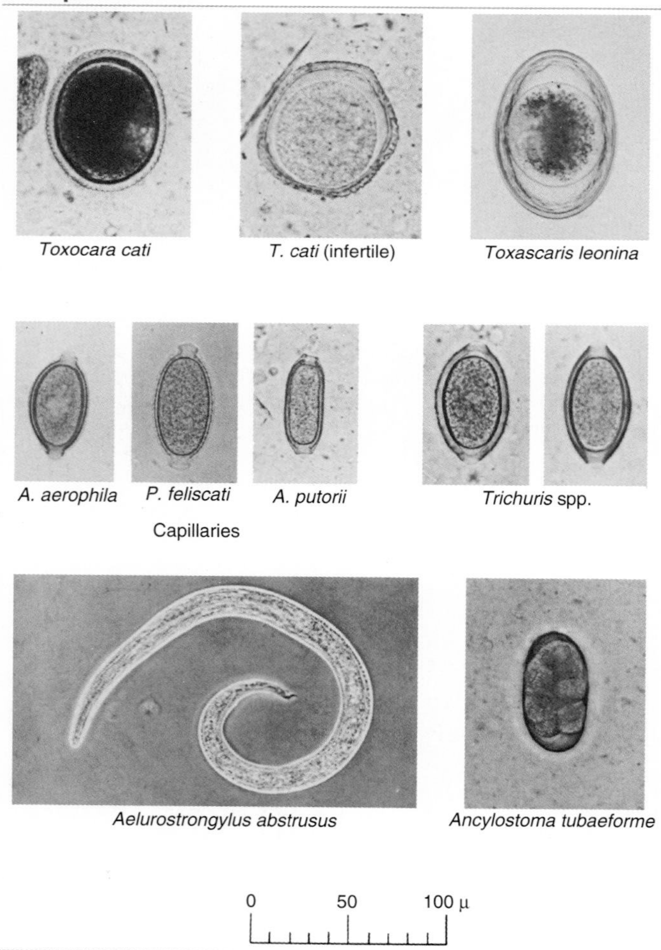	*Trichuris suis*	Diarrhea and unthriftiness Prepatent period is 6 weeks	Eggs in fecal flotation Presence of adults in large intestine at necropsy	Ivermectin, dichlorvos, levamisole, fenbendazole, hygromycin

TABLE 26-3 Common Parasites of Production Animals—cont'd

SWINE				
COMMON NAME/PHOTOGRAPH	**SCIENTIFIC NAME**	**IMPORTANCE**	**DIAGNOSIS**	**TREATMENT**
Threadworm†				
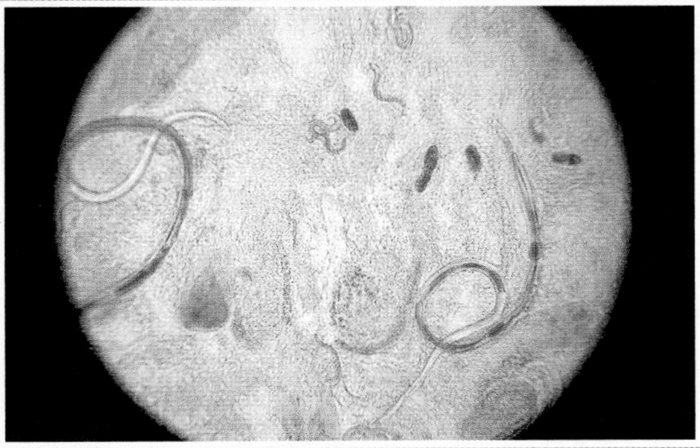	*Strongyloides ransomi*	Severe diarrhea develops between 10 and 14 days of age, with high mortality Prepatent period is 7 days	Fecal flotation Direct observation of mucosal scrapings at necropsy	Ivermectin, fenbendazole, hygromycin, dichlorvos
Coccidia*				
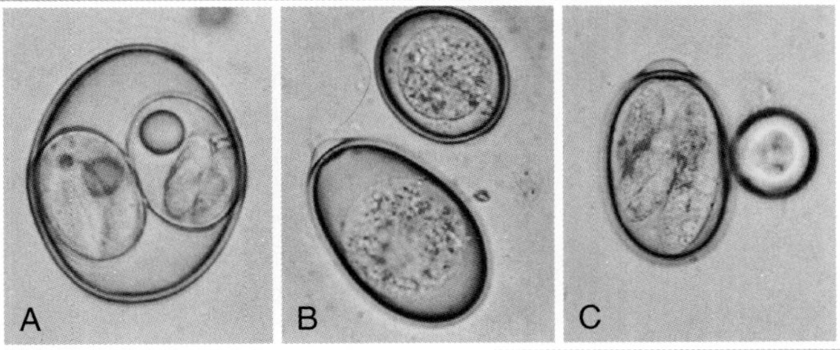	*Eimeria* spp.	In piglets heavy infestations may cause significant enterocolitis Prepatent period is 2 weeks	Oocysts in fecal flotation Oocysts in intestines seen histologically	Sulfamethazine to piglets Decoquinate to sows
Coccidia†				
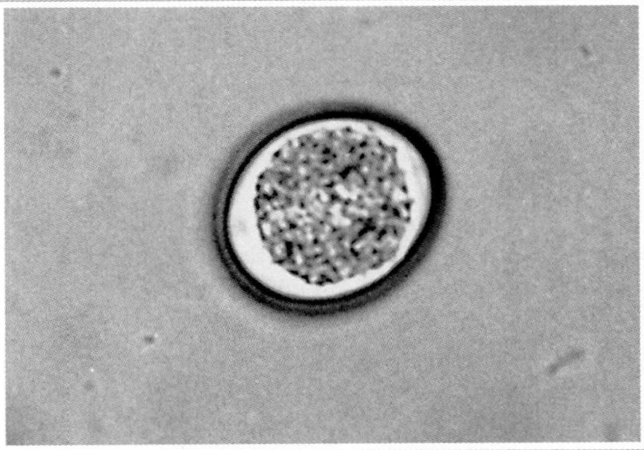	*Cystoisospora suis*	Common in piglets 6–21 days of age Piglets often are stunted, and mortality can be seen Prepatent period is 2 weeks	Oocysts in fecal flotation Oocysts in intestines seen histologically	Sulfamethazine to piglets Decoquinate to sows
Lungworm†				
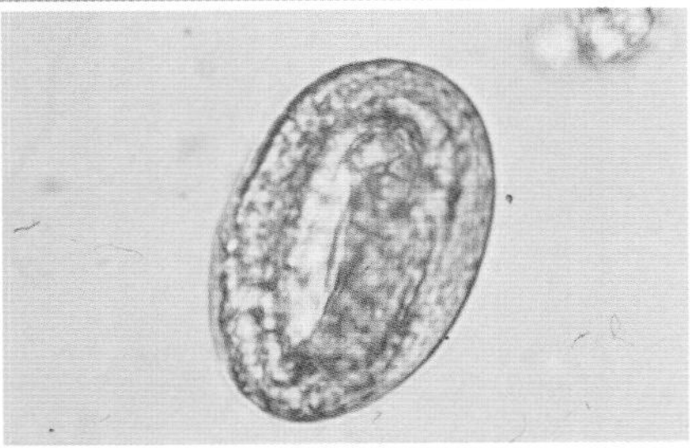	*Metastrongylus* spp.	Coughing, poor growth Prepatent period is 1 month	Larvated eggs in fecal flotation Adults found in lungs at necropsy	Ivermectin, doramectin, fenbendazole, levamisole

Continued

TABLE 26-3 Common Parasites of Production Animals—cont'd

SWINE				
COMMON NAME/PHOTOGRAPH	**SCIENTIFIC NAME**	**IMPORTANCE**	**DIAGNOSIS**	**TREATMENT**
Nodular Worm† 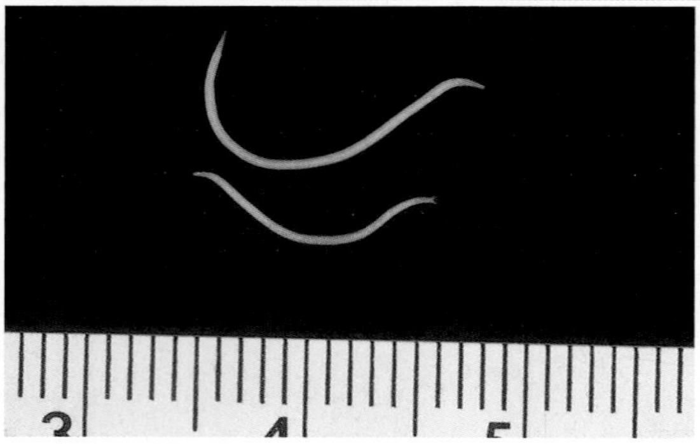	*Oesophagostomum dentatum*	Nodules in gut wall may cause enteritis; however, most infections are asymptomatic Can result in condemnation of intestines at slaughter Prepatent period is 40 days	Eggs in fecal flotation Adults in large intestine at necropsy	Ivermectin, doramectin, levamisole, fenbendazole, pyrantel tartrate, hygromycin, dichlorvos
Stomach Worm† 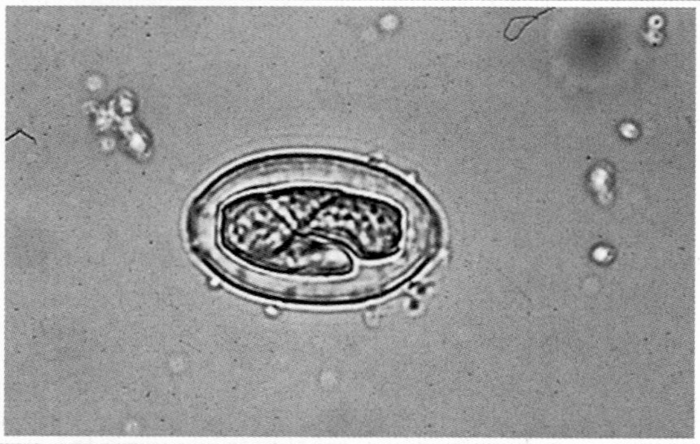	*Ascarops strongylina*	Dung beetle is intermediate host Nonpathogenic unless present in large numbers Prepatent period is 6 weeks	Fecal sedimentation shows embryonated ova Adults found in stomach at necropsy	Ivermectin, doramectin, dichlorvos
Swine Kidney Worm† 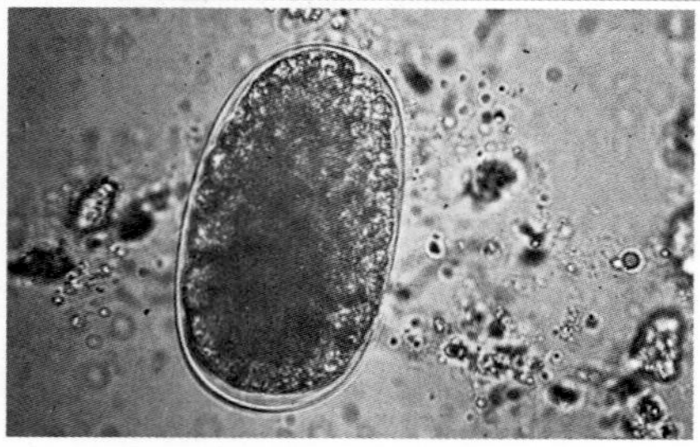	*Stephanurus dentatus*	Loss of weight Condemnation of organs and tissues affected by migrating larvae Prepatent period is 8–16 months	Eggs may be found in urine Adults found in cysts in perirenal fat and pelvis of kidney at necropsy Larvae can be found in liver	Ivermectin, doramectin

TABLE 26-3 Common Parasites of Production Animals—cont'd

SWINE				
COMMON NAME/PHOTOGRAPH	**SCIENTIFIC NAME**	**IMPORTANCE**	**DIAGNOSIS**	**TREATMENT**
Trichina Worm†				
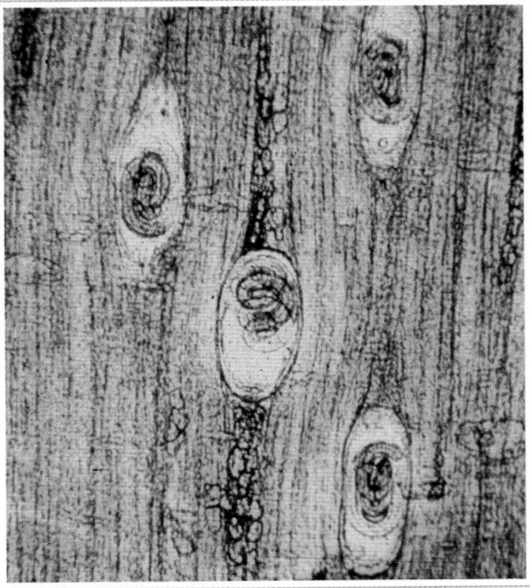	*Trichinella spiralis*	Twenty days for larvae to be infective Larvae to adults in 4 days *Zoonotic:* Infection occurs through ingestion of raw meat	Antemortem diagnosis in animals is rare	No treatment for pigs Do not feed uncooked garbage to pigs; cook all meat to recommended temperatures and for recommended times
Pork Tapeworm				
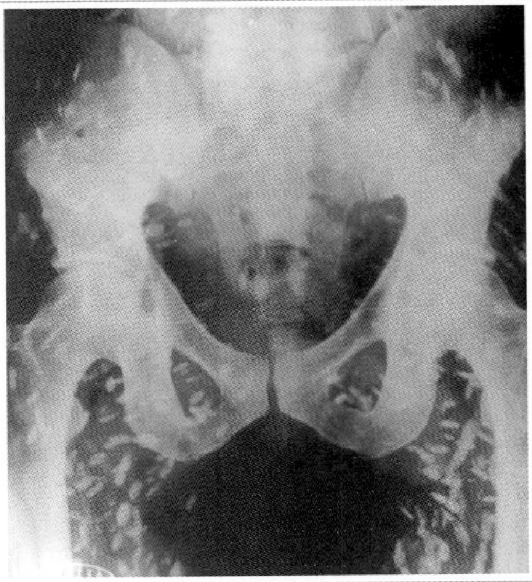	*Taenia solium*	No major pathogenicity to pigs Prepatent period is 2 months *Zoonotic:* Causes taeniasis, cysticercosis Infection occurs through ingestion of raw meat	Observation of cysticerci in pigs at necropsy Serologic tests in humans, pigs Eggs in feces of infected humans	No treatment for pigs Prevent pigs from ingesting human feces; cook all meat to recommended temperatures and for recommended times
Balantidium Coli†				
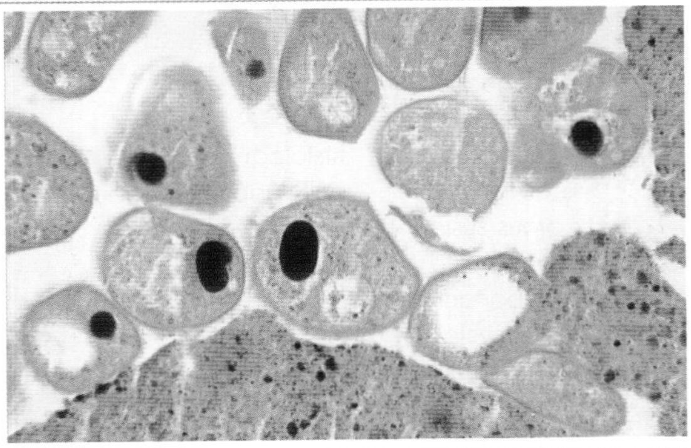	*Balantidium coli*	Mild to severe enteritis Life cycle is 6–14 days Zoonotic	Clinical signs and large numbers of organisms in fecal flotation or smear Lesions seen at necropsy	Tetracycline

Continued

TABLE 26-3 Common Parasites of Production Animals—cont'd

CAMELIDS				
COMMON NAME/PHOTOGRAPH	**SCIENTIFIC NAME**	**IMPORTANCE**	**DIAGNOSIS**	**TREATMENT**
Biting Lice*				
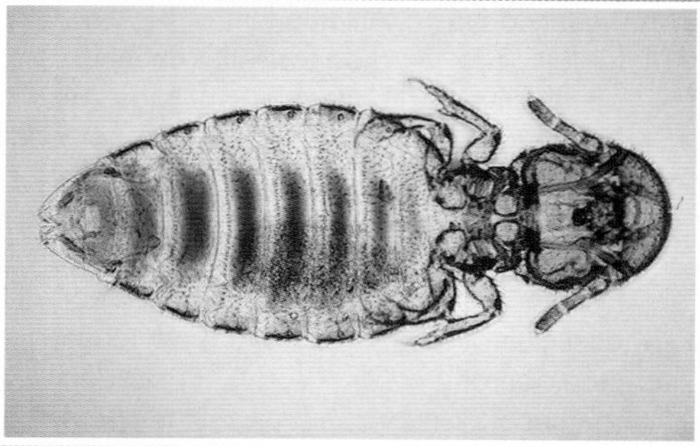	*Damalinia Bovicola* spp.	Often affects llamas during winter Itching and hair loss are often seen Life cycle is approximately 3 weeks	Direct observation of hair	Ivermectin, coumaphos, fenvalerate
Sucking Lice				
	Microthoracius spp.	Often affects llamas during winter Itching and hair loss are often seen Life cycle is approximately 3 weeks	Direct observation of hair	Ivermectin, coumaphos, fenvalerate
Sarcoptic Mange Mite*				
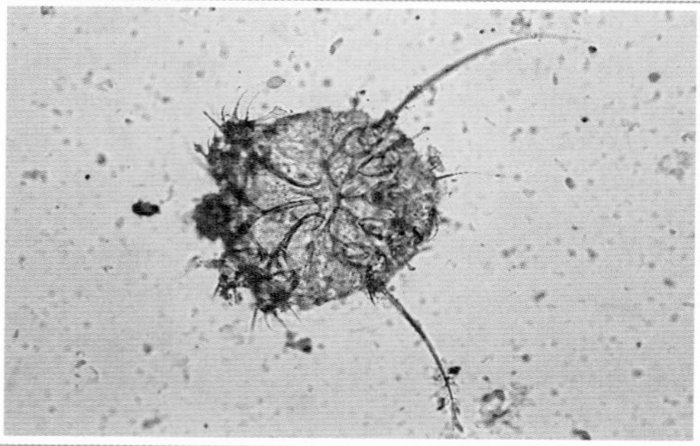	*Sarcoptes scabiei*	Itching and hair loss Life cycle is approximately 3 weeks	Skin scrapings	Ivermectin, doramectin
Meningeal Worm or Brain Worm†				
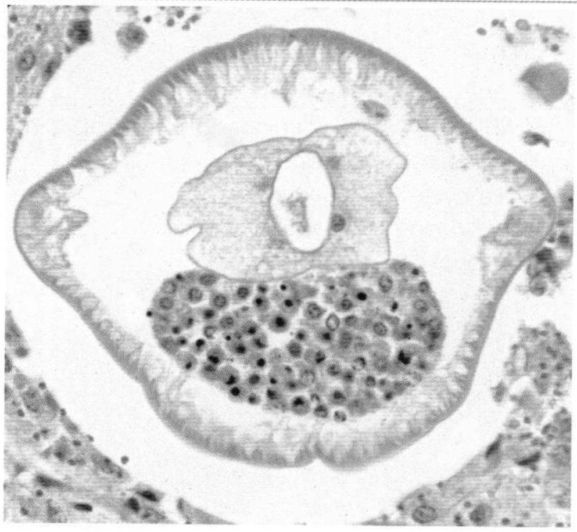	*Parelaphostrongylus tenuis*	Found in white-tailed deer in eastern United States and Canada Causes severe inflammation of central nervous system Snails are important in life cycle Death usually occurs 30–60 days after infection	Evaluation of central nervous system fluid Eosinophilia Seen histologically upon necropsy in brain and spinal cord	Ivermectin

TABLE 26-3 Common Parasites of Production Animals—cont'd

COMMON NAME/PHOTOGRAPH	SCIENTIFIC NAME	IMPORTANCE	DIAGNOSIS	TREATMENT
CAMELIDS				
Strongyles*				
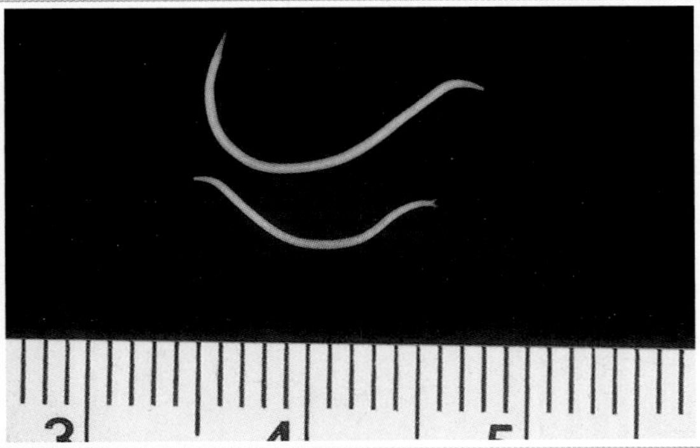	*Camelostrongylus, Cooperia, Haemonchus, Oesophagostomum, Ostertagia, Trichostrongylus*		Eggs in fecal flotation	Ivermectin, doramectin, fenbendazole, levamisole, mebendazole, pyrantel pamoate
Whipworm				
	Trichuris tenuis	Prepatent period is 17–36 days	Eggs in fecal flotation	Ivermectin, doramectin, fenbendazole
Capillary Worm*				
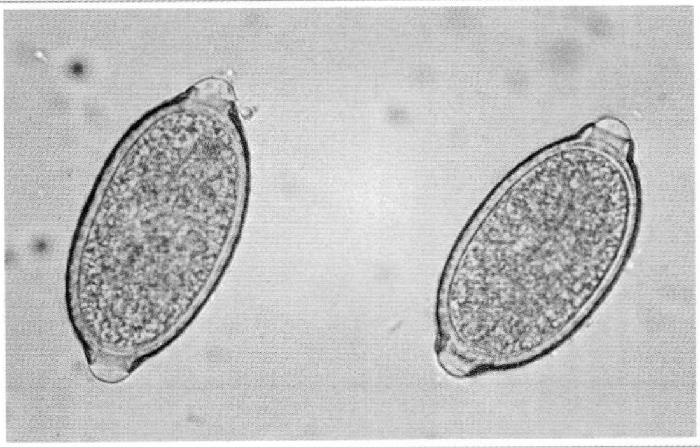	*Capillaria* spp.	Commonly seen at necropsy	Eggs in fecal flotation	Ivermectin, doramectin, fenbendazole
Thin-Necked Intestinal Worm				
	Nematodirus battus, Nematodirus helvetianus	Common in young camelids Prepatent period is 2–3 weeks	Eggs in fecal flotation	Ivermectin, doramectin, fenbendazole, levamisole, mebendazole, pyrantel pamoate

Continued

TABLE 26-3 Common Parasites of Production Animals—cont'd

CAMELIDS				
COMMON NAME/PHOTOGRAPH	**SCIENTIFIC NAME**	**IMPORTANCE**	**DIAGNOSIS**	**TREATMENT**
Coccidia†				
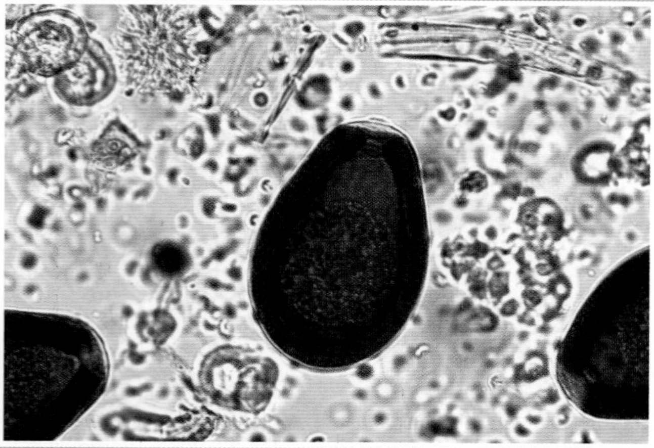	*Eimeria lamae, Eimeria alpacae, Eimeria macusaniensis, Eimeria punoensis*	Common in young camelids Prepatent period in order: 15–16 days, 16–18 days, 33–34 days, 10 days	Oocysts in fecal flotation	Sulfaguanidine, decoquinate, lasalocid, monensin
Crypto*				
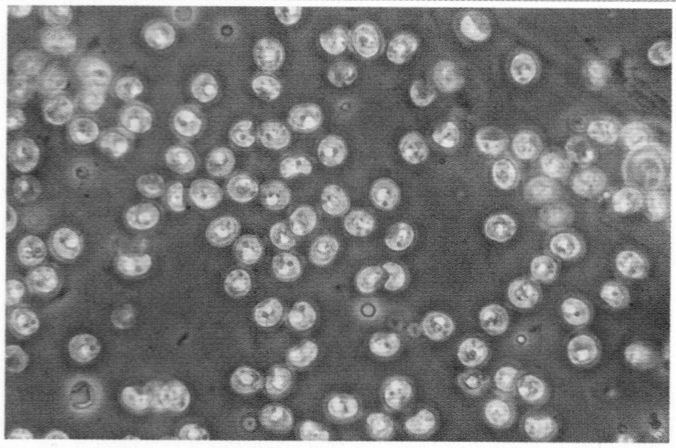	*Cryptosporidium* spp.	Diarrhea Prepatent period is 3–7 days Zoonotic	Oocysts in fecal flotation	None

Note: Some photographs are not of the exact species listed but of similar species.
ELISA, enzyme-linked immunosorbent assay.
*Figure from Bowman DD: *Georgis' Parasitology for veterinarians,* ed 9, St Louis, 2009, WB Saunders.
†From Hendrix CM, Robinson E: *Diagnostic parasitology for veterinary technicians,* ed 3, St Louis, 2006, Mosby.
Table modified from Holtgrew-Bohling, Kristin. *Large animal clinical procedures for veterinary technicians,* ed 3, St Louis, 2016, Mosby.

TABLE 26-4 Bovine Vaccinations*

DISEASE/VACCINATION	CALVES	REPLACEMENTS	FEEDLOT CATTLE	ADULTS	COMMENTS
Anthrax	In the face of outbreak, by state or federal permission	In the face of outbreak, by state or federal permission	In the face of outbreak, by state or federal permission	In the face of outbreak, by state or federal permission	
Bang vaccination	Heifer calves 3-12 months of age				Depends on local and state laws
Bovine respiratory syncytial virus	Weaned calves	Heifers and bulls	Feedlot cattle		
Bovine virus diarrhea type 1 and 2	Calves older than 2 weeks, weaned calves	Heifers and bulls		Cows and bulls	Killed bovine virus diarrhea vaccine must be used in pregnant cows and nursing calves
Clostridial bacteria	Calves older than 10 days, weaned calves	Heifers and bulls	Feedlot cattle	Cows and bulls	Known as 5-, 7-, or 8-way vaccines
Infectious bovine rhinotracheitis	Calves older than 2 weeks, weaned calves	Heifers and bulls		Cows	
Leptospirosis		Heifers and bulls		Cows and bulls	
Parainfluenza 3 virus	Calves older than 2 weeks, weaned calves	Heifers and bulls	On arrival	Cows	
Pasteurella	Weaned calves		Feedlot cattle		
Pinkeye	Calves older than 30 days		Feedlot cattle		
Salmonella	Calves older than 2 weeks		Feedlot cattle		Entire dairy herd in the face of an outbreak
Scour vaccine				Cows 30 days before calving	
Somnus		Heifers and bulls	Feedlot cattle		
Trichomonas				Cows and bulls before breeding	
Vibrio		Heifers and bulls		Cows and bulls before breeding	

*Vaccination protocols should be designed specific to producers by veterinarians.
From Holtgrew-Bohling K: *Large animal clinical procedures for veterinary technicians*, ed 2, St Louis, 2012, Mosby.

TABLE 26-5 Sheep Vaccinations*

DISEASE/VACCINATION	EWES	LAMBS	FEEDLOT LAMBS	RAMS	COMMENTS
Clostridium perfringens type C	4-6 weeks before parturition If animals have never been vaccinated, twice 4 weeks apart with last dose 4-6 weeks before parturition	If born to unvaccinated ewe, at birth and booster in 4-6 weeks Lambs from vaccinated ewes should be vaccinated at 12-16 weeks and booster given in 4-6 weeks	Upon entering feedlot and booster in 2-4 weeks	Annually	

Continued

TABLE 26-5 Sheep Vaccinations—cont'd

DISEASE/VACCINATION	EWES	LAMBS	FEEDLOT LAMBS	RAMS	COMMENTS
Clostridium perfringens type D	4-6 weeks before parturition If animals have never been vaccinated, twice 4 weeks apart with last dose 4-6 weeks before parturition	If born to unvaccinated ewe, at birth and booster in 4-6 weeks Lambs from vaccinated ewes should be vaccinated at 12-16 weeks and booster given in 4-6 weeks	Upon entering feedlot and booster in 2-4 weeks	Annually	
Clostridium tetani	Can be given during pregnancy with *Clostridium* types C and D	At time of castration and tail docking	Annually	Annually	Often combined with *Clostridium* types C and D
Other clostridial diseases (black disease, blackleg, malignant edema, struck, lamb dysentery, botulism)	4-6 weeks before parturition If animals have never been vaccinated, twice 4 weeks apart with last dose 4 weeks before parturition	If born to unvaccinated ewe, at birth and booster in 4-6 weeks Lambs from vaccinated ewes should be vaccinated at 12-16 weeks and booster given in 4-6 weeks	Annually	Annually	Primarily used only in high-risk herds
Leptospirosis					Primarily used only in high-risk herds
Sore mouth	At least 2 months before parturition, booster every 5-12 months depending on risk	1-2 days of age, booster every 5-12 months depending on risk	4 weeks before risk, booster every 5-12 months depending on risk	4 weeks before risk, booster every 5-12 months depending on risk	Live virus Vaccinated sheep can spread the disease for up to 8 weeks after vaccination Use in infected herds only Performed by scratching skin in area without wool (inner ear or under tail in adults and inner thigh in young animals) and then brushing on the vaccine Sores will form at application site
Foot rot	4 weeks before lambing, booster every 4-6 months	4 weeks of age, booster in 4-8 weeks	4 weeks before wet/rainy season, booster every 4-6 months	4 weeks before wet/rainy season, booster every 4-6 months	Vaccinate behind the ear Only reduces infection levels Abscesses are not uncommon, discoloration of the wool at the injection site Booster in 4 weeks from first time of vaccination

TABLE 26-5 Sheep Vaccinations—cont'd

DISEASE/VACCINATION	EWES	LAMBS	FEEDLOT LAMBS	RAMS	COMMENTS
Caseous lymphadenitis	Annually	Annually	Annually	Annually	Primarily used only in high-risk or infected herds Booster in 4 weeks after the first dose
Enzootic abortion in ewes (EAE)	4 weeks before breeding **Do not use in pregnant ewes**				Primarily used only in high-risk or infected herds
Toxoplasma	4 weeks before breeding **Do not use in pregnant ewes** Booster every 2 years				Primarily in only high-risk or infected herds. Vaccine is not available in the United States.
Vibriosis	Annually, 2 weeks before breeding Booster in mid-pregnancy if first vaccination				Primarily used only in high-risk herds
Brucellosis				Rams test positive if vaccinated	
Rabies					Common in pet sheep and possibly in endemic areas
Escherichia coli	4-6 weeks before parturition If animals have never been vaccinated, twice 4 weeks apart	If ewes were unvaccinated, oral antibody can be given at birth			Primarily used only if diarrhea in 1- to 2-day-old lambs is a problem

*Vaccination protocols should be designed specific to producers by veterinarians.
From Holtgrew-Bohling K: *Large animal clinical procedures for veterinary technicians*, ed 2, St Louis, 2012, Mosby.

TABLE 26-6 Goat Vaccinations*

DISEASE/VACCINATION	COMMENTS
Clostridium perfringens types C and D	Use as in sheep
Clostridium tetani	Use as in sheep
Escherichia coli	Use as in sheep, primarily only in high-risk herds
Foot rot	Use as in sheep
Pasteurella	Use as in sheep, primarily only in high-risk herds
Leptospirosis	Primarily used only in high-risk herds
Caseous lymphadenitis	U.S. Food and Drug Administration does not recommend use of the vaccine in goats
Rabies	Use as in sheep, primarily used only in high-risk herds
Enzootic abortion in ewes (EAE)	Use as in sheep, primarily used only in high-risk herds; goats are more sensitive

*Vaccination protocols should be designed specific to producers by veterinarians. These vaccines are used off label.
From Holtgrew-Bohling K: *Large animal clinical procedures for veterinary technicians*, ed 2, St Louis, 2012, Mosby.

TABLE 26-7 Swine Vaccinations*

DISEASE/VACCINATION	PIGLETS	WEANLINGS	REPLACEMENT	BREEDING STOCK
Atrophic rhinitis	7-10 days of age		Gilts and boars	Sows
Mycoplasma	7-10 days of age			Sows
Erysipelas	Preweaning	Postweaning	Gilts and boars	Sows
Contagious pleuropneumonia		Weanlings		
Leptospirosis			Gilts and boars	Sows and boars
Parvovirus			Gilts	
Transmissible gastroenteritis			Gilts	Sows
Escherichia coli		Weanlings		Sows
Glasser disease		Weanlings		

*Vaccination protocols are designed by veterinarians specific to producers.
From Holtgrew-Bohling K: *Large animal clinical procedures for veterinary technicians,* ed 2, St Louis, 2012, Mosby.

TABLE 26-8 Camelid Vaccinations*

DISEASE/VACCINATION	CRIAS	JILLS	ADULTS
Clostridium vaccines	Crias	4 weeks before parturition	All adults
Leptospirosis			All adults
Rhinopneumonitis			All adult
Infectious bovine rhinotracheitis			All adults exposed to cattle
Bovine virus diarrhea			All adults exposed to cattle
Ovine enzootic abortion			All adults exposed to sheep
Rabies	Crias at 3-6 months		All adults in endemic areas

*Vaccination protocols should be designed specific to producers by veterinarians.
From Holtgrew-Bohling K: *Large animal clinical procedures for veterinary technicians,* ed 2, St Louis, 2012, Mosby.

REVIEW QUESTIONS

Matching

Match the described animal type with its associated term.

_______**1.** adult intact male ovine
_______**2.** male adult bovine
_______**3.** young caprines
_______**4.** adult female porcine
_______**5.** young camelid
_______**6.** adult intact male caprine
_______**7.** castrated male porcine
_______**8.** female adult bovine
_______**9.** castrated male ovines/caprines
_______**10.** adult female caprine
_______**11.** male castrated bovine
_______**12.** young ovine
_______**13.** female young adult bovine
_______**14.** young porcine
_______**15.** intact adult male porcine
_______**16.** adult female ovine
_______**17.** young female porcine before farrowing

A. gilts
B. bull
C. piglets
D. doe
E. lambs
F. sow
G. heifer
H. buck/ram
I. boar
J. cria
K. kids
L. billy/ram
M. steer
N. ewe
O. barrow
P. wether
Q. cow

Fill in the chart

Select the appropriate needle or indwelling catheter size from the list below to be used for the species and procedures in the chart.

Animal Species	IM Injection	SC Injection	IV Injection	IV Blood Draw	IV Catheter
Cow					
Bull					
Goat					
Sheep					
Newborn Calf/ Lamb/ Kid					
Pig					
Piglet					
Llama					

Needle Sizes: 14-, 16-, 18-, 20-, 22-, 23-, 25-, 26-gauge (ga)
Needle Lengths: ⅜, ⅝, ¾, 1, 1.5, 2, 3, 4, 6 inch
Catheter Sizes: 14 ga × 2 inch; 16 ga × 2 inch; 18 ga × 2 inch; 20 ga × 2 inch; 22 ga × 2 inch; 16 ga × 6 inch; 18 ga × 6 inch; 20 ga × 6 inch

RECOMMENDED READING

Anderson D, Rings M: *Current veterinary therapy: food animal practice*, ed 5, St Louis, 2008, Saunders.

Cebra C, et al.: *Llama and alpaca care: medicine, surgery, reproduction, nutrition, and herd health*, St Louis, 2013, Saunders.

Fowler ME: *Medicine and surgery of South American camelids*, ed 2, Ames, IA, 1998, Iowa State University Press.

Holtgrew-Bohling K: *Large animal clinical procedures for veterinary technicians*, ed 2, St Louis, 2012, Mosby.

Jensen J, et al.: *Husbandry and medical management of ostriches, emus and rheas*, College Station, TX, 1996, Wildlife and Exotic Animal Consultants.

Pugh DG, Baird AN: *Sheep and goat medicine*, ed 2, St Louis, 2011, Mosby.

Radostits OM, et al.: *Herd health: food animal production medicine*, ed 3, St Louis, 2001, Saunders.

Smith BP: *Large animal internal medicine*, ed 5, St Louis, 2014, Mosby.

Smith MC, Sherman DM: *Goat medicine*, ed 2, Ames, IA, 2009, Wiley-Blackwell.

Tully TN: *Handbook of avian medicine*, ed 2, St Louis, 2009, Saunders.

Tully TN, Shane SM: *Ratite management, medicine, and surgery*, Malabar, FL, 1996, Krieger Publishing.

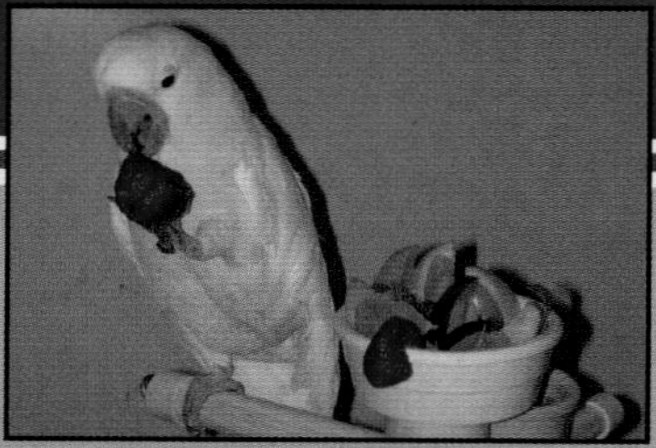

27 Nursing Care of Companion Birds, Reptiles, and Amphibians

OUTLINE

LEARNING OBJECTIVES

After reviewing this chapter, the reader will be able to:

1. Describe the unique features of the anatomy of birds and basic biology of common reptile species.
2. Discuss the basic behavior of birds, reptiles, and amphibians.
3. Discuss the basics of client education, husbandry, and nutrition for the avian, reptile, and amphibian species.
4. Describe how to obtain a complete and thorough history of the avian, reptile, and amphibian patient.
5. Explain the different capture and restraint techniques used for birds, reptiles, and amphibians.
6. Identify methods of sample collection for laboratory analysis.
7. Describe how to obtain quality diagnostic images of avian reptile and amphibian patients.
8. Discuss nursing care and supportive therapy techniques for the avian, reptile, and amphibian patient.
9. Identify and discuss some of the common diseases and presentations of the avian, reptile, and amphibian patient to the veterinary clinic.
10. List the common infectious diseases and zoonoses found in the avian, reptile, and amphibian patient.
11. Describe the routine clinical procedures performed on avian, reptile, and amphibian species.
12. Explain the unique aspects of avian, reptile, and amphibian anesthesia and surgery.
13. Identify and discuss some of the common presentations, emergencies, and critical care.

KEY TERMS

Air sacs
Anisodactyl
Apteria
Basal metabolic rate (BMR)
Cere
Choana
Choanal papillae
Cloaca
Coelom
Columella
Contour feathers
Coprodeum
Coverts
Crop
Diurnal
Down feathers
Ductus deferens
Gavage
Keel
Maintenance energy requirement
Molting
Mouthing
Nocturnal species
Operculum
Passerines
Pneumatized
Primary flight feathers

KEY TERMS—cont'd

Proctodeum
Proventriculus
Psittacines
Pterylae
Secondary flight feathers
Syrinx
Urates
Urodeum
Uropygial gland
Vent
Ventriculus
Zoonotic diseases

BIRDS

As veterinary medicine becomes more specialized, veterinary technicians with specific expertise are increasingly in demand. The field of avian medicine can be challenging, and most veterinary technicians who are new to the profession will need further training and experience to work with birds. There are many resources available to assist with this including attending seminars and becoming members of various exotic species organizations (Box 27-1). These organizations are indispensable sources of knowledge and information on avian medicine and include an international network of approachable experts in these fields.

The common companion birds seen in a small animal veterinary hospital are typically members of the psittacine or passerine family (Box 27-2). These are distinguished by a number of physical characteristics. **Psittacines,** or parrots, make up the majority of avian patients. The psittacines are known as hookbills because of their curved upper beak. Their feet are shaped with the second and third toes facing forward and the first and fourth toes directed backward. This is referred to as zygodactyl. **Passerines** are usually small birds with a pointed or slightly curved beak. Their feet are **anisodactyl;** three toes point forward and one toe points to the rear. Many of these birds are very active and tend to hop or fly about their cage. Most are not trained to sit on their owner's hand and remain inside their cages. Canaries and finches are the most frequently kept passerines.

BOX 27-1 Professional Exotic Species Associations and Journals

- Academy of Veterinary Technicians in Clinical Practice: http://avtcp.org/
- American Association of Zoo Veterinarians: http://www.aazv.org, *Journal of Zoo and Wildlife Medicine*
- Association of Avian Veterinarians: http://www.aav.org, *Journal of Avian Medicine and Surgery*
- Association of Exotic Mammal Veterinarians: http://www.aemv.org, *Journal of Exotic Pet Medicine*
- Association of Reptilian and Amphibian Veterinarians: http://www.arav.org, *Journal of Herpetological Medicine and Surgery*
- International Association for Aquatic Animal Medicine: http://www.iaaam.org, *AAAM News*
- National Wildlife Rehabilitators Association: http://www.nwrawildlife.org, *Wildlife Rehabilitation Bulletin*
- Wildlife Disease Association: http://www.wildlifedisease.org, *Journal of Wildlife Diseases*

AVIAN ANATOMY

Integument

The integument is the largest and most extensive organ system of the body. It protects the underlying structures and forms a physical barrier between the body and the external world.

The body of a bird is covered by skin and its derivatives: the beak, claws, and feathers.

The skin is very delicate and has a dry, slightly wrinkled appearance. Underlying muscles and blood give the skin a reddish appearance in some areas. The skin on the legs resembles the scales of reptiles. The **cere,** or the area around the nostrils, the beak, and the nails, is all modified skin.

TECHNICIAN NOTE The cere is the fleshy structure around the nares in some birds. In budgerigars the cere is generally blue or pink, smooth in males, and brown and lumpy in females.

BOX 27-2 Common Companion Species Seen in an Avian Practice

Psittacines
- Macaw
- Cockatoo
- Amazon
- African Grey
- Love bird
- Conure
- Parakeet
- Cockatiel
- Caique
- Budgerigar
- Lori
- Lorikeet

Passerines
- Finches
- Canaries

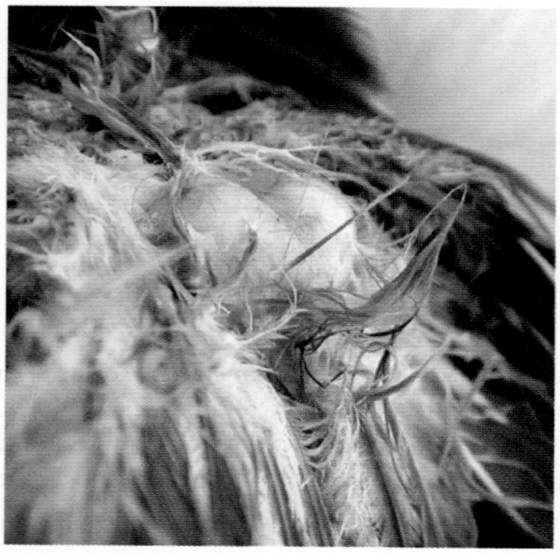

FIGURE 27-1 Uropygial gland of a Meyers parrot located at the base of the tail dorsal to the pygostyle.

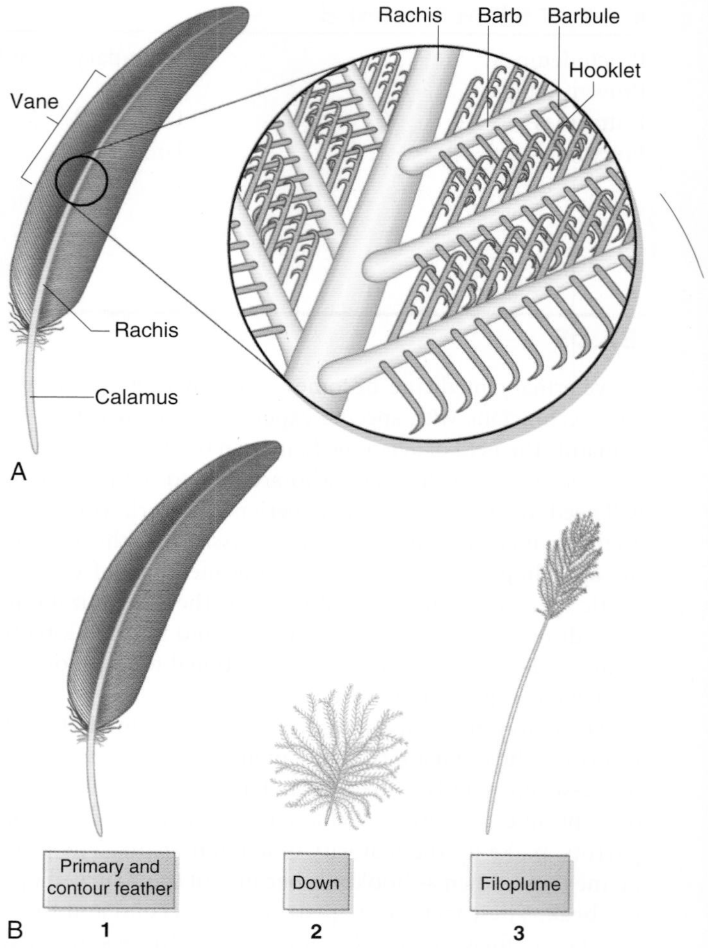

FIGURE 27-2 (A) Feather structure and (B) types of feathers. (From Aspinall V: *The complete textbook of veterinary nursing*, ed 2, St Louis, 2011, Elsevier.)

Sweat glands are absent in birds. The one major skin gland that most birds possess is the **uropygial gland** (Fig. 27-1). This is a bi-lobed gland with one duct opening that empties into a lone papilla, found dorsally at the base of the tail. It secretes a lipoid sebaceous material that is spread over feathers during preening to help with waterproofing. This gland is absent in the ostrich, emu, cassowaries, bustards, frogmouth, many pigeons, woodpeckers, and Amazon parrots.

Feathers are necessary for flight; they protect the skin from trauma and exposure, and assist in thermoregulation, camouflage, and communication. Feather follicles are located in specific tracts over the surface of the body called **pterylae.** These tracts are separated by nonfeathered areas of skin called **apteria.** These tracts overlap each other to give the bird a fully feathered look.

Birds have several types of feathers (Fig. 27-2). The **contour feathers** cover the body and wings and are identified as flight feathers or body feathers. The large, **primary flight feathers** (remiges) are found on the outer end of the wing. The **secondary flight feathers** are located on the wing between the body and the primaries. Body feathers, also known as **coverts,** provide surface coverage over most of the rest of the bird. **Down feathers** insulate the bird and have a soft, fluffy appearance. Cockatoos, cockatiels, and African Greys have powder down, which breaks down to produce a white dusty powder. A healthy bird of these species will have a fine layer of this powder over most of its body and most noticeably on the beak. Birds spend several hours a day preening, or rearranging and conditioning their feathers. **Molting** occurs in all species and results in periodic replacement of old feathers. A new, growing feather has a vascular supply until it reaches full size. The shafts of these "blood feathers" appear dark and bleed profusely if broken, possibly leading to the death of the bird.

Musculoskeletal System

The skeleton of birds is highly modified. Some bones are **pneumatized,** or contain air, which results in a lighter skeleton. The bones have thin walls, which makes them lighter but also more fragile. The skull bones are fused, which strengthens the beak structure. The vertebrae of the neck are shaped in such a way as to create a long, flexible neck. The large sternum, or **keel,** supports the pectoral muscles that are needed for flight. A large portion of the caudal vertebrae is fused to form the synsacrum, which stabilizes the back during flight.

The largest muscles in the body are the pectorals, which account for approximately 20% of the bird's weight. Because of their mass, they are used to determine the body condition of the bird and are ideal for intramuscular injections.

Respiratory System

Birds possess a highly specialized and efficient respiratory system (Fig. 27-3). Air enters the respiratory system through the nares and continues over an **operculum,** which is a cornified flap of tissue located immediately behind the nares in the nasal cavity. Air then travels through the many sinuses in the head, and then enters the oral cavity through the slit-like opening in the roof of the mouth known as the **choana.** The

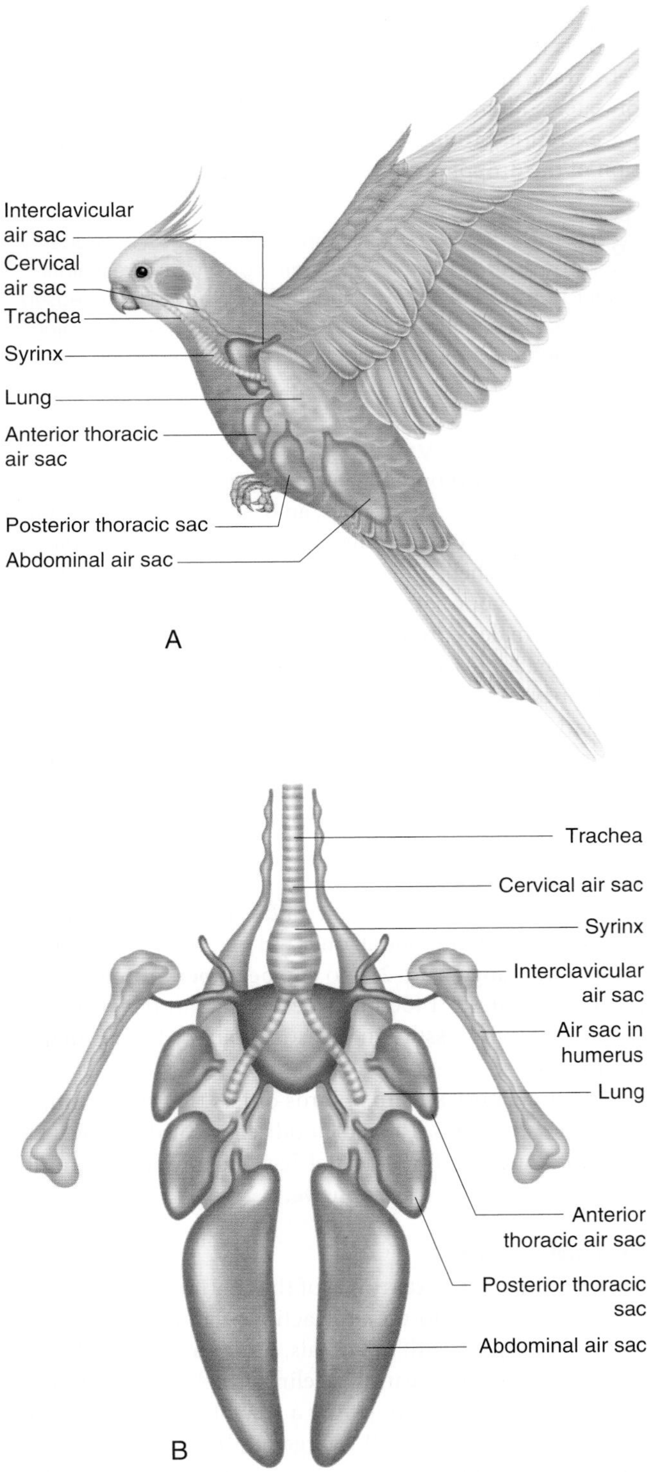

FIGURE 27-3 Respiratory system of a bird. (From Aspinall V: *The complete textbook of veterinary nursing*, ed 2, St Louis, 2011, Elsevier.)

choana is a V-shaped notch in the roof of the bird's mouth that directs air from the mouth and nasal cavities to the glottis. The choana closes during swallowing. This structure should be surrounded by many sharp papillae. If the **choanal papillae** are blunted or absent, this may be indicative of disease or malnutrition.

Birds lack an epiglottis, so air travels through the glottis at the base of the tongue and down the trachea. The trachea is located on the left side of the cervical area, is mobile the entire length of the neck, and consists of complete cartilaginous rings that cannot expand. At the caudal portion of the trachea lies the **syrinx,** and it is the voice box of birds. Birds produce vocalizations by forcing air over the syrinx and vibrating membranes during the expiratory phase of respiration. The complexity of a bird's vocalizations depends on the species and number of muscles in the syrinx.

> *TECHNICIAN NOTE* Birds have complete cartilaginous tracheal rings that cannot expand. Noncuffed endotracheal tubes should be used during anesthesia. If cuffed tubes must be used, the cuff should not be inflated.

The air continues into the small lungs located dorsal near the spine where air exchange takes place. There are no lobes or alveoli, therefore the lungs do not inflate. In the absence of a diaphragm, inspiration of air occurs by extension of the intracostal joints drawing in inspired air with a bellowslike action into the caudal **air sacs.** The **coelom** of a bird is a triangular shaped cavity allowing for the bellowslike action during breathing. Both inspiration and expiration require active muscle contraction.

> *TECHNICIAN NOTE* Birds require the movement of their keel to achieve air exchange. If the keel is not allowed to expand (i.e., as with aggressive restraint) the bird cannot breathe and will go into respiratory arrest, followed closely by cardiac arrest.

Air flows into the air sacs, which are thin walled hollow spaces that are lightly vascularized membranes and are found throughout the bird's body. There are a total of nine air sacs consisting of four paired air sacs: cranial thoracic, caudal thoracic, cervical, and abdominal. The one unpaired air sac is the interclavicular air sac, which is located in the thoracic inlet between the clavicles. Depending on the species, the bird's respiratory tract can communicate with the humerus, femur, clavicles, coracoids, and cervical vertebrae. Gas exchange does not occur in the air sacs. Two complete breath cycles are necessary to move a breath of air completely through the respiratory system. From the caudal air sac the volume of air is pushed into the lungs so that airflow within the lung tissue is predominantly unidirectional, caudal to cranial. Normal respiratory effort in the bird should not be noticeable, and the beak should remain closed. In some cases there may be increased head and tail movement and increased abdominal effort after exercise. The bird should return to normal within a few minutes.

Digestive System

The high metabolism of birds requires ingestion of large amounts of food. The beaks will vary with the diet and foraging strategies. Generally the beak is used to grasp food and crush it with the aid of the tongue. Birds do not have teeth. The mouth consists of a hard upper palate, a soft lower palate, a distinctive tongue, scattered taste buds, and salivary glands. The mouth is relatively dry because little saliva is produced.

When food is swallowed, it travels through the esophagus, a somewhat muscular tube that extends from the pharynx to the stomach along the right side of the neck. In several species the esophagus expands in the interclavicular space to create a **crop.** The crop anatomy varies between species and can be a dilation of the esophagus, a single pouch, or a double pouch. It softens food and allows continuous passage of small amounts of food to the **proventriculus,** or true stomach. The proventriculus is unique to birds; however, it is comparable to the stomach of mammals, containing digestive acid and enzymes.

The food next passes into the **ventriculus,** or gizzard. This is a thickly muscled organ that grinds food into smaller particles. Historically it was thought that companion birds need grit, or small pieces of gravel, in the gizzard to break down hard foods. This is not true and companion birds do not need to be given grit. Grit can be problematic in some birds and they may develop an impaction if they have access to it.

The intestinal tract is comparable to that of mammals (Fig. 27-4). Birds have a pancreas that is a relatively large gland and rests in the loop of the duodenum. The liver is bilobed, with the right side usually larger than the left and produces digestive enzymes and bile. The gallbladder is absent in most parrots but is found in many other avian species. The duodenum or small intestine varies in length and diameter depending on the species and is the major organ responsible for digestion and absorption of nutrients. The large intestine is the segment that extends from the end of the small intestine and terminates at the cloaca.

The **cloaca** is the common terminal chamber of the gastrointestinal, urinary, and reproductive systems. The cloaca is divided in to three compartments: the coprodeum, urodeum, and proctodeum. The **coprodeum** is the cranial portion of the cloaca that receives feces from the rectum. The **urodeum** is the middle part of the cloaca into which the ureters enter dorsolaterally on both sides; in males the **ductus deferens** enters near the ureters, while in females a single oviduct enters the urodeum dorsolaterally on the left side. The **proctodeum** is the caudal part of the cloaca; if a phallus is present, it would be located on the floor of the proctodeum. Psittacines do not have a phallus but it is found in many other avian species.

The external opening of the cloaca is called the **vent,** from which the droppings are passed. In most species the vent is horizontally flattened rather than circumferential as in mammals. Normal bird droppings have three distinct components: liquid urine, semisolid white or cream **urates,** and feces. The droppings will vary in consistency, depending on the diet.

Urinary System

The paired kidneys of birds are closely attached to the vertebrae (see Fig. 27-4, *B*). They empty into the ureters, which carry the liquid urine and semisolid urates to the cloaca. Urine is not concentrated in the kidneys; rather urine moves retrograde into the coprodeum and rectum where resorption of water, sodium, and chloride takes place. Urates are the major excretion product in birds and comprise the white portion of the droppings. Birds do not have a urinary bladder.

> **TECHNICIAN NOTE** Stress droppings—A suddenly stressed bird, such as an avian patient on presentation after transport or an examination, may have an increased urine component to its droppings because the droppings pass before lower intestinal water resorption occurs.

Reproductive System

In the female bird only the left side of the reproductive tract develops fully. As in mammals, an ovary, oviduct, and vagina are present. Various regions of the oviduct produce the egg white and eggshell. The entire process from ovulation to egg laying takes approximately 15 hours. The female lays eggs even if no male is present.

The male bird has paired testes located internally near the kidneys. During periods of active breeding, they enlarge dramatically in size. Sperm cells travel to the cloaca through the epididymis and then the ductus deferens. Most birds do not have a penis or phallus and mating takes place when the vents of the male and female birds come in contact.

Circulatory System

The heart of birds closely resembles that of mammals, but it is proportionally about one and one half times larger. Heart rates range from 250 to 350 beats per minute in large parrots, and up to 1400 beats per minute in the very small species. Blood pressure in birds is typically higher than in mammals.

The circulatory system of birds differs from that of mammals in several ways. The red blood cells of birds are oval and contain a nucleus. Birds do not have lymph nodes, and the lymphatic system is less extensive.

Special Senses

Sensory organs are extensions of the central nervous system that allow animals to monitor actions that occur internally and externally. As with mammals, birds have the traditional five senses: seeing, hearing, feeling, smelling, and tasting. The term "bird brain," implying a small brain, is misleading because the brain of a bird is large in proportion to its body size. The location and control centers within the brain that receive and process stimuli from the senses are comparable to mammals, with a couple of exceptions. In birds the control centers for vision and hearing are larger than those for taste, touch, and smell.

Vision is highly developed in the avian species. The eyes of birds are relatively large, and a significant part of the avian skull is devoted to housing and protecting the eyes (Fig. 27-5). The shape of the eyes is determined by the orbits. Bird eyes can be round, flat, or tubular, depending on the

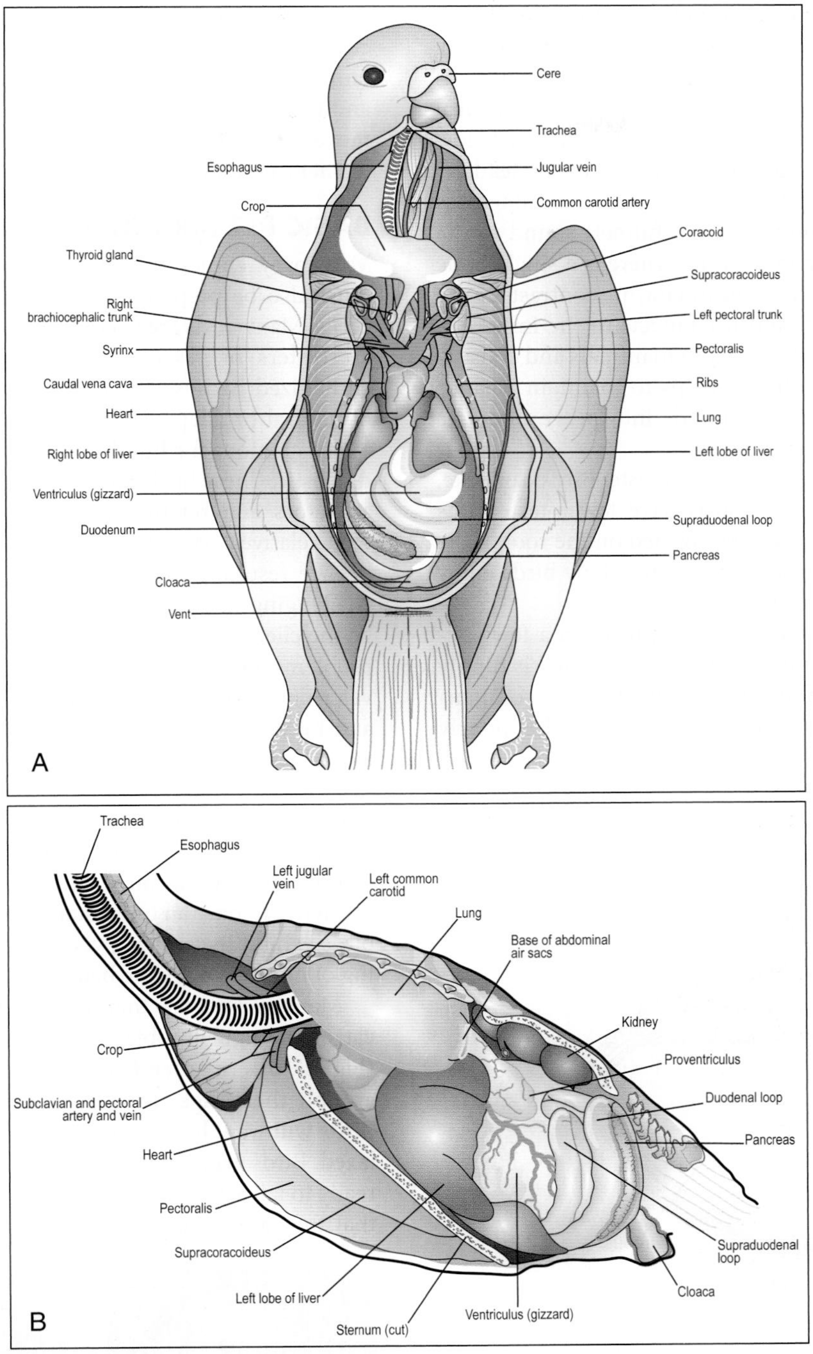

FIGURE 27-4 A, Internal anatomy of a bird, ventrodorsal view. B, Internal anatomy of a bird, lateral view. (From O'Malley B: *Clinical anatomy and physiology of exotic species*, Oxford, 2005, Saunders.)

species. **Diurnal** birds (birds that forage or hunt in the daytime) have round or relatively flat eyes, whereas **nocturnal species** (those that forage and hunt at night) have tubular eyes. Tubular eyes have a pupil with a larger diameter than the retina allowing more light into the eye.

The lens and anterior chamber of the avian eye are comparable to those of mammals with the exception of the presence of a highly vascular, ribbonlike structure called the pecten. The pecten is believed to provide nutrition to the eye.

Bird vision is very acute and they can perceive color. Birds often look closely at something with one eye, tilting their head for a better view. In many species the color of the iris is darker in young birds. The iris contains striated muscles that allow voluntary control over the size of the pupils. Thus pupillary light response is not a good diagnostic indicator in birds; however, this should always be part of a thorough physical examination. Blinking is done using the nictitating membrane, or third eyelid. This structure is mostly transparent. Most birds completely close their eyes when they sleep.

Hearing is an extremely important sense for birds. Hearing can be critical for hiding from predators, defending territories, communication, and finding food. The avian ear is simpler than in mammals, but has exceptional acoustical ability. Located on the sides of the head and slightly below the eyes, the ears of birds are hidden from view by feathers that protect the ear during flight and yet allow sound to pass through. The external auditory canal funnels sound to the middle ear and tympanic membrane. There is a single bone in the middle ear called the **columella,** in contrast to the three bones in mammals, and it connects to the inner ear. The inner ear is comparable to that in mammals and consists of a membranous labyrinth that helps to maintain balance and equilibrium and converts sounds into nerve impulses that are sent to the brain.

Birds have a relatively poor sense of taste. Birds can taste, but it is unknown how well. Birds have fewer taste buds than most mammals and these are located on the roof of the mouth and scattered over the soft palate. Many birds enjoy eating highly spiced or sweet foods.

The sense of smell varies greatly in bird. In a few species such as the turkey vulture, the sense of smell is highly developed for locating food, but in the average companion species it is thought that the sense of smell is poorly developed.

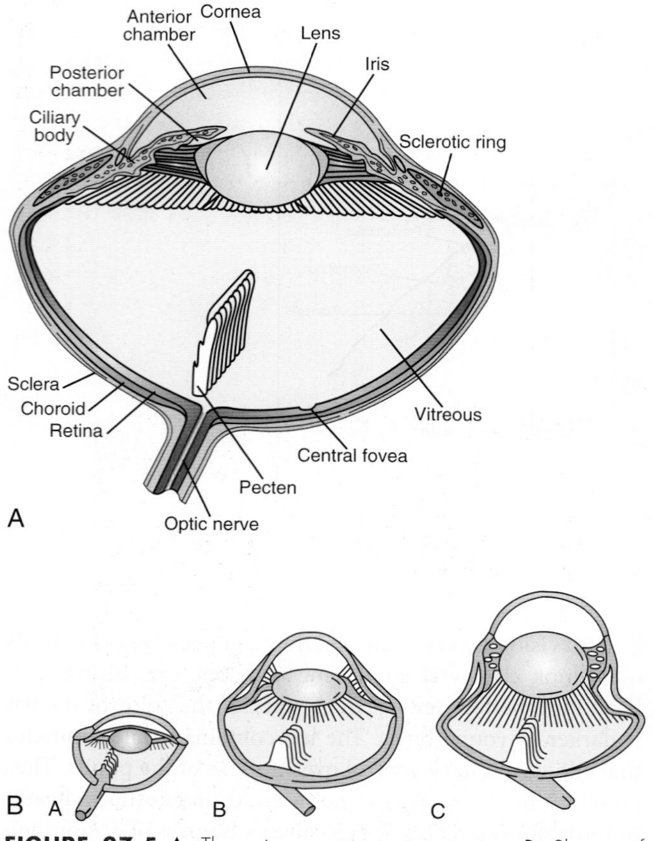

FIGURE 27-5 **A,** The avian eye, transverse section. **B,** Shapes of the avian eye. *A,* Flat. *B,* Round. *C,* Tubular. (From Colville T, Bassert JM: *Clinical anatomy and physiology for veterinary technicians*, ed 2, St Louis, 2008, Mosby.)

The sense of touch is an important sense in many species for finding food and for defense. The skin of birds contains sensory nerve endings that respond to pain, heat, cold, and touch. Some are very responsive to the slightest feather movement and some birds will respond when the tips of the feathers are touched.

BASIC PET BIRD BEHAVIOR

Veterinary clinics that provide care for companion birds must also be prepared to assist clients with behavior concerns. Many birds are needlessly abused, ignored, abandoned at shelters or rescue societies, put up for adoption, or euthanized because the client has a lack of understanding of natural or adapted bird behaviors. Birds have been kept as companions for hundreds of years, but they are far from domestic. These birds are genetically very close to their wild ancestors and retain many of the characteristics of their wild relatives. Most birds have a higher than average intelligence resulting in a patient that is both entertaining and challenging to alter behaviors. The veterinary clinic should be the client's first credible authority for correcting behavior problems and not the local pet or feed store personnel. The veterinary clinic staff must know the basics of bird behavior and be prepared to assist clients or refer problem cases to avian behaviorists.

Common Behaviors

Many of the behaviors that owners wish to modify are the result of instinctive avian reactions or related to the stresses of captivity. To have an understanding of the problem behaviors birds exhibit in captivity, you must have a clear understanding of normal psittacine behavior.

Many parrots use their agile feet to hold food while they eat or manipulate objects they are interested in exploring (Fig. 27-6). They tend to be good climbers, often moving around their cage using a combination of beak and feet. Birds will wag their tail back and forth when happy and relaxed. Birds grind their beak when they are comfortable and ready to fall asleep. Some birds will regurgitate food for those that they are closely bonded to, whether it is the owner or

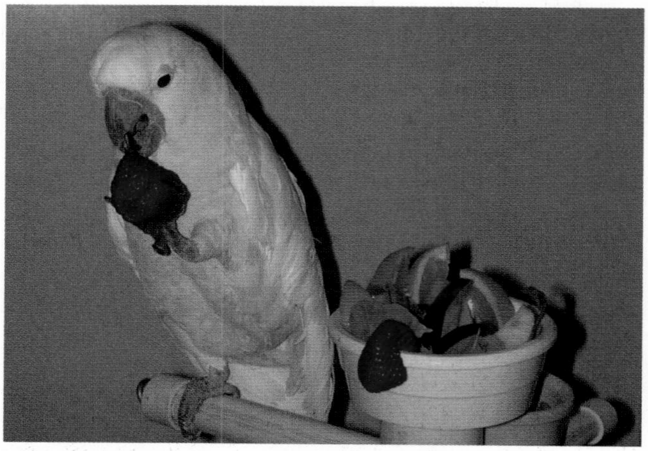

FIGURE 27-6 Birds are very agile and use their feet as utensils for eating.

another bird. The typical behavior that indicates defecation in a calm bird is a slight wiggle of the tail, followed by a squat and an uplifted tail. All birds defecate frequently and more often when afraid or stressed.

Fear is common when the bird is in the clinic and personnel should be aware of this and take appropriate measures to reduce the stress involved with the visit. When a bird is frightened, it may fling itself about the cage, struggle violently, flap its wings, scream loudly, or take flight in response to sudden movements or unfamiliar sights or sounds (Fig. 27-7). This is common during capture and restraint. Birds may easily be injured in their efforts to get away.

Clients often seek help with such problems as biting, chewing, screaming, or destructive feather behavior.

Chewing. **Mouthing** is a term used to describe a juvenile parrot using the tongue to explore surfaces. Juvenile parrots pass through an innocent "beaking" phase, in which they attempt to taste or chew almost anything, somewhat like puppies do. Contrary to puppies, birds do not grow out of this behavior (Fig. 27-8). Clients should be counseled to supervise the parrot when out of its cage and provide the pet with well-designed safe toys to destroy. Toys that are safe to destroy such as paper-based manufactured or homemade, or natural wood toys embedded with nuts provide much needed enrichment for these intelligent confined creatures.

Biting. Birds bite to exhibit dominance, express fear, exhibit jealousy, or as a result of hormonal fluctuations during puberty or the breeding season. Biting may not be an instinctual behavior but rather one that captive birds have developed in the confined world created for our companion birds. In the wild the beak is used primarily for eating, preening, and communication. If a conflict arises, most birds generally fly away rather than using their beak as a weapon. Some protective birds may bite the owner in an effort to communicate with the person to move away from perceived danger. It is important for the owner to realize that the bird must not be allowed to bite as a way of controlling any situation. Mature parrots are more likely to bite during handling as a method of defense.

The larger psittacines, such as macaws, can exert up to 300 pounds of pressure per square inch, inflicting deep bruises and lacerations. Birds such as cockatiels and budgies have the potential to draw blood with their bites. Biting is a common behavior problem and identifying why the bird is biting is the first step to a resolution.

Dominance. Psittacines may attempt to become dominant over their flock and in the captive companion bird world, the flock is their human family. It is important that the owner and other household members use certain techniques to maintain the dominant position in the home. Birds should be taught to consistently step up on or down from the owner's hand when asked. Clipping the bird's wings to limit its flying ability can diminish dominance behaviors, such as flying down from a curtain rod to attack members of the household. When holding the bird, keep it at midchest level. Never allowing it to sit on the head or shoulders keeps it from attaining the highest perch, a position of great power. Situating the cage or perches so that the bird is below eye level also discourages dominant behavior.

Vocalization. Parrots are naturally loud creatures and vocalize for many reasons: communication, entertainment, exercise, and in response to discomfort or restraint. Birds tend to be very noisy at dawn and dusk and feeding time. Noise levels vary between species and parrots can scream loud enough to damage human hearing, so hearing protection is recommended when working with companion birds. Some of these birds have the ability to repeat what they hear. Some will recite any unsavory word or derogatory phrase and bodily function sounds if these scenarios are repetitive. Vocalizations may become a problem in some insecure or dependent birds that call constantly to their owner. Some species are relatively quiet, but all birds make a certain amount of noise. Owners may inadvertently encourage the bird to make more noise by

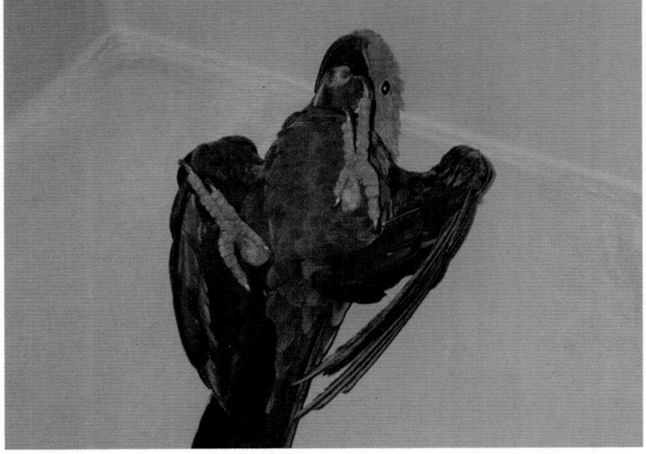

FIGURE 27-7 This bird is frightened and objecting to the clinic visit by throwing himself on his back, flapping and screaming to avoid capture.

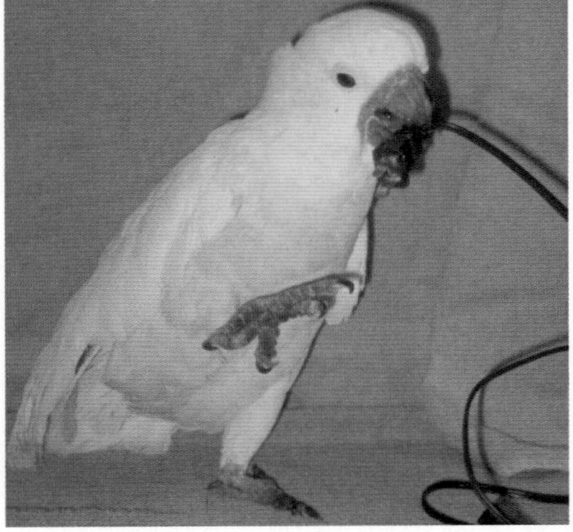

FIGURE 27-8 Birds are naturally curious and will chew on almost anything.

responding to the bird's loud calls with anger or shouting in an effort to quiet the bird.

Self-Mutilation and Feather Destructive Behavior. Feather destructive behavior, also called feather picking or plucking, is a well-known but poorly understood condition. The bird uses its beak to chew on and pull out any feathers that are accessible, including any that start to grow back. Some birds remove all but the feathers on their heads and some may damage muscle as well as skin (Fig. 27-9). Some affected birds may have an underlying medical condition that initiates plucking, but some healthy birds respond to stress with self-mutilation (Fig. 27-10). Stresses can be in the form of separation anxiety from their owner or a change in the cage location or the addition of a new pet or family member. This is a difficult problem to solve and may become a chronic condition. It is most common in cockatoo species and African Grey parrots (Fig. 27-11). The most important first step in correcting this behavior is a thorough medical workup to rule out any underlying pathologic conditions. Once a medical condition has been ruled out or treated, the behavior modification and training can be implemented. Once feather destructive behavior has been established, behavior modification and training may decrease the severity of the disorder but will rarely stop the habit completely.

Inappropriate Bonding. Some owners will unintentionally allow a parrot to form a sexual bond with them by inappropriate petting. Petting the bird repeatedly over its back and tail sends a message to that bird that is comparable to the courtship behaviors performed in the wild. Cuddling and feeding the bird warm foods by hand or mouth can have similar inappropriate bonding results. The bird may pant and masturbate. This is especially common in cockatoos. Chronic masturbation can lead to a chronic prolapsing cloaca (see below) and a dilated vent that may require corrective surgery. This is a difficult situation for the owner to correct, because it involves disrupting the owner's tight bond with the bird using behavior modification.

Correction of behavior problems takes time, an understanding of the underlying cause, and judicious use of behavior modification. Prolonged physical or mental isolation of the bird, withholding food or water, and physical punishment are totally unacceptable methods of dealing with these problems. All may result in permanent emotional or physical damage to the bird.

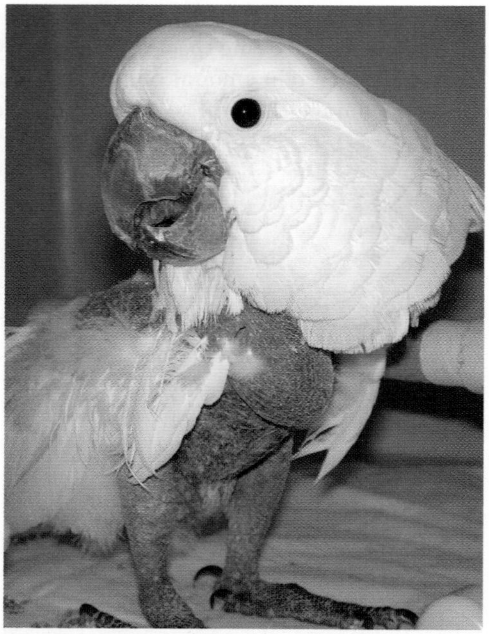

FIGURE 27-9 Some birds will remove all the feathers they can reach, which produces an image such as this cockatoo with a featherless body and fully feathered head.

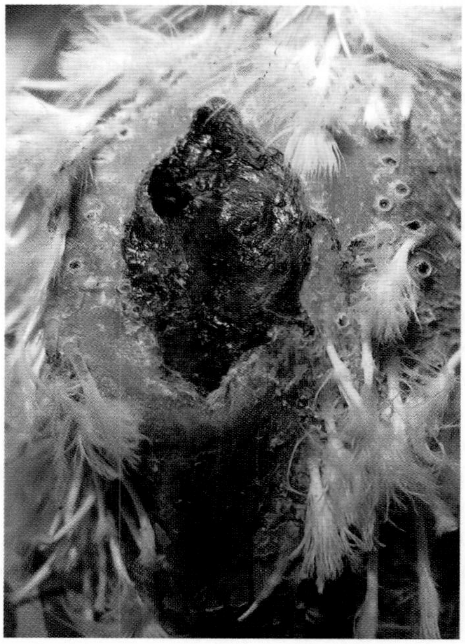

FIGURE 27-10 Cervical self-mutilation wound on a cockatoo. Feather mutilation and plucking can often times go a step further and the bird can start to destroy the skin and muscle and eventually internal structures.

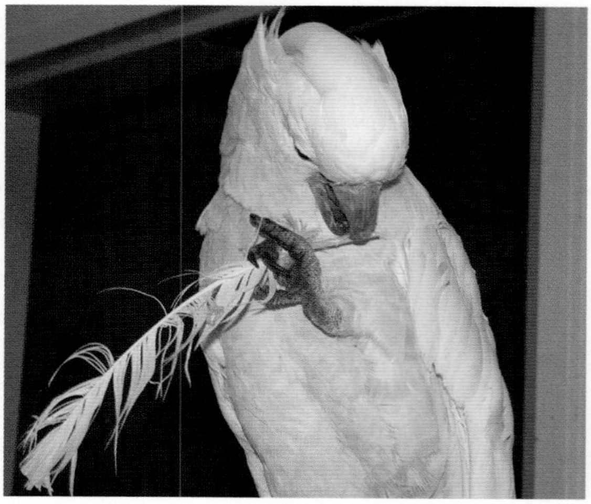

FIGURE 27-11 Feather mutilation and plucking is a common behavior in cockatoos.

Client Education

Client education is a vital service you must provide to ensure the well-being of your avian patients. The majority of birds that present to your clinic for the first time will have medical problems related to improper diet and husbandry provided by poorly educated clients. You need to be the foremost authority of avian care in your clients' minds and encourage them to seek you out when they have a question or concern about their pets. Unfortunately clients will sometimes turn to less informed and educated personnel in pet and feed stores for information, often with disastrous results.

Client education needs to be available for a vast range of topics including proper cages and perch dimensions, substrate, safe transport, nutrition, and disease prevention, just to name a few. Handouts are easy to create on these various topics and appointments can be made with knowledgeable technicians to discuss the topics and address any problem areas.

Enclosures for birds come in many shapes and sizes that are designed to appeal to the client but may fail to address the needs of the bird. The enclosure should be spacious, and the minimum size would allow the bird to spread its wings without touching the sides of the cage. It should be easy to clean and disinfect regularly and be constructed of a durable, nontoxic material. Newspapers or paper towels are inexpensive and very safe substrates for birds, and don't promote the growth of pathogens as do other organic substrates such as wood shavings and corncob bedding. Some of the latter substrates can also be ingested and create a gastrointestinal foreign body with the possibility of obstruction. The position of the enclosure should be in a draft free area, partially out of direct sunlight, and in an area of the house where the family routinely congregates.

Perches should be made from branches of clean, nontoxic hardwood trees and shrubs free of pesticides, mold, or wood rot. Birds need varying sizes, textures, and irregularly shaped perches to decrease the pressure placed on any one point of the foot and decrease the potential for pododermatitis.

Food dishes, toys, mirrors, and other accessories should be provided without overcrowding the bird. If there is insufficient room for the bird to move about, then the bird may not exercise appropriately and may become entrapped in parts of the accessories or toys and be injured. Toys should be made of nontoxic substances and of appropriate size for the bird so as not to allow for ingestion of the pieces.

Nutrition is a very important subject and requires a handout for routine enquiries. Fresh water should be provided at all times. The water dish should be placed high in the bird's cage and not below any perches, to decrease the possibility of fecal contamination. Birds should be offered fresh food on a daily basis. The optimal diet consists of a variety of pellets (70%) and fresh fruits and vegetables (30%). Feeding the bird at the dinner table and from the client's mouth should be discouraged, because some human foods are too high in salts and sugars and some can be toxic to the bird, such as chocolate and avocado. Conversion from seeds to pellets is encouraged, and clients may need assistance with this task in the form of a handout and face-to-face or phone consultations.

> TECHNICIAN NOTE For birds on an all-seed diet, the hospital stay is not the time to convert from seeds to pellets. If the patient is ill and will only eat seeds, then don't force the issue; let the patient get well first. It is a good idea to try a healthier diet with fortified pellets; you may be pleasantly surprised and the patient may instantly take a liking to the pellets or even some fresh fruits and vegetables.

PHYSICAL EXAMINATION

History

The physical examination occurs in three unique steps. The first is a thorough history combined with a brief visual examination, followed by the complete hands-on physical examination. One of the most important first steps when evaluating an avian patient is to obtain a detailed history (Fig. 27-12). Husbandry-related problems are very common findings with the first visit to an avian practitioner. Many medical conditions can be directly related to poor diet and husbandry. Client education handouts are essential in these situations to help correct any problems at home. During the patient's first visit the inquiry may take 10 to 15 minutes of your time, but it is well worth it in the long run. Try to streamline your questions, and make sure to take good notes. Utilize a history form for the client to fill out while waiting to see the doctor. This may reduce the amount of time needed for the inquiry, and the document should be part of the medical record for future reference.

Examination—Before Capture and Restraint

The physical examination is not all hands on. A great deal of information can be obtained simply by observing the bird's behavior and physical appearance before capture and restraint. Companion birds are commonly a prey species with survival instincts and frequently alter their behavior when they are in a stressful environment, such as a clinic. Birds will mask their symptoms in order to not stand out in their "flock" so they will not be eliminated by a predator or members of their own flock. Evaluate the bird's ability to recover from the stress of transport to the clinic. The respiratory rate should be smooth and regular and a healthy bird should show no signs of increased effort. If the bird is exhibiting a tail bob, forward movement of the head, or open beak breathing, this could be a sign of respiratory distress and may need immediate attention.

Evaluate the mentation and stance. If the is bird trying to sleep, is droopy eyed, wobbling, or barely hanging on to the perch, then immediate medical attention may be necessary. After evaluating the patient, take a moment to evaluate the droppings in the cage.

When a bird is stressed or excited, the droppings may be mostly urine. Seed eaters will have drier droppings than those with a diet supplemented with fruits. If the bird is anorexic, then the droppings will be fewer. Look for blood, parasites, or undigested seeds, because these findings may be indicative of disease. The feces may be green or light brown,

AVIAN HISTORY FORM

General History

Bird's Name____________________ Sex: M____ F____ UNK________
How was bird sexed? Blood Test____________ Surgical?____________
Any Specific Identification? (ie: tattoo, band, microchip)____________
If bird is female, has she produced eggs in the past? (if yes, please describe)____________
Bird is a : Pet________ Breeder________
How did you acquire the bird? Store_____ Breeder_____ Other (describe)____________
Date acquired? ____________
Do you have any other pets? Y_____ N_____
If yes, please specify including ages and when acquired____________

Housing

Is this bird kept: Indoors_____ Outdoors_____ Both_____ (if both, please specify % time in each)
____
Is the bird housed alone? Y_____ N_____ If no, describe ____________
If bird is caged, what type of cage? ____________
What do use on the bottom of the cage? ____________
How often is the cage cleaned?____________
Method/ frequency of cleaning food/ water dishes ____________
Any toys in the cage? Y_____ N_____ If yes, describe ____________
Has the bird's environment changed recently? Y_____ N_____ If yes, describe____________
At night, do you cover the bird? Y_____ N_____
How many hours of darkness does the bird have each day? ____________

Diet:

What foods are offered to your bird/ in what total percentages? (ie: 50% seed, etc) ____________
What percentages of these foods do you remove from the cage at night? ____________
Any supplements offered? Brand name? ____________
Any treats offered? Type? How often?____________
Any recent diet changes or new foods? Y_____ N_____ If yes, describe ____________
How is water offered? (ie: sipper bottle, bowl)____________

Reason For Today's Visit:

What signs have you noticed that prompted today's visit? ____________
How long have you noticed the problem?____________
Has your bird been sick previously? ____________
Has the bird ever been seen by any other veterinarian? Y_____ N_____ If yes, when/ why?
____
Have any tests been performed previously on your bird? Please circle all that apply:
Psittacosis; CBC; Psittacine Beak and Feather Disease; Polyoma Disease; Parasites; Other bloodwork;
Other (please describe) ____________

Additional comments (your comments regarding the reason for this visit):

FIGURE 27-12 Avian history form filled out by clients annually or as needed.

and may vary in consistency between species and diet. The color of the droppings can be affected by the color of the food consumed. The urine should be clear and the urates can appear white to a pale tan. In addition to the species and any disease considerations, water intake and diet influence the appearance of droppings.

Capture and Restraint

Restraint is often required for the safety of the patient and the personnel working with the bird. You must learn how to safely and confidently capture and restrain your avian patient to perform various procedures such as a thorough physical examination and many different diagnostic and therapeutic procedures. Competent knowledge about birds and handling of the avian patient in the clinic will inspire confidence in your client.

Capturing a bird needs to be done in a room that can be sealed and has no escape route or hiding places for the bird to get to. Close and lock the door, close window blinds, turn off any exhaust fans, and remove any cage accessories. Darkening the room may help reduce the stress of capture in some cases, mainly smaller birds that otherwise try to fly around in their cages. When working with critically ill patients it is best to perform your physical examination in stages, giving the patient time to recover between each stage.

A terry cloth towel is often useful when capturing and restraining birds ranging in size from the cockatiels or conures to the largest parrots (Fig. 27-13). Paper towels are sometimes used when restraining budgies, cockatiels, or conures. The bird should be allowed to chew on the towel if it wishes, which keeps its beak busy and makes it less likely for the holder to be bitten. The use of a towel to capture a bird helps keep the bird from developing a fear of hands. When the animal returns home after being captured by a human hand, the bird may have a fear of its owner's hands, possibly creating a dissatisfied client. The use of gloves is discouraged because this too will create a fear of hands. The use of gloves also reduces the handler's tactile sensation and ability to feel the patient's most subtle movements and reactions to the stress of restraint.

Small pet birds, such as finches, canaries, and budgerigars, are sometimes transported to the veterinarian in their own cage. They must be safely and gently removed for a hands-on physical examination. Slow and deliberate movements minimize stress to the bird, accompanied by a quiet tone of voice for reassurance. It may be helpful to dim the room lights before proceeding, because this calms some birds. Place the towel over the patient, gain control of the head, pin the wings to the body, and pick the patient up.

Larger parrots may be caught in the cage, in the carrier, on the floor, or from a table top. Never capture a bird from the owner's shoulder. This is dangerous as the bird may bite the owner. As with small birds, a slow and deliberate approach works best. A quiet, soothing tone of voice should be used when approaching the bird. In most cases a towel is used during capture to avoid injury to the bird or technician. It is extremely important to exhibit confidence in the approach to large birds, because they may become aggressive when they detect uncertainty.

Once the bird is captured, the towel can be wrapped around the bird to form a "birdy burrito" to control the wings and the legs. With or without a towel, the body of the bird can be tucked under your arm once you have control of the head. This will aid in restraint of the wings. As with all methods of restraint, you must monitor the patient carefully for stress, hypoxia, and hyperthermia.

The restrainer is the primary person monitoring the bird's condition and stress level during the examination. This allows the person performing the physical to proceed in a timely fashion. The restrainer should keep the bird from injuring itself and others and should assist the person performing the physical examination by readjusting his or her hands to allow access to the bird.

A restraint board is used for procedures that require the bird to remain completely still, such as for radiographs or implantation of microchips for identification, or in other situations when both hands may be needed to perform complicated tasks. Restraint boards should not be used except for radiographs, and only in heavily sedated or anesthetized companion birds. Proper hand-held restraint allows for better observation of the bird's condition and a faster reaction time to return the bird to its cage or carrier if the patient is becoming too stressed during restraint (Fig. 27-14).

Restraint can be a very stressful experience for a bird. It is not unusual for the bird to show signs of extreme distress when released. The bird will typically pant and exhibit open beak breathing, have hot feet, hold its wings away from its body, and fluff the feathers to allow air to cool the skin. Birds with featherless areas on the faces, such as African Grey parrots and macaws, will blush occasionally. One restraint method that may be useful is what appears to be a choke hold. The bird is gripped around the cervical region while extending the neck. This prevents the bird from dropping its head down and biting your fingers. This looks like a choke hold, but it is

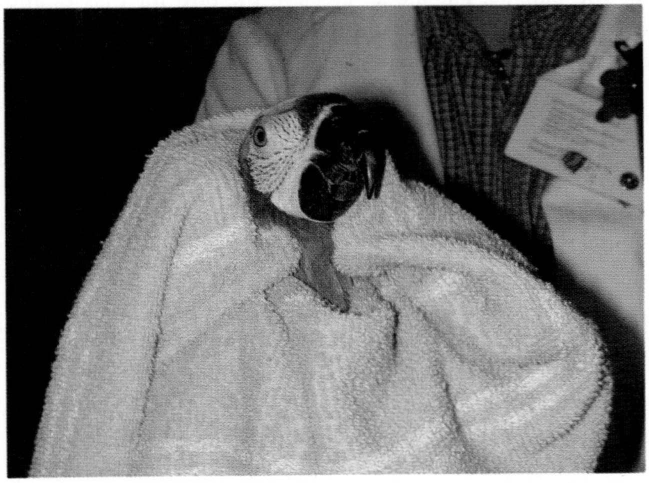

FIGURE 27-13 Small macaw captured by a terry cloth towel.

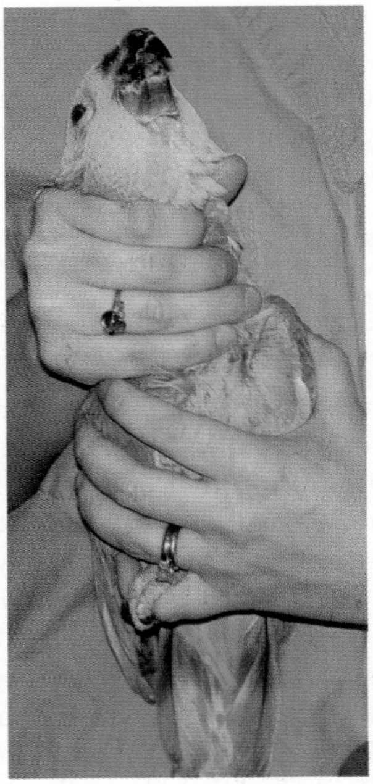

FIGURE 27-14 This image illustrates the improper method of restraint. The restrainer is compressing the keel and the patient is unable to breathe properly.

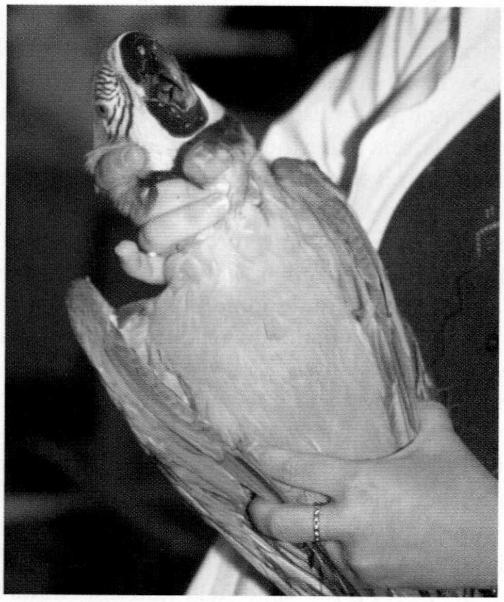

FIGURE 27-15 Choke-hold restraint of a blue and gold macaw.

a great way to restrain macaws or other birds that have fragile facial skin that bruises easily with traditional restraint methods. With the other hand, keep the wings pinned to the sides of the body (Fig. 27-15). After restraint these same birds may develop bruises in these featherless areas on the face.

Physical Examination

Table 27-1 contains some physiologic data for common avian species. When performing the physical examination, you should be systematic and proceed in a timely manner. Develop a routine and apply it consistently (Box 27-3).

A typical physical examination routine is as follows: Examine the eyes, external auditory canals (or ears), nares, beak, and oral cavity. Palpate the crop and esophagus, neck, pectoral region, coelom and pelvic region, wings, legs, feet and back. Evaluate the feather quality and check the preen gland. Auscultate the heart, air sacs, lungs, and sinuses. Examine the cloaca, and evert the mucosa to examine for lesions.

> TECHNICIAN NOTE The average adult bird has a core body temperature of 38° to 42.5° C.

Weighing the Patient. It is very important to obtain an accurate weight of your patient at every visit. Some birds will sit on the scale very nicely while others may require that you place them in box or small cage to weigh them (Fig. 27-16). Weigh the patient every time it comes in to your clinic, even if the bird is not sick. You will be able to monitor trends.

Examination of the Head. Eyes should be clear and bright, bilaterally symmetrical, and free of discharge. Evaluate the eyes with a focal light source and note the patient's pupillary light response. Birds may have voluntary control over this reflex (Fig. 27-17). Periophthalmic swelling or conjunctivitis can be indicative of ocular or sinus abnormalities and require further workup.

Birds lack a pinna. The ears or external auditory canals are located on the sides of the head, behind and slightly below its eyes and consist of three chambers, external, middle, and inner. The ears appear as a hole in the head and should be free of debris (Fig. 27-18). A transilluminator may be used to illuminate the canal or a small otoscope can be used to look into these auditory canals, if necessary.

The head of the bird should be examined for symmetry, feather condition, swellings, and any evidence of trauma. Nares should be smooth, evenly colored, and symmetric. Birds have a keratinized plate inside the nostril called an operculum. These are normal; do not attempt to pick them out. The beak should be smooth and shiny and free of dry flaky regions. In some species such as cockatoos, a fine powder layer on the beak is a normal finding and if absent may be a sign of disease. *Knemidokoptes* spp. infections are presented as proliferate growths on the beak and feet and are commonly found in Budgies (Fig. 27-19). In any species a beak that is malformed, growing excessively, or is found to be in poor condition may be a sign of disease and these birds should be evaluated further. Healthy birds should not need regular beak trimmings.

Oral Examination. The oral examination is a crucial part of the examination. The oral cavity is the window to the gastrointestinal and respiratory systems and much information can be gathered from this examination. The bird should be in an upright position and the oral cavity exposed by using gauze or tape strips to gently fatigue the powerful muscles controlling the beak (Fig. 27-20). In smaller birds you can use small speculums like a hemostat or paper clips or small tape strips.

While looking in the oral cavity observe the color, texture, and moisture of the mucosa; look for swellings, ulcerations, erosions, or plaques. Closely examine the choanal slit and its papillae. The choanal slit is the V-shaped notch on the roof of the mouth. The papillae should be sharp; if they are absent or blunted, this could be a sign of disease and will require a further workup. Assess the hydration status while looking in the mouth. If the bird is dehydrated, it will have tacky oral mucosa.

Palpation. Evaluate the overall condition of the bird as you palpate. Palpate all areas of the bird for masses and swellings, evidence of trauma or self-mutilation, or any other abnormalities.

If you find the crop is distended when you palpate, you may want to quicken the examination or postpone it until the crop has time to empty. This is to prevent regurgitation of the crop contents and potential aspiration.

Using a transilluminator to shine through the crop, you can evaluate the general thickness of the mucosa and evaluate the air sacs for air sac mites (in passerines).

Palpate the pectoral mass which is an indicator of the bird's overall health. The ratio of muscle mass to sternum is measured on a scale from 1 (very thin) to 9 (obese) with 5 being ideal. The pectoral muscles should be solid, well formed, and rounded. The normal appearance will vary between species. For example, the average Amazon will have more rounded pectoral muscles than the average conure.

TABLE 27-1 Physiologic Data for Common Avian Species

BIRD	AVG WT	HEART RATE BPM	RESP RATE BPM	SEXUAL MATURITY	AVG CAPTIVE LIFE SPAN
Budgerigars	30 g	500-600	60-70	6 months	6 years
Love birds	38-56 g	400-600	60-80	8-12 months	4 years
Cockatiels	75-125 g	400-500	40-50	6-12 months	6 years
Conures	80-100 g	500-600	60-70	1-3 years	10 years
Lories	100-300 g	300-500	35-50	2-3 years	3 years
Cockatoos	300-1100 g	150-350	20-30	1-6 years (species dependent)	15 years
Eclectus parrots	380-450 g	160-300	20-30	3-6 years	8 years
Amazon parrots	350-1000 g	160-300	20-30	4-6 years	15 years
Macaws	200-1500 g	120-300	15-32	4-7 years (species dependent)	15 years
African Greys	400-550 g	200-350	25-30	4-6 years	15 years

BOX 27-3 Aspects of Avian Physical Examination

Visual Examination of
- Eyes
- External auditory canals (or ears)
- Nares (nostrils)
- Beak and oral cavity
- Feather quality
- Preen gland
- Plantar surface of the feet
- Cloaca
- Feces

Auscultation of
- Heart
- Air sacs
- Lungs
- Sinuses

Palpation of
- Crop
- Esophagus
- Neck
- Pectoral region
- Coelom
- Pelvic region
- Wings
- Legs
- Feet
- Back

Evaluation of the abdomen is very limited or impossible in small birds. In larger birds, abdominal palpation is used to detect organs that feel hard or unusually shaped. The abdomen or coelom should be concave or flat. In all birds, the vent should be clean and covered by dry feathers. Palpate the pelvic region and extremities for symmetry and masses.

Both wings should be gently examined, with care taken to curve the wing in the direction of the body at all times. Some birds are very sensitive and struggle when their wings are manipulated. If a stressed bird is struggling too much, release the wing and start again when the struggling ceases. It is very

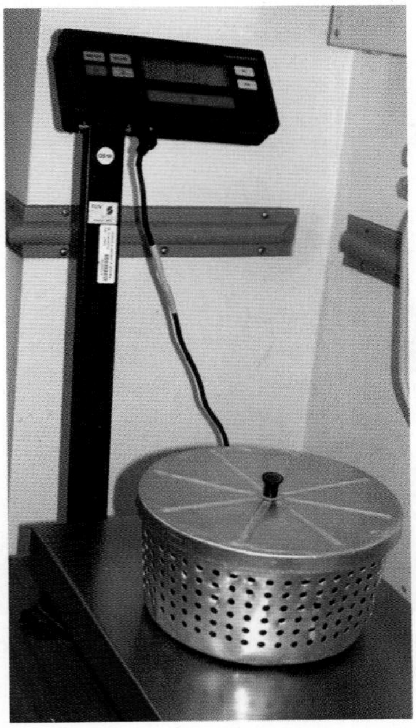

FIGURE 27-16 Weighing your patients is a vital part of monitoring health status of your health examinations and your hospitalized patients. The scale should be able to read to ± 1 gram.

easy to break the wing at this stage of the examination. The remaining musculoskeletal system that was not previously palpated should be checked at this time.

Skin and Feather Condition. Examine skin and feather quality. The delicate skin is usually white, and underlying structures such as muscle or blood vessels are somewhat visible. Evaluate the feet and legs for any lesions or masses and pododermatitis (Fig. 27-21). The feathers should be clean, symmetric, smooth, and structurally sound. Evidence of blood feathers (i.e., growing feathers) should be noted. The presence of the powder down, which is produced by cockatoos, cockatiels, and African Grey parrots, should be evaluated. The nails and skin on the legs should be inspected for overall condition and presence of any abnormal growth. Feather condition is a good indicator of overall health. Stress bars are sometimes found and these represent a

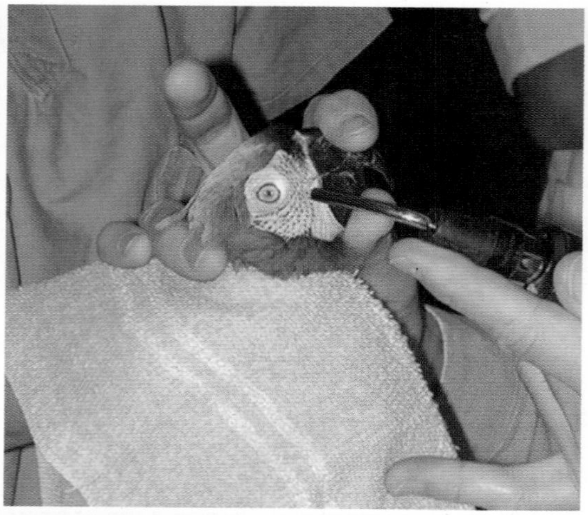

FIGURE 27-17 The sphincter and dilator muscles of the pupil are striated; therefore, unlike mammals, voluntary control may be possible.

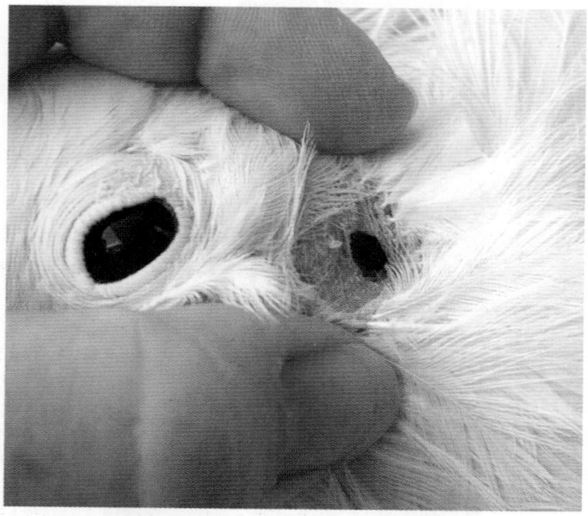

FIGURE 27-18 The short horizontal canal is protected by contour feathers that can be gently swept forward to expose the ear for examination.

period of malnutrition or stress while the feathers were being developed. These bars are symmetrical and segmental malformations in the barbs and barbules (Fig. 27-22).

Examination of the Uropygial Gland. The uropygial gland, also known as the preen gland, should be located and examined. It is located on the dorsal portion of the bird's tail base at the end of the pygostyle. It is absent in Amazon species. This bi-lobed gland should be smooth and evenly colored and excrete a creamy material that the bird will use during preening for waterproofing the feathers. Neoplasia, impactions, and infections are common abnormal findings with this gland.

Auscultation. To auscultate the avian patient, use a pediatric or neonatal stethoscope. Auscultate the heart from the ventral midline along the keel (Fig. 27-23). Heart rates vary with excitation and species but range from 100 to 600 bpm. Auscultate dorsal midline between the shoulder blades to evaluate the lungs, which are a located dorsal near the spine in the coelomic cavity (Fig. 27-24). If the heart cannot

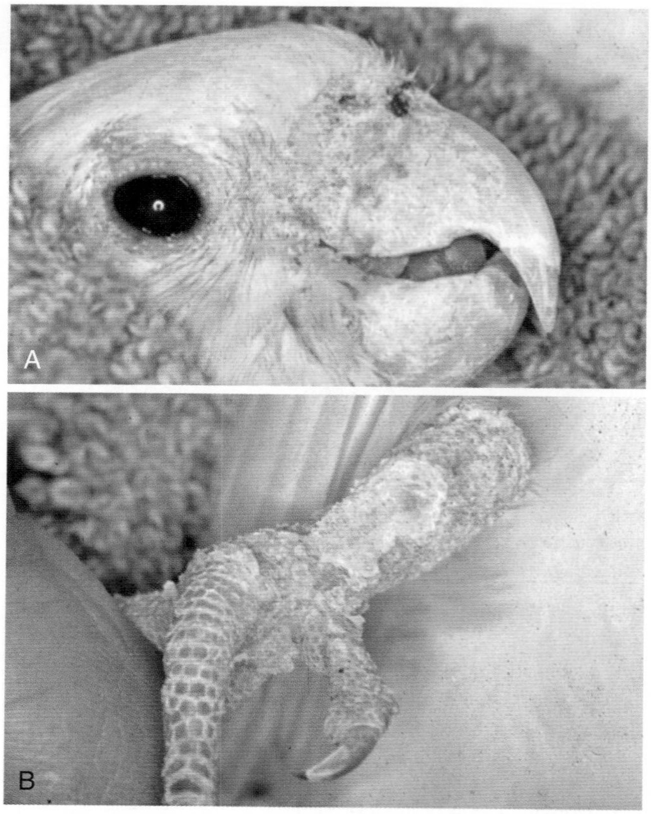

FIGURE 27-19 **A,** Cockatiel with *Knemidokoptes pili* mite infestation, known as the scaly leg and face mite (side view). **B,** view of plantar surface of foot. (From Hnilica KA: *Small animal dermatology*, ed 3, St Louis, 2011, Saunders.)

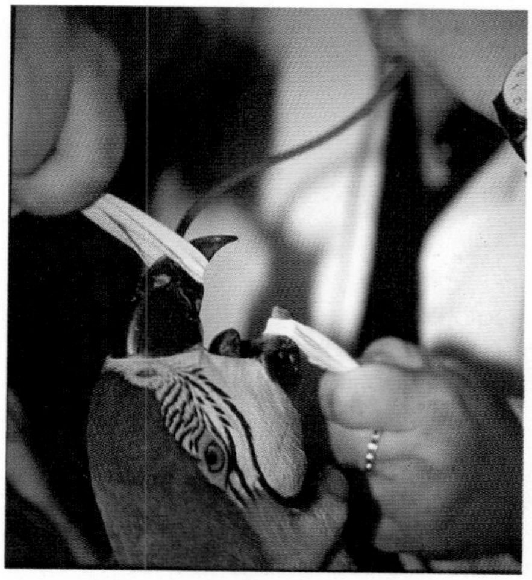

FIGURE 27-20 Oral examination method.

be auscultated in the region, this may be a sign of lung pathology. Listen to the top of the bird's head (Fig. 27-25). You should not hear anything; if you do, sinus problems may be present.

Cloacal Examination. Examination of the cloaca is important because this is where the terminal openings for the urinary, gastrointestinal, and genital tracts empty. Tissue should not protrude from the cloaca. The tissue in this

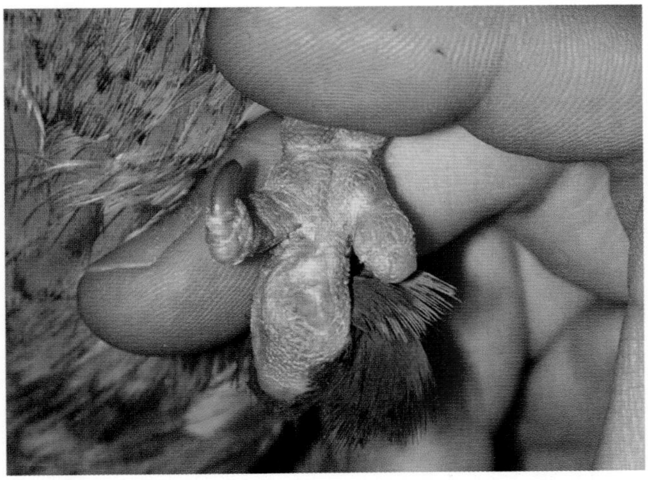

FIGURE 27-21 A thorough physical examination should include evaluating the legs and feet for lesions and pododermatitis as seen here.

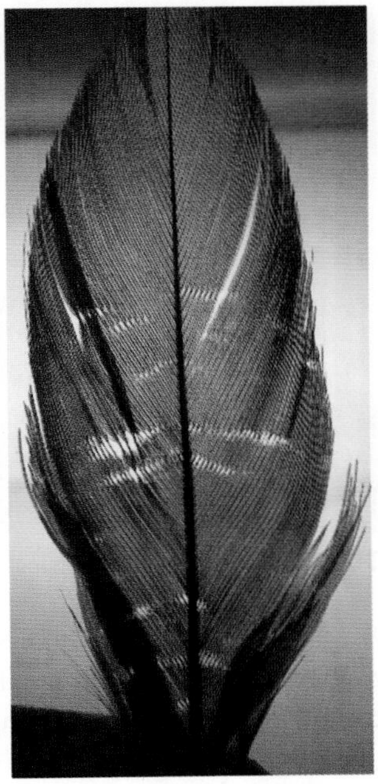

FIGURE 27-22 Stress bars and feather discolorations are signs of potential stressors in the bird's life during feather development, such as malnutrition. Stress bars are normally perpendicular to the feather shaft.

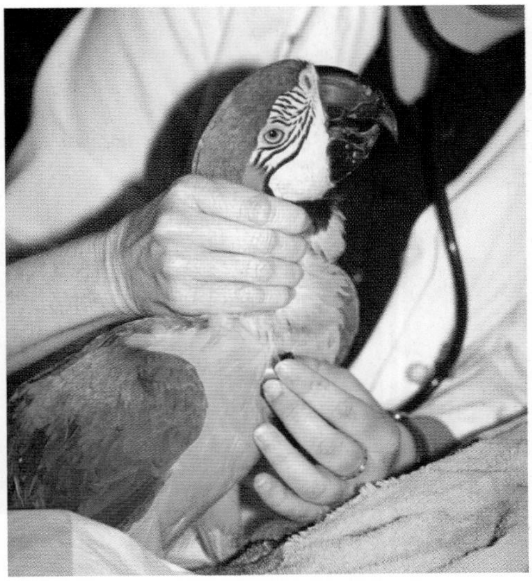

FIGURE 27-23 Auscultate the heart by placing pediatric or neonatal stethoscope ventral midline over the keel.

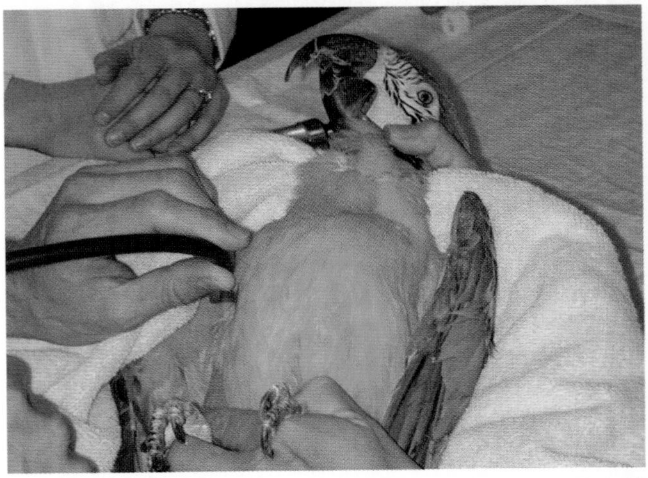

FIGURE 27-24 Auscultate air flow through the air sacs near the axillary region along the lateral dorsal body wall. This is the best place to detect signs of air sac pathology.

area may be distended if the bird is developing an egg, is constipated, or has a cloacal mass. Examine the cloaca for any lesions or masses.

To examine the cloacal mucosa properly, it must be everted. First place the bird in dorsal recumbency. To evert the cloaca, gently insert a slightly moistened cotton tipped applicator into the cloaca. Slowly remove the applicator angling the tip ventrally, everting a small sampling of mucosa for examination (Fig. 27-26). Do this procedure in all four quadrants of the cloaca as if you were looking at a clock: 12 o'clock, 3 o'clock, 6 o'clock, and 9 o'clock. Examine the cloacal tissue closely for evidence of papillomatous growths. Applying 5% acetic acid (apple cider vinegar) will cause papillomas to blanche. This is not definitive because other abnormalities can blanche as well. The only way to truly diagnose papillomatosis is by tissue biopsy.

Hydration Status. Hydration can be assessed by evaluating the eyes, skin turgor, filling time, and lumen size of the ulnar and jugular veins. The condition of the oral and cloacal mucous membranes, packed cell volume, and total solids are other areas for assessing hydration status.

In a dehydrated patient the eyes may appear dull, dry, and sunken, and the skin around them may appear withered and wrinkled. Assess skin turgor around the eye and covering the keel. When muscles of the keel are moved to the side, they will be slow to shift back into position in a dehydrated bird. This is comparable to skin tenting in dehydrated mammals. Refill time of the ulnar and jugular veins will be slow, greater than 1 second to refill, and the vessels will appear undersized if hydration is inadequate. The oral and cloacal mucosa will be tacky or dry in appearance in dehydrated animals.

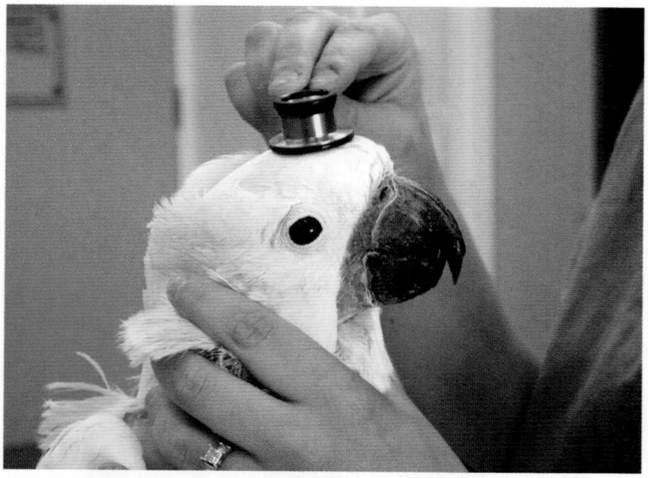

FIGURE 27-25 Auscultate the top of the head; you should not hear anything. If you do hear noises that are not associated with the bird's movement, that could be indicative of sinus problems or pathology.

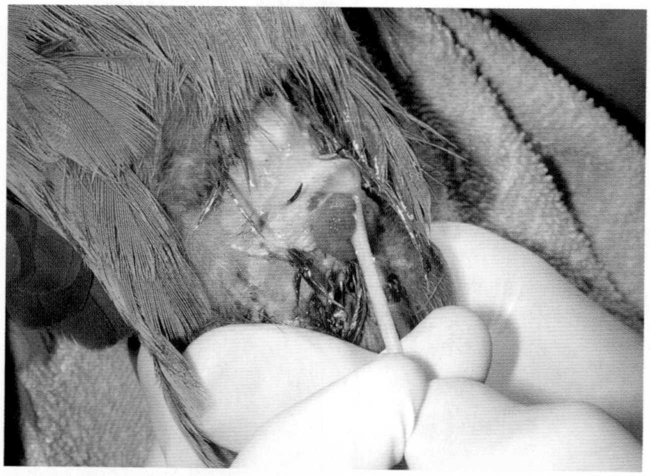

FIGURE 27-26 Everting the cloaca with a cotton-tipped applicator.

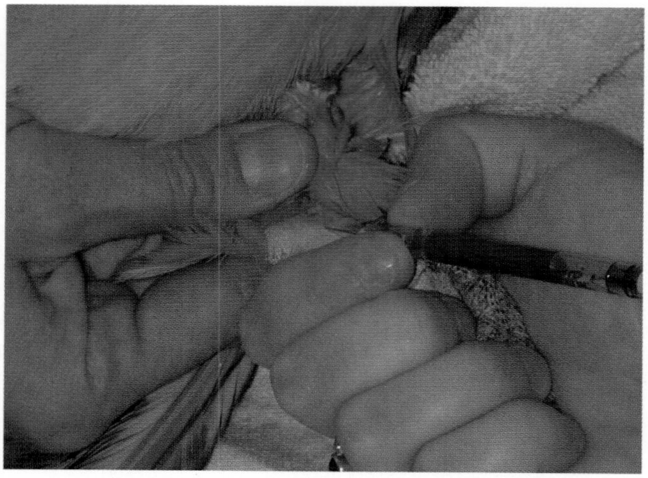

FIGURE 27-27 Venipuncture of the medial metatarsal vein.

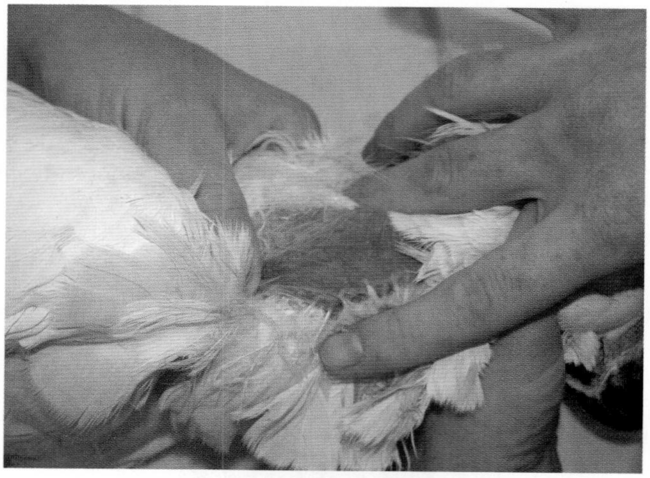

FIGURE 27-28 Jugular venipuncture.

DIAGNOSTIC SAMPLING TECHNIQUES

Blood Collection

Obtaining blood from a severely trimmed toenail is not acceptable. This is painful, stressful, and can yield abnormal cell distributions and cellular artifacts. A venous blood sample should be obtained. You must have a highly skilled restrainer when collecting blood samples from birds. The person collecting the sample must have a steady hand and once in the vessel, not require repositioning the hand to draw the sample.

The medial metatarsal vein or leg vein is the vessel of choice for collecting blood in medium to large birds (Fig. 27-27). The medial metatarsal vein is located on the medial side of the distal tibiotarsus at the tibiotarsal-tarsometatarsal joint. This is an excellent venipuncture site because it is a very stable vessel with little to no mobility, which helps reduce the risk of hematoma formations. Grasp the leg and syringe in one hand while collecting the sample; this will give you more control if the patient moves. Hemostasis can be achieved by bandaging. For best results, a tuberculin syringe with a 25- or 26-gauge needle should be used.

The jugular vein is method of choice for small birds such as budgies and lovebirds (Fig. 27-28). In small birds this is the method of choice for obtaining a blood sample, because the other vessels are usually too small. Birds do have two jugular veins; however, the right jugular is more prominent than the left. Usually a 1-cc tuberculin syringe with a 25- or 26-gauge needle is used for the small birds and a 3-cc syringe equipped with a 25-gauge needle can be used in larger birds. The restrainer should hold the bird in left lateral recumbency. The phlebotomist should arch and extend the neck, part the feathers, lightly wet them with alcohol, and find the featherless track and the jugular. Once the sample is collected, pressure must be applied by the restrainer and is crucial to prevent large hematomas and possible bleed out.

With appropriate restraint the ulnar or basilic vein (also referred to as the wing vein) is an easily accessible vessel for venipuncture (Fig. 27-29). Because of the severity of the complications that can occur, it is recommended to attempt this only on anesthetized patients! Patients that are not anesthetized have an increased chance of forming a large hematoma and/or fracturing the wing. This vein is located on the medial surface of the wing and is most obvious as it runs across

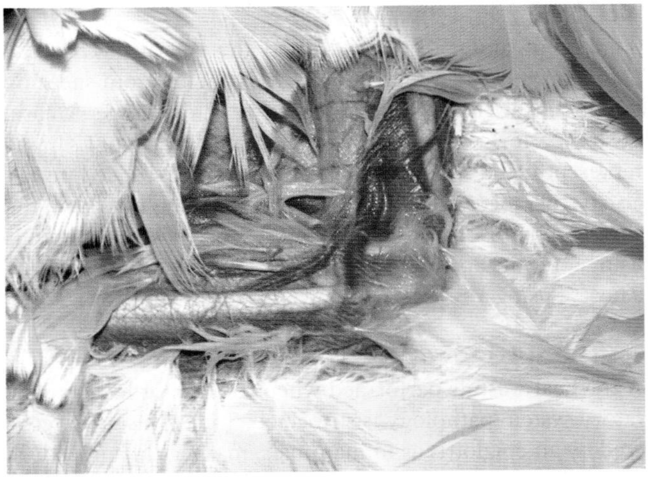

FIGURE 27-29 The ulnar or basilic vein should not be used routinely for blood collection because of hemostasis and traumatic injury concerns.

BOX 27-4 Calculating Blood Volume

To determine the maximum amount of blood that can safely be taken, you can do a simple calculation.

Body Weight (grams) × 0.01 = amount of blood that can safely be taken in healthy birds

and

Body Weight (grams) × 0.005 = amount of blood that can be taken from sick birds

For example, Melanie the Moluccan cockatoo is an 800-gram patient. The urine cup represents her total blood volume of approximately 80 ml. The red-topped tube demonstrates the 8.0 ml that can be safely taken from her for diagnostics, assuming she is not critically ill. If she is critically ill, then you should only take 4.0 ml. In most cases laboratories can run a CBC and chemistry profile with less than 1.0 ml whole blood.

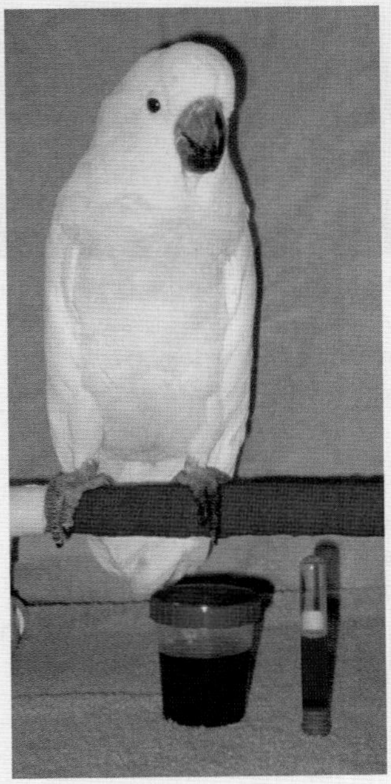

FIGURE 1

the radius and ulna. Place the patient in dorsal recumbency and lightly wet the feathers at the distal end of the humerus. Because of its location it is difficult to bandage this area for hemostasis, thus requiring that the bird be restrained until the bleeding has stopped. It can take 3 to 5 minutes or more to control the bleeding. This is, however, an excellent site to place IV catheters during anesthesia.

Once you have obtained your blood sample, the needle must be removed from the syringe before dispensing the blood into the appropriate tube for sampling. Cell lysis can occur if the blood is dispensed through the needle into the collection tube. If you are not running the samples in your clinic, understand the requirements of the lab you are submitting them to. Develop a rapport with the lab and have a list handy of the minimal sample and submission requirements.

Blood Tubes. Using blood collection tubes such as Microtainer (BD, Franklin Lakes, NJ) that are specially designed for small samples helps eliminate any anticoagulant dilution problems. Samples for a hematology should be collected in ethylenediaminetetraacetic acid (EDTA), because heparin will cause clumping and staining artifacts. A blood film should be made if the blood is going to stay in the EDTA for any length of time. Biochemistry testing can be run using plasma in most laboratories. A large plasma yield can be achieved by using a Microtainer containing lithium heparin.

Blood Volume. Birds come in a wide range of sizes and therefore have a wide range of blood volumes. The smaller the bird the more limited you may be with your blood-work options. You should calculate how much blood you can safely take from your patient. Blood volumes in birds range from 6% to 12% of body weight, depending on the species of bird. It is safe to approximate a bird's blood volume to be 10% of the body weight measured in grams. You can safely take 10% of the bird's total blood volume for diagnostic sampling. Therefore, you can safely take approximately 1% of the bird's body weight in grams in healthy birds and 0.5% in sick birds (Box 27-4).

Fecal Examinations. Examination of the feces is essential for any thorough workup. All that is needed is a very fresh sample with little to no contaminants. A direct smear of the feces is the method for detection of protozoa. Fecal flotation is needed to detect helminths. Gram's stain should be included in any workup to detect yeast and bacteria. Grain- and fruit-eating psittaciformes should have a gram-positive bacterial flora with potentially some yeast. A few yeast or gram-negative bacteria per high-power field could be considered normal, but budding yeast are not normal. Carnivorous or insectivorous passeriformes, raptors, galliformes, and anseriformes will have some gram-negative bacteria in their cloaca. A fecal occult blood test can also be performed.

Respiratory System Diagnostics

Obtaining a culture from this area will be representative of organisms in the sinuses of the bird. Excellent restraint and light are required to obtain the proper amount of exposure to get your sample. Rigid metal speculums can damage the beak of the larger birds which generate a high PSI with every bite. Opening the oral cavity with tape or gauze strips is usually safer for the patient. Gently fatigue the jaws with the strips of gauze or tape, use a tongue depressor or similar object to keep the tongue out of your way, and aim the culturette or sterile cotton-tipped applicator at the choanal slit (Fig. 27-30). Gently advance the culturette into the rostral portion of the slit to collect the sample.

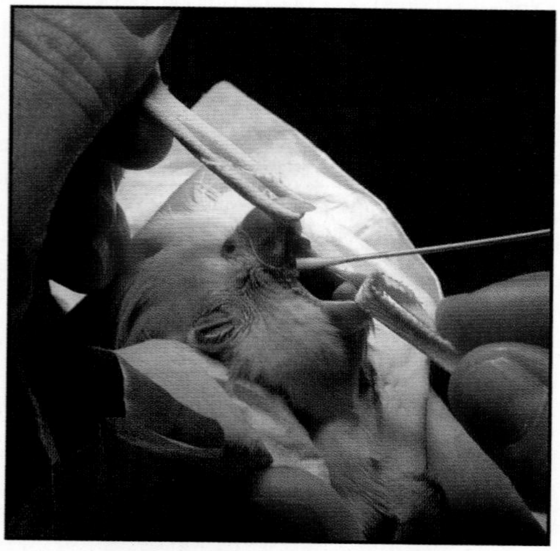

FIGURE 27-30 Obtaining a culture from the choanal slit of a cockatiel.

Nasal Flush

Some companion birds present to the veterinary hospital with sinusitis, which may cause signs ranging from sneezing to regional swelling of the head and nasal discharge. A nasal flush is performed when you wish to obtain a cytology sample representing the organisms of the sinuses. This procedure can also be therapeutic, flushing any debris or rhinoliths out of the sinuses or nares. The solution is injected directly into the sinus using a needle and syringe or flushed into the sinus through a nostril using a syringe without a needle (Procedure 27-1).

Tracheal Lavage

A tracheal wash is performed when tracheal or lower respiratory system pathology is suspected. The glottis is not covered by an epiglottis as in mammals, making this procedure relatively simple (Procedure 27-2). After collecting a tracheal wash sample, be sure to flush through the collection tube. Sometimes debris can accumulate at the tip but never make it to the syringe, therefore flushing back out will push the debris into your sample container.

IMAGING

Radiographs

Radiographs are an excellent diagnostic tool and give valuable information. The diagnostic value of a radiograph is dependent

PROCEDURE 27-1 Nasal/Sinus Flush

Materials

- 3-cc, 6-cc, 12-cc, 20-cc syringe, depending on the size of the bird, and no needle
- Preservative-free saline
- Sterile container to collect the sample

It is best to wear protective eye gear and masks to prevent contaminated liquid from splashing into your face and eyes.

Procedure

- Depending on the size of the bird, fill the appropriate syringe with the saline, position the tip of the syringe so that it completely occludes one of the nares (Fig. 1).

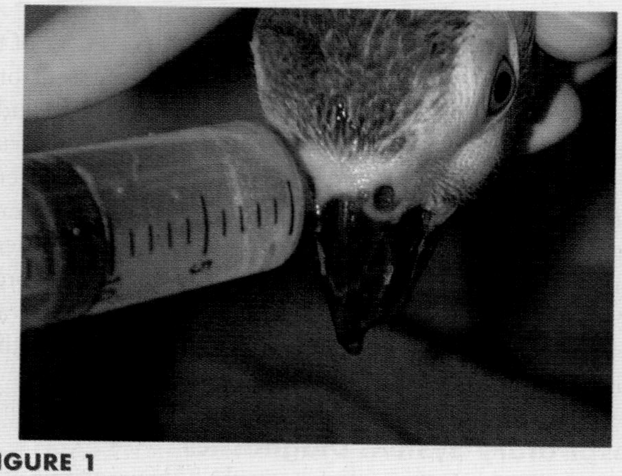

FIGURE 1

- Hold the patient in ventral or lateral recumbency and have the head pointing downward slightly.
- Flush with moderate force.
- The restrainer should monitor the eyes closely; sometimes you will have periorbital swelling during the flush. If this happens, decrease the amount of pressure you are using to flush the fluid through.
- As the sinus flush is performed fluid should come out of the opposite naris and the choanal slit.
- Another person should be ready to collect the sample in a sterile container as it exits the bird (Fig. 2).

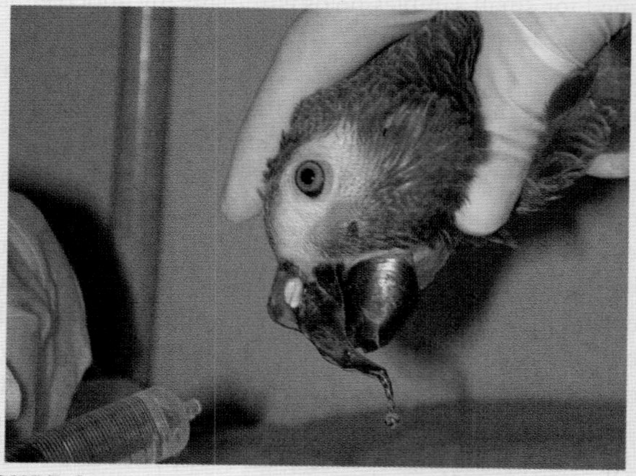

FIGURE 2

- In normal situations you will get fluid from the opposite naris and the choanal slit. Noninsectivorous passeriformes have no connection between the sinuses, so you will only collect fluid from the choanal slit.
- If you feel that the patient has severely packed sinuses, then nebulization before flushing might help loosen up the debris and increase your yield during the flushing.

on the quality of the technique and positioning of the patient. Most companion psittacine birds will require anesthesia or heavy sedation for diagnostic radiographs. When performed on an awake animal, there is a risk of injury such as tissue trauma and fractures from aggressive flapping. Digital radiology is quickly becoming the standard in most clinics and will yield the best results. However, if digital radiology is not yet available in your clinic, then high-detail, rare earth cassettes with single emulsion film provide desired results. Mammography film will produce even better detail, but does require modification of x-ray machine settings. A technique can be extrapolated from the tabletop technique used on most feline patients. For extremely small patients, you can use a dental radiograph unit. Consult with a radiologist to update your technique chart if needed.

The positioning of the patient is crucial for a diagnostic radiograph. The standard whole-body views are a ventrodorsal (VD) and a right lateral. It is vital to always take both views. Plexiglas restraint boards which assist with patient positioning can be used and usually provide excellent results (Fig. 27-31). For the VD, place the bird on its back, legs stretched down to expose the coelomic cavity, wings stretched out symmetrically to the sides, and two pieces of masking tape or paper tape in the form of an X across each carpus. Palpate the keel to ensure it is in line with the backbone. If the patient is not positioned correctly, this can cause misinterpretation because of superimposition of tissues and organs.

Positioning for the lateral view has the patient placed in right lateral recumbency, legs stretched downward, and wings pulled back together. Paper or masking tape is placed across the carpus to keep the wings back, and tape or gauze is used to keep the legs stretched downward. Once the plain films are reviewed, it may be necessary to isolate limbs for an individual shot, or perform a contrast study of the gastrointestinal system or an ultrasound.

The above-mentioned VD and lateral views reveal the same lateral view of the wing. When two views are necessary, then a palmarodorsal (PaD) view needs to be obtained. The PaD can be obtained by placing the bird in a "dive-bombing" position, head on the plate, body up in the air. Extend the wing out as close to the plate as possible and collimate to the desired area (Fig. 27-32).

The Standing Radiograph. The critically ill bird or one in respiratory distress may not be able to survive the stress of restraint required for a routine diagnostic radiograph. The bird can be placed in a cardboard box, induction chamber, or allowed to stand on a low perch to obtain a standing radiograph. If your machine has horizontal beam capabilities then you can obtain a lateral standing view as well. These views are useful to evaluate for heavy metal densities, radiopaque foreign bodies, and bone density.

PROCEDURE 27-2 Tracheal Lavage

Materials

- Gauze or tape strips for opening the mouth
- Focal light source
- Syringe
- Polypropylene catheter or red rubber feeding tube
- Sterile preservative-free saline (0.5-1.0 ml/kg)
- Sterile gloves

Procedure

- The patient should be restrained in an upright position.
- Expose the oral cavity by gently retracting the beak with gauze or tape strips.
- Avoid oral contamination as you advance a sterile plastic or rubber tube down the trachea until resistance is met.
- Administer the calculated amount of fluid and immediately aspirate the contents.
- Place contents into a sterile container.
- This sample can be submitted for cytology as well as culture.

Gastrointestinal Contrast Study

Contrast studies are often done when abnormalities are indicated on the plain films. These are done with the exact same positioning as mentioned previously for the plain films with the addition of barium. The preferred dose is 25 to 50 ml/kg of straight barium sulfate or Iohexol (240 mg/ iodine/ml) diluted 50:50 with water. The barium will need to be administered via a gavage tube into the crop. Because of the fast transit time through the GI tract in an avian patient, an immediate radiograph may be taken with subsequent views taken at 15-, 30-, 60-, and 90-minute intervals. To reduce the risk of aspiration of barium from the crop, the patient can be elevated on the restraint board during positioning (Fig. 27-33). The board can be placed level for the radiograph and then elevated again for patient repositioning.

> **TECHNICIAN NOTE** To help prevent passive reflux of barium into the mouth during a gastrointestinal contrast study, place a small Vetrap bandage around the bird's neck close to the mandible.

Fluoroscopy

Fluoroscopy can be used to create real-time imaging of the gastrointestinal tract. This is the method of choice for

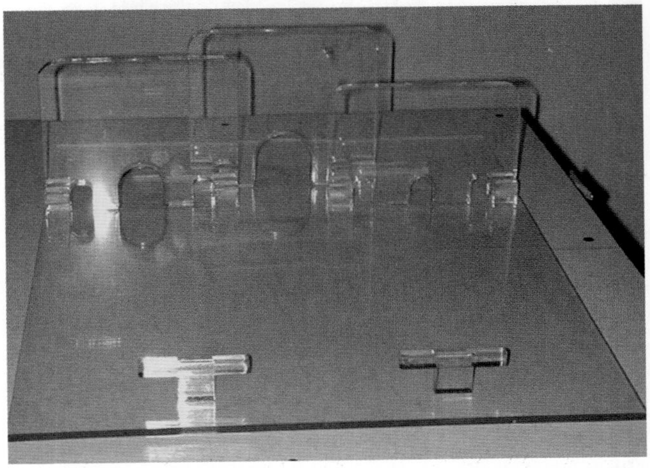

FIGURE 27-31 Avian restraint boards are used to assist with proper positioning for a radiograph. Most companion birds do not tolerate placement on such a device without heavy sedation or anesthesia.

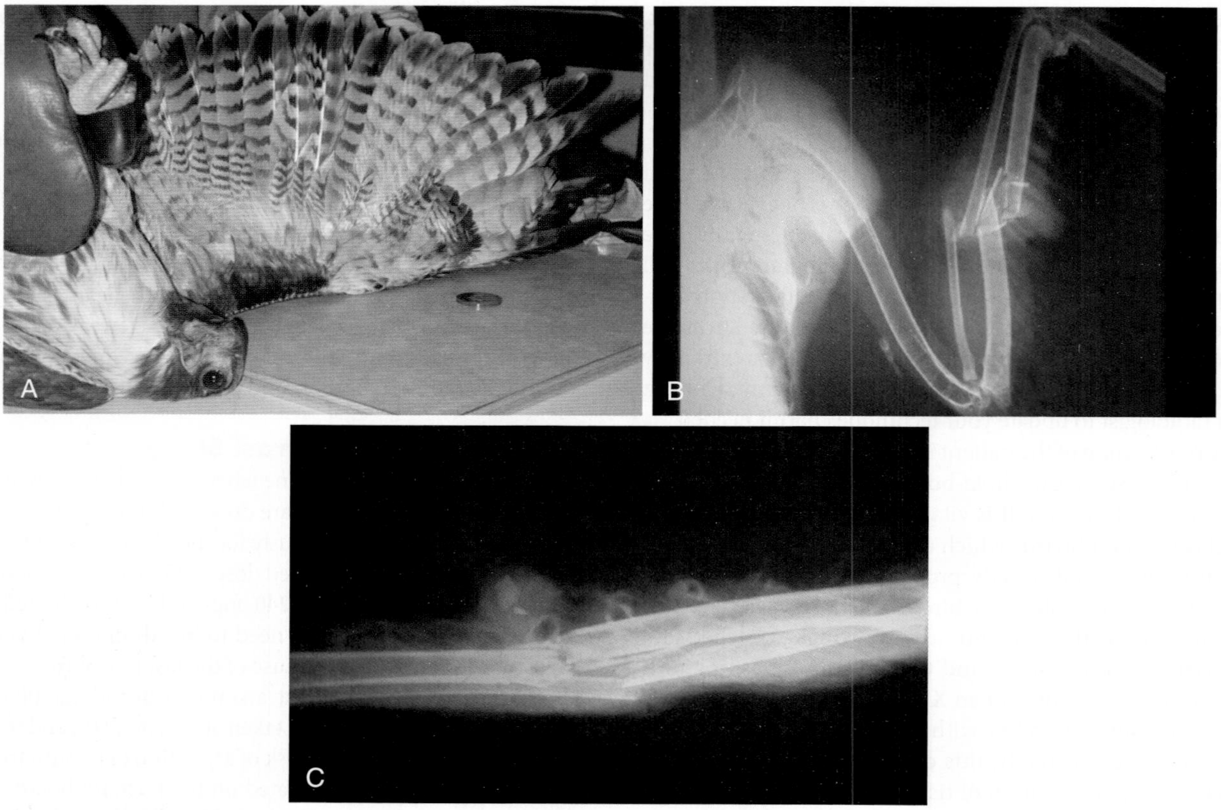

FIGURE 27-32 A, A red-tailed hawk in palmarodorsal (PaD) wing position for radiographs. B, Lateral view of the wing with a fracture. C, Palmarodorsal (PaD) view of the wing with the same fracture.

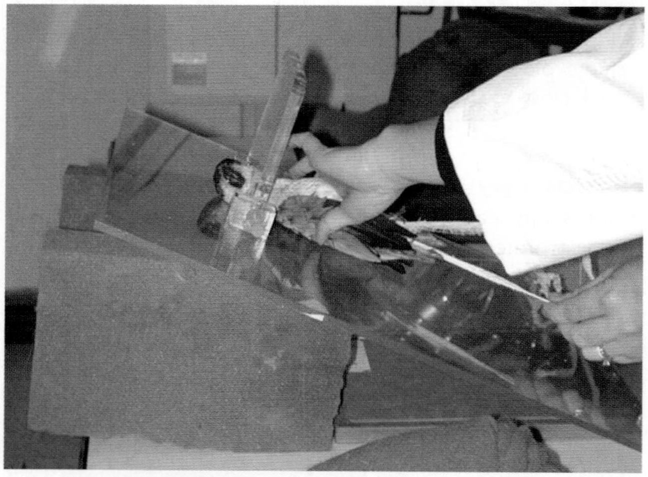

FIGURE 27-33 Elevated restraint board.

evaluating the patient's gastrointestinal motility time and overall function. This can be achieved by placing the patient on a perch or if stressed in a darkened box and placed in front of the fluoroscopy unit. These images can be recorded for further evaluation.

Ultrasound

Ultrasound studies can be fairly limiting in the avian species because ultrasound waves cannot penetrate gas-filled air sacs throughout the bird's body and in some cases the patient is just too small to achieve a diagnostic image. Ultrasound can be used to appreciate organomegaly and coelomic fluid, and masses such as soft-shelled eggs and tumors.

Endoscopy

Endoscopes are fiberoptic probes that use magnification that can provide direct visualization of body structures. There are many different types of endoscopes and the most common are flexible and rigid endoscopes. In avian medicine the rigid endoscopes are an essential piece of equipment. Many veterinarians use the 2.7-mm rigid fiberoptic endoscope, as it can be successfully used in almost all size birds (Fig. 27-34). Most endoscopic procedures are minimally invasive and patient recovery time is more rapid than with exploratory surgeries. The endoscopy can be used for the visual examination of any part of the body that has an orifice large enough to allow the insertion of the instrument. Laparoscopy, tracheoscopy, rhinoscopy, and cloacaloscopy are common diagnostic procedures. Using endoscopy the veterinarian can obtain tissue biopsies, apply interlesional and topical treatments and surgical interventions, in addition to sexing of nondimorphic species.

Proper positioning of the bird for the procedure is very important. The organs or system to be studied determine whether the right or left side will be the site of entry for the scope. The bird will need to be anesthetized and the scope insertion site aseptically prepped and draped. The standard approach for diagnostic evaluation of the internal organs is

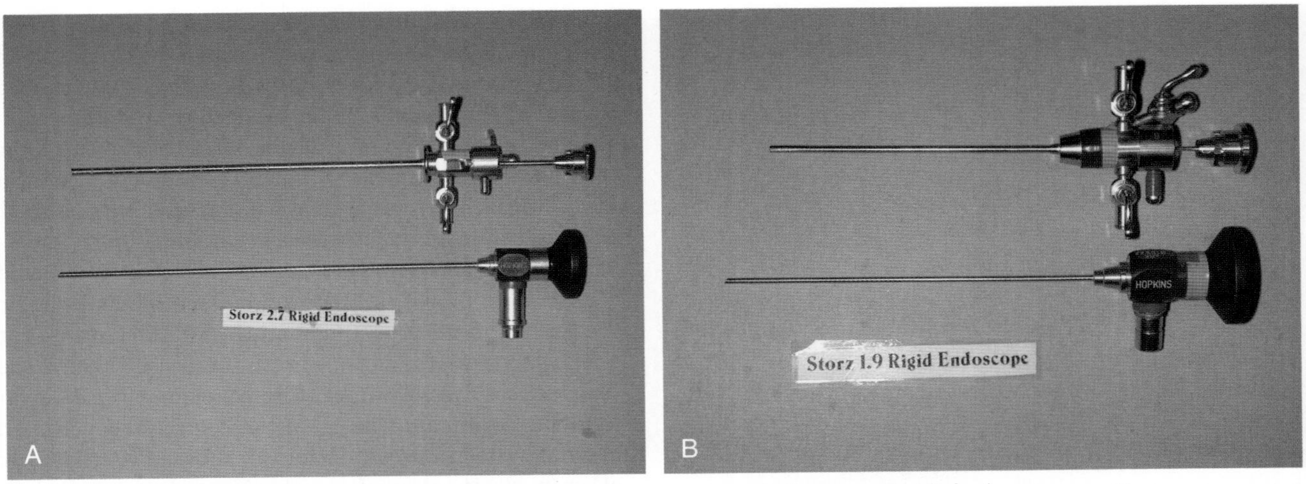

FIGURE 27-34 Common rigid endoscopes in an avian practice. **A,** The most valuable for the avian practitioner is the 2.7 mm rigid. **B,** The 1.9 mm Storz rigid endoscope.

right lateral recumbency. There are two approaches that can be used, one with the left leg pulled caudal and the other with the left leg pulled cranially. The specific position depends on the clinician's preference. A small incision is made in the skin and the muscle layer is bluntly dissected with forceps. The scope and cannula are introduced into the incision through the cranial thoracic or abdominal air sac and organs can be viewed. Lung, reproductive organs, kidney, adrenal glands, ventriculus, and other organs will typically be visualized during this examination. Once the endoscopy is complete, the area will need to be sutured.

Organs may be sampled using the endoscope's biopsy instrument. The tissues obtained in this manner will be very small and easily lost. After collection, they are often arranged on filter paper or closely woven cloth, which is then immersed in fixative solution. Alternatively, biopsy samples may be placed in fixative in a plain blood collection tube that does not contain anticoagulant.

The endoscope is very delicate and must be picked up by the eyepiece. Scope maintenance is essential. Proper cleaning and disinfecting will not only provide higher quality diagnostics, but also increase the longevity of the scope. Make sure to read the manual and follow the manufactures instructions for the proper care of each scope. More information on endoscopy is located in Chapter 6.

NURSING CARE

Hospitalization

Housing the avian patient can be a challenge if you have a small clinic. A separate room is needed for birds. The room should have its own thermostat and able to maintain 85° to 90° F. The cages and perches should be easy to disinfect, and you should have a way to isolate patients suspected of carrying infectious diseases (Fig. 27-35).

For the patient with special requirements such as oxygen, supplemental humidity, or nebulization, you may need to get a little creative. Heat lamps and water circulating heating pads are a great way to provide extra heat to the debilitated patient, but the enclosure needs to be monitored closely so the patient does not become overheated or destroy the pads. An investment in manufactured incubator/oxygen cages is recommended (Fig. 27-36). Many types of these cages are available and are an invaluable addition to your avian practice. These cages can supply heat, humidity, and oxygen and are easy to disinfect.

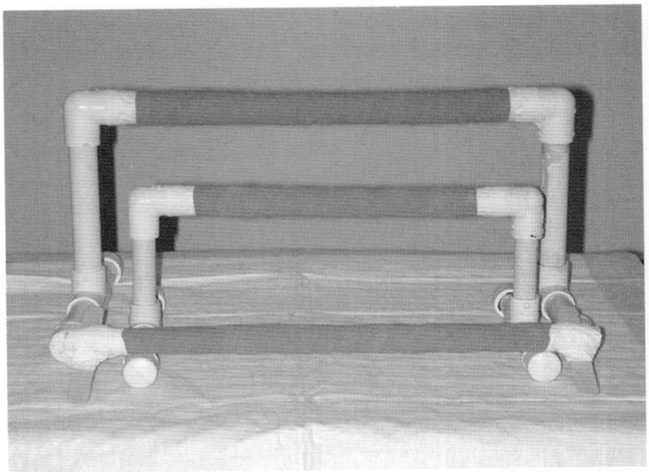

FIGURE 27-35 Perches can be made with inexpensive PVC pipe in a variety of sizes and heights. To these you can add padding as needed per patient.

Avian patients are extremely intelligent and when hospitalized can become very bored and stressed. Patient enrichment is an important part of a patient's road to recovery. This can be achieved by providing the patient with nontoxic and safe disposable toys and mirrors or playing a radio or television for the patient to enjoy. If the patient is willing and receptive you can spend a little time talking quietly and hand feeding the bird in its hospital cage.

Infectious Disease and Zoonoses

Infectious and **zoonotic diseases** are critical problems for bird owners and veterinarians (Box 27-5).

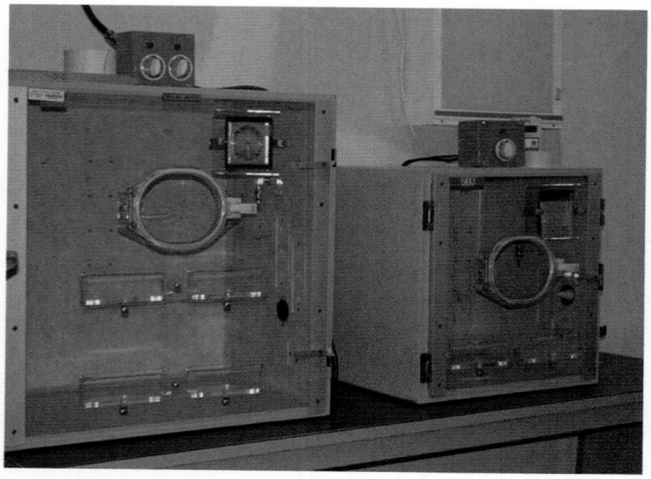

FIGURE 27-36 An oxygen cage is a valuable part of the avian practice.

BOX 27-5 Infectious and Zoonotic Diseases of Birds

- *Chlamydophila psittaci* (Zoonotic)
- Psittacine Beak and Feather Disease Virus (PBFDV); Circovirus
- Avian Polyoma Virus (APV)
- Psittacid Herpes Viruses (PsHVs) or Pacheaco's Disease
- Paramysovirus 3 (PMV-3)
- Exotic Newcastle Disease Virus
- Psittacine Proventricular Dilatation Disease (PDD)
- Papillomaviruses
- Adenoviruses
- Avian Influenza
- West Nile Virus (WNV)
- Eastern Equine Encephalitis (EEE)
- Poxviruses
- *Mycobacterium* sp. (Zoonotic)
- Fungal infections such as aspergillus sp.

Chlamydiosis. Chlamydiosis is caused by the obligate intracellular bacterium, *Chlamydophila psittaci.* This is a zoonotic disease that causes psittacosis in humans and chlamydiosis in avian species. The lungs, air sacs, liver, spleen, central nervous system (CNS), and heart may all be affected. Pneumonia, ocular and nasal discharge, greenish-yellow diarrhea, dehydration, and weight loss are typical signs. Some birds may be asymptomatic carriers of the disease and may shed the organism. Clinical signs and numerous clinical tests are used to diagnose chlamydiosis. Unfortunately, no single test will determine whether the bird is acutely ill, a carrier, or uninfected. Doxycycline is the drug of choice for treatment for duration of a 45-day treatment regimen.

Polyomavirus. The avian polyomavirus (APV) was first discovered in 1981 in fledgling budgerigars. It is a nonenveloped virus that infects primarily young birds, causes acute death in psittacines, and is the most common viral cause of death in breeding facilities. Older affected birds may show lack of blood clotting and gastrointestinal signs such as vomiting, diarrhea, and crop stasis. Surviving birds grow poorly, have abnormal feather development, and produce excessive and watery feces. Recovered asymptomatic birds shed the virus, keeping the facility contaminated. A test and vaccination are available for polyomavirus. Some veterinarians recommend vaccinating all susceptible birds in a breeding facility, or as soon as possible after purchasing the bird and before it is taken into a new home.

Proventricular Dilatation Disease. Proventricular dilatation disease, also known as PDD, can be seen in any psittacine species but occurs most frequently in African Grey parrots, eclectus, cockatoos, and conures. The disease is first seen as early as 10 weeks of age. Clinical signs of disease vary significantly. Inflammations of the central and peripheral nervous systems are responsible for the characteristic signs of crop stasis, anorexia, cachexia, and incoordination. A virus is suspected to cause this disease, and the avian bornavirus (ABV) has been significantly linked to the disease. No diagnostic test is available. Treatment trials with the NSAID drugs have shown promise in slowing progression of the disease. Nutritional support and fluid therapy are also needed in acutely ill birds.

Psittacine Beak and Feather Disease. Psittacine beak and feather disease (PBFD) is a viral disease that may first be seen in neonates in an infected nursery. The large majority of birds with the chronic form first develop lesions between 6 months and 3 years of age. Abnormal feather growth and lack of powder on the beak are the main signs and it is easily spread by feather dust, dander, and feces to other birds. The germinal tissues of the beak are also affected, resulting in a misshapen and crumbly beak. Birds are most susceptible up to age 2 or 3. Diagnostic testing is available. Young birds that test positive must be removed from the flock. All young birds must be tested before they are transferred to new owners or into a breeding situation. New birds are often tested when they receive their post purchase veterinary examination.

Poxvirus. There are many poxviruses and each one has its own host range. Poxviruses need an injury or vectors such as mosquitoes to allow the virus to enter the body. Poxvirus is most often associated with imported Amazons and macaws, but other species such as canaries may be infected if housed outside in temperate or subtropical climates. Clinical presentation of this disease can be lesions around the face, eyelids, and commissures of the mouth, on the feet, and under the wings. Treatment is supportive therapy.

West Nile Virus. The West Nile Virus is a mosquito-borne disease that primarily infects horses, humans, and birds. It has spread rapidly throughout the United States in the past few years. Psittacines appear to be somewhat resistant, because only a few cases have been reported from endemic areas. However, keeping pet birds inside or in screened areas is suggested to prevent exposure. No avian vaccine is available, but zoo and avian veterinarians are using the equine killed West Nile Virus vaccine in an attempt to create immunity in exotic species.

BOX 27-6 Resources for Information on Infectious Diseases

- Center for Disease Control and Prevention, http://www.cdc.gov
- World Health Organization, http://www.who.int
- National Institute of Allergy and Infectious Diseases, http://www3.niaid.nih.gov
- Occupational Safety and Health Administration, http://www.osha.gov

Preventing the Spread of Disease in the Clinic

Patients suspected of having infectious diseases must be isolated from other patients. Isolation areas must be out of the mainstream of the clinic, where there is minimal foot traffic. Ideally the isolation room should have a ventilation system separate from the main clinic system. Disposable protective shoe covers or foot baths must be used when exiting this room to prevent carrying any infectious agent out of the isolation area.

All veterinary team members who handle animals suspected of having a zoonotic or any infectious disease must wear personal protective equipment, not only to protect themselves against infection but also to prevent transmission to other animals and people. Personal protective equipment includes disposable outer garments, lab coats or coveralls, disposable head or hair covers and gloves, safety goggles, and disposable particulate respirators approved by the National Institute for Occupational Safety and Health. Disposable equipment should be considered contaminated and properly disposed of after use. Nondisposable items such as lab coats and goggles should be cleaned and disinfected between uses. When removing contaminated protective equipment, personnel should remove their outer garments—except for gloves—first and discard them. They should then remove their gloves, wash their hands with soap and water, remove their goggles and particulate respirators, and immediately wash their hands again. If soap and water are not available, an alcohol-based hand gel is sufficient. Using these protective measures will help prevent the spread of disease in your clinic and protect those working with the patients. A number of web sites are available that provide reliable, accurate, and timely information about infectious diseases and personal protection (Box 27-6).

Preparedness while Providing Supportive Care. Preparation and efficiency are essential when providing supportive care to the avian patient. Try to develop a systematic routine that you consistently follow. Before capturing and restraining any patients, determine exactly what needs to be done and which patients you should start with. Prepare each patient's medications, fluids, and food before capture. Make sure to treat the infectious disease suspects last, wear disposable attire (or change your lab coat or scrub top after handling), and wash your hands well after handling all your patients to prevent the spread of disease. Evaluate the patient and determine the potential limitations, and perform the patient treatments in stages if needed. If the patient is critical, be prepared to administer oxygen; have an endotracheal tube ready; calculate and prepare resuscitation drugs such as atropine, epinephrine, and glycopyrrolate. If the patient is so ill that you feel it might die within the first minute of treatment, then it may be best to postpone or cancel the scheduled treatments until the patient is more stable.

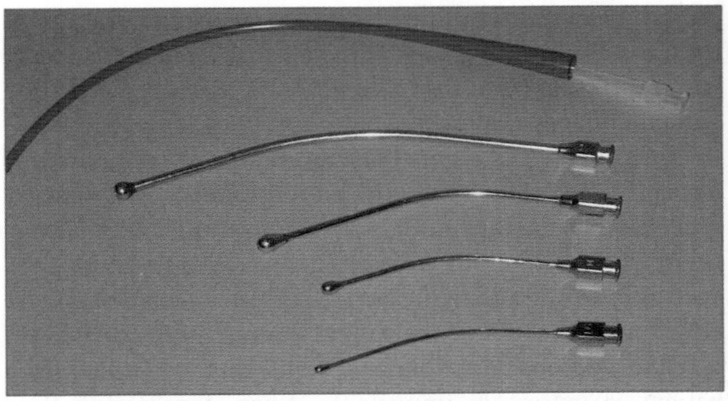

FIGURE 27-37 Gavage needles and red rubber feeding tubes can be used to provide fluid nutritional support and medications to hospitalized birds.

Oral Administration. Medication and fluids may be administered to birds orally if the patient is alert and active. Primary regurgitation or vomiting, poor patient reflexes or recumbency, or oral and upper gastrointestinal trauma may exclude this method. This route of administering medication is practically stress free if the patient is tolerant. Some birds will love the attention of being hand fed and medicated. Medications mixed in mashed banana or fruit baby foods are often well accepted.

Medication of the feed and water is unreliable for the majority of the patients you will see in practice. This method should not be used. This is, however, the major method of administering drugs to poultry and others in large flock situations.

Gavage Feeding. Fluid therapy, nutritional support, and medication administration can be provided by gavage or tube feeding. Limiting factors may include patients with crops stasis, ileus, gastrointestinal impactions, or other gastrointestinal abnormalities that reduce motility or absorption. A variety of flexible and rigid feeding needles and tubes are available (Fig. 27-37).

Gavage feeding will require multiple people to complete in larger birds, but with the smaller birds a skilled person can usually do it alone (Fig. 27-38). In larger birds one person holds the patient in an upright position, another opens the mouth, and another person advances the tube into place and administers the medications and food. Care must be taken that the patient does not bite the tube and ingest it. To place the tube, enter the oral cavity from the patient's right commissure of the mouth, pass the tube/needle along the right side of the tongue, avoiding the glottis and advancing into the esophagus. Palpate the tube in the crop or visualize the glottis before administering any food or medications to verify that you did not place the tube in the trachea. While administering the medications or food, watch the back of the mouth. If food or liquid material appears in the oral cavity, the bird should be immediately placed back into its enclosure without further handling to prevent the risk of regurgitation and potential aspiration.

An estimate of the energy requirement of an animal is needed to determine how much food to feed. Daily energy requirements are the number of calories needed to maintain the animal's weight. An increase in the patient's activity level, such as preening and flying or stressors in the form of disease or trauma will increase the patient's caloric need (Box 27-7).

Fluid Replacement Therapy. Fluid therapy in the avian patient is extremely important. When considering fluid therapy for your patients, you and your clinician will be considering many variables when calculating a fluid dose (Box 27-8). Consider maintenance requirements, sensible losses, insensible losses, and contemporary losses. Most of the birds presented with urgency have a history of inadequate water consumption so we assume most of the avian emergencies to be at least 5% dehydrated. On physical examination the patient may present with dull sunken eyes, tacky oral mucous membranes, increased venous refill time, and increased skin turgor. Monitoring body weight twice daily is important for evaluation of hydration in birds.

Half of the fluid deficit is given over the first 24 hours and the remaining half is given over the next 48 hours. A crystalloid fluid such as lactated Ringer's solution (LRS) is usually sufficient; however, hemodilution can be a limiting factor to LRS use. When proteinemia is present in a critical patient, colloids such as plasma or hetastarch may be a better choice. The routes of fluid administration are oral, subcutaneous, intravenous, and intraosseous.

Subcutaneous Injection Sites. Subcutaneous sites are found in the inguinal, axillary, and dorsal regions. The inguinal region is the preferred site to administer subcutaneous fluids and medications (Fig. 27-39). With the patient restrained in dorsal recumbency, pull the legs straight down; apply a small amount of alcohol to the medial side of the most proximal portion of the leg, parting the feathers. Using a small gauge needle, preferably 25-gauge to 26-gauge, insert the needle

BOX 27-7 Energy Requirements for Birds

Basal Metabolic Rate (BMR)

The BMR is the minimum amount of energy required for daily maintenance while the body is at rest. BMR differs between species. An estimation for BMR can be calculated by using the formula: BMR = K (W $kg^{0.75}$) where W = weight in kg, K = a theoretical constant for kcal/24hrs, and BMR = kcal/kg/day.

K = (non-passerines) = 78 ; passerines = 129

The following simplified calculations can be used to determine the energetic requirements of birds:

$$\text{Passerine BMR Kcal/day} = 114.8 \times kg^{0.726}$$

$$\text{(Non-passerine) BMR Kcal/day} = 73.5 \times kg^{0.734}$$

Maintenance Energy Requirement (MER)

The MER is the BMR plus the additional energy needed for normal physical activity.

MER is measured in kcal/day and is approximately 1.5 × BMR.

MER needs to be adjusted for health status:

Physical inactivity 0.7-0.9 × MER = adjusted kcal/day
Starvation: 0.5-0.7 × MER = adjusted kcal/day
Elective surgery 1.0-1.2 × MER = adjusted kcal/day
Mild trauma 1.0-1.2 × MER = adjusted kcal/day
Severe trauma 1.1-2.0 × MER = adjusted kcal/day
Growth 1.5-3.0 × MER = adjusted kcal/day
Sepsis 1.2-1.5 × MER = adjusted kcal/day
Burns 1.2-2.0 × MER = adjusted kcal/day
Head injuries 1.0-2.0 × MER = adjusted kcal/day

BOX 27-8 Calculating Fluid Replacement Therapy

Maintenance fluid rate is 50 ml/kg/24 hrs + deficit.

Estimated dehydration (%) × body weight (grams) = deficit.

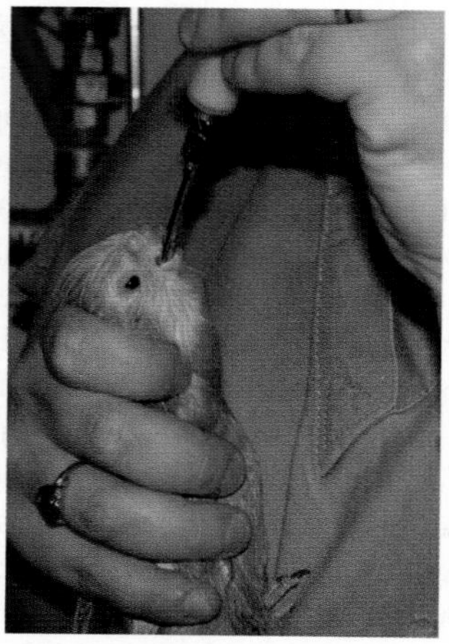

FIGURE 27-38 This experienced technician is able to gavage feed this cockatiel alone, which is the standard accepted method.

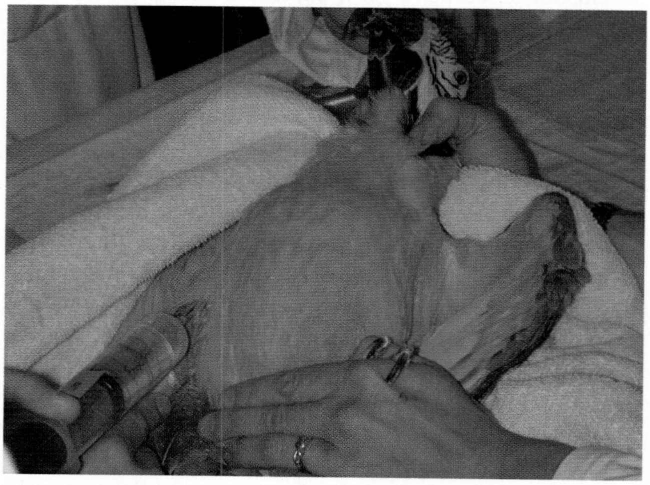

FIGURE 27-39 A blue and gold macaw is receiving a dose of subcutaneous fluids in the right inguinal region.

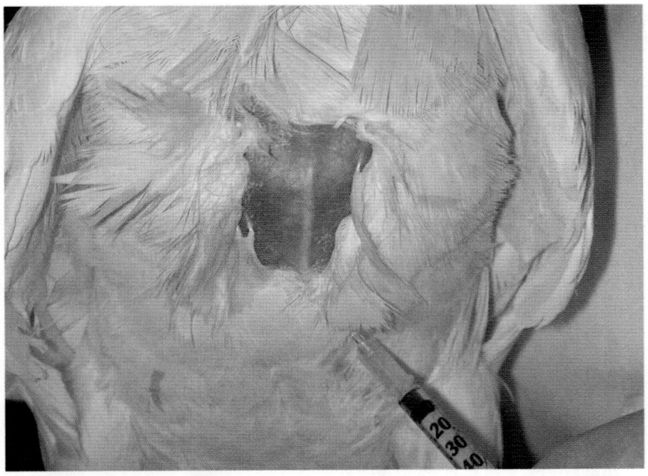

FIGURE 27-40 The pectoral muscles are the optimum injection site for IM injections in birds.

just under the skin and administer some fluids and a bubble should form. Similar administration techniques are used for the axillary and dorsal regions; however, you cannot get as much fluid into these areas.

Intramuscular Injections. For intramuscular injections the pectoral muscles are most commonly used. These represent the largest muscle mass on the bird and are found on both sides of the keel (Fig. 27-40). Always use a small-gauge needle (25- to 26-gauge) to reduce the amount of muscle damage and don't use the same area of muscle every time. Palpate the keel and don't mistake the crop or abdominal region for the pectoral muscles. Have the patient in an upright position then wet the feathers slightly so you can visualize the skin. A maximum of 0.2 to 0.3 ml can be administered in one site for a large bird. If you need to administer a large volume via this route, then use multiple sites and alternate these sites each treatment time to decrease the chances of muscle necrosis. Birds, like reptiles, do have a renal portal system so drugs administered in the caudal third of the body may go through the kidneys before reaching the rest of the body. Keep this in mind when administering potentially nephrotoxic drugs.

Intravenous Catheter Placement. In most veterinary hospitals, the placement of an intravenous catheter ensures reliable venous access that can remain in place for a number of days. This is true for the average small animal patient; however, for the avian patient this can be quite a challenge. IV catheters are normally placed for anesthetic procedures but not routinely used for daily venous access. In the anesthetized patient IV catheters are fairly easy to secure with tissue glue or sutures. Once the patient has recovered from anesthesia, it is very difficult to maintain a patent catheter. The avian patient is more apt to chew out the IV catheter within seconds of placing the patient back into its cage. If the patient is extremely debilitated, it is possible to secure the catheter well enough for a few days and the same sites can be used as previously discussed for venipuncture. Aseptic catheter care must be performed on a daily basis with all catheters placed for long-term medication administration, and the site of the catheter is usually changed every 3 days. Birds in advanced stages of disease do not have very forgiving veins, so you may be limited to the number of potential IV catheter sites. If you are unable to secure an IV catheter for fluid and medication administration, the more feasible option is an intraosseous catheter.

Intraosseous Catheter Placement. Intraosseous (IO) catheters can be used in the same manner as an IV catheter to administer fluid therapy, blood, antibiotics, and other medications. IO catheters can be placed in any bone that has a marrow cavity such as the distal ulna and proximal tibia. Pneumatic bones such as the humerus and femur cannot be used, because these communicate with the respiratory system. Placement in the distal ulna is fairly well tolerated and easier to maintain in debilitated birds than placement in the proximal tibia. Depending on the size of the patient, 20-gauge to 22-gauge spinal needles are used. These are preferred because the stylet feature prevents bone cortex material from occluding the cannula during placement. In small birds such as cockatiels and conures a 25-gauge needle can be placed in the distal ulna. To place a cannula in the distal ulna, the patient will need to be anesthetized and sterile technique used (Procedure 27-3).

Bandaging. The figure-of-eight bandage is used when a patient is presented with fractures or soft tissue injuries distal to the elbow or when you need to stabilize a wing with an intraosseous catheter. Soft roll gauze followed by a layer of self-adherent bandage material will provide the best results. With the wing in a flexed position, start the bandage at the carpus; wrap the gauze around the carpus, thus creating the top of the 8 in the figure 8. Roll the gauze toward the elbow and wrap the gauze around the area proximal to the elbow. Make sure the gauze is high in the axillary region; this will help prevent slipping. This will create the lower end of the figure 8. Be careful not to make the wrap too tight or bulky or constrict the pytagium. If necessary, cut a V-shaped slit in the bandage over the pytagium to help release pressure in that area and prevent injury to the pytagium.

A body wrap is added in addition to the figure-of-eight bandage when the patient has a humeral or pectoral girdle fractures. When placing a body wrap, care must be taken not to place tension on the keel, which can impede breathing. Also ensure that the body wrap is directly over the keel and not putting pressure on the crop or coelomic cavity, or interfering with the movement of the legs. Use caution when placing a body wrap on anesthetized birds, because of the potential respiratory depression that can occur if the body wrap is placed too tight. Once the bandage is in place the bird should be monitored for increased stress, dyspnea, and chewing or destroying the bandage. An Elizabethan collar or a sedative may be necessary in some cases.

Elizabethan Collar Placement. Elizabethan collars (E-collars) and other mechanical barriers are placed for many reasons including prevention of self-trauma such as feather picking and self-mutilation or to protect a bandage or wound (Fig. 27-41). You can make these collars out of old x-ray film, insulation pipe found at the hardware store, or you can purchase very small versions of the ones used for canine and

PROCEDURE 27-3 Intraosseous Catheter Placement

- Pluck a few feathers over the dorsal, distal ulna, and surgically prep the area (Fig. 1).

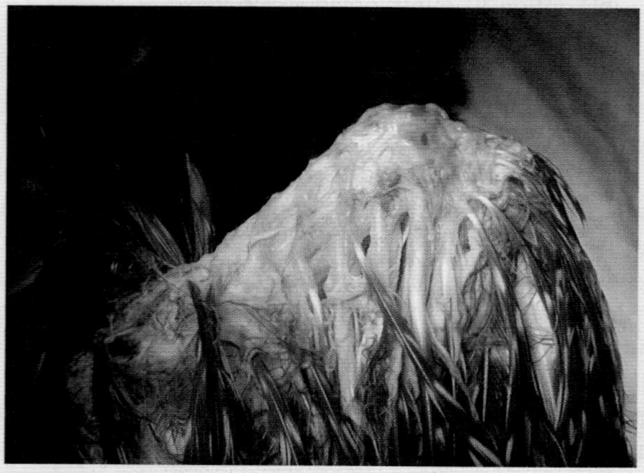

FIGURE 1

- Grasp the ulna with one hand and insert the cannula with the other.
- Palpate the dorsal condyle of the distal ulna and insert the cannula just above this condyle (Fig. 2).

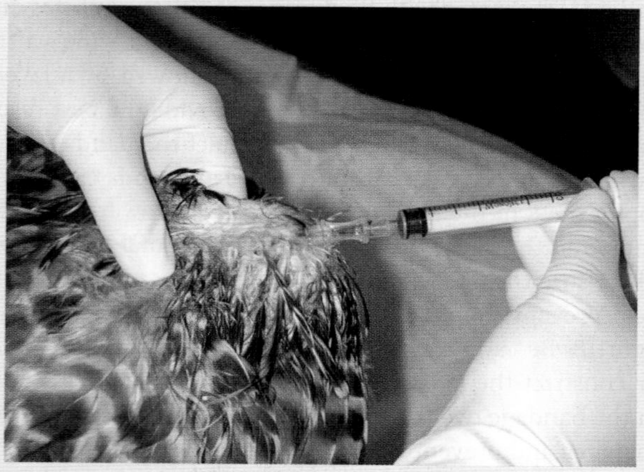

FIGURE 2

- Advance the cannula into the medullary cavity by applying steady firm pressure, with a slight rotating motion, on the cannula as it is positioned in a straight line with the ulna aiming toward the elbow.
- Once the cannula is in place remove the stylet (Fig. 3).

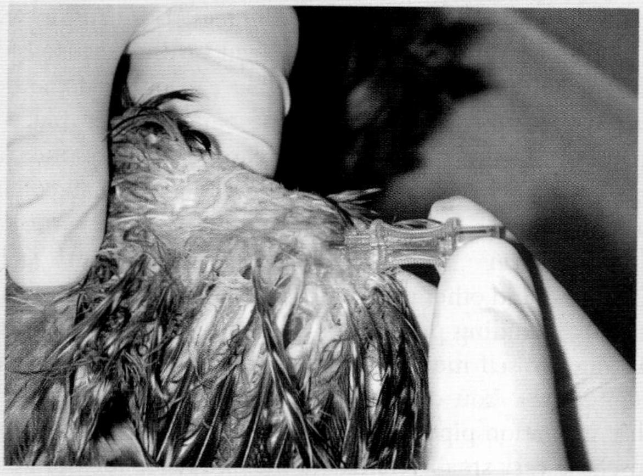

FIGURE 3

- Cap off the cannula with a sterile infusion plug.
- Flush with heparinized saline and you will notice little to no resistance.
- As you flush the catheter, visualize the ulnar vein; it should be clear demonstrating that you are in the correct location.
- The cannula should now be sutured into place (Fig. 4).

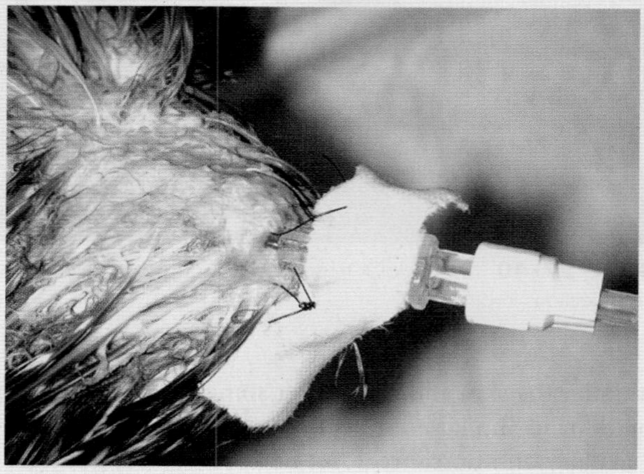

FIGURE 4

- The wing should be wrapped with a figure-of-eight bandage to secure the wing and keep the insertion site clean (Fig. 5).

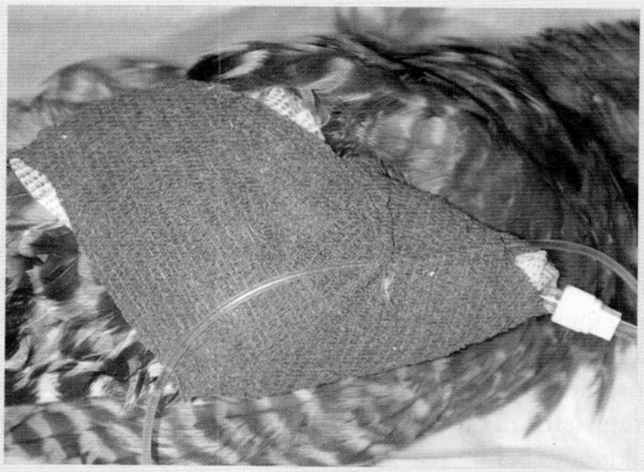

FIGURE 5

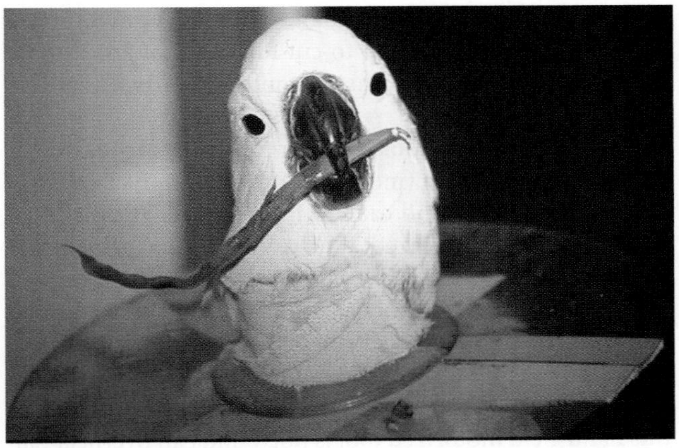

FIGURE 27-41 Some birds adapt very well to life in an Elizabethan collar. Every bird will need to be monitored for proper hydration and ability to eat.

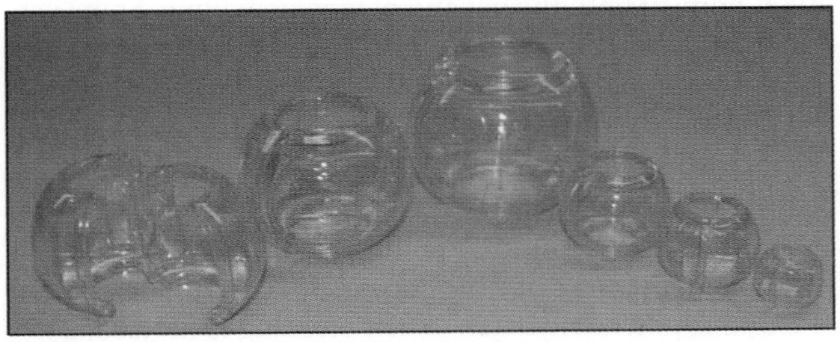

FIGURE 27-42 Commercially available bubble-style Ecollars.

feline patients. If you make a collar, the edges must be padded to prevent sores from forming and ensure that the bird cannot chew at the outside rim of the collar. Crib type collars have an attachable disk. This collar prevents the bird from dropping its head far enough to pick at the upper and lower portions of the body. In some cases the bird can still reach the area just below the lower rim of the crib collar, and the tips of the wings. The disk can be added to prevent any picking altogether; however, you should monitor the bird closely to ensure that it can still eat and drink. Commercially available bubble-style E-collars can be used, but may not be as effective at keeping the bird from reaching the back half of its body (Fig. 27-42).

When a collar is first placed on the bird, sedation and cage padding may be required until the collar is accepted. Some birds are highly stressed after the collar is placed, and begin flipping in all different directions along with flapping uncontrollably and screaming. Once the bird has adjusted to the collar you can return the bird to its owner, providing you counsel the owner on the possible complications regarding the collar. Possible complications include trouble eating and drinking, trouble with balance and navigating around the normal environment, and pressure sores or abrasions from the collar.

HUSBANDRY RESPONSIBILITIES OF TECHNICIANS

Beak Trimming

Overgrowth of the beak in psittacines is a common deformity that will be presented to your clinic for correction (Fig. 27-43).

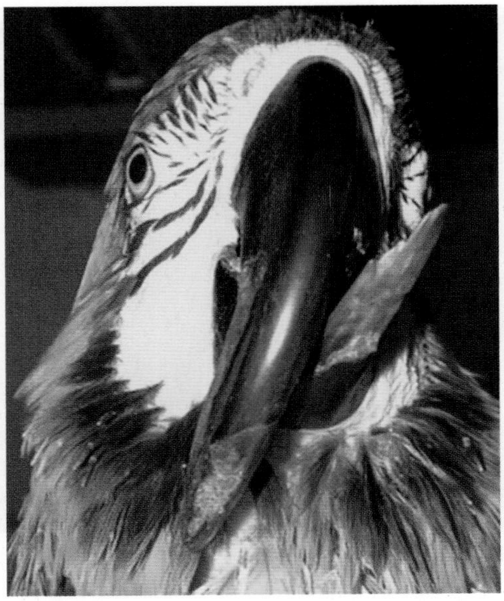

FIGURE 27-43 The need for a beak trim will be obvious in some patients.

It is very important that you know (or have a reference for) the normal lengths of the beaks you are trimming before you trim. It is also very important to try and determine why the beak is overgrown. In some cases overgrowth results from malocclusion resulting in insufficient wear on the beak; liver disease can be another cause. Any patient presenting for beak overgrowth should be required to have a complete workup to determine the cause.

Reducing the length and grooming the beak can be done with a Dremel motor tool (Dremel, Inc, Racine, Wisconsin). Cone-shaped aluminum oxide grinding stones work great on beaks as well as toenails. To prevent the spread of disease, it is best to have a separate grinding stone per patient, which you can sell to the owner and the owner can bring to each visit. To perform this procedure, the restrainer holds the bird in an upright position. The person performing the trim holds the beak closed with one hand, and applies the Dremel with the other. Care should be taken not to cover the nares as you hold the beak shut (Fig. 27-44). Monitor the patient closely for hypoxia and hyperthermia. Once you have achieved the desired length or shape, a small amount of mineral oil can be applied to remove the dust and make the beak aesthetically pleasing.

Wing Trimming

Trimming a bird's wings is one method to decrease the bird's ability to fly. This is done by selectively trimming some of the primary and secondary feathers. The flight feathers are numbered from the inside-out, 1 through 10. There is a natural break in the direction of the feathers with the feathers of the manus (primaries—P-1 to P-10) angled out, and the feathers on the brachium and antibrachium (secondaries—S-1 to S-10) angled in.

It is very important to question the client to determine how much flight is needed and how aesthetically pleasing

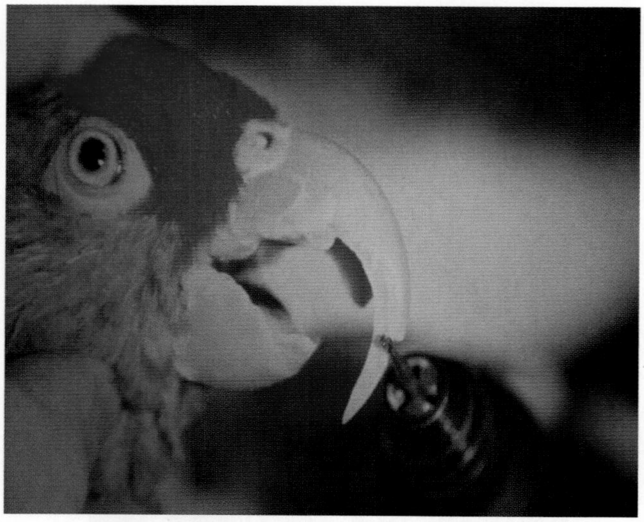

FIGURE 27-44 Trimming a beak with the Dremel.

they want the trim. A nice aesthetically pleasing trim leaves the distal 2 primary feathers intact, trimming only 4 to 8 feathers on each wing. The recommendation is to trim both wings evenly for balance. The general rule of wing trim is that the heavier bodied a bird is, the fewer feathers are removed.

The trim is done up high under the coverts, so that the jagged edges of the cut feathers are not showing. You should evaluate the feather to be trimmed and ensure that it is not a blood feather; these should be avoided and if one is located, the mature feather on either side should be left as support. Flying ability should be tested in the clinic before the bird is sent home. Flight distance should be limited to less than 25 feet, and lift to less than 2 feet. Additional feathers can be trimmed after a flight test if necessary.

Instruments used to perform a wing trimming are varied and include suture scissors, cat nail trimmers, wire cutters, and sharp-sharp scissors. Prevent the spread of disease by sterilizing the trimmers after each use.

> *TECHNICIAN NOTE* Always test flying ability in the clinic after trimming flight feathers.

Nail Trimming

A regularly requested service is trimming of long or sharp nails. Nail trimming is an important preventative care procedure. Excessive nail length can result in improper perching and the nail could be traumatically avulsed. An overgrown nail could get caught in the grate commonly found in the bottom of most birdcages, or on the carpet as the bird wanders around the house. Untrimmed nails can grow into the pad of the foot causing cellulitis or abscess formation. The size and temperament of the bird determines the number of people required to perform the trim (Fig. 27-45). Towel restraint is commonly used.

Birds with light-colored nails have easily visible blood vessels, improving the chances of a nail trim without any bleeding. In birds with black nails, an understanding of the structure of the nail is important. However, even with extreme care it is not unusual to cut the quick of at least one nail, causing bleeding. Owners should be warned that this might happen.

The most common tools used for nail trims include Resco trimmers, the Dremel (motorized) tool, files, nail scissors, fingernail trimmers, and cautery instruments. These should be disinfected or sterilized after using to help prevent the spread of disease between birds. Each clinic and veterinarian prefers certain instruments for nail trims. The typical small animal practice could easily trim bird nails without purchase of additional equipment. The Dremel tool, typically used on large birds, uses a grinding tip to blunt the tips of the nails. This hand-held motorized tool is noisy and can overheat nail tissues if applied too long. Flat or rounded fine tooth files are preferred by some for nail trims of birds of any size. This method slowly blunts the nail tips, causing some birds to become impatient and struggle. Clients can be trained to do this at home if both the pet and owner are willing. Some veterinarians use electrocautery instruments to trim nails and prevent bleeding at the same time. Many birds exhibit pain reactions to this procedure, presumably related to the high heat of the instrument. This method of nail trimming should be done primarily on anesthetized animals.

Any blood loss in birds should be considered serious. In very small birds, loss of what appears to be a minute amount of blood is potentially fatal. When bleeding is noticed, a hemostatic powder must be pressed immediately onto the nail.

Determination of Gender

Pet birds often have spectacularly colorful plumage. However, it is important to realize that it is virtually impossible to determine the gender of the majority of companion birds by appearance, because males and females of each species look identical. One major exception to this rule is the eclectus parrot, in which the female is a deep reddish color with a dark beak, and the male is bright green with an orange beak (Fig. 27-46). The gender of a bird can be determined by endoscopy; however, DNA sexing is a safer alternative to the surgical approach and is available through some labs around the country. With a very small amount of whole blood (a drop or two), the gender of a bird can be determined within a few days. DNA sexing uses the polymerase chain reaction (PCR) to analyze the DNA from the sex chromosomes of the bird.

Microchipping

Microchipping is an identification method that you may already offer your clients. The microchip is a tiny computer chip which has an identification number programmed into it and is encapsulated within a biocompatible material. The whole device is small enough to fit inside a hypodermic needle and can be simply injected intramuscularly, where it will stay for the life of the bird. This provides a permanent, positive identification which cannot be lost, altered, or intentionally removed. The microchip devices are sold as a disposable syringe and large needle unit for one-time use. Before anesthetizing the bird for placement of a microchip it is best to

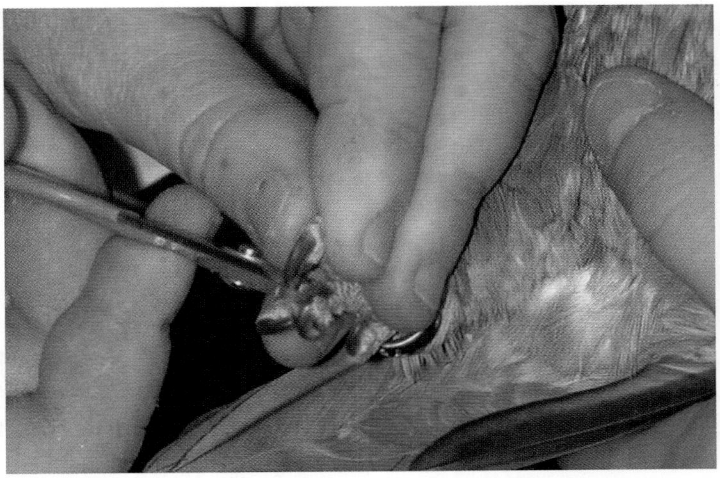

FIGURE 27-45 Grasp one toe at a time, keeping the other toes safely away from the trimmer so that the other toes or toenails will not be cut by mistake.

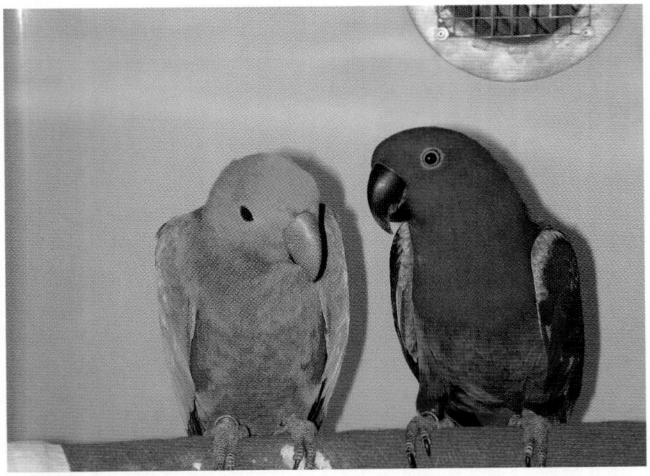

FIGURE 27-46 A pair of eclectus parrots demonstrate sexual dimorphism.

scan the patient to verify that there is not already a chip present. Scan the chip as well to ensure it works. The bird should be anesthetized for the procedure because the microchip is injected into the pectoral muscle via a 15-gauge needle and can be a very painful and stressful procedure. The site should be aseptically prepared. After the chip has been inserted, scan the bird to verify that the chip is functioning correctly.

AVIAN EMERGENCIES AND COMMON PRESENTATIONS

An emergency can be defined as a sudden or unforeseen situation that requires immediate action (Box 27-9). Emergency care of the avian patient can be challenging. Birds are primarily a species that is preyed upon and tend to mask signs of illness as a means of self-preservation. Instinctually birds hide these symptoms so they will not be killed by members of their own flock or by a predator for being the weakest link in the flock. By hiding their illnesses birds can be in an advanced state of debilitation by the time they are brought into the clinic. In some cases handling for examination can be contraindicated, and supportive therapy should be considered a priority. The bird that is having trouble perching or is "fluffed" may be an indication that the bird is very ill and should be considered an emergency. Fluffing (elevating the body feathers to trap warm air near the body) is a bird's response to loss of body heat (Fig. 27-47).

BOX 27-9 Avian Emergencies

- Dyspnea, gasping for air
- Bleeding
- Generalized weakness
- Sudden depression
- "Fluffed Bird"
- Trauma
- Trouble perching
- Regurgitation/Vomiting/Inappetence
- Coelomic distension
- Prolapsed cloaca

Initial Assessment/Stabilization and Supportive Care

Birds are often presented with nonspecific signs such as "fluffed up," sitting on cage bottom, loss of appetite, untidy appearance, lethargic/weakness, droopy eyelids, and loss of interest in surroundings. The bird that is simply not doing well is a challenge. The patient size often limits the diagnostic and treatment options. Because avian patients are sometimes too critical to perform a thorough physical examination or laboratory sampling, start by evaluating the bird in its cage environment and obtain a detailed history. If the patient is dyspneic or appears stressed, don't handle the bird. Place the bird in a quiet, warm, oxygen cage and observe from a distance. Unfortunately, most avian patients decompensate quickly, so prioritize what needs to be done such as physical examination, fluid or antibiotic therapy, radiographs, etc. Once the patient is determined to be stable then these treatments/diagnostics can be done in stages if needed.

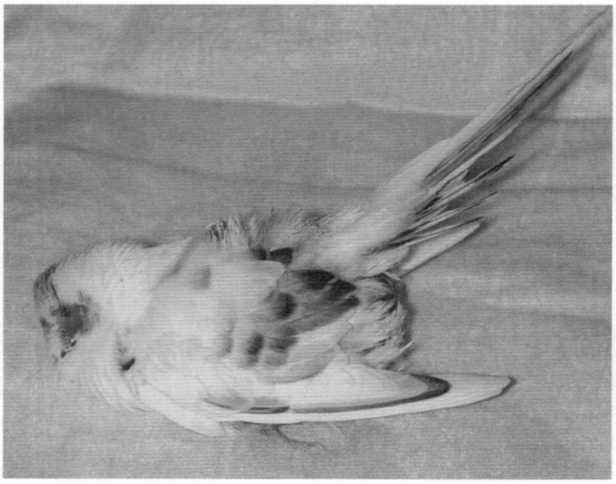

FIGURE 27-47 When a bird is cold or does not feel well, it will elevate the body feathers to trap warm air near the body to conserve energy for other vital functions such as metabolism.

Respiratory Emergencies

A bird in respiratory distress can present to your clinic for a variety of reasons including inhaled toxins, space occupying masses in the coelomic cavity, foreign body aspiration, tumors or other growths in the airway, or respiratory disease. A bird in distress should be handled as little as possible to avoid further stress or death. Diagnosis and treatment is critical in acute onset of respiratory problems, and differentiating between upper airway and lower airway ailments can be challenging. Normal respiratory patterns should be slow and regular and in the healthy bird, virtually unnoticeable (Box 27-10). The respiratory rate can vary from 10 to 40 breaths per minute depending on the size of the bird.

Upper Airway Emergencies. Upper airway emergencies can result from aspirated foreign bodies such as seeds, splinters from wooden toys, or other pieces from toys in the cage. Any condition that results in tracheal obstruction can lead to an upper airway emergency (Box 27-11).

In cases of tracheal or syringeal obstruction, emergency placement of an air sac tube is necessary (Fig. 27-48). The air sac tube is placed directly into the caudal thoracic or abdominal air sac (Procedure 27-4). Air sac cannulas are contraindicated in lower airway diseases. An air sac cannula simply bypasses the obstructed upper airway by entering into the airway via an air sac, comparable to a tracheotomy tube in mammals.

Lower Airway Emergencies. Airborne toxins are dangerous to birds. They may die within a few minutes of exposure or develop chronic problems. Examples include overheated Teflon pans (polytetrafluoroethylene), hairspray, tobacco smoke, paint fumes, strong cleaning chemicals, carbon monoxide, and dust from leaded paint (Box 27-12).

Treatment for aerosol toxicity includes removing the source of the toxin or removing the bird from the toxic environment. Once in the clinic the patient should be placed in an oxygen cage. If the lungs are already compromised or damaged, an air sac tube may have little to no effect. These cases are best managed with minimal stress/restraint of the patient, and supportive care such as nutritional, fluid, and oxygen therapy with nebulization.

BOX 27-10 Signs of Respiratory Distress

- Tachypnea
- Labored respiration
- Open mouth respiration
- Audible respirations
- Change in vocalizations
- Tail bobbing
- Collapse

BOX 27-11 Upper Airway Emergencies

Tracheal Obstructions with
- Tumors
- Papillomas
- Granulomas
- Transtracheal membranes

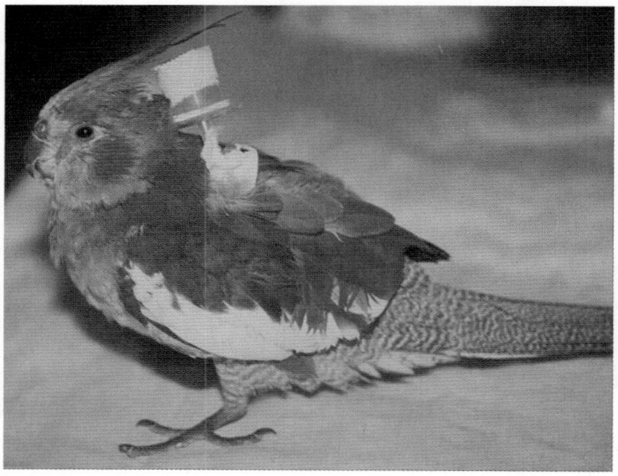

FIGURE 27-48 This cockatiel presented in respiratory distress with a history of changes in vocalization. An air sac cannula was placed in the abdominal air sac with immediate improvement in the respiratory rate and effort. Tracheal endoscopy was performed, and a granuloma was discovered in the trachea at the level of the syrinx, blocking 90% of the bird's airway.

Space Occupying Masses

Some respiratory emergencies may be caused by a space-occupying mass in the coelomic cavity. This can be the result of egg stasis, tumors, organ enlargement, or fluid buildup in the coelom (Fig. 27-49). Birds need air to move through their air sacs to breathe, so if a space-occupying mass is putting pressure on the air sacs, the bird will present in respiratory distress. Obese birds will often present in respiratory distress because their adipose tissue is compressing the air sacs, causing difficulty breathing.

PROCEDURE 27-4 Air Sac Cannula Placement

- Anesthetize the patient and place in right lateral recumbency to utilize the left abdominal or caudal thoracic air sacs.
- Remove the feathers in the region of the last rib and caudal to the last rib.
- Three anatomical landmarks form a triangle that surrounds the insertion site: the latissimus dorsi muscle dorsally; cranial iliotibialis muscle, which is the ventral portion of the triangle; and the last rib.
- Aseptically prepare the insertion site.
- Make a small skin incision caudal to last rib in the flank region.
- Using curved hemostat forceps, bluntly dissect muscle.
- Open the hemostats and feed the tube into place.
- Check for airflow through the tube by listening or holding a feather over the opening of the tube and watch for the airflow to move the feather. Alternately you can use a cover slip or microscope slide, hold it over the end of the tube, and watch for fogging.
- Secure the tube to the body by applying some tape in a butterfly formation and suture the tabs to the skin.
- Place an endotracheal adapter to the end of the tube and cover with a piece of HEPA filter cut from a surgery mask. This will prevent debris from entering the air sac.
- A piece of Tegaderm or other light bandage can be placed over the insertion site.

In an emergency situation the patient may be placed in right lateral recumbency, the feathers saturated with alcohol, the landmarks located, and an 18-gauge IV catheter placed for an immediate airway. The filter will need to be changed daily, and the surgical site will need aseptic wound care daily. The airflow should be evaluated and, if necessary, the cannula should be aspirated to remove any mucus, which commonly accumulates at the distal end of the tube.

BOX 27-12 Causes of Lower Airway Avian Emergencies

- Cigarette smoke
- Overheated polytetrafluoroethylene
- Pesticides
- Paint fumes
- Carpet cleaning solutions
- Wood burning stoves
- Hairspray and perfume
- Scented candles

Bleeding Emergencies

A variety of conditions may cause bleeding emergencies (Box 27-13). Broken blood feathers will often be the result of a traumatic fall or injury to the bird. The bird may be covered in blood from flapping or with an area covered with matted bloody feathers. Immediately locate the broken blood feather. You may need to clean the site with saline or water while trying to locate the feather in question. If the bird is stable, apply direct pressure, with or without styptic powder, to stop the bleeding and try to save the feather from removal. If the bleeding will not cease, then remove the feather using hemostats or needle-nosed pliers. With one hand hold the wing stable and pull in the same direction that the feather is growing. Apply direct pressure to the feather follicle if bleeding continues.

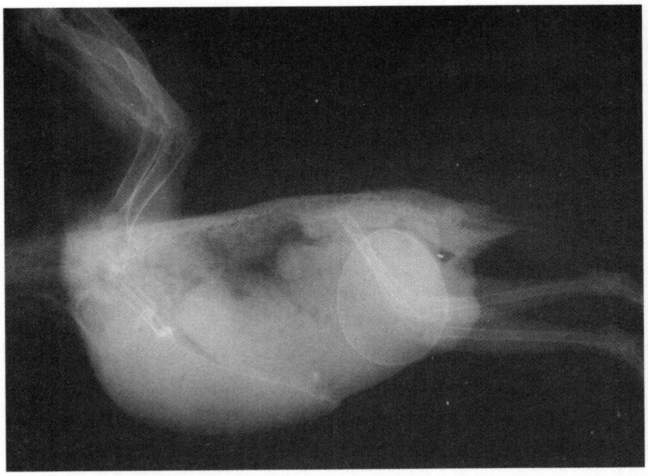

FIGURE 27-49 Space-occupying masses, such as the egg in the bird, can displace air sacs that are needed for air exchange. This can cause a bird to present to your clinic in respiratory distress.

BOX 27-13 Avian Bleeding Emergencies

- Broken blood feathers
- Broken toe nails
- Wounds/Big cat-little bird syndrome
- Open fractures

Egg Stasis or Binding

Egg retention is defined as the failure of an egg to pass through the oviduct at a normal rate. This is a commonly seen emergency in budgies, canaries, cockatiels, finches, and lovebirds. These birds typically have been laying eggs for some time, thus depleting their calcium stores. This causes decreased muscle activity in the oviduct, and the egg becomes trapped. Signs can include abdominal distention and straining, lack of droppings, depression, sitting on the cage bottom, tail wagging, and walking with wide-spread legs. In some cases the bird may be limping because of the pressure placed upon the pelvic plexus.

The causes of egg stasis can be numerous and include malformed eggs, excessive egg production, nutritional insufficiencies that lead to calcium or metabolic disorders, vitamin deficiencies, obesity, and previous oviduct damage or infections. The treatments for egg retention are case dependent. Some cases can be medically managed and some will need surgery. These patients may need supportive care such as oxygen therapy and nutritional support and will need to be monitored closely until the egg is removed.

Prolapsed Cloaca

Occasionally birds will present to your clinic with a prolapsed cloaca (Fig. 27-50). The most important immediate

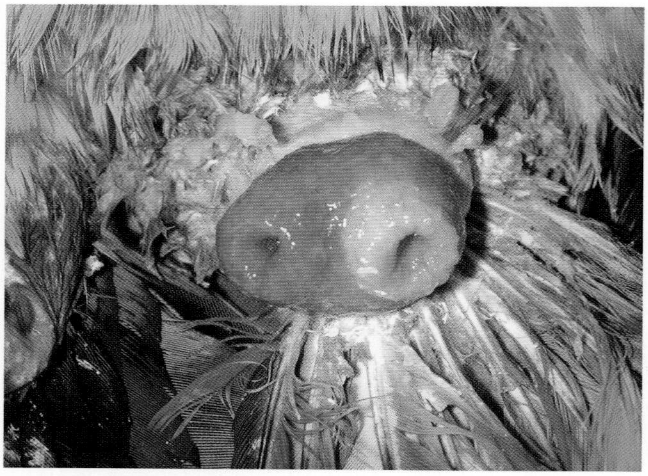

FIGURE 27-50 Prolapsed cloaca may occur secondary to chronic straining from egg laying, space-occupying masses, inappropriate social behavior, and masturbation.

therapy is to keep the prolapsed tissue moist and clean. If the patient is too stressed to restrain, place the patient in a cage lined with clean towels or gauze moistened with sterile saline. There are many aliments that can lead to a prolapsed cloaca such as egg stasis, papillomas, chronic masturbation, and coelomic masses. It is very important to determine the cause of the prolapse to ensure that it will not be a recurring problem.

Animal Bites

This accident normally occurs when a larger animal attacks the smaller bird, and in some cases, when a bird is attacked by another bird (Fig. 27-51). Mammal bites are usually from a pet dog or cat and are true emergencies. Oral bacteria from dogs and cats can be detrimental to the avian patient. The oral cavity of the cat is especially dangerous because they carry *Pasteurella multocida* on the gingival tissue and teeth. Immediate antibiotic therapy is commonly indicated. Evaluating a patient that has been attacked by a cat or dog can be challenging. The puncture wounds may be very small and concealed by the multiple layers of feathers. Gently blow on the feathers to part them enabling you to view the skin beneath. Use a small amount of saline to wet and part the feathers, but be sure that the patient does not get excessively wet as this can cause hypothermia. When a wound is located it will need to be cleaned up. Remove any surrounding feathers by plucking. Be careful when attempting a flush while cleaning the wound, because of the possibility that the puncture may communicate with an air sac. When in doubt, clean the wound but don't flush.

Beak Injuries and Repair

Some birds inflict severe injuries to other birds if given the opportunity. They may destroy the upper or lower beak of their victim and fractures of the mandible can occur. Even seemingly minor injuries may lead to permanent damage. After hemorrhage is controlled, the patient is evaluated for the type of repair that will be required.

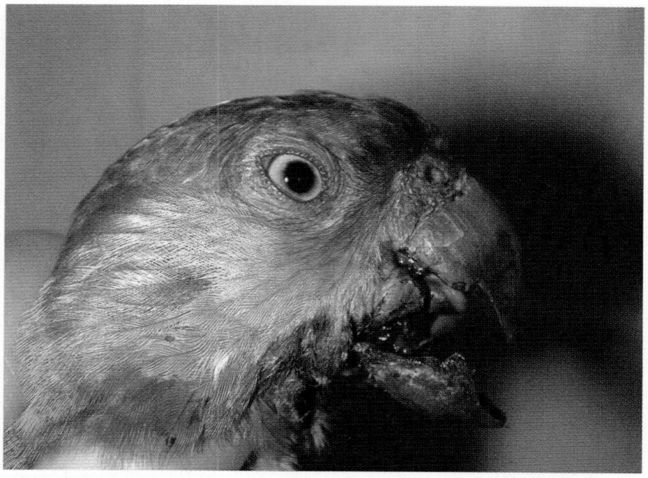

FIGURE 27-51 This Meyer's parrot was attacked by a large bird and has severe trauma to the lower beak.

Injuries that result in minor defects can be filled with acrylic material that hardens and is shaped to match the contours of the rest of the beak. This will eventually be replaced as the beak grows out. Mandibular fractures can be repaired using acrylic with pinning techniques. Depending on the fracture the patient may require weeks of recovery.

In cases in which damage is extensive or involves the growth center of the beak, a prosthetic may have to be created. This is fashioned out of acrylic and formed into a "false beak." It is attached somewhat like a fake fingernail and will need to be replaced regularly.

Clients need to be informed of the disadvantages of beak repairs, which include pressure necrosis, impaction of food at the attachment site, and development of gaps. Some developmental beak disorders such as twisting or underbite may have to be corrected surgically if they do not respond to manipulation. In some developmental or traumatic cases, routine correction of the beak deformity with beak trimming will need to be provided.

Foreign Bodies

Foreign bodies ingested by a curious bird that has been roaming and chewing are very similar to scenarios seen with mammals. Potential ingested foreign materials are toys or parts of toys, bedding, metallic items (wire, hair pins), string, fish bones, splinters, and tough plant fibers.

A thorough physical examination and radiographs often determine the problem, but specialized studies may be required. Endoscopic techniques and/or surgical removal may be required to retrieve the objects.

Fractures

Birds are commonly presented with a number of different scenarios that have resulted in fracture. Scenarios such as being attacked by a larger animal, getting caught in its cage or cage toys, a leg band entrapped in toys or other objects, flying into a window or ceiling fan, or being stepped or sat on are not uncommon. When this type of patient presents to your hospital, place the patient in a quiet, dark, well-padded environment until stable enough to restrain. Provide analgesics and determine the best method to stabilize the fracture.

The veterinarian must make a number of decisions before proceeding with fracture treatment. The condition, age, and personality of the bird have to be considered. The patient should be evaluated for any preexisting or concurrent medical conditions that could prevent immediate repair.

Each individual's fracture is different, and plans for repair may change during the diagnostic process. The client should be consulted to determine acceptable outcomes. It is also necessary to access the client's willingness and ability to comply with aftercare of the fracture repair. Healing time will be about 3 to 8 weeks. This will depend on the repair method selected, fracture location and complexity, extent of associated soft tissue injury, and nervous tissue damage. The least invasive, most effective correction method is desired.

Bandages and splints are used when some support of the fracture is all that is necessary (Fig. 27-52). This method will make the bird more comfortable, but may not allow proper healing and return to full function. Fractures commonly stabilized with this treatment are some wing and foot breaks. Alternatively, there are many different surgical methods and approaches to fracture repair that will be chosen depending on the specific details of the case.

In extreme cases a traumatized leg or wing cannot be salvaged. In this instance amputation may be the only choice. Most psittacines do quite well after losing a leg because they can use their beaks to move around. Most birds will perch comfortably but do run the risk of developing pododermatitis on the remaining foot. In pet birds, removal of a wing may cause some loss of balance, but most seem to manage rather well. The majority of birds are not troubled by toe amputations.

Wing Fractures. Fractures of the wing usually are immobilized with a figure-of-eight bandage. This holds the flexed wing snug against the body. If the humerus is fractured, a body wrap is also applied.

An open fracture should also be cleaned and flushed, using caution to avoid introducing fluid into the airway via the pneumatic bones. Appropriate supportive, antimicrobial, and analgesic therapies should be implemented as soon as possible.

Most broken wings will need to be bandaged for 3 to 5 weeks with routine changes. The bandage should be removed as soon as healing is complete.

Complications include stiffness, muscle atrophy from disuse, and loss of flight feathers. Physical therapy will help the bird become limber and recover muscle mass.

Some severe fractures are best treated by surgery. The wing will need to be stabilized until surgery can be performed.

Leg Fractures. Some lower leg fractures are stabilized with a splint until healing occurs, usually in 4 to 6 weeks. Because of the bird's anatomy, splints will often worsen fractures of the femur and upper tibiotarsus. These often require prompt surgical repair. Toe fractures can be treated in large birds by taping the broken toe to the neighboring intact toe.

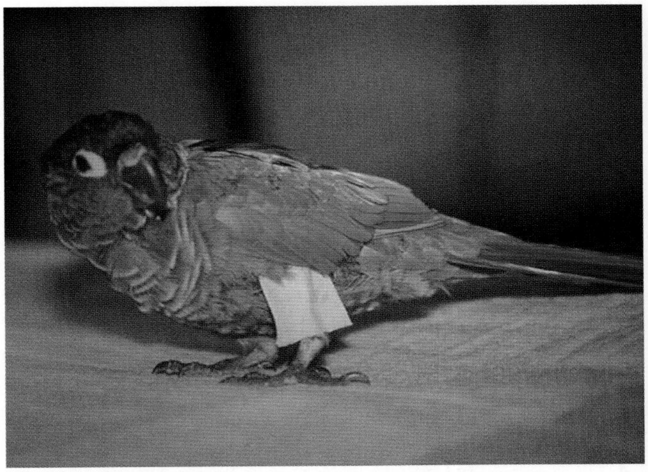

FIGURE 27-52 Tape splints are a lightweight alternative to traditional bulkier bandages for smaller birds.

An open fracture should also be cleaned and flushed using caution to avoid introducing fluid into the airway via the pneumatic bones. Appropriate supportive, antimicrobial, and analgesic therapies should be implemented as soon as possible. Surgical correction will generally be required. Splints will be used to support the repaired break.

The Schroeder-Thomas splint can be used to treat fractures of the lower third of the tibiotarsus and the entire tarsometatarsus. The bandage is changed every 1 to 2 weeks and is accompanied by passive physical therapy. A Robert Jones bandage can be used for simple lower leg fractures. Although these are heavily padded, additional splinting materials such as tongue depressors may be needed. The bandage needs to be changed at least every 2 weeks. A ball bandage is used for broken toes or pododermatitis. A ball formed of gauze sponges is placed so the toes curl around it. The foot is covered with cotton padding and wrapped with stretchy self-adherent bandaging. Very small birds can be difficult to splint. Materials such as pipe cleaners, toothpicks, paperclips, and wooden applicator sticks are used to stabilize their fractures.

With all splints it is necessary to assess circulation in the foot. Look for swelling of the toes, blue coloration, and coldness. The bandage will need to be changed if any of these occur.

Bandages need to be checked often for signs of chewing or moisture. Clients should be advised to bring the bird in to the clinic for a bandage change. Removal of leg bands is advised because they may cause fractures when they become caught on the cage or other objects.

Head Trauma

Head trauma cases in which the bird flies into a window or a ceiling fan require immediate supportive therapy and evaluation. Evaluate for signs of shock, check neurologic signs, and closely examine the eyes, ears, nose, and nares for hemorrhage or bruising. Place the patient in a dark, quiet, and (contrary to other situations) a cool environment to prevent vasodilation of the intracranial vessels. Provide supportive care as needed. Mannitol and furosemide can be helpful in these situations, as with small mammal patients. If the patient is possibly in shock, steroids may be indicated. The chronic use of corticosteroids can delay wound healing and be immunosuppressive. The veterinarian will devise a plan that will be in the patient's best interest. Monitor the patient closely for neurologic symptoms such as circling, head pressing or tremors, and seizures.

Burns

Burns on birds commonly occur on the feet and legs. Birds that are left to free fly through the house can run the risk of landing in a pot of boiling hot liquid or the burners of the stove causing severe burns to the legs and feet. Burns to the oral cavity and tongue may occur by biting electrical cords. Treatment for burns is comparable to treating burns in any other patients. Flush areas with copious amounts of cool water or saline and remove surrounding feathers. Don't use greasy or oily medications because these can accumulate in the feathers and affect thermoregulation. Using silver sulfadiazine topically has antibacterial, antifungal, and analgesic properties.

Crop Burn and Crop Trauma

Owners or breeders may bring in a baby bird that has "food leaking from its chest." A crop burn is normally caused by poorly mixed microwave foods that are fed to neonates. Once the burn has occurred, normally in the right ventral portion of the crop, the crop and skin necrose and form a fistula (Fig. 27-53). Food will leak from this fistula, creating a very alarming situation for the client and this may be an emergency. If the bird is not able to retain enough food or water, there is a risk of dehydration and starvation. This will require anesthesia and a surgical closure, but the recovery is usually fairly quick. Client education on how to properly heat the food is essential to prevent future crop burns.

Timing of surgery on damaged crops will depend on the severity of injury. Birds with extreme trauma from ceiling fans or animal bites must be operated on immediately to stabilize the patient. Surgery on baby birds whose crops were burned with excessively hot formula often is deferred for 7 to 10 days until a fistula develops and the extent of the injury is obvious. After surgery the birds are fed small volumes of formula more frequently until healing occurs.

Seizures

Seizures from exposure to toxins, hyperthermia, liver failure, hypoglycemia, CNS inflammation, hyperglycemia, neoplasia, and cardiac instability all look identical. Seizures in birds are comparable to mammals and manifest in similar ways (Box 27-14).

When a bird presents while seizing, keep it from injuring itself or others. House the bird in a quiet, dark, cool place. Diazepam at a dose of 0.6 mg/kg can be given IV or midazolam at a dose of 0.6 mg/kg IM. When the patient is stable, obtain a detailed history from the client followed by a complete physical examination and try to determine the cause of the seizure.

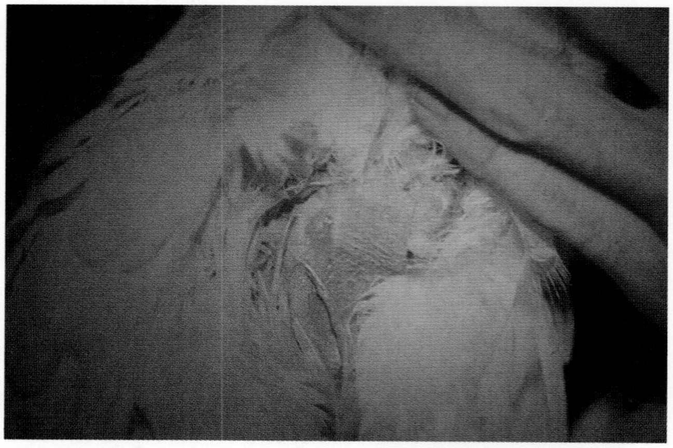

FIGURE 27-53 Crop fistula leaking food in a hand-fed juvenile cockatoo.

BOX 27-14 Manifestations of Seizures in Birds

- Mild seizure: disorientation, inability to perch
- Generalized seizing: vocalizing, wing flapping, and paddling
- Partial seizure: persistent twitching

Heavy Metal Toxicosis

Birds are naturally curious and like to investigate unfamiliar objects with their mouths. When this behavior is combined with the bird given free run of the house, the potential for ingesting foreign objects is increased. Unfortunately this poses numerous hazards, one of which is heavy metal toxicosis. Some materials used to create the patient's cage or toys are made of zinc or lead. Because there is no quality control for toys manufactured for birds, the toys themselves can be made from toxic materials and the client is unaware. Client education is a necessity.

Lead and zinc are the two most common heavy metal poisonings encountered with avian patients. Typically, ingestion of curtain weights, lead clappers from bells, old-style solder, lead-based paints, plaster, foil from wine bottles, and calcium-rich dolomite or bone meal can result in signs of lead poisoning. Galvanized cage wire is the usual source of ingested zinc. Treatment for lead and zinc toxicosis is supportive and chelation therapy with calcium EDTA and removal of the foreign body if possible. Response to therapy is usually rapid, and improvement may be seen in a few hours or days.

Diagnosis may be based on signs and radiographic findings of heavy metal densities within the body (Box 27-15). Whole blood samples can be sent to an outside lab to analyze for heavy metals. Consult with your lab about sample testing requirements. Some labs use serum or heparinized plasma for their zinc evaluation and a separate sample is submitted in lithium EDTA for lead evaluation. Because testing may take a number of days, treatment should be started before the blood levels are received if radiographs and clinical signs suggest poisoning.

BOX 27-15 Signs of Heavy Metal Toxicosis

- Lethargy
- Depression
- Anorexia
- Weakness
- Weight loss
- Anemia
- Regurgitation
- Polyuria
- Polydipsia
- Diarrhea
- Emaciation
- Ataxia
- Convulsions and paresis/paralysis.
- Regenerative anemia

Amazon parrots are the only species that will develop hematuria in acute cases. Eclectus will characteristically show biliverdinuria (greenish staining of urine). Other parrots have no urinary color changes.

Ingested Poisons

As discussed previously, birds often explore new items by mouthing them and feeling their texture with their tongues. This exposes them to possible poisoning with lethal effects. It is imperative to prevent contact of the pet bird with any common household items and other potentially lethal substances listed below. The client must be advised to bring the bird, and container (if any) of the item ingested, in for evaluation as soon as possible. To ascertain the correct treatment, consult a pharmacology reference book and call the poison control center.

Cleaners. Cleaners can cause skin eruptions, gastrointestinal upsets including vomiting and diarrhea, respiratory tract irritation, and esophageal damage.

Polishes. Hydrocarbon-based compounds such as furniture polish and other petroleum products lead to central nervous system effects such as disorientation and depression, pneumonia, gastrointestinal upset, kidney and liver damage, and mucous membrane and skin damage.

Prescription Drugs. Prescription drugs cause a wide variety of signs. The client must bring the container or remaining contents for identification.

Toiletries (Shampoo, Deodorant, Perfume). Perfumes and deodorants may cause damage to the skin and mucous membranes, respiratory tract, kidneys, liver, and central nervous system. Shampoos lead to irritation of the eyes and diarrhea.

Tobacco. Even small amounts of tobacco products can result in vomiting, diarrhea, convulsions, and sudden death.

Fireworks and Matches. Eating fireworks or matches can result in vomiting, diarrhea, blood in the stools, and increased respiration. Cyanosis may also occur.

Poisonous Plants. Many plants have been blamed for illness in birds, but plant poisoning is actually rare. Birds often will tear leaves without eating them, decreasing the amount ingested. The avian gastrointestinal tract empties quickly, further reducing chances of poisoning. Owners may unintentionally expose their birds to poisonous plant materials through feeding, use of poisonous plants for perches, or keeping of certain house plants for house decoration (Box 27-16).

BOX 27-16 Toxic Plants

- Avocado
- Black locust (should not be used for perches)
- Oak (should not be used for perches)
- Oleander (should not be used for perches)
- Rhododendron (should not be used for perches)
- Clematis
- Dieffenbachia
- Foxglove
- Lily of the valley
- Lupine
- Philodendron
- Poinsettia
- Yew
- Crown vetch

If owners call the clinic with a bird showing unusual signs after exposure to any plant, they should be asked to bring the bird in for evaluation. Clients should be advised that poisonings can be lethal without prompt intervention. The offending plant or a sample should be brought to the clinic. The client should try to estimate the amount ingested.

Treatment is supportive and, depending on the agent consumed, activated charcoal may be administered.

AVIAN ANESTHESIA

Anesthesia is an essential skill that every veterinary technician should master. Many advances in monitoring techniques and equipment have helped to provide better control of apnea, hypothermia, and hypoventilation. Birds are often anesthetized for quick diagnostic procedures such as radiographs in addition to major surgical procedures. The avian patient will need to be monitored more closely than the average small animal patient because of the anatomical and physiological differences in birds.

Circuits and Gas Anesthesia

Most models of anesthesia machines are adequate for anesthetizing the avian patient; all that is required is an out-of-circuit vaporizer for administering isoflurane or sevoflurane in oxygen and a non-rebreathing circuit. Non-rebreathing circuits such as Magill, Ayre's T-piece, Mapleson systems, Jackson-Rees, Norman mask elbow, and Bain circuits are adequate for companion bird anesthesia. These non-rebreathing circuits provide less resistance to breathing and almost instantaneous response to changes in the vaporizer settings. In most practices, isoflurane is preferred over sevoflurane because of cost. Sevoflurane tends to cost more than isoflurane. Sevoflurane does produce a faster induction and recovery than isoflurane and may be a safer choice for high-risk patients.

Patient Preparation

In preparation for anesthesia the crop should be empty. Birds have a high metabolic rate and poor hepatic glycogen storage, and it has been recommended that birds be fasted no more than 2 to 3 hours, depending on the size and condition of the patient. Regurgitation can occur if the patient is not properly fasted. Fasting will help decrease the probability of aspiration of crop contents. In emergency situations, when there is no time for fasting, aspirate the crop contents and intubate to reduce the possibility of aspiration.

Preanesthetics, Analgesics, and Sedatives

Routine use of parasympatholytic agents such as atropine and glycopyrrolate are thought to be unnecessary unless there is a predetermined need. Use of these drugs will thicken the salivary, tracheal, and bronchial secretions, creating a greater risk for airway obstructions during anesthesia. Benzodiazepines such as diazepam and midazolam will reduce anxiety and are useful tranquilizers before induction. These drugs have no analgesic properties, so if the procedure will be painful, an analgesic is required. Opioids are commonly used for premedicating small mammals, which use primarily μ opioid receptors. Birds, however, appear to have primarily κ opioid receptors. Butorphanol has both μ and κ agonist properties and seems to be the better analgesic in birds. Table 27-2 lists some common emergency drugs used on avian species.

TABLE 27-2 Emergency Drugs Used in Avian Practice

EMERGENCY DRUG	DOSAGE
Atropine for bradycardia	0.01-1.0 mg/kg SC, IM
Atropine for CPR	0.5 mg/kg, SC, IM, IV, IC
Epinephrine for CPR	0.5-1.0 mg/kg IM, IV, intratracheal, IC
Doxapram	5-10 mg/kg IM, IV, intratracheal
Glycopyrrolate	0.01 mg/kg SC, IM
Midazolam	0.1-0.5 mg/kg, SC, IM, IV
Butorphanol	0.5-2.0 mg/kg, SC, IM, IV
Diazepam	0.2-0.5 mg/kg, IV

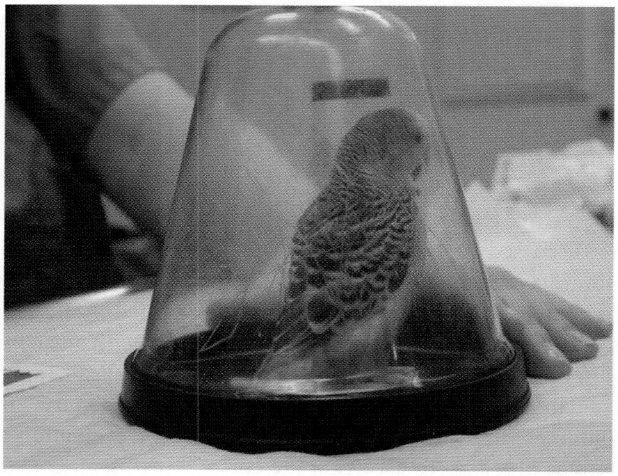

FIGURE 27-54 Small birds can be placed inside a large canine face mask for a chamber induction. The only disadvantage to this induction method is the lack of cardiac monitoring.

Chamber Induction

Consider the patient's stress level when planning the anesthesia. Most patients can be restrained and masked with gas anesthetics. In some cases the patient may need to be induced in a chamber (Fig. 27-54). This type of induction is not without risks. This form of induction prevents monitoring the heart rate of the patient, there is a risk the patient can injure itself if the chamber is not padded adequately, and high concentrations of gas anesthetic are released into the clinic environment when the patient is removed from the chamber. When chamber-inducing a patient, the chamber should be covered to create a calming effect, leaving a small opening for monitoring the patient. Start the isoflurane percentage at 3% to 4% and oxygen flow rate of 4 to 5 L/min and watch the patient closely. The patient can display any of the following: droopy wings, eyes closing, loss of equilibrium. Watch the patient's respiratory rate and effort very closely and once the patient begins to show major effects of the anesthetic, lower the percentage of isoflurane to 2% to 3%. When the patient is sedated, remove the patient from the chamber and continue the induction with a mask. If the patient shows any signs of respiratory distress during chamber induction, remove the patient from the chamber immediately and place an oxygen mask over the beak and nares.

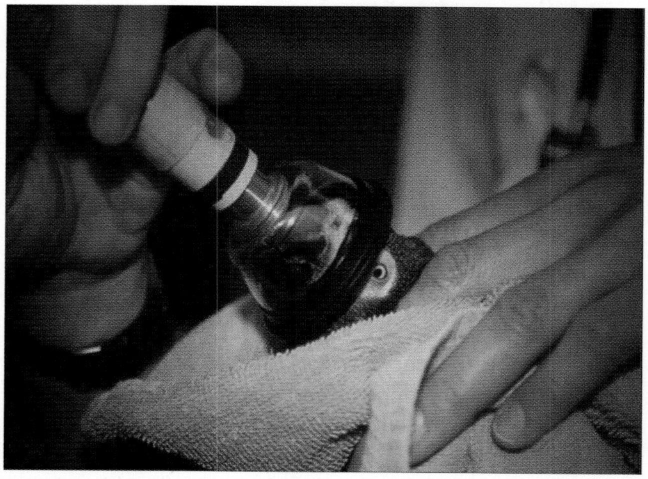

FIGURE 27-55 During mask induction, the patient should be held in an upright position and the mask placed over the nares and entire beak. Monitor the heart rate with a stethoscope and respiratory rate at all times.

Mask Induction

Place the mask over the beak and nares, or with smaller birds, place the entire head inside of the mask (Fig. 27-55). A slow induction is the safest, starting with a low percentage of the anesthetic and working up until the desired depth of anesthesia is reached. Monitor the heart rate with a stethoscope and watch the respiration rate and depth during the entire induction; bradycardia and apnea are common if induction is too quick. The eyes will close, the wings will drop,

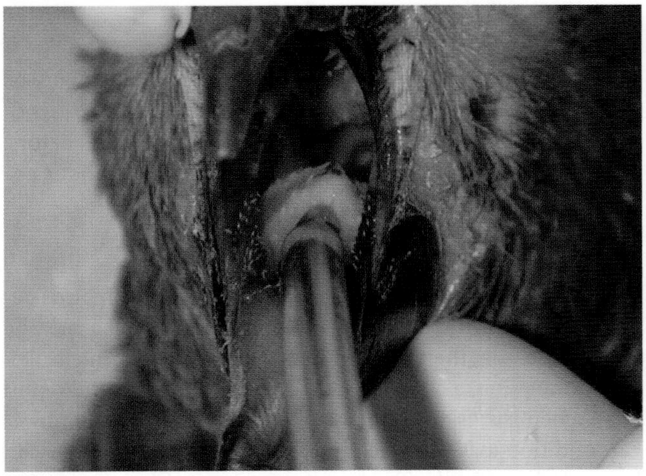

FIGURE 27-56 Tracheal intubation is not difficult in most companion birds, but tracheal trauma is easy to cause and cuffed endotracheal tubes should not be used.

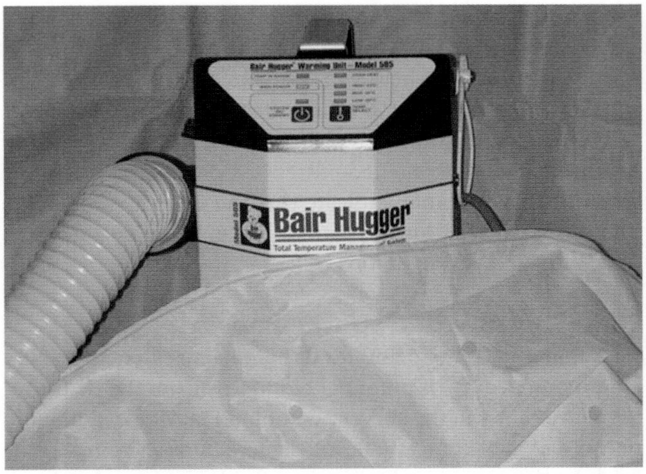

FIGURE 27-57 Forced air heating blankets are a good way to provide supplemental heat to the anesthetized patient.

and the legs will become more relaxed when the patient is feeling the effects of the anesthetic and is ready to be intubated. If bradycardia or apnea occurs, immediately turn off the gas anesthetic and administer oxygen until the patient's vital signs stabilize.

Intubation

Intubation is fairly easy to do in birds and should always be done with long procedures and high-risk patients. This provides the ability to perform mechanical ventilations since birds do not breathe adequately on their own when anesthetized. Birds have complete cartilaginous tracheal rings, so tracheal necrosis can occur if the cuffs on cuffed endotracheal tubes are inflated. Cuffed endotracheal tubes should not be used. Once the patient is relaxed from mask induction (lacking in jaw, wing, and leg tone) and the risk of biting has diminished, the patient can be intubated. Open the beak and either gently pull the tongue out with a pair of hemostats or place a laryngoscope blade on the tip of the tongue. This will expose the glottal opening. Gently place the noncuffed endotracheal tube lubricated with sterile K-Y jelly into the opening (Fig. 27-56). When the tube is in the trachea, secure it by taping once around the tube and then tape the tube to the lower beak. This allows easy access to the mouth for placement of monitoring equipment and removing any regurgitated material. If the patient presents with a tracheal obstruction and an air sac cannula is placed, anesthesia can be administered via the cannula in the same manner as through the trachea.

Oxygen Flow Rate and Ventilation

Safe oxygen flow rates can range from 500 ml/min to 1 L/min; flow rates more than 1 L/min can damage the tracheal mucosa. Normal respirations should be slow, deep, and regular, approximately 10 to 40 breaths/min, depending on the size of the patient. Regardless of how the patient is ventilating or the length of the procedure, monitoring the patient's respiratory rate and effort is vital. For instance, when small endotracheal tubes are used there is a chance that the mucoid secretions may thicken and consolidate inside the tube and block the airway.

Applying pressure to the bag in the anesthetic circuit and forcing air into the patient by hand produces manual ventilation. Watch the patient's keel expansion to ensure that you are not applying too much pressure. Air sacs can be ruptured if the respirations are too aggressive. The amount of pressure applied to the system should range from 5 to 8 cm H_2O. The rate can range between 8 and 20 breaths per minute. This method of ventilation can be too time consuming for the busy veterinary technician, so a positive pressure ventilator can be very useful. The ventilator should never take the place of proper monitoring because equipment can fail. Always be mindful of how the equipment is functioning.

Manual ventilation, high oxygen flow rates, and high-pressure ventilation can cause tracheal mucosal damage if improperly used. Protect the trachea by keeping it moist. Humid-Vents can be placed between the endotracheal tube and the breathing circuit during the procedure. This device helps retain moisture in the trachea to prevent tracheal damage.

Monitoring Body Temperature

Loss of heat during anesthesia can delay recovery, so any attempt to keep the patient's core body temperature up is to the patient's advantage (Fig. 27-57). Normal body temperature for birds ranges from 105° to 112° F. It is not unusual for the core temperature to drop dramatically during surgical procedures, especially when feathers have been plucked and alcohol used in preparation for surgery. An esophageal temperature probe placed as far as the proventriculus is usually needed for monitoring core body temperature; the crop and cloaca will not be representative of the patient's core body temperature, but will provide information on trends.

Monitoring the Patient

In some cases the only piece of monitoring equipment you will be able to place on your patient will be a stethoscope to listen for cardiac changes and a pair of eyes to watch for any respiratory changes. You may not have any specialized monitoring equipment to help you evaluate your patient's status, so you will have to learn how to watch for the subtle changes in your patient's respiratory and cardiac patterns. Slowing heart rate and/or weakened pulses or slowing and shallower respiratory efforts may indicate that the patient is too deep. The reverse is true for the patient that may be on the verge of waking up.

Fluid Therapy during Anesthesia

IV catheter placement and fluid therapy are essential for any lengthy procedure. If potential blood loss from the IV catheter placement and the surgery combined may be detrimental to the patient, then catheter placement should be reconsidered. In those cases subcutaneous fluids are in order. In all other cases IV fluids should be a part of your anesthetic protocol. A fluid rate of 10 ml/kg is normally used, administered by continuous rate infusion with a syringe pump; however, because the average avian patient is relatively small, hemodilution can be a potential problem. The veterinarian will choose administration of either crystalloids or colloids based on the results of preanesthetic blood work. In some cases a blood transfusion may be required. Fresh whole blood is best; however, if there are no eligible donors available, blood replacement products have been used safely.

During anesthesia two sites are optimal for placing an IV catheter: the wing (cutaneous ulnar vein) and the leg (medial metatarsal). These catheters can be secured with tissue glue, tape, or suture.

Recovery

Recovery of the patient from any anesthetic procedure is a very critical time. During recovery some birds will regain consciousness, vocalize, and try to bite, then fall back into a stupor, become apneic, bradycardic, and potentially suffer cardiac arrest if not monitored closely. Once the bird is extubated, supplemental oxygen can be provided by face mask for a few more minutes, and you must continue to monitor heart rate and respiratory rate until the patient is able to ambulate in the cage. Continue to monitor the patient for at least one half hour after any anesthetic procedure, from outside of the recovery cage.

Cardiopulmonary Resuscitation

If the patient goes into cardiopulmonary arrest, follow the same ABC's of emergency medicine that you would use for your other patients. If the patient stops breathing, an endotracheal tube should be placed and positive pressure ventilation must be started at a rate of 1 breath every 4 to 5 seconds. Once you have established an airway, the pulse and heartbeat should be assessed. If no heartbeat can be found on auscultation, firm and rapid compressions of the sternum should be used to massage the heart. CPR in birds usually results in an unfavorable outcome; however, CPR should always be attempted, especially in previously healthy animals that have suddenly collapsed or had adverse reactions to routine anesthesia.

AVIAN SURGICAL TECHNIQUES

Birds are challenging surgical patients. Anesthesia can be complex. The physical characteristics of birds make hypothermia, hypoglycemia, and blood loss significant factors. Surgeries are carefully planned to minimize time under anesthesia and complications.

Presurgical Evaluations

A thorough physical examination should be done on birds before anesthesia. If a patient is new or has never been seen by the veterinarian, then a routine workup may be indicated: a fecal examination, a complete blood count (CBC), radiographs, blood chemistries. Birds that are extremely ill or in poor physical condition may have elective surgery delayed until they can be treated medically. Treatments can range from improving the bird's diet to managing underlying infections.

Surgical Site Preparation and Drapes

The first step in preparation of the surgical site is plucking of feathers to provide 2 to 4 cm of bare space surrounding the proposed incision. Once the bird is anesthetized, feathers are pulled individually in the direction of growth. If possible, removal of flight feathers is avoided. There is the possibility of damage to the feather follicle, resulting in growth of deformed or misdirected feathers.

Once the patient is anesthetized, it will need to be positioned and prepared for surgery. To assist both the anesthetist and the surgeon, the patient can be secured with masking tape on a plastic board or acrylic heating pad (Fig. 27-58). Using a board such as this allows you to elevate portions of the bird easily, change the patient's direction for the surgeon's accessibility, and move the patient from the prep room to the surgery room without disrupting the masking tape used to position the bird and the monitoring equipment. Masking tape or painter's tape works very well for positioning birds because the adhesive is not too sticky but strong enough to hold the bird or feathers in position. Regular white porous or other tape can damage or remove more feathers than necessary when removed or leave a residue.

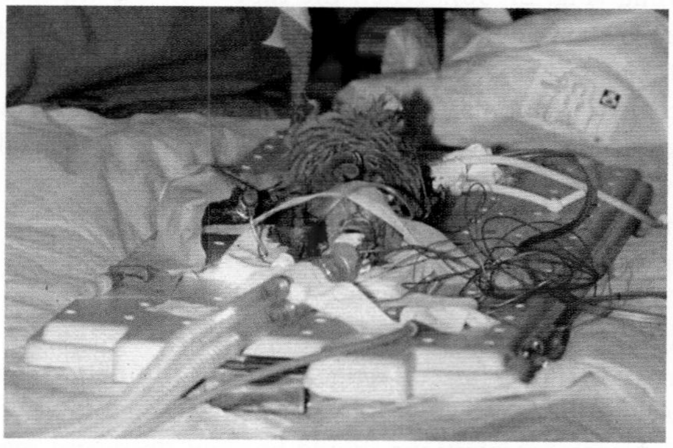

FIGURE 27-58 Once anesthetized, patients can be taped to a restraint board to aid in keeping the monitoring equipment and catheters in place during preparation, moving to the surgical suite, and during surgery.

Any feathers adjoining the surgical site are held away from the incision site by holding them down with masking tape or sterile water-soluble lubricating gels. The surgical site is prepped using dilute chlorhexidine or povidone iodine solution. Sterile saline, rather than alcohol, is used to flush the disinfectant solution away. Alcohol is avoided because its use may trigger hypothermia to develop as it evaporates from the skin.

Transparent adhesive disposable surgical drapes are often used in birds. They adhere directly to the prepped skin and the incision is made through the plastic drape material. Other advantages include ease of monitoring, conservation of body heat, and low cost. The drape must be removed carefully to minimize trauma to the bird's skin.

Suture material in avian surgery needs to be minimally reactive and of a smaller size, 4-0, 5-0, and 6-0. Nylon and stainless steel are nonabsorbable materials that fit that description but are too stiff and may be mechanically irritating to the surrounding tissues. Monofilament suture material is often preferred and has the advantage of minimizing trauma and cutting of tissue when compared to multifilament material. Taper-point needles are less traumatic than cutting needles and are used because avian skin is thin and very friable. Cutting needles can be used for tougher skin such as the skin found on the feet of larger birds.

When the patient is recovering from a medical or surgical procedure it is very important to provide analgesia, thermal support, a nice padded cage with a towel ring if necessary, and in some cases supplemental oxygen therapy.

Ethical Euthanasia Techniques

Euthanasia is sometimes necessary to alleviate patient suffering and should be done in a humane manner. Having to make the decision to end a pet's life is never easy. Many people do not want to talk about it until they have to; then it becomes a decision made under emotional stress. It is important to have the ability to discuss this issue with compassion and explain the details of the procedure with empathy.

Acceptable methods should include anesthesia to create an environment in which the patient is unaware of the injection. In some cases the patient may be incoherent enough that only heavy sedation is necessary and in others gas anesthesia is required. When the patient is unconscious, a commercially available euthanasia solution can be administered. Routes of administration are intravenous, intracardiac, or intraperitoneal. The patient must be anesthetized if intracardiac or intraperitoneal routes are to be used, and in all cases the patient must be monitored until the heart stops. If the client is present, you must make them aware that some patients may experience agonal breaths, muscle twitching, or vocalizations, the eyes may not close, and gastrointestinal contents may release through the cloaca. In most cases the patient will have a peaceful release of tension, as if going to sleep. Because of the animal's individual level of health and stress, each case of euthanasia will be an individual experience.

REPTILES

Reptiles are a diverse group of animals that have become popular pets over the last several years. The Class Reptilia contains four orders of which only two are commonly seen in the private clinical setting. These two orders include Squamata—snakes and lizards—and Testudines—turtles and tortoises. The most common lizards kept as pets in North America include iguanas, bearded dragon, geckos, chameleons, monitors, and water dragons. The most common snakes kept as pets in North America include boas, pythons, king snakes, rat snakes, corn snakes, and gopher snakes. The most common chelonians kept as pets in North America include box turtles, red-eared sliders and other water turtles, and various tortoises. It is important to remember that these are unique animals and not just small dogs and cats. If the veterinary hospital decides to treat reptiles, the staff must become knowledgeable about proper capture, restraint, diagnostic techniques and procedures, anesthesia, husbandry, and common diseases. The veterinary staff must be properly trained to handle reptiles because this can prevent injuries to both the staff and the patient. Box 27-17 lists basic equipment needed to care for reptiles.

REPTILE BIOLOGY

Reptiles are ectothermic, meaning they cannot generate their own body heat. Instead, heat is obtained from the environment. Reptiles are able to regulate their body heat by moving in and out of the heat or shade. Each species has a specific temperature range at which they thrive. This is referred to as the preferred optimum temperature zone (POTZ).

Reptiles have a protective layer of keratinous scales covering the skin. The outermost layer of the skin is shed on a regular basis. Species such as snakes shed their skin all at once. Just before the shed, the skin becomes very sensitive and turns an opaque color (Fig. 27-59). It is suggested that the snake not be handled during this time unless absolutely necessary. The snake may become aggressive and anorexic just before and during the shed.

> **TECHNICIAN NOTE** Handling snakes should be kept to a minimum about 1 week before and during a shed because the skin is delicate and can be easily damaged.

BOX 27-17 Basic Equipment Needed for Reptile Patients

- 1-inch tape, roll gauze, and elastic wrap
- 3-0 to 6-0 suture material
- 25- to 27-gauge needles and butterfly catheters
- Infant and cat toenail trimmers
- Mammography and/or high-detail radiograph film
- Microtainer blood collection tubes
- Ophthalmology instruments
- Tuberculin and insulin syringes
- Various mouth speculums

Unlike snakes, lizards and chelonians shed the skin in pieces. Some reptiles will have problems shedding the skin. This is called dysecdysis. If the patient is having problems shedding the skin, the humidity in the cage should be increased or the animal can be soaked in a warm water bath (Fig. 27-60). You should always examine the toes of lizards such as leopard geckos if they are having problems shedding their skin as the skin can become wrapped around the digits, cutting off circulation and causing necrosis.

Like birds, reptiles lack a diaphragm to separate the thoracic and abdominal cavities. They have one visceral cavity called the coelom. Most reptiles have a renal portal system. This is a network of vessels associated with the kidneys. The renal portal system is clinically significant because medications injected caudal to the kidneys can be carried directly back to the kidneys before being distributed to the rest of the body. This can result in damage to the kidneys if the drug is nephrotoxic or excretion of the drug before it has been distributed throughout the body.

Reptile excrement includes three components: urine, urates, and feces. This is very similar to birds. The cloaca is the common opening through which the urinary, digestive, and reproductive systems empty.

HUSBANDRY

One of the most common reasons a reptile patient is brought to the veterinary hospital is because of illness caused by poor husbandry and diet. It is therefore extremely important that clients are properly educated. The veterinary hospital should provide the client with accurate educational handouts or information. An appropriate website to recommend to clients is www.anapsid.org. An excellent website and association that veterinary professionals can access is the Association of Reptilian and Amphibian Veterinarians, www.arav.org.

Reptile Housing

Many pet reptiles can be housed in a simple terrarium. The cage should be appropriately sized for the animal (in most cases, the larger the better). The terrarium should be easy to clean and disinfect. Appropriate cage furniture should be placed in the terrarium as well. Cage furniture will vary based on the species, but often includes items such as logs, plants, hide boxes, rocks, etc. Cage furniture is often used by the animal to help them shed. Reptiles rub against cage furniture such as logs, rocks, plants, etc. to loosen skin.

TECHNICIAN NOTE Placing appropriate cage furniture in the reptile's enclosure is important not only for providing hiding places and visual barriers, but to also help the animal shed.

It is important to choose the appropriate bedding or substrate for the cage bottom. The substrate should be easy to remove for cleaning and replacement. Indoor/outdoor carpet is easy to clean and inexpensive enough to throw away when necessary. Other appropriate substrates include newspaper, butcher paper, hay, and commercial recycled newspaper bedding. Some people use wood chips and sand, but these can cause intestinal foreign bodies if eaten by the animal. Shavings should not be used as they can cause irritation to the respiratory tract.

Appropriate lighting is important for reptiles. Without the proper ultraviolet (UV) lighting, many species of reptiles cannot metabolize nutrients or synthesize vitamin D adequately. The light should be full-spectrum with the light source being about 18 to 24 inches from the animal. UV bulbs need to be changed about every 6 months even if they are not burnt out, because the UV portion of the light does not usually last more than 6 months. Light cycles will vary by species.

Proper heating is critical for reptiles because they are ectothermic. Because reptiles thermoregulate using their surrounding environment, a basking spot (using various types of bulbs) providing increased heat should be provided as well as a nonheated spot. The reptile will move between the two spots to regulate its own body temperature. The basking spot should be positioned so the animal cannot come in contact

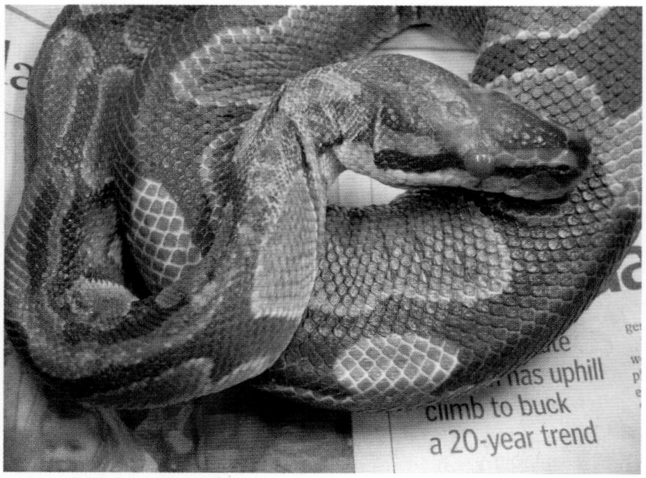

FIGURE 27-59 Just before shedding, the snake's skin and eyes turn an opaque, blue color. The snake should not be handled just before and during the shed, as this can damage the delicate, new skin.

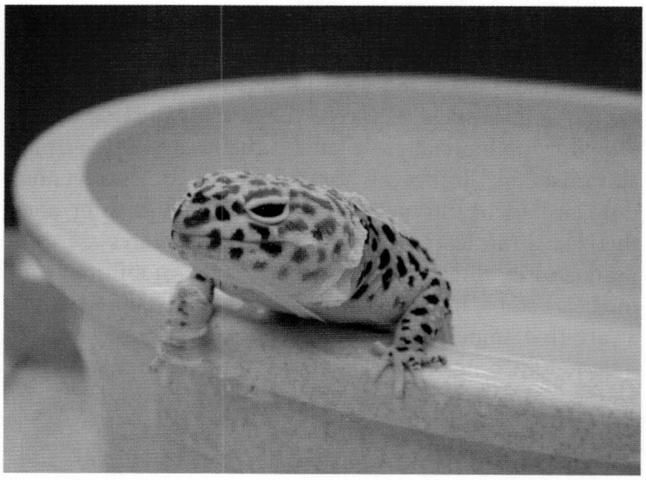

FIGURE 27-60 This leopard gecko has dysecdysis and is being soaked to help shed the skin.

with the heat source. Hot rocks or sizzle stones should not be used to provide heat because they often have uncontrolled hot spots causing thermal burns (Fig. 27-61). Under-tank heaters can be useful in providing additional heat to the cage, but they should only be used under half of the cage so the animal can escape the heat if necessary. Under-tank heaters can cause thermal burns if not used properly.

> TECHNICIAN NOTE Hot rocks and sizzle stones can cause thermal burns and should never be used in reptile enclosures.

Humidity requirements vary among different species of reptiles. Some tropical species such as the green iguana *(Iguana iguana)* require extremely high levels of humidity to stay healthy. This is very difficult to provide in captivity, especially in dry areas of the United States.

Proper sanitation of the reptile enclosure is very important. The cage should be cleaned thoroughly and disinfected on a routine basis. Excrement should be picked up daily. Owners should be aware that all reptiles have the ability to shed *Salmonella* spp. if they are positive carriers of the bacteria. Owners should take precautions by wearing examination gloves during cleaning and handling of the pet. Handling the animal and cleaning of the enclosure should never take place near food areas where food for human consumption is prepared or stored.

Feeding

Improper diet and nutrition is a common cause of disease in pet reptiles. Diets are generally species specific and are beyond the scope of this chapter. Commercial diets are available for some species, but are generally not recommended. Water should be available at all times and changed daily because reptiles often defecate in the dish.

Snakes. All snakes are carnivores and feed on whole prey items. The digestive system of snakes has evolved to digest whole prey and defecate the parts of the prey that are not digested, such as fur. Ingesting the entire carcass provides added nutrients such as calcium from the bone. Further supplementation is not needed when feeding whole prey. Common whole prey items include rats, mice, rabbits, guinea pigs, etc. It is never appropriate to feed meat such as chicken breast, hot dogs, raw beef, etc. as this does not provide a complete diet.

It is suggested that prekilled or stunned food is offered to snakes so they will not be harmed by the prey item. Prekilled food can be ordered frozen from several companies. If frozen mice/rats are offered, they must be thawed before being offered as food.

Lizards. Feeding requirements vary with different species of lizards. Is the lizard a carnivore, herbivore, insectivore, or an omnivore? Herbivores should be fed various types of dark leafy greens and vegetables. Proper leafy greens include kale, chard, turnip greens, escarole, etc. Most insectivores can eat meal worms, silk worms, crickets, etc. Carnivorous lizards should be fed whole prey. Whole prey includes all the bones, GI contents, muscle, and fur. Whole prey items include mice, rats, fish, etc. (depending on the species you are feeding). Omnivores should be offered a variety of both dark leafy greens and in most cases insects. The quality and variety of food offered is important. Animals should not be fed the same food day after day.

Chelonians. Most aquatic turtles are omnivorous; they generally consume fish, invertebrates, algae, leafy greens, etc. Commercial diets are acceptable to feed in moderation but it is important to make sure they contain essential nutrients needed to maintain good health. Tortoises are herbivores. They eat a variety of leaves, grasses, flowers, etc. in the wild. In captivity a healthy diet includes dark leafy greens, rose petals, hay, and vegetables. Commercial diets can be fed in moderation and should be appropriate for herbivores. Do not feed dog food, tofu, monkey biscuits, or anything that has animal protein in it.

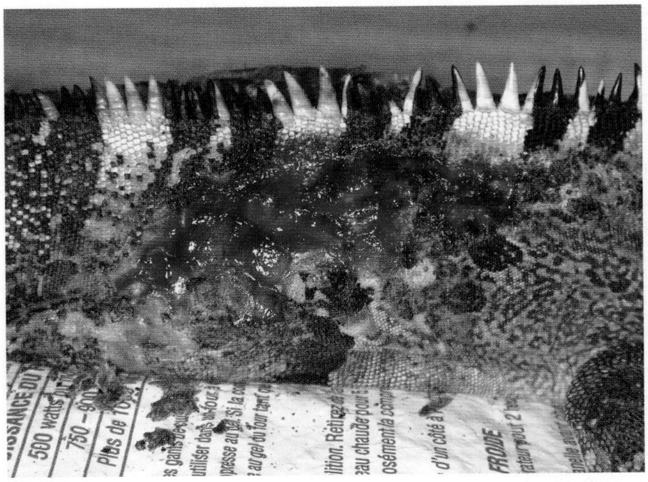

FIGURE 27-61 This lizard has a thermal burn caused by a light in the cage.

OBTAINING A HISTORY

A thorough history should be obtained from the owner before performing a physical examination. The owner can be given a history form to fill out while waiting to be called back into the examination room. An example of a complete history form is shown in Figure 27-62. The owner should be asked to bring in pictures of the patient's regular enclosure. This will give the veterinary staff a good idea of the type of husbandry practices being used.

> TECHNICIAN NOTE Reptiles can intermittently shed *Salmonella* spp. if they are carriers of the bacteria. Vinyl or latex examination gloves should be worn anytime you are working with reptiles to help prevent spread of *Salmonella* spp.

CAPTURE, RESTRAINT, AND HANDLING

Snakes

Most snakes can be easily captured directly out of the carrier or cage they are in. When dealing with nonaggressive snakes, the restrainer can simply pick the animal up and pull it out of the cage. If the snake is aggressive, it may be necessary to use a towel along with leather gloves to safely capture it. In these cases it is easiest to gently toss the towel over the snake and find the head. Once the head has been isolated and restrained, the snake can be safely taken out of the enclosure. If the snake is extremely aggressive or if it is a venomous snake, a snake hook should be used to pin down the head of the snake long enough to safely grasp its head and body. Improper use of the snake hook can cause trauma to the patient; therefore extreme caution should be taken.

Snakes are commonly brought into the clinic in pillowcases (Fig. 27-63). It is important that the veterinarian or technician does not just open the pillowcase and quickly pull the snake out (especially if unfamiliar with the patient). It is important to first know what type of snake is in the pillowcase. To safely remove the snake from the pillowcase, first find the snake's head and gently grasp it from the outside of

REPTILE HISTORY FORM

UC Davis School of Veterinary Medicine
Companion Avian and Exotic Pet Medicine Service
One Garrod Drive
Davis, CA 95616
(530) 752-1393

General History

Species
Reptile's Name ____________ Sex: M____ F____ UNK ________
How was your reptile sexed? (Visual, Blood Test, Surgical or Probes) ____________
Any specific identification? (ie: tattoo, microchip) ____________
If your reptile is female, has she produced eggs or given birth to young in the past? (if yes, please describe)
____
Reptile is a: Pet ________ Breeder ________
How did you acquire your reptile? Store ____ Breeder ____ Other ____ (describe) ____________
Date acquired? ____________
Do you have any other pets? ________ If yes, please specify, including ages and when acquired
____
When did your reptile last shed its skin? ____________
Did the shed appear normal (describe)? ____________

Housing

Is your reptile kept: Indoors ____ Outdoors ____ Both ____ Roam free in house ____________
(please specify % time for each location) ____________
Describe your reptile's enclosure (size, material) ____________
____
Is your reptile housed alone? ________ If no, describe ____________
What is/are the heat source(s)? ____________
Enclosure temperatures; High temperature (day/night) ________ Low temperature (day/night) ________
Basking site temperature ________
What is the humidity? ____________
How are the heat and humidity measured in the cage? ____________
What is/are the light source(s)? Please describe hours of use ____________
Is there a UV or full spectrum light source? Please describe (including hours of use) ____________
____
What substrate and other objects are in the cage (sand, gravel, newspaper, PVC, wood, hiding spots)?
____
How often is the cage cleaned? Using what products? ____________
Method/ frequency of cleaning food/ water dishes ____________
Does your reptile hibernate (if applicable)? ________ If yes, where and for what time period?
____
Has the reptile's environment changed recently? ________ If yes, describe ____________
Do you soak your reptile? ________ If so, how often? ________ Where? ________

FIGURE 27-62 Example of a history form used for reptile patients.

REPTILE HISTORY FORM

Diet:

What foods are offered to your reptile/ in what total percentages? (i.e.: 50% green leafy vegetables, 30% crickets, etc) ______

If live insects are fed, are they offered food at home ("gut loaded") before being fed to your reptile? ______

If so, with what product? ______

Any vitamin or mineral supplements offered? Brand name? ______

Any treats offered? Type? How often? ______

Any recent diet changes or new foods? ______ If yes, describe ______

How is water offered? (ie: sipper bottle, bowl, dropper) ______

Reason For Today's Visit:

What signs have you noticed that prompted today's visit? ______

How long have you noticed the problem? ______

Has your reptile been sick previously? ______

Has any other veterinarian ever seen your reptile? ______ If yes, when/why? ______

Have any tests been performed previously on your reptile? Please circle all that apply:
Bloodwork, fecal parasite test, skin parasite test, radiographs (X-rays); Other (please describe) ______

Additional comments (your comments regarding the reason for this visit): ______

ARE YOU AWARE THAT REPTILES CAN CARRY THE SALMONELLA BACTERIA?
IF NOT, PLEASE ASK US TO EXPLAIN.

FIGURE 27-62, cont'd

the pillowcase. Once the snake is restrained, the restrainer should put his or her free hand into the pillowcase and transfer the head to the "free hand." After this is accomplished, it should now be safe to take the entire snake out of the pillowcase.

It is important to gently hold the snake directly behind the head with one hand (so it cannot turn around and bite!) and support the body with the other hand (Fig. 27-64). If the snake is large, more than one person may be needed to restrain it. A good general rule is one person should be restraining per 3 ft of snake.

Chelonians

Although chelonians are usually the easiest to capture, they are the hardest to restrain. Unless working with extremely large tortoises, most chelonians can just be picked up with both hands and placed on the examination table. When examining large tortoises (i.e., several kilograms), it is easiest to set up an examination area within the animal's enclosure or on the floor in the clinic's examination area. Because there is such a great deal of variation in size and strength, restraint techniques may vary between small and large chelonians. Once the animal's body is under control, it is imperative that the head is properly restrained. Although this is relatively easy when the animal is sick, it can be difficult on strong healthy chelonians, especially large tortoises and box turtles.

There are several ways the restrainer can gain control of the animal's head. Many turtles and tortoises are very curious. If they are set down on the table or the ground, they may just start walking around to check things out. If this is the case, the technician can just walk up to them and grasp the head with one hand while restraining the body with the

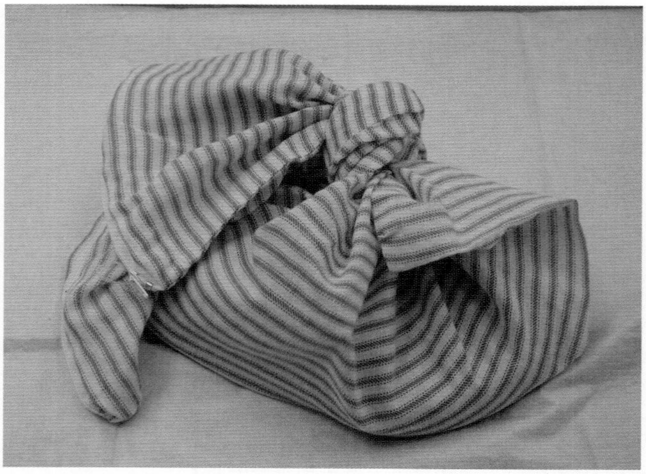

FIGURE 27-63 Snakes are commonly transported to the veterinary hospital in a pillowcase.

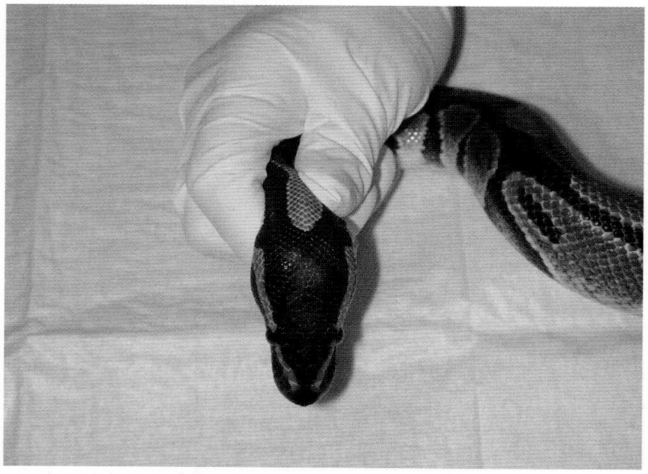

FIGURE 27-64 The snake's head is restrained by placing your hand behind the base of the skull. This will keep the snake from turning around and biting you.

other hand. To keep control of the head, it is best to position your thumb on one side of the cranial portion of the neck and position the rest of your fingers (or just the index finger for smaller species) on the other side of the neck just behind the base of the skull (Fig. 27-65). Healthy chelonians are strong so it may take a lot of constant but gentle force to keep the turtle or tortoise's head out of the shell. If the animal is extremely active, an additional person may be necessary to help restrain the limbs and body.

Another way to gain control of the head is by trying to coax the animal out of its shell. Many chelonians will extend their head out of the shell if food is offered to them or if they are placed in a container of shallow warm water. Once the head is extended, the same techniques mentioned above can be used to gain and keep control of the animal's head. If these techniques fail, it may be possible to slip a small blunt ear curette or spay hook under the horny portion of the upper beak, known as the rhinotheca. Once the probe has been placed, it can be gently pulled back to extend the neck to a position for

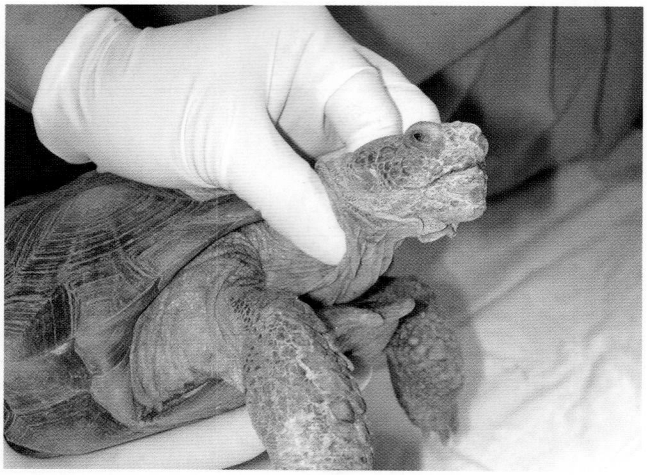

FIGURE 27-65 The tortoise is restrained by placing one hand behind the base of the skull to help keep the head and neck extended. The other hand should be used to support the body.

the restrainer to grasp. It is important to note that this technique can be dangerous. The beak can be chipped or broken if the animal struggles or is in poor health. If a spay hook is the tool of choice, it is a good idea to pad the hooked portion of the instrument. Padding can simply consist of tape or an elastic wrap cut to the appropriate size. Caution should be taken when dealing with any aquatic turtle, especially snapping turtles. These species of turtles have a tendency to bite, and many of the larger turtles can cause serious bodily harm to the people working with them.

Box turtles can be the most challenging chelonians to properly restrain. Because box turtles have a hinge on their plastron, many species are able to completely tuck themselves into their shells. The easiest way to extend their head is to gently prop open the cranial portion of the carapace (upper shell) and the plastron (lower shell). Use a well-padded object and exercise extreme care when trying to prop the shell open. This will help avoid traumatizing or fracturing the shell. Another way to extend a box turtle's head is to grasp one of the forelimbs, keeping the leg extended out of the shell until the head can be successfully pulled out and properly restrained. This method works well because once the leg is extended, the turtle will usually not close its shell down on its own leg. It is important to remember that any of these capture and restraint techniques can potentially cause a fair amount of stress to the turtle or tortoise. If initial attempts at capture and restraint are not successful, chemical restraint may be necessary for any reptile, especially large tortoises and box turtles.

Lizards

Lizards can be challenging animals to both capture and restrain. Smaller lizards are generally easy to capture but can be difficult to restrain because they tend to wiggle and squirm while they are being held. Most small lizards can simply be picked up with both hands and taken out of the enclosure. This is also true of the larger lizard species as well. However, some of the larger lizards can be both

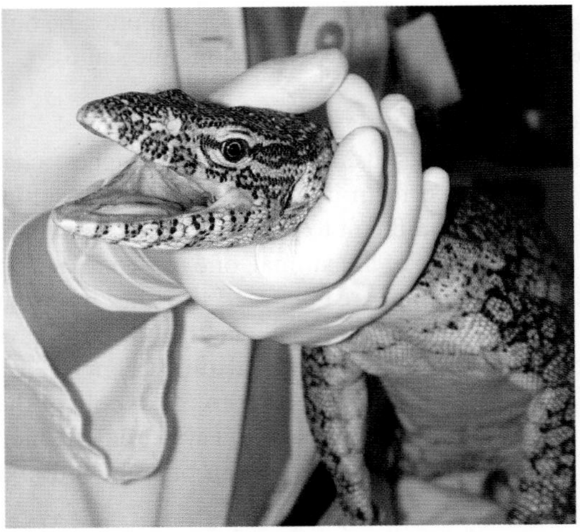

FIGURE 27-66 Long-necked lizards such as monitors should be restrained by placing one hand behind the base of the skull and the other hand supporting the body. Placing your hand behind the skull base will help keep the animal from biting you.

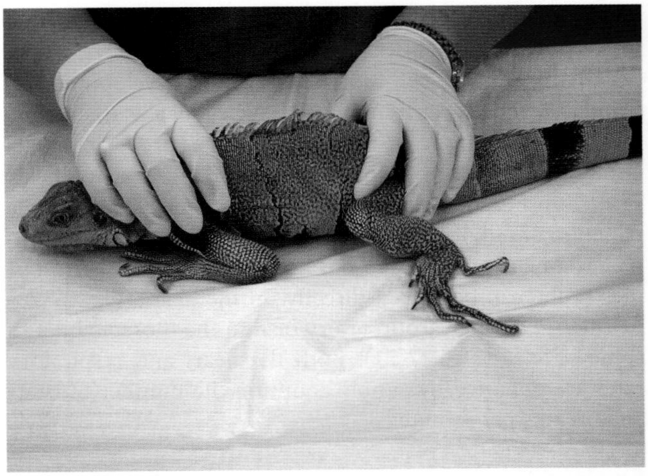

FIGURE 27-67 Restraint of a large lizard, with one hand around the pectoral girdle and the other hand around the pelvic girdle.

difficult to capture and restrain, especially if they are aggressive. If the lizard is aggressive, a towel or blanket along with leather restraint gloves should be used. It is important to remember that lizards can scratch and bite when they are scared or nervous. Therefore it is a good idea to wear long sleeves when possible and always keep track of where the head is. Long-necked lizards like monitors can easily turn around and bite if their head is not properly restrained during capture. Keeping one hand on the neck, just behind the base of skull, will help prevent getting bitten (Fig. 27-66). Many species of lizards have a natural predatory response to voluntarily "drop" or autotomize their tail in an attempt to escape predation. Never capture any species of lizard by the tail.

Generally, lizards can be restrained by placing one hand around the neck and pectoral girdle region while the other hand can be used to support the body near the pelvis (Fig. 27-67). Although it is sometimes difficult, try to avoid pressing down and damaging the dorsal spines of lizards such as iguanas when they are being restrained. It is also important to remember that not all lizards have durable and tough skin. Some lizards such as geckos have extremely delicate skin that can easily be damaged by capture and restraint. Make sure only soft towels are used on geckos.

REPTILE PHYSICAL EXAMINATION

Performing a physical examination on reptiles is comparable to performing a physical examination on most mammalian species. When working with any exotic species, all items needed for the physical examination should be ready and within reach. This will help decrease the time that the patient must be restrained and hopefully provide a less stressful experience for both the animal and the veterinary staff. Perform a visual precapture and restraint examination. This can give you are good idea of the animal's attitude and mentation before it has been potentially stressed by handling.

> TECHNICIAN NOTE It is important to perform a precapture and restraint examination. Observing the animal before stressing it for a physical examination can give you a good idea of mentation and attitude.

One of the easiest ways to perform a thorough physical examination is to start at the head and work your way down to the tail. This method will help ensure that nothing is overlooked. During the physical examination, the eyes, ears, and oral cavity should be thoroughly examined. The eyes should be bright, clean, and free of any discharge. A pen light and ophthalmoscope should be used to visually observe and examine the eyes. The sclera should be observed for any signs of redness or irritation. Any opacity should also be noted during the ophthalmologic examination. The ears or tympanic membranes should be observed with a pen light during the physical examination. They should be clean, clear, and free of any debris.

A thorough examination of the oral cavity is an important part of performing a complete physical examination. The oral cavity can be safely opened with either porous tape stirrups or a soft plastic instrument such as a spatula (Fig. 27-68). Metal specula can be used, but caution should be taken to avoid causing trauma to the mouth. The oral cavity should be moist, pink, and free of any lesions. Sometimes mucous membranes in snakes are paler than one would expect. Pale mucous membranes could be a sign of a medical problem, but many times this coloration is considered "normal." During the oral examination the mouth should be observed for any signs of erythema, stomatitis, fractured teeth, and any evidence of plaques on the mucous membranes.

As you move down the body, the coelomic cavity should be palpated (Fig. 27-69). Palpation of the extremities and tail should then follow. The same techniques used to palpate dogs and cats can be used to palpate most reptiles. It is important to note any abnormalities such as soft tissue swellings, space-occupying masses such as urinary calculi, developing eggs, neoplasia, and any current or old injuries such as fractures.

During the physical examination, make sure to get an accurate heart rate and respiratory rate (Table 27-3). A heart rate is most easily obtained by using a Doppler. Most reptile patients cannot be auscultated with a stethoscope, so a Doppler is an essential tool to have in your practice. The Doppler probe can be placed directly on the heart (Fig. 27-70) or either over the carotid artery or into the thoracic inlet in some species (Fig. 27-71). Both the heart and respiratory rates are obtained by simply counting the number of beats and breaths per minute.

Snakes

In snakes it is difficult to palpate many of the organs. In most snakes you can palpate the heart, gall bladder, and a prey item or feces if present. If the animal has a systemic infection or is septic, petechiae and ecchymosis can often be observed on the ventral aspect of the snake along the scutes.

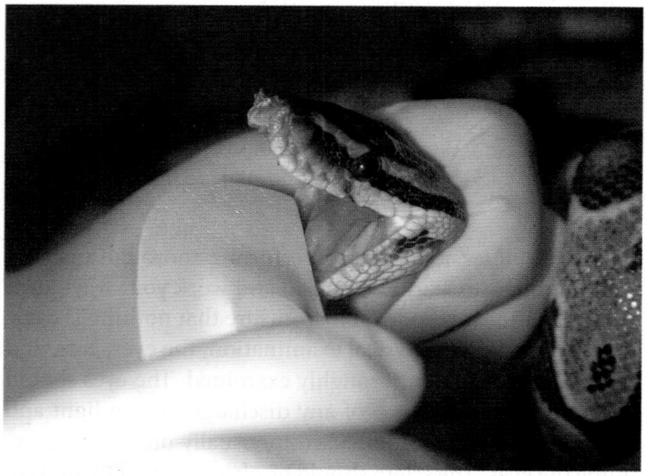

FIGURE 27-68 An oral examination should be performed as part of a complete physical examination. A soft plastic spatula is commonly used to gently open the mouths of snakes.

Chelonians

Turtles and tortoises usually present the biggest challenge when trying to perform a complete physical examination. The shell makes it difficult to palpate most of the organs. Depending on the size of the animal, one or two fingers may be placed in the inguinal area between the hind limbs and the shell. This will enable you to palpate the coelomic cavity for any abnormalities such as cystic calculi, foreign bodies, neoplasia, or eggs. It is also important to make note of the shell quality and color. If the animal has a systemic infection or is septic, petechiae and ecchymosis can often be found on the shell, especially the plastron.

Lizards

In lizards it is sometimes difficult to palpate many of the organs. In some of the larger lizards, the kidneys can be palpated via a rectal examination. If you can palpate the kidneys without a rectal examination, there is usually a problem. The kidneys sit in the pelvic girdle and are almost impossible to palpate unless they are enlarged or mineralized. If the animal has a systemic infection or is septic, petechiae and ecchymosis can often be observed. In some lizards such as iguanas, petechiae and ecchymosis are commonly seen on the dorsal spines along the animal's back.

> TECHNICIAN NOTE In lizards the kidneys are palpated by performing a rectal examination. This can only be performed on medium to large lizards. The kidneys cannot be palpated externally unless they are enlarged.

Normal Physiologic Values

Generally, normal physiological values in reptiles have an extremely large range. Many reptiles can have a heart rate that ranges from approximately 10 beats per minute to

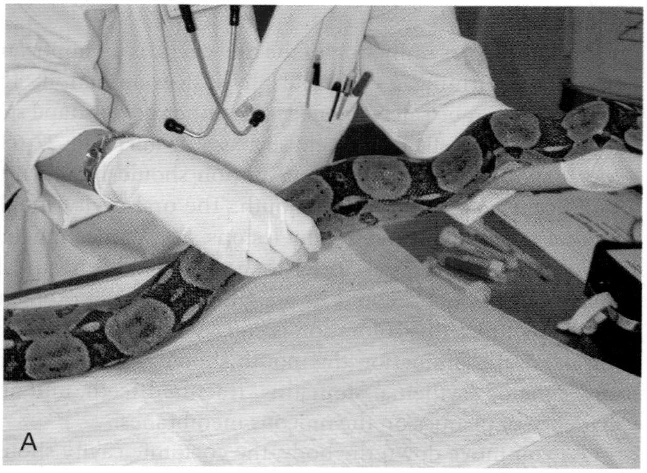

A

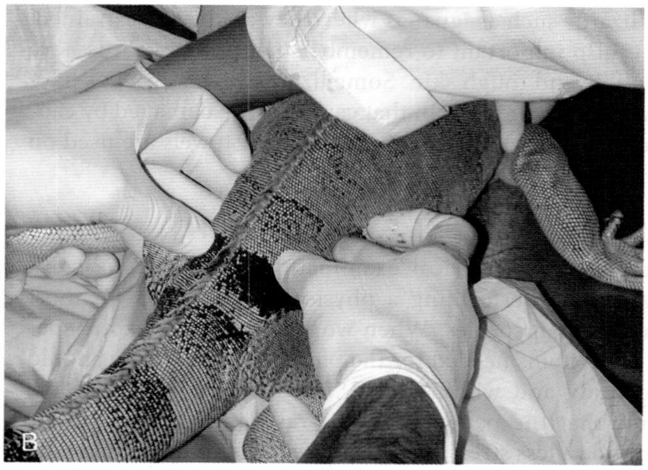

B

FIGURE 27-69 A, The entire length of the snake should be palpated while performing a complete physical examination. B, The coelom of lizards can be easily palpated and is done in a comparable manner as dogs and cats.

TABLE 27-3 Obtaining a Heart Rate with a Doppler

SPECIES	PLACEMENT OF THE DOPPLER
Lizards	Lateral cervical region over the carotid artery Cranial thorax over the heart Medial aspect of thigh over femoral artery Ventromedial aspect of the carpus over the artery
Snakes	Ventral aspect of the body directly on the heart Carotid artery Tail artery
Chelonians	Directly over the carotid artery Doppler probe placed directly into the thoracic inlet
Amphibians	Ventral aspect of the body directly over the heart

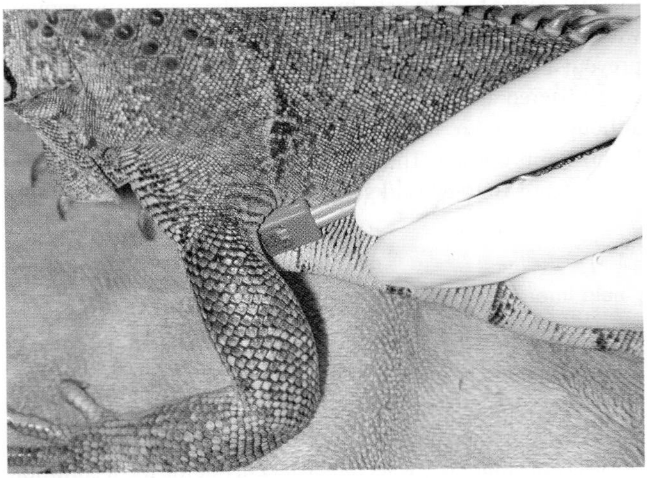

FIGURE 27-70 The Doppler probe is placed in the axillary region to obtain a heart rate on most lizard species.

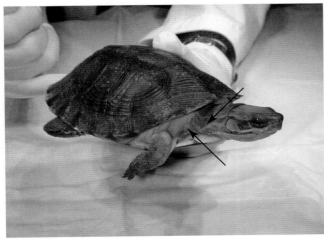

FIGURE 27-71 The Doppler probe is placed either over the carotid artery or into the thoracic inlet as indicated by the two black arrows.

about 80 or more beats per minute. Heart rates and respiratory rates can vary depending on ambient temperature, age, species, and health status. The respiratory rate may range from just a few breaths per minute to 20 or more breaths per minute depending on the previously mentioned factors. The body weight of the patient will also vary depending on age, gender, nutritional status, and species. Patients can range from as little as a few grams to several kilograms. A scale that weighs to the nearest gram should always be used to obtain an accurate weight on the patient. Body condition scoring is also performed on reptiles and follows the same guidelines that are used in mammalian medicine. The scale ranges from 1 to 9 with 1 being emaciated and 9 being grossly obese.

Determination of Gender

For many species of reptiles, determination of gender is relatively easy. For example male iguanas and bearded dragons have very large femoral pores compared with females (Fig. 27-72). Many species of male tortoises have a concave plastron making it easier to mount the female. Several male water turtles have elongated nails which are used to dangle in front of the female to impress her. Some species of male box turtles have brilliant red eyes. These are just a few examples.

The gender on snakes can be determined using a well lubricated metal or plastic probe inserted into the cloaca and then directed caudolaterally (Fig. 27-73). In male snakes the probe will enter the cavity where the inverted hemipenis (one of the two reproductive organs) is located. In female snakes the probe will enter a blind diverticula. Once the probe has been inserted, it is slowly and gently advanced until it will not advance any further. Your thumb should be placed on the scale where the end of the probe is located. You can now pull the probe out and count the number of scales from the cloacal opening to your thumb. If the number is greater than 7, it is a male and if it is less than 5, it is a female. If the number

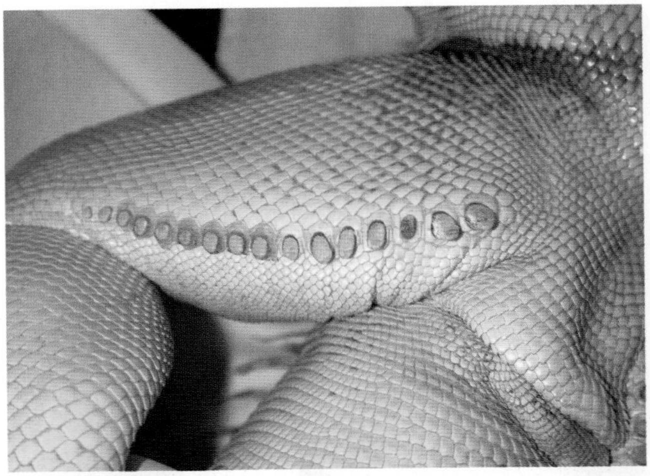

FIGURE 27-72 The femoral pores are commonly used to sex lizards such as iguanas and bearded dragons. The males (pictured) have large femoral pores, while females have tiny femoral pores.

is in between, it is very hard to say whether the animal is a male or female.

Assessing Dehydration and Fluid Therapy

Assessing dehydration in reptiles is comparable to assessing dehydration in dogs and cats. First look at the mucous membranes. Note whether they appear dry or pale, are moist and pink, or have mucous strands draping from the top to the bottom of the mouth (Fig. 27-74). Some reptiles, especially snakes, may have paler mucous membranes than mammals. Evaluate the skin to determine if it is wrinkled or lacks normal elasticity. You should also tent the skin (if possible) to assess dehydration. The same techniques used on dogs and cats can be used for most reptiles. Evaluate the eyes to determine if they appear sunken in and whether the skin around the eye stands up when touched. If the animal is dehydrated, fluid therapy should be considered and a percentage of dehydration should be estimated for the animal. Accurately estimating percent dehydration for any reptile is based on experience and using the above mentioned methods such as skin tenting, looking at the eyes, and examining the mucous membranes.

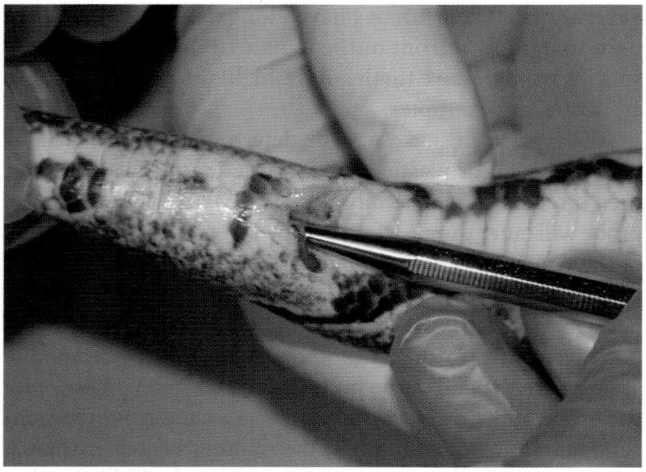

FIGURE 27-73 Gender of snakes can be determined using a well-lubricated metal or plastic probe inserted into the cloaca.

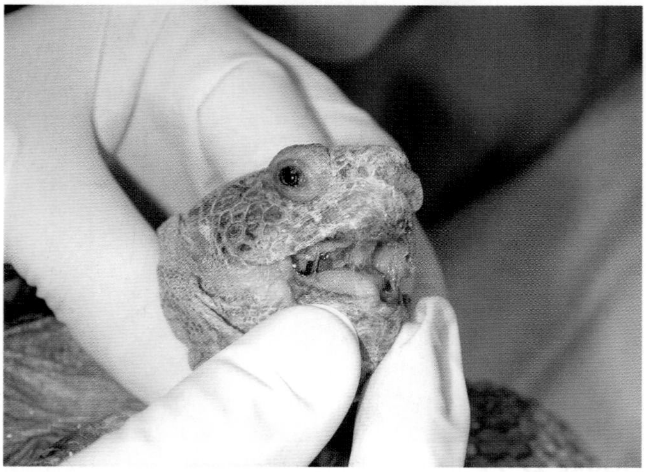

FIGURE 27-74 The stringy saliva in the mouth of this desert tortoise indicates severe dehydration.

Fluid therapy routes in reptiles include oral, subcutaneous, intracoelomic, intraosseous, and intravenous (although IV fluid therapy can be difficult) fluid administration. Subcutaneous fluid therapy can be easily given to reptiles when hospitalized. In lizards and snakes a butterfly catheter is placed under skin between two scales. You must aspirate the syringe before giving any injection. This is to ensure the needle has not been placed into a blood vessel, bladder if present, or the lungs. Butterfly catheters are generally used as it is easier to administer fluids to a moving patient with a butterfly catheter (Fig. 27-75). Subcutaneous fluids are commonly given into the inguinal or axillary region of chelonians. Either a butterfly catheter or hypodermic needle can be used to administer fluids. You must aspirate the syringe before administering the fluids. This will help ensure the fluids are not given into a blood vessel, the bladder, or the lung. Soaking the animal in a shallow tub of warm water (appropriate temperatures will depend on the species) can also be used in conjunction with other fluid therapy routes to help with hydration. The water must remain warm and the patient should be watched the entire time to prevent accidently drowning. The most common types of fluid administered are lactated Ringer's solution and Normosol-R, although there are many different opinions about what fluid is most appropriate. The daily fluid maintenance for reptiles ranges from 10 to 30 ml/kg/day.

> TECHNICIAN NOTE Daily soaking of reptiles can help improve overall hydration.

DIAGNOSTIC TECHNIQUES

Reptile Venipuncture

Venipuncture is a common diagnostic tool used in pet reptiles. A variety of laboratory tests can be taken, but the most common are the complete blood count (CBC) and chemistry panels.

Venipuncture sites vary with different species (Table 27-4). When you draw blood from most reptiles you need to

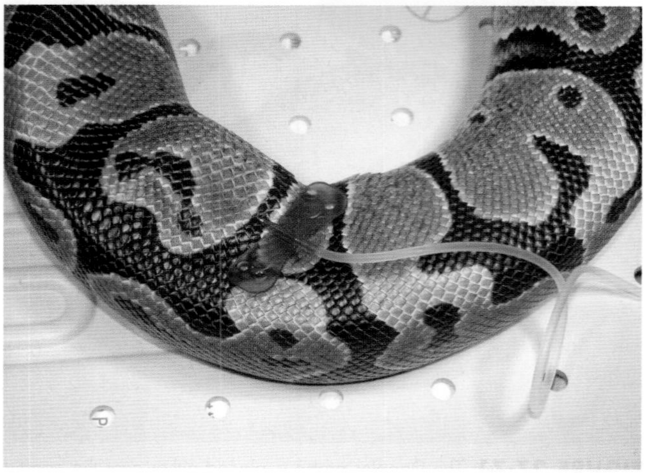

FIGURE 27-75 Subcutaneous fluid therapy using a butterfly catheter.

TABLE 27-4 Common Venipuncture Sites in Reptiles

SPECIES	VENIPUNCTURE SITES
Chelonians	Radialhumoral plexus sinus (brachial sinus) Dorsal venous sinus (coccygeal vein) Jugular vein Subcarapacial venous sinus Femoral vein
Lizards	Ventral and lateral aspects of the caudal tail vein
Snakes	Heart Ventral aspect of the caudal tail vein

evaluate the patient weight, determine how much blood you need to take for diagnostic sampling, and the total blood volume of the patient. It is estimated that the blood volume of most reptiles ranges between 5% and 8% of their total body weight. It is usually safe to calculate circulating blood volume using 8% unless the patient is very sick, anemic, or has lost a substantial amount of blood. Many reptiles can tolerate a loss of up to 10% of their total blood volume without any obvious detrimental effects to their health; however, it is generally unnecessary to take 10% of the total blood volume unless the lizard is very small (100 grams or less).

A few simple calculations can be used to determine how much blood can be safely drawn. First, the lizard's total circulating blood volume is calculated as follows:

$$\text{Body weight (grams)} \times \text{Percentage of total blood volume} = \text{Total circulating blood volume}.$$

Once the reptile's total blood volume has been calculated, 10% of the circulating blood volume can be withdrawn safely. This amount is determined as follows:

$$\text{Circulating blood volume (ml)} \times \text{Maximum percentage of blood that can be safely drawn} = \text{Maximum safe sample size (ml)}$$

For example: Let's determine how much blood can be safely drawn from a lizard that weighs 500 grams. For this calculation, the total blood volume is calculated at 8%:

$$500 \text{ grams} \times 0.08 \text{ total blood volume} = 40 \text{ ml of circulating blood}$$

The blood samples can contain up to 10% of the 40 ml of circulating blood. The amount (ml) that can be safely drawn from this patient for blood sampling is calculated as follows:

$$40 \text{ ml of circulating blood} \times 0.10 = 4 \text{ ml of blood}$$

Therefore, up to 4 ml of blood can be taken from this lizard, which is more than enough blood to run a CBC and a chemistry panel.

> **TECHNICIAN NOTE** It is important to become familiar with your commercial laboratory. Have a list available of the minimum amounts of blood needed for common diagnostic panels.

As with dogs and cats, blood collected from reptiles needs to be placed into an anticoagulant. Because only a small amount of blood is generally obtained, blood collection tubes such as Microtainers should be used. These tubes are made specifically for small amounts of blood and the anticoagulant is powdered rather than liquid. This helps to avoid dilution out the blood sample. The most common anticoagulants are EDTA (ethylenediaminetetraacetic acid), the "purple top tube," and lithium heparin, the "green top tube." EDTA is generally used for the CBC, while heparin is generally used for the chemistry panel. Heparin is preferred over a nonadditive tube such as a "red top tube" because the yield is higher.

Some species of reptile blood will clot or hemolyze when placed into EDTA. If this happens, the blood will not be able to be used for a CBC. For these species, the blood must be placed directly on a slide with no additive used or placed into a heparin tube. A CBC can be run from the heparinized sample, but the heparin will interfere with the staining of the cells.

Clipping toenails to obtain a blood sample is a method that some veterinary professionals may use either on very small lizards or when attempts to access other venipuncture sites have failed. Cutting toenails to the point of bleeding should not be used as a means for obtaining a blood sample. This can be very painful for the animal and may introduce infection. Blood from a clipped toenail also has the potential to skew blood chemistry levels (i.e., uric acid). Reptiles produce uric acid as their primary nitrogenous waste product. When reptiles release their urates (which are primarily made up of uric acid), they have a tendency to walk through the waste, thereby contaminating their feet and toenails. Even with a good scrubbing, the potential still exists for contamination of blood collected from this area.

Snakes. There are two common venipuncture sites in snakes which include the caudal tail vein and the heart. The palatine vessels are not appropriate for drawing samples of blood in snakes. Drawing blood from the tail vein is best accomplished in large snakes as it can be difficult in small snakes because of the size of the vessel. The same method used to draw blood from the ventral midline approach in lizards is used in snakes as well (see lizard section below). Obtaining a blood sample from the heart (also called cardiocentesis) is generally the quickest method, which will yield a large amount of blood. A 27- to 22-gauge needle on a 1- or 3-cc syringe is used for blood collection (size of needles and syringes will depend on the size of the snake). To obtain a blood sample, the snake should first be placed in dorsal recumbency. The heart can then be located in the cranial third of the body. The heart can move both cranially and caudally, so it is best to place your thumb and index finger on either side of the heart. Look for the caudal portion of the beating heart. The needle insertion site should be two scutes (scales) below that. To obtain blood from the heart, the needle should be inserted between two scutes at a 45-degree angle (Fig. 27-76).

Chelonians. The radial-humoral plexus (brachial plexus sinus), subcarapacial venous sinus, dorsal venous sinus (coccygeal vein), and jugular vein are the major sites where

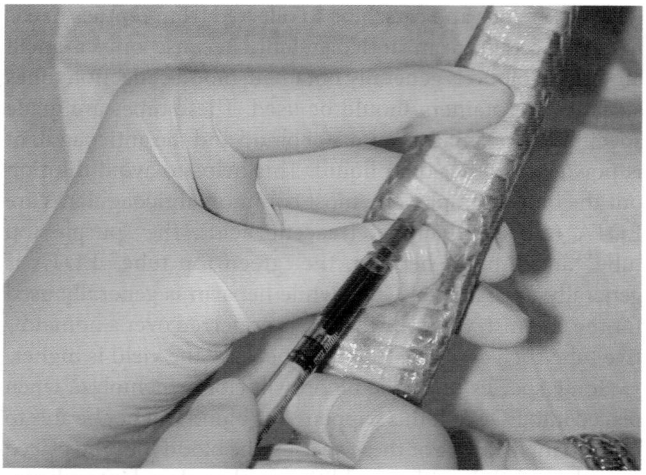

FIGURE 27-76 Cardiocentesis. The needle should be inserted about two scutes caudal to the last beating scale.

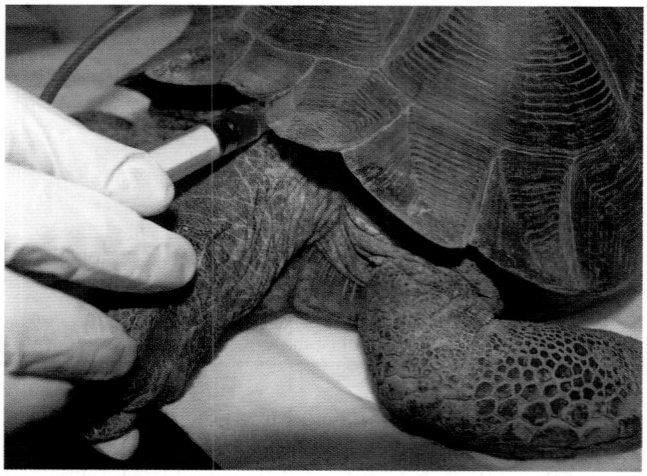

FIGURE 27-77 Blood collection from the subcarapacial venous sinus.

blood can be obtained from a turtle or tortoise. The venipuncture site will depend on the size and species of the patient and the preference of the phlebotomist. If drawing blood from the jugular vein, the turtle/tortoise should be placed in lateral recumbency. The head and neck should be pulled away from the shell. The jugular vein can be found in the same plane as the eye and the tympanum. To obtain the sample, the phlebotomist will hold the head while the restrainer will keep the patient in lateral recumbency. A 27- to 20-gauge needle attached to a 1- to 3-cc syringe is used and will vary depending on the size of the patient.

The subcarapacial venous sinus is generally used when jugular venipuncture is not an option (Fig. 27-77). Depending on the size of the patient, a 1- to 1½-inch, 27- to 20-gauge needle or a 2-inch spinal needle attached to a 1- to 3-cc syringe is used to obtain the blood sample. The needle is inserted upward at about a 60-degree angle just dorsal to the neck. Slight negative pressure should be applied on the syringe until either blood enters the syringe or bone is encountered. If bone is encountered, back away from the bone and redirect the needle.

The radial-humoral plexus sinus is generally used in larger chelonians. You must pull the front limb away from the body and palpate the tendon near the radiohumeral joint. A 22- to 20-gauge needle attached to a 1- to 3-cc syringe is inserted at a 90-degree angle to skin and angled toward the radiohumeral joint.

When drawing blood from the dorsal venous sinus, the patient should be placed in sternal recumbency. The tail should be held as straight as possible and the needle should be inserted on midline. A 1- to 1½-inch 27- to 20-gauge needle attached to a 1- to 3-cc syringe should be used. The size of the syringe and needle will depend on the size of the patient. The needle should be inserted at a 45-degree angle into the tail. Slight negative pressure should be placed on the syringe and the needle should be inserted until either the needle is in the vein or the needle touches bone. If bone is hit, slowly back the needle off the bone until blood enters the syringe.

Lizards. The cephalic, jugular, and ventral abdominal vessels can be used to obtain a blood sample from various species of lizards you may encounter in your clinic. However, these vessels are not commonly used for several reasons. The cephalic vein is usually extremely small, and because this is a "blind stick," a surgical cut-down may be necessary. The ventral abdominal vein is not generally used (especially in awake animals) because of the inability to both properly restrain the animal and control hemorrhage. Last, the jugular vein is not commonly used because in many species it is also a "blind stick" and may also require a surgical cut-down to access the vessel. Lymphatic fluid contamination is also common when performing venipuncture from the jugular vein. Lymph contamination can alter blood test results.

The most common vessel used for lizard venipuncture is the caudal tail vein, also called the ventral coccygeal vein. There are two different techniques commonly used to obtain blood from this vessel. These techniques include a lateral and ventral approach. To successfully obtain a blood sample from either approach, a 1- or 1½-inch 27- to 20-gauge needle attached to a 1-ml or 3-ml syringe should generally be used. The size of the needle and syringe will depend on the size lizard you are drawing blood from. Insulin syringes can be used on very small lizards, but remember to cut the needle off before putting the blood into the appropriate tubes. The small needle size can cause lysis of the blood cells if pushed through the needle (the same is true for 26- or 25-gauge needles). It is important that the tail is gently restrained during the blood draw. The left hand can be used to restrain the caudal portion of the tail, while the right hand is used to perform the blood draw. If you are left-handed just obtain your blood sample from the other side of the tail using your left hand to draw blood and your right hand to gently restrain the tail.

For a lateral approach, the needle should be inserted into the tail (between two scales) at approximately a 90-degree angle. Slowly insert the needle into the tail, keeping slight negative pressure on the syringe until either blood enters the syringe or the needle touches the vertebrae. If the needle is touching the vertebrae, slowly back the needle off the bone (still keeping slight negative pressure on the syringe) and redirect the needle into the vessel. It is important to put only slight negative pressure on the syringe while obtaining the blood sample. Too much negative pressure may collapse the vessel.

The technique for the ventral midline approach is very similar to the lateral approach. The needle should be inserted into the tail (between two scales) at approximately a 90-degree angle. The needle should be slowly inserted into the tail, keeping slight negative pressure on the syringe until either blood enters the syringe or the needle touches the vertebrae. The blood vessel is located just ventral to the vertebrae. If you touch the vertebrae first, slowly back off of the bone until your needle is seated within the vessel.

Lizards usually struggle when they are placed on their backs, making it difficult to draw blood from them. Therefore, it is important to keep the animal in sternal recumbency while obtaining the blood sample. During the blood draw, it is also important that the phlebotomist gently restrains the caudal portion of the tail with one hand and obtains the blood sample with the other.

Endoscopy

Rigid endoscopy can be performed in many reptiles by passing the endoscope through the oral cavity and into the stomach. Endoscopy is primarily used to obtain gastric biopsies or to retrieve foreign bodies from the stomach.

Cloacal Wash

Cloacal washes are used to collect feces for laboratory analysis. This is very common as fresh stool is often not available. A red rubber feeding tube of appropriate size is attached to a 1-ml syringe. The tube is well lubricated with a water based jelly and placed into the cloaca. Saline is infused into the cloaca and aspirated back out. This lavage will often yield enough fecal material for microscopic analysis.

Skin Scrape and Touch Smears

Performing skin scrapes or touch (impression) smears is an easy way to obtain information on potential bacterial and fungal infections of the skin. A cover slip edge in gently scraped across the skin and then placed on a slide with saline making a wet mount. This sample should be analyzed immediately to obtain accurate results. Skin scrapes should not be performed on specific lesions as this can cause more damage to the skin. A touch or impression smear is primarily used on specific lesions such as ulcers or other damaged tissue. A microscope slide is touched to skin in an attempt to collect histological data. The smear is then stained for analysis.

Tracheal Wash

The mouth is gently opened using an appropriate mouth speculum. Using aseptic technique, the tracheal wash is performed by inserting a sterile red rubber feeding tube or polypropylene urinary catheter into the trachea. The patient must be anesthetized for the procedure because it can be very stressful and the tissues are very delicate. Generally, a small amount of saline is infused and then aspirated from the trachea. The volume will depend on the size of the patient. The sample should be smeared onto a slide and stained for analysis.

PARASITOLOGY

Reptiles can be affected by a wide variety of parasites. There are several different ways to check for parasite load including direct fecal examination, fecal flotation, and cloacal wash. The direct fecal examination and flotation are done in the same manner as a dog or cat. The cloacal wash is accomplished by inserting a soft rubber feeding tube attached to a syringe into the cloaca. Saline is then flushed into the cloaca and suctioned out, obtaining a diagnostic sample.

RADIOLOGY

Good radiographs are an important tool used as part of your diagnostic workup. The diagnostic value of a radiograph depends on the quality of the technique and positioning of the patient. Digital radiology is quickly becoming the standard in most hospitals and will yield the best results. However, if digital radiology is not yet available in your hospital then high-detail, rare earth cassettes with single emulsion film provide desired results. Mammography film will produce even better detail, but does require modification of x-ray machine settings. A technique can be extrapolated from the tabletop technique used on most of your feline patients. For extremely small patients you can use a dental radiology unit.

Snakes

Two views are normally taken which include a dorsoventral (DV) or ventrodorsal (VD) and a lateral. Radiographs are taken in sections from head to tail and labeled with numbered lead markers to delineate each section. In most cases the snake will need to be heavily sedated or anesthetized to obtain good radiographs, unless the snake is very sick. A plastic snake tube can be used to obtain radiographs, but often diagnostic films are not produced unless the snake is unable to move within the tube and remains completely straight.

Chelonians

Three views are normally taken, which include a dorsoventral (DV), horizontal lateral, and horizontal craniocaudal views. The craniocaudal view is taken to evaluate the left and right lung fields. A horizontal beam is essential to obtain good radiographs. Because chelonians do not have a diaphragm, placing them in lateral recumbency causes shifting of the organs into the lung cavity, which leads to poor radiographs. Most chelonians do not need to be sedated for radiographs, but chemical restraint can be used if necessary. In most cases the patient will just sit there, or it can be placed on a plastic dish with its feet hanging in the air.

Lizards

Two views are normally taken which include a dorsoventral (DV) and horizontal lateral. A horizontal beam is essential to obtain good radiographs. Because reptiles do not have a diaphragm, placing them in lateral recumbency causes shifting of the organs into the lung cavity which leads to poor radiographs. Most lizards do not need to be sedated for radiographs, but chemical restraint can be used if necessary. In most cases the patient will just sit there while the radiographs are being taken. You can also use vagal stimulation or the "vagal response" to calm the patient if needed. The vagal response in iguanas and other medium to large lizard species can be induced by gently applying digital pressure to both eyes for a few seconds to a few minutes. The patient will usually respond with a decrease in heart rate and blood pressure. The vagal response can also be induced by placing cotton balls over the eyes (Fig. 27-78). The vagal response induces a short-term trance-like state, allowing time to take radiographs and in some cases even draw blood.

HOSPITALIZATION AND NURSING CARE

HOSPITALIZATION

Critically ill patients will need to remain in the hospital for intensive care and treatments. Common daily treatments include fluid therapy, soaking, force or syringe feeding, and administration of any needed medications.

Providing the proper cage setup is extremely important. Reptiles need external heat, therefore an incubator or cage with an external heating source is an excellent way to provide this environment. Additional humidity can also be provided by misting the cage. This can be done either several times per day or a continuous drip system can be set up. Temperature and humidity will vary by species and should be monitored using a thermometer and hygrometer. Cages should also be easy to clean and escape proof. When possible, reptiles should be housed in a separate room from dogs, cats, and other exotic pets. This will help reduce the spread of disease and unnecessary stress to the reptile.

FORCE-FEEDING

Patients frequently present to the veterinary hospital for anorexia or lethargy. Nutritional supplementation and fluid therapy are often required. Animals that are not eating are in a catabolic state. Decreased food intake results in the breakdown of protein and fat for energy. This can contribute to hepatic lipidosis, azotemia, muscle wasting, impaired gastrointestinal function, and decreased immunity.

Patients that are not eating on their own will need to be tube or syringe fed. Syringe feeding is relatively easy. Tube feeding is comparable to that in birds. The mouth is opened with a speculum such as a plastic spatula. The tube is premeasured to estimate where the stomach is located before inserting it into the patient. Unlike metal tubes that are usually used in birds, a red rubber feeding tube is usually used with most reptile species (Fig. 27-79). An esophagostomy tube can be placed in chelonians that will need long-term assisted feeding. Tube placement is done in a similar manner as it is in mammalian species.

> *TECHNICIAN NOTE* Veterinary technicians can easily teach owners to syringe feed or assist feed via an esophagostomy tube.

It is important to use proper syringe feeding diets such as Oxbow Carnivore Care for carnivores or Oxbow Critical Care for herbivores. Omnivorous animals can be fed a mixture of the two. Other diets can be used as well, as long as they are complete and balanced. Insectivores can be fed an appropriate meat-based baby food.

ADMINISTRATION OF FLUIDS AND MEDICATIONS

The intramuscular and subcutaneous routes are the most common routes for administration of medications. Because of the renal-portal system, only the front limbs should be used for intramuscular and subcutaneous injections.

The intravenous route is rarely used, but administration of fluids and some medications can be given into the caudal tail vein in reptiles or the jugular vein in chelonians (Table 27-5). This can be accomplished by either a single injection

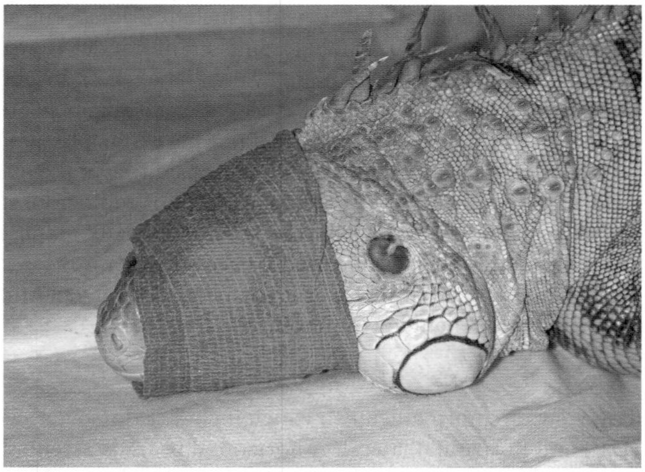

FIGURE 27-78 To induce the vagal response, place cotton balls over the eyes and lightly wrap an elastic wrap around the head. This wrap takes the place of digital pressure.

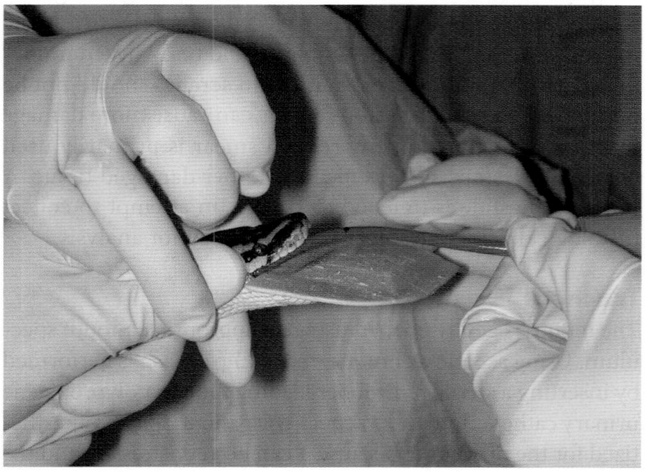

FIGURE 27-79 Tube feeding is best accomplished by opening the mouth with a soft plastic spatula, plastic card, or tape stirrups.

or by placing an indwelling catheter. The needle and catheter size generally ranges from 27 to 20 gauge, depending on the size of the patient.

Intraosseous fluids can be given in many lizard species (Fig. 27-80). In lizards a 25- to 20-gauge spinal needle is placed into the distal portion of the femur or humerus or into the proximal portion of the tibia. A spinal needle is preferred because the stylet will help keep the needle from becoming clogged with bone core fragments. The catheter is placed using aseptic technique and is sutured to the skin for stability. It is then bandaged to protect the catheter site. This procedure is painful and requires either sedation with analgesia, general anesthesia, or the use of a local anesthetic.

The intracoelomic route can be used for administration of fluids. The patient should be placed in lateral recumbency, with the hind leg extended away from the body. The needle is then placed under the skin and into the coelomic cavity. You must aspirate before administering any fluids. If the needle is placed into the wrong spot, fluids could accidentally be given into the bladder or into the lungs, both of which are detrimental.

The oral route is often used to administer medications. Oral medications can be given using a feeding tube or just titrated in with a syringe.

COMMON DISEASES AND PRESENTATIONS

There are a myriad of diseases commonly seen in clinical practice (Box 27-18). It is beyond the scope of this chapter to talk about each disease. Therefore it is suggested that a reptile medicine textbook be consulted to learn more about common disease processes.

TABLE 27-5 Common Intravenous Catheter Sites in Reptiles

SPECIES	CATHETER SITES
Chelonians	Jugular vein
Lizards	Ventral and lateral aspects of the caudal tail vein
Snakes	Ventral aspect of the caudal tail vein

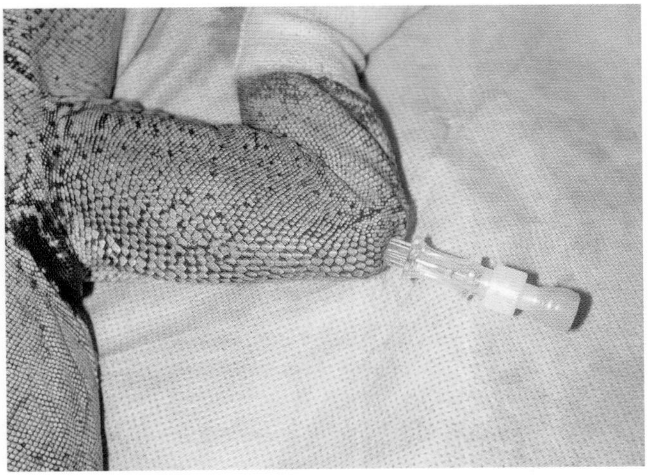

FIGURE 27-80 Intraosseous fluids in a lizard.

Metabolic Bone Disease

Metabolic bone disease (MBD) affects both reptiles and amphibians and is usually the result of long-term dietary deficiency of calcium or vitamin D, a lack of exposure to UV light, and/or a negative dietary calcium to phosphorus ratio. Common dietary causes include a lack of bone in the diet of carnivorous animals and a lack of calcium with excess phosphorus in herbivorous diets. Common clinical signs include, but are not limited to, a pliable mandible or maxillae, kyphosis, scoliosis, fractures, tremors, lameness, abnormal shell development and pyramiding of the shell in chelonians, or the overall inability to move.

EMERGENCY AND CRITICAL CARE

Chelonians, lizards, and snakes commonly present on emergency for traumatic injuries. Common emergencies include hit by car, attacked by another animal, stepped on, dropped, and thermal burns (Fig. 27-81). Wounds are treated with the same medical techniques used to treat small mammals.

BOX 27-18 Common Diseases and Conditions of Reptiles

- Egg binding
- Foreign body obstruction
- Gout
- Hypocalcemia
- Hypovitaminosis A (chelonians only)
- Metabolic bone disease
- Parasitic infestations
- Poor husbandry and diet
- Respiratory disease
- Reproductive organ prolapse
- "Shell rot" (chelonians only)
- Stomatitis
- Thermal burns
- Trauma
- Variety of bacterial, viral, and fungal infections

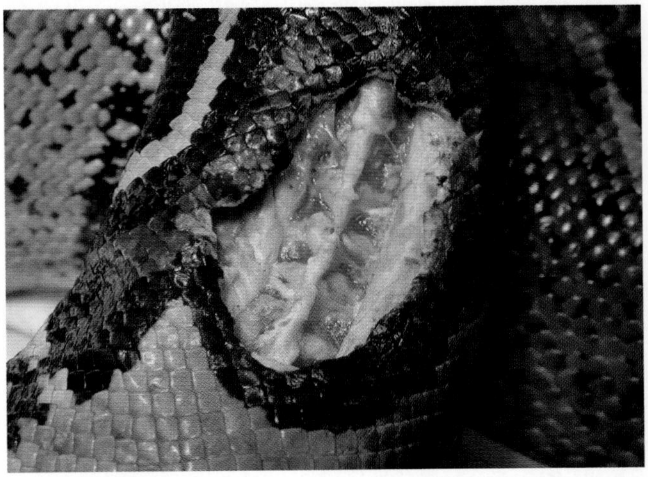

FIGURE 27-81 This wound was caused by offering live prey. The snake did not eat the rat and was left alone with it for a few days. When the owner returned, the rat had caused severe damage to the flesh and vertebrae.

Wound care, fluid therapy, nutritional support, and pain medications should be provided as necessary.

Anesthesia

Anesthesia can be challenging in reptiles. Premedications should always be given before any anesthetic induction. Common premedications include butorphanol, morphine, midazolam, ketamine, and dexmedetomidine used in various combinations. Premedications are given intramuscularly cranial to the kidneys (because of the renal portal system) and should be given at least 30 to 60 minutes before anesthetic induction. It is important to keep the patient warm, enabling it to properly metabolize the drugs.

While the premedications are taking effect, the anesthetist should prepare for the anesthetic procedure. All instrumentation should be organized and ready to place once the patient has been anesthetized (Box 27-19). Common instruments used for reptiles during anesthesia include an electrocardiogram (ECG), Doppler, end-tidal carbon dioxide monitor, and a temperature probe. The ECG is placed in the same manner as in mammals. The end-tidal carbon dioxide monitor is attached to the endotracheal tube and the temperature probe is placed either rectally or into the esophagus. Pulse oximetry is not reliable in reptiles and is therefore not commonly used. An intravenous catheter should be placed when possible, although this can be very difficult. In snakes the most common site for catheterization is the caudal tail vein, or you can perform a surgical cut-down and place a catheter in the jugular vein. In chelonians the most common site for catheterization is the jugular vein. In lizards the most common site for catheterization is the caudal tail vein.

Propofol is the most common injectable induction agent used in reptiles. Propofol is given intravenously slowly over a few minutes. Once the patient has been induced, it should be intubated and placed on isoflurane in oxygen at an appropriate percentage. Snakes do not have an epiglottis, making it very easy to intubate them after anesthetic induction. Once the endotracheal tube is placed, it is taped around either the mandible, maxilla, or around the back of the head to properly secure it (Fig. 27-82).

BOX 27-19 Basic Anesthetic Equipment and Supplies Needed for Reptile Patients

- 24- to 26-gauge intravenous catheters
- Ambu bag
- Electrocardiogram
- End-tidal CO_2 monitor (capnograph)
- Esophageal and rectal temperature probes
- Heating pad or forced hot air unit
- Pediatric anesthetic face masks
- Pediatric blood pressure cuffs and sphygmomanometer
- Pediatric fluid administration sets (60 drops/min)
- Pediatric fluid extension sets
- Pediatric intubation tubes 3.0 mm and smaller; noncuffed tubes should be available
- 14- to 24-gauge intravenous catheters can be adapted into an endotracheal tube
- Pediatric intravenous fluid therapy T-ports
- Positive pressure ventilator
- Syringe pump
- Ultrasonic Doppler flow detector

The patient should be placed on a ventilator or bagged by hand to provide intermittent positive pressure ventilation (IPPV) throughout the procedure because reptiles do not breathe well on their own while under anesthesia. It is very important to keep the patient at an appropriate temperature during the surgical procedure. For most species of reptiles, core body temperature should be kept between about 80° and 90° F (although this varies by species). If the patient is kept too cold, the drugs will take hours to metabolize and the patient will have a prolonged recovery time. Lactated Ringer's solution or Normosol-R is commonly given intravenously at a rate of 5 ml/kg/hour.

> **TECHNICIAN NOTE** It is essential to keep reptiles warm while under anesthesia. Cold animals have a prolonged recovery time and drugs will not metabolize very quickly. Each species has a specific ideal body temperature.

Once the procedure is over, the inhalant anesthetic should be turned off and the patient should be taken off of pure oxygen. The reptile's respiratory drive to take a breath is more oxygen driven rather than carbon dioxide driven as in mammals. If kept on pure oxygen, the reptile patient has little drive to take a breath on its own and recovery will be very prolonged. An Ambu bag should be attached to the endotracheal tube and the patient should be given a breath about 4 to 6 times per minute until the patient is awake and can be extubated.

Postoperative analgesic medications should be given at the conclusion of the surgical procedure. The most common postoperative drugs include butorphanol, morphine, meloxicam, and tramadol.

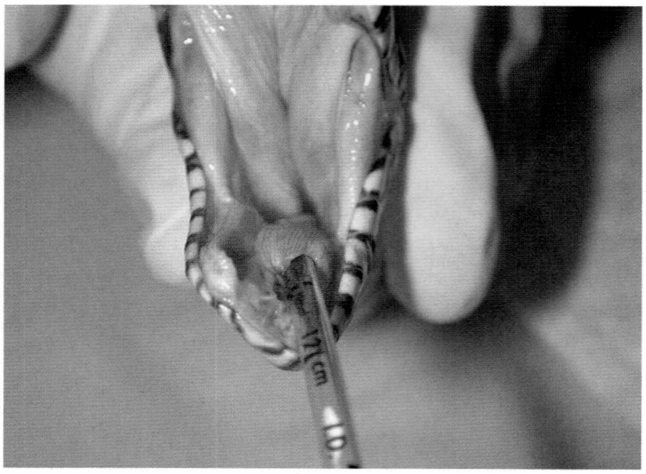

FIGURE 27-82 Endotracheal intubation in a snake.

Euthanasia

Euthanasia can be difficult because it can sometimes be hard to access a vessel. A euthanasia barbiturate solution can be given into any vessel, the heart, or into the coelomic cavity. If injecting into the heart, the patient must be anesthetized before the injection. The heart may take several minutes to several hours to completely stop, even though the patient may be clinically dead. A Doppler can be used to check for a heartbeat. The patient should be kept in the clinic for several hours or overnight to ensure the patient has been properly euthanized before sending it home with the owner if that is the owner's preference.

AMPHIBIANS

Amphibians are a diverse group of animals that have become popular pets over the last several years. The class Amphibia contains three orders, which include Anura—frogs and toads; Caudata—salamanders, newts, and sirens; and Gymnophiona—caecilians. While there are over 4000 species alive today, only a few are commonly seen in most clinical practices.

Amphibians can be difficult animals to work with, so it is extremely important for the veterinary technician to become properly educated on the common aspects of amphibian medicine and techniques, including physical examination, handling, venipuncture, common diagnostic procedures, common diseases and presentations, husbandry, and water quality parameters.

HUSBANDRY

An entire book can be dedicated to husbandry alone, but for the purposes of this chapter, only the very basics of amphibian husbandry will be discussed.

> **TECHNICIAN NOTE** The veterinary hospital can make client education handouts to provide owners with appropriate husbandry and diet information. The clinic name, address, and phone number can be placed at the top of the document, helping advertise the clinic as well.

The terrarium setup will vary based on the species of amphibian you are working with and whether it is aquatic or terrestrial. Regardless of the type of enclosure or species, the native habitat should be mimicked whenever possible. The best way to provide a proper habitat is to do ample research about the species involved. For example, a terrestrial cage may consist of mosses, various plants, rocks, logs, and a small amount of water in the cage. An aquatic cage will have a completely different set of criteria. If the amphibian is arboreal, you must provide height in the cage so it can climb into a planted canopy. Many species also need a temperature and humidity gradient in the cage. Whether the cage is set up for an aquatic species or a terrestrial species, you must maintain proper lighting, heating, humidity, water quality parameters, and cleanliness. Most diseases in exotic animals are caused from poor husbandry and improper diet.

Water Quality

Water quality and care is one of the most important aspects of caring for amphibious pets. Amphibians are very sensitive to poisoning from nitrogenous waste buildup and disinfectant residues. Frequent water changes and having a good filtration system on the terrarium will help keep water parameters under control. There are several parameters that should be checked on a regular basis including temperature, pH, salinity, water hardness, alkalinity, dissolved oxygen, carbon dioxide, un-ionized ammonia, nitrite, nitrate, and chlorine (Box 27-20). A specific amphibian care book can give more detailed information regarding each of these parameters. Many parameters will vary based on the species involved. This is especially true for pH and temperature. Chlorine should be undetectable for all species.

Nutrition

An entire book can be written for amphibian nutrition. This section will only discuss the very basics. It is important to remember that amphibians are not domesticated animals. In many cases, they have been taken from the wild and sold into the pet trade. There is not a simple commercial diet available for owners to feed amphibious pets like there is for dogs and cats. It is almost impossible to provide them with their native diet, but we can and must replicate it as much as possible. Most amphibians are carnivorous or insectivorous as adults. It is important for owners to do research regarding exactly what food is recommended and how often to feed before purchasing a specific amphibian species. The key to providing a healthy diet is offering a variety of different types of food. For example, just crickets or just neonatal mice should not be offered every single day. Providing an improper diet will lead to severe life-threatening nutritional disorders. Some species eat daily while others do not. Some species will only eat in the water, other species may only eat flying insects, and still others will only eat prey that is alive and moving around. It is also important that reputable resources are used to find this information.

PHYSICAL EXAMINATION

Amphibians will present to the veterinary clinic for a multitude of reasons ranging from trauma to a variety of different diseases or infections. It is very important to be able to

BOX 27-20 Important Water Quality Parameters for Amphibians

- Alkalinity
- Carbon dioxide
- Chlorine
- Dissolved oxygen
- Nitrate
- Nitrite
- pH
- Salinity
- Temperature
- Un-ionized ammonia
- Water hardness

properly handle and perform a quick yet thorough physical examination on these unique species. Before the physical examination is performed, a complete history should be taken from the client. This should be very detailed and should include information about the husbandry, water quality, and diet of the patient. When possible, ask the client to provide you with pictures of the animal's terrarium. This will give you an insight to the animal's normal living conditions.

Amphibians can be challenging animals to both capture and restrain. It is important to keep stress to a minimum therefore the patient should only be handled when necessary. You should always wear nonpowdered gloves when handling and keep the patient moist to avoid dehydration. This will protect both you and the patient. Some amphibians can release toxins from their skin that cause irritation or illness in humans, and amphibians can absorb substances through their skin, so anything on your hands can be potentially harmful to the patient.

Generally amphibians can be restrained by placing one hand around the neck and pectoral girdle region while the other hand can be used to support the body near the pelvis. In some cases the patient may need to be anesthetized to perform a physical examination. This is especially true with aggressive animals or extremely stressed animals.

Performing a physical examination on amphibians is comparable to performing a physical examination on most mammalian species. When working with any exotic species, all items needed for the physical examination should be ready and within arm's reach. This will help decrease the time that the patient must be restrained and hopefully provide a less stressful experience for both the animal and the veterinary staff. Always perform a visual precapture and restraint physical examination. This can give you a good idea of the animal's attitude and mentation before it has been potentially stressed by handling. Note how it is reacting to the current surroundings, whether it is alert, and whether any signs of increased respiratory effort are present.

One of the easiest ways to perform a thorough physical examination is to start at the head and work your way down to the tail or back end. This method will help ensure that nothing is overlooked. During your physical examination, the eyes and oral cavity should be thoroughly examined. The eyes should be bright, clean, and clear of any discharge. A pen light and ophthalmoscope should be used to visually observe and examine the eyes. The sclera should be observed for any signs of redness or irritation. Any opacity should also be noted during the ophthalmologic examination.

A thorough examination of the oral cavity is an important part of performing a complete physical examination. The oral cavity can be safely opened with either porous tape stirrups or a soft plastic instrument such as a spatula. Metal specula can be used, but caution should be taken to avoid causing trauma to the mouth. The oral cavity should be moist, pink, and free of any lesions. During the oral examination, the mouth should be observed for any signs of erythema, stomatitis, fractured teeth, and any evidence of plaques on the mucous membranes. As you move down the body, the thoracic and coelomic cavities should be palpated. Palpation of the extremities and tail (if present) should then follow. The same techniques used to palpate dogs and cats can be used to palpate most amphibians. It is important to note any abnormalities such as soft tissue swellings, space-occupying masses, developing eggs, neoplasia, and any current or old injuries such as fractures. In amphibians, it is very difficult to palpate many of the organs. If the animal has a systemic infection or is septic, petechiae and ecchymosis can often be observed.

During the physical examination, make sure to get an accurate heart rate and respiratory rate. A heart rate is most easily obtained by using a Doppler. Most amphibian patients cannot be auscultated with a stethoscope, so a Doppler is an essential tool to have in your practice. In amphibians the Doppler probe should generally be placed in the same area a stethoscope would be placed on a dog or cat. You will need to place the probe on the caudal aspect of the thoracic cavity. Both the heart and respiratory rates are obtained by simply counting the number of beats and breaths per minute.

TECHNICIAN NOTE Nonpowdered latex or vinyl examination gloves should always be worn when working with amphibian patients.

Venipuncture Techniques

Blood collection can be very challenging in amphibians. Alcohol should not be used to clean the venipuncture site. This can irritate and/or desiccate the patient's skin. A 1:40 diluted 2% chlorhexidine solution should be used to cleanse the site instead.

Venipuncture in salamanders is generally performed using the caudal tail vein. This is the same technique described in this chapter for both lizards and snakes. It is important to remember that the vessel is very small and can collapse easily, therefore do not place a large amount of negative pressure on the syringe during collection. A 25- to 27-gauge needle attached to a 1-ml syringe should be used. An insulin syringe can also be used for very small patients. The blood sample should be placed in a heparinized Microtainer tube for analysis.

Venipuncture sites in frogs and toads include the femoral vein, ventral abdominal vein, and the lingual vein. The femoral and lingual veins are rarely used. The ventral abdominal vein is by far the easiest vessel to obtain a blood sample from. The frog or toad is gently positioned on its back with the restrainer holding the pectoral girdle. The person drawing blood can hold the pelvic girdle with one hand and draw blood with the other hand. Some amphibians will need to be anesthetized for venipuncture. A 1-ml syringe with a 25- to 27-gauge needle is generally used to obtain the sample although an insulin syringe can be used as well. The blood sample should be placed into a heparinized Microtainer tube for analysis.

Blood volume needs to be considered in these small patients. No more than 1% of the body weight should be taken in blood volume from healthy patients and no more than 0.5% should be taken from sick patients. For example, if you need to take blood from a 200-gram patient, you can only take 2.0 ml. This is plenty of blood for a CBC and chemistry panel.

COMMON DISEASES AND PRESENTATIONS

There are a myriad of diseases commonly seen in clinical practice (Box 27-21). It is beyond the scope of this chapter to talk about each disease; therefore, it is suggested that an amphibian medicine text book be consulted to read about common disease processes.

DIAGNOSTIC AND TREATMENT TECHNIQUES

Common routes for administration of medications to amphibians are located in Table 27-6. It is important to check a current exotic animal drug formulary for the most appropriate proper drug administration routes. Intravenous and intraosseous routes are not generally used in amphibians.

Celiocentesis

Celiocentesis is an important diagnostic technique used to analyze fluid retained within the coelomic cavity. Fluid accumulation can occur for a variety of different reasons and is usually secondary to cardiac, renal, or hepatic diseases or osmotic imbalances. The patient should be placed on its back and gently restrained. Anesthesia may be required for this procedure. The site should be cleansed with a 1:40 diluted 2% chlorhexidine solution. Generally a 25- to 27-gauge needle attached to a 1-ml syringe is used to aspirate the fluid. Do not aspirate aggressively as this can cause damage to the internal organs. After the fluid has been obtained, it should be immediately smeared onto a slide or placed into a heparinized Microtainer tube for analysis. Celiocentesis is not only diagnostic, but therapeutic as well.

Cloacal Wash

Cloacal washes are used to collect feces for laboratory analysis. This is very common as fresh stool is often not available. A red rubber feeding tube of appropriate size is attached to a 1.0-ml syringe. The tube is well lubricated with a water-based jelly and placed into the cloaca. Isotonic saline (0.6%) is infused into the cloaca and aspirated back out. In most species, approximately 0.5 to 1.0 ml of fluid is used. This lavage will often yield enough fecal material for microscopic analysis.

BOX 27-21 Common Diseases and Presentations in Amphibians

- Cutaneous bacterial infection (red leg)
- Egg binding
- Foreign body obstruction
- Metabolic bone disease
- Mycobacteriosis
- Parasitic infestations
- Poor husbandry and diet
- Toxin exposure
- Trauma
- Ulcerative dermatitis
- Various bacterial and fungal infections

Culture Collection

Culture collection is accomplished by simply swabbing the area in question with a sterile culture swab. Both bacterial and fungal cultures can be performed. Blood cultures can be performed in amphibian species provided they have enough blood to take for the sample.

Endoscopy

Rigid endoscopy can be performed in many amphibians by passing the endoscope through the oral cavity and into the stomach. This is generally only done in larger amphibians that are under anesthesia. Endoscopy is primarily used to obtain gastric biopsies or to retrieve foreign bodies from the stomach.

Fecal Examination

Performing a fecal examination in amphibians is done in the same manner as in dogs and cats. The two most common fecal examinations include the fecal flotation and direct smear. For a fecal flotation, the feces are examined using standard commercial fecal flotation solutions. To perform a direct fecal smear, the feces are smeared onto a slide and 0.9% saline is applied to examine the feces under a microscope. Common ova include nematodes, trematodes, coccidian, protozoans, and lung worm larvae.

Skin Scrape and Touch Smears

Performing skin scrapes or touch (impression) smears is an easy way to obtain information on potential bacterial, fungal, or protozoal infections of the skin. A coverslip edge is gently scraped across the skin and then placed on a slide with saline making a wet mount. This sample should be analyzed immediately to obtain accurate results. Skin scrapes should not be performed on specific lesions as this can cause more damage to the skin. A touch or impression smear is primarily used on specific lesions such as ulcers or other damaged tissue. A

TABLE 27-6 Routes of Medication Administration in Amphibians

ROUTE	COMMENTS
Intracoelomic route	Injections can be given into the coelom in larger amphibians.
Intramuscular route	Medications can be given IM, but some medications can cause damage to the muscle or internal organs.
Oral route	If the GI tract works, use it. Oral medications can be given using a feeding tube or just titrated in with a syringe.
Subcutaneous route	Subcutaneous injections can be given if needed. This is usually performed in large toads and salamanders.
Topical route	Many medications can be given topically owing to systemic absorption.

microscope slide is touched to skin in an attempt to collect histological data. The smear is then stained for analysis.

Radiology

Good radiographs are an important tool used as part of the diagnostic workup. Two views are normally taken which include a dorsoventral (DV) and horizontal lateral (Fig. 27-83). A horizontal beam is essential to obtain good radiographs. In most cases the patient will just sit there while the radiographs are being taken.

Tracheal Wash

A tracheal wash is performed in the same manner as described in the reptile section in this chapter. The patient must be anesthetized for the procedure as it can be very stressful and the tissues are very delicate. Generally 0.25 to 0.5 ml of isotonic saline (0.6%) is infused and aspirated from the trachea. The volume will depend on the size of the patient. The sample should be smeared onto a slide and stained for analysis.

Urinalysis

Urine can be collected with a good amount of success in many amphibian species. Many frogs and toads will urinate when you pick them up. If the patient will not urinate, it can be stimulated by placing a red rubber feeding tube into the cloaca. Samples should be taken with aseptic technique. Every species is different so it is important to have normal values from the same species you are working with. The urinalysis is performed in a similar manner to dogs and cats.

ANESTHESIA

Anesthesia is not only necessary for surgical procedures, it may be necessary for physical examinations as well. The most common anesthetic used in amphibians is tricaine methanesulfonate (MS-222). MS-222 is a white crystalline powder that must be mixed with water to anesthetize both fish and amphibians. This solution is then buffered with sodium bicarbonate. Amphibians are placed into the water with the MS-222 until the proper anesthetic plane is achieved. Once anesthetized, the animal can be removed from the water to perform the examination or procedure. If surgery is being performed, a continuous stream of water with MS-222 can be run over the patient. For long procedures the animal can be intubated and maintained on isoflurane.

Monitoring vitals can be difficult, but a Doppler can be placed on the heart if possible and/or an electrocardiogram can be placed on the animal using platinum needle probes.

Force-Feeding

Patients that are not eating on their own will need to be syringe fed or tube fed. Syringe feeding is relatively easy. The patient will first need to be restrained. The syringe can be placed into the corner of mouth and the food can be slowly titrated into the patient. Tube feeding is similar to that in birds. The mouth is opened with a speculum such as tape stirrups or a plastic spatula. The tube is premeasured to estimate where the stomach is located before inserting it into the patient. Unlike metal tubes that are generally used in birds, a red rubber feeding tube is generally used with most amphibian species. It is important to use proper syringe feeding diets. It is also important to realize that this is very stressful for most patients.

Euthanasia

Euthanasia can be difficult because it can be hard to access a vessel. The patient can be given ketamine for sedation or placed into a bath of MS-222 to anesthetize before giving the injection of euthanasia solution. Euthanasia solution can be given into any vessel or into the coelomic cavity. The heart may take several minutes to several hours to completely stop even though the patient may be clinically dead. A Doppler can be used to check for a heartbeat. The patient should be kept in the clinic for several hours or overnight to ensure the patient has been properly euthanized before sending it home with the owner, if that is the owner's preference.

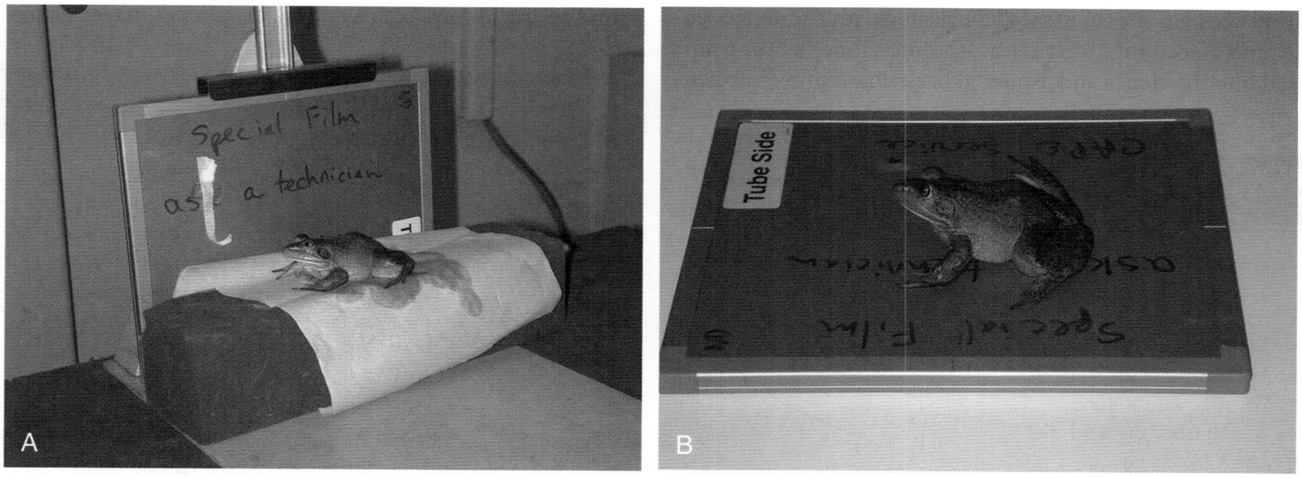

FIGURE 27-83 **A,** Horizontal lateral view is preferred over a traditional lateral because the patient does not generally have to be anesthetized. They will often just sit on the plate. **B,** A dorsoventral view (DV) is also part of a complete radiographic series taken of amphibians. In some cases the animal will need to be anesthetized. It is important to keep the animal moist during this time.

REVIEW QUESTIONS

Matching—Anatomy Terms

Match the anatomy term with its definition.

_____ **1.** anisodactyl
_____ **2.** coprodeum
_____ **3.** coracoid
_____ **4.** coverts
_____ **5.** proctodeum
_____ **6.** pygostyle
_____ **7.** remiges
_____ **8.** supracoracoideus
_____ **9.** urodeum
_____ **10.** uropygial
_____ **11.** zygodactyl

A. caudal part of the cloaca
B. cranial portion of the cloaca that receives feces from the rectum
C. a plate-like bone at the distal vertebrae, consisting of fused caudal vertebrae
D. middle part of the cloaca; most of the bird
E. another term for large primary flight feathers
F. a paired bone part of the shoulder
G. arrangement of feet with second and third toes facing forward and the first and fourth toes directed backward
H. located at the end of the pygostyle
I. arrangement of feet so that three toes point forward and one toe points to the rear
J. body feathers that provide surface coverage over most of the bird
K. the muscle ventral to the pectorals

Matching—Diseases and Disorders

Match the disease or disorder with its definition.

_____ **1.** avian polyomavirus (APV)
_____ **2.** chlamydiosis
_____ **3.** lead and zinc
_____ **4.** poxviruses
_____ **5.** proventricular dilatation disease (PDD)
_____ **6.** psittacine beak and feather disease (PBFD)
_____ **7.** *Salmonella* spp.
_____ **8.** West Nile virus

A. seen as early as 10 weeks of age in African Grey parrots, cockatoos, and conures
B. psittacines appear to be somewhat resistant to this mosquito borne virus
C. most often associated with imported Amazon parrots and macaws
D. easily spread by feather dust, dander, and feces to other birds
E. intermittently shed by reptiles if they are carriers of this bacteria
F. two heavy metals most commonly encountered with avian patients
G. zoonotic disease that causes psittacosis in humans
H. most common viral cause of death in budgerigar's breeding facilities

True or False

Indicate whether each of the following statements is True or False.

_____ **1.** The average adult bird has a core body temperature of 38-42.5° C (105-112° F).
_____ **2.** If a blood feather needs to be removed it should be pulled in the opposite direction that the feather is growing.
_____ **3.** When flushing a wound, care needs to be taken that the puncture is not communicating with an air sac.
_____ **4.** The uropygial gland is absent in the ostrich, emu, cassowaries, bustards, frogmouth, many pigeons, woodpeckers, and Amazon parrots.
_____ **5.** Since birds have complete cartilaginous tracheal rings that cannot expand, inflated cuffed tubes are best used. Manual ventilation, high oxygen flow rates, and high-pressure ventilation are safe to use.
_____ **6.** The proventriculus or true stomach is very similar to the stomach of mammals, containing digestive acid and enzymes.
_____ **7.** The largest muscles in the avian body are the pectorals.
_____ **8.** Grit is required in the gizzard to properly digest hard foods.
_____ **9.** When a bird is stressed there is an increased fecal component to the droppings because the droppings pass before lower intestinal water resorption occurs.

_____**10.** In most birds, ovulation to egg laying takes approximately 15 hours.

_____**11.** Amazon parrots are the only species that will develop hematuria in acute cases of heavy metal toxicosis.

_____**12.** When examining a turtle, one or two fingers may be placed in the inguinal area between the hind limbs and the shell so that you are able to palpate the coelomic cavity.

_____**13.** In order to examine the cloacal mucosa properly it must be everted and all four quadrants of the cloaca must be examined.

_____**14.** When surgically preparing a bird, all feathers, including flight feathers, should be removed by pulling in the direction of their growth.

_____**15.** Alcohol is the agent of choice when flushing the dilute chlorhexidine from a surgical site.

_____**16.** Most diseases in exotic animals are caused from poor husbandry and improper diet.

_____**17.** When differentiating between genders, male iguanas and bearded dragons have very large femoral pores compared to females.

_____**18.** Many species of male tortoises have a concave plastron making it easier to mount the female.

_____**19.** When determining the gender of a snake, the probe will advance further into the cloaca for a female snake.

_____**20.** EDTA is the anticoagulant used for chemistry evaluation while lithium heparin is the anticoagulant generally used for CBC evaluation in birds and reptiles.

_____**21.** For accurate core body temperature during avian anesthesia an esophageal temperature probe should be placed as far as the proventriculus.

RECOMMENDED READING

Ballard B, Cheek R: *Exotic animal medicine for the veterinary technician*, ed 2, Ames, IA, 2010, Wiley-Blackwell.

Carpenter JW: *Exotic animal formulary*, ed 4, St Louis, 2012, Saunders.

Companion Parrot Quarterly: P.O. Box 2428, Alameda, CA, 94501, www.members.companionparrot.com.

Fowler M: *Zoo and wild animal medicine*, ed 6, St Louis, 2008, Saunders.

Harcourt-Brown C: *BSAVA manual of psittacine birds*, Gloucester, UK, 2005, British Small Animal Veterinary Association.

Harrison G, Lightfoot T: In *Clinical avian medicine*, vol I & II. Palm Beach, FL, 2006, Spitz Publishing.

Johnson-Delaney CA, et al.: *Exotic companion medicine handbook for veterinarians*, Lake Worth, FL, 1996, Wingers Publishing.

Mader D: *Reptile medicine and surgery*, ed 2, St Louis, 2006, Saunders.

Mitchell M, Tully T: *Manual of exotic pet practice*, St Louis, 2009, Saunders.

O'Malley B: *Clinical anatomy and physiology of exotic species*, Oxford, UK, 2005, Elsevier Saunders.

Ritchie BW, Harrision GJ, Harrison LR: *Avian medicine: principles and application*, Lake Worth, FL, 1994, Wingers Publishing.

Silverman S, Tell LA: *Radiology of birds: an atlas of normal anatomy and positioning*, St Louis, 2010, Saunders.

Wright KM, Whitaker BR: *Amphibian medicine and captive husbandry*, Malabar, FL, 2001, Krieger Publishing.

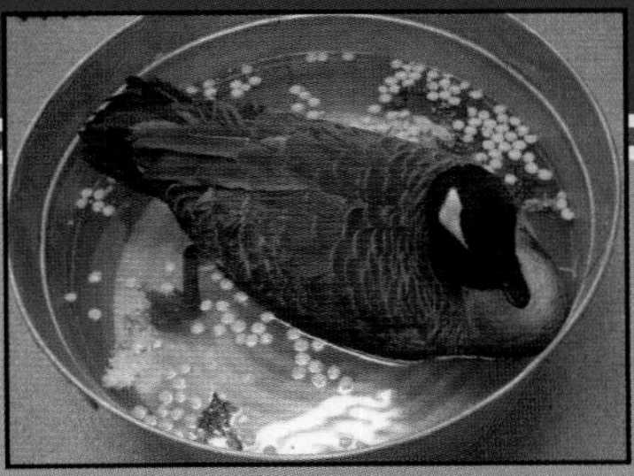

28 Nursing Care of Orphaned and Injured Wild Animals

OUTLINE

LEARNING OBJECTIVES

After reviewing this chapter, the reader will be able to:

1. Discuss ways to provide nursing care of wildlife.
2. Discuss regulations and laws concerning wildlife care.
3. Discuss appropriate ways to take a thorough history.
4. Describe ways to perform a physical examination.
5. Assess the condition of orphaned or injured wild animals
6. Discuss ways to provide supportive care to wild animals.
7. Describe methods of sample collection and diagnostic testing for laboratory analysis.
8. Describe how to obtain diagnostic imaging of wildlife.
9. Identify routes of administration of medication.
10. Discuss the ethical treatment and releasability of wild animals.
11. Identify potential zoonotic and infectious diseases in common wild animal species.
12. Describe the proper use of personal protective equipment.

KEY TERMS

Air sac	Crop	Nares	Snake hook
Autotomize	Ecchymosis	Petechiae	Uropygial gland
Carapace	Hemostasis	Plastron	Venipuncture
Chelonian	Lavage	Releasability	
Cloaca	Lysis	Rhinotheca	
Coelom	Mentation	Scutes	

PREPARING YOUR CLINIC FOR WILDLIFE TRIAGE AND CARE

It is not uncommon for a Good Samaritan to find an injured or orphaned native or nonnative wild animal on the ground. Generally these are well-meaning individuals who want to help the animal get healthy so it can be released back into the wild. If the veterinary hospital decides to take in injured or orphaned wild animals, not only must it be prepared to provide proper housing and diet, but also it must provide the animals with experienced staff to safely handle and care for each individual species.

If the veterinary hospital wishes to receive injured or orphaned wildlife from the public or animal control, a specific list of protocols and standard operating procedures (SOPs) needs to be written and followed. All clinic members, including the front office staff, should be aware of the protocols and SOPs. It is very important that all members of the veterinary hospital understand that dealing with injured wildlife can be emotionally taxing. Staff members must be very practical and not become attached to the animals brought into the hospital. Wildlife medicine can be very sad. Many animals will have to be euthanized because of injuries that will keep them from returning to the wild. This can be very hard for some people to handle. Some wildlife can certainly be placed in permanent wildlife sanctuaries, zoos, or educational centers, but this is rare, as many places are already overloaded with common species of wild animals.

The staff should also be aware of common zoonotic diseases carried by wildlife species. You must be able to recognize zoonotic diseases and protect yourself against them. Latex or vinyl exam gloves should be worn while working with wild animals. Proper hygiene as well as keeping the housing facility clean is very important. Wildlife should not be housed with client-owned pets, not only because of zoonotic disease potential, but also because of the stress placed on the patients being housed together.

If the veterinary hospital chooses not to accept wild animals into the clinic, individuals should be directed to appropriate resources, such as licensed wildlife rehabilitators, wildlife centers, or other veterinary hospitals that do accept these animals.

One of the most important services a veterinary hospital can provide is accurate and timely advice over the phone. Several members of the veterinary staff should be trained to deal with concerns and questions about injured, sick, and/or orphaned wildlife from the public. If an adult wild animal can be easily captured and/or picked up by an untrained person, it is very likely that it is sick or injured in some way. This animal needs to be examined by a veterinary professional. Box 28-1 lists conditions that require immediate medical attention.

It is not uncommon for a member of the public to bring in a healthy, young baby animal that is not necessarily orphaned or injured. Many times people think they are doing the right thing, but in fact they are taking the baby away from the parents when it is not necessary. If the baby is cold,

BOX 28-1 Conditions Requiring Immediate Medical Attention

Unconsciousness
Bleeding
Cold body temperature
Fractures
Weakness or inability to stand
Swelling on head or body
Seizures
Eyes closed or matted shut
Shock
Puncture wounds
Maggots present (Fig. 1)

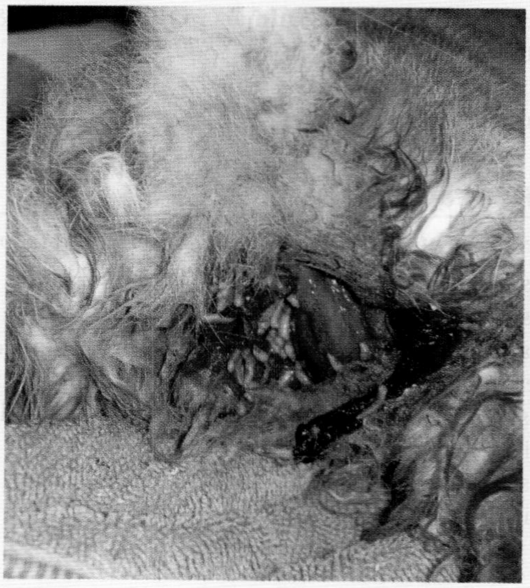

FIGURE 1 This rabbit has been infested by maggots.

skinny, weak, or if there are dead siblings nearby, the baby is most likely orphaned and needs medical attention. It is important to note that mothers will not abandon their babies simply because humans have touched them. This is a false belief. If the baby seems to be warm and strong, it should be returned to the place where it was found (Fig. 28-1).

If the veterinary hospital is only going to give medical advice over the phone, the staff must provide advice that is medically sound and legal. Some individuals will ask for advice about how to care for the wildlife themselves. It is the responsibility of the veterinary technician or other veterinary staff member to advise these individuals that it is illegal and dangerous for them to take care of the wild animal. They should be advised about zoonotic disease potential and that untrained people taking care of wild animals can actually cause harm to them. Giving the wrong food can suppress growth, causing metabolic diseases, whereas imprinting the wild animal will cause it to become nonreleasable.

CAPTURING AND TRANSPORTING WILDLIFE

Capturing a wild animal sometimes can be dangerous. In some cases it may be as easy as simply picking up the animal and placing it in a carrier, but in other instances it may be difficult, and you may need leather gloves, nets, snares, traps, or towels/blankets.

A variety of transport cages are available to safely transport a wild animal to a veterinary hospital or wildlife center. Anything from a cardboard box to a dog or cat carrier can be used, depending on the size and type of the animal being transported. For example a songbird can be placed in a small box, whereas a raccoon should be placed in a dog carrier of an appropriate size. When possible, the cage or box should be lined with a towel, indoor/outdoor carpet, or newspaper to help prevent the animal from slipping around in the carrier. A towel or blanket can be placed over the carrier to make the environment dark.

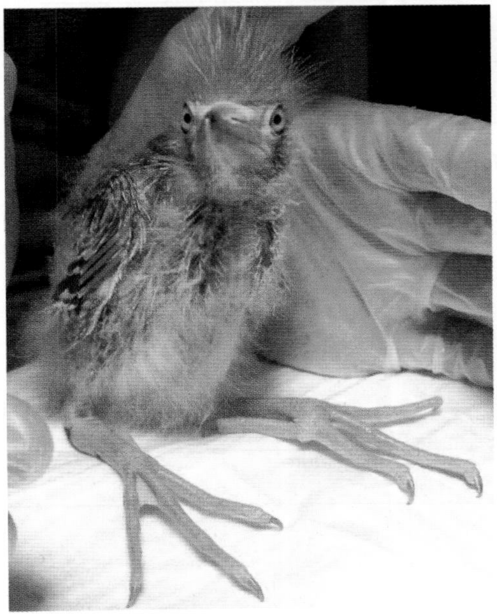

FIGURE 28-1 This baby wading bird has been unnecessarily removed from its nest.

LEGAL CONCERNS

Native wild animals are protected under a variety of local, state, and federal regulations and laws. It is important for the veterinary hospital to become aware of these regulations and make sure they are followed. Every state has a specific agency responsible for regulating possession of native wildlife. Under many circumstances, a permit is required to work with or possess native wildlife, especially those that are endangered, threatened, or are protected under the migratory bird act. The easiest way to provide veterinary care for native wildlife is to develop a relationship and closely work with a permitted and licensed rehabilitator or wildlife facility. If the veterinary hospital is not working under these circumstances, the veterinarian must obtain the proper permits. This can be accomplished by contacting the state wildlife agency. Wildlife laws vary by state; therefore the veterinarian should contact the local game warden for specific information.

> *TECHNICIAN NOTE* Be sure you are well versed in the state and local laws related to wildlife that might be seen in your clinic.

INTAKE PROCEDURES AND HISTORY

The person brining the animal to the clinic should fill out a form giving information about the wild animal they found (Fig. 28-2). This paperwork should include the address or area where it was found, how it was captured, how long the individual has had the animal, whether the animal was fed, whether dead wildlife was found in the area, etc. A release form should be signed stating that he or she does not own the animal and will not be receiving the animal back. The wild animal should also have a medical record generated just as if it were a client-owned animal. All physical exam findings, medical procedures, and treatments should be entered into the medical record.

Once the animal has been brought into the hospital or wildlife center, it should not be handled or looked at between treatments or feedings. The animal should never be petted, talked to, or played with at any time.

CAPTURE AND RESTRAINT OF WILDLIFE

Most of the wild animals presented for evaluation are victims of trauma and may have multiple injuries. A complete physical examination is essential. When examining, providing supportive care, or obtaining diagnostics, restraint is required for the safety of the patient and the personnel working with the animal. Wild birds have defensive weapons such as beaks and talons and use them when stressed. Many reptiles and mammals can inflict severe bites and scratches.

VETERINARY MEDICAL TEACHING HOSPITAL
UNIVERSITY OF CALIFORNIA-DAVIS
WILDLIFE FORM

First name: __________ Home phone: __________
Admission date to VMTH: _____ Time: _____ Date found by Good Samaritan: _____ Time: _____
WNV form received __________ (Initials)

A Where found:

1 Address, street and city: __________

2 Number of miles from nearest city: __________

3 Description of area or facility found in: (Ex: side of road? In an orchard? Spraying orchard? Barn? A working farm?) __________

4 Was any other wildlife noted in the area at the time? Any interaction with this animal? __________

B Additional information for stray birds:

1 Species: __________

2 Type of terrain where bird was found: (PLEASE CIRCLE ONE)
Park   Lake   Urban area   Wooded area   Agricultural area   River   Residential area

3 If known-proximity (miles) to sentinel chicken flock: __________
Nearest city or residential area where bird was found: __________
Zip code of bird location: __________ County: __________

4 Were any dead birds seen in area where bird was found? YES NO
If yes, what species? __________

C Circumstances of acquisition?

1 What was the animal doing? How was it acting? Attitude? __________

2 How was it caught? __________

D Was the animal fed?

1 What and how much was offered? __________

2 What and how much did it eat? __________

3 Offered water? __________

4 How much did it drink? __________

E Any other information or history you can give to help us care for this animal? __________

ACKNOWLEDGMENT
I certify that I do NOT own this animal and understand that the university has sole authority and responsibility for the care and disposition of this animal. I further understand that this animal will NOT be returned to me.

____
Signature

FIGURE 28-2 Sample intake form.

Terry cloth towels, leather welder's gloves, nets, and protective eye wear are valuable tools to neutralize these weapons.

> TECHNICIAN NOTE Proper restraint is essential when handling wildlife to protect you and keep from injuring the animal.

Capturing a wild animal from a cage needs to be done in a room that can be sealed and has no escape route or hiding places. The door should be locked and the window blinds should be closed. Darkening the room may help reduce the stress of capturing many wild animals. Before capturing any animal, assess the patient. Some critically ill patients may need time to recover from transport and may need supplemental oxygen before restraint. When working with these critically ill patients, it is best to perform your physical exam in stages, giving the patient time to recover between those stages. Depending on the species, general anesthesia may be needed to perform a complete physical examination (Fig. 28-3).

RAPTOR CAPTURE AND RESTRAINT

Welder's gloves and a terry cloth towel are often useful when capturing birds of prey. You should first approach the bird cautiously and place the towel over the patient's head and body. Grasp the bird's body on both sides over the wings and work your hands down to the legs until you have a firm hold on both legs and control of the feet. With the towel remaining over the head, and the feet directed away from you, bring the bird to your torso and maintain control of the feet and wings. A stockinette or leather raptor hood can be used to cover the head to reduce stress and restrict vision. The legs can be bound together with homemade Velcro wraps to help retain control of the legs and talons. The use of gloves reduces the handler's tactile sensation and ability to feel the patient's most subtle movements and reactions to the restraint; therefore once the patient is captured and properly restrained, the leather gloves may be removed (Fig. 28-4).

SMALL WILD BIRD CAPTURE AND RESTRAINT

Small wild birds, such as finches, house sparrows, and scrub jays, frequently present with traumatic injuries after presumably flying into a window or being attacked by a cat. They must be safely and gently restrained for a hands-on physical examination. A small terry cloth or paper towel can be used combined with slow and deliberate movements to minimize stress to the bird. It may be helpful to dim the room lights before proceeding, as this calms some birds. To capture, place the towel over the patient, gain control of the head, pin the wings to the body, and pick the patient up.

MAMMAL CAPTURE AND RESTRAINT

Capture and restraint techniques used with wild mammals depend on the species with which you are working. In many cases, the animal will need to be anesthetized to perform a complete physical examination. If this is the case, the animal is either anesthetized in the carrier or cage it is in, or given an intramuscular injection using a syringe pole to sedate or tranquilize it. Anesthesia is discussed in further detail later in this chapter. Once the animal is tranquilized it can be removed from the cage and fully anesthetized. Common wild mammals that must be anesthetized before performing a physical examination include raccoons, canids, most rodents, bats, and any large or potentially aggressive mammal.

A large towel should be used to help capture wild hares and rabbits. A towel is generally placed on top of the rabbit. Once you have done this, you can scoop the rabbit into your arms while it is still wrapped in the towel. It is

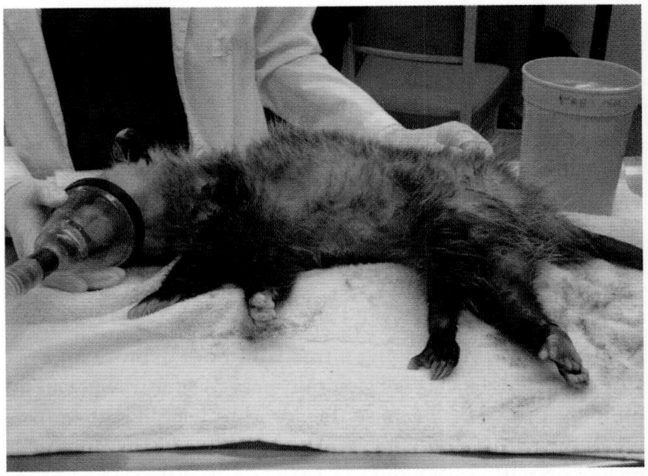

FIGURE 28-3 Wild mammals are generally anesthetized in a chamber or box before physical examination unless they are extremely debilitated. Very sick mammals can be mask-induced, as pictured.

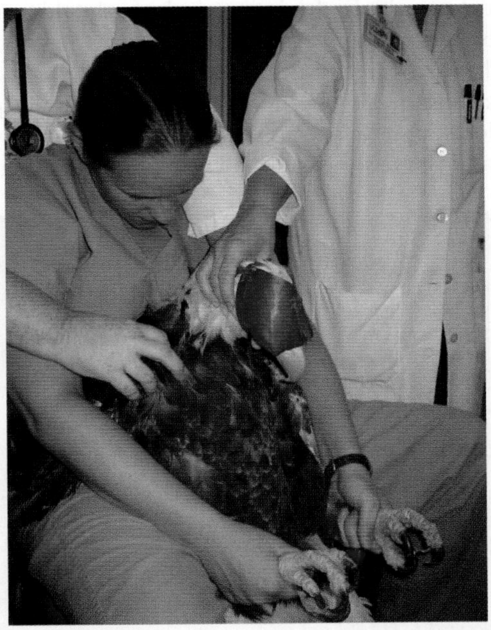

FIGURE 28-4 A leather hood should be placed over the head of the bird to reduce vision and overall stress. The restrainer should sit in a nonrolling chair during the physical examination. This helps prevent injuries to the animal and the veterinary staff because you have more control over the restraint of the animal.

important to note that with improper restraint, rabbits can kick out their hind legs and fracture their backs. In some cases the physical examination can be done with the rabbit covered with the towel. This helps reduce stress to the rabbit. The towel is simply removed from each section of the body as the examination is being performed. The rabbit may need to be anesthetized to perform a proper examination. If the rabbit is very sick, young, or calm, all of this may not be needed and the rabbit can be simply restrained by tucking the head between the side of your body and your arm. The other arm should support the rest of the rabbit's body against your own body. Essentially it looks like you are tucking a football against your body (Fig. 28-5). Wild hares and rabbits are very stressed animals. Dimmed lights and low voices should be used when possible, as this can help reduce stress.

REPTILE CAPTURE AND RESTRAINT

Restraint techniques vary based on the type of reptile with which you are working. Exam gloves should be worn when handling these patients, as reptiles can shed *Salmonella* spp. intermittently if they are positive for the bacteria.

Lizards

Lizards can be challenging animals to both capture and restrain. Smaller lizards are generally easy to capture but can be difficult to restrain because they tend to wiggle and squirm while they are being held. Most small lizards can simply be picked up with both hands and taken out of the cage. This is also true of the larger lizard species. However, some of the larger lizards can be difficult to capture and restrain, especially if they are aggressive. If the lizard is hostile, a towel or blanket along with leather restraint gloves should be used. It is important to remember that lizards can scratch and bite when they are scared or nervous. Therefore, it is a good idea to wear long sleeves when possible and always keep track of the location of the head. Keeping one hand on the neck, just behind the base of skull, will help prevent getting bitten.

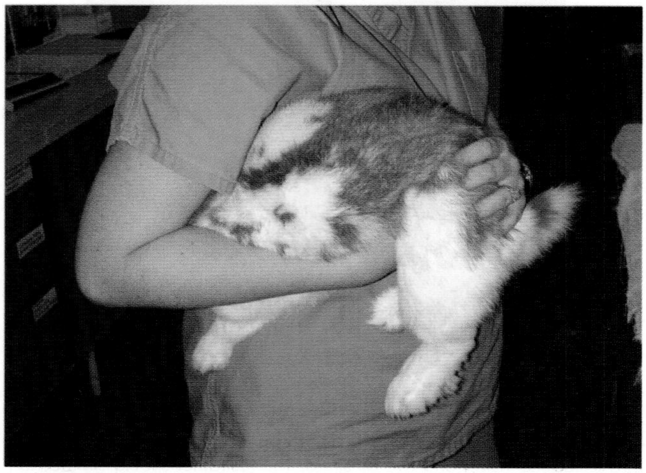

FIGURE 28-5 Although the rabbit pictured in this image is a domestic pet rabbit, restraint is performed in the same manner on calm, young, or sick wild hares and rabbits.

Many species of lizards have a natural predatory response to voluntarily "drop" or **autotomize** their tail in an attempt to escape predation. Therefore, it is a good guideline to never capture any species of lizard by the tail.

Generally lizards can be restrained by placing one hand around the neck and pectoral girdle region while the other hand is used to support the body near the pelvis. Although it is sometimes impossible, try to avoid smashing down and damaging the dorsal spines of lizards when they are being restrained. It is also important to remember that not all lizards have durable and tough skin. Some lizards, such as geckos, have extremely delicate skin that can be damaged easily by capture and restraint. Make sure only soft towels are used on geckos.

Snakes

Most snakes can be captured easily directly out of the carrier or cage. When dealing with nonaggressive snakes, the restrainer can simply pick the animal up and pull it out of the cage. If the snake is aggressive, it may be necessary to use a towel or **snake hook,** along with leather gloves to safely capture it. In these cases, it is easiest to gently toss the towel over the snake and find the head. Once the head has been isolated and restrained, the snake can be safely taken out of the enclosure. If the snake is extremely aggressive or venomous, a snake hook should be used to pin down its head long enough to safely grasp its head and body. Improper use of the snake hook can cause trauma to the patient; therefore extreme caution should be taken.

Snakes are commonly transported to the hospital in pillowcases. It is important that the veterinarian or technician does not just open the pillowcase and quickly pull the snake out. To safely remove the snake from the pillowcase, first find the snake's head and gently grasp it from the outside of the pillowcase. Once the snake is restrained, the restrainer should put his or her free hand into the pillowcase and transfer the head to the "free hand." After this is accomplished, it should now be safe to take the entire snake out of the pillowcase (Fig. 28-6).

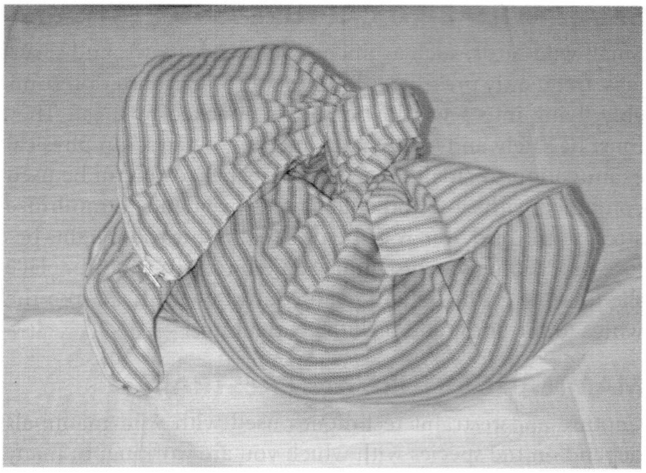

FIGURE 28-6 Snakes are commonly transported to the hospital in pillowcases.

It is important to gently hold the snake directly behind the head with one hand (so it cannot turn around and bite!) and support the body with the other hand. If the snake is large, more than one person may be needed to restrain it. A good guideline is one person per 3 ft of snake.

Chelonians

Chelonians are turtles and tortoises. Although chelonians are usually the easiest to capture, they are the hardest to restrain. Unless working with extremely large tortoises, most chelonians can just be picked up with both hands and placed on the exam table. When examining large tortoises (i.e., several kilograms), it is easiest to set up an exam area within the animal's enclosure or on the floor in the hospital's exam area. Because there is such a great deal of variation in size and strength, restraint techniques may vary between small and large chelonians. Once the animal's body is under control, it is imperative that the head is properly restrained. Although this is relatively easy when the animal is sick, it can be difficult in strong healthy chelonians, especially large tortoises and box turtles.

There are several ways the restrainer can gain control of the animal's head. Many turtles and tortoises are very curious. If set down on the table or the ground, it may just start walking around to check things out. If this is the case, the technician can walk up to it and grasp its head with one hand while restraining the body with the other hand. To keep control of the head, it is best to position your thumb on one side of the cranial portion of the neck and position the rest of your fingers (or just the index finger for smaller species) on the other side of the neck just behind the base of the skull. Healthy chelonians are strong, so it may take a lot of constant but gentle force to keep the turtle or tortoise's head out of the shell. If the animal is extremely active, an additional person may be necessary to help restrain the limbs and body.

Another way to gain control of the head is by trying to coax the animal out of its shell. Many chelonians will extend their head out of the shell if food is offered to them or they are placed in a container of shallow warm water. Once the head is extended, the same techniques just mentioned can be used to gain and keep control of the animal's head. If these techniques fail, it may be possible to slip a small blunt ear curette or spay hook under the horny portion of the upper beak, known as the **rhinotheca.** Once the probe has been placed, it can be gently pulled back to extend the neck to a position for the restrainer to grasp. It is important to note that this technique can be dangerous. The beak can be chipped or broken if the animal struggles or is in poor health. If a spay hook is the tool of choice, it may be a good idea to pad the hooked portion of the instrument. Padding can simply consist of tape or an elastic wrap cut to the appropriate size. Caution should be taken when dealing with any aquatic turtle, especially snapping turtles. These species of turtles have a tendency to bite, and many of the larger turtles can cause serious bodily harm to the people working with them.

Box turtles can be the most challenging chelonians to properly restrain. Because box turtles have a hinge on their **plastron,** many species are able to completely tuck themselves into their shells. The easiest way to extend their head is to gently prop open the cranial portion of the **carapace** (upper shell) and the plastron (lower shell). Extreme care must be taken when trying to prop the shell open. It is suggested that a well-padded object be used when attempting this. This will help avoid traumatizing or fracturing the shell. Another way to extend a box turtle's head is to grasp one of the forelimbs, keeping the leg extended out of the shell until the head can be successfully pulled out and properly restrained. This method works well because once the leg is extended, the turtle will usually not close its shell down on its own leg. Any of these capture and restraint techniques can potentially cause a fair amount of stress to the turtle or tortoise. If initial attempts at capture and restraint are not successful, chemical restraint may be necessary for any reptile, especially large tortoises and box turtles.

PHYSICAL EXAMINATION OF WILDLIFE

As with other exotic species, an initial visual physical examination should be performed before the hands-on physical examination. You should observe the animal in its cage or box. Note its **mentation** and whether any normal feces/urine is present in the cage. Note the presence of any vomit or regurgitation in the cage. Examine for the presence of a wing droop or obvious injury. Once the visual examination has been completed, you can move on to the hands-on physical examination.

Before starting the hands-on physical examination you must have everything out and within reach. This will help the physical examination move along smoothly and quickly. Performing a physical examination on a wild animal is very similar to performing a physical examination on other exotic animals. When performing the physical examination you should be systematic, proceed in a timely manner, and try to complete the physical portion of the examination quickly. Again, because of the high stress of many wildlife species, general anesthesia is often required to perform a complete physical examination.

AVIANS

The physical examination is not all hands on. Much information can be obtained simply by observing the bird's behavior and physical appearance before capture and restraint. Some wild birds are prey species with survival instincts and frequently alter their behavior when they are in a stressful environment, such as a hospital. In some cases these birds will mask their symptoms so as to not stand out in their "flock" so they will not be eliminated by a predator or members of their own flock. Covertly evaluate the bird if possible. If the bird does not know it is being watched, it may not hide signs of illness. The respiratory rate should be smooth and regular. A healthy bird should show no signs of increased effort. If the bird is exhibiting a tail bob (forward movement of the head or open beak breathing), this could signal respiratory distress, which requires immediate attention. Evaluate the mentation and stance. If the bird is trying to sleep, not interested in your presence, or laterally recumbent, then immediate medical attention is necessary.

After obtaining a body weight, a typical physical examination routine is as follows. Examine the eyes, external auditory canals (or ears), nares, beak, and oral cavity. Palpate the crop and esophagus, neck, pectoral region, coelom and pelvic region, wings, legs, feet, and back. Evaluate the feather quality and check the uropygial gland. Auscultate the heart, air sacs, lungs, and sinuses. Examine the cloaca and evert the mucosa to examine for lesions. Some wild birds may have multiple lesions because of traumatic injuries; therefore do not stop the examination after finding one lesion.

MAMMALS

The wild mammal physical examination is performed similarly to that for other small animals such as dogs and cats. Wild mammals can become easily stressed, so it is essential to minimize the length of time during which restraint is necessary. Before you start the hands-on portion of your examination, perform a visual examination. It is important to note the mentation of the patient. Obtaining the patient's weight and temperature should be the first part of the physical examination. Because many wild mammal patients are very small, it is best to use a scale that weighs to the nearest gram (Fig. 28-7). Obtaining a temperature can be challenging in smaller species. Using a digital thermometer is generally the quickest and best method, but only if it is small enough not to cause any damage.

> TECHNICIAN NOTE Use a systematic approach when performing the physical examination.

A general guideline for performing a physical examination is to start at the head and work your way down to the tail. This helps to ensure that nothing is overlooked. It is a good idea to obtain both a heart and respiratory rate as soon as the animal is removed from the cage. If the respiratory rate seems exaggerated, recount the rate upon completion of the examination and after the animal has been placed back into the cage.

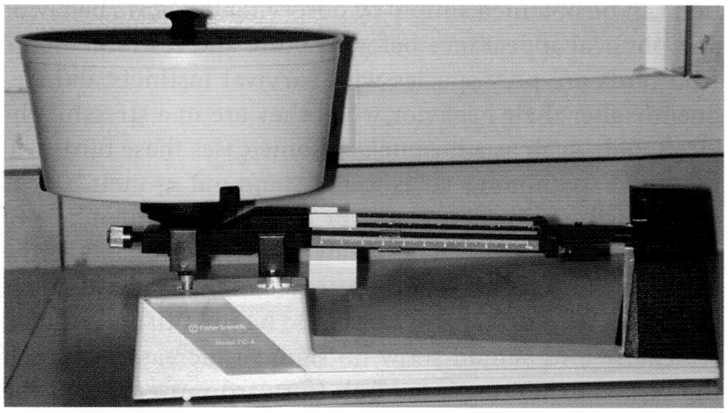

FIGURE 28-7 A gram scale should be used to weigh small wildlife patients.

Continue the examination by looking at the eyes, ears, and nares. They should be clean, clear, and free of any discharge. Any signs of discharge or debris from the eyes, ears, and/or nares can be a sign of an underlying disease process and should be investigated further.

The oral exam in nonrodent and rabbit species is performed in the same manner as with a dog or cat. Because rabbits and rodents have unique dentition and their mouths do not open widely, a special instrument must be used to properly perform an examination. A mouth speculum with a light source is one of the most helpful instruments that can be used when performing an oral examination (for rodents and rabbits only and done only under heavy sedation or general anesthesia). A few different mouth specula can be used (Fig. 28-8). A long otoscope cone attached to the otoscope handle can be used to examine the mouth. A small vaginal speculum and a pen light can also be used. One of the most effective ways to perform an oral examination on a small mammal is with a bivalve nasal speculum. This instrument has a light source and attaches to a battery hand piece. Examine the gums, tongue, and all of the teeth, including the incisors.

It is important to palpate the limbs and the abdomen during your physical examination. Palpation should include checking for any masses, old wounds or lesions, or any other potential abnormalities on the body. After palpating the abdominal cavity, examine the feet and genitalia. Examine the skin and look for any signs of dermatophytes or ectoparasites.

The heart and lungs should be auscultated. Note the presence of any potential heart murmurs, arrhythmias, harsh lung sounds, or anything that may sound abnormal. This is performed in the same manner as would be performed on a dog or cat. A body condition score should also be assigned to the patient. The same system used with dogs and cats is also used with wild mammals, with 1 out of 9 being emaciated and 9 out of 9 being grossly obese.

The hydration status of the patient should be evaluated during the physical examination. This is done similarly to

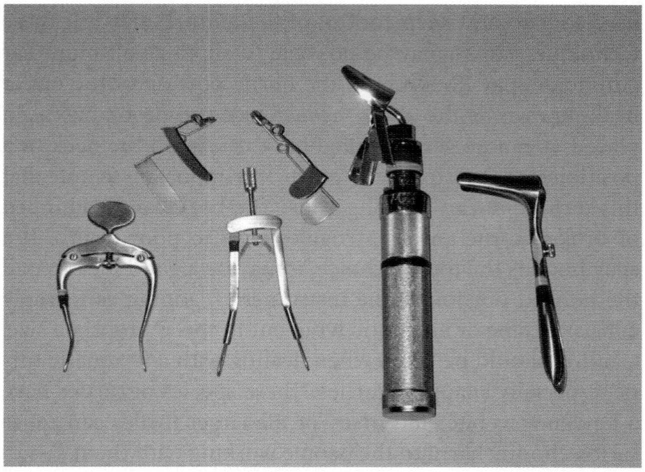

FIGURE 28-8 A variety of mouth specula should be available for rodent and rabbit oral examinations.

a dog or cat. The mucous membranes should be moist and pink. As with most other mammals, the capillary refill time should be between 1 and 2 seconds. A common sign of dehydration is dry or tacky mucous membranes. Another sign of dehydration is sunken eyes and lack of skin turgor. The skin should be tented or pulled upward to assess dehydration.

Remember that many wild mammals must be heavily sedated or placed under general anesthesia to perform a complete physical examination.

REPTILES

Performing a physical examination on reptiles is similar to performing a physical examination on most mammalian species. As with other species, it is a good guideline to perform a visual precapture and restraint physical examination. This can give you are good idea of the animal's attitude and mentation before it has been potentially stressed by handling.

One of the easiest ways to perform a thorough physical examination is to start at the head and work your way down to the tail. This method helps to ensure that nothing is overlooked. During your physical examination, the eyes, ears, and oral cavity should be thoroughly examined. The eyes should be bright, clean, and clear of any discharge. The ears or tympanic membranes should be observed with a pen light during the physical examination. The ears or tympanum should be clean, clear, and free of any debris.

A thorough examination of the oral cavity is an important part of performing a complete physical examination. The oral cavity can be safely opened with either porous tape stirrups or a soft plastic instrument such as a spatula. Metal speculums can be used, but caution should be taken to avoid causing trauma to the mouth. The oral cavity should be moist, pink, and free of any lesions. During the oral examination, the mouth should be observed for any signs of erythema, stomatitis, and any evidence of plaques on the mucous membranes. As you move down the body, the thoracic and coelomic cavities should be palpated. Palpation of the extremities and tail should then follow. The same techniques used to palpate dogs and cats can be used to palpate most reptiles. It is important to note any abnormalities, such as soft tissue swellings, space-occupying masses such as urinary calculi, developing eggs, neoplasia, and any current or old injuries such as fractures.

Turtles and tortoises usually present the biggest challenge when trying to perform a complete physical examination. The shell makes it difficult to palpate most of the organs. Depending on the size of the animal, one or two fingers may be placed in the inguinal area between the hind limbs and shell. This will enable you to palpate the coelomic cavity for any abnormalities, such as cystic calculi, foreign bodies, neoplasia, or eggs. It is also important to make note of the shell quality and color. If the animal has a systemic infection or is septic, **petechiae** and **ecchymosis** can often be found on the shell, especially the plastron.

In lizards, it is difficult to palpate many of the organs. In some of the larger lizards, the kidneys can be palpated via a rectal examination. If you can palpate the kidneys without a rectal examination, there is usually a problem. The kidneys sit in the pelvic girdle and are almost impossible to palpate unless they are enlarged or mineralized. If the animal has a systemic infection or is septic, petechiae and ecchymosis can often be observed on the dorsal spines along the animal's back.

It is difficult to palpate many of the snake's organs. In most snakes you can commonly palpate the heart, gall bladder, and a prey item or feces if present. If the animal has a systemic infection or is septic, petechiae and ecchymosis often can be observed on the ventral aspect of the snake along the scutes.

During the physical exam, make sure to get an accurate heart and respiratory rate. A heart rate is most easily obtained by using a Doppler (Fig. 28-9). Most reptile patients cannot be auscultated with a stethoscope; therefore a Doppler is an essential tool to have in your practice. In lizards, the Doppler probe generally should be placed in the same area a stethoscope would be placed on a dog or cat. In chelonians, the Doppler probe is placed either into the thoracic inlet (on the left or right side) or on the neck over the carotid artery. In snakes, the Doppler is placed directly over the heart. In most species of snake, the heart is located in the cranial third of the body. Both the heart and respiratory rates are obtained by simply counting the number of beats and breaths per minute.

SAMPLE COLLECTION AND DIAGNOSTIC TESTING

Diagnostic procedures that may be needed when working with wildlife include:

- Cloacal wash
- Fecal flotation and direct smear
- Skin scrape and touch smear
- Gram stain
- Nasal flush
- Tracheal lavage
- Blood collection
- Stomach lavage
- Dermatologic tape preparation

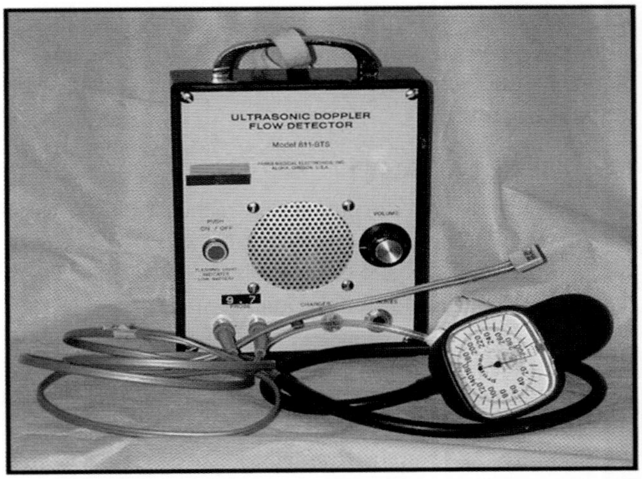

FIGURE 28-9 A Doppler is an essential instrument used to obtain a heart rate in reptilian species.

CLOACAL WASH

Cloacal washes are used to collect feces for laboratory analysis. This is very common, as fresh stool is often not available. A red rubber feeding tube is attached to an appropriate-sized syringe. The tube is well lubricated with a water-based jelly and placed into the cloaca. Saline is infused into the cloaca and aspirated back out. This **lavage** often yields enough fecal material for microscopic analysis. This is primarily performed in reptile species.

FECAL EXAMINATION

A fecal examination is performed in the same manner as in dogs and cats. The two most common fecal examinations include the fecal flotation and direct smear. For a fecal flotation, the feces are examined using standard commercial fecal flotation solutions. To perform a direct fecal smear, the feces are smeared onto a slide and 0.9% saline is applied to examine the feces under a microscope. See Chapter 10 for more details.

SKIN SCRAPE AND TOUCH SMEARS

Performing skin scrapes or touch (impression) smears is an easy way to obtain information on potential bacterial and fungal infections of the skin. Skin scrapes and touch smears are performed in the same manner as with traditional domestic species. Skin scrapes should not be performed on specific lesions, as this can cause more damage to the skin. A touch or impression smear is primarily used on specific lesions such as ulcers or other damaged tissue.

A microscope slide is touched to the skin in an attempt to collect histologic data. The smear is then stained for analysis. See Chapter 9 for more details.

GRAM STAIN

A Gram stain is a good diagnostic tool used to identify gram-negative and gram-positive bacteria. Chapter 10 contains more information on performing the test and interpreting results.

NASAL FLUSH

A nasal flush is performed to obtain a cytologic sample representing the organisms of the sinuses. This procedure can be therapeutic, flushing any debris or rhinoliths out of the sinuses or nares.

TRACHEAL LAVAGE

A tracheal lavage is performed when tracheal or lower respiratory system pathology is suspected.

All of these diagnostic procedures are performed in the same manner as in traditional domestic species.

BLOOD COLLECTION

After the physical examination, diagnostic testing such as blood work may be required for further evaluation. Obtaining blood from a severely trimmed toenail is not acceptable. This is painful, stressful, and can yield abnormal cell distributions and cellular artifacts. A venous blood sample should be obtained. You must have a highly skilled restrainer when collecting blood samples from wild animals.

Avians

The medial metatarsal vein is located on the medial side of the distal tibiotarsus at the tibiotarsus-tarsometatarsus joint. This is an excellent **venipuncture** site because the vessel is very stable. This helps reduce the risk of hematoma formations. Grasp the leg and syringe in one hand while collecting the sample with the other hand. This will give you more control if the patient moves. **Hemostasis** can be achieved by bandaging the venipuncture site. For best results a 1-ml tuberculin syringe with a 26- to 25-gauge needle should be used.

This is the method of choice for obtaining a blood sample in small birds because the other vessels are usually too small. Birds have two jugular veins; however, the right jugular is more prominent than the left. Usually a 1-cc tuberculin syringe with a 26- to 25-gauge needle is used for the small birds and a 3-cc syringe equipped with a 25-gauge needle can be used in larger birds. The restrainer should hold the bird in left lateral recumbency. The phlebotomist should arch and extend the neck and lightly wet and part the feathers with alcohol and find the featherless track and the jugular. Once the sample is collected, hemostasis must be applied, and it is crucial to prevent large hematomas and possible bleed out.

Because of the severity of the complications that can occur, it is recommended to only attempt this on anesthetized patients. Patients that are not anesthetized have an increased chance of forming a large hematoma and/or fracturing the wing. This vein is located on the medial surface of the wing and is quite obvious, as it runs across the radius and ulna. Place the patient in dorsal recumbency; lightly wet the feathers at the distal end of the humerus. Because of its location, it is difficult to bandage this area for hemostasis, thus requiring that the bird be restrained until the bleeding has stopped. It can take up to 3 to 5 minutes to control the bleeding. This is, however, an excellent site to place IV catheters during anesthesia.

Mammals

Venipuncture sites vary among different species, but the most common venipuncture sites include the cephalic, lateral saphenous, auricular (rabbits and hares), and jugular veins. The jugular veins can be difficult to obtain blood from in rabbits that have large dewlaps. Obtaining blood samples from the mentioned venipuncture sites is accomplished in the same manner as with dogs and cats. The needle and syringe size vary based on the size of the patient with which you are working.

Reptiles

Snakes. The two venipuncture sites in snakes include the caudal tail vein and the heart. The palatine vessels are not appropriate for drawing samples of blood in snakes. Drawing blood from the tail vein is best accomplished in large snakes; it can be difficult in small snakes because of the size of the vessel. The same method used to draw blood from the ventral midline approach in lizards is used in snakes as well (see the lizard section that follows). Obtaining a blood sample from the heart (also called cardiocentesis) is generally the quickest method that will yield a large amount of blood. A 27- to 22-gauge needle on a 1- or 3-cc syringe is used for blood collection. (The size of the needles and syringes depends on the size of the snake.) To obtain a blood sample, the snake should first be placed in dorsal recumbency. The heart can then be located in the cranial third of the body. The heart can move both cranially and caudally, so it is best to place your thumb and index finger on either side of the heart. Look for the caudal portion of the beating heart. The needle insertion site should be two scutes (scales) below that. To obtain blood from the heart, the needle should be inserted between two scutes at a 45-degree angle. It is important not to poke around searching for the heart.

Lizards. The cephalic, jugular, and ventral abdominal vessels can be used to obtain a blood sample from various species of lizards you may encounter in your hospital. However, these vessels are not commonly used for several reasons. The cephalic vein is usually extremely small, and because this is a "blind stick," a surgical cut-down may be necessary. The ventral abdominal vein generally is not used (especially in awake animals) because of the inability to both properly restrain the animal and control hemorrhage. Lastly, the jugular vein is not commonly used because in many species it is also a "blind stick" and may require a surgical cut-down to access the vessel. Lymphatic fluid contamination is also common when performing venipuncture from the jugular vein. Lymph contamination can alter blood test results.

The most common vessel used for lizard venipuncture is the caudal tail vein, also called the ventral coccygeal vein. There are two different techniques commonly used to obtain blood from this vessel. These techniques include a lateral and ventral approach. To successfully obtain a blood sample, a 1-inch or 1½-inch 27- to 20-gauge needle attached to a 1- or 3-ml syringe generally should be used. The size of the needle and syringe depends on the size of the lizard from which you are drawing blood. Insulin syringes can be used on very small lizards, but remember to cut the needle off before putting the blood into the appropriate tubes. The small needle size can cause lysis of the blood cells if pushed through the needle. (The same is true for 26- or 25-gauge needles.) It is important that the tail is gently restrained during the blood draw. The left hand can be used to restrain the caudal portion of the tail, while the right hand can be used to perform the blood draw. If you are left-handed, just obtain your blood sample from the other side of the tail using your left hand to draw blood and your right hand to gently restrain the tail. For a lateral approach, the needle should be inserted into the tail (between two scales) at approximately a 90-degree angle. Slowly insert the needle into the tail, keeping slight negative pressure on the syringe until either blood enters the syringe or the needle touches the vertebrae. If the needle is touching the vertebrae, slowly back the needle off the bone (still keeping slight negative pressure on the syringe) and redirect the needle into the vessel. It is important to put only slight negative pressure on the syringe while obtaining the blood sample. Too much negative pressure may collapse the vessel.

The technique for the ventral midline approach is very similar to the lateral approach. The needle should be inserted into the tail (between two scales) at approximately a 90-degree angle. The needle should be slowly inserted into the tail, keeping slight negative pressure on the syringe until either blood enters the syringe or the needle touches the vertebrae. The blood vessel is located just ventral to the vertebrae. If you touch the vertebrae first, slowly back off the bone until your needle is seated within the vessel.

Lizards usually struggle when they are placed on their backs, making it difficult to draw blood from them; therefore it is important to keep the animal in sternal recumbency while obtaining the blood sample. During the blood draw, it is also important that the phlebotomist gently restrains the caudal portion of the tail with one hand and obtains the blood sample with the other.

Chelonians. The radial-humoral plexus (brachial plexus sinus), subcarapacial venous sinus, dorsal venous sinus (coccygeal vein), and jugular vein are the major sites where blood can be obtained from a turtle or tortoise. The venipuncture site depends on the size and species of the patient and the preference of the phlebotomist. If drawing blood from the jugular vein, the turtle/tortoise should be placed in lateral recumbency. The head and neck should be pulled away from the shell. The jugular vein can be found in the same plane as the eye and the tympanum. To obtain the sample, the phlebotomist holds the head while the restrainer keeps the patient in lateral recumbency. A 27- to 20-gauge needle attached to a 1- to 3-cc syringe is generally used, and varies depending on the size of the patient.

The subcarapacial venous sinus is generally used when jugular venipuncture is not an option. Depending on the size of the patient, a 1- to 1½-inch 27- to 20-gauge needle or a 2-inch spinal needle attached to a 1- to 3-cc syringe is used to obtain the blood sample. The needle is inserted upward at about a 60-degree angle just dorsal to the neck. Slight negative pressure should be applied on the syringe until either blood enters the syringe or bone is encountered. If bone is encountered, back away from the bone and redirect the needle.

The radial-humoral plexus sinus is generally used in larger chelonians. You must pull the front limb away from the body and palpate the tendon near the radiohumeral joint. Generally a 22- to 20-gauge needle attached to a 1- to 3-cc syringe is inserted at a 90-degree angle to skin and angled toward the radiohumeral joint.

When drawing blood from the dorsal venous sinus, the patient should be placed in sternal recumbency. The tail should be held as straight as possible and the needle should be inserted on midline. A 1- to 1½-inch 27- to 20-gauge needle attached to a 1- to 3-cc syringe should be used. The size of the syringe and needle depend on the size of the patient. The needle should be inserted at a 45-degree angle into the tail. Slight negative pressure should be placed on the syringe, and the needle should be inserted until either the needle is in the vein or the needle touches bone. If bone is hit, slowly back the needle off the bone until blood enters the syringe.

Once you have obtained the blood sample, regardless of the species the needle must be removed from the syringe before dispensing the blood into the appropriate tube for sampling. Cell lysis can occur if the blood is dispensed through the needle into the collection tube. If you are not running the samples in your hospital, understand the requirements of the lab to which you are submitting them. Develop a rapport with the lab and have a list handy of the minimal sample and submission requirements.

Blood Tubes

Using blood collection tubes such as Microtainer that are specially designed for small samples helps eliminate any anticoagulant dilution problems (Fig. 28-10). In most species the complete blood count should be collected in ethylene diamine tetra-acetic acid (EDTA), since heparin will cause clumping and staining artifacts. In others, EDTA can cause clumping and hemolysis and a heparinized sample should be obtained. A blood film should be made if the blood is going to stay in the EDTA for any length of time. EDTA exposure may cause increased disruption of cells in the blood film. Biochemistries can be run on plasma in most laboratories. A larger plasma yield can be achieved by using a Microtainer containing lithium heparin.

Blood Volume

Safe diagnostic sampling can be achieved by taking a percentage of the patient's total blood volume. This percentage varies depending on the species and the condition of the patient. In healthy birds it is safe to take 10% of the total blood volume or 1% of the total body weight for diagnostic sampling. In reptiles and mammals it is safe to take up to 8% of

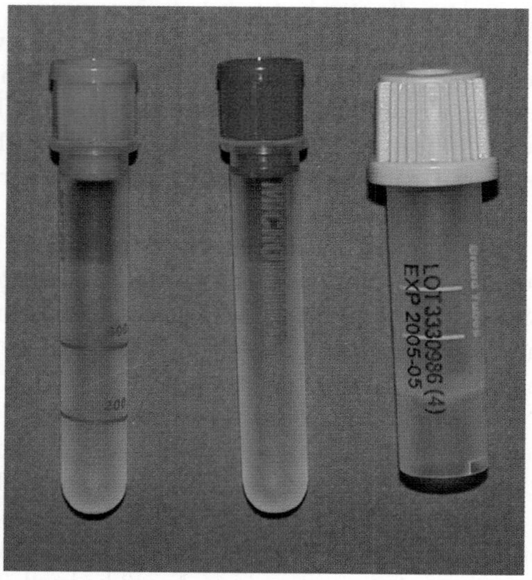

FIGURE 28-10 Microtainer brand blood collection tubes are often used for wildlife diagnostic sampling because of the small volume of blood available.

total blood volume or 0.8% of the total body weight. Because the vast majority of wildlife patients are presented to the veterinary hospital because of illness or traumatic injury, it is advisable to take only half of the mentioned percentages of the patient's blood volume.

Before collecting blood from a patient you must first determine what tests are to be run and the minimum amount of blood needed for sampling. If your hospital is not equipped with an in-house blood analyzer, it is best to consult with your lab about the minimum requirements for sampling.

A few simple calculations can be used to determine how much blood can be safely drawn. This can be used for any species so long as the correct percentage of total blood volume is used. For example, 10% is used for birds, whereas 8% is generally used for mammals and reptiles.

Example: In the lizard, total circulating blood volume is calculated as follows:

$$\text{Body weight (grams)} \times \text{Percentage of total blood volume} = \text{Total circulating blood volume.}$$

Once the reptile's total blood volume has been calculated, 10% of the circulating blood volume can be withdrawn safely. This amount is determined as follows:

$$\text{Circulating blood volume (ml)} \times \text{Maximum percentage of blood that can be safely drawn} = \text{Maximum safe sample size (ml)}$$

For example: Determine how much blood can be safely drawn from a lizard that weighs 500 grams. For this calculation, the total blood volume is calculated at 8%:

$$500 \text{ grams} \times 0.08 \text{ total blood volume} = 40 \text{ ml of circulating blood}$$

The blood samples can contain up to 10% of the 40 ml of circulating blood. The amount (ml) that can be safely drawn from this patient for blood sampling is calculated as follows:

$$40 \text{ ml of circulating blood} \times 0.10 = 4 \text{ ml of blood}$$

Therefore, up to 4 ml of blood can be taken from this lizard, which is more than enough blood to run a CBC and a chemistry panel.

DIAGNOSTIC IMAGING

Radiographs are excellent diagnostic tools that yield valuable information. The diagnostic value of a radiograph depends on the quality of the technique and positioning of the patient. Most species require anesthesia or heavy sedation for diagnostic radiographs. When done with the animal awake, there is a risk of injury such as tissue trauma and fractures from aggressive struggling. However wild birds seem to be more tolerant of the restraint required for radiographs than other wild animals. Digital radiology is quickly becoming the standard in most hospitals and yields the best results. However, if digital radiology is not yet available in your hospital, then high-detail, rare-earth cassettes with single emulsion film provide desired results. Mammography film produces even better detail, but requires modification of x-ray machine settings. A technique can be extrapolated from the tabletop technique used on most of your feline patients. For extremely small patients, you can use a dental radiology unit. If you have the luxury of a digital radiology machine, then you can use similar techniques with a few adjustments. Consult with a radiologist to update your technique chart if needed.

Avians

The positioning of the patient is crucial for a diagnostic radiograph. Standard whole-body views are a ventrodorsal (VD) and a right lateral. It is vital to always take both views. Plexiglas restraint boards that assist with patient positioning can be used and usually provide excellent results. For the VD place the bird on its back, legs stretched down to expose the coelomic cavity, wings stretched out symmetrically to the sides, and two pieces of masking tape or paper tape in the form of an X across each carpus. Palpate the keel to ensure it is in line with the backbone. If the patient is not positioned correctly, this can cause misinterpretation from superimposition.

For the lateral view the patient is placed in right lateral recumbency, legs stretched downward, and wings pulled back together. Paper or masking tape is placed across the carpus, keeping the wings back, and tape or gauze is used to keep the legs stretched downward (Fig. 28-11). Once the plain films are reviewed, it may be necessary to isolate limbs for an individual shot, or perform a contrast study of the gastrointestinal system or perform an ultrasound examination.

The mentioned VD and lateral views reveal the same view of the wing, a lateral. When two views are necessary, a palmarodorsal (PaD) view needs to be obtained. The PaD can be obtained by placing the bird in a dive-bombing position, head on the plate, body up in the air. Extend the wing out as close to the plate as possible and collimate to the desired area.

Mammals

Sedation or general anesthesia is often needed to take good diagnostic radiographs of wild mammals. If radiographing small patients such as most rabbits and rodents, whole-body radiographs are usually taken. The patient is gently taped down to the x-ray table or directly onto the plate and positioned as necessary. Positioning is the same as with dogs and cats. The most common radiographic views include a VD and right lateral. Obliques and extremity views can also be taken as needed.

Reptiles

Snakes. Sedation or general anesthesia is needed to take good diagnostic radiographs of snakes. Whole-body radiographs are usually taken of the patient. This is accomplished by gently taping down to the patient to the x-ray table or directly onto the plate and positioned as necessary. Because of the length of snakes, radiographs are generally taken in sections labeled with lead numbers for identification purposes. The most common views include a VD and right lateral for each section of snake. If sedation or anesthesia is not going to be used, a plastic snake tube can be used to position the awake snake for radiographs. Snake tubes work well only if they are of the appropriate size, making it impossible for the snake to move or become obliqued.

Chelonians. Three views are normally taken which include a dorsoventral (DV), horizontal lateral, and horizontal craniocaudal views (Fig. 28-12). The craniocaudal view is taken to evaluate the left and right lung fields. A horizontal

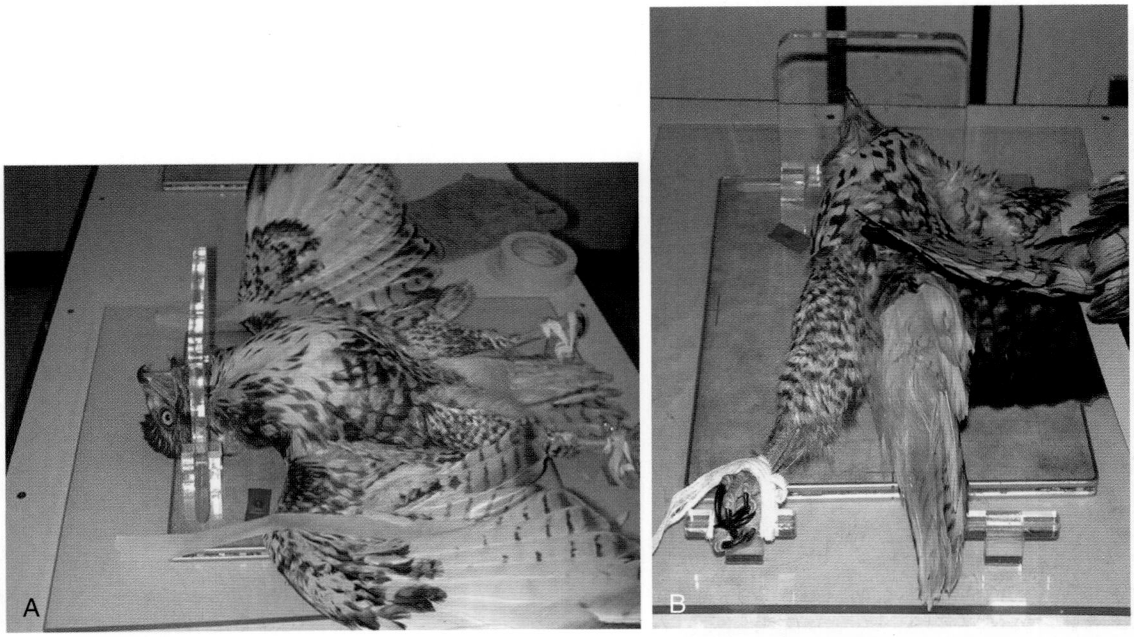

FIGURE 28-11 The avian restraint board is used to properly position the patient for a ventrodorsal (**A**) and lateral (**B**) radiograph.

beam is essential to obtain good radiographs. Because chelonians do not have a diaphragm, placing them in lateral recumbency causes shifting of the organs into the lung cavity, which leads to poor radiographs. Most chelonians do not need to be sedated for radiographs, but chemical restraint can be used if necessary. In most cases the patient will just sit there or can be placed on a plastic dish with its feet hanging in the air.

Lizards. Two views are normally taken, which include a DV and horizontal lateral. A horizontal beam is essential to obtain good radiographs. Because reptiles do not have a diaphragm, placing them in lateral recumbency causes shifting of the organs into the lung cavity, which leads to poor radiographs. Most lizards do not need to be sedated for radiographs, but chemical restraint can be used if necessary. In most cases the patient will just sit there while the radiographs are being taken. You can also use vagal stimulation or the "vagal response" to calm the patient if needed. The vagal response in iguanas and other medium to large lizard species can be induced by gently applying digital pressure to both eyes for a few seconds to a few minutes. The patient usually responds with a decrease in heart rate and blood pressure. The vagal response induces a short-term trancelike state allowing time to take radiographs and in some cases even draw blood.

Ultrasound

Ultrasound is a superb diagnostic tool and can be used when evaluating wildlife. Keeping in mind the anatomic differences among species, the same techniques used for the majority of domestic species can be used on wildlife. Ultrasound studies can be fairly limiting in the avian species because ultrasound waves cannot penetrate gas-filled air sacs throughout the bird's body and in some cases the patient is just too small to achieve a diagnostic image. In reptiles ultrasound can also be limiting because of the thickness of scales and shells in chelonian species.

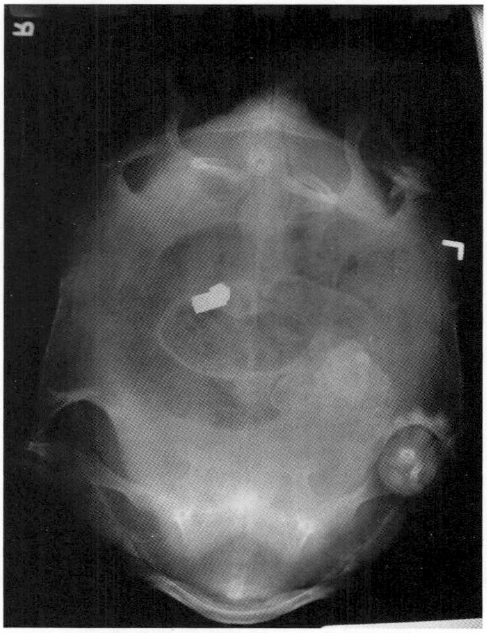

FIGURE 28-12 A tortoise has ingested two metal foreign bodies.

ROUTES OF ADMINISTRATION OF MEDICATIONS AND FLUIDS

AVIANS

The intramuscular and subcutaneous routes are the most common paths for administration of medications. Because of the renal-portal system, injections should only be given cranial to the kidneys. Injections are most often given into the pectoral muscles.

The intravenous route can be used as needed in many species. An indwelling catheter or single injection can be given into the medial metatarsal, cutaneous ulnar, or jugular veins (Fig. 28-13).

The oral route is often used to administer medications. If the gastrointestinal tract works, then feel free to use it. Oral medications can be given using a feeding tube or just titrated in with a syringe.

MAMMALS

Intramuscular injections are given in the same manner as in dogs and cats. Remember to aspirate the syringe to ensure you are not in a vessel before giving the injection.

Subcutaneous injections are given in the same manner as in a dog or cat. Larger volumes of fluids can be given in this site. The injection is usually given in the subcutaneous space between the shoulder blades. The patient must be held by another technician before giving the injection. It is preferred to use a butterfly catheter instead of a regular needle. A 27- to 19-gauge needle can be used based on the size of the patient. The skin should be tented with one hand while the other hand places the needle under the skin and then gives the injection. It is important to aspirate back before giving the injection to ensure you are in the correct spot. You should not aspirate blood or air. If this happens, you need to start over.

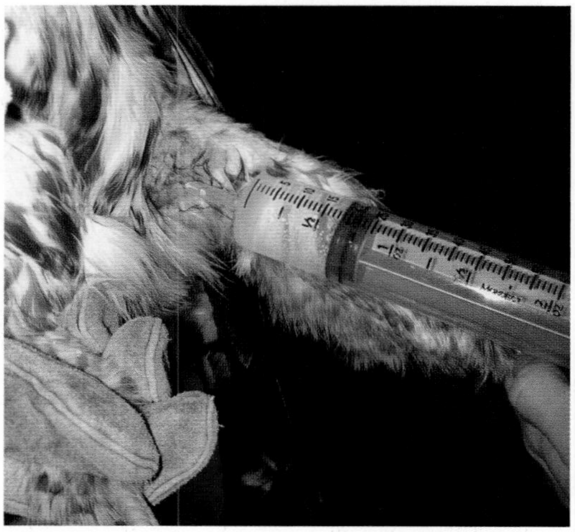

FIGURE 28-13 Subcutaneous fluids are generally given in the inguinal area in most species of birds.

Intravenous injection of drugs can be difficult in most awake wild mammals. Intravenous injections can be given in the cephalic, saphenous, jugular, or auricular (usually rabbits only) veins. It is important to have the proper syringe and needle size for the injection you are giving. In most cases, a 1-ml or insulin syringe with a 27- to 25-gauge needle should be used. Intravenous injections are given in the same manner as in dogs and cats.

Intramuscular injections are commonly given in the lumbar or quadriceps muscles. Another technician should properly restrain the patient while the injection is given. Oral medications can be mixed with food or just given orally via a syringe. Putting medications in food is often the best way to medicate wild animals as this causes the least amount of stress.

REPTILES

The intramuscular and subcutaneous routes are the most common routes for administration of medications. Because of the renal-portal system, only the front limbs should be used for intramuscular injections.

The intravenous route is rarely used, but administration of fluids and some medications can be given in reptiles. An indwelling catheter can also be placed for continuous fluid therapy replacement, but this can be very difficult.

The intracoelomic route can be used for administration of fluids. The patient should be placed in lateral recumbency with the hind leg extended away from the body. The needle is then placed under the skin and into the coelomic cavity. You must aspirate before administering any fluids. If the needle is placed into the wrong spot fluids could accidentally be given into the bladder or lungs, both of which are detrimental.

Intraosseous fluids can be given in many lizard species. In lizards, a 25- to 20-gauge spinal needle is placed into the distal portion of the femur or humerus or the proximal portion of the tibia. A spinal needle is preferred because the stylet will help keep the needle from becoming clogged from a bone core fragment. The catheter is placed using aseptic technique and is sutured to the skin for stability. It is then bandaged to protect the catheter site. This procedure is painful and requires sedation with analgesia, general anesthesia, or the use of a local anesthetic.

The oral route is often used to administer medications. If the gastrointestinal tract works, then feel free to use it. Oral medications can be given using a feeding tube or just titrated in with a syringe.

SUPPORTIVE CARE OF WILD ANIMALS IN THE HOSPITAL

RAPTORS

Raptors receive most of their water intake from the prey they eat; therefore if they are not readily eating, they can become dehydrated. Fluid therapy and/or force feeding should be considered while in the hospital if the patient is not eating on its own. The most common fluid given to raptors is lactated Ringer's solution (LRS) subcutaneously at a dose of 50 to 60 ml/kg/day. Fluids are generally given in the inguinal area. In some cases, IV fluid therapy can be initiated. If the patient is not eating on its own, it needs to be force fed. This can be done by either defrosting and chopping up (if necessary) pieces of mice, rats, fish, or chicks (it depends on the species you are working with) or using a manufactured food such as Oxbow Carnivore Care. Prey is fed by either using tongs to offer the prey or just using your finger to place the prey into the mouth (Fig. 28-14). If a commercial formula is used, it is delivered using a feeding tube. This is done in the same manner as with a pet parrot, although a rubber feeding tube is generally chosen over the use of the metal tubes usually used with parrots. The mouth is opened and the tube in placed into the distal esophagus. The food should be delivered at a slow pace, watching the back of the mouth to ensure the food is not coming back up the esophagus. If this happens the tube should be pulled out and the bird immediately placed back into the cage. When pulling the tube out of the mouth, the tube should be pinched off so that any residual food is not draped across the glottis, causing aspiration. Ideally, babies should be fed using a bird puppet.

If the raptor is going to be in the clinic for several days, the tail should be wrapped. Tail feathers are only replaced about once per year, so it is very important that they are not damaged. Wrapping them with paper packing tape or x-ray film protects them from getting broken.

Most metal dog and cat cages can be used for short-term housing of raptors in the veterinary clinic. The cage should be lined with newspaper and most commonly bricks covered with indoor/outdoor carpet are used as perches (Fig. 28-15). Bricks are easy to clean and the indoor/outdoor carpet can be thrown away after the patient has left. The front of the cage should be covered with newspaper as well. This provides a visual barrier between the patient and the rest of the hospital. Adults can be kept at room temperature, but small babies need to be kept much warmer.

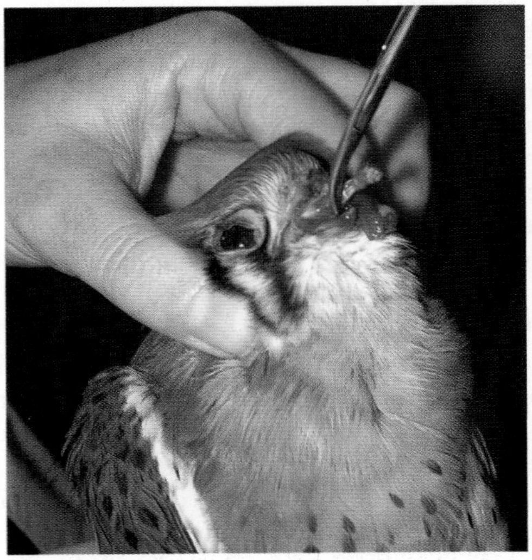

FIGURE 28-14 Wild birds can be fed using a syringe, pipette, forceps (as seen in this picture), or be tube fed using a red rubber feeding tube or metal feeding tube.

FIGURE 28-15 A common raptor cage setup includes a perch covered in indoor/outdoor carpet. The cage is lined with newspaper.

NONRAPTORIAL BIRDS

There are many diets and formulas that can be used to provide nutrition to growing songbirds and waterfowl. A maintenance soaked dog food can be used for short-term feeding in songbirds, but a more nutritional formula should be used for long-term care. Forceps, syringes, pipettes, tongue depressors, and toothpicks can all be used to feed small songbirds. Most babies are easy to feed because movement or tapping them on the beak will cause them to gape their mouths open. Care must be taken not to overfeed the bird during each feeding. If the patient is dehydrated, fluids such as LRS should be given at a dose of 50 to 60 ml/kg/day subcutaneously in the inguinal area. In some cases IV fluid therapy can be initiated.

Songbirds should be housed in cages that either have small wire mesh or a dog/cat carrier that they cannot get stuck in or fly through. Perches such as covered bricks, wood branches, or covered PVC pipes can be used. The fronts and sides of the cages should also be covered with newspaper to help keep the stress level down and provide a visual barrier. If you are housing water birds such as ducks, geese, and swans, you must provide a swim tank or pool of some sort for them (Fig. 28-16).

MAMMALS

Mammals can be kept in either a dog/cat carrier (small mammals) or a regular metal dog/cat cage. Again the front and/or sides of the cage should be covered to reduce stress and provide a visual barrier for the animal. Diets depend on the species you are working with; many diets and formulations are available. Each veterinary hospital and wildlife center often uses a slightly different formula. It does not really matter what formula is used so long as it is nutritionally sound. It is important for mammalian patients to maintain normal hydration while hospitalized. Assessing dehydration is done in the same manner as in dogs and cats. Fluid therapy should be initiated if the patient is dehydrated. Administering subcutaneous fluids is the most common route used with wild mammals. The fluid rate ranges from 60 to 100 ml/kg/day. LRS is the most commonly administered fluid. Intravenous fluid therapy can be initiated under some circumstances.

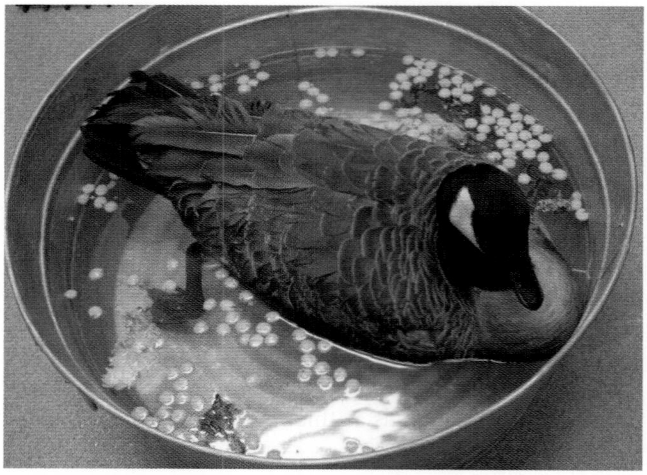

FIGURE 28-16 Waterfowl kept in the hospital should have an area in which to swim on a daily basis.

REPTILES

Snakes

All snakes are carnivores and feed on whole prey items. The digestive system of snakes has evolved to digest whole prey and defecate the parts of the prey that are not digested, such as fur. Ingesting the entire carcass provides added nutrients such as calcium from the bone. Further supplementation is not needed when feeding whole prey. It is never appropriate to feed meat such as chicken breast, hot dogs, raw beef, etc., as this does not provide a complete diet.

It is suggested that prekilled or stunned food is offered to snakes so they will not be harmed by the prey item. Prekilled food can be ordered frozen from several companies. If frozen mice/rats are offered, they must be thawed first (Fig. 28-17).

Lizards

Feeding requirements are based on the type of lizard with which you are working. Lizards can be carnivores, herbivores, insectivores, or omnivores. You should also know what diet is most appropriate for the individual species. Herbivores should be fed various types of dark leafy greens and vegetables. Proper leafy greens include, but are not limited to, kale, chard, turnip greens, escarole, etc. Most insectivores can eat meal worms, silk worms, crickets, etc. Carnivorous lizards should be fed whole prey. Whole prey includes all the bones, GI contents, muscle, and fur. Whole prey items include mice, rats, rabbits, guinea pigs, fish, etc., depending on the species you are feeding. Omnivores should be offered a variety of both dark leafy greens and in most cases insects. The quality and variety of food offered is important. Animals should not be fed the same food day after day.

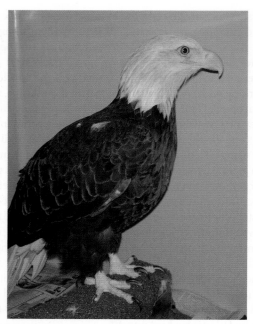

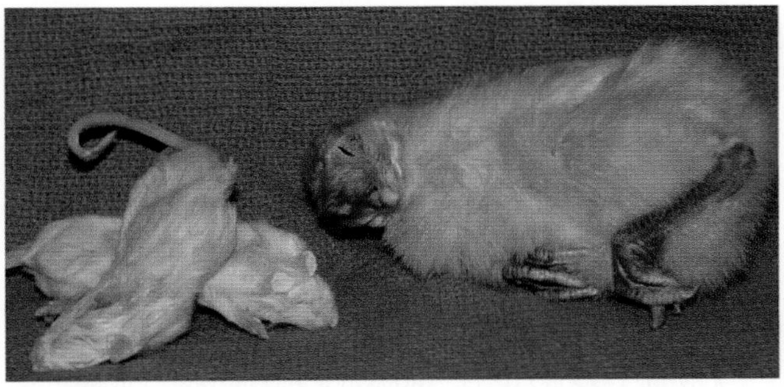

FIGURE 28-17 Prekilled prey items rather than live prey should always be offered to patients such as snakes or carnivorous lizards.

Chelonians

Most aquatic turtles are omnivorous, eating fish, invertebrates, algae, leafy greens, etc. Commercial diets are acceptable to feed in moderation, but it is important to make sure it contains essential nutrients needed to maintain good health. Tortoises are herbivores and eat a variety of leaves, grasses, flowers, etc. in the wild. In captivity a healthy diet includes dark leafy greens, rose petals, hay, and vegetables. Commercial diets can be fed in moderation and should be appropriate for herbivores. Do not feed dog food, tofu, monkey biscuits, or anything that has animal protein in it.

If a reptile patient is dehydrated, fluid therapy should be implemented. Assessing dehydration in reptiles is very similar to assessing dehydration in dogs and cats. First look at the mucous membranes. Are they dry, pale, and have mucous strands draping from the top to the bottom of the mouth or are they moist and pink? Note that some reptiles, especially snakes, may have paler mucous membranes than mammals do. Is the skin wrinkled or does the skin lack a normal elasticity? You should also tent the skin (if possible) to assess dehydration. The same techniques used on dogs and cats can be used for most reptiles. Lastly, take a look at the eyes. Are they sunken? Does the skin around the eye stand up when touched? If the animal is dehydrated, fluid therapy should be considered and a percentage of dehydration should be estimated for the animal. Accurately estimating percent dehydration for any reptile is based on experience and uses the mentioned landmarks such as skin tenting, looking at the eyes, and examining the mucous membranes. Fluid therapy routes in reptiles include oral administration, subcutaneous, intracoelomic, intraosseous, and intravenous (although IV fluid therapy can be difficult) fluid administration. Soaking the animal in a tub of warm water (appropriate temperatures depend on the species) can also be used in conjunction with other fluid therapy routes to help with hydration. Common fluids used for reptiles include LRS and Normosol-R. Maintenance fluid rates in reptiles range from 10 to 30 ml/kg/day.

IMMOBILIZING FRACTURES

Any fracture should be immobilized as soon as possible and pain medications should be provided. The same rules of fracture stabilization used with dogs and cats are used with wild animals as well. The joint above the fracture site and the joint below the fracture site must be stabilized to properly stabilize the fracture. A tape splint can be used to stabilize leg fractures in small songbirds. Figure-eight bandages are used in birds that either have a wing fracture or an injury to the wing causing a droop. The figure-eight bandage by itself is used to stabilize a fracture of the radius and/or ulna because the bandage supports the elbow and wrist joints. If the bird has a fracture of the humerus, a body wrap must be placed because the shoulder joint must be stabilized. Stabilization of fractures in mammals and reptiles employs similar techniques to those used in dogs and cats.

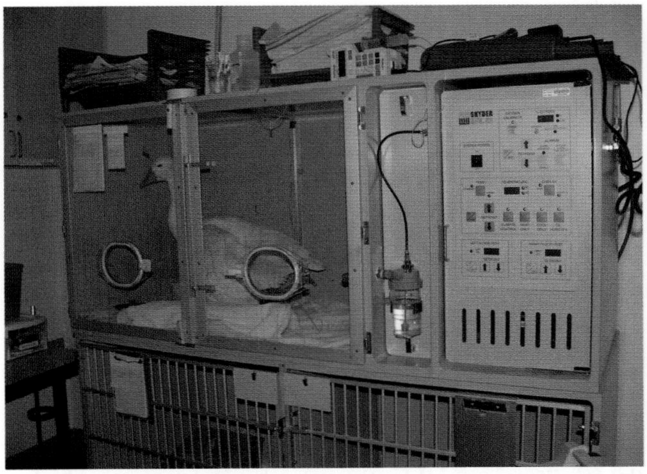

FIGURE 28-18 Large oxygen cages often used for dogs and cats can be used for wildlife such as the goose pictured here.

LONG-TERM REHABILITATION

Most veterinary hospitals are not set up for long-term rehabilitation, and most places do not have the proper permits to house wild animals for more than a few days (Fig. 28-18). Long-term rehabilitation should only take place if the hospital has a quiet area for the animal to rest, recover, and/or grow. Short-term care, meaning a few days or so, can be provided by many hospitals. Once the animal is brought into the clinic, it should be stabilized and then sent to a licensed wildlife rehabilitation center or rehabilitator as soon as possible. It is very important that the clinic has a clear understanding of the role it is going to play.

FOOD PREPARATION

All food should be made just before feeding. Even food that sits in the refrigerator can become a haven for bacterial growth. It is also essential to have proper diets for each species with which you are working.

FEEDING FREQUENCY

Baby birds are fed sunup to sundown by the parents. Although it may be hard to feed babies frequently during the day in a busy hospital, it is very important that time is made.

- Hatchlings should be fed every 10 to 20 minutes.
- Nestlings should be fed every 20 to 30 minutes.

- Fledglings should be fed every 45 to 60 minutes.
- Juveniles should be fed every 2 hours.

Birds may not eat at every feeding, but you should still offer food.

ETHICAL TREATMENT AND RELEASABILITY OF WILD ANIMALS

EUTHANASIA VS. RELEASE OF A WILD ANIMAL

The concept of **releasability** must be considered for every wild animal that is triaged in the veterinary hospital. The overall goal of wildlife medicine and rehabilitation is to release the animals back to the wild so that it can thrive and continue to breed. During the physical examination, one must consider the injuries sustained by the animal and determine whether this animal will be successfully returned to the wild.

It is important to know what types of injuries warrant euthanasia and what types of injuries warrant rehabilitation. Some injuries are much more obvious than others. It is important to remember that saving a life for the sake of saving a life is not the appropriate way of thinking. You must remember that the patient must be releasable and be able to thrive in the wild. Box 28-2 lists common injuries that may require euthanasia. Some of these injuries may be more detrimental for specific species (Fig. 28-19).

The same euthanasia techniques used with other exotic and domestic animals are used on wildlife as well. The animal should be sedated or anesthetized before giving the intravenous injection of the barbiturate euthanasia solution. The euthanasia can also be given intraperitoneal (IP) or directly into the heart. Giving the euthanasia solution IP takes longer to become effective. If you are giving the euthanasia solution into the heart, the animal must be anesthetized. It is unethical to give a cardiac injection of euthanasia solution into an animal if it is not anesthetized. If you are working with threatened or endangered species that require euthanasia, you should contact the state fish and wildlife department for permission, as there may be rules and regulations regarding euthanasia of these species.

It is unlawful for people to possess bald or golden eagles or their parts. If a bald or golden eagle is euthanized in a veterinary hospital, it should be sent to the national eagle repository for use by federally recognized Native American tribes (national eagle repository: www.fws.gov/le/Natives/EagleRepository.htm).

If an animal is determined to be nonreleasable, it can be placed into a zoo, wildlife education center, or raptor center if they have the proper permits. This can be a daunting task, as many facilities already have common species of wild animals.

BOX 28-2 Common Injuries That May Require Euthanasia

- Compound or open fracture that is more than 24 to 48 hours old
- Complete loss of sight or hearing in any wild animal species
- Impaired vision in one or both eyes
- Nocturnal owls with hearing impairment in one or both ears
- Amputation or partial amputation of wing or leg
- Any injury to the foot or digits that impair raptors from hunting and catching prey
- Fractures near a joint such as the elbow or shoulder
- Open fractures with a significant piece of bone missing
- Severe head trauma
- Back injuries that result in loss of limb function
- Animals that have imprinted to humans
- Animals that have an incurable infectious disease
- Mammals with two or more nonfunctional legs
- A rabies vector species from a rabies endemic area
- Rodents or rabbits with a fractured jaw or trauma to the teeth
- Electrocution
- Avian pox virus (Fig. 1)

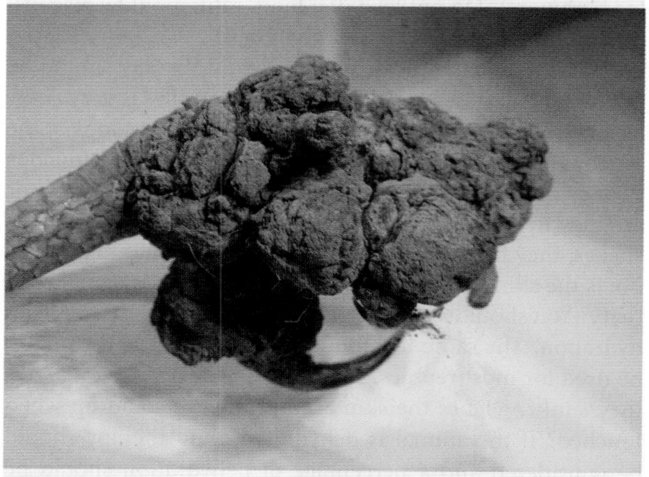

FIGURE 1 This hawk is showing classic signs of avian pox virus.

CHEMICAL RESTRAINT AND ANESTHESIA

It is important to become comfortable with chemical restraint and anesthesia in common wildlife patients that may present to the veterinary clinic. When possible, premedication should be used to sedate or tranquilize the patient before inducing general anesthesia. This generally produces a smoother induction. Because of the high stress experienced by these patients, the most common way to induce anesthesia is by chamber or box induction. Isoflurane and sevoflurane in oxygen are the two most common inhalation agents used to rapidly and safely induce anesthesia. Mask induction can be used for patients such as birds that can be physically restrained. Many reptile species can be induced using propofol intravenously. Injectable drugs such as ketamine, dexmedetomidine, xylazine, telazol, full μ-opioids, buprenorphine, butorphanol, and midazolam can be used alone or in combination with each other to sedate or induce anesthesia. The type of species and procedure being performed will determine the appropriate drug combination. A current exotic animal formulary should be consulted before giving any anesthetic agent.

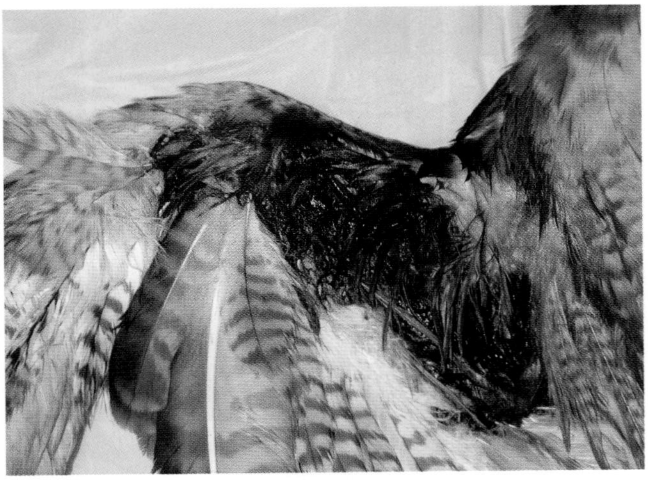

FIGURE 28-19 This red-tailed hawk *(Buteo jamaicensis)* exhibits classic signs of electrocution. Electrocution carries a poor prognosis.

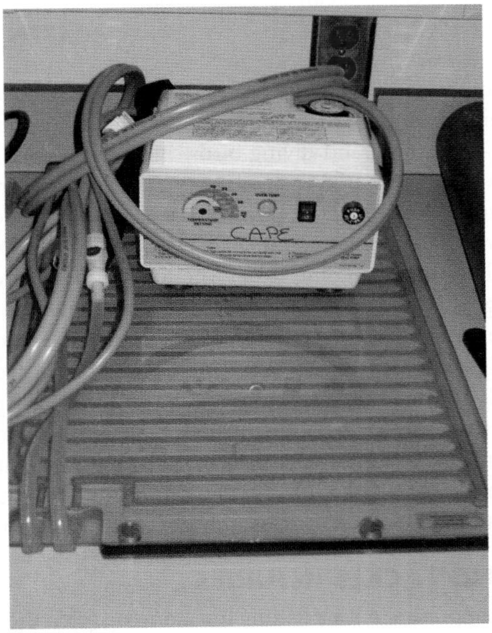

FIGURE 28-20 A hard plastic heating pad is ideal for wild animals because it is easy to clean and hard to damage.

Once induced, endotracheal intubation is performed when possible and an intravenous catheter is placed to provide fluid therapy throughout the anesthetic period. Please refer to the anesthesia sections in Chapter 27 for more in-depth information about maintenance of general anesthesia, as this is similar for wild birds and reptiles. Anesthetic maintenance for wild mammals is similar to that of dogs and cats. At minimum, the blood pressure (direct or indirect), heart rate, respiratory rate, and temperature should be monitored. Other monitoring techniques include the use of a pulse oximeter, end-tidal CO_2, and electrocardiogram.

Anesthetic recovery can be very stressful for wild animals. Recovery should take place in a dark, warm, and quiet room (Fig. 28-20). The area should be padded to help prevent further injury to the patient. Recovery is generally quick when maintaining on isoflurane or sevoflurane in oxygen. Injectable drugs such as xylazine and dexmedetomidine can be easily reversed. Postoperative pain medications should be administered to provide analgesia in patients recovering from painful procedures. Common postoperative pain medications include butorphanol, buprenorphine, nonsteroidal anti-inflammatory drugs, and full μ opioids. Food and water should be offered to the patient once it has recovered from the anesthetic procedure.

BOX 28-3 Common Diseases Diagnosed in Wildlife

Viral Diseases
- Avian pox
- Polyomavirus
- Paramyxovirus
- Herpesvirus
- Cytomegalovirus
- Circovirus
- Avian influenza
- West Nile virus

Bacterial Infections
- *Aeromonas* spp.
- *Campylobacter fetus*
- *Chlamydophila psittaci*
- *Enterococcus faecalis*
- *Mycobacterium avium*
- *Mycoplasma* spp.
- *Pseudomonas* spp.
- Salmonellosis (paratyphoid)
- *Pasteurella multocida*
- *Yersinia pseudotuberculosis*
- *Staphylococcus*

Mycotic Infections
- Candidiasis
- *Aspergillus* spp.

Parasitic Infections
- Coccidiosis
- *Toxoplasma gondii*
- Cryptosporidiosis

Protozoal Infections
- *Cochlosomosis* spp.
- *Giardia*
- *Trichomonads*

Ectoparasites
- *Mallophaga* spp.
- *Anoplura* spp.

COMMON DISEASES AND INJURIES OF WILD ANIMALS

Wildlife present to the veterinary clinic for a variety of reasons including various bacterial, fungal, and viral infections (Box 28-3); ingesting toxins; trauma, including being hit by a car (Fig. 28-21); electrocution; attack by another animal; gunshot wounds; and fractures (Fig. 28-22). Treatment varies based on

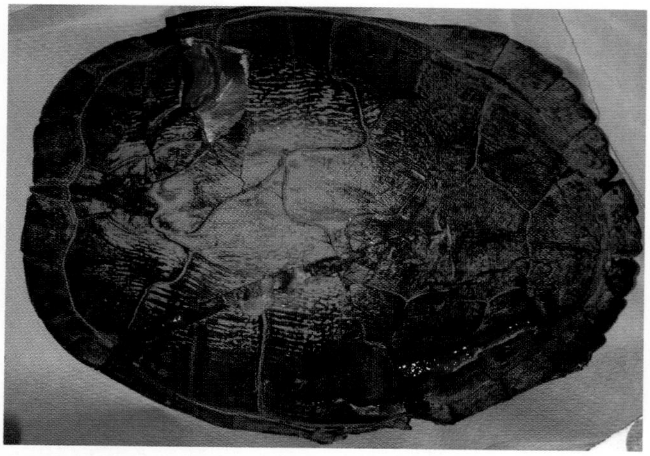

FIGURE 28-21 This pond turtle was hit by a car. Injuries to this extent warrant euthanasia.

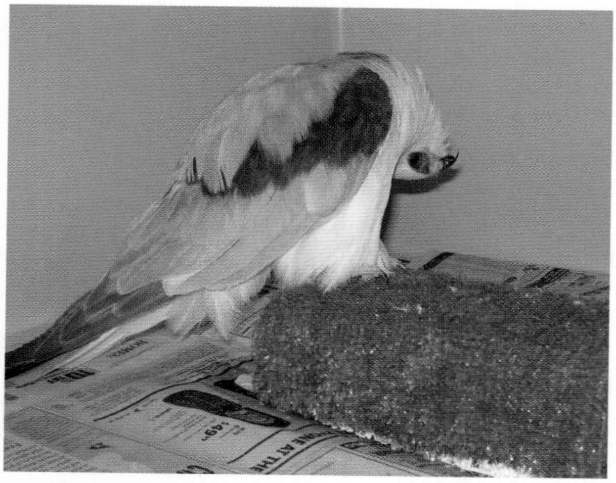

FIGURE 28-22 This white-tailed kite *(Elanus leucurus)* has sustained head trauma.

the extent of the injuries and the species with which you are working. Listed in the following are some of the common diseases and presentations of various wildlife species.

TOXICOSIS

Heavy Metal Toxicosis

Lead poisoning is common and is caused by ingestion of lead shot used by fishermen's weights or shotgun pellets from the wetlands. Lead shot in other tissues, such as from a gunshot wound, is not a cause of systemic lead toxicosis. Zinc toxicity can occur from ingesting galvanized metal or some coins.

Botulism

The causative agent of botulism is *Clostridium botulinum* and is an intoxication rather than an infectious disease. It is contracted by ingestion of the toxin and can be responsible for large die-offs of migrating waterfowl.

Algal Toxins

Freshwaters exposed to warm temperatures can suffer explosive blooms of toxin-producing phytoplankton, usually

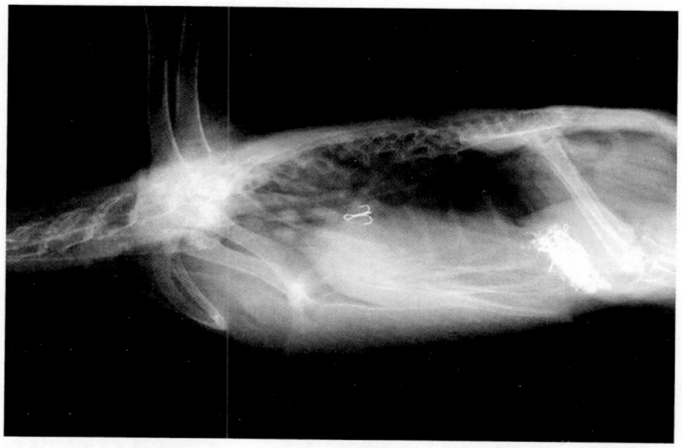

FIGURE 28-23 A treble hook was swallowed by a wild duck. It was later removed using a flexible endoscope.

referred to as blue-green algae. Very high concentrations of toxins can occur and can be neurotoxic and hepatotoxic.

Oiled Birds

Major oil spills that pollute the sea with crude or heavy fuel (bunker oil) are major environmental problems that affect the surface-swimming and diving birds. Birds that swim into an oil slick can get covered with oil, coating the feather structure, and causing loss of waterproofing, insulation, and buoyancy. Birds will vigorously preen their feathers in an attempt to remove the oil and become toxic. The toxicity of different oils varies greatly and the degree of toxic effect depends on the volume ingested. Hypothermia, dehydration, emaciation, and electrolyte imbalances can occur and need to be treated. Only when the bird is stable can the bathing begin, as the process itself is stressful. The recommended detergent used worldwide is Dawn dish soap (Procter & Gamble) as a 2% solution. A good source for further information can be found through the International Bird Rescue Research Center at www.ibrrc.org/.

FISHING TACKLE INJURIES

Birds that present with a fishing line hanging from the mouth should be examined for entanglements externally around the limbs, neck, or beak. Patients should then be radiographed to determine what the bird ingested: hook, weight, or lure (Fig. 28-23).

WILDLIFE COMMONLY SEEN IN THE CLINIC

RAPTORS

Birds of prey commonly present to the veterinary hospital for a variety of different traumatic injuries, including gunshot wounds, being hit by a car, flying into a window, being attacked by another animal, and electrocution (Figs. 28-24 to 28-27). Other presentations may include bacterial, viral, fungal, or parasitic infections.

Bumblefoot

Bumblefoot is a degenerative, inflammatory condition affecting the plantar surface on the feet of raptors and is a byproduct of captive management, not an infectious disease

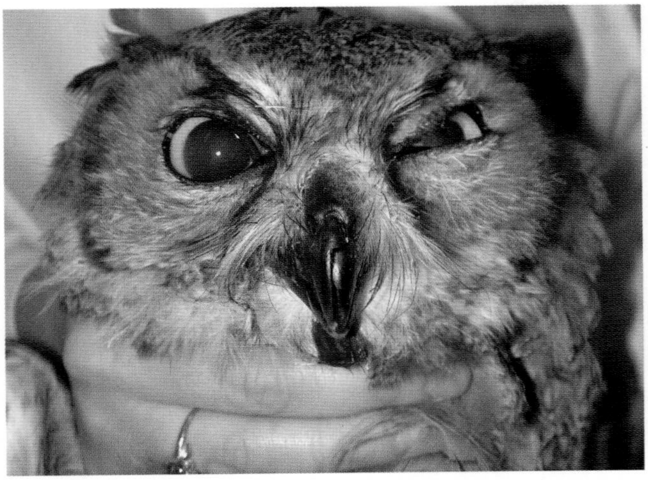

FIGURE 28-24 This great horned owl *(Bubo virginianus)* has sustained a beak fracture from an unknown trauma.

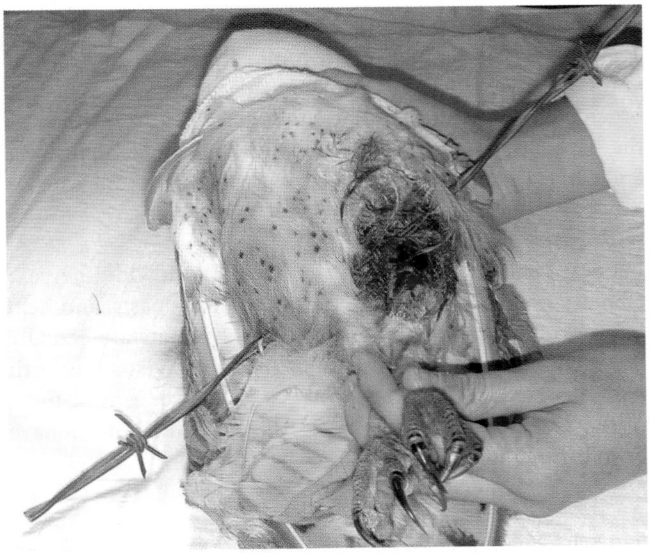

FIGURE 28-25 This barn owl *(Tyto alba)* has sustained trauma by flying into barbed wire. These traumatic injuries often produce a poor prognosis.

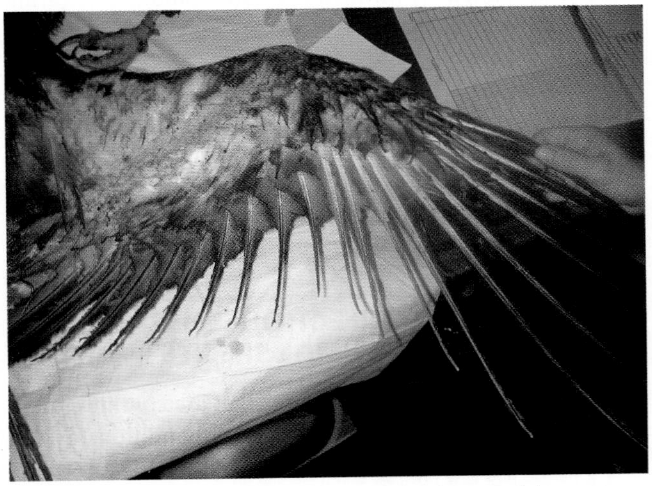

FIGURE 28-26 This golden eagle *(Aquila chrysaetos)* shows classic signs of electrocution.

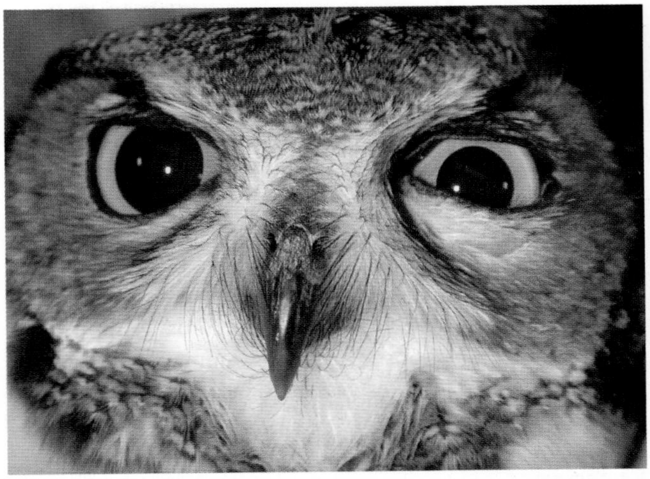

FIGURE 28-27 This great horned owl is exhibiting anisocoria (uneven pupil size) commonly caused by head trauma.

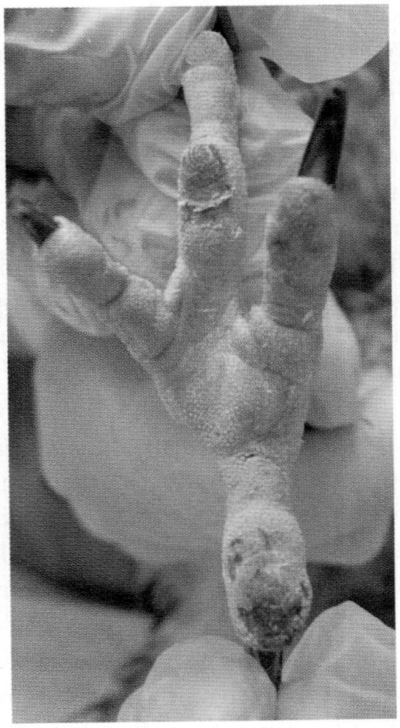

FIGURE 28-28 The feet should always be examined during the physical examination. This raptor is exhibiting signs of pododermatitis, also call bumblefoot.

(Fig. 28-28). This is a rare finding in wild birds. This condition is created by abnormal pressures placed on the plantar surfaces of the feet, such as uneven weight distribution because of the opposite foot or leg injury.

NONRAPTORIAL BIRDS

The most common presentation for nonraptorial birds is trauma. Common traumatic injuries include flying into a window, being attacked by a cat or dog, and gunshot wounds. Other common presentations include ingestion of toxic substances such as Avitrol poisoning in pigeons and other species of birds.

REPTILES

Common presentations for reptiles include trauma such as being hit by car, being attacked by another animal, fractures, open wounds, etc. All reptiles can carry the *Salmonella* species of bacteria. Contact with reptiles has been directly implicated in human Salmonellosis outbreaks, and the reptiles typically exhibit no signs of illness themselves. Other zoonotic disease potential exists but is not common. Latex or vinyl gloves should be worn at all times when handling reptile species.

MAMMALS

Mammals present to the veterinary hospital for a variety of different reasons, including trauma, bacterial, viral, fungal, and parasitic infections. Common traumatic injuries are caused by being hit by a car, attacked by another animal, and wounded by a gunshot.

Raccoons

Proper infectious disease precautions should be implemented when allowing a raccoon into your clinic. Raccoons act as a reservoir for rabies in the United States. No parenteral vaccine is approved for use in raccoons, so care must be taken not to be bitten in the clinic.

Raccoons are carriers of *Baylisascaris procyonis,* an intestinal roundworm that is zoonotic to humans. People become infected when they accidentally ingest infected soil, water, or objects contaminated with raccoon feces. Once ingested, the eggs hatch into larvae and travel throughout the body, affecting the organs and muscles. This infection can be fatal.

Raccoons are susceptible to contracting canine and feline distemper. Care should be taken not to carry this disease to your other patients in the hospital. *Trypanosoma cruzi, Rickettsia rickettsii,* leptospirosis, and *Salmonella* spp. are organisms also commonly found in raccoons. Because of the zoonotic potential of many common diseases carried by raccoons, personal protective equipment including gloves, gowns, and goggles should be worn during handling.

Opossums

Opossums have an impressive immune system, and a lower than average body temperature. Because of this, they do not carry many of the standard zoonotic diseases that other animals carry. Although an opossum might carry rabies, it is very unlikely. However, opossums do often carry fleas and other parasites, and the potential diseases that go along with those.

Squirrels

Like all animals, squirrels can carry a multitude of parasites. Their droppings are associated with *Leptospirosis* spp. and *Salmonella* spp. Squirrels can also be vectors for the rabies virus; therefore care must be taken when handling. Bubonic plague is caused by the bacterium *Yersinia pestis* and can be found in rodents. Fleas transmit plague from animal to animal.

Rabbits and Hares

One common zoonotic disease found in wild rabbits and hares is tularemia (also known as rabbit fever). Tularemia is a serious infectious disease caused by *Francisella tularensis* spp. This disease is found in lagomorphs in North America and is highly virulent for humans and domestic rabbits. The organism can penetrate intact undamaged skin. In humans the bacteria rapidly grow in the blood, produce high fever, and can lead to death if it goes undiagnosed and untreated.

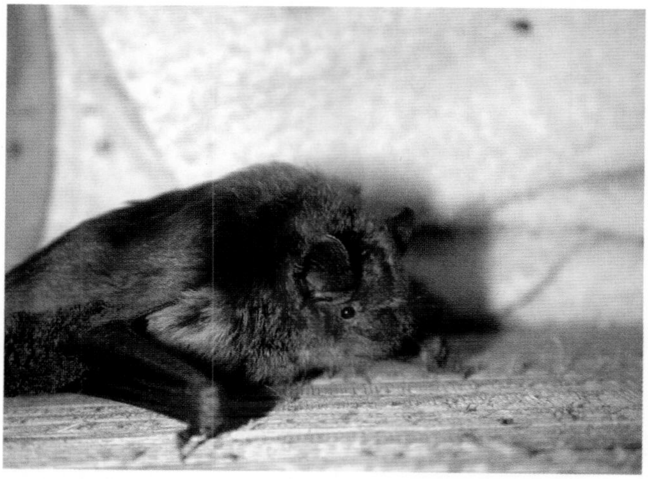

FIGURE 28-29 Bats should be given a place to hide and cling to while kept in the hospital.

Bats

Bats are the only true flying mammal. Worldwide they are primary predators of a vast number of insect pests, and help to control insect populations (Fig. 28-29). Bats are actually the most common transmitter of the rabies virus in North America. According to the Centers for Disease Control, most of the recent human rabies cases in the United States have been caused by rabies virus from bats.

Armadillos

Armadillos are not really a concern for infectious diseases in people except for one curious note. Many wild armadillos have been known to be infected with *Mycobacterium leprae,* the bacterium that causes leprosy (Hansen's disease). Transmission to humans is through excessive handling or eating the armadillo meat.

Wild Canids

Common diseases found in various wild canids include sarcoptic mange, rabies, canine distemper, and parvovirus. Proper precautions should be taken not only to yourself protect against these diseases, but also to protect domestic species hospitalized in the clinic.

ZOONOTIC AND INFECTIOUS DISEASES IN COMMON WILD ANIMAL SPECIES

Zoonotic diseases are those diseases that are communicable from animals to humans under natural conditions. Many zoonotic diseases are known to exist and wildlife serves as a reservoir for many of those diseases common to domestic

BOX 28-4 Common Zoonotic Diseases Associated With Wildlife

Bacterial Diseases
- *Chlamydophila psittaci*
- *Salmonella* spp.
- *Campylobacter* spp.
- *Escherichia coli*
- *Staphylococcus aureus*
- *Bacillus anthracis*
- *Streptococcus* spp.
- *Mycobacterium* spp.
- *Leptospira interrogans*
- *Clostridium* spp.
- *Francisella tularensis*
- *Yersinia pestis*
- *Yersinia pseudotuberculosis*
- *Rickettsia rickettsii*
- *Borrelia burgdorferi*

Fungal Diseases
- *Aspergillus* spp.
- *Histoplasma* spp.
- *Blastomyces* spp.

Viral Diseases
- Rabies
- West Nile virus
- Avian influenza
- St. Louis encephalitis
- Eastern equine encephalitis

Parasitic Diseases
- *Giardia* spp.
- *Cryptosporidium parvum*
- *Baylisascaris procyonis*
- *Ancylostoma* spp.
- *Sarcoptes* spp.
- *Encephalocytozaoon cuniculi*
- *Toxoplasma gondii*

animals and humans (Box 28-4). As professionals in the field of veterinary medicine, we should be alert to the potential for disease transmission from animals. It is important to educate ourselves and the public of this concern. In most cases you should have no reason to be alarmed or frightened, but should respect the potential for disease transmission and use sound preventive measures. In general disease is more easily prevented than treated. Some diseases are listed in Box 28-4 and grouped according to their causative agent or mode of transmission.

RABIES

Rabies is an infectious viral disease that affects the nervous system of humans and other mammals. This virus causes acute encephalitis and eventual death. People get rabies from the bite of a rabid animal. Any wild mammal, such as a raccoon, skunk, fox, coyote, or bat, can have rabies and transmit it to people. It is also possible, but quite rare, that people may get rabies if infectious material from a rabid animal, such as saliva, gets directly into their eyes, nose, mouth, or a wound.

SALMONELLOSIS

Salmonellosis is a bacterial disease caused by *Salmonella* spp. bacteria. *Salmonella* spp. exist in virtually all wildlife droppings, and several serotypes are pathogenic to humans and other animals. Salmonellosis can lead to severe cases of gastroenteritis, enteric fever septicemia (blood poisoning), and death. One common means of transmission is through food tainted by the feces of animals contaminated with the *Salmonella* spp.

CHLAMYDIOSIS

Chlamydiosis is caused by the obligate intracellular bacterium *Chlamydophila psittaci*. This is a zoonotic intracellular bacterial organism that causes the disease psittacosis in humans and avian chlamydiosis in avian species. The infectious agent is often transmitted by inhaling the organism from dried feces or feather dust from the infected bird.

LEPTOSPIROSIS

Leptospirosis is caused by bacteria in the genus *Leptospira*. It affects a wide variety of wildlife species, including rodents, skunks, and raccoons. Human cases of leptospirosis usually occur with exposure to urine of infected animals. In some cases, this disease can be very serious and life threatening. Symptoms include fever, headaches, weakness, and vomiting.

HANTAVIRUS PULMONARY SYNDROME

Hantavirus pulmonary syndrome (HPS), first discovered in 1993, is a deadly disease contracted from rodents caused by the hantavirus. Rodents such as rats and mice are the primary vectors for viruses in this group, and these viruses are found across the United States. Humans can contract the disease by coming into contact with the urine, feces, and saliva of infected rodents. The droppings from infected rodents are believed to be the source of both airborne and direct transmission to other rodents and humans.

BUBONIC PLAGUE

Bubonic plague is the best known manifestation of the bacterial disease plague caused by the bacterium *Yersinia pestis*. Bubonic plague is an infection of the lymphatic system resulting from a bite of an infected flea. These fleas can be found on wild rodents, most commonly rats. Fleas transmit plague from animal to animal. Early symptoms of bubonic plague include fever, confusion, and fatigue. Untreated bubonic plague has a relatively high fatality rate.

TULAREMIA

Tularemia is caused by *Francisella tularensis* and is a severe bacterial disease carried by rodents that is readily transmissible to humans who come into contact with contaminated food or droppings. The organism can penetrate intact undamaged skin. In humans the bacteria rapidly grow in the blood, produce high fever, and can lead to death if undiagnosed and untreated.

WEST NILE VIRUS

West Nile Virus is a virus of the family Flaviviridae. This virus is a mosquito-borne disease that infects horses, humans, birds, dogs, cats, bats, chipmunks, skunks, squirrels, and domestic rabbits. It has spread rapidly throughout the United States in the past few years. This can be a serious, life-altering, and even fatal disease. Clinical signs may include depression, anorexia, weakness, recumbency, weight loss, and neurologic signs.

ISOLATION CAGING AREA—PREVENTING THE SPREAD OF DISEASE IN THE CLINIC

Wildlife patients have a high risk of exposure to infectious diseases and can harbor various bacterial, fungal, viral, and parasitic diseases that can be transmitted to domestic pets. It is imperative that you disinfect well between patients. Wildlife suspected of having infectious diseases must be isolated from other patients. Isolation areas must be out of the mainstream of the clinic, where there is minimal foot traffic. Ideally the isolation room should have a ventilation system separate from the main clinic's system. Disposable protective shoe covers or foot baths (sodium hypochlorite 10% solution) must be used when exiting this room to prevent the tracking of infectious diseases throughout the hospital. Foot baths should be changed daily or as needed, as organic debris can accumulate in the bath and render the foot bath useless.

All veterinary team members who handle animals suspected of having a zoonotic or any infectious disease must wear personal protective equipment, not only to protect themselves against infection, but also to prevent transmission to others. Personal protective equipment includes disposable outer garments or coveralls, disposable head or hair covers and gloves, safety goggles, and disposable particulate respirators approved by the National Institute for Occupational Safety and Health. Disposable equipment should be considered contaminated and be properly disposed of after use. Nondisposable items such as lab coats and goggles should be cleaned and disinfected between uses. When removing contaminated protective equipment, personnel should remove their outer garments—except for gloves—first and discard them. They should then remove their gloves, wash their hands with soap and water, remove their goggles and particulate respirators, and immediately wash their hands again. If soap and water are not available, an alcohol-based hand gel is sufficient. NOTE: Washing your hands is the number one way to prevent the spread of disease, so do it between each patient regardless of whether the patient is suspected of carrying infectious diseases. Using these protective measures will help prevent the spread of disease in your clinic and protect those working with patients.

REVIEW QUESTIONS

Matching

Match the disease or condition with its description.

___**1.** botulism
___**2.** bubonic plague
___**3.** bumblefoot
___**4.** chlamydiosis
___**5.** *Cryptosporidium parvum*
___**6.** *Giardia*
___**7.** hantavirus pulmonary syndrome
___**8.** lead poisoning
___**9.** leptospirosis
___**10.** rabies
___**11.** salmonellosis
___**12.** trauma
___**13.** tularemia
___**14.** West Nile virus
___**15.** zinc toxicity

A. Human symptoms include fever, headaches, weakness and vomiting.
B. Highly virulent for domestic rabbits and humans.
C. Exists in virtually all wildlife droppings with several serotypes being pathogenic to humans and other animals.
D. Caused by ingestion of matter left by fishermen or guns.
E. Occurs from ingesting galvanized metal or some coins.
F. Caused by *Yersinia pestis.*
G. The most common presentation for nonraptorial birds.
H. Parasite.
I. A mosquito-borne disease.
J. A zoonotic intracellular bacterial organism.
K. This virus causes acute encephalitis and eventual death.
L. Affects the plantar surface on the feet of avians in captive management.
M. Rodents such as rats and mice are the primary vectors of viruses in this group.
N. Etiological agent is *Clostridium botulinum.*
O. Protozoa.

True or False

Indicate whether each of the following statements is True or False.

__**1.** If a fledgling or hatchling is touched by humans the mother bird will abandon it.
__**2.** Under many circumstances, a permit is required to work with or possess native wildlife, especially those that are endangered, threatened, or are protected under the Migratory Bird Act.

__3. Depending on the species you are working with, general anesthesia may be needed to perform a complete physical examination.

__4. To capture a bird, place the towel over the patient, gain control of the head, pin the wings to the body, and pick the patient up.

__5. Towels are not useful to capture wild hares and rabbits.

__6. It is acceptable to pick up any species of lizard by the tail.

__7. Some lizards such as geckos have extremely delicate skin that can easily be damaged by capture and restraint.

__8. When being handed a pillowcase that contains a snake it is not important to first find the snake's head and then gently grasp it from the outside of the pillowcase.

__9. Although chelonians are usually the easiest to capture, they are the hardest to restrain.

__10. To keep control of the head of a chelonian, it is best to position your thumb on one side of the cranial portion of the neck and the rest of your fingers just behind the base of the skull.

__11. Snapping turtles will not actually bite and if they do, they will not cause serious harm.

__12. When performing a physical examination on birds or reptiles, it is a good idea to covertly evaluate the species if possible to view signs of illness that it may be hiding.

__13. As with the physical examination of dogs and cats use a systematic approach, start at the head and work your way down to the tail, and obtain both a heart and respiratory rate as soon as the animal is removed from the cage.

__14. When performing an oral examination on rodents and rabbits, sedation or general anesthesia may still be required even with the use of a mouth speculum and light source.

__15. The same system used to assess body score in dogs and cats may be used with wild mammals, with 9 out of 9 being emaciated and 1 out of 9 being grossly obese.

__16. A visual precapture and restraint physical examination is not necessary in wild animals to determine the animal's attitude and mentation before it has been potentially stressed by handling.

__17. A systemic infection or sepsis will not be evident on the plastron of a turtle or the dorsal spines of a snake.

__18. Most reptile patients can easily be auscultated with a stethoscope.

__19. In most species of snake, the heart is located in the center third of the body.

__20. Depending on the species, common collection and diagnostic testing for laboratory analysis include fecal flotation, impression smears, Gram stain, nasal flush, and tracheal lavage.

__21. Obtaining blood from a severely trimmed toenail is acceptable in birds.

__22. Snake tubes only work well for radiographing snakes if the tubes are of appropriate size, making it impossible for the snake to move or become obliqued.

__23. It is not uncommon for healthy snakes to have pale mucous membranes.

__24. The goal of wildlife medicine should be to treat the species regardless of whether the patient is releasable and able to thrive in the wild.

__25. Injectable drugs such as ketamine, dexmedetomidine, xylazine, telazol, full μ opioids, buprenorphine, butorphanol, and midazolam can be used alone or in combination with each other to sedate or induce anesthesia.

RECOMMENDED READING

Carpenter JW: *Exotic animal formulary*, ed 3, St Louis, 2005, Saunders.

Fowler M: *Zoo and wild animal medicine*, ed 5, St Louis, 2003, Saunders.

Fowler M: *Zoo and wild animal medicine current therapy*, ed 6, St Louis, 2008, Saunders Elsevier.

Fowler M: *Zoo and wild animal medicine current therapy*, ed 4, St Louis, 1999, Saunders.

Harrison G, Lightfoot T: *Clinical avian medicine*, vol. I & II. Palm Beach, FL, 2006, Spitz Publishing.

Mader D: *Reptile medicine and surgery*, ed 2, St Louis, 2006, Saunders.

Mitchell M, Tully T: *Manual of exotic pet practice*, St Louis, 2009, Saunders.

O'Malley B: *Clinical anatomy and physiology of exotic species*, St Louis, 2005, Elsevier.

Quesenberry K, Carpenter J: *Ferrets, rabbits, and rodents: clinical medicine and surgery*, ed 2, St Louis, 2004, Saunders.

Ritchie BW, Harrison GJ, Harrison LR: *Avian medicine: principles and application*, Lake Worth, FL, 1994, Wingers Publishing.

Silverman S, Tell LA: *Radiology of birds: an atlas of normal anatomy and positioning*, St Louis, 2010, Elsevier.

Silverman S, Tell L: *Radiology of rodents, rabbits and ferrets: an atlas of normal anatomy and positioning*, St Louis, 2005, Elsevier.

Stocker L: *Practical wildlife care*, Malden, 2000, Blackwell Science.

West G, et al.: *Zoo animal and wildlife: immobilization and anesthesia*, Ames, IA, 2007, Blackwell Publishing.

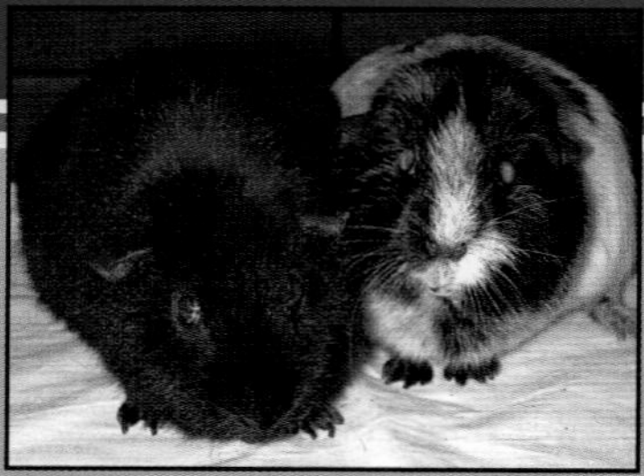

29 Nursing Care of Laboratory Animals

OUTLINE

LEARNING OBJECTIVES

After reviewing this chapter, the reader will be able to:

1. Discuss how biomedical research affects the lives of people and animals.
2. Describe the positive and negatives aspects of biomedical research.
3. Describe the views of the animal rights and animal liberationist groups.
4. List and describe the laws that protect animals from abuse.
5. Explain the principles of the 3 Rs.
6. Describe the role of mice and rats in biomedical research.
7. State the general characteristics of mice, rats, hamsters, gerbils, guinea pigs, chinchillas, rabbits, and ferrets.
8. Discuss husbandry and principles of sanitation for laboratory animals.
9. Describe techniques for general nursing care of rodents, rabbits, and ferrets.
10. Describe techniques used for diagnosing and treating disease in small mammals.
11. List and describe methods of sample collection in laboratory animals.
12. State routes of administration of medication in laboratory animals.
13. Describe identification methods used in research animals.
14. Discuss anesthesia of rodents, rabbits, and ferrets.

KEY TERMS

Ad libitum	Bumblefoot	IACUC	Rodents
Alopecia	Cavys	Jill	Sentinel
Animal model	Doe	Lagomorphs	Sow
Barbering	GEM	Malocclusion	Transgenic
Boar	Hobs	Murine	Zoonotic
Buck	Husbandry	Pruritus	

This chapter has two major objectives. First we address the field of biomedical research. Biomedical research, which uses live animals as research models, is explained, defined, and evaluated. Our discussion includes both the positive results of biomedical research and the negative aspects that must be considered, including the arguments of those groups that oppose the use of animals for this purpose. The role of the general public and the legislation that governs biomedical research is looked at closely to understand the current status of this important segment of medical research. Our discussion includes the different species used most often in research, with special emphasis given to the role of mice and rats. Finally we discuss the opportunities of trained veterinary technicians within the biomedical community.

Our second objective is to discuss specific species of small mammals that are used both as research animals and domestic pets. Our discussion includes the important aspects of **husbandry** for each species, and when applicable, the use of the species in research.

THE USE OF ANIMALS TO ADVANCE MEDICAL KNOWLEDGE: THE PROS, THE CONS, AND THE LAWS

The use of animals in biomedical research is a controversial subject. During the past century many of the advances in human medicine can be directly attributed to research done with animals. We all benefit from biomedical research every day of our lives. Anyone who has ever taken an antibiotic, been given a general anesthetic, or knows a diabetic who takes insulin has seen the benefit of animal research. Today, recipients of heart bypass surgery and heart and kidney transplants can all thank animal research for developing these life-saving procedures. Animals have benefited as well; our pet animals now live longer happier lives because of the vaccines and other drugs that were developed through biomedical research.

The list of the positive ways biomedical research has changed our lives is extensive and grows each year. However, with every positive there are negatives that must also be considered, and therein lies the controversy. Many of the progressive accomplishments of biomedical research required the sacrifice of animal life. To people who consider themselves animal activists, this is totally unacceptable, regardless of the benefits.

Two of the most active well-funded animal rights and animal liberation groups in the United States are the Animal Liberation Front (ALF) and People for the Ethical Treatment of Animals (PETA). The feelings of these groups were summed up by Ingrid Newkirk, a founder of PETA, in her famous quote:

> Animal liberationists do not separate out the human animal, so there is no rational basis for saying that a human being has special rights. A rat is a pig is a dog is a boy. They are all mammals. (*Vogue*, September 1, 1989)

Hence animal rights and animal liberation groups look at human life and animal life as equal, and they believe that animals deserve the same rights as people. Therefore they conclude that any activity that uses animals for the benefit of humankind should be stopped. These include:

1. Animals kept in zoos and the circus
2. Animals raised for food and/or clothing
3. Animals used in sport, such as horse and dog races
4. Purebred animals sold as pets and those that compete in shows
5. The euthanasia of unwanted animals
6. Pet ownership
7. The use of animals in biomedical research and teaching

Specifically, in their opposition to biomedical research they argue that if we do not conduct research on people without their consent, we should not do research on animals that are unable to give their consent. Their doctrine simply states that any activity that is seen as unsuitable for humans should not be used on animals.

Significant funds are spent each year by PETA and other groups in an effort to enlist people from the general public to their cause. Students, beginning in elementary school, are targeted, as are pet owners, and anyone with an emotional tie to animals. How would you feel, they ask, if your pet was used in animal research? The fact that the likelihood of a family pet ending up in a research facility is infinitesimally small does not enter into the picture. Emotions sometimes carry more weight than facts.

We live in a free society, and debates of the ethical and moral aspects of biomedical research are legitimate topics for debate. Thankfully the majority of persons who call themselves animal liberationists are law-abiding citizens who enter debates, petition their legislators, and demonstrate legally. However, small groups of animal advocates exist whose actions are considered terroristic. These individuals resort to illegal and sometimes violent acts in the name of animal rights, which have led to arrests and jail sentences. Unfortunately, during the last decade, incidents of vandalism, cybercrimes, physical violence, and even death threats have increased. Many law-abiding animal liberationists have questioned if these acts of violence have helped or hindered the animal rights movement in the mind of the general public. How then does the average citizen feel about using animals as research subjects?

When the general public is polled on the propriety of using animals in biomedical research, a significant majority approves. Most individuals in our culture understand the value and necessity of biomedical research, but they also insist that animal subjects should never be mistreated or abused. Americans, as a society, believe that animals should always be treated with care and consideration. Throughout the years these feelings have been backed up by laws that protect against animal abuse. The ownership of an animal is considered a privilege. Hence pet owners who abuse their animals face strict legal consequences.

What then are the obligations of the research community? Animal welfare organizations such as the American Society for the Prevention of Cruelty to Animals (ASPCA) accept the necessity of using animals in biomedical research but demand that these animals be treated with kindness and compassion. The animal welfare groups have successfully lobbied legislatures to enact legislation specifically written for the biomedical industry. These laws protect research animals and make the scientists responsible for any abuses that may occur.

In the field of biomedical research, all personnel are guided by the concept of the three Rs. The concept was developed by William Russell and Rex Burch in 1959. The three Rs stand for Reduction, Replacement, and Refinement. Let us take a quick look at how these three basic concepts are put to use by the biomedical profession.

REDUCTION

The concept of reduction is the simplest to understand. Reduction means that the number of animals requested must be the minimum needed to show scientific accuracy. However, it also means that enough animals must be requested to make the results scientifically meaningful; if not, the animals may have been sacrificed for naught. Each animal life is important and none should be wasted unnecessarily.

REPLACEMENT

Replacement requires the scientist to show that a nonanimal model cannot be used to obtain the required data. The use of computer models, tissue cultures, or other synthetic systems has replaced many animal models in the past decades. Replacement can also mean that the lowest form of life that can be used is employed as the research model. Scientists have placed all animals on a relative scale in consideration of their evolutionary closeness to humans; with single-cell organisms such as the amoeba at one end and our closest relatives, nonhuman primates, at the other. A scientist is obligated to use the lowest-scale animal possible. For example, a scientist who proposes a research project using nonhuman primates would be permitted to perform the experiments only if there is significant evidence that no other alternative model exists.

REFINEMENT

Refinement includes three major aspects:

1. The research cannot be trivial and must be of obvious benefit to humankind. The profession rightfully discourages the use of animals in any project that cannot show significant scientific value.
2. Secondly, refinement demands that only the most qualified and trained persons are permitted to do research with live animals. The use of animals in high school science projects, for example, is seldom approved.
3. Most importantly, refinement ensures that pain and discomfort to the animals will be eliminated or minimized whenever possible. This is an obligation that is taken very seriously.

Almost all federal laws on the care and use of animals within the biomedical industry originate from two sources: the Animal Welfare Act, under the direction of the Secretary of the U.S. Department of Agriculture (USDA), and the Health Research Extension Act, directed by the Secretary of Health and Human Services. The National Institutes of Health (NIH), a division of Health and Human Services, establishes rules for compliance with the federal laws. The NIH has a sub-branch called the Office of Laboratory Animal Welfare (OLAW) that publishes the Public Health Services (PHS) Policy on Humane Care and Use of Laboratory Animals. The National Research Council publishes "The Guide for the Care and Use of Laboratory Animals," The Guide, which establishes standards for animal care and use. Both the USDA and the NIH require research institutions to conform to the regulations found in the publication The Guide.

> *TECHNICIAN NOTE* Remember the 3 Rs: Reduction, Replacement, and Refinement.

In very specialized situations, other laws and agencies come into play. Research sometimes requires the capture of animals from the wild. In such cases, other agencies, including the U.S. Fish and Wildlife Service and the Department of the Interior, must be involved. Some of the laws enforced by these agencies include the Endangered Species Act, the Lacy Act, and the Marine Mammal Protection Act. International treaties intended to protect endangered species and migratory birds are also invoked to enforce specific requirements in certain research projects.

The Animal Welfare Act and the Health Research Extension Act set specific guidelines concerning review of all animal activities by an Institutional Animal Care and Use Committee (IACUC). The American Welfare Act (AWA) first passed by Congress in 1966 has been amended on several occasions. The laws are very objective. They empower the IACUC to address every aspect of animal use, including a review of the specific research that will be conducted, housing of the animals, specific enrichment plans, pain management, and training of research personnel. Since there is great variation in research projects, each institution is allowed to develop its own Animal Care Policy based on its specific needs and the federal legal requirements. In all cases, the IACUC includes a veterinarian and at least one outside member, a nonscientist with no association with the company or institute of learning. In this way, the law ensures that the IACUC addresses the needs of the animals and the concerns of the general public.

During the past four decades all legislation and official policy decrees have had one simple goal: the betterment of the life of research animals. Today, the biomedical profession is the third most regulated industry in the United States. The image of the mad scientist doing terrible experiments on animals in his basement is a mere Hollywood fantasy. True biomedical research is carefully regulated, institutionalized, and supervised. The veterinary profession applauds this progress. The biomedical industry can be proud of its accomplishments and the high ethical standards it maintains.

THE ROLE OF THE VETERINARY TECHNICIAN IN BIOMEDICAL RESEARCH

A career in the biomedical sciences appeals to a certain type of person. A genuine interest in advancing science is essential. Each experiment offers new challenges, which appeals to many people. Workers in the profession must feel that what is being done to gain scientific knowledge is important, necessary, and done in a way that shows compassion for the animals. Feeling good about the path you have chosen is essential for a technician's success.

Successful laboratory animal technicians are always careful and meticulous persons, who will record what they see and do it with candor and accuracy. They understand the rules and are willing to abide by them. Compensation for technicians in the biomedical industry is usually higher than in private practice. Other benefits not always seen in private practice include regular hours, health and pension benefits, and the opportunity for advancement. Many persons, who began as laboratory animal caretakers, advance to laboratory animal technicians, then laboratory animal technologist, and vivarium supervisors. With advancement comes an increased financial reward as well as the satisfaction of knowing that they are an essential part of the biomedical research team.

ANIMALS USED IN BIOMEDICAL RESEARCH

Everyone hopes that the day will come when animals are no longer used as research subjects. It is the hope of the future and a realistic goal. However, the reality of the present is that animal research still represents the best way for humankind to solve its medical problems.

Over the years, hundreds of different species have been used as research subjects, from the fruit fly to the zebra fish to the armadillo, to large farm animals such as sheep and goats. The public accepts most species as research animals without emotion, but the exceptions are dogs, cats, and nonhuman primates. No one, including scientists, really wants to work with these animals, so for many years the research community has developed alternatives to their use, and today the three species combined make up only about 3% of the total number of animals used in research. Where then does the remaining 97% come from? Approximately 90% of all animals used as biomedical models are mice and rats. The remaining 7% is made up of all the other species, including many of the animals discussed later in this chapter, but first we will examine the role rats and mice now occupy in biomedical research.

> **TECHNICIAN NOTE** More than 90% of all animal research is done with rodents.

MICE AND RATS: CREATING THE ULTIMATE RESEARCH ANIMALS

Since early in the 20th century scientists have studied mice and rats with great care and precision. We know more about mice and rats' genetic makeup than that of any other species. This wealth of information is available to every scientist, permitting them to begin their work at the highest level possible.

WHY MICE AND RATS ARE POPULAR EXPERIMENTAL MODELS

Rats and mice have become the most commonly used research animals for the following reasons:

1. Both species are mammals, sharing many genetic traits with humans.
2. Both species are relatively inexpensive to obtain, house, and maintain.
3. Mice and rats breed easily with short gestation periods and large litters that mature quickly.
4. These two species are relatively easy to handle and adjust well to housing in a research facility.
5. Decades of research with these species have created the largest data base for any animal model, shortening the time and animal numbers that a scientist needs to establish normal values.
6. Extensive variations within the species have been developed. As an example a researcher who is studying diabetes can choose a strain of mouse or rat that has a predisposition for this condition.
7. Both species can be genetically engineered to create animals with specific conditions that mimic human diseases.
8. The general public finds it easier to accept mice and rats as research models in preference to using cats, dogs, and nonhuman primates.

TYPES OF MICE AND RATS AVAILABLE TO RESEARCHERS

As the knowledge of these two species developed, colonies of specialized animals were created that satisfied specific needs of research scientists. The following are some of the most commonly used varieties of mice and rats.

1. *Inbred Strains:* After 20 or more generations of inbreeding, all members of this group are close to genetically identical. *Uses in Research:* Used to study a specific condition (such as leukemia) because all the subjects are genetically the same.
2. *Outbred Stock:* Compared with a race of people, each member of an outbred stock is part of a large group in which all the animals have a natural bond, but each is individually unique genetically. *Uses in Research:* Used in toxicology studies because outbred animals represent the natural mix found in the general population.
3. *Mutant Strains:* Colonies of animals have been developed from individuals who underwent spontaneous mutations that gave them a predisposition for specific unique traits. Here are some examples of existing mutant strains:
   a. Immunodeficient animals
   b. Animals with a high rate of mammary tumors
   c. Obese animals
   d. Animals with high blood pressure

Uses in Research: These animals become specific models for the human diseases which correspond to the predisposition of the animal.

GENETICALLY ENGINEERED ANIMALS

Since the 1980s scientists have been developing techniques that can successfully change the genetic makeup of animals. Scientists can now introduce human genetic DNA into a nonhuman fertilized egg or a developing zygote and have the human DNA become part of the mature animal. For example, it is now possible to purchase human milk that was produced by a goat.

Mice are the animals most used for genetic engineering, and these animals are called **GEM,** which stands for genetically engineered mice. The procedures to produce these animals are complicated, expensive, and not always successful, but the animals that have been successfully created have revolutionized biomedical research. These are unique animals that have never existed before and are specific to study particular human genetic diseases. Here are the most common types of GEM seen in research:

1. **Transgenic** Mice: Animals containing foreign DNA that was injected directly into the pronucleus of a mouse zygote. This DNA will be passed on to offspring.
2. Knock-Out Mice: The animals have a nonfunctional section of their DNA produced by targeting embryonic stem cells.
3. Knock-In Mice: This refers to a gene overexpression produced when a transgene is inserted directly into the existing DNA.

Genetic engineering is still in its infancy. Most scientists believe that in the future biomedical research will rely more and more on these procedures. Indeed, GEM may eventually replace the vast majority of other animal models.

ANIMAL MODELS

To study a specific human disease, research scientists look for an animal whose anatomy and/or physiology closely resembles the human condition. The animals chosen are called **animal models.** Many different factors enter into the choice of a model. For example, the nine-banded armadillo is a unique animal that is susceptible to human leprosy and is therefore the perfect model to study this disease. In other cases animals are chosen as models if their specific body structures, physiologic values, or life expectancies are significant to the study.

The remainder of this chapter discusses the following species: mouse, rat, hamster, guinea pig, rabbit, chinchillas, and ferrets. These small mammals are popular pets and are often referred to as "pocket pets" because of their small size. We address the needs and requirements of these pet animals in some detail; however, these small mammals can also function as research subjects. To understand some of their values in biomedical research please refer to Table 29-1, in which

TABLE 29-1 Animals in Biomedical Research

SPECIES	USE IN RESEARCH	RATIONALE FOR USE
Mice and rats	Research that requires specific genetic variations Drug testing Toxicity studies	Adaptable to extensive genetic engineering Physiology and organ function similar to human Physiology and organ function similar to human
Chinchillas	Dental diseases Audio research Chagas' disease (American trypanosomiasis)	Very susceptible to dental disease Chinchilla has similar middle ear anatomy to humans Species is native to South America, where this protozoon parasite is commonly found
Guinea pigs	Immunology, nutrition, audiology Anaphylaxis studies	Physiology and organ anatomy similar to human Often respond to histamine release with bronchial constriction
Rabbits	Antibody production Drug toxicology studies Draize Eye Test: Evaluates the adverse effects of commercial products, such as cosmetics, if they should accidentally get into the eye. Note: Whenever possible this test is replaced with procedures that do not require live animals, such as the use of cell lines.	Easily assessable veins and arteries in ear Physiology and organ anatomy similar to human The prominent rabbit eye
Hamster	Cancer studies Hypothermia studies Diabetes mellitus studies	Human tissue can be transplanted in hamster cheek pouches without rejection. Species can exist in hibernated state with very low body temperature. The Chinese hamster has a naturally occurring form of diabetes mellitus.
Gerbil	Epilepsy Stroke research	High incidence of spontaneous seizures. An incomplete Circle of Willis allows arterial manipulation in the brain simulating a stroke in people.

specific research areas are listed. Please understand that this table contains only some common examples of how each species is used and is not a complete listing of all the uses of the species as a research subject.

SMALL MAMMALS KEPT AS PETS AND USED IN RESEARCH

Small mammals are popular pets. These "pocket pets" include ferrets, rabbits, mice, rats, hamsters, gerbils, guinea pigs, and chinchillas. Although small mammals are relatively easy to care for, they require care that is different from that of dogs and cats. Prospective owners should be encouraged to read about a species they have never cared for before. Sometimes success or failure in raising and animal will depend on the knowledge an owner has about the pet.

Small mammals are often purchased as first pets for children. Small mammals can make acceptable pets for children, but children should always be supervised when handling these delicate creatures. Small mammals can bite, and children should be made aware of this and told that these pets are "real live creatures" and not stuffed animals. All pets should be handled with care. Small mammals should not be allowed free run of the house, because this can prove fatal to them. Because the life span of most small mammals is only 2 to 4 years, children should be counseled so that an "early" death is not unexpected. Allergies to animal dander, saliva, and urinary proteins occur commonly in humans. Cutaneous and upper respiratory allergies to small mammals, especially rats and guinea pigs, are very common.

Special anatomic and physiologic traits in different species make them valuable for specific research projects. The mice and rats that are most commonly used in research are produced by commercial breeders specifically for research. These animals are raised in special environments, using pathogen-free barriers that prevent the introduction of disease agents. The use of small mammals as research models has made valuable contributions to science and has advanced the medical care of humans and animals alike.

HOUSING

Caging must be escape-proof to prevent injury or fatality. **Rodents** can be housed in plastic or metal cages with slotted bars or wire mesh lids. Shoebox-type cages made of plastic materials are popular for housing rodents (Fig. 29-1). Cages hung from a supporting frame are frequently seen in research settings. Several individual cages can be placed on a shelving unit called a rack (Fig. 29-2). Cage flooring can be either solid bottom or wire mesh. Solid flooring with bedding material is generally preferred. If mesh flooring is used, care must be taken to prevent foot injury and loss of neonates through the flooring. Aquariums are adequate to house pet rodents, but should have a screen-type top with locking device. This type of housing unit allows easy access to the pet; however, it is heavy and can be difficult to clean. When aquariums are used for housing, care should be taken to ensure that rodents have access to food and water. Conventional cages such as those purchased from pet stores should have a large door to facilitate easy removal of the animal and be easy to disassemble and clean. Rabbits, chinchillas, and ferrets can be housed in wire or front-opening cages with catch pans to collect urine and feces. Pet ferrets and rabbits can also be housed in large cat or dog carriers with a litterbox. Some owners build rather elaborate "condos" for their pet rabbits and ferrets. Rabbits and ferrets can be housed outdoors, but care must be taken to prevent heat stroke, myiasis, and dog and cat attacks. Animals maintained outdoors should be provided with shelter from direct sunlight, rain, snow, and wind.

In a research setting, The Guide, mentioned previously, should be used to determine minimum cage size requirements. In research facilities, different species are housed in

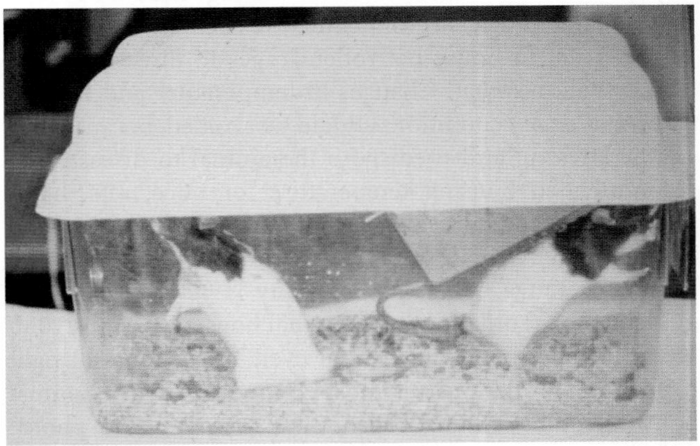

FIGURE 29-1 Shoebox-type cage with microisolator top.

FIGURE 29-2 Rack of individual shoebox cages.

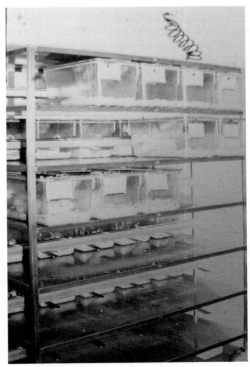

separate rooms to meet experimental requirements, prevent interspecies disease transmission, and reduce anxiety because of interspecies conflict. In addition, in certain cases special housing may be required. Immunocompromised rodents are housed in microisolator cages or ventilated cage racks in which air is HEPA-filtered to reduce their exposure to viruses or bacteria. Metabolic cages allow for collection of urine and feces, and inhalation chambers provide a way to expose an animal to various agents.

Animals should be housed in caging that is appropriate for the animal's size and weight and in accordance with current regulations or guidelines. Some animals, such as chinchillas, are very acrobatic and active and should be provided with a large cage to allow for exercise. Cage height should allow an animal to make normal postural adjustments. For example, gerbils frequently sit upright, so the height of their caging should allow them to do so. The cage should be located in an area protected from climatic extremes. Care should be taken not to house pet rodent cages in direct sunlight, as they will overheat. Changes in temperature and humidity and/or drafty conditions should be avoided, because they can be stressful and predispose the animal to disease. The recommended housing temperature for mice, rats, hamsters, gerbils, and guinea pigs is 18° to 26° C, for rabbits and chinchillas is 16° to 22° C, and for ferrets is 4° to 18° C. The acceptable range of relative humidity is 30% to 70%. The guideline for ventilation in an animal housing room is 10 to 15 air changes per hour. A light cycle of 12 hours of light to 12 hours of darkness is most commonly used in animal housing rooms. Albino rodents are susceptible to phototoxicity, so care should be taken to ensure safe illumination levels in their housing area. Noise should be minimized in animal housing areas because excessive sound exposure can be stressful and produce untoward effects. It is important to remember that many species can hear frequencies of sound that are inaudible to humans and some rodents are prone to sound-induced seizures.

Bedding used for solid-bottom caging should be absorbent, comfortable, nonnutritive, nontoxic, and disposable. A variety of bedding material can be used, including paper, sawdust and soft pine, aspen, cedar, corncob, or hardwood chips. Cedar and soft pine shavings are frequently used for pet rodent bedding because of their pleasant aroma. These should be avoided in a research setting because they emit aromatic hydrocarbons that induce liver changes and cytotoxicity. Burrowing rodents such as the rat and gerbil should be provided with deeper bedding to allow for this behavior.

Cage toys can provide psychological stimulation as well as exercise for small mammals. Tubes, mazes, and exercise wheels are popular. Timid animals such as guinea pigs and chinchillas are more comfortable if they are given a place to hide. Polyvinyl chloride plumbing pipes, especially elbows and Y and T sections, make ideal hiding places. These pipes can be sanitized in the dishwasher. Cardboard tubes, softwood pieces, and small Nylabones can be given to rodents to gnaw on. Paper tissues or towels can be given to rodents who build nests, such as mice, gerbils, and hamsters. Metallic items like washers can be suspended in a rabbit's cage to encourage nudging, playing, and investigative behaviors. Paper bags, hard plastic or metal toys, or cloth toys made for cats or babies are safe for ferrets. Ferrets love to run through cylindrical objects such as large mailing tubes and dryer vent tubing. Latex rubber toys that are intended for dogs or cats should not be given to ferrets.

SANITATION

Sanitation involves bedding changes, cleaning to remove dirt and debris, and disinfection to reduce or eliminate microorganisms. All animal caging and bedding must be cleaned or changed as often as necessary to prevent accumulation of odor and waste, and to keep the animals clean and dry. A major cause of respiratory disease in small mammal pets is poor environmental ventilation, which allows ammonia from accumulation of urine to irritate the pet's airways. Caging is usually cleaned once or twice a week. After removal of gross dirt, urine, and feces, cages should be disinfected by washing all surfaces with hot water (82° C) or by applying a disinfectant solution. A good, safe, readily available disinfectant for animal cages is laundry bleach (5% sodium hypochlorite), prepared by mixing 30 ml in 1 L of water. A fresh mixture should be prepared before using, because it deteriorates upon standing. Rabbit, guinea pig, and hamster urine is alkaline and contains crystals. Urine crystals accumulate, forming a scale on the cage that can be difficult to remove. Acidic products available commercially or white vinegar can be used to remove the scale. It is important to thoroughly rinse detergents and disinfectants from cleaned cages and feeders, because residues may cause health problems. Deodorizers should not be used to mask animal odors, because they can be toxic to the animal or add a variable to a research study.

DIET

The rat and mouse are omnivorous, whereas the guinea pig, rabbit, chinchilla, and gerbil are herbivorous. The hamster is primarily granivorous. Ferrets are carnivorous and depend upon meat protein and fats for their dietary requirements. Animals should be fed a clean, wholesome, and nutritious diet **ad libitum,** free choice. It is important to feed a balanced diet, freshly milled and formulated for that particular species. Pelleted foods are available commercially. These diets are complete and do not require supplementation. Block-style pellets work well for rodents such as mice, rats, hamsters, and gerbils. Much of the rodent feed found in pet stores and sold as seed mixes or treats is inadequate in protein for these species. Smaller pelleted foods work well for guinea pigs, chinchillas, and rabbits. Rabbits should be fed a high-fiber rabbit chow to prevent obesity and hairball formation. Rabbits, guinea pigs, and chinchillas can be fed small amounts of grass or alfalfa hay. Hay not only provides them with fiber, but helps reduce boredom. Ferrets can be fed ferret chow or commercial cat food. As with dogs and cats, periodontal disease is common in ferrets. Feeding dry food can help reduce tartar accumulation. In most instances, the food should be placed in a feeder hung in the animal's cage. This prevents soiling of the food with urine and feces, keeping it dry and clean. If vegetables or fruit are offered to supplement the diet, they should be fresh and washed before feeding them. Any uneaten vegetables or fruits should be removed daily. Supplements should not make up more than 10% of the animal's daily food ration. Animals should have access to fresh water via an automatic watering system or water bottles with sipper tubes.

In the research environment specialized diets may be required. Often the nature of the study will determine the contents of the diet, resulting in the addition or subtraction of one or more components. As examples a pregnant female may be fed a diet with a higher protein content, and diets that can be autoclaved are used to feed barrier-housed animals.

RODENTS

Mice, rats, gerbils, hamsters, guinea pigs, and chinchillas are rodents. The word *rodent* is derived from a Latin verb that means to gnaw. Rodents have four continuously erupting chisel-like incisors and powerful jaw muscles that contribute to their gnawing ability. They are nocturnal for the most part, being more active at night rather than during the day. The sex of most rodents can be determined by anogenital distance, the distance being longer in males and shorter in females (Fig. 29-3). Rodents are usually prolific breeders. Pet owners need to be aware of the potential for overpopulation when housing animals of the opposite sex together. The term **murine** specifically refers to mice and rats. Guinea pigs and chinchillas are hystricomorph, or hedgehog-like, rodents related to porcupines.

> *TECHNICIAN NOTE* Mice, rats, and rabbits cannot vomit.

Although rodents do not require annual vaccinations, an annual examination is recommended to ensure good health and husbandry. Owners should be encouraged to bring their new pet in for a visit to the veterinarian. The pet can be examined to ensure health, maintain the "health guarantee" that might accompany the purchase, and allow the technician and doctor to educate the owner on proper feeding, housing, and handling of the species.

MICE

The mouse *(Mus musculus)* is a small rodent, easily housed and handled, and relatively inexpensive to purchase and maintain as a pet. It is the animal most commonly used in research. The exact number of mice used annually in research is not known but it has been estimated in the millions. Balb/c (albino), C57BL (black), and C3H (agouti) are common inbred strains of mice. Swiss and ICR are outbred stocks of mice. Mutant and genetically altered mice provide researchers with a wide variety of animal models to study diseases. Indeed, genetically engineered mice (GEM) are fast becoming the biomedical research scientists' most valuable tool.

Mice may live up to 3 years. They weigh 20 to 40 g and have a rapid heart rate (approximately 500 to 600

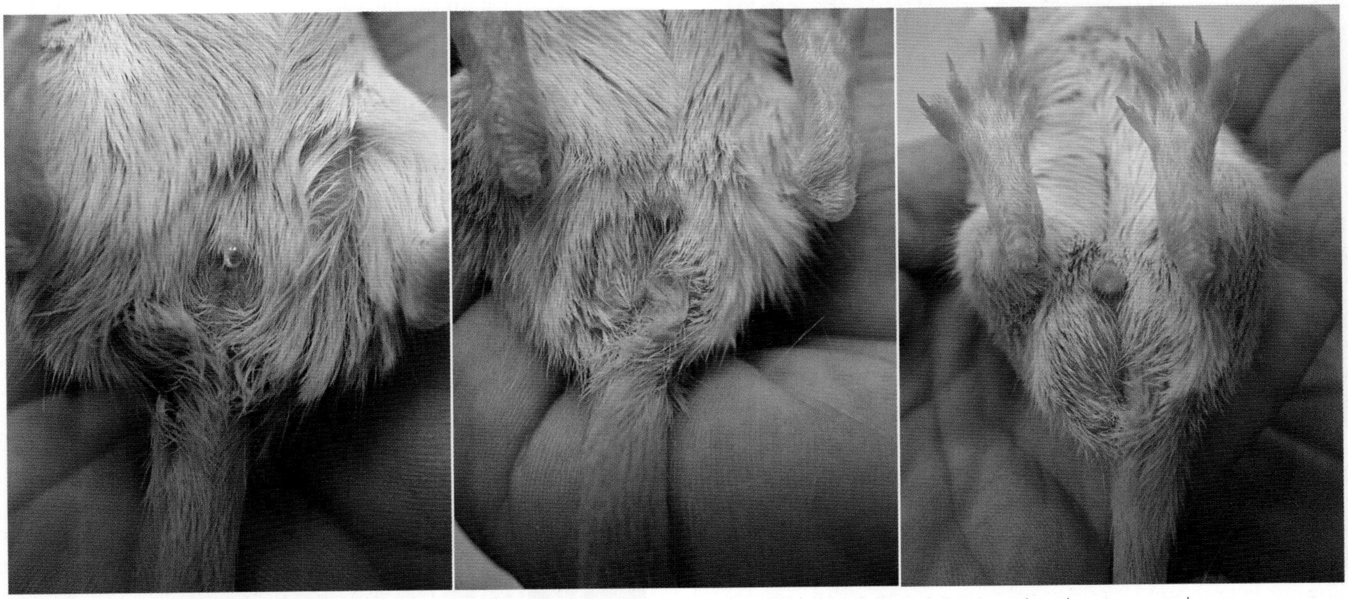

FIGURE 29-3 External genitalia of the male *(right, middle)* and female *(left)* gerbil. Note that the anogenital distance of the female is shorter than that of the male. The adult male can also be determined by the presence of testicles in the scrotum *(right)*, but the frightened gerbil may retract the testicles from the scrotum *(middle)*. (From Mitchell M, Tully TN, Jr: *Manual of exotic pet practice*, St Louis, 2008, Saunders.)

beats/min), a rapid respiration rate, and a body temperature of 36.5° to 38° C. Mice have a high metabolic rate and are constantly active. They spend much of their time grooming and keeping their environment organized. Their mammary glands are extensive, reaching from the ventral midline to the back and neck. Like most rodents, the gender of mice is determined by anogenital distance. Mice are continuously polyestrous, with an estrous cycle lasting only 4 days. The female mouse should always be taken to the male, because a female will defend her living space and may injure the male. The male is less defensive and will accept the presence of the female more readily. Mating can be confirmed by the presence of a white, waxy vaginal plug 12 to 24 hours after breeding. The gestation length is 21 days, with pups born hairless and helpless. Young mice are weaned at 21 days of age.

Mice can be caught and safely picked up by grasping the scruff of the neck with forceps or by grasping the base of the tail with the fingers (Fig. 29-4). For manipulation or examination, the animal is caught by the base of the tail and placed on a surface it can grasp, such as the cage lid. The scruff of the neck is then grasped by the thumb and forefinger (Fig. 29-5), and the mouse is inverted to lie on its back with the tail positioned between the palm of the hand and the little finger. Clear plastic restraint devices can also be used for restraint and manipulation (Fig. 29-6).

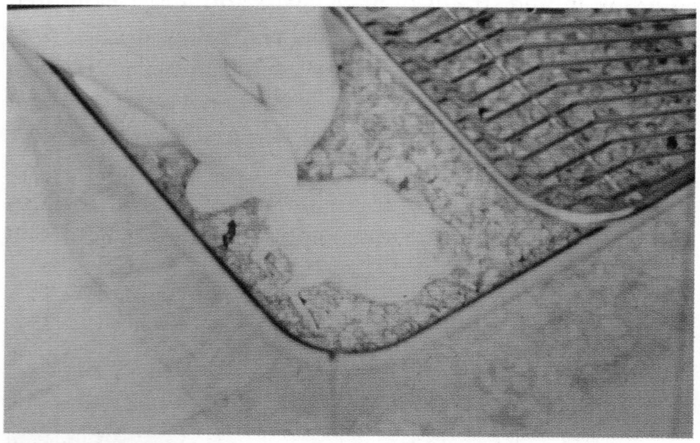

FIGURE 29-4 Proper technique for removal of a mouse from its cage.

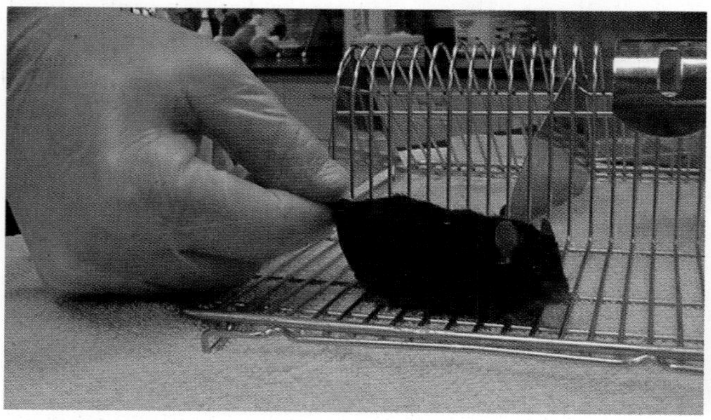

FIGURE 29-5 Proper technique for picking up a mouse. Grasp the loose skin over the back of the neck when the animal grabs the bars of the wire cage lid. (From Sheldon CC, et al: *Animal restraint for veterinary professionals*, St Louis, 2006, Mosby.)

A dominant mouse sometimes chews the fur off a subordinate mouse in the facial area. This harmless behavior is called **barbering.** Unlike female mice, male mice housed together frequently fight. Bite wounds are inflicted on the back and rump. Mite infestation can also produce areas of **alopecia** around the facial area, and is accompanied by **pruritus.** *Syphacia* and *Aspiculuris* are common endoparasites. These pinworms are generally considered nonpathogenic. Diarrhea is often of viral origin. Mouse hepatitis virus (MHV) infection is widespread and highly contagious. It can produce respiratory and/or gastrointestinal disease.

RATS

The common rat *(Rattus norvegicus)*, found in pet stores or research laboratories, was developed from the wild brown Norway rat. Rats are easily maintained and make excellent pets if handled gently. They are burrowers and communal critters. Several females and males may be housed together, as fighting rarely occurs among adults. They are the second most commonly used laboratory animal. Hooded or Long-Evans rats have pigmented eyes and are white with darker hair (tan to black) over portions of the head and back. They tend to be smaller than albino rats, such as Sprague-Dawley and Wistar.

The life span of the rat is 2½ to 3½ years. Rats weigh 250 to 500 g, with females being smaller than males. Their body temperature is 36° to 37.5° C. Rats have continuously erupting incisors and cheeks that close into the diastema, a space that separates the incisors from the oral cavity. They have no gall bladder. The Harderian gland, a lacrimal gland located caudal to the eyeball, secretes a red porphyrin-rich secretion that lubricates the eye. In times of stress or illness, red tears overflow and stain the face and nose. The stomach is divided into two parts, a nonglandular forestomach and a glandular pyloric portion. The esophagus enters through a fold of the ridge that separates the two parts of the stomach. This fold is responsible for the rat's inability to vomit. This inability to vomit is a major reason why rats have been useful research subjects in toxicology studies.

Rats are continuously polyestrous, with an estrous cycle length of 4 to 5 days. Mating can be confirmed by the presence

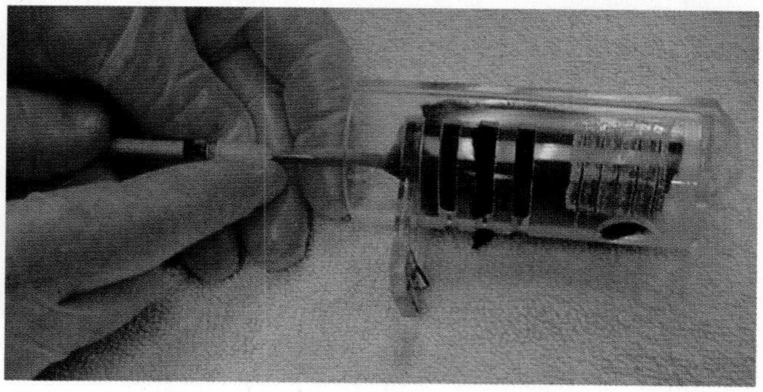

FIGURE 29-6 Mouse restraining device. (From Sheldon CC, et al: *Animal restraint for veterinary professionals*, St Louis, 2006, Mosby.)

of a plug in the vagina 12 to 24 hours postbreeding. The vaginal plug can also be discharged in the cage or litter pan. Females are usually separated from the male before parturition. Gestation is 21 days in length, with pups born hairless and helpless. Young rat pups are weaned at 21 days of age.

TECHNICIAN NOTE Most rodents' incisors grow continuously, so they need hard food to prevent overgrowth.

Rats can be caught and safely picked up by grasping the base of the tail to transport them a short distance, such as when changing cages. When rats are held upside down, they are more interested in righting themselves than in biting the handler. To restrain for manipulation or examination, pick up the rat by placing the hand firmly over the back and rib cage and restraining the rat's head and shoulders with one's thumb and forefinger (Fig. 29-7). If additional control is needed, the base of the tail may be restrained with the other hand. An alternative method is to pin the rat with your free hand while pulling on the base of the tail. Position your index and third fingers to firmly grasp either side of the rat's neck caudal to the mandible; the thumb and other fingers are used to gently restrain the chest.

Overgrowth of the incisors can occur when the jaw is maloccluded or if the diet is too soft. If rat pups are housed in low humidity, ringtail can occur. Ringtail is characterized by annular constrictions that may progress to necrosis and spontaneous amputation of a portion of the tail. Nonspecific signs of illness in rats include rough hair coat, weight loss, and red ocular discharge. Rats are susceptible to respiratory disease caused by *Mycoplasma pulmonis* and cilia-associated respiratory bacillus. Mammary gland tumors are common. Aged rats are frequently affected by chronic renal disease.

HAMSTERS

The Syrian or golden hamster *(Mesocricetus auratus)* originated in the Middle East. It is the most common hamster in the pet trade and research. It is noted for its ease of taming, low waste production, and lack of odor. The golden hamster is stocky and short-tailed, weighs approximately 120 g, and has a reddish-golden brown body color with a gray ventrum. Other color varieties, such as cinnamon, cream, white, piebald, albino, and the long-haired teddy bears, are popular as pets. The Chinese or striped hamster *(Cricetulus griseus)* is gray-brown with a dark strip down its back and is smaller than the golden, weighing 35 g. They tend to be more difficult to handle and thus are not as popular as pets. Female Chinese hamsters are belligerent and must be housed individually. Caging should be selected with the knowledge that hamsters are adept cage chewers and escape artists. Plastic tubes frequently sold as cage extensions are easily chewed through. Hamsters do seem to enjoy running on exercise wheels placed in their cages.

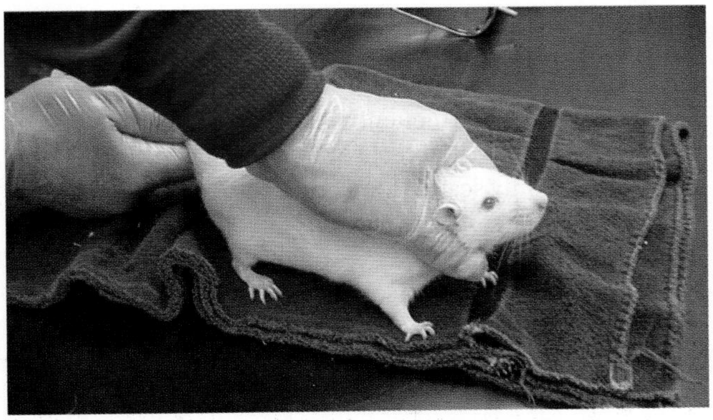

FIGURE 29-7 Restraining a rat. (From Sheldon CC, et al: *Animal restraint for veterinary professionals*, St Louis, 2006, Mosby.)

Hamsters usually have a life span of 1½ to 2 years. Females are usually larger than males and, unlike most mammals, they tend to fight more readily and are generally more aggressive. Males, therefore, live longer than females. On occasions hamsters are cannibalistic. Hamsters have cheek pouches that can transport an amazing amount of food and bedding. A female hamster sometimes packs her whole newborn litter in her pouches to move them to another location. The hamster's cheek pouches are considered an immunologically privileged site; therefore they have been used in research settings for the study of transplanted tumors. Hamsters have extremely loose skin. Marking glands, called flank or hip glands, are located in the skin of both flanks and are more prominent in males. Hamsters are permissive hibernators, so when temperatures fall below 8° C, some hamsters become inactive for periods of 2 to 3 days. During this transient state of hibernation, they have a reduced body temperature and reduced heart and respiratory rates. Hamsters have some control over whether they will hibernate or not. When hamsters are group housed, on occasion the nonhibernating hamsters will cannibalize the sleeping hamsters.

TECHNICIAN NOTE Hamsters have cheek pouches, and they can hibernate in very cold weather.

Hamster urine is normally turbid and milky because it contains a large amount of crystals.

The gender of hamsters is determined by anogenital distance, as with rats and mice. Females have an estrous cycle length of 4 days. They are commonly belligerent toward the male unless sexually receptive. During the winter, hamsters have a normal seasonal breeding quiescence. Hamsters have a gestation length of 16 days, the shortest of the laboratory animals. Cannibalism is common during the first pregnancy and in the first week postpartum. Care should be taken not to disturb a new litter during this period. Providing nest material such as paper tissue several days before delivery of young helps the female feel more secure. Newborn hamsters have fully erupted incisor teeth. Hamsters are weaned at 21 days of age.

Hamsters are sound sleepers and on casual observation may appear dead. An important point to remember when handling a hamster is to avoid surprising it. Make sure the hamster is awake and knows the handler intends to pick it up. Startled or awakened hamsters often bite. Hamsters are most

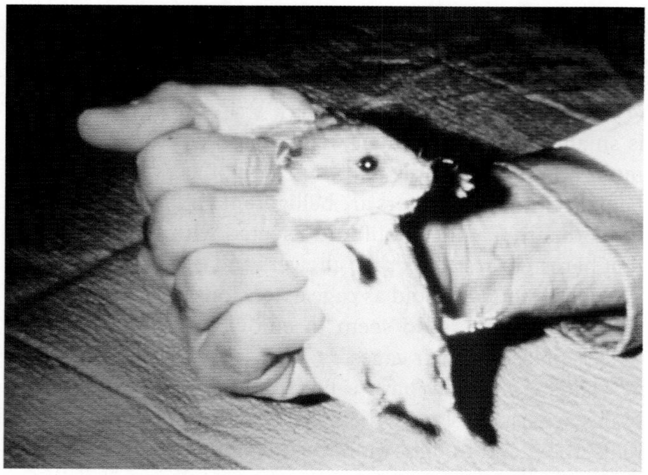

FIGURE 29-8 Holding the hamster.

easily moved by grasping the loose skin across the shoulders or using the hands as a scoop to transfer the hamster from one cage to another. They can also be picked up in a small can or cup. To restrain a hamster, gently grasp the loose skin across the back by curling the fingers and thumb around opposite sides of the animal to gather in as much loose skin as possible. Grasp the skin, not the body, of the hamster (Fig. 29-8). An alternative method is to reverse your hand so that your thumb and forefinger hold the skin at the base of the tail.

Hamsters do well on pelleted food, but pet owners are cautioned not to buy a large quantity because a deficiency of vitamin E may be seen in food that is not used within a 6-month period.

Proliferative ileitis, or wet tail, is caused by a bacterial infection and is the most common spontaneous disease of hamsters. Young animals are affected most often and produce foul-smelling, watery diarrhea, hence the term wet tail. Aged hamsters are frequently affected with cardiomyopathy and amyloidosis, a metabolic disease. Lymphocytic choriomeningitis virus (LCMV) can infect hamsters. LCMV is **zoonotic** and of public health concern. Sedation or anesthesia is usually required if a blood sample is required. When using antibiotics, avoid those that target the gram-positive organisms, such as penicillin, ampicillin, erythromycin, lincomycin, and cephalosporin. These antibiotics allow the gram-negative organisms to take over, which may kill the animal.

GERBILS

The Mongolian gerbil *(Meriones unguiculatus)* is a native to desert regions of Mongolia and northeastern China. It is an active, burrowing, social animal that tends to be more exploratory than other rodents. The gerbil is clean and produces little waste, making it one of the simplest laboratory animals to maintain. It is relatively odorless, nonaggressive, and easy to handle, making it a good "pocket pet." The agouti or mixed-brown gerbil is the color variety most commonly seen, but black and other colors, such as piebald, white, and cinnamon, are available.

The gerbil, or jird, as it is sometimes referred to, has an average life span of 3 years and weighs less than 100 g when mature. It has long hind limbs adapted for leaping and, unlike most other rodents, has a hair-covered tail. When threatened or excited, gerbils will drum their hind legs on the cage flooring. They have large adrenal glands, adaptive mechanisms for temperature extremes, and a unique ability to conserve water. Gerbils have high cholesterol levels and lipemic serum. These can be accentuated by feeding sunflower seeds. Both sexes have a distinct dark orange midventral sebaceous gland, which is used for territorial marking. Gerbils form stable lifelong monogamous arrangements and breed throughout the year. The female is polyestrous and has an estrous cycle of 4 to 6 days in length. Gestation normally lasts 24 days but can be as long as 48 days. The male participates in care of the young and can be left in the cage. Gerbils are weaned at 21 days of age.

A gerbil can be safely picked up by cupping both hands under it or by grasping the base of the tail to lift it from its cage. To restrain the gerbil for examination or injection, the loose skin at the nape of the neck is grasped with one hand and the base of the tail is grasped with the other hand. Extreme care must be taken not to grasp the tip of the tail because the skin may tear and slip off, exposing the underlying muscle and vertebrae. Alternatively, an over-the-back grip can be used. Gerbils resist being placed on their back.

Spontaneous seizures frequently occur when gerbils are stimulated by loud noises, rough handling, or a novel environment. The seizure is usually short, lasting from a few seconds to more than a minute. During a seizure, the gerbil freezes and holds its legs stiffly extended, while the body trembles. No treatment is necessary. Humidity in excess of 50% will cause a gerbil's coat to mat. Sorenose, or rednose, is common in gerbils. This nasal dermatitis is associated with excessive burrowing activity, porphyrin secretion, and staphylococcal infection. Gerbils are very susceptible to Tyzzer's disease caused by *Clostridium piliforme.*

GUINEA PIGS

Guinea pigs *(Cavia porcellus),* often referred to as "**Cavys,**" are tailless rodents, with a compact, stocky body and short legs. They originated in South America and are a hystricomorph rodent related to chinchillas and porcupines. The guinea pig makes a nice children's pet because it is docile and seldom bites or scratches. Guinea pigs have a variety of vocalizations and frequently whistle and squeak when a caregiver approaches their cage. They are messy housekeepers and commonly scatter food and bedding. The guinea pig has been associated with research for so long that a human volunteer for an experiment is often called a "guinea pig." Guinea pigs can be monocolored, bicolored, or tricolored. The most common pet and laboratory variety is the English, American, or short-haired guinea pig (Fig. 29-9). The Abyssinian has short, rough hair arranged in whorls or rosettes; the Peruvian or "rag mop" variety has long, silky hair (Fig. 29-10).

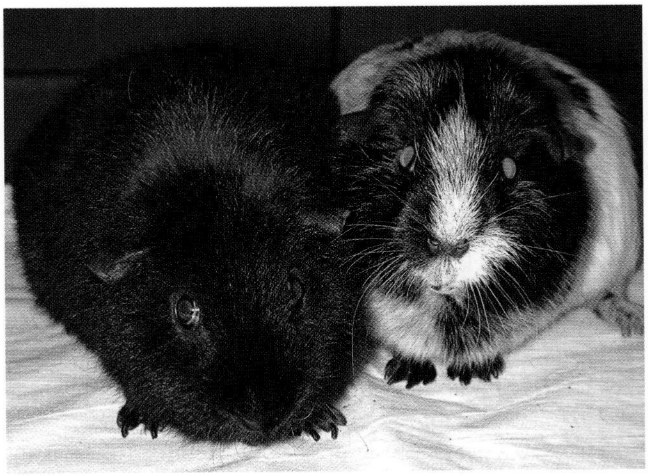

FIGURE 29-9 Two common guinea pig breeds: Teddy *(left)* and American *(right)*. (From Mitchell M, Tully TN, Jr: *Manual of exotic pet practice*, St Louis, 2008, Saunders.)

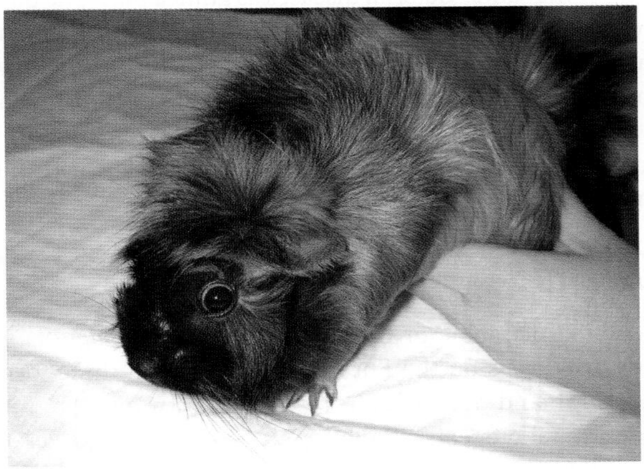

FIGURE 29-10 Abyssinian guinea pig. (From Mitchell M, Tully TN, Jr: *Manual of exotic pet practice*, St Louis, 2008, Saunders.)

The guinea pig weighs 700 to 1200 g as an adult. It has a normal body temperature of 37.2° to 39.5° C and a life span of 4 to 5 years. Guinea pigs have four digits on their front limbs and three digits on their hind limbs. All teeth are open rooted and erupt continuously. They have a large cecum and a long colon. Guinea pigs are actively coprophagic. Their urine is normally opaque and creamy yellow, and contains crystals. Large, mononuclear lymphocytes called Kurloff cells are seen in the blood, especially during times of estrogen stimulation. Marking glands are located around the anus and on the rump. Both male and female guinea pigs have inguinal nipples. Sexing is difficult because, unlike other rodents, there is little difference in the anogenital distance in males and females. The female has a Y-shaped anogenital opening and vaginal membrane that remains intact and closed except during the few days of estrus and at parturition. Males have scrotal pouches lateral to the anogenital line and a penis that can be protruded by manual pressure. The guinea pig usually responds to danger in one of two ways, either by becoming immobile for up to

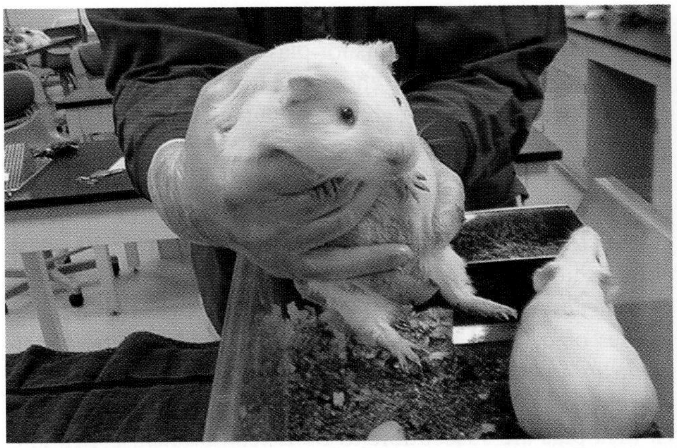

FIGURE 29-11 Remove the guinea pig from its cage by lifting it up while supporting its body with your hand. (From Sheldon CC, et al: *Animal restraint for veterinary professionals*, St Louis, 2006, Mosby.)

20 minutes, or by the scatter response in which they run for their lives.

TECHNICIAN NOTE Antibiotics that target gram-positive organisms can kill hamsters and guinea pigs.

Female guinea pigs are called **sows;** males are called **boars;** and the act of giving birth is called farrowing. The sow is polyestrous throughout the year and has an estrous cycle of 15 to 17 days. A sow should be bred for the first time before 6 months of age, before fusion of the pubic bones, to prevent dystocia. The gestation period is lengthy, averaging 68 days. Larger litters have shorter gestation periods. Neonates are precocious and nearly self-sufficient. They are born fully furred, with eyes and ears open and teeth erupted. Young guinea pigs eat solid food within the first few days postpartum and can be weaned at 14 to 21 days.

To restrain a guinea pig, lift the animal by grasping under the trunk with one hand while supporting the rear quarters with the other hand (Fig. 29-11). It is especially important to use a two-hand support method with adult and pregnant animals. An alternative method is to place one hand over the shoulder area, with the thumb and forefingers just caudal to the front legs, while the other hand supports the rear quarters. Use care not to overly compress the chest with this method.

Like the rabbit, the guinea pig is herbivorous. Food preferences are established very early in life. Guinea pigs have rigid eating habits, and any change in food or water may cause them to stop eating. Dietary vitamin C must be provided to guinea pigs because, like primates, they cannot synthesize their own vitamin C. Lack of vitamin C causes scurvy. Guinea pigs with scurvy have swollen joints and are reluctant to move. Even under ideal storage conditions, the vitamin C content of food deteriorates rapidly, so it is important to use freshly milled food within a 90-day period. Commercial rabbit and guinea pig foods look alike; both are small pelleted chows, but they differ in vitamin C content. Citrus fruits, cabbage, peppers, and kale can be fed to supplement vitamin C. Guinea pigs are notorious for playing with sipper tubes of their water bottle, causing the bottle to empty. They will also blow chewed food through the sipper tube and block it or foul the water supply.

Lower premolar teeth are frequently maloccluded and overgrown and can cause excessive salivation or slobbers. Pododermatitis, also called **bumblefoot,** is found in obese animals housed on wire. Animals have pressure sores on the palmar and plantar surfaces of their feet. Subcutaneous abscesses or cervical "lumps" caused by *Streptococcus zooepidemicus* are common in guinea pigs. Respiratory disease is frequently accompanied by nasal and ocular discharge. Guinea pigs are susceptible to *Bordetella bronchiseptica* and should not be housed with rabbits, dogs, cats, or other species that carry this bacteria subclinically. Conjunctivitis is commonly caused by a bacterial infection. All antibiotics should be used with caution for this species, and avoided whenever possible. Guinea pigs are sensitive to antibiotics that change their gastrointestinal flora. Similar to hamsters, penicillin and other gram-positive antibiotics should not be used in guinea pigs, because it often allows a potentially fatal overgrowth of gram-negative organisms, especially *Clostridium* sp., which produces a lethal enterotoxin. Streptomycin is toxic to the species.

CHINCHILLAS

The chinchilla *(Chinchilla laniger)* has a compact body, delicate limbs, large eyes, large round ears, long whiskers, and a bushy tail. It has a soft, very dense hair coat that is normally bluish-gray with yellow-white underparts. It originated in South America like its relative the guinea pig. Chinchillas are quiet, shy animals that adapt well to humans when handled at a young age. They rarely bite and are virtually odorless. Chinchillas are very active, agile, and like to climb and jump. They require a larger cage than do guinea pigs, who tend to be less active.

The chinchilla weighs 400 to 600 g as an adult. It has a normal body temperature of 37° to 38° C and a life span of 10 years. Its life span is much longer than that of other pet rodents. Chinchillas have four toes on their front and rear feet. Like the guinea pig, all their teeth are open rooted and evergrowing. They have a long gastrointestinal tract and are coprophagic. The female has a vaginal closure membrane that remains intact and closed except during a few days of estrus and at parturition. The anogenital distance is the best criterion for sexing. The female has a large urinary papilla that can be confused with a penis. The penis can be protruded by manual pressure to confirm the sex. Males do not have a true scrotum. The testes are contained within the open inguinal canal or abdomen.

Chinchillas can be housed in pairs or larger units. Females tend to be highly selective in their choice of mate and can be aggressive. If housed in pairs, the male can remain with the female if she tolerates him during parturition and raising of the young. Chinchillas are seasonally polyestrous and have a lengthy gestation period of 111 days. Unlike the guinea pig, dystocias are uncommon. The young are precocious, being fully furred with teeth and eyes open at birth. The female chinchilla stands, rather than lying on her side, when nursing young. Young chinchillas begin to eat solid foods at 1 week and can be weaned at 6 to 8 weeks. They are sexually mature at 8 months.

A tamed chinchilla will willingly come out of its cage. To restrain it, place one hand under the abdomen or around the scruff of the neck and hold it by the base of the tail with the other hand. If the chinchilla escapes from its cage, you must be fast to catch it. Use care, because a frightened chinchilla can lose a patch of fur where it is grasped. This condition is called fur-slip and is a predator avoidance mechanism. It takes 6 to 8 weeks for the hairless patch to fill in.

Access to a dust bath should be provided for 1 hour daily to prevent matted fur. Commercial chinchilla dust or a mixture of silver sand and Fuller's earth can be used. One inch of dust is placed in a pan that is big enough for the chinchilla to roll around in and fluff its fur. Chinchillas are susceptible to many of the same bacterial diseases as guinea pigs. The bones of chinchillas are thin and fragile. It is common to see traumatic fractures. The tibia is particularly fragile, being longer than the femur, and has little soft tissue covering it. Chinchillas are prone to heat stroke at environmental temperature in excess of 28° to 30° C, especially when coupled with high humidity.

RABBITS

The domestic rabbit, or European rabbit *(Oryctolagus cuniculus),* still exists on the European continent in three forms: wild, feral, and domestic. In North America only feral and domestic rabbits exist. Rabbits can be divided by size. The Flemish Giant is a large breed weighing 6 to 7 kg, the New Zealand and Californian are medium-size breeds weighing 2 to 5 kg, and the Dutch and Polish are small breeds weighing 1 to 2 kg. The albino New Zealand is popularly used for meat production and research. The smaller breeds are kept as pets and in research. Rabbits make good pets. They are mild tempered, seldom bite, and can be house trained.

Rabbits are **lagomorphs,** differentiated from rodents by the presence of two upper pairs of incisors that continuously grow. The second set of upper incisors is smaller and occurs behind the large front incisors. They are called peg teeth or wolf teeth. The rabbit has a life span of 5 to 6 years or more, body temperature of 38.5° to 40° C, heart rate 130 to 325 beats per minute, and respiratory rate of 30 to 60 breaths per minute. Rabbits have a wide field of vision, can readily detect motion, and see well in dim light. Their ears are highly vascular and function in heat regulation.

Rabbits have several unusual features to their intestinal tract, including a sacculus rotundus located at the terminal end of the ileum, a large cecum that terminates in a vermiform process or appendix, and a colon with regular sacculations called haustra. Rabbits are coprophagic and pass two types of feces. Soft, moist "night feces" are rich in vitamins and protein and are eaten directly from the anus. Firm, dry pellets are passed during the daytime. Hairballs can be a serious, potentially fatal problem in rabbits because they cannot vomit. The addition of proteolytic enzymes such as those found in papaya or pineapple-type products help prevent this condition. High-fiber diets are of value in trying to prevent hairballs and also tend to prevent obesity, hair chewing, and enteritis. The color of rabbit urine varies from orange-red to brown; the pH is greater than 8 and therefore very basic. A small amount of protein in the urine is normal. Crystals of calcium carbonate and magnesium phosphate can be expected to be found in rabbit urine.

TECHNICIAN NOTE Never pick up a rabbit by its ears.

Male rabbits are called **bucks** and female rabbits are called **does.** Sexing can be accomplished by gently pressing the skin back from the genital opening. Females have an elongated vulva, with a slit opening; males have a rounded, protruding penile sheath. The dewlap, a heavy fold of skin at the throat, is more prominent in females. Rabbits do not have a true estrous cycle but have periods of sexual receptivity. They are induced ovulators, meaning that they only ovulate after coitus. Because the doe is territorial, she is taken to the buck's cage for breeding. Mating usually occurs within minutes. Gestation is approximately 31 days. As with guinea pigs, larger litters are carried for a shorter period of time. Parturition in the rabbit is called kindling and the young are called kits or, more commonly, bunnies. Young rabbits are born naked and helpless, yet they require little maternal care. Does nurse young rabbits only for a few minutes once or twice daily. Weaning occurs at 6 to 8 weeks of age.

Rabbits have a small skeletal mass compared with similar-sized animals, and large hindquarter muscles that make them prone to back fractures. Fractures of this type are considered incurable and the animal must be euthanized. Most fractures of the spinal column result from poor handling techniques. When carrying a rabbit longer distances, its head should be tucked into the crook of the arm that is supporting the hindquarters (Fig. 29-12). Rabbits that are incorrectly handled may injure themselves by struggling and can also scratch their handler with their powerful hind legs. A towel wrapped around the rabbit works well for restraint, especially if the eyes are covered. Mechanical devices made of plastic or metal are frequently used for restraint during minor procedures, such as blood collection from an ear vein, IV injections, or treatments. The restraining device holds the head in place and has a sliding partition that fits snugly against the rabbit's rump (Fig. 29-13). Rabbits should never be lifted or restrained by grabbing their ears, because the ears are sensitive and fragile. When returning a rabbit to its cage, place it in the cage rump first to prevent injury to the rabbit or handler. A rabbit has a tendency to leap toward the cage if allowed to enter the cage head first.

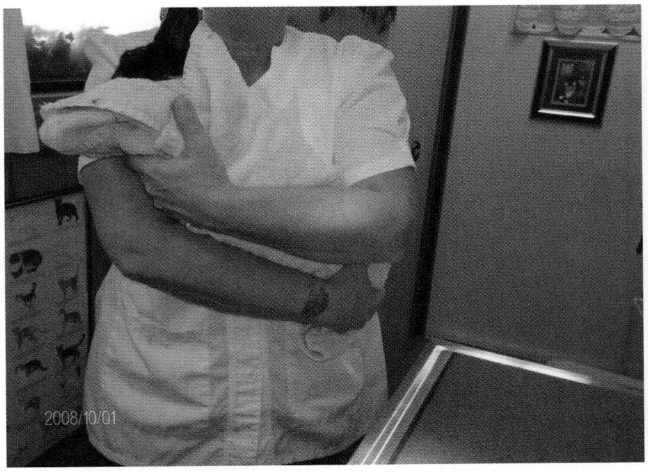

FIGURE 29-12 Rabbits can be carried by supporting the body while directing the head into the crook of the elbow.

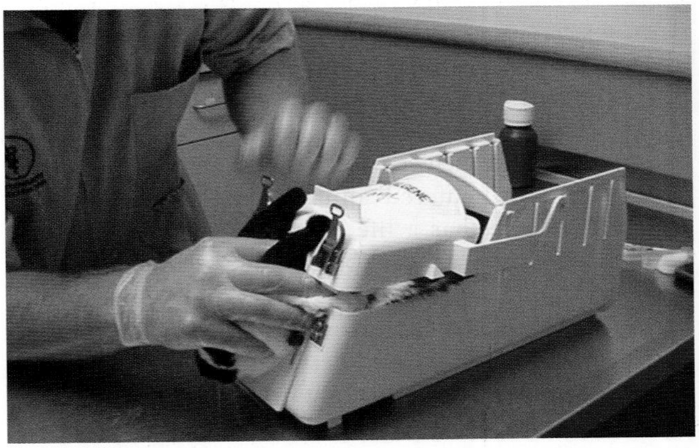

FIGURE 29-13 Rabbit in restraining device. (From Sheldon CC, et al: *Animal restraint for veterinary professionals*, St Louis, 2006, Mosby.)

TECHNICIAN NOTE Rabbit urine is very basic, and calcium and magnesium crystals are found in normal urine.

Malocclusion can result in overgrown incisors that may need to be trimmed every 2 to 3 weeks. Ear mite infections with *Psoroptes* are common in pet rabbits. The mites characteristically cause a dry, brown, crusty material to accumulate on the inner surface of the ears. Pododermatitis, a pressure necrosis of the plantar surface of the metatarsal area, commonly called sore hocks, is seen in heavy, obese rabbits. Rabbits are very susceptible to infection with *Pasteurella multocida*. Several clinical forms of the disease occur; the most common are rhinitis *(snuffles)* and pneumonia. Stressed or recently weaned rabbits are frequently affected with coccidia.

FERRETS

The domestic ferret *(Mustela putorius furo)* belongs to the same family as weasels, mink, otter, and skunks. Ferrets were initially used as hunting animals for the control of rabbits and rodents and raised for their pelts. They have become popular pets because of their small size, ease of care, and comical engaging personalities. Keeping domestic ferrets as pets is not legal in all states and/or cities. Thus, it is important to be aware of legislation in your locality regarding the keeping of ferrets as pets. The natural color of ferrets is fitch, also known as sable. Fitch-colored ferrets have black guard hair with a cream-colored undercoat, black feet and tail, and a black mask on the face. Two other natural colors that are seen are albino and cinnamon. In addition, more than 30 color variations are recognized. Ferrets have long tubular bodies with short legs and very flexible spines. This allows them to get into small openings and turn around easily. Ferrets leap, jump, and can climb. Pet owners need to keep a ferret in a secure, escape-proof cage. If a ferret is allowed to run loose in the house it should be "ferret proofed" to close up any holes or areas from which a ferret cannot be retrieved.

> **TECHNICIAN NOTE** Ferrets are susceptible to canine distemper and require vaccinations against it.

Ferrets that are neutered early weigh from 0.8 to 1.2 kg when adult. Unneutered animals are larger, especially males. The ferret has a life span of 5 to 8 years of age, body temperature of 37.8° to 40° C, heart rate 180 to 250 beats per minute, and a respiratory rate of 33 to 36 breaths per minute. A ferret's skin is remarkably thick, especially over the neck and shoulders. Ferrets experience a seasonal change in body fat, losing weight in the summer and gaining it back in the winter. They also molt in the spring and fall. Ferrets do not have sweat glands in their skin and thus are prone to heat stroke. Their claws are not retractable, as in cats, and need to be trimmed. The canine teeth are prominent as they are in other carnivorous animals. Ferrets have a simple stomach and short small intestine. They do not have a cecum. Ferrets have well-developed anal glands that produce a foul-smelling liquid when they are frightened. The anal gland secretion, however, is not responsible for the musky body odor of ferrets. The sebaceous secretions of their skin produce the animals' odor. Ferrets originating from large breeding farms are routinely descented and neutered when they are 5 to 6 weeks of age before entering the pet market.

Female ferrets are called **jills** and males are called **hobs.** Young are called kits. A neutered female is called a sprite and a neutered male a gib. It is easy to sex a ferret. The preputial opening in male ferrets is located on the ventral abdomen as in male dogs and the os penis is readily palpable. The urogenital opening in female ferrets is located in the perineal region ventral to the anus. The breeding season for ferrets is from March to August in most climates. Females are seasonally polyestrous. During estrus, the vulva becomes swollen and protuberant. Gestation is 42 days and young ferrets are weaned at 6 to 8 weeks of age.

> **TECHNICIAN NOTE** Cats, ferrets, and rabbits are induced ovulators.

Most ferrets are quite docile and can be easily examined without undue restraint. Assistance is usually needed to give medications. Tractable ferrets can be lightly restrained on the exam table. An active ferret can be restrained by scruffing the loose skin on the back of the neck and suspending it off the table. Many animals can be distracted by feeding Nutri-Cal with a syringe or placing a small amount of it on their fur for them to lick.

Ferrets are highly susceptible to canine distemper. They must be vaccinated against this virus, because canine distemper is typically a fatal disease in ferrets. Ear mites are common in ferrets. Ferrets are susceptible to human influenza virus. Influenza causes upper respiratory disease in ferrets as it does in humans. Adrenal gland disease and insulinomas are common conditions seen in older pet ferrets. If female ferrets are not spayed, they frequently remain in estrus if they are not bred. They can develop estrogen toxicity with bone marrow suppression and severe anemia.

GENERAL NURSING CARE

Because of the cost involved in hospitalization and intensive care, most pet rodents are treated on an outpatient basis, whereas rabbits and ferrets are often hospitalized. As with any other sick pet, proper nursing care is vital to maximize the pet's chances for full recovery.

Pet rodents that must be hospitalized are usually critically ill. Fluid therapy, antibiotics, forced feeding, and proper environment are important. These patients should be handled as little as possible. The proper ambient temperature must be maintained. Incubators serve this function well; however, care must be taken not to overheat small mammals. The temperature should be kept no warmer than 80° F. Temperatures above this often results in death from heat stroke. When necessary, oxygen can be supplemented through a port on the incubator. Food and water should be offered even if forced feeding is needed.

When possible, small mammals should be isolated from other hospitalized animals, not only because of the risk of disease spread (e.g., *Bordetella* passed from dogs, cats, or rabbits to guinea pigs), but also because these sick pets are extremely stressed. Remember that most small mammals are prey in the wild. Housing them near a natural predator such as a dog or cat may increase their stress levels.

DIAGNOSTIC AND TREATMENT TECHNIQUES

Techniques used to diagnose disease in companion and food animals are used in small mammals. Some techniques such as skin scrapings can be more challenging in rodents because they are very mobile and can be difficult to restrain. Diagnostic testing is important, as many of these pets are presented with vague complaints such as lethargy and lack of appetite.

Although certain syndromes are more common in certain species, diagnostic testing can help determine a definitive diagnosis and proper treatment plan. Unfortunately, many owners of some less expensive small mammals, particularly rodents, may not allow diagnostic testing because of the cost involved. In addition, the small size of these animals makes it more difficult to obtain adequate laboratory samples. In the research setting, the health status of the rodent colony is often more important that the health status of an individual animal. Health status is frequently monitored by serologic testing of sentinel animals that are placed in the colony.

VENIPUNCTURE

Venipuncture is a technique commonly used in ferrets and rabbits and infrequently used in pet rodents. Venipuncture is used for withdrawing blood for hematologic and biochemical analysis, administration of certain medications, and catheterization for administration of fluids. Anesthesia may be required when performing venipuncture on small mammals. Although each diagnostic laboratory has specific requirements for the volume of blood required for various tests, most laboratories can perform a mini-battery of tests (CBC, chemistries, electrolytes) on 0.5 ml of blood collected in a green top (lithium heparin) tube. Special blood collection tubes (Microvette), which hold a maximum of 0.3 ml, are available commercially. These are particularly useful when collecting samples from small rodents. Except for mice and gerbils, 0.5 ml is a realistic amount of blood to collect from a small mammal; 0.2 ml of blood could be routinely collected from a mouse or gerbil. To prevent volume depletion in pet rodents, some clinicians replace the volume of blood withdrawn with an equal volume of balanced electrolyte solution.

RODENTS

Small blood samples can be collected from rodents by superficial venipuncture. The lateral saphenous vein is a good superficial vessel to use. Other superficial vessels that can be used include the cephalic vein, jugular vein, and tail vessels in rodents that have long tails (Fig. 29-14). The central vena cava of guinea pigs is easily accessible, but they must be anesthetized first. The orbital sinus is frequently used to collect blood from anesthetized rodents in research but rarely used with pet animals. Cardiac puncture can also be used in an anesthetized rodent, but it is not recommended except for collection before euthanasia.

RABBITS

The marginal ear veins and central ear artery of the rabbit are easily visualized and can be used to collect blood (Fig. 29-15). Blood can be collected with a syringe and needle or by cannulating the vessel and collecting the blood in a blood tube or heparinized microhematocrit tube as it drips freely from the vessel. Jugular venipuncture is also fairly easy. The rabbit is placed in ventral recumbency and the blood is collected in a similar manner to dogs and cats. The cephalic vein tends to be a more difficult vessel from which to collect blood.

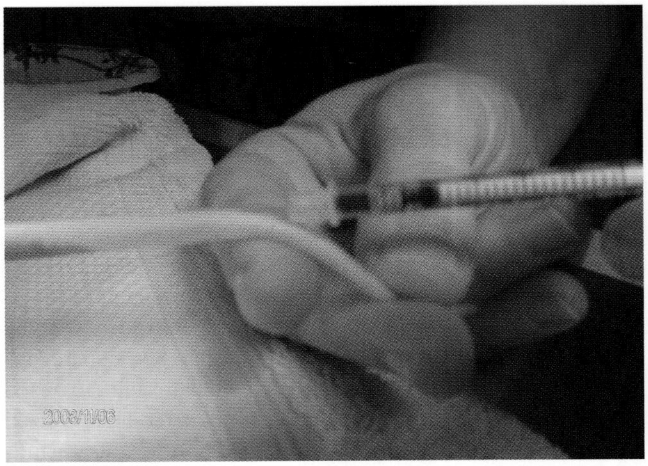

FIGURE 29-14 Blood collection from the tail vein of a rat.

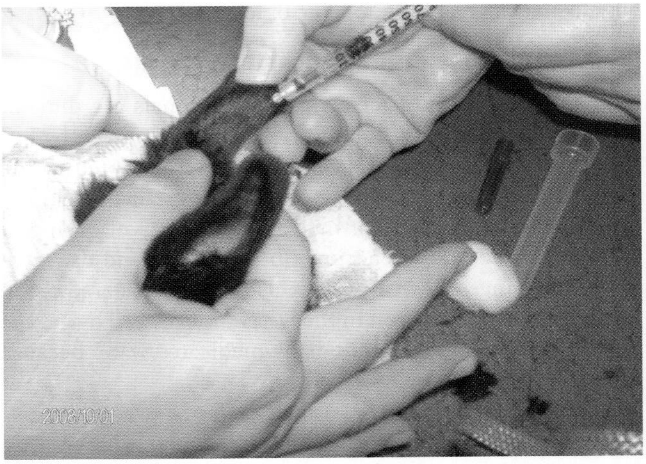

FIGURE 29-15 The marginal ear vein can be used for blood collection or small-volume intravenous injections in rabbits.

FERRETS

The cephalic vein, jugular vein, cranial vena cava, and lateral saphenous vein can be used to collect blood samples in ferrets. Venipuncture is most easily performed under isoflurane anesthesia maintained by face mask. When obtaining a jugular sample, the ferret is placed in dorsal recumbency, with the legs pulled caudally while the head and neck are extended dorsally. Venipuncture can be done in an awake cooperative ferret. Obtaining small volumes of blood from larger ferrets is possible using the central artery of the tail.

FORCE FEEDING

Many small mammals are presented for veterinary care because of anorexia and lethargy. In addition to the need for rehydration, nutritional supplementation is often required but overlooked. Small mammals such as rodents have high metabolic rates and thus high energy requirements. Animals that are not eating are in a catabolic state. Decreased food intake results in breakdown of protein and fat for energy. This can contribute to hepatic lipidosis (especially in rabbits), acidosis, azotemia, muscle wasting, impaired gastrointestinal function, and decreased immunity. To prevent or correct these complications, supplementation with food is important. Force feeding can be done in the hospital or by the owner at home if the pet will be treated on an outpatient basis.

High-energy paste supplements can be given to all small mammals on a short-term basis. Sick rabbits often eat hay or greens, such as carrot tops and parsley, even if they refuse pellets. These can be offered free choice. Apples and yogurt can also be used. A nasogastric or gastric tube can be used to deliver a mixture of powdered pellets and water. Rodents can be supplemented with apples and peanut butter. Sweetened condensed milk is also a favorite. Pedialyte or Gatorade can be fed via small syringe for hydration along with water. Hospitalized ferrets can be force fed any of the diets suitable for cats, including Hill's a/d or CliniCare. Meat-based baby foods can also be used. The food can be offered to the ferret to eat voluntarily or given with a syringe or through a tube. Warming the food slightly may increase the appetite of ferrets.

ADMINISTRATION OF MEDICATIONS

With the exception of ferrets, small mammals are difficult to medicate with pills. Liquid oral medication given by eye dropper or small syringe is generally better accepted by the pet. Because of the small size of rodents, medications usually have to be diluted. For increased accuracy of dosing, it is important to have an accurate body weight and use a tuberculin syringe. Medication can also be administered orally by mixing the medication in the water or feed, and by gavage needle. Rodents often do not drink medicated water because of its unpleasant taste.

Injectable medications are usually preferred over oral medications in hospitalized small mammals. Extremely ill pets may have reduced intestinal function, making absorption of oral medication erratic and unpredictable. Using the parenteral route of drug administration rather than oral also decreases the possibility of gastrointestinal problems in these small mammals.

The standard routes of injection (IV, IM, SC, ID, IP) are used in laboratory animals. Rodents have few readily accessible veins, making it difficult to administer drugs IV. Tail veins can be used in the mouse and rat. The margin ear veins, located on the lateral sides of the pinna in the rabbit, are accessible and can be used for IV injections. Because it is difficult to do venous catheterization in small mammals, intraosseous catheterization to administer fluids to critically ill exotic pets is often preferred. The trochanteric fossa of the femur is the preferred site for intraosseous catheterization. The subcutaneous route is frequently used for fluid supplementation. SC fluids are given over the dorsal neck, back, and flank of small mammals. Fluids can also be given intraperitoneally (IP) in rodents. The small muscle mass of rodents makes it difficult to inject drugs IM. For this reason the IP route is more commonly used in rodents. When giving IP injections, it is best to use the caudal left abdominal quadrant and tilt the animal's head and forequarters ventrally. This helps to avoid accidental puncture of the large cecum in these animals (Fig. 29-16).

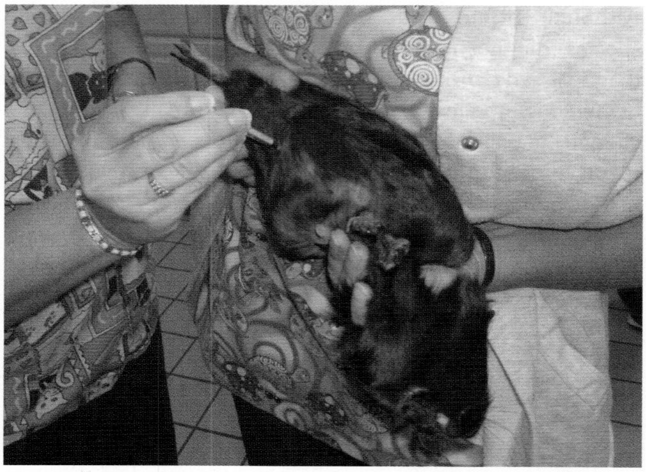

FIGURE 29-16 The guinea pig should be held with its head pointed downward when administering an IP injection.

Antibiotics

Caution must be used when administering antibiotics to rodents and rabbits. These animals have a predominantly gram-positive gastrointestinal flora and are very sensitive to antibiotics that change the balance of the flora. Guinea pigs and rabbits are particularly prone to antibiotic-associated enterotoxemia. Drugs such as ampicillin and penicillin will destroy susceptible gram-positive organisms and allow overgrowth of *Clostridium difficile* and production of its toxin. Safe antibacterials for use in rabbits and rodents include enrofloxacin, ciprofloxacin, trimethoprim-sulfas, and chloramphenicol. If diarrhea develops, drug administration should be stopped immediately and the animal examined. Ferrets can be treated safely with most antibacterials used in cats.

Vaccines

Rodents and rabbits do not currently require annual vaccines. Ferrets must be vaccinated against canine distemper virus with an appropriate vaccine. Never use canine combination vaccines or vaccines of ferret cell origin because of the possibility of vaccine-induced disease. Give ferrets a series of vaccines at 6 to 8 weeks, 10 to 12 weeks, and 14 weeks of age, then annually. Vaccination against rabies is highly recommended for ferrets, especially in rabies-endemic areas. An inactivated rabies vaccine approved for use in ferrets should be given SC at 3 months of age and annually.

FECAL ANALYSIS

Microscopic fecal analysis is used to evaluate animals with diarrhea and any nonspecific complaint. The method is similar to that used in dogs and cats. A fresh fecal smear and flotation should be performed. A cellophane tape test can be used on the anal region to check for the presence of pinworms in rodents.

URINE SAMPLES

Urine samples can be obtained by gentle manual expression of the bladder or cystocentesis. Rodents can be placed on a cold surface or in a cooled plastic bag until urine is voided.

IDENTIFICATION METHODS USED IN RESEARCH ANIMALS

Identification of individual animals is important in a research setting as many animals appear identical. The researcher frequently needs to tell individual animals apart. Rodents are identified by ear tag or by an ear notch or punch pattern. Ear tags or ear tattoos are used in rabbits. A microchip can be implanted subcutaneously in laboratory animals for quick electronic identification.

ANESTHESIA

Many factors, such as species, strain, ingesta content, weight, and nutritional and health status, affect the response of rabbits and rodents to anesthesia. Small rodents are not fasted before inducing anesthesia. Food, but not water, should be withheld for 3 to 6 hours from guinea pigs, chinchillas, and rabbits before inducing anesthesia. Young ferrets, like dogs and cats, are fasted for 8 hours. Food is withheld from older ferrets for no more than 4 hours. A small scale should be used to obtain an accurate weight of the animal to calculate the dose when using injectable anesthetic agents. Inhalation agents, such as isoflurane, can also be used; however, they should be delivered using a calibrated vaporizer to prevent anesthetic overdose. Inhalation agents are commonly administered via chamber, face mask, or nose cone because it is difficult to intubate most small mammals. Ferrets can be intubated in a similar fashion to cats. It is essential to monitor the animal closely and keep it warm to prevent hypothermia. Hydration, nutritional support, and analgesia are important postoperative considerations.

REVIEW QUESTIONS

Matching

Match the disease or condition with its description.

____**1.** *Bordetella bronchiseptica*
____**2.** canine distemper
____**3.** coccidia
____**4.** heat stroke
____**5.** lymphocytic choriomeningitis
____**6.** MHV
____**7.** *Mycoplasma pulmonis*
____**8.** *Pasteurella multocida*
____**9.** proliferative ileitis
____**10.** *Psoroptes*
____**11.** rednose
____**12.** ringtail
____**13.** *Streptococcus zooepidemicus*
____**14.** *Syphacia* or *Aspicularis*

__**A.** common pinworm of mice
__**B.** spontaneous bacterial infection of young hamsters
__**C.** subcutaneous abscess or cervical lumps
__**D.** rabbit ear mite
__**E.** common endoparasite in rabbits
__**F.** zoonotic virus of hamsters
__**G.** contagious respiratory/GI disease
__**J.** susceptibility in guinea pigs
__**K.** chinchillas prone to this with increased humidity
__**L.** "snuffles"
__**M.** respiratory disease common in rats
__**N.** fatal disease of ferrets

Fill in the Chart

Provide answers to complete the following chart.

	Genus Species	Adult Weight (grams)	Gestation (days)	Estrous Cycle (days)	Body Temperature °C	Life Span (years)	Fill in the Blank
Mice						3	Subordinate mice often show evidence of ____________
Rat						2½-3½	____________tumors are quite common
Syrian hamster					38.9		Cheek pouches are ____________
Mongolian gerbil	*Meriones unguiculatus*			4-6	37.4-39.0	3	Female gerbil: ______
Guinea pig						4-5	Vitamin ______requirement
Chinchilla	*Chinchilla longer*			30-50		10	Access to a ____________ should be provided as part of the husbandry

	Genus Species	Adult Weight (grams)	Gestation (days)	Estrous Cycle (days)	Body Temperature °C	Life Span (years)	Fill in the Blank
RABBIT (New Zealand White)				induced ovulator			Young are called ___________
FERRET	*Mustela putorius furo*	0.8-1.2 kg		induced ovulator		5-8	Susceptible to and should be vaccinated for___________________

RECOMMENDED READING

American Association for Laboratory Animal Science assistant laboratory animal technician (ALAT) training manual, Cordova, TN, 2009, AALAS.

American Association for Laboratory Animal Science assistant laboratory animal technician (ALAT) training manual, Cordova, TN, 2012, AALAS.

Field JF, Sibold AL: *The laboratory hamster & gerbil: a volume in the laboratory pocket reference series*, Boca Raton, FL, 1999, CRC Press.

Flecknell P: Anesthesia of rodents and rabbits. In Thomas JA, Lerche P, editors: *Anesthesia and analgesia for veterinary technicians*, ed 4, St Louis, 2011, Mosby.

Harkness JE, et al.: *Harkness and Wagner's the biology and medicine of rabbits and rodents*, ed 5, Ames, IA, 2010, Wiley-Blackwell.

Hrapkiewicz K, Medina L, Homes D: *Clinical laboratory animal medicine: an introduction*, ed 4, Ames, IA, 2013, Wiley Blackwell.

Macrina FL: *Scientific integrity: text and cases in responsible conduct of research*, ed 3, Washington, DC, 2005, ASM Press.

Quesenberry KE, Carpenter JW: *Ferrets, rabbits, rodents: clinical medicine and surgery*, ed 3, St Louis, 2011, Saunders.

Sharp PR, LaRegina MC: *The laboratory rat: a volume in the laboratory pocket reference series*, Boca Raton, FL, 1999, CRC Press.

Sirois M: *Laboratory animal medicine: principles and procedures*, ed 2, St Louis, 2015, Mosby.

Glossary

A

Abduction Movement of a limb or part away from the median line or middle of the body.

Abrasion An injury in which the epithelium is removed from the tissue surface.

Absolute value The number of each type of leukocyte in peripheral blood; calculated by multiplying the relative percentage from the differential count by the total white blood cell count.

Absorption The movement of drug molecules from the site of administration into the systemic circulation.

Academy Establishes its own bylaws, leaders, application committee, testing committee, and credentialing committee, testing only those candidates who meet specific requirements.

Acariasis Infestation with mites.

Accuracy The closeness with which test results agree with the true quantitative value of the constituent.

Acid-fast A staining procedure for demonstrating presence of microorganisms that are not readily decolorized by acid after staining; a characteristic of certain bacteria, particularly *Mycobacterium* and *Nocardia*.

Acidosis A condition in which the blood pH is less than 7.35.

ACTH stimulation Test designed to evaluate the response of the hormone that stimulates adrenocortical growth and secretion (adrenocorticotropic hormone).

Activated clotting time A test of the intrinsic and common pathways of blood coagulation that uses a diatomaceous earth tube to initiate clotting.

Active immunity An animal's production of antibody as a result of infection with an antigen or immunization.

Acupressure Use of finger pressure instead of needles on acupoints along body meridians.

Acupuncture Placing of small, sharp, sterile needles into specific points on the body.

Ad libitum Free choice, as much as desired.

***Ad libitum* feeding** Offering food at all times so the animal can eat at its leisure.

Adaptive immunity A component of the immune system that responds to specific antigens.

Adduction Movement of a limb or part toward the median line or middle of the body.

Aerobic In the presence of oxygen.

Aerosolized The form of ultramicroscopic solid or liquid particles dispersed or suspended in air or gas.

Agammaglobulinemic Without immunoglobulins.

Agar A seaweed extract used to solidify culture media.

Agglutination Clumping of particles.

Aggression Behavior that is intended to harm another individual.

Agonist A chemical substance that can combine with a cell receptor and cause a reaction or create an active site.

Agonistic Behaviors shown in situations of social conflict to diffuse aggressive behavior.

Agranulocyte White blood cell group that has no visible cytoplasmic granules.

Air sacs In avian species; nine thin, transparent membranes that are connected to the primary and secondary bronchi and act as reservoirs for air entering and leaving the lungs.

ALARA As Low As Reasonably Achievable; a program in place by the National Committee on Radiation Protection that ensures that radiation exposures are a low as possible by wearing of safety protection and use of nonmanual restraint for veterinary patients.

Albumin A group of plasma proteins that comprises the majority of protein in plasma.

Alcohol Disinfectant that must remain in contact with the site for 15 to 20 minutes so as to be effective.

Alkaline phosphatases A group of enzymes that functions at alkaline pH and catalyzes reactions of organic phosphates.

Alkalosis A condition in which the blood pH is higher than 7.45.

Allergen An antigen that evokes an allergic or hypersensitivity reaction.

Allopathic medicine Another term used to describe Western medicine.

Alopecia Loss of hair.

Alpha hemolysis Characterized by partial destruction of blood cells on a blood agar; evident as a greenish zone around the bacterial colony.

Alphanumeric system A dental charting system that identifies each tooth with letters that directly correlate with the type of tooth and numbers that correlate to the placement of the tooth in the dental arcade.

ALT Alanine aminotransferase; cytoplasmic enzyme of hepatocytes released when hepatocytes are damaged.

Alternative therapies Practices that deviate from the Western approach.

Alveolus Tiny grapelike clusters of thin cells, the site of gas exchange in the lungs.

American Animal Hospital Association (AAHA) An organization that has set standards for veterinary practice facilities. Approximately 3000 veterinary hospitals hold AAHA accreditation designation.

American Association for Laboratory Animal Science (AALAS) Organization founded in 1950 and dedicated to the humane care and treatment of laboratory animals and quality research that leads to scientific gains that benefit people and animals.

American Society for the Prevention of Cruelty to Animals (ASPCA) Organization founded by Henry Bergh in 1866 to enforce animal anticruelty laws.

American Veterinary Medical Association/Professional Liability Insurance Trust Company that provides service that protects the assets and reputations of the participants and enhances the image of the profession. May, in the near future, offer professional insurance to technicians.

Amylase Enzyme derived primarily from the pancreas that functions in the breakdown of starch.

Anaerobic In the absence of oxygen.

Analgesia Pain relief, in the form of oral, transdermal, or injectable medication; the inability to feel pain while still conscious. Derived from the Greek *an-*, meaning without, + *algesis*, meaning sense of pain.

Analgesics Drugs that reduce the perception of pain without loss of other sensations.

Anamnesis Information gained from the patient and others regarding the patient's medical history. Derived from the Greek meaning loss of forgetfulness.

Anaphylaxis A severe hypersensitivity reaction characterized by profound hypotension, pulmonary edema, and collapse, caused by massive exposure to an antigen.

Anatomic timed scrub Surgical personnel preparation accomplished by repeating scrub protocol for 5 minutes.

Anechoic Used to describe a tissue that does not reflect ultrasound waves back to the transducer

Anemia Reduction in the oxygen carrying capacity of blood because of a reduced number of circulating red blood cells, reduced packed cell volume, or a reduced concentration of hemoglobin.

Anesthesia Loss of feeling or awareness. Literally means no feeling and may be local, regional, spinal/epidural, or general (supraspinal).

Angiotensin-converting enzyme (ACE) inhibitors Medications that block the angiotensin-converting enzyme and prevent formation of angiotensin II and aldosterone.

Angiotribes Large crushing instrument used to clamp blood vessels.

Animal model An animal whose anatomy and/or physiology make it suitable for studying a specific human disease.

Animal Welfare Act Federal law in the United States that regulates the treatment of animals in research, exhibition, and transport and by dealers. Other laws, policies, and guidelines may include additional species coverage or specifications for animal care and use, but all refer to the Animal Welfare Act as the minimum acceptable standard.

Anion Negatively charged ion.

Anisocoria Uneven pupil size.

Anisodactyl The foot shape of passerines; three toes point forward and one toe points to the rear.

Anisokaryosis Variation in the size of the nuclei in cells of a sample.

Anisonucleoliosis Variation in size of nucleoli.

Annular array Type of transducer with the crystals in concentric rings

Anode A positively charged electrode within the x-ray tube that consists of a tungsten target that produces x-rays when hit with electrons from the cathode.

Antagonist A drug or other chemical substance capable of reducing the physiologic activity of another chemical substance; refers especially to a drug that opposes the action of a drug or other chemical substance on the nervous system by combining with and blocking the nerve receptor.

Anthelmintic General term used to describe compounds that kill various types of internal parasites.

Anthropomorphism Attributing human characteristics and emotions to animals.

Antibiotic See antimicrobial; the terms are interchangeable.

Antibloat medications Act by reducing numbers of gas-producing rumen microorganisms or breaking up the bubbles formed in the rumen with frothy bloat.

Anticholinergic The action of certain medications that inhibit the transmission of parasympathetic nerve impulses and thereby reduce spasms of smooth muscle (such as that, for example, in the bladder).

Anticonvulsants Drugs that are used to control seizures.

Antiemetic A drug given to prevent vomiting. Derived from the Greek *emesis,* meaning vomiting.

Antigen Any substance capable of eliciting an immune response.

Antigenic determinant (epitope) The particular part of the antigen that binds the antibody.

Anti-inflammatory drugs A drug that relieves pain or discomfort by blocking or reducing the inflammatory process.

Antimicrobial Drugs that kill or inhibit the growth of microorganisms such as bacteria, protozoa, or fungi.

Antisepsis The prevention of infectious agent growth on animate (living) objects; the destruction of most living pathogenic microorganisms on animate (living) objects.

Antiseptics Chemical agents that kill or prevent the growth of microorganisms on living tissue.

Anuria Absence of urine.

Anxiolysis A drug given to prevent anxiety. Suffix derived from the Greek *lysis*, meaning breakdown, destruction, separation.

Aortic thromboembolism An aggregation of platelets and fibrin that acutely migrates and lodges at a distant site in the circulatory system.

Apnea Suspension of external breathing.

Apnea monitor Sensor placed between an endotracheal tube connector and breathing circuit to determine whether the patient is breathing or not.

Apteria The featherless tracts of birds.

Arch Row of teeth, such as the mandibular/maxillary arch.

Aromatherapy Therapeutic use of pure essential oils derived from aromatic plants to help balance and heal the mind, body, and spirit.

Arrhythmia Any abnormal pattern of electrical activity in the heart; abnormal heart rhythm; irregular heartbeat.

Arthropod Ectoparasite belonging to the phylum Arthropoda (insects).

Artifact A structure or feature not normally present, but visible, that diminishes the quality of a diagnostic image.

Asepsis A condition of being free from infection.

Aseptic technique All precautions taken to prevent contamination and ultimately infection.

Aspartate aminotransferase (AST) An enzyme of hepatocytes found free in the cytoplasm and attached to the mitochondrial membrane that is released when hepatocytes are damaged.

Assertive communication Acting confidently, confident in stating a position or claim.

Ataxia A wobbly or uncoordinated gait.

Atelectasis The lack of gas exchange within alveoli, usually caused by alveolar collapse or fluid consolidation.

Atlas First cervical vertebra.

Audition Listening carefully.

Auditory sense A mechanical sense. Through a complex set of auditory passageways and ear structures, vibrations of air molecules are converted into impulses that the brain decodes as sounds.

Auscultation Listening to heart and lung sounds using a stethoscope; listening to sounds produced by the body, directly (with the ear and no instrument) or indirectly (using a stethoscope to amplify sounds).

Autoclave A sterilization unit that creates high-temperature, pressurized steam.

Autoimmune disease Humoral or cell-mediated response against antigens found in a bodies own cells; examples include systemic lupus erythematosus or rheumatoid arthritis.

Autoimmunity Any condition that results in production of antibody against a body's own tissues.

Autotomize Breaking away of part of the lizard tail at points of fracture planes of cartilage through the vertebral bodies.

AVMA Accreditation Policies and Procedures Manual Guidelines created by the CVTEA for veterinary technician programs to follow, outlining standards for education of veterinary technicians. Can be found on www.avma.org.

Axons Conduct impulses away from the cell body, to other neurons or the effector organs, such as muscle cells.

Ayurveda East Indian philosophy of diet, herbs, and exercise used to promote health and vitality.

Azotemia An increase in waste products in the blood, specifically BUN and creatinine; increased retention of urea in the blood.

B

Bacilli Rod-shaped bacteria.

Bactericidal Kills bacteria.

Bacteriology Study of bacteria.

Bacteriostatic Inhibits bacterial replication.

Baermann technique Parasitology test used to recover larvae.

Bain coaxial circuit A type of nonrebreathing circuit, also referred to as the modified Mapleson D system, in which the tube supplying fresh gas is surrounded by the larger, corrugated tubing that conducts gas away from the patient.

Balanced anesthesia A technique for general anesthesia involving two or more drugs.

Balanced fluid solution Fluid that is similar in composition to plasma.

Balfour retractor Self-retaining retractor with a set screw to maintain tension on tissues, commonly used to retract abdominal wall.

Ballottement Rhythmically pressing the fist into an area of the abdomen in an attempt to "bump" any large underlying masses or organs.

Band cell Immature granulocyte with parallel sides and no nuclear lobed or indentations.

Bandage scissors Scissors with a blunt tip that can safely be introduced under a bandage for removal.

Barbering When a dominant mouse chews the fur of a subordinate mouse.

Barotrauma Respiratory system injury after excessive circuit pressure changes; may also refer to injury to the eustachian tube, eardrum, and stomach.

Basal metabolic rate (BMR) The minimum amount of energy necessary for daily maintenance.

Base narrow canines When the angle of the canine growth is directed inward from a normal occlusion.

Base wide canines When the angle of the canine growth is directed outward from a normal occlusion.

Basophilia Increase in numbers of basophils in a cell; also refers to the bluish-gray appearance of cells or components of cells that have high affinity for stains with alkaline pH (e.g., methylene blue).

Beer's law Describes the relation between light absorbance, transmission, and concentration of a substance in solution.

Behavior Any act done by an animal; exhibited for a reason and with purpose.

Benign A tumor or growth that is not malignant; can refer to any condition that is not life threatening.

Beta hemolysis Complete destruction of red blood cells on a blood agar that creates a clear zone around the bacterial colony.

Bile acids Group of compounds synthesized by hepatocytes from cholesterol that aid in fat absorption.

Bilirubin Insoluble pigment derived from the breakdown of hemoglobin, which is processed by hepatocytes.

Biologics Wide range of medicinal products such as vaccines, blood and blood components, allergenics, somatic cells, gene therapy, tissues, and recombinant therapeutic proteins created by biological processes (as opposed to chemically). Biologics can be composed of sugars, proteins, or nucleic acids or complex combinations of these substances, or may be living entities such as cells and tissues. Biologics are isolated from a variety of natural sources—human, animal, or microorganism—and may be produced by biotechnology methods and other technologies.

Biopsy Removal of cells or tissues for microscopic or chemical examination.

Biosafety level I Substances that ordinarily do not cause disease in humans, include most soaps and cleaning agents, vaccines administered to animals, and infectious diseases that are species specific. It should be noted, however, that these otherwise harmless substances may affect individuals with immune deficiency.

Biosafety level II Substances that have the potential to cause human disease if handled incorrectly. At this level, specific precautions are taken to avoid problems. The hazards in this level include mucous membrane exposure, possible oral ingestion, and puncture of the skin.

Biosafety level III Substances that can cause serious and potentially lethal disease. The potential for aerosol respiratory transmission is high.

Biosafety level IV Substances that pose a high risk of causing life-threatening diseases. Facilities that handle these substances exercise maximum containment. Personnel shower-in and shower-out and dress in full body suits equipped with a positive air supply.

Biotransformation The alteration of a drug by the body before eliminated.

Bisecting angle technique A radiographic technique in which the film is placed as close to the intended tooth as possible. (The shape of the oral cavity usually prevents parallel placement.) The cone is then directed midway between the angle of the tooth and the film.

Bladderworm Fluid-filled larval stage of some cestodes.

Blend Combinations of herbs.

Blood agar An enriched medium that supports the growth of most bacterial pathogens; usually composed of sheep blood.

Blood cross-match Complex testing that is performed before a blood transfusion to determine if the donor's blood is compatible with the blood of an intended recipient.

Blood group antigens Antigens on the surface of red blood cells that characterize the blood as being of a certain type.

Blood type A classification of blood based on the presence or absence of inherited antigens on the surface of red blood cells.

B lymphocyte (B cell) A type of lymphocyte that can be transformed into plasma cells on antigenic stimulation to produce antibodies.

Boar A male guinea pig or pig.

Board of Veterinary Medical Examiners A state body interpreting the practice act governing the practice of veterinary medicine reviewing cases brought against a veterinarian or lay person performing surgery, prescribing medicine, or diagnosing disease. The board is charged with protecting consumers and their pets and livestock. They review cases to determine if the standard of care has been met and if there has been negligence or malpractice, causing injury or death to an animal.

Body condition scoring Method of subjectively quantifying subcutaneous body fat reserves.

Body language Body mannerisms, postures, and facial expressions that can be interpreted as unconsciously communicating somebody's feelings or psychological state.

Bolus A drug given intravenously as a single volume at one time; a large tablet or ball of food that is intended to be swallowed or a large amount of fluid or liquid medication given quickly, intravenously (as opposed to being given slowly, or titrated).

Brachycephalic A condition of having a short face; more specifically, a short, wide muzzle (i.e., short-nosed dogs).

Brachygnathism Maxillary underbite; the mandibular arcade is longer than maxillary the arcade.

Bradyarrhythmia Any disturbance of the heart's rhythm resulting in less than normal heartbeats. The prefix is derived from the Greek *brady-*, meaning slow.

Bradycardia Abnormally low heart rate; decreased heart rate.

Brain stem Forms the stem to which the cerebrum, cerebellum, and spinal cord are attached; maintains the vital functions of the body such as respiration, body temperature, heart rate, gastrointestinal tract function, blood pressure, appetite, thirst, and sleep/wake cycles.

Breathing circuit That part of the anesthetic machine in which the flow of gases is directed through two unidirectional valves, one in an expiratory and one in an inspiratory tube. The rebreathing bag and the canister of soda lime for CO_2 absorption are located between the two tubes.

Bronchial sounds Produced by movement of air through the trachea and large bronchi; usually heard over the area of the trachea and carina, most noticeably during expiration.

Bronchoalveolar lavage Procedure using an infusion of saline into the respiratory tree to aspirate a sample for evaluation.

Bronchodilator Drug that inhibits bronchoconstriction.

Brown-Adson tissue forceps Tissue forceps with small serrations on the tips that cause minimal trauma but hold tissue securely.

Buccal Referring to the cheek.

Buck A male rabbit.

Bucky Sliding metal tray under the x-ray table that holds the cassette and grid.

Buffy coat A layer of material above the packed erythrocytes after centrifugation; consists primarily of leukocytes and thrombocytes.

Bulk laxatives Substances that act to pull water into the bowel lumen via osmosis or help to retain water in the feces.

Bumblefoot (pododermatitis) An inflammation of the ball of the foot of birds and guinea pigs; usually caused by infection with *Staphylococcus* sp.

Bursa of Fabricius The lymphoid organ in birds in which B lymphocytes were first discovered.

Byproduct feeds Residues of the feed-processing industry; span a wide array of feedstuffs.

C

Calculus Hardened, or calcified, plaque.

Capillary refill time The time required for blood to refill capillaries after displacement by finger pressure.

Capnometer A device that determines respiratory rate and the end-tidal CO_2 by estimating partial CO_2 in bloodstream at the end of expiration, when CO_2 levels of the expired gas are approximately equal to alveolar and arterial CO_2 ($Paco_2$).

Capnophilic An organism requiring high levels of carbon dioxide for growth or for enhancement of growth.

Capsid Protein coat that surrounds the genetic material of viruses.

Carapace The upper or dorsal shell of chelonians.

Carcinoma Tumors of epithelial cell origin.

Cardiopulmonary arrest (CPA) The cessation of functional ventilation and effective circulation.

Caseous exudate Exudate formed when a purulent material changes into a thick, pasty material.

Cast Structure formed from protein precipitate of degenerating kidney tubule cells; may contain embedded materials.

Castroviejo needle holders Needle holders with a spring and latch mechanism for locking.

Catabolic A destructive metabolic process by which complex substances are converted by living cells into simpler compounds, with release of energy.

Catalase An enzyme that catalyzes the breakdown of hydrogen peroxide to oxygen and water.

Catchpole Rigid pole with a loop at one end used to move an aggressive or fearful dog to or from a run or cage.

Cathode A negatively charged electrode that produces electrons in the x-ray tube.

Caudal Pertaining to the tail end of the body, or denoting a position more toward the tail or rear of the body than another reference point (body part).

Cavys A common name for guinea pigs.

Celiotomy An incision into the abdominal cavity, also called a laparotomy.

Cell-mediated immunity An immune system mechanism involving actions of the cells of the immune system rather than antibodies.

Cementoenamel junction (CEJ) The division of the tooth between the crown and root of the tooth.

Cementum The substance that covers the root of the tooth. Is more similar to bone (45% to 50% inorganic) and is formed by cementoblasts. The cementum is able to regenerate.

Centers for Disease Control and Prevention (CDC) One of the major operating components of the Department of Health and Human Services. It serves as the national focus for developing and applying disease prevention and control, environment health, and health promotion and education activities designed to improve the health of the people in the United States. The CDC's top organizational components include the Office of the Director, six Coordinating Centers and Offices, and the National Institute for Occupational Safety and Health.

Centesis The act of puncturing a body cavity or organ with a hollow needle to draw out fluid.

Central catheter A long catheter left in place for extended periods and composed of materials designed to produces little if any tissue reaction.

Central nervous system The brain and spinal cord.

Central venous pressure (CVP) The pressure of blood in the thoracic vena cava, near the right atrium of the heart. CVP reflects the amount of blood returning to the heart and the ability of the heart to pump the blood into the arterial system.

Cercaria Life cycle stage of trematodes that develops in the intermediate host.

Cere The flesh-colored skin located at the base of the upper beak in many bird species.

Cerebellum Located just caudal to the cerebrum. The cerebellum does not initiate movements but serves to coordinate, adjust, and generally fine-tune movements directed by the cerebrum.

Cerebrovascular accident A stroke.

Cerebrum The largest, most rostral part of the brain. It is the center of higher learning and intelligence, and it functions in perception, maintenance of consciousness, thinking and reasoning, and initiating responses to sensory stimuli.

Certification This is generally kept by a private or professional organization such as a state veterinary technician association.

Cervical vertebrae Located in the neck region.

Cervix The round, muscular structure that separates the uterus (cranially) from the vagina (caudally).

Cesarean section The surgical removal of newborns via an abdominal incision.

Cestode Organism in the order Cestoda; tapeworms.

Chelonian Referring to turtles and tortoises.

Chemical name Describes the chemical composition of a drug.

Chemical sterilization indicators Generally, paper strips or tape that change color when a certain temperature, pressure, or chemical exposure has been reached, indicating that conditions for sterility have been met.

Chief complaint The reason the client has sought veterinary care for the animal; the primary medical problem.

Chiropractic Spinal adjustments performed to reverse a variety of nerve, muscle, and motion problems.

Chisel Instrument used to shape bone and cartilage.

Choana The V-shaped notch in the roof of the mouth of birds that provides communication between the nasal cavity and the oropharynx.

Choanal papillae Small, rounded projections that surround the choanal slit in birds.

Cholestasis Any condition in which bile excretion from the liver is blocked.

Cholesterol Plasma lipoprotein produced primarily in the liver as well as ingested in food; used in the synthesis of bile acids.

Chromic surgical gut Surgical gut suture that has been exposed to chrome or aldehyde to slow absorption.

Chylomicron A small fat globule composed of protein and lipid.

Cicatrix A scar; the contracted area of fibrous tissue that remains under the dermis after the healing of a wound.

Cloaca In birds, the terminal end of the urinary, reproductive, and gastrointestinal tracts.

Closed-suction drains Uses vacuum bottles and plastic conduits to draw fluid away from the wound by producing a negative pressure.

Cocci A bacteria with a round shape.

Coccygeal vertebrae Vertebrae found in the tail.

Coelom A body cavity; in birds and reptiles, the coelom makes up the thoracic and abdominal cavities.

Colic Severe abdominal pain of sudden onset caused by a variety of conditions, including obstruction, twisting, and spasm of the intestine.

Collimator A device on an x-ray machine that is used to restrict the x-ray beam to reduce scatter.

Colloidal gold assay A type of immunochromatographic test that uses a colloidal gold/antibody conjugate in the test system.

Colonic Drugs or functions related to the colon.

Colostrum Thin, milky fluid secreted from the mammary glands just before and immediately after parturition; important for transfer of passive immunity.

Colostrometer A tool that measures the specific gravity of the colostrum.

Columella The middle ear bone in birds.

Coma An unconscious patient that does not respond to any stimuli.

Combining form A word or root word that may or may not use the connecting vowel *o* when it is used as an element in a medical word formation. The combining form is the combination of the root word and the combining vowel.

Combining vowel A vowel, usually an *o*, used to connect a word or root word to the appropriate suffix or to another root word.

Commissure Location where two things are joined.

Committee on Veterinary Technician Education and Activities A group of individuals having varying backgrounds in veterinary medicine and veterinary technology who oversee the curricula and guidelines outlined in the AVMA Accreditation Policies and Procedure Manual.

Common law Laws developed by judges through decisions of courts and similar tribunals (called case law), rather than through legislative statutes or executive action, and to corresponding legal systems that rely on precedent case law.

Companion Animal Parasite Council Organization that fosters animal and human health, while preserving the human-animal bond, through recommendations for the diagnosis, treatment, prevention, and control of parasitic infections.

Complement A group of plasma proteins that function to enhance the activities of the immune system.

Complementary therapies Practices used in conjunction with or as complements to the Western approach.

Compound word Two or more words or root words combined to make a new word.

Comprehensive Drug Abuse Prevention and Control Act A law created in 1970 by the US Congress to regulate the manufacture, distribution, dispensing, and delivery of certain drugs that have the potential for abuse.

Compress Cold herbal tea on a cloth.

Computed tomography (CT) A modality that uses an x-ray tube that freely rotates around a patient, creating a dataset of images that can be manipulated in a sagittal, transverse, and axial plane.

Concentrates Feeds that are low in fiber and high in energy and/or protein.

Conclusions The results or outcomes.

Concussion A violent shock or jarring of the tissue.

Congenital disease A disease present at birth.

Congestive heart failure Increased pulmonary or systemic venous capillary pressure, resulting in fluid leakage and subsequent pulmonary edema or effusion.

Consent forms An educational tool explaining treatments, procedures, anesthesia, risks, and the possibility of death. When signed by the educated client, the form acts as a tool providing some evidence that the client understood diagnosis, treatment, and outcome as well as payment methods acceptable at end of services rendered if litigation arises.

Contamination The presence of microorganisms within or on an object or wound.

Continuous rate infusion Drugs given over a long period ranging from hours to days as a slow injection or drip.

Contour feathers The largest feathers that form the external appearance of adult birds. These are found on the wings, tail, and body surface and are the feathers of flight.

Contrast In radiography, the differences in radiographic density between adjacent areas on a radiographic image

Control A biologic solution of known values used for verification of accuracy and precision of test results.

Controlled substance A drug that has been deemed by the DEA as potentially abusive; a substance with potential for physical addition, psychological addiction, and/or abuse. Also referred to as a schedule drug.

Controlled Substance Act (CSA) A law most applicable to the veterinary community regarding the drugs used by veterinarians.

Contusion A bruise or injury with no break in the surface of the tissue.

Coombs test An immunologic test designed to detect antibodies on the surface of erythrocytes (direct Coombs test) or antibodies in plasma against erythrocytes (indirect Coombs test).

Co-pay A specified dollar amount of a covered service that is the policy holder's responsibility.

Coprodeum The terminal end of the rectum in the cranial compartment of the cloaca.

Corticosteroid A glucocorticoid.

Cortisone A glucocorticoid.

Cotton suture An organic nonabsorbable suture material with less tissue reaction than silk; cotton supports bacterial growth.

Counted brush stroke method A surgical personnel prep accomplished by dividing skin into surface areas and applying a set number of brush strokes to each surface.

Coupage A technique used in conjunction with nebulization to promote removal of respiratory secretions.

Coverts Smaller feathers that cover the remiges and rectrices. They are for covering the body and play no role in flight.

Computed radiography (CR) A type of digital radiography that uses a cassette screen (imaging plate) system.

Cranial Pertaining to the cranium or head end of the body, or denoting a position more toward the cranium or head end of the body than another reference point (body part).

Cranial cruciate ligament repair The surgical stabilization of the stifle joint after cranial cruciate ligament rupture.

Cranial sacral A subtle manipulation of the skull and spine to relax and align the body for optimal energy flow.

Cream A semisolid dosage form that is applied to the skin.

Creatinine Waste product formed during normal muscle cell metabolism.

Credentialed veterinary technician A person who has graduated from an AVMA-accredited program and passed the Veterinary Technician National Exam, and maintains certification, registration, or licensure in the state in which he or she lives or works.

Crile forceps Hemostatic forceps with transverse serrations that extend the entire jaw length.

Critical care Intensive monitoring and treatment of an unstable patient with a life-threatening or potentially life-threatening illness or injury.

Crop In birds, an outpocketing of the esophagus; the outcropping or dilatation of the esophagus located at the base of the neck just cranial to the thoracic inlet.

Crossbite, anterior Maxillary incisors are caudal to mandibular incisors.

Crossbite, posterior The mandible is wider than the maxilla.

Crown The exposed, or visible, portion of the tooth above the gingival tissue.

Cryoprecipitate A blood product that is prepared from plasma and contains von Willebrand factor, factor VIII, fibrinogen, and fibronectin.

Cryosupernatant plasma Plasma from which cryoprecipitate has been removed.

Crutched Removal of wool from the perineal area in pregnant ewes.

Curettes An instrument used to scrape surfaces of dense tissue.

Curved needles Suture needles that are manipulated with needle holders.

Cusps Flaps.

Cutaneous exudate See serous exudate.

Cut-down Procedure for surgically exposing superficial blood vessels.

Cutting needles Suture needles with two or three opposing cutting edges; used in tissues that are difficult to penetrate.

Cyanosis A blue coloration of the skin and mucous membranes because of the presence of deoxygenated hemoglobin.

Cyclozoonosis A zoonosis in which several cycles of disease usually occur sequentially in several different vertebrate species, one of which is human.

Cysticercus A larval form of tapeworm consisting of a single scolex enclosed in a bladderlike cyst.

Cytokines Soluble molecules that serve as mediators of cell responses.

Cytotoxic T cell A type of lymphocyte that searches for and destroys pathogens in infected body cells on stimulation by cytokines.

D

Direct digital radiography (DDR) A type of digital radiography that uses an imaging plate of detectors that is connected directly to a computer system.

Debridement phase Entering of the neutrophil into the wound to scavenge debris and kill bacteria and therefore decontaminate the wound from foreign debris.

Deciduous teeth The primary, or first set of teeth; often referred to as baby teeth. They fall out and are replaced by permanent teeth.

Declawing Onychectomy, the surgical removal of a claw.

Decongestant Reduces congestion of the mucous membranes.

Decubital ulcer Pressure sores exacerbated by recumbency, increased skin moisture, and irritation; pressure sores (bedsores) that result from an animal lying on a bony prominence for too long.

Deductible The dollar amount an individual must pay for services before the insurance company's payment. Clients may have a choice of per-incident deductible or annual deductible with a pet health insurance policy.

Definitive host The host that harbors the adult, mature, or sexual stages of a parasite.

Delta foramina The entry point for the nerves and blood vessels into the pulp cavity; also called the apical delta, because it is located at the apex, root tip, of the tooth.

Dendrites Parts of a neuron that conduct impulses received from other neurons toward the nerve cell body.

Dental pad An area of dense tissue that replaces the upper incisors in most ruminant species.

Dentin The layer beneath the enamel and cementum (70% inorganic, 30% organic collagen and water); formed by odontoblasts from pulpal tissue continue to manufacture dentin in a tubular pattern throughout the life of the tooth.

Department of Labor The federal agency that fosters and promotes the welfare of job seekers, wage earners, and retirees, administering a variety of labor laws, including those that guarantee workers' rights to safe and healthful working conditions; a minimum hourly wage and overtime pay; freedom from employment discrimination; unemployment insurance; and other income support.

Depressed When patient is conscious but slow to respond to stimuli.

Differential diagnoses Diagnostic possibilities.

Dermatophyte A group of cutaneous mycotic organisms commonly known as ringworm fungi.

Developer A chemical solution that converts the exposed silver halide crystals of an exposed x-ray film to black metallic silver.

Diabetic ketoacidosis (DKA) A potentially life-threatening complication in patients with diabetes mellitus, wherein the body switches to burning fatty acids and produces harmful ketone bodies.

Diapedesis The process by which cells, especially neutrophils, exit the blood vessels usually at a site of inflammation by "squeezing" through the microscopic space between the endothelial cells lining the blood vessels.

Diastema A gap in the dental arcade, as seen between incisors and cheek teeth of some species.
Diastole Relaxation of heart chambers to receive the blood.
Diastolic blood pressure The minimum force during the relaxation phase, or when the aortic and pulmonic valves are closed; the pressure of blood in the artery when the heart relaxes between beats.
Differential cell count Procedure for classifying cells to determine relative percentages of each cell type present in a peripheral blood or bone marrow sample.
Differential media Bacterial culture method that allows bacteria to be identified based on their biochemical reactions on the medium.
Diffusion Movement of molecules across a semipermeable membrane from an area of high concentration to low concentration of solutes.
Digital imaging and communications in medicine (DICOM) The universal method in which medical images are stored and transferred.
Diptera An insect of the taxonomic order Diptera (flies); most adults contain a single pair of wings.
Direct exposure film High-detail film that does not require the use of intensifying screens.
Direct marketing The most popular form of marketing. The Yellow Pages are a classic example of direct marketing.
Disinfectants Chemical agents that kill or prevent growth of microorganisms on inanimate objects.
Disinfection The destruction of pathogenic microorganisms or their toxins; the destruction of vegetative forms of bacteria on inanimate or nonliving objects; may not necessarily include spores or spore-forming bacteria.
Dispensing fee A fee added to medication that is dispensed through the hospital to recover the cost of the pill vial, label, and team members' time to fill the prescription.
Disseminated intravascular coagulation (DIC) Also referred to as consumption coagulopathy and defibrination syndrome; it is an acquired, secondary coagulation disorder characterized by depletion of thrombocytes and coagulation factors.
Distal Farther from the center of the body relative to another body part or a location on a body part relative to another closer location; away from the center of the dental arch.
Distance enhancement Phenomenon that describes the appearance of ultrasound image when the sound beam traverses a cystic structure
Distraction technique The use of mild pain to distract the attention of an animal so a procedure can be performed.
Distribution Movement of a drug from the systemic circulation into the tissues.
Diuretic A drug that increases urine formation and promotes water loss.
Diurnal Pertaining to those species that forage or hunt in the daytime.
Doe A female rabbit.
Dolichocephalic The condition of having a long face; more specifically, a long, narrow muzzle.
Dorsal Pertaining to the back area of a quadruped (animal with four legs), or denoting a position more toward the spine than another reference point (body part).
Dorsal recumbency Restraint technique whereby the animal is held in position resting on its back; may require use of a V-trough to keep the patient in position.
Dosage form The form in which the drug is supplied; solid, semisolid, liquid.
Dosage interval The time between administrations of separate drug doses.
Dosage regimen The dose and dosage interval of a specific drug.
Dose The amount of drug administered at one time.
Dosha The metabolic body type used in Ayurveda to determine balances and imbalances.
Dosimetry badge Used for monitoring cumulative exposure to ionizing radiation.
Down feathers The layer of fine feathers under the exterior feathers.
Drenching Administration of small volumes of liquid using a dose syringe
Drug elimination Removal of a drug from the body.
Drug Enforcement Agency (DEA) The primary federal law enforcement agency responsible for combating the abuse of controlled drugs.
Drug metabolism The alteration of a drug by the body before elimination.
Dry cow A dairy cow that is not being milked during her dry period. The dry period usually consists of a 60-day window between the end of one lactation cycle and the expected birth of another calf, which will start a new lactation cycle.
Ductus deferens A convoluted structure in which sperm storage and maturation occur.
Dullness A thudlike sound produced by encapsulated tissue, such as the liver or spleen.
Dysphagia Difficulty eating.
Dyspnea Increased respiratory effort or difficulty breathing.
Dystocia An abnormal or difficult labor.

E

Ecchymosis A small hemorrhagic spot, larger than petechiae, in the skin or mucous membrane, forming a nonelevated, rounded or irregular, blue or purplish patch.
Echoic Used to describe a tissue that reflects most ultrasound waves back to the transducer.
Economic order quantity Method for determining the correct amount of inventory to order.
Ectoparasite A parasite that resides on the surface of its host.
Ectropion Condition in which the eyelid turns outward.
Effective renal plasma flow (ERPF) A clearance study to evaluate kidney function; uses test substances eliminated both by glomerular filtration and renal secretion.
Effector cell Collective term for the lymphocytes that function in the immune system to enhance the functions of other cells.
Effleurage A massage technique using palm and fingers in a light and slow motion.
Effusion Excess fluid in a tissue or body cavity.
Electrocautery A device containing a needle tip or scalpel that is heated before it is applied to tissue, to provide hemostasis in vessels less than 2 mm.
Electrocoagulation A process that involves generating heat in tissue with a high-frequency current, to provide hemostasis in vessels less than 2 mm.
Electrolyte Any substance that dissociates into ions when in solution.
Elimination The passing of urine or feces.
ELISA Enzyme-linked immunosorbent assay, an immunologic test.
Elixir A solution of drug dissolved in sweetened alcohol.
Emasculatome A castrating instrument to accomplish closed castration, keeping the skin intact.

Emasculator An instrument used to perform open castration by crushing and severing the spermatic cord.
Emergency care An action directed toward the assessment, treatment, and stabilization of a patient with an urgent medical problem.
Emetics Drugs that induce vomiting.
Employee handbook A document created in well-managed veterinary hospitals to outline policies and procedures (including labor expectations, sexual harassment, overtime, vacation, benefits, etc.); hospital philosophy; and mission, vision, and value statements. At time of hire and annually the employee handbook is reviewed with employee and updated.
Enamel The substance that cover the crown of the tooth. It is the substance in the body (96% inorganic) and is made of hydroxyapatite crystals.
End tidal Occurs at the end of expiration, when CO_2 levels of the expired gas are approximately equal to alveolar and arterial CO_2 ($Paco_2$).
Endemic Refers to a disease that is commonly found in a given geographic area.
Endoparasite A parasite that resides within a host's tissues.
Endospore The dormant form of a bacterium; intracellular refractile bodies resistant to heat, desiccation, chemicals, and radiation; formed by some bacteria when environmental conditions are poor.
Endotoxin A chemical substance that causes disease; produced in the cell walls of gram-negative bacteria and often stimulate the release of pyrogens by the host's cells.
Energy-producing nutrient Substances that have a hydrocarbon structure that produces energy through digestion, metabolism, or transformation.
Enrichment media A type of culture media formulated to meet the requirements of the most fastidious pathogens.
Ensiling A harvesting process by which forage is chopped and placed into a storage unit (e.g., silo) that excludes oxygen.
Enteric Drugs or functions related to the duodenum, jejunum, or ileum (small intestines).
Enteric bacteria Bacteria inhabiting the intestinal tract.
Enteric-coated tablet A tablet that has a special covering that protects the drug from the harsh acidic environment of the stomach and prevents dissolving of the tablet until it enters the intestine.
Enterotomy An incision into the intestine.
Entropion Condition in which the eyelid turns inward.
Enzootic A normal level of animal disease over time in a given geographic area.
Eosinophil A cell of the inflammatory system that contains pink to reddish-orange staining granules when stained with Wright-Giemsa stain; usually prominent in inflammation associated with parasitic infestations and allergic reactions.
Eosinophilia An increase in circulating eosinophils; also used to describe the reddish appearance of cells or components of cells that have high affinity for stains with acid pH.
Eosinophilic exudates Exudates composed primarily of eosinophils.
Epidemic An increase over the normal expected number of disease cases in a geographic area or a certain period of time.
Epidemiology The study of the occurrences of disease and the risk factors that cause disease in a population.
Epidural anesthesia A form of regional anesthesia involving injection of drugs through a catheter placed into the subarachnoid or epidural space of the spinal cord to block the transmission of signals through nerves in or near the spinal cord.
Epiglottis A flap of cartilage that acts as a "trap door" to cover the opening of the larynx during swallowing.
Epitheliotropic A term used to characterize pathogens, especially viruses, that infect epithelial cells, such as the respiratory, intestinal, or urinary epithelium.
Epizootic An increase over the normal expected number of animal disease cases in a geographic area or a certain period of time.
Epizootiology The study of the occurrences of disease and the risk factors that cause disease in an animal population.
Equal Employment Opportunity Law that promotes equal opportunity in employment through administrative and judicial enforcement of the federal civil rights laws and through education and technical assistance.
Erythrocyte indices Calculated values that provide the average volume and hemoglobin concentrations of erythrocytes in a peripheral blood sample.
Eschar Necrotic layers of tissue that slough off.
Esophageal stethoscope An instrument placed in the esophagus during anesthesia at the level of the heart to amplify the heartbeat, audible from a distance.
Essential amino acids Amino acids that cannot be synthesized in the body and so must be supplied by the diet.
Estrogen A steroid compound, named for its importance in the estrous cycle, functioning as the primary female sex hormone.
Ethics The system of moral principles that determines appropriate behavior and actions within a specific group.
Ethmoturbinates Delicate bony scrolls located in the nasal cavity of some species.
Ethology The study of animal behavior.
Ethylene oxide The organic compound with the formula C_2H_4O; carcinogenic. It is used to sterilize substances that would be damaged by high-temperature techniques. The gas kills bacteria (and their endospores), mold, and fungi.
Etiologic diagnosis The causal description of a lesion, such as "enteric salmonellosis."
Etiology The study of causes of disease.
Eukaryote An organism whose cells have a membrane-bound nucleus; includes most plant and animal cells.
Euthanasia The act of ending a patient's life in a humane manner.
Evaluation Sorting data to determine which is important and which is irrelevant.
Eviscerate The protrusion of an organ (viscera) through an incision.
Excretion The removal of a drug from the body.
Exempt employee Those who are exempt from certain wage and hour laws (i.e., overtime pay); usually applies to administrative, executive, or professional employees.
Exfoliative cytology The study of cells shed from body surfaces.
Exotoxin A chemical substance that causes disease; often produced by gram-positive bacteria and secreted into the surrounding medium.
Expectorants Compounds that increase the fluidity of mucus in the respiratory tract by generating liquid secretions by respiratory tract cells.
Extension The act of straightening, such as a joint; also, the act of pulling two component parts apart to lengthen the whole part
External marketing A marketing technique that targets potential clients.
Extracellular fluid (ECF) Body fluid outside the cells, such as plasma and interstitial fluid.

Exudate The visible product of the inflammatory process; usually composed of cellular debris, fluids, and cells that are deposited in tissues and on tissue surfaces.

Eyed needles Suture needles onto which suture material must be threaded.

F

Facial Referring to both labial and buccal surfaces.

Facultative anaerobe Bacteria that do not require oxygen for metabolism but can survive in the presence of oxygen.

Fair Debt Collection Practices Act An act that was passed to protect the public from unethical collection procedures.

Fair Labor Standards Act A federal law that sets minimum wage and overtime regulations.

Fastidious A bacterial species with complex growth or nutritional requirements.

Fat-soluble vitamins Metabolized in a manner similar to fats and stored in the liver.

Federal law A law established by the United States government and legislators (congressmen and senators), enforced by different departments and agencies.

Feed analysis A chemical analysis that determines the proportion of specific components of a feedstuff.

Feedstuff Any dietary component that provides some essential nutrient or serves some other function.

Femoral head ostectomy The surgical amputation of the femoral head.

Fever (pyrexia) An abnormal increase in body temperature caused by the release of agents that increase the body's biological setting to a higher temperature.

Fiberoptic A type of endoscope that uses glass fiber bundles for transmission of images.

Fibrin An insoluble protein that is essential to the clotting of blood.

Fibrinous exudate An exudate composed mostly of fibrin, which is derived from a plasma protein, fibrinogen.

Fibrosis Scarring; the end result of tissue repair.

Film-focal distance (FFD) The distance that is measured from the target of the x-ray tube to the radiographic film or plate. Now commonly referred to as source-image distance (SID).

Film latitude X-ray film's inherent ability to produce shades of gray.

Finochietto retractor A self-retaining retractor with a set screw to maintain tension on tissues; commonly used to retract the thoracic wall.

First-intention healing Also called primary healing; the healing of injured tissue directly without intervention of granulation tissue.

Fixer A chemical solution that clears the unchanged silver halide crystals on the x-ray film after developing and hardens the gelatin layer.

Flank incision An incision oriented perpendicular to the long axis of the body, caudal to the last rib.

Flanking Placing a calf in lateral recumbency.

Flatness An extremely dull sound produced by very dense tissue, such as muscle or bone.

Flexible endoscope An instrument used for gastrointestinal endoscopy, duodenoscopy, colonoscopy, and bronchoscopy.

Flexion The act of bending, such as a joint.

Flowmeter Part of the anesthetic machine that receives medical gases from the pressure regulator. The purpose is to measure and deliver a constant gas flow to the vaporizer, the common gas outlet, and the breathing circuit.

Fluoroscopy An imaging technique that uses an x-ray tube and image intensifier that produces a continual stream of images.

Focused grids X-ray grid with lead strips placed at progressively increasing angles to match the divergence of the x-ray beam.

Fomentation A hot compress.

Forages Feeds made up of most or all of the plant.

Formaldehyde/formalin A chemical compound with the formula CH_2O; it exists in water as the hydrate $H_2C(OH)_2$. Aqueous solutions of formaldehyde are referred to as formalin; exposure to formaldehyde is a significant consideration for human health because it is carcinogenic.

Fractional clearance of electrolytes A mathematic manipulation that describes the excretion of specific electrolytes relative to the glomerular filtration rate.

Fresh frozen plasma The liquid portion of blood that has been harvested and frozen within 8 hours from the time of blood collection, preserving all coagulation and other proteins in the plasma.

Fresh whole blood A unit of blood that was collected less than 8 hours before and has been kept at room temperature, preserving all components in the blood.

Friction massage A fast, invigorating circular massage.

Fructosamine A molecule formed as a result of the irreversible reaction of glucose bound to protein.

Fungicidal A substance that kills fungi.

Furcation The junction at which multiple roots join the neck of the tooth.

G

Gait The manner of walking, stepping, or running.

Gastric Drugs or functions related to the stomach.

Gastroenteropathies Any disease of the stomach and intestines.

Gastropexy The surgical fixation of the stomach to the abdominal wall.

Gastrotomy An incision into the stomach.

Gauntlets Heavy leather gloves used to restrain animals.

Gavage Feeding with a feeding tube passed through the oral cavity into the stomach.

Gelpi retractor A self-retaining retractor with a box lock to maintain tension on tissues, commonly used in orthopedic surgeries.

GEM Genetically engineered mice.

General anesthesia A purposeful derangement of a patient's normal physiologic processes to produce a state of unconsciousness, relaxation, analgesia, and/or amnesia.

General appearance The patient's facial expression, size and position of the eyeballs, general body condition (flesh and hair coat), response to commands, and temperament.

General senses Tactile, temperature, kinesthetic, and pain. They are distributed generally throughout the body or over the entire skin surface.

Generic equivalent A copycat drug that has properties equivalent to the original compound.

Gestation The period of pregnancy.

Gingival margin An epithelial collar often not directly attached to the tooth. Also called the free gingiva.

Gingival sulcus The space between the free gingiva and the enamel of the tooth; often called a pocket. A pocket is the abnormal or additional depth to the sulcus.

Gingivitis Inflammation of the gingiva.

Globulin A complex group of plasma proteins designated as alpha, beta, or gamma; includes immunoglobulins, complement, and transferrin.

Glomerular filtration rate (GFR) The rate at which substances are filtered through the glomerulus and excreted in urine.

Glucose A monosaccharide that represents the end product of carbohydrate metabolism.

Gonadotropin Protein hormones secreted by gonadotrope cells of the pituitary gland, including follicle-stimulating hormone (FSH) and luteinizing hormone (LH).

Granulation tissue Highly vascularized connective tissue produced after extensive tissue damage.

Granulocyte Any cell with distinct cytoplasmic granules.

Granulomatous An inflammatory condition characterized by high numbers (more than 70%) of macrophages.

Gray (Gy) The measured unit of radiation dose that is absorbed because of ionized radiation.

Grid A device made up of lead strips interspaced with a radiolucent material that allows most of the primary radiation to pass through and absorbs the scatter radiation.

Gustatory sense A chemical sense that detects substances that are in the mouth and dissolved in saliva.

H

Hahnemann, Samuel German physician that researched homeopathic remedies.

Hands-on therapy Practitioners use their own hands or body to move, adjust, or manipulate the patient to help facilitate the healing process.

Hay Forage that is cut and allowed to dry before being collected into bales for storage.

Hazardous materials plan An identified, detailed plan explaining how toxic materials are to be tended to; may include safety training and contact numbers for local Hazardous Materials Teams, authorities, and physicians.

Healing crisis A temporary worsening of symptoms followed by overall improvement.

Heel effect An incidence in which there is greater radiation intensity on the cathode side because of the angle of the target on the anode side.

Helper T cell A type of lymphocyte that binds to the antigen on a macrophage surface and then secretes specific cytokines to activate other elements of cell-mediated immunity.

Hematuria The presence of intact erythrocytes in the urine.

Hemoglobinuria The presence of free hemoglobin in the urine.

Hemolysis The rupture of a red blood cell; the destruction of erythrocytes.

Hemoprotozoa Parasites located in peripheral blood.

Hemorrhagic exudate Exudates that consist primarily of erythrocytes that have collected in a tissue after disruption of the vascular system.

Hemostasis The arrest of bleeding by the physiologic properties of vasoconstriction and coagulation.

Herbal therapy The use of specific plant leaves, roots, and/or flowers to assist healing.

Herniorrhaphy The surgical repair of a hernia by suturing the abnormal opening closed.

Heterophil A leukocyte of avian, reptile, and some fish species containing prominent eosinophilic granules; functionally equivalent to the mammalian neutrophil.

Hexacanth The infective stage of some cestodes.

Histopathology The evaluation of tissue samples; the microscopic study of diseased tissues.

Hob A male ferret.

Hobbles A device used to fasten together the legs of an animal to prevent straying.

Hog snare A mechanical restraint device consisting of a metal pipe with a cable loop on one end.

Homeopathy Remedies based on "like curing like." A system of healing that uses dilute substances known to cause the same symptoms as the illness.

Homeostasis A constant internal environment in the body.

Horizontal nystagmus Recurrent flickering back-and-forth eye movements.

Host A living being that offers an environment for maintenance of the organism; not always necessary for the organism's survival.

Human-animal bond The interaction between humans and animals, the special interactive bond that actually enhances human quality of life.

Human carcinogen Any substance, radionuclide, or radiation that is an agent directly involved in the promotion of cancer or the increase of its propagation.

Humoral immunity An immune response involving production of specific antibody.

Husbandry The production, housing, and management of animals.

Hyaline cast A structure formed from protein precipitate of degenerating kidney tubule cells with no imbedded materials.

Hydatid cyst Larval cyst stage of the tapeworms *Echinococcus granulosus* and *E. multilocularis,* which contains daughter cysts, each of which contains many scolexes.

Hydrocephalus An abnormal buildup of cerebrospinal fluid in the brain.

Hydrosols Water left behind after the steam distillation process of aromatherapy. Hydrosols are dilute, gentle, and only subtly aromatic.

Hydrotherapy Use of water as physical therapy; can be passive hydromassage or active walking or swimming therapy.

Hypercapnia Derived from the Greek, *hyper + kapnos,* meaning vapor. It is the excess of carbon dioxide in the blood, indicated by an elevated Pco_2 as determined by blood gas analysis, and resulting in respiratory acidosis. Also known as hypercarbia or hypercarbemia.

Hypercarbemia Excess carbon dioxide in the blood.

Hypercarbia Excess carbon dioxide in the blood.

Hyperechoic A structure in an ultrasound image that appears bright or white compared with adjacent structures.

Hyperkalemia An increased concentration of potassium in the blood.

Hypermotility An increased frequency or intensity of intestinal sounds.

Hypernatremia An increased concentration of sodium in the blood.

Hyperplasia An increased number of cells of an organ or tissue.

Hyperresonance A "booming" sound heard over a gas-filled area, such as an emphysematous lung.

Hypersegmented A neutrophil with more than five nuclear lobes.

Hypersensitivity Immune system reactions that damage a body's own tissues.

Hyperthermia An increase above the body's normal temperature caused by drugs, toxins, or external temperatures, such as in heatstroke; increased body temperature.

Hypertonic A solution that has a greater solute concentration than cells located in it that causes cells to lose water as a result of osmotic pressure.

Hyphae The body of a fungus created as a result of the linear arrangements of cells that form multicellular or multinucleate growth.

Hypoadrenocorticism A deficiency in the production of mineralocorticoid and/or glucocorticoid steroid hormones.

Hypochlorite A sanitizing agent found in products such as laundry bleach, which has a wide spectrum of antimicrobial activity.

Hypochromic Erythrocytes with decreased staining intensity because of decrease in hemoglobin concentration.

Hypoechoic Tissues that reflect less sound back to the ultrasound transducer than surrounding tissues.
Hypokalemia A decreased concentration of potassium in the blood.
Hypomotility A decreased frequency or intensity of intestinal sounds.
Hyponatremia A decreased concentration of sodium in the blood.
Hypothermia Decreased body temperature.
Hypothermic Abnormally low body temperature.
Hypotonic A solution that has a lower solute concentration than cells located in it that causes cells to gain water (swell); caused by osmotic pressure.
Hypovolemia Abnormally low circulating blood volume.
Hypovolemic shock Physiologic compensatory mechanisms that result from decreased intravascular volume.
Hypoxemia Deficiency in the amount of oxygen reaching body tissues.

I

IACUC The Institutional Animal Care and Use Committee.
Icterus Abnormal yellowish discoloration of skin, mucous membranes, or plasma as a result of increased concentration of bile pigments.
IgA An isotype of antibody important in mucosal immunity; secreted onto the mucosal surface of such organs as the lungs and gastrointestinal tract and found in secretions as milk and tears.
IgE The primary immunoglobulin associated with allergic and parasitic reactions.
IgG The most common antibody, found in the highest concentration in the blood.
IgM The second most common antibody in the blood; major immunoglobulin isotype produced in a primary immune response.
Ileus Lack of bowel motility
Immunodeficiency The inability to build up a normal immune response; a state in which the immune system's ability to fight disease is compromised or entirely absent.
Immunodiffusion An immunologic test performed by placing reactants in an agar plate and allowing them to migrate through the gel toward each other.
Immunoglobulin An antibody; plasma proteins produced against specific antigens.
Immunologic tolerance A state of nonresponsiveness to antigens, whether self or foreign.
Implants A solid dosage form of drug that is injected or inserted under the skin and dissolves or releases that drug over an extended period.
Imprinting A rapid learning process that enables a newborn animal to recognize and bond with its owner.
Inactivated vaccine A vaccine that consists of a noninfectious agent, such as whole killed pathogens or selected antigenic subunits; enough to induce immunity.
Indemnity insurance A structure of pet health insurance in which the client is reimbursed for services after they have been provided.
Indirect marketing A marketing technique that is used by practitioners on a daily basis—clean facilities, genuine service, and excellent customer care are a few examples.
Infection Microorganisms in the body or a wound that multiply and cause harmful effects.
Inflammatory phase Healing phase in which bacteria and debris are phagocytized and removed, and factors are released that cause the migration and division of cells involved in the proliferative phase.
Informed consent A person's agreement to allow something to happen, such as a medical treatment or surgery, which is based on full disclosure of the facts necessary to make an intelligent decision.
Injectable A medication that is administered via a needle and syringe.
Innate immunity The nonspecific components of the immune system that function the same way regardless of which antigen is present.
Inquiry Probing into the significant areas requiring more clarification.
Insensible water loss Water loss that is difficult to measure and/or cannot be seen (e.g., losses from the respiratory tract).
Inspection An active process in which the technician visually examines the patient's entire body in a systematic manner for structure and function, paying close attention to deviations or abnormalities.
Instincts Inherited or genetically coded responses to environmental stimuli.
Integrative veterinary medicine (IVM) A combination of natural and holistic therapies with conventional veterinary therapies.
Intensifying screens Plates within the x-ray cassette that are composed of phosphorescent crystals (phosphors) that function to emit light.
Interdental space A space, void of teeth, found in both the upper and lower arcades and that extends from the corner incisors to the first premolars.
Interferons Small soluble proteins that enhance the function of the immune system.
Intermediate host The host that harbors the larval, immature, or asexual stages of a parasite.
Intermediate-acting glucocorticoids Glucocorticoids that exert an anti-inflammatory effect for 12 to 36 hours.
Internal marketing A marketing technique that targets current or existing clients for services offered within the practice.
Interproximal The surface between two teeth.
Interstitium Between cell layers.
Intervertebral disk fenestration The surgical removal of prolapsed intervertebral disk material causing pressure on the spinal cord.
Intestinal anastomosis A surgical procedure designed to restore continuity of the bowel segments.
Intestinal resection and anastomosis The surgical removal of a segment of intestine, followed by suturing together of the cut ends.
Intra-arterial Into an artery.
Intracellular fluid (ICF) Fluid located within the cells.
Intradermal injection (ID) Injecting a drug within (not beneath) the skin with very small needles.
Intramedullary bone pinning The surgical insertion of a metal rod or pin into the medullary cavity of a long bone to fix fracture fragments into place.
Intramuscular (IM) administration Injecting a drug into a muscle mass.
Intraosseous Referring to route of injection directly into the marrow of the bone.
Intraperitoneal (IP) injection Injecting a drug into the abdominal cavity.
Intravenous (IV) injection Injecting a drug into a vein.
Inventory turns per year The number of times an item must be reordered within a stated period; 8 to 12 turns per year should be a goal of each practice.
Iris scissors Delicate scissors designed for fine, precise cuts, often used in ophthalmic procedures.

Irritant laxatives Substances that act to irritate the bowel to increase peristaltic motility.

Isoechoic Tissue that appears on ultrasound to have the same echotexture as surrounding tissues.

Isoenzymes A group of enzymes with similar catalytic activities but different physical properties.

Isoerythrolysis An uncommon, complex disorder of newborns that results from a blood group incompatibility between mother and offspring resulting in destruction of the red blood cells of the offspring.

Isosthenuria A condition in which urine specific gravity approaches that of the glomerular filtrate.

Isotonic A solution with the same solute concentration as cells so that the cells neither gain nor lose water.

Isotype A class of antibody based on molecular weight; examples include IgG, IgM, IgA, IgE, and IgD.

J

Jackson-Rees circuit A type of nonrebreathing circuit also referred to as the Mapleson F system. As with other Mapleson circuits, it contains a fresh gas flow that is used to remove exhaled carbon dioxide, a fresh gas inlet at the patient end of the breathing tube, and a reservoir bag at the opposite end. As with an Ayre's T-piece, the fresh gas inlet of a Jackson-Rees circuit enters the breathing tube at a 45- to 90-degree angle.

Jill A female ferret.

K

Karyolysis Degeneration or dissolution of a cell nucleus.

Karyorrhexis Fragmentation of a cell nucleus.

Keel The bony ridge on the sternum of birds where the flight muscles attach.

Kelly forceps Hemostatic forceps with transverse serrations that extend over only the distal portion of the jaws.

Ketoacidosis Accumulation of ketone bodies in the body tissues and fluids.

Ketonuria The presence of detectable ketone bodies in urine.

Kilovoltage peak (kVp) The maximum voltage applied across an x-ray tube that determines the energy of the electrons produced

Kinetic assay A chemical test that measures the rate of change of a substance in the test system.

kVp (kilovoltage peak) The maximum voltage applied across an x-ray tube that determines the energy of the electrons produced.

L

Labial The surface toward the lip.

Laceration A tear or jagged wound.

Lagomorphs Gnawing mammals that have two pairs or incisors in the upper jaw, one behind the other; rabbits.

Laminitis Inflammation of the hoof lamina; a cause of lameness; also called founder.

Laparotomy An incision into the abdominal cavity, also called celiotomy.

Laryngoscope A medical instrument that is used to obtain a view of the vocal folds and the glottis, which is the space between the cords. Often used to help place the endotracheal tube.

Laryngospasm An uncontrolled/involuntary muscular contraction (spasm) of the laryngeal cords. The spasm can happen often without any provocation, but tends to occur after tracheal extubation.

Larynx Commonly called the voice box, a short, irregular tube of cartilage and muscle that connects the pharynx with the trachea and controls airflow to and from the lungs.

Latent image The invisible image that is within the emulsion of an x-ray film produced after the film has been exposed to light.

Lateral Denoting a position farther from the median plane of the body or a structure, on the side or toward the side away from the median plane, or pertaining to the side of the body or of a structure.

Lateral ear resection The surgical removal of the lateral wall of the vertical portion of the external ear canal.

Lateral intercostal thoracotomy An incision into the lateral thorax, oriented between two ribs.

Lateral recumbency A restraint technique whereby the animal is held in position resting on the side of the body.

Lavage To irrigate or wash.

Laws These set the maximum limits from which we can deviate from the acceptable norm; enforced by authorized officers.

Left shift The presence of increased numbers of immature cells in a peripheral blood sample.

Lethargy Sluggish or drowsy.

Leukemia The presence of neoplastic cells in the blood or bone marrow.

Leukopenia A decreased number of leukocytes in blood.

Leukocyte A white blood cell.

Leukocytosis Increased numbers of leukocytes in the blood.

Licensure Maintained by the state government or veterinary state board and may be mandatory.

Lignin An inert compound that increases rigidity of the plant cell wall.

Lingual A surface toward the tongue.

Lipase A pancreatic enzyme that functions in the breakdown of fats.

Lipemia The presence of fatty material in plasma or serum.

Local/municipal law Legislation created by townships, counties, or cities that governs the rules and regulations within a municipality authorizing enforcement offers to enforce the laws.

Long-acting glucocorticoids Glucocorticoids that exert an anti-inflammatory effect for more than 48 hours.

Loop diuretics Medications that produce diuresis by inhibiting sodium resorption from the loop of Henle in nephrons.

Lumbar vertebrae Bones located in the abdominal region; they serve as the site of attachment for the large sling muscles that support the abdomen.

Lymphadenitis Inflammation of one or more lymph nodes.

Lymphocyte A leukocyte involved in the inflammatory process; also has roles in humoral and cell-mediated immunity.

Lymphokine A type of cytokine produced by T lymphocytes.

Lysis The destruction or decomposition, as of a cell or other substance, under the influence of a specific agent or force.

M

M:E ratio Relative percentages of myeloid and erythroid cells in the bone marrow.

mA (milliamperage) The current produced by the x-ray tube during an exposure.

Macrophage An important cell in the inflammatory process; functions to phagocytize pathogens, then presents antigen on its surface for recognition by immune cells; a phagocytic cell derived from the monocyte.

Magill circuit An example of a semiclosed breathing circuit, also known as the Mapleson A system, in which rebreathing is prevented by having the gas flow rate from the cylinders slightly in excess of the patient's minute respiratory volume.

Maintenance energy requirement (MER) The BMR plus the additional energy needed for normal physical activity.

Maintenance fluid solution Fluids with a composition different than plasma; low-sodium, high-potassium concentration.

Major blood crossmatch Detects antibodies in the recipient plasma against the donor red blood cells.

Malocclusion The improper positioning of teeth.

Malpractice/professional negligence A type of negligence in which a physician fails to follow generally accepted professional standards, causing injury to the patient.

Mandible The lower jaw or arcade of teeth.

Margin The difference between the selling price and the cost per unit.

Markup A term commonly used to price a product based on a percentage of cost, such as per tablet, per milliliter, or per bottle.

Mast cell Tissue cell characterized by abundant, small, metachromatic cytoplasmic granules that functions in the immune system.

Mastectomy The surgical removal of part or all of one or more mammary glands.

Material Safety Data Sheet Informational material that must be kept in all businesses; contains detailed product safety information on hazardous materials found in that place of a business; an OSHA mandate.

Mathieu needle holders Needle holders with a ratchet lock at the proximal end of the handles of the holder, permitting locking and unlocking simply with a progressive squeezing of the instrument.

Maturation phase Wound healing process during which collagen is remodeled and realigned along tension lines and cells that are no longer needed are removed by apoptosis.

Maxilla The upper jaw or arcade of teeth.

Maximum permissible dose (MPD) The radiation dose for occupationally exposed persons; cannot exceed 5 REM per year.

Mayo scissors Tissue scissors designed for cutting heavy tissue such as fascia.

Mayo stand An instrument stand that is moveable and has a removable tray top.

Mayo-Hegar needle holders Needle holders with a ratchet lock just distal to the thumb, with a blade for cutting suture.

Mean arterial pressure Defined as the average arterial pressure during a single cardiac cycle and considered to be the perfusion pressure seen by organs in the body.

Medial Denoting a position closer to the median plane of the body or a structure, toward the middle or median plane, or pertaining to the middle or a position closer to the median plane of the body or a structure.

Median sternotomy An incision along the midline of the ventral thorax.

Megakaryocyte Bone marrow cell from which blood platelets arise.

Mentation The mental state or status of a patient; the patient's attentiveness or reaction to its environment; mental function.

Meridians Rivers or channels that travel throughout a body connecting and regulating different body parts and organs.

Merozoite Life cycle stage of a protozoal parasite that results from asexual reproduction.

Mesaticephalic A condition of having a medium face; more specifically a medium length and width muzzle; mesiocephalic.

Mesenchymal Cells or tissues derived from the embryonic mesoderm.

Mesial Toward the center of the dental arch (rostral).

Mesophiles Organisms with an optimal growth temperature between 25° and 40° C.

Mesothelial Cells that line body cavities; derived from the embryonic mesoderm.

Metabolite An altered drug molecule.

Metastasis Neoplastic cells present in areas other than the location where they originated.

Metazoonosis A zoonosis that is maintained by both invertebrate (tick or mosquito) and vertebrate species.

Metzenbaum scissors Delicate scissors designed for cutting fine, thin tissue.

Microaerophilic An organism requiring oxygen for growth at a level below that found in air.

Microbial fermentation Process by which herbivores break down cellulose.

Microfilaria Larval offspring of the group of filarial worms in the phylum Nematoda.

Milliamperage (mA) Controls the number of electrons in the electron cloud generated at the filament of the cathode and thus the quantity of x-rays produced.

Minimum prescription fee The minimum amount charged to a client for a prescription fill; for example, if a client only needs two pills, a minimum prescription fee may be instituted.

Minor blood crossmatch Detects antibodies in the donor plasma against the recipient red blood cells.

Miracidium Ciliated larval stage of a digenic trematode.

Mirror-image Ultrasound artifact produced in areas with strongly reflective interfaces.

Mixed nerves A combination of both sensory and motor nerves.

Modified-live A vaccine that consists of a weakened version of the pathogen, which will induce an immune response but is attenuated enough so that it will not cause disease.

Molting The process of feather replacement that occurs one to several times a year, species depending.

Monocyte A precursor cell in the stage of development of tissue macrophage; after a monocyte leaves the bloodstream and enters tissue at a site of inflammation, it becomes an activated macrophage.

Monofilament suture A suture made of a single strand of material, creating less tissue drag than multifilament suture.

Monokine A type of cytokine produced by macrophages.

Morphologic diagnosis A physical description of a lesion, such as "acute necrotizing enteritis."

Mosquito hemostats A small hemostatic forceps with transverse jaw serrations.

Mother tincture A natural source combined with alcohol; a term used in homeopathy and flower essences.

Motor nerves Carry instructions from the central nervous system out to the body.

Mott cell Plasma cells containing multiple globular cytoplasmic inclusions composed of immunoglobulin (Russell bodies).

Mouthing A beaking phase of neonatal development.

Magnetic resonance imaging (MRI) A modality that uses a magnetic field that recognizes the natural resonance of the atoms within the body to produce images.

Mucogingival line The border between the attached gingiva and the looser mucosa.

Mucopurulent exudate This consists of a mixture of purulent and mucous exudates.

Mueller-Hinton media Standard culture media used to evaluate susceptibility of microorganisms to antimicrobial agents.

Multifilament suture A suture made of several strands of material twisted or braided together, more pliable and flexible than monofilament.

Multimodal therapy The use of several analgesic drugs, each with a different mechanism of action resulting in lower dosages and thus increasing safety for the animal.

Murine Pertaining to mice or rats.

Muzzle Nylon, leather, or gauze covering placed over an animal's mouth to prevent biting.

Mycology The study of fungi.

Myelography An exam that involves injecting a contrast media in the subarachnoid space to visualize the spinal cord.

Myiasis Infestation with larvae (maggots) of dipterans.

Myoclonus A brief, involuntary twitching of a muscle or a group of muscles.

Myopathy A muscular disease in which the muscle fibers do not function for any one of many reasons, resulting in muscular weakness. Derived from the Greek *myo-*, meaning muscle, and *-pathy,* meaning suffering.

N

Narcosis Unconsciousness induced by a narcotic drug.

Nares The nostrils; the external openings of the nasal cavity.

Nasogastric Pertaining to the nose and stomach, particularly placement of a feeding tube into the stomach via the nares.

National Fire Protection Association An authority on fire, electrical, and building safety.

Natural immunity An immunity conferred to the body by exposure to a pathogen by natural means rather than through vaccination.

Natural killer (NK) cell A subpopulation of lymphocytes capable of direct lysis of cells infected with antigen.

Nebulization Humidification of inspired gases to promote mobilization and removal of unwanted secretions in patients with respiratory disease.

Necropsy Postmortem examination of an animal body.

Negative contrast agents Gases such as oxygen or carbon dioxide that are radiolucent on radiographs that are used to outline organs during diagnostic imaging procedures.

Negligence Finding that a practitioner's actions were below the level of competence expected of the professional.

Negri body Eosinophilic staining inclusion body found in cells that have been infected with rabies.

Neoplasia The process of abnormal and uncontrolled growth of cells; generic term to describe any growth; often used to describe a tumor, which may be malignant or benign.

Neuroleptanalgesia A state of central nervous system depression (sedation or tranquilization) and analgesia induced by a combination of a sedative, tranquilizer, and analgesic.

Neuron Nerve cell; the basic structural and functional unit of the nervous system.

Neuropathic pain A complex, chronic pain state that usually is accompanied by tissue injury in which the nerve fibers may be damaged, dysfunctional, or injured, and send incorrect signals to other pain centers.

Neurotransmitter Molecules diffuse across the synapse to contact the cell membrane of the adjacent nerve cell.

Neurotropic A term used to characterize pathogens, especially viruses, which infect cells of the central nervous system.

Neutropenia Abnormal decrease in the number of neutrophils in a peripheral blood sample.

Neutrophil Leukocyte that functions to phagocytize infectious agents and cellular debris; plays a major role in the inflammatory process.

Neutrophilia An abnormal increase in the number of neutrophils in a peripheral blood sample.

Nitrogen-free extract (NFE) The nonfiber carbohydrate portion of the feed.

Nit The egg stage of lice bound to hair or feather shaft of the host.

Nociception The neural processes of encoding and processing noxious stimuli. It is the afferent activity produced in the peripheral and central nervous system by stimuli that have the potential to damage tissue, initiated by nociceptors, or pain receptors.

Nocturnal species Those that forage and hunt at night.

Non–energy-producing nutrients Play an important role throughout the body system and are often called the "gatekeepers of metabolism."

Nonessential amino acids Building blocks of proteins that are synthesized in the body.

Nonexempt employee Receives hourly wages; subject to wage and hour laws (i.e., overtime pay); usually applies to nonprofessional employees not in administrative positions.

Nonnutritive feed additives Buffers, hormones, binders, and medications added to feeds.

Nonproductive cough A dry and hacking cough with no mucus produced.

Nonproprietary name Also known as generic name; a concise name given to a specific compound.

Nonrebreathing system Anesthetic breathing circuits in which exhaled gases are discharged to the environment and do not pass back to the patient.

Nonsuppurative exudate An exudate composed primarily of lymphocytes and monocytes; usually restricted to exudates in central nervous system and the integumentary system (skin).

Nonsystemic antacids Medications that directly neutralize acid molecules in the stomach or rumen.

Nonverbal communication Communication by means other than by using words (e.g., through facial expressions, hand gestures, and tone of voice).

Norman mask elbow A nonrebreathing circuit that is almost identical to a Jackson-Rees, except that the endotracheal tube connector is at right angles to the breathing tube. This is considered a Mapleson F system. This circuit may slightly reduce mechanical dead space compared with an Ayre's T-piece or Jackson-Rees.

Normochromic Cells that stain with their characteristic color.

Normocytic Cells that appear with their characteristic morphology.

Normothermia Normal body temperature.

Nosocomial infection A hospital-acquired infection.

NSAIDs Nonsteroidal anti-inflammatory drugs.

Nuclear medicine A modality that uses a gamma camera and radioisotopes to image the metabolic, physical, and functional processes.

Nuclear molding A deformation of nuclei by other nuclei within the same cell or adjacent cells.

Nutrient Any constituent of food that is ingested to support life.

Nystagmus Involuntary eye movement.

O

Object-film distance (OFD) That distance between the object being radiographed and the film or plate. Object-image distance (OID) is the term now in use.

Oblique At an angle, or pertaining to an angle.

Observation Observing nonverbal communication, body language, and facial expressions.

Occlusion The surface of the tooth that touches the opposing tooth.

Occupational Safety and Health Act (OSHA) A federal law designed to provide a safe workplace for all persons working in any business effecting commerce.
Ointment A semisolid dosage form that is applied to the skin.
Olfactory sense A chemical sense that detects chemical substances in inhaled air.
Oliguria Decreased urine production.
Olsen-Hegar needle holders Needle holders with a ratchet lock just distal to the thumb.
Onychectomy Declaw; surgical removal of a claw.
Oocyst The resistant spore phase of some parasitic protozoans.
Operant conditioning A behavioral theory based on the principle that the consequences of a behavior will influence its frequency.
Operculum A lid or flap covering an opening; common structure on the eggs of some trematodes; a keratinized flap of tissue inside the nares of some birds.
Opisthotonus A state of a severe hyperextension and spasticity in which a patient's head, neck, and spinal column enter into a complete "arching" position.
Opsonization The coating of the outer surface of pathogens by antibodies to allow easier phagocytosis by macrophages.
Orally administered Drugs given by mouth.
Orchiectomy The surgical removal of the testes.
Organophosphates Compounds that are commonly used as insecticide dips and may result in toxicity if used inappropriately.
Orogastric administration Delivery of medication or nutritiona support via an orogastric tube.
Orogastric tube A flexible tube that is passed through the mouth (*oro-*), down the esophagus and into the stomach (*-gastric*) for the purpose of delivering fluids and liquid medication directly into the stomach.
Oropharynx The oral cavity in birds.
Oscillometer An instrument used for measuring the changes in pulsations in the arteries, especially of the extremities.
Osmolality The concentration of particles in a solution, expressed as mOsm/kg.
Osmosis The movement of water across a semipermeable membrane from the side with high water concentration to low water concentration.
Osmotic diuretic A medication that helps retain water in the renal tubular lumen via osmosis by altering the solute concentration.
Osmotic pressure The pressure required to stop the movement of water into a solution containing solutes when the solutions are separated by a semipermeable membrane.
Osteotome An instrument designed to cut or shape bone and cartilage.
Outstanding accounts Client accounts that owe money to the veterinary practice; money owed to a creditor.
Ovariohysterectomy The surgical removal of the uterus and ovaries.
Overtime Any time accumulated while on the time clock; more than 40 hours in any 1 week (7 consecutive days).
Oxidase An enzyme present in some groups of bacteria that is involved with the reduction of oxygen during normal bacterial metabolism.
Oxygen saturation A relative measure of the amount of oxygen that is dissolved or carried in a given medium; also known as dissolved oxygen (DO).

P

Packed cell volume Ratio of red blood cells to total plasma volume.
Packed red blood cells A unit of packed red blood cells begins as a volume of whole blood, from which platelets and plasma have been removed, leaving a preparation of mostly red blood cells.
Pain An unpleasant sensory or emotional experience associated with actual or potential tissue damage. Classified as peripheral (visceral or somatic), neuropathic (originating from damaged nerves), clinical (ongoing pain), and idiopathic (unknown cause).
Palatal A surface toward the mouth.
Palisade A parallel arrangement of some species of bacteria; often described as looking like a picket fence.
Palmar The caudal surface of the front foot distal to the antebrachiocarpal joint; also pertains to the undersurface of the front foot.
Palpation Using the hands and the sense of touch to detect tenderness, altered temperature, texture, vibration, pulsation, masses or swellings, and other changes in body integrity; can be classified as light or deep.
Pancytopenia Decreased numbers of all blood cells and platelets in a peripheral blood or bone marrow sample.
Paracostal incision An incision oriented parallel to the last rib.
Parakeet Various small slender parrots, usually having long tapering tails and often kept as pets; also referred to as budgerigars.
Parallel technique A radiographic technique in which the film is placed in the mouth parallel to the teeth and the cone is aimed perpendicular to the film and tooth.
Paramedian incision An incision located lateral and parallel to the ventral midline of the animal.
Parasite An organism that has adapted to live on or within a host organism, deriving all its nutrients from that host, ideally without killing the host.
Parasympathetic system The "rest and restore" system. It predominates during relaxed, routine, business-as-usual states.
Parenterally administered Drugs given by injection.
Parthenogenic A condition in which female organisms produce eggs that develop without fertilization.
Partial intravenous anesthesia (PIVA) Combining intravenous and inhalation anesthesia to achieve balanced anesthesia.
Parturition The act of giving birth
Passerinines Pertaining to or relating to birds of the order Passeriformes, which includes perching birds and songbirds such as canaries, finches, and sparrows.
Passive exercise No voluntary muscle activity is used during this type of physical therapy.
Passive immunity Receiving antibodies from colostrum or synthesized antibodies.
Paste A semisolid dosage form that is given orally.
Pathogen An infectious organism that can cause disease in a host.
Pathologist One who studies disease.
Pathology The study of disease.
Pecten A dark ribbonlike structure attached to the retina and extending into the vitreous humor and thought to provide nourishment to the eye.
Pediculosis Infestation with lice.
Peer assistance Veterinary professional organizations offering wellness programs to veterinary professionals in the midst of substance abuse challenges.
Penrose drain A surgical device placed in a wound to drain fluid. It consists of a soft rubber tube placed in a wound area.
Penumbra effect The partial or imperfect shadow of an object outside of the complete shadow where the light from the source of light is partly cut off.
Per os By mouth.
Percussion Tapping of the body's surface to produce vibration and sound; commonly used on the thorax for examining the heart and lungs; the creation of waves of air to loosen secretions in the

lungs, typically accomplished by clapping hands across the thorax to elicit a cough.

Perfused Having a blood supply.

Perfusion Blood flow across all tissues in an individual body; derived from the Latin *perfundere*, meaning to pour over; refers to the passage of oxygenated blood through body tissues.

Perianal Pertaining to the area around the anus.

Perineal urethrostomy An incision into the urethra and suturing of the splayed edges to the skin to create a larger urethral orifice.

Periodic parasite A parasite that lives part of its life cycle on its host and part off the host.

Periodontal ligament A ligament that holds the tooth into the alveolar bone. It is attached to cementum and to the alveolar socket. It absorbs the shock of pressures applied to the occlusal surface of the tooth.

Periodontitis Inflammation of the periodontium.

Periodontium The supporting structures around the tooth.

Periosteal elevator An instrument designed to remove the periosteum.

Peripheral Pertaining to or situated near the periphery, the outermost part, or surface of an organ or part.

Peripheral nervous system Carries impulses between the central nervous system and the rest of the body.

Peritonitis An infection in the abdominal cavity.

Perivascular Pertaining to around a blood vessel.

Permanent teeth A secondary, or second set of teeth; often referred to as adult teeth.

Personal Protective Equipment (PPE) Any item used to protect against undue harm; includes ear plugs, lead gloves, lead apron, safety glasses, exam gloves, and hot mitts.

Petechia Small red or purple spots on the body, caused by minor hemorrhage or broken capillary blood vessels.

Petrissage A deep massage used on the back, flank, and chest in which the skin is lifted, pulled, and kneaded.

Phagocytosis The ingestion of substances, including pathogens, by cells.

Pharmacokinetics Description of how a drug moves into, through, and out of the body.

Pharynx The throat, a common passageway for both the digestive and respiratory systems.

Phenols Disinfecting products that kill vegetative forms of many gram-negative and gram-positive bacteria.

Pheromone A natural or synthetic chemical that may influence the behavior of an animal.

Phlebitis Local venous inflammation.

Phosphors A substance that phosphoresces or emits light when exposed to electromagnetic radiation.

Photostimulable Being able to store a latent image that may be freed as light when stimulated by a scanning laser such as a CR or DDR plate.

Picture Archival Computing System (PACS) Dedicated computer systems (servers) that are used for storage, retrieval, transferring, and manipulating of images.

Pili A component of some bacterial cells that allows bacteria to more easily attach to and colonize host tissues and minimize the host's immune response.

Plain surgical gut A suture material made from the submucosa of sheep intestine or serosa of bovine intestine.

Plantar The caudal surface of the back foot distal to the tarsocrural joint; also pertains to the undersurface of the rear foot.

Plaque A soft mixture of bacteria and mucopolysaccharides (carbohydrates) that adheres to the tooth.

Plasmacyte (plasma cell) Antibody-producing cells. A cell derived from a B lymphocyte that has been transformed to produce and secrete antibodies.

Plastron The lower or ventral shell of chelonians.

Platelets Irregular, disc-shaped fragments of megakaryocytes in the blood that assist in blood clotting.

Pleuritis An infection in the thoracic cavity.

Pneumatized Filled with air.

Pneumonia Inflammation of the lungs with tissue consolidation.

Poikilocytosis Any abnormal cell shape.

Pollakiuria Increase in the frequency of urination.

Polychromasia A variable staining pattern; basophilia.

Polycythemia An increase in the numbers of circulating erythrocytes.

Polymerase chain reaction The method used to replicate and amplify DNA molecules in a sample.

Polyuria An increase in the total volume of urine produced.

POMR Problem-oriented medical record; a common type of record system in which each entry follows a distinct format; the defined database, the problem list (also referred to as master list), the plan, and the progress section. Within the progress section, a standard SOAP format is followed.

Porous adhesive tape A tape that allows evaporation of fluid from the bandage and also allows movement of fluid into the wound.

Positive contrast media Compounds such as barium or iodine that are radiopaque on radiographs used to visualize organs in the body.

Positive inotropic drugs Drugs that increase the strength of contraction of a weakened heart.

Posture The position or carriage of the body.

Potassium-sparing diuretics Drugs that promote secretion of sodium and conservation of potassium in the body.

Potentiometers A type of electrochemical analyzer used to evaluate ionic concentration in a solution.

Poultice A wet herbal pack.

Precision The magnitude of random errors and the reproducibility of measurements.

Preemptive analgesia Taking steps to predict and prevent pain before it occurs.

Prefix A syllable, a group of syllables, or a word joined to the beginning of another word to alter its meaning or create a new word.

Preliminary data Information gathered from the client such as patient characteristics (e.g., age, breed, sex, reproductive status).

Premium The amount paid annually or monthly for a policyholder to maintain an insurance policy for a pet.

Prepatent period The time interval between infection with a parasite and demonstration of the infection.

Preprandial samples Samples from an animal that has not eaten for some time.

Prescription An order from a licensed veterinarian directing a pharmacist to prepare a drug for use in a client's animal.

Presenting complaint What the client perceives the patient's problem to be; the primary medical problem.

Pressure manometer A device that measures the pressure of gases within the breathing circuit and the patient's lungs.

Presumptive diagnosis To make a diagnosis without having all of the facts or proof.

Primary flight feathers Also known as remiges area, the contour feathers on a bird's wing and emerge from the periosteum of the metacarpus; numbered from carpus distally; numbered from the carpus proximally.

Primary healing Also called first-intention healing; the healing of injured tissue directly without intervention of granulation tissue.
Primary hemostasis The formation of the primary platelet plug after injury to the vessel, involving the blood vessel, platelets, and certain adhesive proteins (e.g., von Willebrand factor, collagen).
Primary hyperalgesia Describes pain sensitivity that occurs directly in the damaged tissues.
Proctodeum The caudal part of the cloaca, which empties contents into the vent.
Productive cough A cough that produces mucus and other inflammatory products that are coughed up into the oral cavity.
Progestin A reproductive hormone similar to progesterone.
Proglottid Segments that comprise the body of a cestode.
Prognathism, maxillary Overbite; the maxillary arcade is longer than the mandibular arcade.
Prokaryote A single-celled organism, usually a bacterium; contains a cell wall, lacks a nucleus and organelles; DNA consists of one double-stranded chromosome.
Prophylaxis The process by which the teeth are cleaned to prevent disease.
Proprietary name Also known as trade name; a unique drug name given by a manufacturer to its particular brand of drug.
Proprioception The sense of body part position.
Proteinuria An abnormal presence of protein in the urine.
Protozoistatic Inhibits protozoal replication.
Proud flesh Excess granulation tissue formation on the leg of a horse; the formation of excessive granulation tissue.
Proventriculus The glandular portion of the stomach responsible for production of the gastric juices and propulsion of food into the ventriculus (gizzard).
Proximal Nearer to the center of the body, relative to another body part, or a location on a body part relative to another, more distant, location.
Proximate analysis Determinations of dry matter (DM), crude protein (CP), ether extract (EE, crude fat), crude fiber (CF), and ash.
Pruritus Itching.
Psittacines Birds belonging to the family Psittacidae, which includes the parrots, macaws, and parakeets.
Psychrophiles Organisms with optimal growth at cold temperatures (15° to 20° C).
Pterylae The feather tracks on the skin of birds; specific tracts located on the surface of the body where feather follicles are located.
Public health A community's effort to prevent disease and promote life and health
Pulp cavity Consisting of the pulp chamber, in the crown and the root canal, in root. Is the cavity surrounded by the dentin. Contains blood vessels, nerves, and connective tissue.
Pulse deficit Presence of a difference between the heart rate and the pulse rate, as in atrial fibrillation.
Pulse oximeter A device that detects changes in oxygen saturation of hemoglobin by calculating the difference between levels of oxygenated and deoxygenated blood. Also determines heart rate.
Pulse oximetry A noninvasive technique that continuously measures arterial oxygen saturation in the blood.
Pulse pressure The difference between systolic and diastolic arterial pressures.
Pulse quality A series of pressure waves within an artery caused by contractions of the left ventricle and corresponding with the heart rate that is easily detected over certain superficial arteries.
Punishment Something that decreases the likelihood of a behavior occurring.
Purulent Containing, discharging, or causing the production of pus; a cytology sample characterized by the presence of neutrophils representing more than 85% of total nucleated cells in the sample.
Pyknosis Condensed nuclear chromatin in a degenerating cell.
Pyogenic A characterization of bacteria that causes the host to produce a purulent or suppurative exudate.
Pyogranulomatous A cytology sample characterized by the presence of macrophages representing more than 15% of total nucleated cells in the sample.
Pyometra An infection in the uterus.
Pyrexia Fever.
Pyrogen An agent within the body that increases the body's biological setting to a higher temperature.

Q

Qi The Chinese term for central life force.
Quaternary ammonium compound A sanitizing agent most effective against gram-positive bacteria but less effective against gram-negative bacteria.
Queen A female cat, intact; mother cat.

R

Radiographic density The degree of blackness on a radiograph.
Radiolucent Dark (black) appearance of air-filled structures on a radiograph.
Radiopaque Light (white) appearance of dense structures on a radiograph.
Rare-earth elements Photosensitive elements such as lanthanum oxybromide and gadolinium oxysulfide that are in a x-ray intensifying screen.
Rebreathing system Anesthetic breathing circuits in which the exhaled gas is recirculated to the patient with CO_2 removed.
Receiver In communications, the person listening to a message.
Receptor A specific protein molecule on or in the cell with which a drug will combine.
Recipe The full chemical compound of the drug being prescribed.
Recombinant vaccine A vaccine that consists of a live, nonpathogenic virus into which the gene for a pathogen-related antigen has been inserted.
Recumbent Lying down; a modifying term is needed to describe the surface on which the animal is lying.
Redia A secondary larval form of some digenic trematodes that develops within a mollusk intermediate host.
Reflexology The use of hand and finger pressure to massage and stimulate pressure points located in the paws.
Refractive index Measure of the degree of light bending as it passes from one media to another, relative to air; function of the dissolved material in the sample.
Refractometer Instrument used to measure the refractive index of a solution.
Regional or segmental anesthesia Achieved by blocking the nerve or nerves that supply a region or segment of the body by injecting an anesthetic around the nerves that supply the area to block conduction from the area.
Registration Maintained by the state government, veterinary state board, or state veterinary technician association and may be mandatory.
Reiki A Japanese hands-on energy healing practice that promotes the flow of energy to aid in the healing process.

Reinforcement Something that increases the likelihood of a behavior occurring.

Releasability The ability for a wild animal to be released upon recovery based on the injuries sustained.

Remiges Contour feathers found on the wing of a bird.

Reorder point The inventory level at which additional product is ordered.

Repair phase Wound healing phase characterized by angiogenesis (blood vessel formation), collagen deposition, granulation tissue formation, epithelialization, and wound contraction.

Replacement fluid solution Fluids with a composition similar to plasma; high-sodium, low-potassium concentration.

Rescue Remedy A combination of five flower essences used to calm an individual experiencing shock, trauma, panic, or mental paralysis.

Reservoir A location in which a pathogenic agent is maintained prior to transmission; a reservoir is often a living organism.

Reservoir bag A rebreathing bag that provides a gas volume sufficient for the patient to inhale maximally without creating negative pressure in the circuit.

Residue An accumulation of a drug or chemical or its metabolites in animal tissues or food products, resulting from drug administration to animal or contamination of food products.

Resonance A hollow sound, such as that produced by air-filled lungs.

Respiration The transport of oxygen from the outside air to the cells within tissues, and the transport of carbon dioxide in the opposite direction.

Respondeat superior An employer who is responsible for the actions of the employees performed within the course of their employment.

Rete pegs Interdigitations of connective tissue that provide a firm attachment to the periosteum of the alveolar bone.

Reticulocyte An anuclear, immature erythrocyte.

Reticulopericarditis ("hardware disease") A disease that can occur when a cow ingests a metallic foreign body that penetrates the forestomach, diaphragm, and pericardium.

Retrices Contour feathers found on the tail of a bird.

Rhinotheca The upper beak of a bird or chelonian.

Right to Know Law A federal law mandating that all work places educate employees regarding the hazards they will encounter while on the job.

Rigid endoscope Instrument comprised of a metal tube, glass rods, lenses, and a light source better used for rhinoscopy, cystoscopy, laparoscopy, arthroscopy, vaginoscopy, colonoscopy, and thoroscopy.

Rochester-Carmalt forceps A large crushing instrument often used to control large tissue bundles.

Rodents Relatively small, gnawing mammals that have a single pair of incisors with a chisel-shaped edge in the upper jaw (e.g., mice and rats).

Roentgen equivalent mean (REM) Expresses the dose equivalent that results from exposure to ionizing radiation.

Rongeurs An instrument designed to cut and remove bone pieces.

Root The unexposed, or submerged, portion of the tooth below the gingival tissue.

Root word The "subject" part of the word consisting of a syllable, group of syllables, or word that is the basis (or word base) for the meaning of the medical word.

Rostral Pertaining to the nose end of the head or body, or toward the nose.

Rouleaux The arrangement of erythrocytes in a column or stack.

Rumenotomy An incision into the rumen.

Ruminatorics Drugs used to stimulate an atonic rumen.

S

Sacral vertebrae Fused vertebrae in the pelvic region; sacrum.

Saddle thrombus An embolus that breaks loose and occludes one or more branches of the aorta at the aortic trifurcation.

Safelight Light produced that will not affect radiographic film; consists of a low-wattage light bulb and special filter.

Sanitizer Another term for either antiseptics or disinfectants.

Saprozoonosis A zoonotic disease that depends on an inanimate reservoir to maintain the cycle of infection.

Sarcoma A generic term to describe any cancer arising from cells of the connective tissues.

Scatter radiation Radiation that is created as a result of the interaction of primary beam x-ray photons and body parts or matter that travel in a different direction and are comprised of lower energies.

Scavenging system Component of an anesthetic machine that functions to properly discard excess gas; some are located on machines as a filter canister; others are set up as a central unit with a fan to direct gases out of the building.

Schedule drug See controlled substance.

Schistocyte Fragmented erythrocytes usually formed as a result of shearing of the red cell by intravascular trauma.

Schizont Life cycle stage of some protozoal organisms; arises from multiple asexual fission.

Scolex The head of a cestode by which it attaches to its host.

Scutes Pertaining to chelonians; the bony shell covered by a superficial layer of keratin shield; pertaining to snakes; the large scales found on the ventral aspect of the body.

Secondary container labeling Mandated by OSHA, all materials dispensed out of the primary storage unit must be properly identified with MSDS information, to include: health hazard, flammability, reactivity, and personal protection.

Secondary flight feathers Also known as remiges area, the contour feathers that emerge from the ulna and are numbered from the carpus proximally.

Secondary hemostasis Formation of fibrin, involving certain coagulation factors in the extrinsic, intrinsic, and common coagulation pathways.

Second-intention healing Closure of a wound using granulation tissue.

Sedation A mild to profound degree of central nervous system depression in which the patient is drowsy but may be aroused by painful stimuli.

Seizures Periods of altered brain function characterized by loss of consciousness, altered muscle tone or movement, altered sensations, or other neurologic changes.

Selective media A type of culture media that contains antibacterial substances that inhibit or kill all but a few types of bacteria.

Semiclosed breathing system A circle system in which some rebreathing occurs, there is adequate fresh gas flow, and the pop-off settings are at intermediate values.

Sender In communications, the person delivering a message.

Senn (rake) retractor Double-ended retractor, one end with finger-like curved prongs (sharp or blunt); the other end is a flat, curved blade.

Sensible water loss Water loss that is easy to measure and can be seen (urine).

Sensitivity test A method used to determine the resistance or susceptibility of a microorganism to specific antimicrobials.

Sensory nerves These nerves only carry information toward the central nervous system.

Sentinel A surveillance animal housed for the purpose of identifying abnormal occurrences.
Serology The study and application of antibody detection in the serum.
Serous exudate An exudate that consists primarily of fluid with a low protein content.
Schistocyte Fragmented erythrocyte
Short-acting glucocorticoid A glucocorticoid that exerts an anti-inflammatory effect for less than 12 hours.
Shrinkage The unexplained loss of inventory.
Sievert (SV) The dose of radiation equivalent to the absorbed dose by tissue; 1 sievert equals 100 REM.
Sig On a written prescription, this indicates directions for the client in treating the animal.
Signalment Patient characteristics, including age, breed, gender, reproductive status, markings.
Silage A partially fermented forage state.
Silk suture Braided multifilament organic nonabsorbable suture material.
Sinus arrhythmia Fluctuation of heart rate with respiration
Sinus rhythm The normal conduction sequence of the heart.
Slice thickness Ultrasound artifact that occurs when the transducer receives echoes with different amplitudes from the same area at the same depth.
Snake hook A piece of equipment used to temporarily restrain the head of an aggressive or venomous snake for the purpose of capturing it.
Snubbing A restraint technique in which the animal is held in position using a leash through a wall anchor or the hinges or the bars on a low cage.
SOAP An acronym that identifies the most common data entry formats used by veterinary practices: Subjective, Objective, Assessment, and Plan.
Socialization The exposure of a young animal to new experiences, people, other animals, and places with the goal of preventing fearful or anxious behavior as adults.
Society Group of individuals with a common interest in a veterinary technician discipline.
Solid Powdered drugs compressed into pills, discs, or capsules.
Soluble factor An enzyme or protein produced by bacteria that inhibit host functions and provide the bacteria a "foothold" within the host.
Solution A drug dissolved in a liquid vehicle that does not settle out if left standing.
Somatic pain Generally well-localized pain that results from the activation of peripheral nociceptors without injury to the peripheral nerve or central nervous system.
Sonolucent Tissues that transmit most of the sound to the deeper tissues, with only a few echoes reflected back to the ultrasound transducer.
Source-image distance (SID) Film-focal distance.
Sow A female guinea pig or pig.
Special senses Gustatory, olfactory, auditory, vestibular, and visual senses. These are concentrated in certain areas, rather than being generally distributed.
Specific Any herb known for its effectiveness in the treatment of a particular condition.
Specific gravity The weight (density) of a quantity of liquid compared with that of an equal amount of distilled water.
Specificity The ability of a test to evaluate a given parameter correctly.
Spectrophotometers These instruments are designed to measure the amount of light transmitted through a solution.
Sphygmomanometer Also called a blood pressure meter, it is a device used to measure blood pressure. It comprises an inflatable cuff to restrict blood flow and a mercury or mechanical manometer to measure the pressure. The word comes from the Greek *sphygmós* (pulse) plus manometer (pressure meter).
Spinal nerves Nerves of the peripheral nervous system that originate from the spinal cord.
Splenectomy The surgical removal of the spleen.
Spoilage The forage harvested at a given stage of development and fed directly.
Sporocyst The larval stage of a digenic trematode that develops in a mollusk intermediate host.
Sporozoite The infective stage of some protozoal parasites.
Squeeze chute A capture device made of metal or wood that restrains cattle.
Standard A nonbiologic solution of an analyte, usually in distilled water, with a known concentration.
Standard Operational Procedure (SOP) A written set of directions and policies; a practice may abbreviate medical record annotations; however, an SOP must be kept on premises detailing the procedure.
Stasis The congestion of blood vessels caused by "sludging" of blood flow in the vessels from fluid loss through exudation.
Sterilization The destruction of all organisms, including bacteria and spores.
Sterilization indicators Objects that undergo a chemical or biologic change with some combination of time, temperature, or chemical exposure, allowing for monitoring of effectiveness of sterilization.
Sterilizer Another term for either antiseptics or disinfectants.
Sternal recumbency A restraint technique in which the animal is held in position resting on its breastbone.
Stimulus An internal or external change that exceeds a threshold causing stimulation of the nervous or endocrine systems.
Stock A small, square restraining pen with a front and back gate.
Stored whole blood A unit of blood that was collected more than 8 hours before and that has been refrigerated, adversely affecting certain components in blood.
Strabismus A condition in which the eyes are not properly aligned with each other.
Straight (Keith) needles A suture needle used in accessible places where the needle can be manipulated directly with the fingers.
Stretch pressure massage A massage technique that combines pressure on a muscle with a stretching motion.
Struvite A common crystal seen in alkaline to slightly acidic urine; sometimes referred to as triple phosphate crystals or magnesium ammonium phosphate crystals.
Stupor A semiconscious patient that can respond to noxious (painful) stimuli.
Subcutaneous injection (SQ or SC) Injecting a drug deep to (beneath) the skin, into the subcutis.
Subgingival Below the gingiva.
Subluxations Misalignment of vertebrae causing compensation in posture or movement.
Substrate Material selected or preferred by an animal for urination and defecation.
Subtherapeutic level A dose of a drug that is below the ideal range of concentration and therefore does not achieve a beneficial effect.
Suffix A syllable, a group of syllables, or a word added at the end of a root word to change its meaning, give it grammatical function, or form a new word.

Superficial Situated near the surface of the body or a structure; the opposite of deep.
Supine Lying face up, in dorsal recumbency.
Suppository A drug that is inserted in the rectum, dissolved, and released to be absorbed across the membranes of the intestinal wall.
Suppurative Purulent.
Supragingival Above the gingiva.
Surgical biopsy The evaluation of tissue that has been surgically removed from the body.
Suspension A drug in which the particles are suspended but not dissolved in the liquid vehicle.
Suture Any strand of material that is used to approximate tissues or ligate blood vessels.
Sutures Immovable joints in the skull.
Suture scissors Scissors with a concavity at the top of one blade, designed for removing skin sutures after wound healing.
Swaged needles Suture needles that are joined with suture into a continuous unit.
Symmetry To observe closely for complementary ("balanced") or noncomplementary conformation of the thorax and abdomen. Note any difference in size or shape of the extremities.
Sympathetic system This produces the "fight or flight" reaction in response to real or perceived threats.
Sympatholysis Inhibition of the postganglionic functioning of the sympathetic nervous system (SNS).
Synapse The junction of an axon with another nerve cell.
Syrinx The voice box of birds; analogous to the mammalian larynx.
Syrup A solution of drug with water and sugar.
Systemic antacids Medications that decrease acid production in the stomach.
Systole The contraction of heart chambers to pump the blood into body tissues and lungs.
Systolic blood pressure The maximum force caused by contraction of the left ventricle of the heart.

T

Tachyarrhythmia An abnormally rapid heartbeat accompanied by an irregular rhythm. Derived from the Greek *tachy,* fast, and *a* + *rhythmos,* rhythm.
Tachycardia Abnormally rapid beating of the heart.
Tachypnea Rapid breathing.
Tail jacking Restraint technique used to relax the hindquarters for rectal palpation and tail bleeding of cows whereby the base of the tail is lifted straight up.
Tapered needles A suture needle with a sharp tip that pierces and spreads tissues without cutting them.
Target cells Leptocyte with a peripheral ring of cytoplasm surrounded by a clear area and a dense central rounded area of pigment.
Tellington Touch A gentle manipulation therapy used as a realignment technique.
Telodendron The branched end of an axon.
Tenesmus Straining to defecate.
Tenotomy scissors Delicate scissors designed for ophthalmic procedures.
Therapeutic Index The lethal dose of a drug for 50% of the population (LD_{50}) divided by the minimum effective dose for 50% of the population (ED_{50}); also known as the therapeutic ratio.
Therapeutic range The ideal range of a drug concentration in the body.
Thermal therapy The use of heat or cold to facilitate circulation and pain relief.
Thermophiles Organisms with optimal growth at elevated temperatures.
Third-intention healing The treatment of a grossly contaminated wound by delaying surgical closure until after contamination has been markedly reduced and inflammation has subsided.
Thoracic vertebrae Bones in the chest region that form joints with the dorsal ends of the ribs.
Thoracotomy An incision into the thorax.
Thorax The area located between the neck and the diaphragm.
Thrombocyte Platelet; cytoplasmic fragment of bone marrow megakaryocyte.
Thrombocytopenia Decrease in circulating platelets.
Thrombophlebitis The inflammation of a vein associated with clotting.
Thrush A degenerative condition of the hoof that may occur secondary to a bacterial infection and appears as black, malodorous material in the region of the frog.
Thymus A lymphoid organ of birds and mammals.
Tick paralysis A condition resulting from introduction of a neurotoxin into the body during attachment of and feeding by the female of several tick species.
Tidal volume The lung volume representing the normal volume of air displaced between normal inspiration and expiration when extra effort is not applied.
Time gain compensation Ultrasound control that modulates the amount of returning echoes.
Tincture An alcohol solution meant for topical application; liquid herbal extracts usually preserved with alcohol or vegetable glycerin.
Tisane An herbal infusion.
Titer The greatest dilution at which a patient sample no longer yields a positive result for the presence of a specific antibody.
T lymphocyte (T cell) A type of lymphocyte involved in cell-mediated immunity.
Tonicity The osmotic pressure between two solutions determined by solute concentration.
Topical anesthesia Numbing of the area by reversibly block nerve conduction near their site of administration, thereby producing temporary loss of sensation in a limited area.
Topical application/administration Applied onto the skin.
Total body water (TBW) The total water content of the body; accounts for 60% of lean body weight.
Total daily dose The amount of drug delivered to the animal in 24 hours.
Total intravenous anesthesia (TIVA) Uses two or more injectable drugs in combination to achieve balanced anesthesia.
Toxic Containing or being poisonous material, especially when capable of causing death or serious debilitation, toxic waste, radiation, or chemical.
Toxic neutrophils A neutrophil characterized by the presence of cytoplasmic basophilia, Döhle bodies, vacuoles, heavy granulation, and/or giantism.
Toxoid Inactivated antigenic toxin molecules that stimulate development of the animal's own antibodies.
Trachea Also known as the windpipe; carries air from the larynx to the lungs.
Trade name See proprietary name.
Traditional Chinese Medicine (TCM) The ancient practice of acupuncture and herbal therapy originating in China.
Tranquilization A state of relaxation and calmness characterized by a lack of anxiety or concern without significant drowsiness.
Transducer A device on an ultrasound machine that emits and receives a sound wave signal that converts the waves into electrical impulses.

Transduction Part of the nociception and pain pathway. The signal begins with tissue trauma where the nociceptors are stimulated, and is converted into electrical impulses once the threshold is exceeded.

Transgenic Animals containing foreign DNA that was injected directly into the pronucleus of the zygote.

Transmission Part of the nociception and pain pathway in which noxious stimulus exceed nociceptor's threshold, and travel along peripheral nerves to the spinal cord (dorsal horn) and the brain (thalamus).

Transudate An effusion characterized by low protein concentration and low total nucleated cell counts.

Trematode Organism in the phylum Trematoda; commonly referred to as a fluke.

Trephine An instrument designed to bore holes in bone.

Triadan Charting System A method of dental charting that identifies each tooth with a three-digit number that corresponds to each tooth.

Triage From the French for "to sort"; used to classify patients according to the severity of illness or injury determine their relative priority for treatment.

Trophozoite The motile form of a protozoal parasite.

Twitch A rope, strap, or chain that is tightened over a horse's lip as a restraining device.

Tympany A musical or drumlike sound produced by an air-filled organ, such as with gastric dilatation-volvulus.

U

Ultrasonic Doppler A device that monitors heart rate and rhythm by detecting flow of blood through small arteries.

Ultrasonography Imaging technique that uses echoes of sound to delineate structures.

Ultrasound A modality that uses sound waves that interact with tissues and are reflected back to create an image.

Unbalanced fluid solution Fluid that differs in composition from plasma.

Urates The end product of nitrogenous waste production from the liver that is excreted by the kidney as a pasty white to yellow material found in bird droppings.

Urea The principal end product of amino acid breakdown in mammals.

Urethrotomy An incision into the urethra.

Uric acid A metabolic byproduct of nitrogen catabolism.

Urochromes Pigments that impart color to a urine sample.

Urodeum The middle compartment of the cloaca that is the terminal end of the ureters and genital ducts.

Urolithiasis The presence of calculi (stones) in the urinary tract.

Uropygeal gland In the bird, an oil-producing gland used to waterproof feathers; a bilobed gland with one duct opening that empties into a lone papilla, found dorsally at the base of the tail; secretes a lipoid sebaceous material that is spread over feathers during preening to help with water proofing.

Urticaria A relatively mild cutaneous hypersensitivity reaction such as hives.

V

Vaccine A biological product representing a pathogenic organism that stimulates immunity toward the pathogen.

Vaporizer A component of the anesthetic machine that produces a controlled and predictable concentration of anesthetic vapor in the carrier gas by delivering a diluted anesthetic to the patient.

Vasoconstriction Narrowing of the blood vessels resulting from contraction of the muscular wall of the vessels, particularly the large arteries, small arterioles, and veins.

Vasodilation The dilation of blood vessels.

Vasodilator Any substance that opens (dilates) constricted vessels.

Vector Any organism that transmits a disease-causing organism to new hosts.

Vehicle A mode of transmission of an infectious agent from the reservoir to the host.

Venipuncture Puncture of a vein for the purposes of withdrawing blood.

Ventilation Measured as the frequency of breathing multiplied by the volume of each breath. It maintains normal concentrations of oxygen and carbon dioxide in the alveolar gas and, through the process of diffusion, also maintains normal partial pressures of oxygen and carbon dioxide in the blood flowing from the capillaries.

Ventral Pertaining to the underside of a quadruped, or denoting a position more toward the abdomen than another reference point (body part).

Ventral midline incision An incision located on the ventral midline of the animal.

Ventriculus The second stomach of birds and is the site of protein digestion and mechanical breakdown of food.

Vent The external opening of the cloaca.

Vermicide An anthelmintic that kills a parasitic worm.

Vermifuge A drug that paralyzes a worm but does not kill it.

Vertebrae A series of individual bones in the spinal column.

Vertebral canal A long, flexible tube formed by the vertebrae.

Vesicular sounds Heard over normal lung parenchyma and are produced by movement of air through small bronchi, bronchioles, and alveoli; best heard on inspiration.

Vestibular disease Disorders of the body's balance system in the inner ear.

Vestibular sense A mechanical sense that monitors balance and head position.

Veterinarian A person who has graduated from a 4-year AVMA-accredited program receiving a Doctor of Veterinary Medicine degree.

Veterinary assistant A person with the training of a clinical aide, less than that required of a veterinary technician.

Veterinary behaviorist A veterinarian who is board certified in animal behavior by the American College of Veterinary Behaviorists.

Veterinary Medical Association A not-for-profit professional organization of veterinarians establishing bylaws, nominating officers, and enhancing the professional experience through volunteerism.

Veterinary Practice Act A statute enacted as an exercise of the powers of the state to promote the public health, safety, and welfare by safeguarding the people of the state against incompetent, dishonest, or unprincipled practitioners of veterinary medicine.

Veterinary State Practice Act Law that describes which persons may practice veterinary medicine and surgery in the state and under which conditions.

Veterinary team Usually consists of a veterinarian, technician, assistant, receptionist, and hospital manager.

Veterinary technician A person who has graduated from an AVMA-accredited veterinary technician program.

Veterinary Technician Association A not-for-profit professional organization of veterinary technicians establishing bylaws, nominating officers, and enhancing the professional experience through volunteerism.

Veterinary technician specialist A technician who is credentialed and has met all the requirements established by the testing agency and passed the exam according to the organization's guidelines; must be a member in good standing of the specialty group.

Veterinary technologist A person who has graduated from a 4-year AVMA-accredited program.

Veterinary technology The science and art of providing professional support service to veterinarians.

Virology The study of viruses.

Virucidal Kills viruses.

Virus An extremely small, nonliving infectious agent, ranging from 30 to 450 nm in diameter, which can cause disease in a wide variety of animals.

Visceral larva migrans The migration of certain nematode through an organisms tissues and organs.

Visual sense An electromagnetic sense (sight). Its receptor organ, the eye, has a complex organization of component parts that function together to gather and focus light rays on photoreceptor cells.

Vomiting center The group of neurons in the medulla of the brainstem that control the complex process of emesis.

W

Warble Common name for the larva of some species of flies; often in swollen, cystlike subcutaneous sites, with a fistula or pore communicating to the outside environment.

Water-soluble vitamins Those vitamins that are passively absorbed from the small intestine, and excess amounts are excreted in the urine.

Weitlaner retractor A self-retaining retractor with a box lock to maintain tension on tissues, commonly used in neurologic surgeries.

Wheal A fluid-filled, raised area on the surface of the skin that is the result of an allergic or hypersensitivity reaction to an irritant; a small, but palpable, amount of fluid that was injected into the top layers of the skin by using a syringe and a small-gauge needle.

Withdrawal time The minimum length of time that must pass from the last administration of the medicine until the time that the animal is slaughtered for food or the milk is collected for human consumption.

Wound An injury caused by physical means, with disruption of normal structures.

Wry bite Right and left, mandible and maxilla, are different lengths and widths.

X

X-ray A form of electromagnetic radiation.

Y

Yang energy Traditional Chinese Medicine term describing male energy—insistent, unyielding, activity, brightness, fire, and sun.

Yin energy Traditional Chinese Medicine term describing female energy—calm, yielding, stillness, darkness, water, and moon.

Z

Zone of inhibition An area of no bacterial growth around an antimicrobial disk; indicates some sensitivity of the organism to the particular antimicrobial.

Zoonoses Any disease or infection that is naturally transmissible between vertebrate animals and humans.

Zoonotic diseases Infectious agents shared by humans and animals. Approximately 150 zoonotic diseases exist.

Zoonotic infection Capable of being transmitted between animals and human beings.

Zygodactyl The foot shape of psittacines; the second and third toes face forward and the first and fourth toes are directed backward.

Index

Note: Page numbers followed by "f" indicate figures; "t" indicate tables, and "b" indicate boxes.

X

Y

Z